W9-CZK-228

Introduction
to
PATIENT CARE

A Comprehensive Approach to Nursing

4th Edition

Beverly Witter Du Gas
R.N., B.A., M.N., Ed.N., LL.D. (Honorary)

Coordinator of Continuing Education
Associate Professor
School of Nursing
Faculty of Health Sciences
University of Ottawa

with special editorial assistance from

Barbara Marie Du Gas Dymond, B.A.

Professional Teaching Certificate
Diploma in Translation (French)

1983

W. B. SAUNDERS COMPANY

Philadelphia London Toronto Mexico City Rio de Janeiro Sydney Tokyo

W. B. Saunders Company: West Washington Square
Philadelphia, PA   19105

1 St. Anne's Road
Eastbourne, East Sussex BN21 3UN, England

1 Goldthorne Avenue
Toronto, Ontario M8Z 5T9, Canada

Apartado 26370—Cedro 512
Mexico 4, D.F., Mexico

Rua Coronel Cabrita, 8
Sao Cristovao Caixa Postal 21176
Rio de Janeiro, Brazil

9 Waltham Street
Artarmon, N.S.W. 2064, Australia

Ichibancho, Central Bldg., 22-1 Ichibancho
Chiyoda-Ku, Tokyo 102, Japan

Library of Congress Cataloging in Publication Data

Du Gas, Beverly Witter.

Introduction to patient care.

Includes bibliographies and index.

1. Nursing.   I. Title. [DNLM: 1. Nursing care. WY 100
   D866i]

RT41.D75 1983   61o.73   82–42568

ISBN 0–7216–3227–0

Listed here are the latest translated editions of this book together
with the language of the translation and the publisher.

Dutch (*3rd Edition*)—Wolters-Noordhoff bv, Groningen, The Netherlands

French (*3rd Edition*)—Les Editions HRW Ltee., Quebec, Canada

Portuguese (*3rd Edition*)—Editora Interamericana Ltda., Rio de Janeiro, Brazil

Spanish (*3rd Edition*)—Nueva Editorial Interamericana, S.A.

Japanese (*3rd Edition*)—Hirokawa Publishing Company, Tokyo

Introduction to Patient Care   ISBN   0-7216-3227-0

Last digit is the print number: 9   8   7   6   5   4   3   2   1

To my students, past and present, whose enthusiasm and idealism have never failed to inspire me.

PREFACE

Each successive edition of this text has reflected the constantly evolving nature of nursing. Each, it seems, is a little bigger than the last, and each has contained more depth of content as the scientific body of nursing knowledge has expanded and nursing methodology has become more precise.

The purpose of the present edition is the same as that of previous editions, that is, to provide students with an introduction to the practice of nursing and to give them a solid foundation of basic knowledge and skills on which to build in more senior nursing courses. The first unit focuses on the role of the nurse in today's health services. The second unit introduces students to the methodology of nursing and helps them to acquire the tools needed to begin practice. In the third unit the student is assisted in applying the nursing process in the care of patients who need help in meeting their basic needs, regardless of their medical diagnosis.

It is my firm belief that if a textbook is to be used by students, the material in it must be presented in language that is both readable and interesting to them. In this regard, I agree with the noted educator Jerome Bruner that it is possible to present complex ideas in understandable terms in an intellectually honest form, provided one teaches by fundamental concept. This is the approach that has been used in this text.

Fundamental concepts underlying the provision of health care are introduced early in the book, and relevant scientific principles are highlighted in each chapter. Each chapter, except the first, begins with a set of objectives for students to use in evaluating their own progress in learning. A guide for assessing the patient's functional status in regard to each of the basic needs and a guide for evaluating the effectiveness of nursing action have been included at the end of each chapter wherever these are appropriate to the content. In addition, a study situation is included. In this edition, references cited throughout each chapter are listed at the end of the chapter. A suggested readings list provides an additional source of material for those who wish to pursue a particular topic more extensively. Included at the end of the text are a list of prefixes and suffixes used in medical terminology and a glossary of terms defined in the text.

ACKNOWLEDGMENTS

A great many people have contributed to the preparation of the fourth edition of this text, and I would like to express my gratitude to all of them. Firstly, I would like to thank the numerous nurse educators who helped with ideas and suggestions for the inclusion of new content and the revision and reorganization of material that has been retained. Special thanks are due to Barbara Gillies and to Joyce Campkin, who have served as clinical advisors for material included in the text, and to the other faculty members of the Vancouver General Hospital School of Nursing and those of the Douglas College School of Nursing for their helpful suggestions. I would also like to thank the nursing teachers who critiqued new chapters and contributed good suggestions on content and organization of these.

I am also grateful to Sven Fletcher-Berg for his assistance in taking pictures for this edition—and to the many people who were so agreeable to having their pictures taken and allowing them to be used to illustrate material in the text. I would also like to thank the staffs of Vancouver General Hospital; Children's Hospital of Eastern Ontario; Hospital of Ottawa; Rehabilitation Centre of Ottawa, and Shaughnessy Hospital, Vancouver, Canada, for their help in obtaining photographs for use in the book.

The assistance of Valerie Simmons with research for this edition and of Sue Hiscocks with typing of the final chapters of the manuscript is also gratefully acknowledged.

A special word of thanks is due, too, to the editors, artists, and production staff of the W. B. Saunders Company for patience and support throughout the lengthy process of manuscript preparation and production of this book.

Finally, I would like to express my gratitude to my daughter, Barbara Du Gas Dymond, for her help with each successive edition of this text—as a sounding board for level and clarity of content during preparation of the first edition, as typist and reader for the second edition, and as research and editorial assistant during preparation of the third and present editions.

CONTENTS

SECTION THREE   PROTECTION AND SAFETY NEEDS, 508

HEALTH CARE AND THE PRACTICE OF NURSING

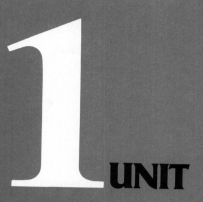

1 UNIT

1

INTRODUCTION TO HEALTH CARE

CHAPTER 1

FOCUS ON HEALTH

Health has been defined by the World Health Organization as *a state of complete mental, physical and social well-being and not merely the absence of disease or infirmity*.[1] And it is health, rather than illness, that is finally becoming the focus of our health services. In the past few years, there has been a major change in the philosophy of health care in North America. We appear at long last, to have swung towards a more positive approach—one that stresses health promotion and the prevention of illness as matters of primary concern, with restoration to optimum health, not merely the curing of disease, as the goal of therapeutic care.

Even the language we use in connection with health care is changing to reflect a more optimistic outlook. Instead of discussing "treatment" levels, people are now talking about levels of health promotion or levels of disease prevention to describe health services. The three levels of health promotion most commonly discussed are:

1. Primary Health Promotion. This is concerned with encouraging people to become as fit and healthy as possible, so that they are able to enjoy life to the fullest.[2] Primary promotion encompasses generalized health promotion as well as specific protection against disease.[3] Services such as nutrition, counseling on exercise and hygiene, and immunizations against specific diseases would be included in primary promotion programs.

2. Secondary Health Promotion. This is concerned with both (a) the early detection of deviations from normal growth and development, or signs of ill health, and (b) prompt intervention either to prevent abnormality or illness or to lessen their severity. Secondary promotion services include screening programs, such as the mass screening of specific population groups to detect persons with tuberculosis or the hypertension (high blood pressure) screening clinics that are often held in shopping malls by the Heart Association and other groups. Also included at the secondary level is the care and treatment of the ill on an inpatient basis in the hospital, on an outpatient basis in a clinic, or in the home.

3. Tertiary Health Promotion. This level is primarily oriented toward rehabilitation, with services designed to restore individuals (and their families) who have been ill or disabled to as full and independent a life as possible within the constraints of their disability. Services at this level include the retraining of individuals in basic life skills—if necessary, to walk or perhaps to talk again, to adjust to their disability, and, sometimes, to reorient their lives to accommodate the residual effects of an illness or to prevent its recurrence.

Although the three levels of health promotion have been described separately, it is important to remember that they exist on a continuum, with many of the services overlapping in actual practice.

REALIGNMENT OF SERVICES

Along with the increased emphasis on promotion of health rather than care of illness, there has been a realignment of health services, with a major shift towards the provision of more ambulatory and home care services in the community. We have seen in the past ten years the rapid growth of Health Maintenance Organizations in the United States and of Family Practice

3

Units and Community Health Centres in Canada, as well as "storefront" and "free" clinics, crisis centers, and other forms of primary care in both countries to give more ready access to health services for people in a community. This trend can be explained in part by the rising costs of hospital care, which have soared astronomically in the past few years. It would seem a better investment economically to keep people healthy and to detect and treat disease early, rather than to permit serious illnesses to develop that require costly institutional care. This approach has, indeed, been utilized effectively in the Health Maintenance Organizations, where it has been shown that the incidence of hospitalization among people enrolled in the HMO is less than in the general population.[4]

Certainly, the concept of health monitoring throughout the life cycle—to promote optimum health, to detect the early signs of illness or abnormality, and to initiate prompt treatment—appears to be becoming more widely accepted. In one program using this approach, health goals and the professional services needed to attain them at various stages of the lifespan have been identified for each of ten different age groups, starting with pregnancy and the perinatal period and ending with old age. For example, in infancy (the first year of life) one goal is to establish immunity against specified infectious diseases. This goal would be achieved in the course of four professional visits with the healthy infant. During these visits, other goals would also be accomplished. The infant would be observed for any deviations from the normal pattern of growth and development and for the early signs of disease, so that treatment could be initiated before irreversible damage was done. The mother, or father, accompanying the infant would be counseled regarding care and feeding to promote the child's optimum physical and psychosocial development.[5]

We are likely to hear much more about health monitoring in the next decade, as health insurance carriers and government agencies begin to recognize the economic value of a preventive approach to health care.

PHYSICAL FITNESS PROGRAMS

There has been a tremendous upsurge in physical fitness programs in North America in recent years. We have suddenly become very conscious of the value of exercise. We are also much more interested in nutrition and more aware of the benefits of sound health practices than previous generations have been. Physical fitness testing has become popular. A "fitness evaluation" usually includes an assessment of your respiratory functioning, an estimation of the percentage of body weight you are carrying in fat, your general strength, and your cardiovascular fitness. This evaluation is often combined with a lifestyle inventory to provide the basis for an analytical and critical look at the risk factors in your lifestyle. Risk factors are habits or existing health states that render a person more vulnerable to major health problems. Cigarette smoking, for example, has been linked to respiratory diseases (such as cancer of the lungs) and is therefore considered a risk factor. Obesity is felt to contribute to the development of such problems as heart disease, diabetes, and hypertension and is therefore also considered a major risk factor.

Many places where people work now have a physical fitness program for their employees, with facilities (and instructors) available so that people can exercise during their lunch or coffee breaks or after working hours. Occupational health programs also often utilize a fitness evaluation and lifestyle inventory as the basis for health counseling of employees. An exercise program tailored to the individual's age and fitness status might be suggested, for example, or a diet might be recommended if the person is overweight. The individual would be referred to his private physician if a serious problem is suspected.

POPULATION CHANGES

Aging. Not only have there been major changes in recent years in the philosophy of health care and in the alignment of services, there has also been a change in the composition of the population to be served. In both the United States and Canada, we have seen a marked slowing down in the rate of population growth. The birth rate in both countries dropped dramatically in the 1970's and this, together with the lengthening of the lifespan, has led to a greater proportion of older people in the population than at any other time in our history.

Family Dispersion. This phenomenon has occurred at a time when there has been increasing fragmentation of the extended family. Grownup children now often live thousands of miles away from their parents and, with more women working outside the home now than ever before, there is often no one at home to look after an aging mother or father. Alternative services have had to be developed to assist older people to remain independent as long as possible, and facilities have had to be built to care for them when they are no longer able to care for themselves.

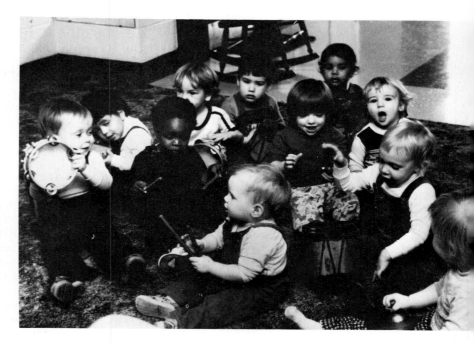

Well-staffed, well-run day care centers provide positive experiences for children of working parents—single and married. In the United States as many as 50 percent of preschool children have mothers who work outside the home. (Courtesy Canadian Nurses Association, Helen K. Mussallem Library. Photo by Victor Wong, Studio Impact, Ottawa, Ontario.)

Single Parent Families. There has also been a striking increase in the number of "single parent" families—there were an estimated 4.2 million in the United States in 1980. This situation, combined with the increased numbers of working mothers, has meant that social institutions, such as day care centers, schools, and community centers, must provide many services that once were provided by parents in the home. The day-to-day management of many transient and chronic problems of children's illnesses may be delegated to the day care worker, the teacher, or the school health nurse. For example, the school nurse may be asked to give a child medication at specified times after the acute phase of an illness is past and the parent must return to work.[6]

Urbanization. Then, too, we are having to cope with the need for rapid expansion of health services in our cities, as the trend toward urbanization continues. All too often, the number of people moving into the city far outstrips the capacity of its health services. This is particularly true in inner city neighborhoods, where overcrowding and poverty frequently coexist—not always peacefully—to compound the situation. It is the inner city neighborhoods, too, that usually have most of the new immigrants. This situation usually results in a rich cultural mix among the inhabitants, but often poses problems for health workers both in overcoming language barriers and in understanding different beliefs and customs in regard to health and illness.

CHANGING NATURE OF DISEASE PATTERNS

As the composition of our population has changed over the years, so has the nature of the diseases and disease patterns affecting us. The twentieth century has witnessed tremendous advances in medical science that have radically altered disease patterns in our Western societies and revolutionized our health care. Most of the communicable diseases that necessitated lengthy hospitalization and took such a toll of human lives at the beginning of the century have been virtually eliminated by improvements in public health measures coupled with the discovery and widespread use of specific immunity-producing agents. The "miracle drugs" of the 1940's and 1950's, the sulfonamides and the antibiotics, radically changed methods of patient care by hastening recovery and lowering fatality rates from infections. The rapid advances in medical therapy and in surgical techniques during the 1960's and 1970's have also contributed to increasing the lifespan of people in our society.

The longer people live, however, the more likely they are to suffer from chronic and degenerative diseases. And, indeed, heart conditions, cerebrovascular accidents (strokes), and cancer are the three leading causes of death in North American today. These disorders also figure prominently on the list of chronic conditions from which people suffer.

Many of our present-day health problems are

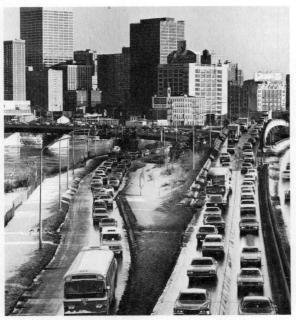

The tensions created by a heightened tempo of life and problems such as overcrowding in urban areas have led to many stress-related health problems. (H. Armstrong Roberts.)

directly attributable to the way in which we live. Faster automobiles, driven at high speed on the nation's roads, have contributed to making accidents the fourth leading cause of death in both the United States and Canada. The care and treatment of accident victims has become a major portion of the workload in our hospitals. The need for rehabilitation services to help restore these people to an active, functioning role in society has greatly increased. Still, the large number of people permanently handicapped as a result of accidents keeps growing, adding greatly to the demand for long-term care services.

The heightened tempo of life in today's world has led to many stress-related health problems. There has been a marked increase in the incidence of mental illness, for example, especially among our young people, and we are also seeing much evidence of the tragic effects of alcohol and drug abuse. Suicide, homicide, and other acts of violence are on the increase, as noted in the health statistics, and also as seen in the people coming into, or being brought into, our health agencies for care.

TECHNOLOGICAL ADVANCES

The latter half of this century has been characterized by a biomedical knowledge explosion. It has been estimated that new information stem-

ming from research in the biomedical sciences in the past 35 years has more than doubled the total amount of knowledge in the field. We have already mentioned the discovery of the sulfonamides and the antibiotic drugs, which so radically and rapidly altered the care of diseases caused by infectious agents. Tranquilizers and mood-changing drugs, which came into widespread use in the mid-1950's, had much the same effect in altering treatment for the mentally ill. It was no longer necessary to put people in straightjackets or otherwise restrain them physically to keep them from harming themselves or others. Tranquilizers can quickly calm a violent patient, making him easier to cope with and, also, more amenable to other types of therapy.

Then, too, advances in the use of anesthetic drugs and new surgical techniques have made extensive heart surgery possible and organ transplant feasible. A new area of treatment has been opened up in nuclear medicine, with radioactive iodine, gold, and phosphorus, for example, being added to the armamentarium of possible treatments for various disorders.

But it has not been in treatment alone that advances in technology have proved useful in the health field. New equipment such as the body scanners, fetal monitoring machines, and the cardiac monitors have helped both in detecting illness and abnormality and in maintaining surveillance of patients undergoing treatment. Nor should we forget the computer, with its tremendous capabilities for the rapid processing of information, which is being used in the diagnosis and continued monitoring of persons with disease.

There have been many changes, too, in the field of rehabilitation. Our knowledge of the functioning of the human body has increased, and we have been able to utilize much of our new knowledge—in nutrition, body chemistry, and the like—in hastening people's recovery from illness and their restoration to health. We have a better understanding, for example, of the physiology of motor activity, and this knowledge has contributed to the development of the new science of *kinesiology*, which deals with the study of human movement and human performance.

New communications technology has made possible alternative methods of delivering health care. In the Australian bushland, a doctor may talk directly to a patient on an isolated sheep station, for example, by radiotelephone to find out what the problem is and to advise on treatment. A person with a pacemaker can receive prompt counsel on the state of his heart and his pacemaker, wherever he or she may be in the world, through the use of a new electronic device. The device, called a "screener," is battery-operated and, when placed on the skin near the

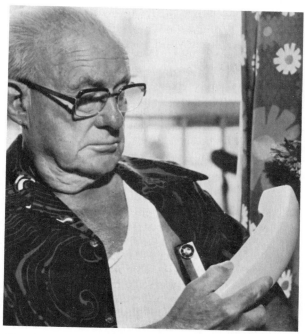

Heart patient Dick Jensen with screener (a battery-operated device that picks up electrical activity of the heart and converts it to an audible tone) in place can telephone the cardiac unit of the hospital to have his cardiac performance monitored. (Courtesy Westworld Publications Ltd., Vancouver, B.C. Photo by Michael Maher.)

top of the left arm and chest, picks up the electrical activity of the heart as an audible tone. The sound can be transmitted by telephone to the cardiac receiving unit of the patient's hospital for interpretation and follow-up counseling.[7]

Television has also proved to be very useful in health work. It has helped to bring the latest in health care to many people far away from major health centers. Health education programs are now being beamed to remote villages in northern Canada via satellite television. Television equipment in the operating rooms of teaching hospitals can allow students and doctors in adjoining rooms and buildings as well as in faraway hospitals to follow the progress of operations. The possibility of monitoring patients by videotelephone no longer seems a futuristic dream.

THE BLENDING OF TRADITIONAL AND WESTERN MEDICINE

Rather ironically, at the same time that Western medicine is being catapulted into the space age in terms of detection and treatment of illness, there has been a resurgence of interest in the ways of traditional healers. We are, in fact, beginning to recognize that perhaps there was something to be said for Grandmother's home remedies after all. For a long time, the Chinese have successfully blended scientific and traditional medicine, and the Western world is starting to take another, less prejudiced, look at some of the folk medicine we scoffed at in the not-too-distant past. Acupuncture, for example, which has been practiced in the Orient for many centuries but was scorned by Western medicine until recently, is now accepted as having a legitimate role in our medical therapy.

In recent years there has also been a great deal of research into plant medicine in such countries as Ghana and Nigeria, where herbalists have long been a part of the traditional health scene. Results from this research are showing that many herbs traditionally used to treat disease do indeed have remarkable curative powers. This is perhaps not so startling when one realizes that digitalis, which is so very important in the treatment of heart disease, was extracted originally from the foxglove plant, although it is now manufactured chemically in the laboratory.

In many countries of the world, including the Philippines, Thailand, and Ghana, to name but a few, traditional birth attendants are being incorporated into the organized system of health care in the country. Training programs sponsored by governments and international agencies help to upgrade the midwives' skills, and they are proving to be very helpful in promoting the health of women, particularly in the rural areas. Another individual now being viewed as a strong potential partner in health care in many developing nations is the witch doctor, or medicine man, whose methods of healing have often included many different forms of treatment, including the use of herbs and massage as well as invocation of the spirits.

IMPLICATIONS FOR NURSING

And what, you may ask, does all this mean for nursing?

Insofar as the emphasis on health promotion and disease prevention these days is concerned, it certainly means that nurses must have a good knowledge base about health, nutrition, exercise, and life skills.[8] Nurses are seen as key figures in health promotion, for several reasons. Health teaching has long been considered a major nursing responsibility, although it has not always received the attention it warrants in nursing education programs. Nurses have earned their acceptance by the public as persons knowledgeable about health matters. Nurses are also more accessible than many other health profes-

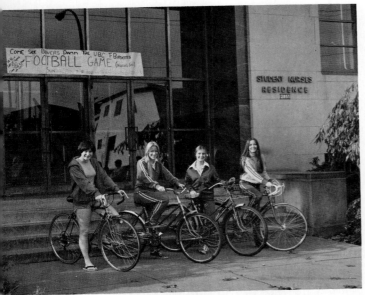

Nurses need exercise and recreation too. These students are combining both in an outing after classes are finished for the day.

sionals to people who want help and advice on health matters. Consider the nurse who is living in the community and raising a family. Even if she is not engaged in active professional practice, her house soon becomes a neighborhood center for the care and treatment of minor illnesses, for first-stop emergency care in many cases, and for general counseling about health problems for people in the community.

Nurses who are in active practice, particularly those in school settings, occupational health, or community health, play a major role in providing information and counseling people about ways and means to promote their health and prevent disease. Many nurses have become involved in starting and, often, operating fitness programs in schools, hospitals, offices, plants, and communities. A great many more are teaching others by example, through their own attitudes toward, and participation in, fitness programs.[9]

Many large companies employ nurses who, in addition to performing routine first-level care functions, act as health counselors. The nurse may undertake fitness evaluations or set up lunchtime exercise programs for employees. She might counsel an employee who suffers from chronic bronchitis, for example, on the hazards of cigarette smoking. Nurses who act as health counselors require effective communication skills as well as a broad knowledge base.

The realignment of our health care system, with the shift toward more ambulatory and home care services, has increased the number of nurses working in the community. Here, nurses are playing an increasingly large role in identifying patient needs, coordinating the various services available, and providing care. They require skills for assessing the health status of individuals and families, for applying techniques to maintain or restore health and to prevent illness, and for helping people to cope with the effects of illness or disability.[10]

Nurses need to be knowledgeable about the resources available in the community in which they work. Many new and innovative programs are developing to fill needs created by the disintegration of the traditional family unit. There are now day care services for senior citizens as well as for children, and drop-in centers for all age groups. Transition houses for battered wives and their children have begun to appear in major urban centers in the United States and Canada, as have halfway houses for the mentally ill and for alcoholics and drug abusers. In inner-city neighborhoods, where language and cultural beliefs of different ethnic groups may pose problems for the nurse, interpreters and other resource persons for the newcomer are often available through neighborhood community centers, local drop-in centers, or churches.

An increasingly large number of nurses are involved in working with older people, who now constitute such a large part of our society. Many nurses are providing health maintenance services for people in senior citizen housing units, helping them to keep well and as active and independent as possible, for as long as possible. Nurses are also the principal providers of care in nursing homes and extended care facilities, where so many of the sick elderly are in residence.

People coming into short-stay hospitals these days are usually acutely ill. Many, like the accident victim with multiple injuries or the person who has just suffered a heart attack or a stroke, require very intensive nursing care. The complexity of care and the highly sophisticated machinery used require specialized skills and, indeed, a large number of nurses are now taking advanced preparation to become clinical specialists.

As so many of the diseases prevalent in our society today are attributable to high-pressure urban living, it is important for nurses to have a good understanding of the nature of stress and the common ways of coping with it. Nurses, as well as their patients, are vulnerable to the effects of stress, and the nurse must examine her own lifestyle carefully to make sure that she plans her activities to include sufficient rest and recreation in order to offset the stress she encounters in her working environment.

Many of our stress-reduction techniques, as, for example, yoga and meditation, have come to us from other cultures. We are beginning to recognize that we have a great deal to learn from the traditional ways of healing of other peoples. An understanding of different beliefs and customs in regard to health and illness has become important for nurses, particularly in view of the multicultural fabric of our North American society.

SUMMARY

All indications point to a greater emphasis on the promotion of health and the prevention of illness in our health care services. Agencies are rapidly developing to provide more ambulatory and home care services, and it is likely that hospitals in the future will be reserved for the acutely ill who require highly specialized services. These trends in health care delivery indicate a greater need for nurses who are able to work in the community, can assume broader clinical responsibilities, and can plan, organize, and carry out health promotion and disease prevention programs for all age groups. Nurses working in hospitals will need even more highly developed skills to care for the acutely ill. The next decade will undoubtedly see a tremendous increase in the numbers of nurses functioning in expanded roles, both in the community and in the hospital setting, as nurse practitioners and clinical specialists.

The explosion in biomedical knowledge that we have seen in the past 35 years has brought about so many changes in the health care field that a major problem is to keep practitioners up to date with the latest developments in their field. For nurses (and others), this means a continuous renewal of knowledge and skills throughout their professional careers. The basic knowledge and skills you will gain from your introductory course in nursing should provide a solid foundation on which to build.

SUGGESTED READINGS

Aiken, L.: Nursing Priorities for the 1980's: Hospitals and Nursing Homes. American Journal of Nursing 81(2):324–330, February, 1981.

American Nurses' Association: A National Policy for Health Care: Principles and Positions. Nursing Dimensions, 7:12–14, Fall, 1979.

Banning, J.: A Personal Commitment to Fitness Results in Healthier Clients. The Canadian Nurse, 76(5):38–41, May, 1980.

Colt, A. M., et al.: Home Health Care is Good Economics. Nursing Outlook, 25(10):632–636, October, 1977.

Dayani, I.: Concepts of Wellness. Nursing Practice, 4:31 +, January-February, 1979.

Galton, L.: Questions Patients Want to Ask about Their Health and How You Can Answer Them. Nursing 77, 7(4):54–59, April, 1977.

Hirshman, A.: "Interested in Preventive Health Care? Try Working in a Health Maintenance Organization." Nursing 78, 8(10):16–18, October, 1978.

Iveson-Iveson, J.: Prevention: How to Stay Healthy.
Part 1: The General Picture and Diet. Nursing Mirror, 149:27, September 13, 1979.
Part 2: Exercise. Nursing Mirror, 149:29, September 20, 1979.
Part 12: Everybody's Business—but Especially the Nurse's. Nursing Mirror, 149:26, November 29, 1979.

Shamansky, S. L., et al.: "Levels of Prevention: Examination of the Concept." Nursing Outlook, 28(2):104–108, February, 1980.

REFERENCES

1. Constitution of the World Health Organization, Geneva, April 7, 1948.
2. Best, P.: The Elderly: A Challenge to Nursing. Health Promotion for the Elderly. Part 13. Nursing Times, 74:111–114, January 19, 1978.
3. Shamansky, S. L., et al.: Levels of Prevention: Examination of a Concept. Nursing Outlook, 28(2):104–108, February, 1980.
4. Hirshman, A.: Interested in Preventive Health Care? Try Working in a Health Maintenance Organization. Nursing 78. 8(10):16–18, October, 1978.
5. Breslow, L., and Somers, A.: Lifetime Health Monitoring Program. Parts 1 and 2. Nursing Practice 4:40 +, May-June 1979, 4:S–ix to S–xii, July-August, 1979.
6. Johnston, M.: Ambulatory Health Care in the 80's. American Journal of Nursing 80(1):76–77, January 1980.
7. Tompkins, J.: "Help Is Just a Heartbeat Away." Westworld, Westworld Publications Ltd. Vancouver, B.C. 7(1):21, January-February, 1981.
8. Bajnok, I.: Perspective (Guest Editorial). The Canadian Nurse, 76(4):6, April, 1980.
9. Macnamara, E. L.: Fitting Nursing into Fitness. The Canadian Nurse, 76(4):33–35, April, 1980.
10. Second Report to the Congress. March 15, 1979 (Revised). Nurse Training Act of 1975. Health Manpower References. U.S. Department of Health, Education and Welfare, Public Health Service. (DHEW Publication No. HRA 79–45). Division of Nursing, Hyattsville, Maryland.

2

The Nurse Should Be Able to:

- Describe the health-illness continuum
- Explain the concept of optimal health
- Discuss the "holistic" approach to health care
- List the five types of basic needs postulated by Maslow
- Explain the concept of homeostasis as it applies to an individual's
     health
- Explain the role of stress in the causation of illness
- List and give examples of various types of stressors
- Explain the general adaptation syndrome
- Explain the local adaptation syndrome
- Describe the flight-fight reaction of the body
- List and give examples of commonly used psychological adaptive
     mechanisms

HEALTH AND ILLNESS

CHAPTER 2

INTRODUCTION

In North America today, we are a highly health-conscious people. For the past decade, our governments and private agencies interested in health have been telling us that, despite the advances in medical science and the tremendous sums of money spent on health care, most of us are not really healthy. We have not compared well with some of our European counterparts on international studies of physical fitness. Furthermore, we are told, much of our ill health is due to our own bad habits. We are eating too much, we are leading lives that are too sedentary, and we are living at too hectic a pace.

The campaigns waged by government agencies and others appear to be having some effect. Millions of North Americans—an estimated 100 million in 1980—now include some form of exercise in their lifestyle. There has also been a tremendous increase in the number of people learning yoga, meditation, and other techniques to assist in reducing tension. We have also become very conscious of the nutritional value of the foods we eat as well as the calories they contain. Although some experts are now saying that we may have emphasized slimness too much and that some people may be healthier with a little extra weight, there is no doubt that "thin" is currently "in."

It is all part of a fitness revolution that has swept across the United States, Canada, Great Britain, Australia, New Zealand, and many other countries in the past few years. Experts are telling us that it is one of the major sociological events of the twentieth century.[1]

As health professionals to whom other people turn for advice on ways to develop a healthy lifestyle, nurses need to have a good understanding of what health and illness are all about. They need also to be aware of current thinking in regard to factors that contribute to good health, as well as those that contribute to ill health.

THE HEALTH-ILLNESS CONTINUUM

Basic to the practice of all of the health professions is an understanding of the health-illness concept. Both health and illness are relative states, and the words themselves mean different things to different people. As a person gets older, he tends to accept a few aches and pains as a normal part of the aging process, whereas a runner may feel that he is not in good health unless he can cover 15 miles easily. Health and illness may indeed be viewed on a continuum that ranges from extreme poor health when death is imminent to peak or high-level wellness.[2]

Neither health nor illness is constant or absolute; both are ever-changing states of being. A person may wake up in the morning, for example, with a headache. He may feel so ill, in fact, that he decides that he is not well enough to go to work, but he remembers that he has an important appointment at nine o'clock. After one or two cups of coffee and breakfast, he may begin to think that he is not so sick as he thought he was, and if his appointment goes well, he may feel in excellent health by lunch time.

What, then, constitutes health and illness? Extreme states of ill-health are usually fairly easy to identify, but a person who is carrying out his normal daily activities may have a serious illness according to his physician and yet appear healthy to other people. Some illnesses that are looked upon as serious deviations from health in our Western society may be highly desirable in other cultures. In some societies, for example, the person who sees visions or hears imaginary voices talking to him may be highly esteemed, whereas we might consider that this individual has a serious mental illness. Worm infestations are so common in some parts of the world that it is rare to see an individual who does not suffer from one.

THE HEALTH CONTINUUM

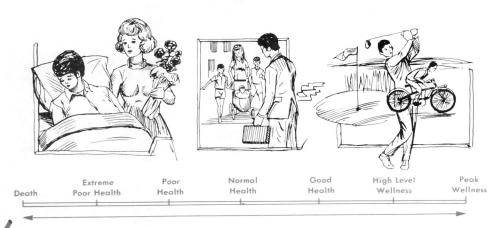

| Death | Extreme Poor Health | Poor Health | Normal Health | Good Health | High Level Wellness | Peak Wellness |

Health may be viewed as a continuum that ranges from extreme states of ill health to peak wellness.

THE MEANINGS OF HEALTH, ILLNESS, AND DISEASE

At one time, health was defined as the absence of illness; a person was considered healthy as long as he was not sick. Statements in the literature of recent years, however, indicate that health is no longer looked upon simply as the absence of illness, but has a positive meaning of its own. Some people have criticized the World Health Organization's definition of health quoted at the beginning of Chapter 1, on the basis that complete well-being for all is an unattainable goal. Still, others feel that it should be looked upon as an ideal toward which we should consciously strive.

In a similar vein to the World Health Organization definition (although not quite so idealistically), the U.S. President's Commission on the Health Needs of the Nation stated that health means "optimum physical, mental and social efficiency."[3]

A working document prepared by the Department of Health and Welfare in Canada entitled A New Perspective on the Health of Canadians also discusses the goal of health care "to increase freedom from disability, as well as to promote a state of well-being sufficient to perform at adequate levels of physical, mental and social activity, taking age into consideration."[4]

Despite the difference in terms used to modify "well-being," these statements express essentially the same thought, that is, that health is a positive state of being that includes physical fitness, mental (or emotional) stability, and social ease.

As health has assumed a more positive meaning for us, the term "illness" has conversely taken on a more negative connotation. We are now inclined to talk of a person as having a "health problem" or a "health deficit," rather than say that he is ill. Illness in this context is looked upon as an interruption in the continuous process of health, manifested by abnormalities or disturbances of functioning. When these abnormalities appear clustered together, they become recognizable as the signs and symptoms of a particular disease, for example, the high temperature, cough, and chest pain that are commonly seen in people with pneumonia.[5]

But definitions of the term "disease" are also changing. The following statement by McHugh is perhaps helpful in this regard:

The term "disease" is difficult to define, because it is a concept and not something given or concrete in nature. As a concept it focuses on patients as organisms and conveys the idea that among all the morbid physical changes in physical and mental health, it is possible to recognize groups of abnormalities as distinct entities or syndromes separable from one another and from the normal. . . .

Abnormalities can as logically be viewed as quantitative changes merging imperceptibly into one another and into the normal.[6]

TWO BASIC CONCEPTS: OPTIMAL HEALTH AND HOLISM

Optimal Health. Implicit in the definitions of health discussed previously are two basic concepts that underlie the framework on which modern health care is based. The first is the concept of *optimal health*, or optimal functioning, as the aim of health care for each individual. This concept is based on the premise that each individual has his own optimal level of functioning,[7] which represents the best state of well-being that is possible for him. Most people have some type of minor health deficit. They may have a minor physical problem, such as an allergy to certain foods, for example, or a small speech impediment. Or, they may be "shy" and have a problem in meeting people. Some people have an unreasonable fear of heights or of cats, which would be examples of problems in the psychological realm of functioning. The point here is that people rarely attain perfection in all aspects of their health—physical, mental, and social—and certainly do not achieve it all of the time, but each individual has his own unique optimum that is attainable for him.

Many people in our society have chronic health problems of a more serious nature than those described above, yet they manage to maintain a normal lifestyle as long as they take certain precautions and respect the limitations imposed by their illness. A person with a condition such as diabetes, for example, may consider himself to be in good health as long as his diabetes is under control and he can carry on with his usual activities. He may have to be careful with his diet and take more precautions than the average person does to guard against infection, but the majority of people with diabetes manage very well, with only occasional disturbances of total functioning. The optimal level of health for a diabetic would, of course, be different for each individual with diabetes, as well as being different from that which is possible for a person without this problem.

To use another example, the person who has suffered a stroke and is paralyzed on one side of his body may not regain total functioning of his affected arm and leg, but he may be able to achieve independence in daily living activities and take an active functioning role in society again. The optimal level of health, in his case, would include the best possible restoration of physical, emotional, and social functioning compatible with his illness.

Holism. The second basic concept is the premise that an individual's health must be considered in terms of his total functioning. That is to say, man must be viewed as a whole; one cannot separate the physical, social, and emotional components of his health. This concept is frequently referred to as the "holistic" approach to health care.

If we again take the example of the person who has had a stroke, it is easy to see that his physical disability will interfere with both his emotional and his social well-being. He will undoubtedly be very anxious and will probably be afraid that he is no longer the person that he was. His illness will perhaps require lengthy hospitalization and he will be cut off from normal social activities with his family and friends. This individual will need considerable help from nursing and other health personnel to regain optimal functioning in regard to all aspects of his health.

Even in the case of minor illnesses, such as a bout of influenza or a short-lived gastrointestinal upset, a person's mental outlook and his interactions with other people are affected. Conversely, an emotional problem, such as anxiety over examinations or an unpleasant social encounter, will affect one's appetite, one's digestion, and perhaps other aspects of physical functioning. In considering a person's health, then, one must look at the whole person, not just his physical fitness, or his mental state, or his social functioning.

BASIC HUMAN NEEDS

If we accept the premise that good health is the ability to function at one's highest level physically, mentally, and socially, it seems appropriate to look next at the conditions that foster good health. What is needed for an individual to attain his optimal level of well-being? This leads us, then, quite logically, to a consideration of basic human needs.

There does not seem to be any doubt that there are certain basic needs that are common to all beings of the human species, and that these needs must be fulfilled if an individual is to attain his optimal level of well-being. The subject of basic needs has been studied in depth by people in the social sciences looking for primary motivating forces underlying human behavior, and by people in the health field seeking to identify factors causing health problems. At one point, it was felt that all human needs could be categorized under two headings, one physiological in derivation and the other psychological. Another group of theorists classified needs on the basis of whether their origin was internal or external. Still others have identified long lists of human needs, all considered basic.

Abraham Maslow's theory of a hierarchy of needs is used in many nursing schools as a conceptual framework for the consideration of human needs. Not everyone agrees with all aspects of his theory, and some have suggested modifications in his hierarchy, but the basic principles outlined in the theory are fairly well accepted.

Maslow has suggested that there are five basic categories of human needs and that these may be arranged in order of priority for satisfaction. According to Maslow's theory, lower level needs must be satisfied (or, at least, mostly so) before the individual attempts to satisfy needs of a higher order. The basic types of needs identified by Maslow, in order of priority, are:

1. Physiological needs
2. Safety and security needs
3. Needs for love and belonging
4. Esteem needs
5. Needs for self-actualization[8]

These will be discussed in detail in Chapter 13.

MAINTAINING EQUILIBRIUM

Throughout life, an individual must continuously adjust to changes both within himself and in his relationships with the world around him. His basic needs must be met, and at the same time he must maintain his equilibrium in a constantly changing world.

Physiological Homeostasis. As we go about the daily business of living, changes are constantly occurring within the body as it adjusts to the demands we make upon it. Our temperature, for example, rises during our waking hours and falls again during sleep. The heart beats faster when we exercise and returns to a lower rate when we rest. Our muscles alternately tense and relax as we engage in various activities. In fact, an infinite number of minor adjustments are continuously being made in the body during the normal process of daily living. However, these adjustments must be kept within certain limits if the individual is to survive.[9] As you proceed with your studies, you will notice that normal ranges have been established for body temperature, for blood pressure, for pulse rate, for the amount of sugar in the bloodstream—in fact, for all of the body processes that are measurable. Deviations outside the normal range usually indicate that the body's internal equilibrium, that is, its physiological homeostasis, has been disturbed.

Environmental Equilibrium. Just as the body must maintain a certain consistency in its internal environment, the human organism must also achieve a balance in its interactions with the surrounding environment. Man's environment is made up of two components: the physical environment, which consists of the natural elements as well as the structures that man has built upon the earth, and the social environment, that is, the people around him and the society in which he lives.

Man has learned both to adapt himself to the

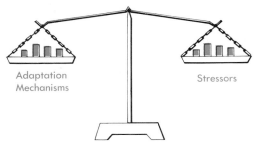

In homeostasis the body attempts to restore a state of equilibrium by counterbalancing the effect of stressors with adaptation mechanisms.

physical environment and to change that environment to suit his needs. In a cold climate, for example, his basal metabolic rate increases in order to maintain his body temperature at a constant level; he eats more energy-giving foods and he wears warm clothing to protect himself from the cold. But man also modifies the environment to meet his requirements. Depending on the climate, he either builds a well insulated home and installs central heating, so that the immediate surroundings are suited to his needs, or he designs a well ventilated house and puts in air conditioning (if he can afford to do so). In some climates, he may need central heating for the winter and air conditioning for the summer.

There are, however, many aspects of man's interaction with the physical environment that are currently giving cause for concern. There is considerable interest in the subject of *ecology* as it applies to man. Ecology is the study of organisms and how they relate to their environment.

Good water is pure water. A sample of this water will be analyzed for pollutants that could endanger the health of people who live in the housing development being built across the bay.

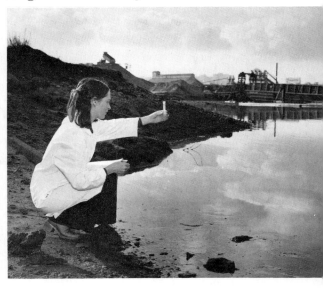

Many people fear that the delicate balance between man and nature is being disturbed: for example, by nuclear explosions, which alter atmospheric conditions, by the pollution of our lakes and rivers, which creates unsanitary living conditions, and by the rapid diminishment of many of our natural resources, to name but a few of the concerns of ecologists.

Psychosocial Equilibrium. Then, there is the social environment. Man is a social animal, and contact with other human beings is essential to his well-being. He is constantly interacting with his family, his friends, his neighbors, the people he meets at work or at school—in fact, with all of the people who inhabit his social world. Most of us have learned to achieve a balance in our relationships with other people, so that our psychosocial equilibrium remains intact. We have learned to use emotional outlets when stress becomes too great. We may use strenuous physical exercise, yoga, or meditation, for example, to get rid of tensions caused by an unpleasant day with people at work. Or, we may go to a movie to forget our troubles with the family temporarily.

In discussing health and illness, it is impossible categorically to separate physiological homeostasis from ecological equilibrium or from psychosocial equilibrium. Each affects the others. A business executive, for example, may be under considerable pressure at work—in his psychosocial environment, if you like—but the ulcer he develops indicates a resultant disturbance in his physiological equilibrium. On the other hand, when a person is physically ill, his relationships with people undergo a change. You have probably found when you had a bad cold or the flu that you did not want to be bothered with other people. The physical environment, too, affects not only a person's physiological state but also his psychosocial equilibrium. A lack of adequate housing, for example, can be a major factor in both physical and mental illness.

STRESS AND STRESSORS

Stresses of any kind upset the delicate balance of the human organism, which reacts by altering certain structures, processes, or behaviors to restore equilibrium. A person may perspire profusely on a very warm day, for example; he then becomes thirsty and increases his fluid intake to restore the fluids he has lost through sweating. The term "stressor" is used to designate any factor that disturbs the organism's equilibrium. There are a number of ways of categorizing

stressors. They may be classified on the basis of whether they are internal or external, or as biological, psychosocial, or environmental (referring to the physical environment). Freeman has suggested four categories of stressors that would seem to be logical and to encompass all types of disturbances that may act as stressors:[10]

1. Deprivational stress
2. Stresses of excess
3. Stresses created by change
4. Stresses of intolerance

Deprivational Stress. In deprivational stress, there is a lack of some essential factor for the well-being of the individual. Deprivational stressors, then, would include the lack of essential items needed to maintain the chemical balance of the body, such as the lack of water, of oxygen, or vitamins, or of food elements. Other types of deprivational stress might be psychological or sociological in nature. A person who is isolated from contact with other human beings suffers considerable stress. The lack of sufficient parental affection in infancy and early childhood is felt to be not only one of the causes of psychological disorders but also a factor in an infant's failure to thrive. Lack of adequate housing, again a basic need, is an environmental factor that could be considered a deprivational stressor.

Stress of Excess. On the other hand, an excess of certain factors may also disturb the organism's equilibrium. Exposure to intense heat causes tissue damage in the form of a burn; intense cold causes frostbite. If a person eats excessively, he usually has disturbances of body functioning; he becomes obese and may suffer from gastrointestinal upsets and other types of physiological disturbances. His interpersonal relationships are affected, and he is usually unhappy because he is fat.

Excessive interpersonal contact may also be a source of stress, as in a family situation where individual members have no opportunity to get off by themselves every once in a while, or in high density residential areas in a city where the neighbors seem to be constantly impinging on the privacy of one another. (The reverse is often quite true, of course, also; one can be very lonely in a crowded city if one does not have friends or close human contact.)

Changes. Changes of any sort may upset the physiological processes of the body as well as an individual's behavior. Even the time change experienced by international travelers creates stress, and an individual may take several days to become adjusted to a different "time clock"

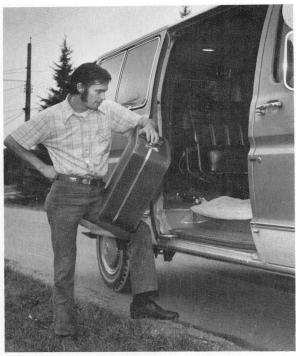

Stress wears many faces. As this young man wonders where to put all the luggage, he is probably unaware of the many stressful situations yet to be encountered on the family vacation.

for the normal body functions of eating, sleeping, and elimination. A number of studies in recent years have shown evidence of a positive relationship between the number of changes in a person's life and his subsequent development of illness. The amount of stress created by different types of change has been assessed for its impact on a person's health, and rating scales have been developed to calculate a person's vulnerability to illness on the basis of the number of major changes in his life in a one-year span of time. The death of a spouse is usually considered to be the change causing the greatest disturbance in a person's life. Other stressful events include losing one's job, changing jobs, moving from one part of the country to another, or even from one neighborhood to another, and changes in one's lifestyle. Happy events, such as marriages, getting a promotion, taking a vacation, and even Christmas, also bring their stresses. If a person has too many changes in his life in too short a period of time, he becomes a likely candidate for major illness.[11]

Stress of Intolerance. Stresses of intolerance are exemplified in the allergic reactions to certain foods, chemical substances, or pollens from which many people suffer. The body's reaction

to poisons or toxins would also illustrate this point. If one eats food that has "gone bad," the body attempts to remove the substance, frequently by vomiting the stomach's contents. An intolerance to psychological factors in the environment, such as an unhappy work situation, is also a source of stress. Moving to a different country where customs and social values are markedly different from those one has been accustomed to may cause stress sufficient to result in what is called cultural shock. Nurses working with minority groups in our own country or in poverty neighborhoods may experience some of this cultural shock when they encounter customs and ways of life that are different from their own.

THE BODY'S REACTION TO STRESS: ADAPTATION MECHANISMS

The nineteenth century French biologist Claude Bernard is credited with first pointing out the body's need to maintain a certain consistency in its internal environment. He described the process of physiological homeostasis, although he himself did not use the term. It was Walter Cannon, an American physiologist of the twentieth century, who coined the word "homeostasis." Cannon wrote of the "wisdom of the body" in bringing into play certain mechanisms if changes in its internal environment threaten to go beyond safe limits.[12] These are frequently referred to as "adaptation mechanisms"; they are the body's counterbalances, in other words.

For example, if body temperature threatens to go too high, the individual usually becomes very flushed and breaks out into a profuse sweat. Both of these reactions are attempts on the body's part to lower its internal temperature. Increased circulation to the tissues underlying the skin (which causes the appearance of flushing) helps to expose more blood to the cooling effects of the surrounding atmosphere. The perspiration from the profuse sweating evaporates on the surface of the skin and, in the process, also helps to carry heat away from the body. The body has a number of adaptation mechanisms, and we will be discussing many of these in later chapters of this text in conjunction with specific body processes.

The General Adaptation Syndrome

Hans Selye, a professor at the University of Montreal, was also interested in the body's reactions to disturbances in its equilibrium and pointed out that there is a general nonspecific response that occurs. He described this originally as the phenomenon of "just being sick" and later elaborated on it in his theory of the general adaptation syndrome (G.A.S.). This syndrome he believed, is the response of the body to any agent that causes physiological stress. The response may be divided into three stages: the alarm reaction, in which the body's defense mechanisms are mobilized; the stage of resistance, when the battle for equilibrium is most active; and the stage of exhaustion, which occurs if the stressor is severe enough, or is present over a long enough period of time, to deplete the body's resources for adaptation.

The early signs and symptoms of disease are remarkably the same for many illnesses; this was Selye's original "just being sick" phenomenon. These symptoms usually include a slight rise in temperature, a loss of energy, a lack of interest in food, and a general feeling of malaise. It is in the second stage of the syndrome, the "stage of resistance," that the signs and symptoms of the body's reaction to specific disorders are seen: the rash erupts on the skin of the child with measles, or the localized pain in the chest and difficulty in breathing occur in pneumonia. If the stress is not relieved, or if it is of sufficient intensity to cause extensive damage to tissues, the body's adaptive mechanisms may not be able to restore equilibrium and exhaustion will set in.

The Local Adaptation Syndrome

In addition to the generalized reaction that occurs in the body as a result of stress, localized reactions occur when a specific part or organ is affected. Probably the most common example of a localized reaction is inflammation, which represents an attempt on the part of the body to barricade or "wall off" a particular section that has been damaged to prevent the spread of the harm-producing agent to other healthy sections of the body. Thus, if you prick your finger with a contaminated needle, you will probably soon have a swollen, painful finger. The finger may be very uncomfortable, but the localization of the inflammation is useful in that it helps to prevent the infection from entering the blood stream and traveling to other parts of the body.[13]

Selye called this local reaction the "local adaptation syndrome" (L.A.S.). It follows the same three-stage pattern as the G.A.S. First, there is a generalized reaction—the whole hand becomes slightly reddened and a little swollen. This is followed by a more localized reaction in the specific finger, which becomes very painful, reddened, and swollen. The inflammation will gradually subside unless the infection is sufficiently potent to overcome the defenses marshaled to stop it. In the latter case, it will surmount the "barricade" and travel up the arm, spreading to other parts of the body.

Reaction to Psychosocial Stressors

Although much of the early work on stress was related to the body's reactions to physiological stressors, there is considerable evidence that stress created by psychological or social factors will also cause physiological damage to the body. This is illustrated in the case of the business executive discussed previously who developed an ulcer as a result of pressure at work.

One well-known response involving physiological reactions to psychological stress is the flight-fight reaction first described by Cannon. This reaction represents the body's response to immediate danger and is called forth whenever the individual is frightened or feels threatened with harm. There is an emergency mobilization of the body's physiological defense mechanisms as the body prepares for instant action (either fight or flight). This, too, is an alarm reaction, but of a different sort from that described by Selye in his G.A.S. When a person is frightened, his heart beats more forcefully and faster; his breathing is increased in rate and depth; blood is withdrawn from surface vessels and the viscera and is shunted to the muscles; the unneeded gastrointestinal tract goes into a temporary slowdown; blood pressure increases, and the muscles become tense in preparation for action. This is the body's emergency mechanism, designed to protect the individual from real or imagined danger. Anxiety, which is a modified form of fear, usually accompanies people to a health agency, and the nurse will often note manifestations of the flight-fight reactions in her patients. She will probably also note them in herself, particularly when she is in new and unfamiliar surroundings or has to do a treatment for the first time. Helping the patient to become familiar with the physical surroundings and providing him with an explanation of routines and procedures in the particular agency will help to allay many of his fears. Fear of the unknown is one of the main sources of anxiety for most people. Nurses tend to become so accustomed to the environment of the agency in which they work that they often forget that everything may be strange and frightening for the patient. (The subject of anxiety is discussed in Chapter 30.)

Individual Differences in the Stress Response

Stress is considered to be the nonspecific response of the body to any demand. It is a normal and useful mechanism but can sometimes be excessive and damaging. The ability to cope with stressors varies from one individual to another and, also, within the same individual from time to time, depending on such factors as the state of one's general health, the time of the day or month, one's mental outlook, and current relationships with other people.[14] Of 20 people in a crowded room, for example, all of whom are exposed to someone who is coughing and sneezing and coming down with influenza, possibly only one or two—or, perhaps, none at all—will subsequently become ill with the flu. It will depend on each individual's vulnerability at the particular time. A person who is overly tired, has just had a run-in with his boss, or has had to cope with too many changes in his life in the last little while is much more likely to become ill.

Evidence suggests that we become ill not so much from the presence of the stressor itself but, rather, from the way we react to it. As Selye himself puts it, "it is not so much what happens to you but the way you take it" that is important in producing stress.[15]

Some people enjoy a high level of stress in their lifestyle and deliberately seek it out. Often these individuals have very great achievement needs and set themselves increasingly difficult goals. Sometimes referred to as "Type A individuals" or "workaholics," these people tend to drive themselves to the brink of exhaustion while ignoring the need for rest and relaxation. These people have been identified as being particularly prone to coronary artery disease.[16]

Some illinesses are not caused by any particular stressor but arise from a faulty adaptive response on the part of the body to the stressor. These are called "diseases of adaptation" and are believed to be brought about by hormonal disturbances. Among the disorders included in this category are insomnia, high blood pressure, indigestion, gastric and duodenal ulcers, and cardiovascular and kidney diseases.[15]

Almost everybody has some particular part of the body that, in him, appears to be most vulnerable to disease. Some people are prone to stomach upsets, for example, and others to chest conditions. The part of the body usually affected depends on a number of factors, such as previous illness in a body organ or a genetic predisposition to certain disorders. After they have had one ear infection, some children seem to get another every time they have a cold. And, if your aunt had a "nervous stomach," this may help to explain your gastrointestinal upsets as examinations draw near, while some of your classmates have symptoms related to other parts of the body.

PSYCHOLOGICAL DEFENSE MECHANISMS

Another level of response to stress is seen in the adaptive defense mechanisms we use to maintain psychosocial equilibrium. These are often referred to as "mental mechanisms" because they represent intellectual processes, or changes, in thought behavior; we use them to protect ourselves from stressors that threaten our self-esteem. If a person is frustrated in his attempts to fulfill his basic needs, he usually becomes angry and may retaliate with aggression toward the person or object that is thwarting his goal-attainment. Open aggression toward other people is not generally acceptable in our society, and by the time a person has reached adulthood, he has usually learned to control his hostility. Adults seldom attack people in a physical sense, as children often do, but they resort to more subtle forms of aggression, such as verbal attacks, against the person or group of persons blocking them from attaining their goals.

If a person fails to gain his objective on the first attempt, he may try again, fighting a little harder this time or seeking alternative means to achieve the same goal. A person who wants to be an executive in his company, for example, may not get the coveted job on first application. He may then decide that he needs to upgrade his qualifications and enroll in night classes to improve his chances for the next opening. Or, he may decide to use every means at his disposal, fair or unfair, to make sure that he gets promoted the next time there is an opening in the executive ranks. Alternatively, of course, he may decide to quit the field and move to a different company, or else to settle for a less prestigious position in the same company.

If a person has used socially unacceptable means to achieve his goals—for example, the executive who has ridden roughshod over others to reach the top—or if he has failed to achieve his goals either by withdrawing from the field completely or by accepting a lesser, more achievable goal, he must somehow protect his self-esteem so that he can continue to live with himself. In order to make his behavior acceptable to himself and to others, he frequently makes use of defense mechanisms.

One of the most commonly used defense mechanisms is rationalization, in which a person gives socially acceptable reasons for his behavior. A student who goes to a movie, for

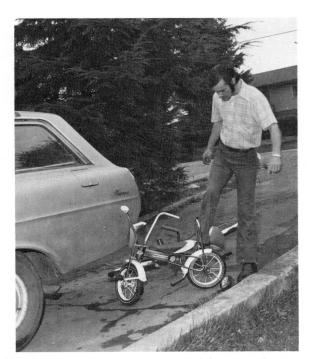

Displacement is a commonly used defense mechanism. A child's tricycle becomes the object on which this young father vents the anger and hostility he would probably like to direct at his employer after a frustrating day at work.

example, instead of staying in to study for exams, may rationalize his behavior by explaining to himself (and to others) that, after all, everyone needs a little relaxation. If he later gets angry at the teacher for not giving him what he considers a high enough grade, he may not be able to express his hostility directly at the teacher. Instead, he may become annoyed with his best friend, or go home and take his anger out on his parents. This is a form of *displacement*, in which aggressive feelings are not directed at the offending person (or object), but are shifted to a substitute; it has often been called the "kick the cat" phenomenon. Another example to illustrate this very common defense mechanism is the man who has had a frustrating day at the office and is angry with his boss. He may, on arriving home, yell at his wife for not having dinner ready, or swear at a child's tricycle that is in his path. If the hostility is frequently directed at one particular person or group of people, it is called *scapegoating*. In a family situation, there is often one member, child or adult, who seems to bear the brunt of the other members' anger. He, or she, is the family scapegoat.

Oftentimes, we ascribe our own unacceptable feelings or attitudes to other people. A person may say that so and so is very ambitious or doesn't want any members of such and such a minority group in his neighborhood, when in actual fact these are his own feelings that he dares not admit to himself. This is called *projection* and is another form of defense mechanism by which we protect our feelings of self-worth.

When people cannot achieve their own goals, they may tend to identify themselves with someone who has. They may adopt his form of dress or his mannerisms and suffer acute distress when their idol is attacked. Children, of course, identify with parents of the same sex as themselves, and this is a necessary part of their development. Students, too, on their way to goal achievement, will frequently select one particular teacher or practitioner in their field as an example of the person they want to become when they graduate, and they try to model themselves upon the image they have of this person. *Identification*, like the other defense mechanisms we use, is not necessarily a bad thing; it is often a help in goal achievement, as long as it is not carried to extreme.

Compensation can also be a constructive defense mechanism. With this mechanism we attempt to make up for real or imagined inferiorities by becoming highly competent in a sphere of endeavor different from the one in which we feel we are not good, or sometimes in the same sphere. The child who has poor motor coordination and does badly at sports in his early school years, perhaps because of his growth pattern, may compensate by becoming a "bookworm" and subsequently a high achiever in the academic field. Alternatively, he may feel that he has to make good at sports whatever the cost in time and energy, and he will then practice night and day until he overcomes his physical problems and becomes skilled at some form of sports. He may choose a highly individualized sport where he can develop his skills at his own rate, and become an expert tennis player, Ping-Pong champion, or long distance runner, for example. Or he may become a physical education teacher with an unconscious (or expressed) desire to help children with problems similar to the ones he had.

When we have feelings or desires that we cannot accept consciously, or when we encounter problems that we do not feel capable of resolving, there are a number of defense mechanisms we use to deal with the situation. We may deny that we have the forbidden motive or problem and unconsciously refuse to acknowledge that it is there, in which case we are using *denial*. We may state, for example, "I would never do that sort of thing," when we may subconsciously be tempted to do just that (whatever it is). A person's first reaction on learning that he has a serious health problem may be to deny that the words he is hearing are true. He does not have venereal disease—he could not possibly—the laboratory has mixed up the test results. Sometimes the denial persists for a long time, and the person has to work through his acceptance of the diagnosis before he will undergo treatment.

At times, a person may attempt to remove a subconscious, and forbidden, motive or desire by vigorously attacking it. Witness the ex-smoker who denounces the evils of smoking to those who still indulge. Then there is the person who jokes about unacceptable feelings, for example, fear, thereby giving the impression that only the weak are afraid—he certainly is not. Such behaviors as proclaiming too loudly against other people's sins and temptations and joking about unacceptable feelings or actions are termed *reaction formation*.

Socially unacceptable motives are, however, often channeled into acceptable forms of behavior. This is called *sublimation*. A person may sublimate his strong aggressive feelings by participating in sports where these feelings are acceptable; he can kick the football as hard as he likes and attack his opponents physically, within the rules of the game, of course.

When we have problems that we cannot resolve or experiences we would prefer to forget, we may unconsciously put them out of our mind; this is called *repression*. Without knowing we are doing so, we forget all about the appointment we do not want to keep, or completely eliminate from our minds all memory of unpleasant events. This has sometimes been called the "old oaken bucket" phenomenon, from the lyrics in which the songwriter describes the fond memories of his childhood; the unplesant ones for most of us are fortunately removed from our memory by the subconscious mechanism of repression. If, however, we consciously decide to forget about something, the behavior is called *suppression*. Like Scarlett O'Hara in *Gone With the Wind*, we decide that we will not think about that unpleasant thing until tomorrow.

Most of us also use *fantasy* in the form of daydreaming to escape temporarily from the realities of our everyday problems. In fantasy we can indulge our secret desires, achieve our goals, and forget our troubles. Daydreaming can, of course, be very productive. When lost in reverie, we may work out the solution to an impossible problem, or develop long-range plans to achieve our goals; sometimes it is very difficult to separate thoughtful reverie from daydreaming.

On occasion, in attempting to reach our goals, we may revert to a form of behavior that was acceptable at one stage of our development but is no longer considered appropriate. The expression "you are acting like a child" succinctly describes this type of mental mechanism, which is called *regression* in technical terminology. People, when they are ill, are often forced to sacrifice their independence in regard to caring for themselves; having to have someone else do for them the things they are accustomed to doing, such as feeding or bathing themselves, is often seen as a form of regression to an earlier dependent stage of their development.

Psychological defense mechanisms serve a useful purpose. They help to reduce the anxieties caused by conflicts or frustration in our attempts to fulfill basic needs; they help us to maintain our equilibrium. It is only when they are overused, or used inappropriately, that illness ensues. As with disturbances of physiological functioning, abnormalities in the use of defense mechanisms may be viewed as quantitative changes that blend imperceptibly into one another and into the normal.

STUDY SITUATION

Mr. Albert is a 45-year-old clerk in a large department store. He has suffered from asthma since early childhood. He and his wife live in a modest bungalow in a working class neighborhood. They have no children, but keep two budgies as pets. Mr. Albert's hobby is growing roses, which he exhibits at the local Horticultural Society's annual show. He has won second prize the last two years in succession. The next show is in June this year. Mrs. Albert is a thin, nervous woman who does not work outside the home. She is an immaculate housekeeper and appears to be a devoted wife, catering to her husband's every whim. Mr. Albert is frequently off work because of his asthma.

Mr. Albert arrived at the Community Health Center one afternoon toward the end of May, saying that he was too ill to work and wanted to see the doctor immediately. He appeared agitated and his breathing was labored. On being told that the doctor was busy and he would have to wait, Mr. Albert became very hostile to the nurse, telling her that he was a very sick man and needed to see the doctor right away, whereupon he collapsed at the nurse's feet.

1. What factors would you take into consideration in determining Mr. Albert's optimal level of health?

2. Which, if any, of Mr. Albert's basic needs do you think are not being met?

3. What factors do you think might be causing stress to Mr. Albert?

4. How would you categorize these factors?

5. Is Mr. Albert showing any signs of the general adaptation syndrome?

6. Is Mr. Albert exhibiting any defense mechanisms? If so, what are they?

7. Can you identify any signs of the flight-fight reaction in Mr. Albert?

SUGGESTED READING

Baldwin, J. E.: Never Jump out of a Perfectly Good Airplane. *American Journal of Nursing,* 80(5):916–917, May, 1980.

Bell, J. M.: Stressful Life Events and Coping Methods in Mental Illness and Wellness Behaviors. *Nursing Research,* 26:136–141, March-April, 1977.

Cole, W. J.: What Can We Do about Stress?" *Nursing Mirror,* 146:39, March 30, 1978.

Jones, P. S.: "An Adaptation Model for Nursing Practice." *American Journal of Nursing,* 79(11):1900–1906, November, 1978.

Milio, N.: "A Broad Perspective on Health: A Teaching-Learning Tool." *Nursing Outlook,* 24(3):160–163, March, 1976.

Pesznecker, B. L., et al.: Relationship among Health Habits, Social Assets, Psychological Well-being, Life Changes and Alterations in Health Status. *Nursing Research,* 24:443–447, November-December, 1975.

Pollitt, J.: Symptoms of Stress.
Part 1: "Types of Stress and Types of People. *Nursing Mirror,* 148:13–14, June 16, 1977.
Part 2: The Effects of Stress. *Nursing Mirror,* 148:24–26, June 23, 1977.

Sanders, M. M.: Stressed? Or Burnt Out? *The Canadian Nurse,* 76(9):33, October, 1980.

Scully, R.: Stress in the Nurse. *American Journal of Nursing,* 80(5):912–915, May, 1980.

Strom, L. M., and Tierney, M. J. G.: Type A Behavior in the Nurse. *American Journal of Nursing,* 80(5):915–918, May, 1980.

REFERENCES

1. Cohn, V.: Alive and Well and Living. *The Vancouver Sun,* January 13, 1981, p. B1.

2. Dunn, H. L.: High-Level Wellness for Man and Society. In Folta, J. R., and Deck, E. S. (eds.): *A Sociological Framework for Patient Care.* New York, John Wiley and Sons, Inc., 1966, pp. 213–219.

3. President's Commission on the Health Needs of the Nation: *Building America's Health: A Report to the President.* Washington, D.C., U.S. Government Printing Office, 1951.

4. *A New Perspective on the Health of Canadians.* A Working Document. Ottawa, Department of National Health and Welfare, April, 1974, p. 8.

5. *Ten Year Health Plan for the Americas.* Final Report of the III Special Meeting of Ministers of Health of the Americas (Santiago, Chile, October 2–9, 1972.) Official document No. 118, January 1973. Washington, D. C., Pan American Health Organization, Pan American Sanitary Bureau, p. 4.

6. McHugh, P. R.: Psychological Illness in Medical Practice. In Beeson, P. B., McDermott, W., and Wyngaarden, J. (eds.): *Textbook of Medicine,* 15th ed., Philadelphia, W. B. Saunders Company, 1979, p. 664.

7. Archer, S. E., and Fleshman, R.: *Community Health Nursing: Patterns and Practices.* North Scituate, Massachusetts, Duxbury Press, 1975, p. 24.

8. Maslow, A. H.: *Motivation and Personality.* 2nd ed. New York, Harper and Row, 1970.

9. Oken, D.: Stress—Our Friend, Our Foe. In *Blueprint for Health.* Vol. 25. Chicago, The Blue Cross Association, 1974.

10. Freeman, V. J.: Human Aspects of Health and Illness: Beyond the Germ Theory. In Folta, J. R., and Deck, E. S. (eds.): *A Sociological Framework for Patient Care.* New York, John Wiley and Sons, Inc., 1966, pp. 83–89.

11. Holmes, T. H. and Holmes, T. S.: How Change Can Make Us Ill. In *Blueprint for Health.* Vol. 25. Chicago, The Blue Cross Association, 1974.

12. Cannon, W. B.: *The Wisdom of the Body.* New York, W. W. Norton and Company, Inc., 1939.

13. Selye, H.: Stress and Nation's Health. In *Proceedings of the National Conference on Fitness and Health, Ottawa, December 4, 5 and 6, 1972.* Department of National Health and Welfare, Canada.

14. Wallace, J. M.: Living with Stress. *Nursing Times,* March 16, 1978, pp. 457–458.

15. Selye, H.: A Code for Coping with Stress. *AORN Journal,* 25(1):35–42, January, 1977.

16. O'Flynn-Comiskey, A. I.: Stress. The Type A Individual. *American Journal of Nursing.* 79(11):1956–1959, November 1979.

3

The Nurse Should Be Able to:

- Describe differences in the way people view health and illness
- Explain factors influencing a person's perception of his health status
- Name the three stages of illness
- Describe reactions of patients in each of these three stages
- Identify some of the needs of patients during each of these stages
- Describe ways in which the nurse may help to meet these needs
- Describe the impact of illness on the family

THE PERCEPTION OF HEALTH

INTRODUCTION

People do not usually think of their health in the scientific terms we have used in the previous chapter. Most people are aware, however, when they are functioning at their highest level mentally, physically, and socially, and they usually know when they are sick—by standards they have established for themselves. Because every person is a unique individual, each interprets his health and illness status according to his or her own particular perspective.

These personal perspectives are, however, considerably influenced by social and cultural factors. In assessing an individual's health, it is important to understand the social context in which he lives. All societies, as well as subgroups within these societies have certain norms, or standards, with regard to health and illness. In some cultures, for example, obesity is considered a healthy and desirable state, whereas in others it is regarded as an affliction.

The customs, traditions, and mores of a society also dictate acceptable behaviors in regard to health and illness. Individuals are expected to take all measures necessary, as approved by that society, to promote and protect their health. In most developed countries, for example, parents are expected to take their infants to the physician or to a well-baby clinic for regular checkups and to see that their children have all of the recommended immunizations to protect their health. We frown on parents who fail to have their children inoculated against typhoid fever, whooping cough, measles, poliomyelitis, and the other communicable diseases for which there are known immunity-producing agents.

When a person is ill, there are also acceptable and unacceptable standards of behaviors laid down by society. The sick person is expected to seek "appropriate" care to restore himself to a healthy state—be it treatment by a witch doctor, shaman, nurse practitioner, or specialist physician. While ill, he is also expected to cooperate with those who are caring for him.

CRITERIA FOR JUDGING HEALTH

Everyone has his own standards for assessing the state of his health. In a study to determine differences in the attitudes of people toward health and illness, Baumann identified three distinct ways in which people establish criteria to judge their health status.[1] One was related to the presence or absence of symptoms. Pain is, of course, one of the most common symptoms by which people judge the state of their health. If a person has pain, particularly of a severe or persistent nature, he usually considers himself ill. Vomiting and fever are two other common symptoms that people usually consider indicative of illness.

A second method by which people judge the state of their health is by the way they feel; they feel "good", "on top of the world" or in "top form," as the British say; or they feel "so-so," they "don't feel well," they "feel poorly," or as Selye put it, they just "feel sick."

A third way of establishing the state of one's health is on the basis of performance. Often, the criteria used relate to the individual's ability to carry out his daily activities. One person may feel that his health is good if he can work all day and still have enough energy to play a round of golf or enjoy a game of bowling in the evening. Another may decide he is ill when he finds he cannot walk up a flight of stairs without experiencing acute distress in breathing.

Now we have another set of performance criteria for assessing our health status. These are related to physical fitness testing. A person's

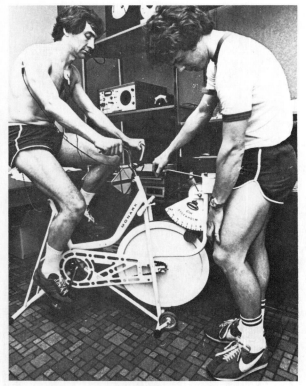

Many agencies today hold fitness testing clinics where individuals come to be tested and to learn how to maintain or improve their level of fitness.

results on the test items (measurements and performance) are compared with established norms based on age, sex, and body frame. He can then find out such things as whether he has an excess amount of fatty tissue, whether his heart responds normally to exercise, whether his respiratory functioning is as good as it should be and whether the strength in his muscles is above average, below average, or normal for his age, sex, and body build.

FACTORS INFLUENCING THE PERCEPTION OF HEALTH

The way a person views his health status tends to vary with a number of factors. Sociologists tell us that our norms for health and illness are determined as much by social and cultural factors as they are by clinical investigation.[2] A person's socioeconomic status influences the way he perceives his health, as does his level of educational attainment. People in higher socioeconomic brackets—like business executives and professionals, college professors and other teachers, and the well-educated in all walks of life—are usually much more knowledgeable about the signs and symptoms of illness than people in lower socioeconomic straits. They are also more inclined to seek the help of a health professional on the basis of symptoms. Studies have shown that poor people are just as concerned over their health as people in higher socioeconomic brackets, but often poverty is associated with a lack of knowledge about health matters as well as, in some instances, a lack of accessibility to health care and, sometimes, a lack of trust in the prevailing health care system.[3] Thus, poor people with little education often have a fatalistic view of illness.

Ethnic orientation is also a factor in how a person views his health. In both the United States and Canada, with their rich multicultural backgrounds, it is important to remember that beliefs about health and about ways of preventing and treating illness in other cultures do not always coincide with those of westernized medicine. North American Indians, for example, view a healthy individual as being in harmony, or balance, with the universe. Illness is seen as an imbalance, often caused by supernatural forces.[4] The traditional Chinese belief in the principles of Yin and Yang is also based on a balance theory. To maintain a state of health, one must balance the Yin (or cold air) forces and the Yang (or warm air) forces. An excess of either Yin or Yang is believed to cause illness. For practitioners of both beliefs, traditional cures consist of restoring a state of balance both within the individual and between the individual and the universe.

Nurses, like many other professionals, are concerned about the need to improve their own health. These young nurses are taking advantage of the recreational facilities of a park near their residence to improve their physical fitness.

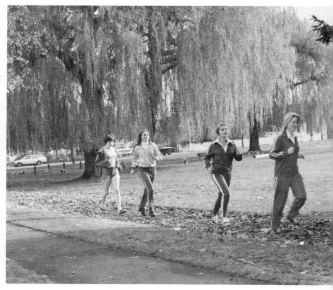

F. that incluence
   perception of health

social
status
cultural
ethnic
Religious
age
Role in family

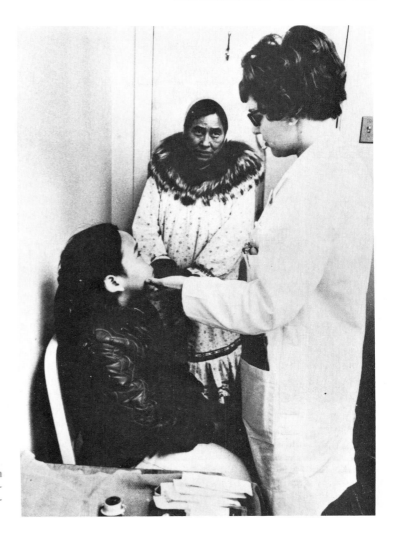

Ethnic orientation is a factor in how a person views health and the health care professional. (Courtesy Canadian Nurses Association, Helen K. Mussallem Library.)

Such beliefs may lead to conflicts with practitioners of Western scientific medicine. For example, a Chinese woman in a hospital to have a baby may be reluctant to leave her bed or participate in exercises after delivery. According to the Yin-Yang theory, her pores remain open for 30 days postpartum, during which time she must concentrate on reducing the Yin (cold air) forces within her body.[5] Other ways in which cultural differences affect our health will be discussed further in later chapters in relation to particular needs.

In many cultures, it is virtually impossible to separate medicine and religion. One very common belief about the cause of illness is that the individual is being punished for his sins. This belief will, or course, affect a person's reaction to illness. He may feel guilty about being sick, or feel that he has to atone for his sins through suffering, and sometimes may feel that he does not deserve to get better. Some religious sects believe in the total efficacy of prayer to help the individual either overcome or accept his illness, and do not believe in intervention by physicians or other health practitioners.

Other factors also affect an individual's perception of his health status. Age, for example, has a great deal to do with it. Older people usually value health as one of the most important assets in life, but they do not expect to enjoy the same level of health as they did when they were younger. The community health nurse may have to persuade them to join in exercise programs designed to improve their physical fitness, because they may think they are too old to derive benefit from them. Many adolescents appear to be particularly concerned with their health and worry over every blemish on their skin.

In most cultures, men are not supposed to complain about pain as much as women are permitted to; hence, they may tend to negate the early signs and symptoms of illness. Also, women who attend well-baby clinics and the

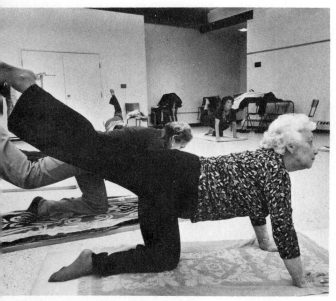

Physical fitness programs are available for people of all ages. These ladies are taking part in an exercise program for senior citizens at their local community center. (*Vancouver Sun* photo. Used with permission.)

like often have more access to health-related information. It is usually the mother in the family who sets the tone for health care, and her attitudes and practices greatly influence those of her children.

Situational factors also play a role in the perception of health. The mother in a family, for example, frequently does not become ill, even though one after another of the children, and the father, take to their beds with a cold or influenza; she is too busy looking after everyone else. Often, it is after a crisis is past that a person succumbs to illness, when the stresses and strains have subsided and the individual has time to rest.

THE STATE OF ILLNESS

The way a person views health and illness determines, to a large extent, the measures he will take to protect and improve his health, as well as the type of care he seeks when he is ill. He is also influenced in this regard by the advice of his family and friends. The person who feels in need of health care usually receives much advice on where to go to obtain it. Today, he has many choices from which to select. He may decide to go to a private physician, to the outpatient section of a hospital, or to a Health Maintenance Organization or a Community Health Center, for example, but he also has the

choice of seeking help from any one of a number of nonmedical practitioners of the healing arts, such as herbalists, naturopaths, or spiritual healers.

An increasing number of people are now seeking the advice of health practitioners to improve their health and to help them with measures to prevent illness. The majority of people seeking such advice, however, are going because they are concerned about their health—they think there is something wrong—or they know they are ill. Often, people have tried all the home remedies they have heard about from family and friends before they seek professional advice.

By the time an individual has made a decision to seek professional help, he is usually quite worried. His first appointment in the office or clinic is fraught with anxiety. He wants to know what is wrong with him—and he doesn't want to know. He would like to begin treatment, yet he may be afraid of what "they" are going to do to him. If he has undergone diagnostic tests or is referred to a specialist for further examinations, his anxiety mounts, and he awaits the final verdict with great trepidation. His fears are usually multiplied if he is told that his condition requires surgery or that he needs to be hospitalized for medical treatment. The hospital, for most people, is an unknown place; many people think of it as a place to die.

The attitude of the nurse in the physician's office or the clinic, and the initial contacts the patient has with the nurse who receives him in an inpatient facility, can do a great deal to help the patient through the difficult initial period of illness. Kindness and patience are essential. It is helpful to remember that people who are the most demanding and critical are usually the most frightened ones. Helping to allay their fears is a large part of the nurse's responsibility. The nurse who takes a personal interest in the patient and shows respect for him as an individual does a great deal to offset the depersonalization the patient so often feels in a busy health agency. Explaining treatments and procedures in simple terms, telling him what is going to be done and the reason for it, can take away much of his fear of the unknown. A knowledge of the physical layout of the agency, and of the routines, will also help the patient to feel more comfortable in a new situation (see Chapter 11).

During the initial stages of an illness, the patient usually remains in his home, although many people are admitted to the hospital for investigation and undergo a series of diagnostic examinations as inpatients. During this period, the patient may experience many of the discomforts that Selye described as "just being sick." He usually does not feel well; he may have distressing symptoms; and he often finds that he cannot keep up with his normal workload without tiring or, perhaps, cannot enjoy his usual leisure-time activities. He may not feel up to going bowling with his friends or participating in the Saturday night card game. People are usually irritable when they do not feel well. This irritability may show itself in easy tears, which seem to come at the slightest provocation, or in anger.

People react to the early signs of illness in a variety of ways. Some attempt to deny that they are ill and "keep going" despite their fatigue, or they may even try to do more than usual to prove to themselves that they are not really sick. Some people respond to the threat of illness with anger; others become very quiet and withdrawn. A few seem to enjoy their symptoms and the attention they receive from other people. If the individual subscribes to the belief that illness is a punishment, or knows he has transgressed some of the laws of health, he probably feels guilty. Cigarette smokers, for example, often are self-conscious and feel guilty if they develop a cough or a chest condition.

The Acute Phase of Illness

A person who is acutely ill has disturbances in all areas of his functioning. If the problem is a physical one, not only is he physiologically in a state of disequilibrium but also his emotional balance is threatened, and his relationships with other people are upset. Physically, he is often weakened by the illness and simply does not have the strength to cope with the daily activities of living, let alone withstand additional stress. He is particularly vulnerable, then, to assault by such stressors as shock, fluid and electrolyte imbalance, or infection. Particular care, then, must be taken to protect the patient from further harm. Extra precautions must be taken against infection, for example, and the patient's physiological responses carefully monitored to assess progress of the disease and the effects of therapy.

Mentally, the patient's energies are focused on his illness. He is usually much concerned with the daily processes that are going on in his body. He wants to know what his temperature and his blood pressure are, and he anxiously

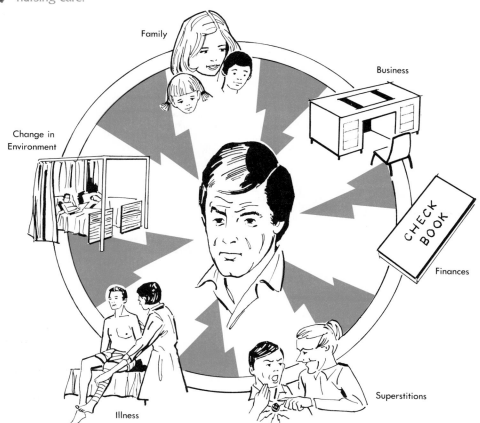

Anxiety usually accompanies illness; it is therefore a major consideration in providing nursing care.

Family

Business

Change in Environment

Finances

Illness

Superstitions

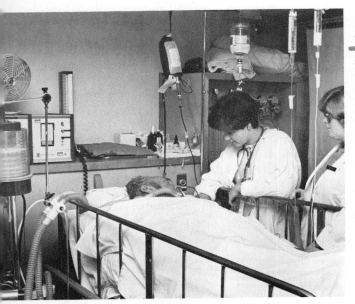

The acutely ill patient is often highly dependent on nursing personnel. This patient's recovery from anesthesia is being carefully monitored by nurses in the Postanesthetic Recovery Room of a large metropolitan hospital. (Courtesy of Vancouver General Hospital.)

awaits the outcome of tests and examinations. The interests of the acutely ill are narrowed; the patient is much more concerned with himself and his immediate environment than with anything that goes on outside the sickroom. Frequently, defense mechanisms the individual has found useful in coping with the initial stages of illness, such as denial, minimization, and repression, continue to be used. It is important that the nurse respect these behaviors, not challenge them. It is essential that the patient maintain his integrity and, if he has found coping strategies that help him to do this, the nurse should support these.[6]

In the social realm, there are certain expectations that go along with being ill. And, we also expect certain things of the ill person. He should want to get well, for example, since illness is not a desirable state of being. Today he is also expected to cooperate with those who are helping him in the process of getting better, and to assume increasing responsibility for his own care.

The acutely ill person often finds himself in a highly dependent role. He may be unable to do many things for himself, and have to rely on others to do them for him. He may need to be bathed, for example, to have his position changed, or to have his dressing reinforced. He may even need the nurse's help in maintaining such a vital body function as breathing. A person who has been independent all of his life may find it difficult to accept this help, and the nurse will need to be very tactful to enable such a person to maintain his self-respect and his dignity. Often, the patient's family can be very helpful during the acute stage in doing things for him, and the nurse should support them in their effort to aid the patient.

The Convalescent Stage

During the convalescent stage of an illness, the patient is recovering his physical and psychosocial balance. Soon, he must leave the sickroom and move back into the everyday world. This is a transition period and, for many patients, it is a difficult time. Most people recovering from an acute illness are irritable. Their strength has not fully returned, yet often new demands are being put upon them. If the person has been hospitalized because of diabetes, for example, and this is his first experience with the disorder, he will probably have to adjust to the fact that there will be many changes in his lifestyle. He may have to learn to give himself an injection of insulin, to test his urine for sugar and acetone, and to modify his eating habits to keep the diabetes under control. Often, people worry about their ability to learn everything they need to know to look after themselves. They may be fearful, too, about resuming their normal activities.

The primary focus of nursing during the convalescent stage is to enhance the patient's ability to care for himself. The nurse's teaching role is important here. Not only must she help the patient to gain new knowledge and skills, but she must also provide him with the support and encouragement he needs to foster a good learning environment. Again, the patient's family, or significant others in his life, are resources to be tapped for assistance to the patient during the convalescent stage. This will often involve the nurse in working with the family, as well as the patient, and supporting them in their efforts to help him.

Stage of Restored Health

After the convalescent stage is over, and the person returns to his normal activities, he enters a stage of restored health. For people who have had a self-limiting illness, such as a bout of pneumonia or surgery to remove a diseased gallbladder, restoration to health ideally means a return to a state of balance in all areas of functioning. For those who have a chronic health problem, such as the newly diagnosed diabetic, and those with a terminal illness such as leukemia (often called cancer of the blood), it means restoration to a state of optimal functioning.

All will, however, require continued supervision by health personnel to make sure that health, once restored, is maintained. The person who has had an episode of acute illness, with no residual problems, will probably need a check-up in a few weeks and, then, perhaps, another in a few months to make sure that all is going well with the healing process. After that, he can usually return to his regular health maintenance program. A person with a chronic health problem will require monitoring throughout the remainder of his lifetime—to assess the individual's responses to his therapeutic regimen and institute changes as needed, and to detect the early signs of any developing imbalance before it reaches critical proportions. The person with a terminal illness also requires continued monitoring to help him maintain an optimal level of functioning for as long as he can, and to provide comfort and support for him and his family as his health deteriorates.

In the stage of restored health, the nurse's focus is again primarily on enhancing the patient's self-care abilities. Once the patient is discharged from a health agency and begins to resume normal daily activities, doubts and fears may arise. The person with diabetes, who was doing well with his injections under the nurse's supervision, may lose some of his self-confidence when he is at home, and require reinforcement of prior teaching. He may also need help in fitting an exercise schedule into his daily routine, or assistance in utilizing health information services in the community. For example, there may be a "Dial-a-Dietitian" service available that could help him if he has any uncertainties about his diet, and the nurse could alert him to the service.

Today, there are many services available in the community to help people with chronic health problems and those who have been discharged from the hospital while still in the convalescent stage. There are "meals on wheels" for those who might otherwise not be able to look after their nutritional needs adequately. Help with the housework can be obtained through homemaker services for those who need it. Indeed, a major part of the nurse's work is often to coordinate the resources that are available to enable patients to care for themselves in the home.

THE IMPACT OF ILLNESS ON THE FAMILY

The illness of a family member has an impact on the total family. If the person who is sick is the breadwinner, there is a natural concern about the loss of ability to maintain financial responsibility for the family; both patient and family may worry about how long the patient will be unable to work and the using up of sick leave from the place of employment. There may be additional concern over the costs of illness, the payment of medical and hospital bills, and the charges for diagnostic and therapeutic services. The head of the household may not be in a position to make decisions about family matters while ill; someone else may have to take over the responsibility for this.

When the mother in the family is sick, household routine is disrupted and other family members must take over the shopping, the planning and cooking of meals, the washing, and the ironing. In our small nuclear families, the relatives who might have done this are often thousands of miles away, and the family may have to rely on friends or "homemaker services" to provide help.

If it is an older member of the family who is ill, there is usually much concern. It may be the first member of the household to be seriously ill, and the family is reminded of the mortality of human life. There may be additional worries over who will care for the patient, and again the costs, particularly of prolonged illness, may be a matter to cause considerable concern.

When one of the children is sick, parents are usually very anxious. They may feel guilty of being in some way responsible for the child's illness. Often they feel helpless, and their anxiety and feelings of helplessness may be expressed in hostility and criticism directed toward those who are caring for the child. Many hospitals today permit open visiting on children's wards and encourage parents to share in the care of their children. If the nurse understands some of the reasons behind the parents' behavior and that of family members, and also realizes her own feelings about this behavior are normal, she is better able to accept hostility and criticism without showing anger and hostility in return.

When a person is hospitalized, his admission has many meanings for him and for his family. While he was ill at home, his care and the responsibility for it probably fell to other family members. After he enters a hospital, the responsibility for his care is transferred from the family to hospital personnel. This transfer of responsibility often produces emotions of mixed relief and guilt on the part of the family: relief because trained people will now provide professional care, and perhaps guilt because members of the family feel that the patient would be happier at home or that they have passed on responsibilities that they should be accepting as a family. These feelings are sometimes expressed verbally to hospital personnel or they may be expressed in activities such as bringing food to the patient or by criticizing the personnel and the institution. If the nurse recognizes the needs of family members and solicits their help in appropriate areas of patient care, such as assisting the patient to eat, the family will feel more comfortable and will be better able to assist in the patient's recovery.

STUDY SITUATION

Mr. Lopez is a 34-year-old man who emigrated from Mexico to California 15 years ago. He was born and raised in a small village, where he attended a school run by Catholic Sisters until the age of 13. He then worked as a migrant farm laborer until the time of his emigration. He now works as a truck driver for a large intercontinental van line. He has come to the doctor's office because his back has been bothering him and he finds it difficult to lift the heavy crates he carries in his truck. He also has pain when he drives for long periods. Mr. Lopez is married and has three small children. He asks whether he will have to go to the hospital.

1. What factors should be considered in assessing Mr. Lopez's perception of his health status?

2. For what reasons might Mr. Lopez be anxious?

3. What factors might affect how Mr. Lopez reacts to his illness if surgery is needed?

4. What are some of the implications of his illness and how might they affect his family?

5. What can the nurse do to help Mr. Lopez?

SUGGESTED READINGS

Hautman, M. A.: Folk Health and Illness Beliefs. *Nurse Practitioner*, 4:23–28, July-August, 1979.
Hodgson, C.: Transcultural Nursing—the Canadian Experience. *The Canadian Nurse*, 76(6):23–25, June, 1980.
Leininger, M.: Cultural Diversities of Health and Nursing Care. *Nursing Clinics of North America*, 12(1):5–18, March, 1977.
Leininger, M.: Suggested Bibiliography on Cultural Diversities and Transcultural Nursing. *Nursing Clinics of North America*, 12(1):85–86, March, 1977.
Primeaux, M. H.: American Indian Health Care Practices. *Nursing Clinics of North America*, 12(1):55–65, March, 1977.
Rosenblum, Estelle H.: Conversation with a Navajo Nurse. *American Journal of Nursing*, 80(8):1459–1461, August, 1980.
Shubin, S.: Nursing Patients from Different Cultures. *Nursing 80*, 10(6):26–29, June, 1980.
Sivarajan, E. S., and Halpenny, C. J.: Exercise Testing. *American Journal of Nursing*, 79:(12):2162–2170, December, 1979.
Speck, P.: East Comes West. *Nursing Times*, 72:662–664, April 29, 1976.
Standard Test of Fitness. Ottawa, Minister of State. Fitness and Amateur Sport Canada, 1979.
White, E. H.: Giving Health Care to Minority Patients. *Nursing Clinics of North America*, 12(1):27–40, March, 1977.
Your Lifestyle Profile. Ottawa, Department of Health and Welfare, Operation Lifestyle. Information Directorate, 1978.

REFERENCES

1. Baumann, B.: Diversities in Conceptions of Health and Physical Fitness. In Skipper, J. K., and Leonard, R. C. (eds.): *Social Interaction and Patient Care*. Philadelphia, J. B. Lippincott Company, 1965, pp. 206–210.
2. Jaco E. G. (ed.): *Patients, Physicians and Illness*. Part III: Socio-cultural Aspects of Medical Care and Treatment. New York, The Free Press, 1967.
3. Olendzki, M. C.: Concerns of the Consumer. Paper presented at the Conference on Education of

Nurses for Public Health, May 23–25, 1973. In *Redesigning Nursing Education for Public Health, Report of the Conference, May 23–25, 1973.* Bethesda, Maryland, U. S. Department of Health, Education, and Welfare Publication No. (HRA) 75–75.

4. Hautman, M. A.: Folk Health and Illness Beliefs. *Nurse Practitioner,* 4:23–28, July-August, 1979.

5. Chung, H. J.: Understanding the Oriental Maternity Patient. *Nursing Clinics of North America,* 12(1):67–75, March, 1977.

6. Miller, J. F.: The Dynamic Focus of Nursing: A Challenge to Nursing Administration. *Journal of Nursing Administration.* 10:13–18, January, 1980.

4

The Nurse Should Be Able to:

- Compare the nature of health problems in North America today with those at the beginning of the century
- Discuss the biologial, environmental, lifestyle, and health care factors affecting health
- List the four principal health status indicators used in international comparisons
- Compare and contrast the health of people in North and South America on the basis of these indicators
- List the five leading causes of death in North America today
- Discuss major causes of death and disability throughout the life span of people in North America
- Identify sources of information the nurse may use to learn about factors affecting health and the principal health problems in a community
- Describe how the nurse can go about gathering this information

MAJOR HEALTH PROBLEMS

INTRODUCTION

Good health is the bedrock on which social progress is built. A nation of healthy people can do those things which make life worthwhile and, as the level of health increases, so does the potential for happiness.[1]

So far, we have been talking about health as it pertains to the individual and, to a certain extent, the family. Nursing students at all levels, however, as well as students in the other health disciplines, need to be aware of the health status and the major health problems of people in the society in which they intend to practice.

In all of the *developed* countries of the world, including the United States and Canada, there has been a marked improvement in health conditions since the turn of this century. Longevity has been increased dramatically, and death rates have been drastically reduced, particularly among mothers and children. The infectious diseases, with the exception of influenza/pneumonia and certain diseases of early infancy, have disappeared entirely from the lists of major causes of death. Indeed, in 1978, the World Health Organization announced that smallpox had been completely eradicated throughout the world.

Still, a large number of problems remain, and others have emerged, many as a result of the longer life span and the changing lifestyles of people in our society. People are living longer, and more of them suffer from chronic and degenerative disorders that impose limitations on their way of life. Industrialization, increasing urbanization, and affluence have all contributed their share of health problems. A faster pace of living, alterations in family structure, and changing social values have also created new stresses that affect our health. We are concerned, for example, about the alarming incidence of mental illness, of alcoholism and drug addiction, par-

ticularly among our young people, and of the premature loss of life resulting from accidents, suicide, and other acts of violence. We are also concerned about the respiratory problems aggravated by environmental pollution and by smoking, and about obesity and lack of exercise as contributing factors in many illnesses. Nor have we entirely eliminated the communicable diseases; the resurgence of the venereal diseases is currently a matter of major concern.

In many of the *developing* countries, longevity and mortality rates are still at about the same level as they were in the developed countries some 75 years ago. Infectious diseases continue to be a major problem in a large part of the world, and maternal and child death rates remain excessively high in the developing countries. Although remarkable progress has been made in many countries, the gap between the rich and the poor nations continues to be a matter of international concern. Even in countries where improvements in health have been considerable, such as our own, there is still a great difference in the health status of different segments of the population—between the rich and the poor, and between majority and minority ethnic groups.

The difference in health status between people in the *developed* countries and people in the *developing* countries of the world is illustrated by comparisons between the various regions of the Americas, where we have countries at different stages of development. In this chapter, we will look at some of these differences and also at some of the differences that exist among various segments of the population in North America. First, however, we will look at the major factors affecting health. Later, we will explore ways the nurse can learn about the health status of people and the factors affecting health in the community in which she is going to work.

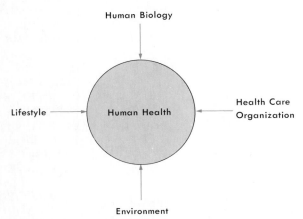

Factors affecting health. (Source: *Community Health Nursing*. Report of a W.H.O. Expert Committee. Technical Report Series 558. Geneva, World Health Organization, 1974, p. 8.)

MAJOR FACTORS AFFECTING HEALTH

The four principal factors affecting both individual and group health are said to be human biology, environment, lifestyle, and health care organization.[1, 2]

Human Biology

The element of human biology includes an individual's genetic inheritance and the processes of maturation and aging (which affect us all), as well as the complex network of structures and systems that compose the human body. We often hear it said that someone has inherited the strong constitution of his father's side of the family, or that another person has the same weak eyes as his aunt. Certainly, we inherit our physical structure, our skin texture and pigmentation, and some say our native intelligence, through the genes we receive from our parents.

A number of specific diseases are known to be passed down through families. One example is Huntington's chorea, a progressive degenerative disorder of the nervous system, which is transmitted through a single, dominant gene and may affect both males and females in the family. Another is hemophilia, the so-called bleeder's disease, which has afflicted several generations of males in the Hapsburg family and other royal families.

The more common disease of diabetes also has an inherited component, although its exact mode of transmission is still not well understood. Then, there are the congenital problems, that is, those present at birth. Although many are caused by difficulties encountered by the unborn infant in utero or by difficulties during delivery, in many congenital problems the genetic factor is clear and has been well documented. The underlying cause of Down's syndrome (mongolism), for example, is considered to be a defective chromosome, although this is not necessarily inherited.

In many other disorders that affect human beings, the effect of genetic inheritance is suspected but the relationship has not yet been fully established. We do not know for certain at this point in time, for example, the extent of the role of heredity as a causative factor in heart trouble, or in hypertension, or in a number of other health problems. Nor do we know why some diseases seem to afflict people of one ethnic group more than another, as, for example, the high prevalence of diabetes among Jewish women, or of glaucoma (increased tension within the eyeball) among people in many of the West Indian ethnic groups.

The processes of maturation and aging also affect an individual's health in many ways. Each stage of development, from conception through maturity to old age, involves changes in the human body and, also, changes in the interactions of the individual with the world around him. Many things can go wrong during the process of change. During the period of growth, for example, the bones or other structures may not develop as they should, and disturbances may occur in the functioning of the endocrine glands. Emotional problems frequently result from the psychosocial stresses on an individual as he moves from childhood to adulthood, to parenthood, to middle age, and then to old age. The number and types of problems related to difficulties associated with the processes of maturation and aging are numerous, and at the present time, we know far too little about many of them.

Then, too, there are all the disturbances that can occur in the complicated systems of the human body, such as the skeletal system, the nervous system, the digestive system, and the like. As you proceed through your nursing course, you will learn about a good many of the systemic disorders that can occur in the human body; we will be touching on some of these in later chapters of this text in connection with common health problems.

The Environment

The environment, as we have mentioned earlier, includes both the physical world that surrounds us and the people who inhabit that world. Man has learned to control many aspects

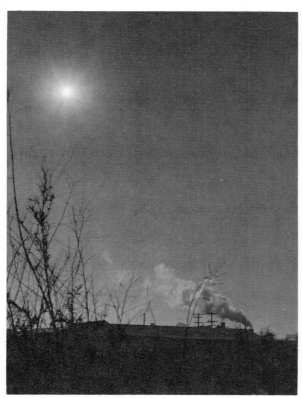

Air pollution is a growing cause for alarm in most major urban centers today.

some homes, there is still no running water or indoor plumbing. Raw sewage still pours into many of our lakes and rivers, and insects, rats, and other disease-carrying pests infest many poverty-stricken neighborhoods.

Then, too, other environmental problems have emerged in recent years, many as a result of industrialization and increasing urbanization. The contamination of our waterways by industrial pollutants is currently a matter of major concern. There is also growing alarm about the potential threat to health of air pollution, particularly in our large urban centers. Many cities have installed monitoring devices and instituted controls to curb industrial activity when air pollution reaches a level considered harmful to health.

Considerable research is currently being done on the effects of weather on people's health. It has been estimated that approximately 30 per cent of the world's population are particularly sensitive to atmospheric changes. These people experience symptoms ranging from mental depression to severe pain with impending changes in the weather.[3]

The effect of increasing urbanization on both the physical and social environment is also causing considerable concern to people in the health field. In many instances, cities and new communities have grown too rapidly to cope with the housing, sewage, and other basic services needed by the population. Overcrowding,

of his physical environment to make it more conducive to healthy living. One of the major factors in the improvement of health in North America in the past 75 years has been the reduction of environmental hazards through the application of known public health measures. These have included such basic measures as standards for housing; provisions to ensure safe water, food, and milk supplies; safety standards for places where people work; and the control of communicable disease.

In many of the developing countries, the lack of a pure water supply, of adequate sanitation, and of effective measures to control communicable disease is held responsible for the continuing prevalence of many health problems, as, for example, the water-borne diseases such as cholera and typhoid fever, the fecally transmitted infectious diarrheas, and the air-borne communicable diseases such as tuberculosis, diphtheria, whooping cough, and the like.

Although we have greatly reduced the effect of environmental factors on health in North America, there is still much lack of uniformity in the application of basic public health measures across the country. Housing for many people is still inadequate or even unsafe. Access to a safe water supply is not guaranteed to all. In

Increasing urbanization is another concern of health workers. New housing developments such as the one in this picture are rapidly being constructed in attempts to meet the needs of the ever-increasing influx of people to metropolitan areas.

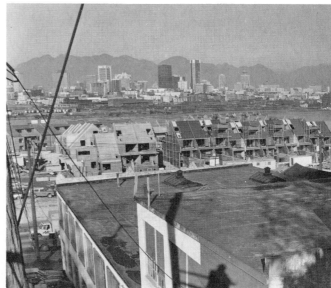

lack of recreational facilities, excessive noise, violence, and solitude are among the social factors resulting from urbanization that contribute to the health problems of city-dwellers.

In looking at factors in the environment that affect health, we must remember that man is a social animal. His relationships with other people are very important to the satisfaction of many of his basic needs. The relationships he has with other people in the home, in the work or school setting, and in the numerous other activities in which he engages, then, contribute positively or negatively to his health, depending on whether or not they are assisting in the satisfaction of his basic needs.

Lifestyle

The ways of life of people in a community, and their individual lifestyles, also have a significant impact on health. Lifestyle is determined in part by circumstance and in part by the decisions made, consciously or unconsciously, by people about the way they choose to live. A child born into a poor family in a ghetto neighborhood in a city in North America, for example, or into a poor family in a remote village in Central America, has little to say in the matter of his lifestyle—during his early years, at any rate. Lifestyle depends to a large extent on the occupation of the head of the

Obesity is considered a major health problem in North America. This individual, who has already lost 50 pounds under her doctor's supervision, shows, for the benefit of this photograph, the kinds of food that formerly made up her diet.

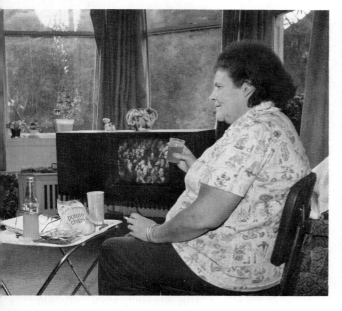

household, the income level of the family, and the things that income can purchase in the way of housing, food, clothing, recreation, and even education and health care. Another major factor contributing to better health for North Americans in this century (in addition to improved public health measures) has been the general overall raising of income levels of the population with its concomitant raising of standards of living, perhaps one of the good things that has come from industrialization.

In much of the developing world, many health problems are directly attributable to a lack of the basic essentials of life, such as adequate nutrition and housing, resulting from widespread poverty among large segments of the population in many countries. Nor is North America entirely exempt from the influence of poverty on the health of its people. The effects of income level on health stand out in startling relief when we look at differences among socioeconomic groups in relation to infant mortality and maternal death rates in both the United States and Canada, as we shall do later in this chapter. The poor are obviously at a disadvantage, healthwise.

In addition to circumstantial factors, there is also the element of personal decision-making that enters into an individual or family lifestyle, regardless of income. One of the byproducts of affluence has been obesity, which is considered a major health problem in North American society. Although other factors contribute to obesity—and we do not know about all of its causes yet—certainly individual choice of diet has a great deal to do with it. Obesity is felt to be a major contributing factor in many of the diseases that afflict large numbers of North Americans today, such as heart conditions, hypertension, diabetes, and the like. Nor should we forget that malnutrition can occur even in the midst of a plentiful food supply, as evidenced by recent studies on nutrition in both the United States and Canada. Malnutrition is most usually associated with poverty, but it may also result from poor choice in the foods eaten, as, for example, the eating of too many snack foods and sweets instead of regular, well balanced meals.

The sedentary way of life among many people in North America (and among people in higher socioeconomic groups in many parts of Central and South·America as well) must also be considered as a lifestyle factor affecting health. It, too, has been a product of the affluent society, with its motor cars for transportation and television sets for entertainment. There is no doubt that a lack of exercise contributes to a generally lowered state of physical fitness. It is encouraging to see so many of our young—and older—

people today engaging in programs of regular exercise.

In discussing health problems resulting from lifestyle factors, we should also mention the terrible toll in human lives from excessive speed and careless driving on the highways, and the heavy burden put on our health care system for the care, treatment, and rehabilitation of countless victims of automobile accidents. The lowering of the speed limit on U.S. highways and in several Canadian provinces that resulted from the energy crisis of 1974, it has been said, probably saved more lives and eliminated more hospital days than any other single factor in recent years.

Numerous other major problems that are causes of increasing concern in the health field today can also be attributed to lifestyle factors. These include alcoholism, drug addiction, the venereal diseases, and mental health problems, including suicide. It is especially troubling that these are affecting increasing numbers of young people.

Health Care Organization

Health care organization is the fourth and last on our list of major factors affecting health. Improvements in health care have been given as one of the main reasons for the reduction in maternal and childhood deaths in North America, and have contributed to increases in the life span in many ways. Yet, many problems remain in the equitable distribution of health care services. We will be going into this topic in more detail in Chapter 5. Suffice it to say here, then, that it is necessary to have comprehensive and accessible care for all, with a full range of services—promotional and preventive, as well as curative—if the highest level of health is to be attained for all of our people. And these services must be acceptable to people, or they will not be utilized.

HEALTH STATUS INDICATORS

The individual health of people and their major health problems are reflected in the statistical information collected and compiled by governments about illness and death in the country. The kinds of statistical information usually compiled on an annual basis by national governments include:

1. the average life span of people in the country (*life expectancy*)
2. the number of deaths relative to the population (*mortality rates*)
3. the reasons for these deaths (*causes of death*)
4. the incidence of illness (*morbidity data*)

These four sets of statistical information are considered the main health status indicators for a given population. They provide a base for identifying major health problems, that is, those problems responsible for the most deaths and those causing the greatest amount of disability to people. They also help to give some insight into the principal factors affecting the health of the population.

Because virtually every country in the world collects information related to these four indicators, it is possible to look at differences between countries, and where statistical information has accumulated over a number of years, to look at trends over time.

Life Expectancy

The average lifespan of people in a given country reflects the total effect of its economic development and its health care programs. In the developed countries of the world, such as the United States and Canada, life expectancy has increased dramatically since the turn of the century—from a little under 50 years in 1900 to 72 years in 1980. The biggest changes in the life span occurred during the first half of the century, with smaller but still significant gains since 1950.

This remarkable extension of the life span in North America during this century has been attributed to a constellation of factors. These include the general overall raising of standards of living, improved sanitation, the development and widespread use of immunity-producing agents to protect people from communicable disease, improvements in health care services, and advances in medical science and technology.

One trend that should be noted in the statistics of life expectancy in North America particularly is the widening gap between men and women. In 1900, women outlived men by an average of approximately 2 years in both the United States and Canada. By 1976, this figure had increased to approximately 7.7 years in the United States and 7.5 years in Canada. The resulting imbalance between the sexes, particularly in the older age group, has brought about changes in the structure of our society. One of the unfortunate results of this trend is that widowhood and loneliness all too often contribute to the health problems of many of our senior citizens.

In the United States, there is a sizeable difference—5 years—in life expectancy between

	1960–65	1980–85
0 5 10 15 20 25 30 35 40 45 50 55 60 65 70 75 80		

	1960–65	1980–85
Northern America	70.1	72.0
Latin America	57.7	65.4
Caribbean	59.6	65.7
Continental Middle America	57.2	65.7
Temperate South America	63.3	68.7
Tropical South America	56.6	64.9

Estimates and projections of life expectancy at birth, by regions of the Americas, 1960–1965 and 1980–1985. Source: *Health Conditions in the Americas 1973–1976.* Washington, D.C., Pan American Health Organization, Pan American Sanitary Bureau, Regional Office of the World Health Organization, 1978, page 14.)

members of the white population and all others. The biggest difference is found among the blacks and North American Indians, among whom mortality rates are much higher, especially in the early and middle years of life. Mortality rates for Asian Americans, however, are below the national average.[4]

The figure above shows estimates and projections of life expectancy at birth in five regions of the Americas for the periods 1960 to 1965 and 1980 to 1985. Even in the region with the lowest life expectancy (Tropical South America), considerable progress has been made in lengthening the life span over the past two decades.

Mortality Rates

A major factor in the lengthening of the average life span in North America has been a dramatic reduction in the number of infant and maternal deaths. Relatively few women in either the United States or Canada die as a result of childbirth these days; the *maternal mortality rate* is now less than 1 per 10,000 live births in Canada and 1.2 in North America overall.

In Middle and South America, the rates were approximately seven to ten times greater than in North America for the year 1975. Trends in maternal death rates in three regions of the Americas, as seen in the figure opposite, show the continuing decline in maternal death rates in North America and the progress made in Central and South America over the period 1960 to 1975.

Maternal deaths are considered to be largely preventable. The importance of early and adequate prenatal care cannot be overstressed. The

reduction in maternal death rates in both the United States and Canada is attributed mainly to improved prenatal care for pregnant women and to hospitalization for the mothers during delivery.

Although the record in North America is very good, there are still differences in the extent of care received by women in different socioeconomic groups. It has been estimated that *early prenatal care*, that is, care during the first 3 months of pregnancy, is received by approximately 77 per cent of white women in the United States and by only 59 per cent of black women, and by far more women with education beyond high school than by those who left school in the primary grades. Unfortunately, it is often the women at highest risk who delay prenatal care until late in pregnancy. These include women who are black, adolescents, older women, those

Maternal deaths per 10,000 live births in the three regions of the Americas, 1960–1975. (Source: *Health Conditions in the Americas 1973–1976.* Washington, D.C., Pan American Health Organization. Pan American Sanitary Bureau, Regional Office of the World Health Organization, 1978, p. 45.)

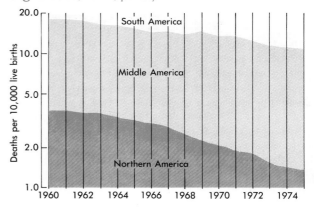

INFANT MORTALITY RATES, SELECTED COUNTRIES, 1977*

Rank	Country	Infant Deaths per 1000 Live Births
1	Sweden	8.0
2	Japan	9.3
3	Netherlands	9.5
4	Switzerland	10.7
5	France	11.4†
6	German Democratic Republic	13.1
7	England and Wales	13.7
8	United States	14.1
9	Canada	14.3
10	Australia	14.3
11	German Federal Republic	17.4
12	Italy	17.6
13	Israel	22.9

*Data for Canada, Israel, and Australia refer to 1975; data for the German Federal Republic and Switzerland refer to 1976; all of the 1977 data are provisional, except for the United States.

†Excludes infants who have died before registration of birth.

Source: *Health United States 1979.* Hyattsville, Maryland, U.S. Department of Health, Education, and Welfare Publication No. (PHS) 80–1232. Public Health Service. National Center for Health Statistics, 1980, p. 142.

who already have a number of children, and those who are unmarried.[4]

Infant mortality is considered one of the most sensitive indicators of a nation's health status. In both the United States and Canada, major accomplishments are reflected in the significant drop in infant mortality rates, from slightly over 100 deaths per 1000 live births in the early 1920's to 14.2 in 1977.* There is, however, still room for improvement, as can be seen when these figures are compared with Sweden's rate of 8.0 per 1000 live births in 1977, and with Japan's rate of 9.3 for the same year. In 1977, the United States ranked eighth and Canada ninth in international comparisons of infant mortality. The grounds for hope of further improvement in the reduction of infant deaths in North America are evident when one looks at the differences between segments of the population divided on socioeconomic and geographic lines. In the United States, for example, the mortality rate is considerably higher for black infants than for white infants. Japanese-Americans and Chinese Americans, on the other hand,

*Although American and Canadian infant mortality rates are not identical, over the years the differences have been slight, and progress in both countries has followed a similar pattern. The following statistics give some indication of trends in North America. In 1921, Canada reported an infant mortality rate of 102 per 1000 live births. In 1949, the rate in the U.S. was reported as 47 per 1000 live births. In the late 1950s and early 1960s, it remained stationary at about 25 deaths per 1000 live births in both countries, but has continued to decline from around 1965 to the present.

have the lowest infant mortality rates of all ethnic groups in the United States. The rate for American Indians has dropped dramatically since 1950—from 82.1 in that year to 15.6 in 1977. Considerable improvement in infant mortality rates has also been seen among the Inuit and native Indian populations in Canada, and this has helped to lower the overall rate for the country.

The majority of early infant deaths (neonatal) are associated with the status of the infant at birth. Later infant deaths (postnatal), with the exception of those caused by congenital anomalies, are more likely to be associated with environmental factors. In the United States and Canada, the decrease in infant mortality has shown a continuous decline in both neonatal and postnatal deaths. In other words, babies are getting a better start in life (an important factor here would be better prenatal care for mothers), and the infant's chances of survival through the first year are better owing to less danger from environmental factors (including, in this instance, improved nutrition and better infant health care).

In both Middle and South America, infant deaths remain excessively high, although considerable improvement has been made since 1960. Rates were reduced in Middle America, for example, from an average of 70 deaths per 1000 live births in 1960 to 48.3 in 1975, and in South America from close to 85 in 1960 to 49.4 in 1975.[5]

It is felt that a large number of these deaths could be prevented by further improvements in disease prevention, environmental sanitation, and better programs of maternal-child health care.[5]

Principal Causes of Death and Disability

Statistical data on the leading causes of death and the prevalence of illness (morbidity data) also help to identify the major health problems in a country. The pattern in leading causes of death in North America has changed considerably since the turn of the century. In 1900, deaths from infectious diseases headed the list. These included pneumonia/influenza, tuberculosis, and diarrhea/enteritis, in that order. Also on the list of major killers at that time were nephritis (for the most part, postinfectious) and diphtheria. By 1940, the noninfectious disorders of heart disease, cancer, and cerebrovascular accidents had become the three leading causes of death, although tuberculosis, pneumonia, and nephritis were still listed among the major causes. By 1970, influenza/pneumonia was the only infectious disease remaining on the list of major causes of death in both the United States and Canada.[6]

The five leading causes of death in North America, as shown in the figure below, are now diseases of the heart, malignant neoplasms, cerebrovascular disease, accidents, and influenza/pneumonia, in that order.

Diseases of the heart are responsible for over one third of all deaths each year. The number of deaths from heart disease has been declining steadily during the past decade. A number of factors are felt to have contributed to this decline, including: decreased smoking, improved

management of hypertension, reductions in dietary intake of saturated fats, more widespread physical activity, improved medical emergency services, and a greater number of coronary care units better equipped to handle acute cases.[4] Heart disease is, however, the leading cause of death in the population. It also accounts for the greatest amount of acute illness and major disability among the total population.

Malignant neoplasms (cancer) cause almost one fifth of the total number of deaths each year. Cancer strikes people of all ages and becomes a principal cause of death and disability among people from the latter half of the young adult years onward. There has, however, been a considerable decrease in cancer mortality among young people since 1950, owing in part to the reduced incidences of breast cancer in younger women and of lung cancer in younger men and improved treatment of Hodgkin's disease (a malignant disease of the lymph glands and nodes) and childhood leukemia.[4]

Cerebrovascular disease is primarily a problem of aging. It is a leading cause of death and of both acute and chronic conditions in people over 65 years of age. The fact that cerebrovascular disease now accounts for more than one tenth of all deaths each year in North America is a reflection of the lengthening life span of people in our country.

Accidents have become the fourth leading cause of death in North America (accounting for more than 6 per cent of the total annual death toll each year). They are the leading cause of death for the population 1 to 34 years of age. They are also the second leading cause of acute hospitalization, surpassed only by heart disease. The residual effects of accidents in the form of long-term disability also constitute a very major health problem.

Despite our progress in the control of other infectious diseases, influenza/pneumonia continues to be a major health problem in North America. It is a principal cause of death in infants under 1 year of age and remains an important cause of death and a major cause of acute illness throughout the life span. The proportion of total deaths in North America attributed to influenza/pneumonia each year is approximately 3 per cent.

The principal causes of death as a percentage of total deaths in three regions of the Americas are shown in the figure on this page. Although enteritis (inflammation of the intestinal tract) and other diarrheal diseases continue to be a major concern in Middle America, other major health problems in Middle America and South America are the same as those in North America, albeit in different rank order.

Principal causes of death as a percentage of total deaths in three regions of the Americas, 1975. (Source: *Health Conditions in the Americas 1973–1976*. Washington, D.C., Pan American Health Organization. Pan American Sanitary Bureau, Regional Office of the World Health Organization, 1978, p. 27.)

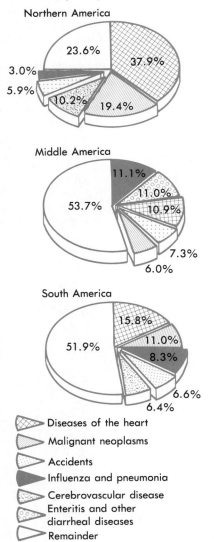

Northern America

23.6%
37.9%
3.0%
5.9%
10.2%
19.4%

Middle America

11.1%
11.0%
10.9%
53.7%
7.3%
6.0%

South America

15.8%
11.0%
8.3%
51.9%
6.6%
6.4%

Diseases of the heart
Malignant neoplasms
Accidents
Influenza and pneumonia
Cerebrovascular disease
Enteritis and other diarrheal diseases
Remainder

MAJOR HEALTH PROBLEMS THROUGHOUT THE LIFE SPAN

The list of the leading causes of death, taken alone, does not give us a full picture of all the major health problems in North America today. From the vast amount of statistical data gathered in both the United States and Canada on the causes of death and the prevalence of illness, it is possible to gain further insight into the nature of these problems, and to look at them from the point of view of the principal age groups affected.

The Childhood Years (Birth to 14 Years)

The period during and immediately after birth is the most critical time for infants. Most of the deaths at this time result from problems in regard to the infant's supply of oxygen or from abnormalities of the placenta (afterbirth), or from both. After the first week of life, congenital abnormalities become the leading cause of infant deaths, and they account for a major portion of the acute conditions requiring care in hospitals. During the first year of life, the infant is particularly susceptible to infections of the respiratory and gastrointestinal tracts. These, together with accidents and nutritional disorders, account for the largest number of remaining deaths as well as acute illnesses in infants.

Once a child has passed his first birthday, his chances of survival are much greater. The age group of 1 to 14 years now has the lowest overall death rate of any period in the life span in North

Percentage of deaths of children under 5 years of age in three regions of the Americas, 1968–1974. (Source: *Health Conditions in the Americas 1973–1976*. Washington, D.C., Pan American Health Organization. Pan American Sanitary Bureau, Regional Office of the World Health Organization, 1978, p. 46.)

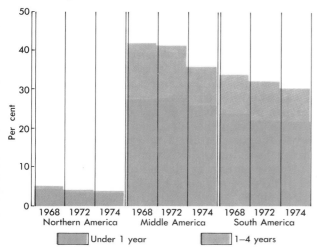

America. The common childhood illnesses continue to be a problem, but the number of deaths resulting from them has been markedly reduced. The only infectious disease that remains a major killer in this age group is influenza/pneumonia, which is the second most common cause of death and the principal cause of hospitalization in children. The leading cause of death in this age group is now accidents, with motor vehicle accidents responsible for approximately one half of these. Accidents are also the second most common cause of acute illness in children and a major cause of long-term disability as well. The most common chronic conditions in children are the respiratory disorders of bronchitis and asthma. Other problems in this age group include the developmental defects and the residual effects of congenital abnormalities, which account for a major portion of both acute and chronic conditions in children.

In contrast to North America, childhood deaths remain disproportionately high in the rest of the Americas, where the communicable diseases, malnutrition, diarrhea, and other infections of the gastrointestinal tract continue to take a heavy toll. (See figure below.) Although malnutrition is not always listed as the principal cause of death, the relationship between it and infections in children has been well documented.[7]

The Young Adult Years (15 to 44 Years)

More young people lose their lives each year from accidents, suicides, and homicides than from any other cause in North America today, with more premature deaths resulting from these among young men than among women. Suicide has become an important cause of death in people as young as 15 years, according to both U.S. and Canadian statistics. In the U.S., it has been estimated that deaths from motor vehicle accidents have increased by one third in the 15 to 24 year age group, and deaths from homicide and suicide have more than doubled since 1950.[8] Combined, these three causes now account for almost half of all deaths in the 15 to 44 year age group. Rates for deaths due to accidents and homicide are particularly high among blacks and American Indians. Accidents are also the principal cause of acute illness, with their resultant head injuries, fractures, burns, and complicating disorders. Probably the most unfortunate aspect of these statistics is that so many accident victims are left with residual long-term disability as well. In the United States, it is estimated that over 1.6 million young adults (aged 15 to 24 years) and 3.7 million people in the 25 to 44 year age group suffer permanent disability resulting from accidents occurring during these age periods or earlier.[8]

The second leading acute condition in young adults is mental illness, which has shown an alarming increase in this age group in recent years. Associated with mental illness are the problems of alcoholism and drug addiction. The rising incidence of alcoholism among very young teenagers, among whom it appears to be replacing the drug problem, is currently causing a considerable amount of concern.

The widespread prevalence of venereal disease is also an alarming problem in adolescents and young adults. Since 1970, gonorrhea has ranked first among the reportable communicable diseases in North America. There was a steady rise in the incidence of this disease from 1950 through the mid 1970's, but indications are that this trend is now reversing itself. Meanwhile, the incidence of other venereal diseases, such as syphilis, has been decreasing.[4]

In the latter half of the early adult years, heart disease begins to assume importance, both as a leading cause of death and as a cause of acute and chronic illness. Although the chronic illnesses are not so prevalent among the younger members of this age group (the 15 to 25 year olds), hypertension and arthritis begin to show up as major disablers in the 25 to 44 year age group.

Obesity has been mentioned several times before as a factor in many acute and chronic conditions. It is of particular concern in young adults because it contributes another risk factor to health in later years. Diabetes, for example, in which the relationship to obesity is currently under considerable study, becomes a principal cause of death and disability in the 15 to 44 year age group (it is one of the leading causes of death in the 25 to 44 year age group).

Cancer also begins to attack a large number of people in the latter half of the young adult years, striking women at an earlier age than it does men.

The Middle Years (45 to 64 Years)

By the middle years of the life span, the chronic diseases have become, and remain, the principal causes of death and disability. Diseases of the heart are by far the most common of these. Other leading causes of death and of acute and long-term illness in this age group include cancer, cirrhosis of the liver (associated with alcoholism), and the chronic respiratory disorders such as emphysema, bronchitis, and asthma. These problems, together with mental illness and accidents, are among the principal disorders requiring hospital care in people during the middle years. Other common causes of hospitalization in this age group are disorders of the reproductive system (in women particularly), disorders of the nervous system, cholelithiasis (stones in the gallbladder), ulcers, hypertension and arteriosclerosis, diabetes, and hernia.

The Older Age Group (65 Years and on)

Among the older age group, it is not surprising to find that the chronic and degenerative disorders are by far the principal causes of death, with heart conditions, cerebrovascular accidents (strokes), and cancer being the most common. These conditions, together with accidents, are also responsible for the largest amount of acute illness in the elderly.

The number of older people being cared for in acute care hospitals is very high in proportion to their numbers in the population. The majority of reasons for their hospitalization usually involve chronic problems or conditions that require a lengthy hospital stay. An increasingly large number of older people are receiving care in nursing homes and extended care facilities, and the residents of these homes usually have multiple chronic problems.

It is important to remember that the chronic disorders have a cumulative effect. As people grow older, more of them tend to suffer from chronic and degenerative diseases, and their numbers add to those in whom chronic condi-

Prevalence of selected chronic conditions per 1000 persons in the United States, all ages. (Source: Adapted from *Health United States 1975*. Rockville, Maryland, U.S. Department of Health, Education, and Welfare Publication No. (HRA) 76–1232. Public Health Service. Health Resources Administration, National Center for Health Statistics, 1976, p. 247.)

	10 20 30 40 50 60 70 80 90 100
Arthritis	92.9
Hearing impairments	71.6
Hypertensive disease	60.1
Heart conditions	50.4
Visual impairment	47.4
Chronic bronchitis	32.7
Diabetes	20.4

tions began to appear at an earlier age, thus accumulating and increasing the proportionate number of people with long-term disability in the older age group. The most common causes of long-term disability among the total population in the U.S. are shown in the figure on page 42.

The picture is, of course, not entirely bleak for our senior citizens. The vast majority of them are not residents of institutions; only about 5 per cent are. A number of innovative programs are being developed to assist older people to maintain as independent a lifestyle as possible; some of these were discussed in Chapter 1.

THE NURSE AND HEALTH PROBLEMS IN THE COMMUNITY

It is important for the nurse to be aware of the major health problems in her country. National statistics and national averages, however, do not necessarily give a representative picture of the problems she will encounter in the community in which she is working. Each community will have its own unique set of problems, and the factors affecting health in each community will vary. The problems will be different, for example, in rural as opposed to urban settings, or between affluent neighborhoods and poor ones, and will also vary with the inhabitants of each community and their lifestyles.

In order to play her part in the promotion and protection of health, the care of the ill, and the restoration of health, the nurse should become knowledgeable about the particular health problems and the factors affecting health in the community in which she is going to practice.

A good first step in learning about a community is to find out what has been written about it. The nurse can often get quite a bit of information about the people who live and work there by reviewing the statistical data published by government agencies. Census data, for example, provide basic information about a given population, such as total number of people, age and sex distribution, ethnic origin of the inhabitants, population density (number of people per square mile), and birth rates. Government health departments—federal, state (provincial), and municipal—usually collect and publish basic health statistics such as life expectancy rates, infant mortality rates, leading causes of death, and major illnesses. These statistics often go down to the county or municipal level. Information about the nature of health services in a community and the financing and utilization of these services is also frequently available in the publications of governmental and other health agencies.

Other written material that the nurse can usually find in a library to increase her knowledge about a community includes maps, encyclopedias, informational brochures (such as those put out by government tourist bureaus), and local newspapers. From these sources the nurse can often learn much about environmental factors affecting health, such as the geographic location of the community, climatic conditions, and the community's transportation and communication systems, and major industries in the area, as well as something about recreational and educational facilities and churches. The community's concern about health matters, such as health care financing and environmental pollution, are often discussed in articles in the local newspapers.

The information obtained from written material can be supplemented by talking with knowledgeable and informed people in the community, such as the medical officer of health and his staff, public health nurses in the area, social workers, clergymen, and teachers. Sometimes, too, the local law enforcement officer may be the best informed person in a community with regard to the assets and liabilities of its health status.

Direct observation, such as that made while walking about the community, gives the nurse who is new to the area an opportunity to note the location of health agencies, particularly in relation to schools, shopping areas, and residential accommodation. It also helps the nurse to gain an insight into local housing conditions,

The nurse can learn much about factors affecting health through observations made while walking about the community. Here, the nurse explores the neighborhood in which she is to work.

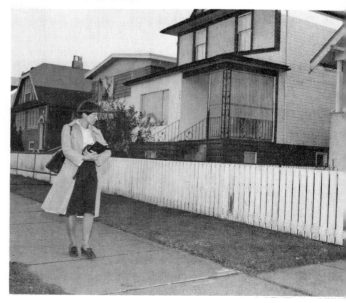

FACTORS AFFECTING HEALTH IN A COMMUNITY

Human Biology	Environment	Lifestyles	Health Care System

Population Data
  Number of people
  Age distribution
  Density/square mile
  Ethnic origins
 	
Health Data
  Life expectancy rates
  Probable birth rates
  Major causes of death
  Major illnesses
	Geographic Data
	  Climate
	  Location (accessibility)
	  Transportation
	  Communication
	  Water supply
	  Food quality control
	  Sewage disposal
	  Environmental
	    pollution
	  Housing
	  Major industries
		Occupational
		  characteristics of
		  population
		Average income level
		Recreational facilities
		Educational facilities
		Churches
		Health care financing
			Preventive health services
			Health maintenance services
			Agencies for diagnosis, treatment
			  and rehabilitation of the sick
			Physician population
			Nursing services available
			Attitudes toward health and health
			  care
			Utilization of services

the presence or absence of parks and other recreational facilities, the number of churches, and the general appearance of the community.

The nurse, in her appraisal of a community, might also talk with individuals who live there in order to gain an appreciation of their knowledge about health care services available in the community, their attitudes toward health and health care, and their utilization of health services.

Some of the types of information that are useful in assessing health problems and the factors affecting health in a community are detailed in the table above.

STUDY SITUATION

You have been offered a summer job in a Neighborhood Health Center in an area of the city with which you are not familiar. In preparation for this assignment, you want to find out something about the factors affecting health and the health problems of the people in the neighborhood.

Outline a plan for obtaining the information you feel would be helpful to you. The following questions are suggested to help you to organize your plan for looking at biological, environmental, lifestyle, and health care organization factors.

Suggested Items to Be Considered Under Biological Factors
1. How many people live in the community?
2. What is the approximate age distribution of the population?
3. What is the population density?
4. What are the predominant ethnic groups?
5. What are the common illnesses of the people who live in the community?
    among infants   among the adults
    among children   among old people

Suggested Items to Be Considered under Environmental Factors
1. What is the general description of the community, e.g., housing, neighborhood conditions, and the like?
2. Is the housing adequate? Safe?
3. What is the state of sanitation in regard to:
    water supply
    sewage
    garbage disposal
    control of animals, insects, and other vectors of disease, e.g., dogs, rats, mice, insects, cows, goats
4. How would you describe the social environment of the community?
5. Are there parks or recreational areas in the community?

Suggested Items to Be Considered under Lifestyle Factors
1. What are the principal occupations of people who live in this community?
2. Where do they work?
3. What is the approximate average yearly income?
4. Do people live in single family dwellings? Multiple family dwellings?

5. What do people do in their leisure time?
   children   middle aged adults
   youth   older people
   young adults

Suggested Items to Be Considered under Health Care Organization
1. What health services are available in the community?
   health promotion services
   hospitals, health centers, or clinics
   physicians' offices
   nursing services
   preventive health services
   rehabilitation services
2. Where do people go when they are sick?
3. How do they feel about the health services that are available?
4. How do they pay for their health services?

SUGGESTED READINGS

Ahern, C.: I Think I Have V.D. *Nursing Clinics of North America,* 8(1):77–89, March, 1973.

A New Perspective on the Health of Canadians. A Working Document. Ottawa, Department of National Health and Welfare, 1975.

Ardell, D. B.: Prevention. High Level Wellness Strategies. *Health Education,* 8:2–4, July-August, 1977.

Atwater, J. B.: Adapting the V.D. Clinic to Today's Problem. *American Journal of Public Health,* 64:433–437, May, 1974.

Begin, M.: Health: An Integral Part of Human Development. *Canadian Journal of Public Health,* 69:271–275, July-August, 1978.

Canadian Nurse, November, 1980. Includes a series of articles on alcoholism and drug abuse.

Diekelmann, N. L.: The Young Adult: The Choice Is Health or Illness. *American Journal of Nursing,* 76(8):1272–1277, August, 1976.

Health Conditions in the Americas 1973–1976. Washington, D.C., Pan American Health Organization, 1978.

Health United States 1979. Hyattsville, Maryland. U.S. Department of Health, Education and Welfare. Public Health Service. DHEW Publication No. (PHS) 80–1232, 1980.

Hoyman, H. S.: Rethinking an Ecologic System Model of Man's Health, Disease, Aging, Death.

American Journal of Public Health, 66:516, 1975.

Krepick, D. S., et al.: Heroin Addiction: A Treatable Disease. *Nursing Clinics of North America,* 8(1):41–52, March, 1973.

Long, B. L., et al.: "New Perspectives on Drug Abuse." *Nursing Clinics of North America,* 8(1):25–40, March, 1973.

Louria, D. B.: A Critique of Some Current Approaches to the Problem of Drug Abuse. *American Journal of Public Health,* 65:581–583, June, 1975.

Milo, N.: A Framework for Prevention: Changing Health Damaging to Health Generating Patterns. *American Journal of Public Health,* 66:435, 1976.

Murray, R., et al.: Guidelines for More Effective Health Teaching. *Nursing 76,* 6(2):44–53, February, 1976.

Overfield, T.: Biological Variation Concepts from Physical Anthropology. *Nursing Clinics of North America,* 12(1):819, March, 1977.

Pender, N. J.: A Conceptual Model for Preventive Health Behavior. *Nursing Outlook,* 23:385–390, June, 1975.

Stewart, M., and White, L.: Nursing the Community. *The Canadian Nurse* 77(1):32–33, January, 1981.

REFERENCES

1. *A New Perspective on the Health of Canadians.* A Working Document. Ottawa, Department of National Health and Welfare, 1974.
2. *Community Health Nursing.* Report of a W.H.O. Expert Committee. Technical Report Series 558. Geneva, World Health Organization, 1974.
3. Claire Gerus. Wind, Weather and Work. *Financial Post Magazine,* December, 1979.
4. *Health United States 1979.* Hyattsville, Maryland, U.S. Department of Health, Education, and Welfare, Public Health Service, Office of Health Research, Statistics and Technology, DHEW Publication No. (PHS) 80–1232, p. 30.
5. *Health Conditions in the Americas, 1973–1976.* Washington, D. C., Pan American Health Orga-

nization. Pan American Sanitary Bureau, Regional Office of the World Health Organization, 1978.
6. J. H. Dingle: The Ills of Man. *Scientific American,* 229:77–84, September, 1973.
7. Puffer, R. R., and Serrano, C. V.: *Patterns of Mortality in Childhood.* Scientific Publication No. 262. Washington, D.C., Pan American Health Organization, 1973, pp. v–vi.
8. *Health United States 1975.* Rockville, Maryland, U.S. Department of Health, Education, and Welfare Publication No. (HRA) 76–1232. Public Health Service, Health Resources Administration, National Center for Health Statistics, 1976, p. 161.

5

The Nurse Should Be Able to:

- Discuss health care as social policy
- Differentiate between explicit and implicit health policies
- Discuss factors contributing to the increased demand for health services
- Discuss the effects of escalating costs and increased demand on health care services
- Compare and contrast the health care systems in the United States and in Canada
- Describe the spectrum of health care services in a community
- Describe the functions of official and voluntary agencies, with particular reference to their role in health promotion and protection
- Discuss the principal providers of primary care services in a community
- Explain the various functions of a hospital
- Describe the functions of various departments within a hospital
- Discuss the nature of home care programs
- Discuss the nature of extended care facilities
- Discuss the nature of hospices
- Describe the nature of rehabilitation services
- Discuss the role of the nurse in rehabilitation
- Describe the usual procedure for admitting a patient to hospital
- List principles relevant to the care of newly admitted patients
- Describe measures the nurse can take to assist the patient to adjust to the hospital
- Describe measures the nurse can take to assist the patient when he is being discharged from the hospital

HEALTH CARE AGENCIES

CHAPTER 5

INTRODUCTION

Health is said to be a human right, that is, a condition to which everyone has a just claim. The very acceptance of the notion of human right implies that society assumes a responsibility and will give a high priority to carrying it out.[1]

As discussed in the previous chapter, health is affected by a number of social and economic factors as well as health care per se. In order to develop and maintain good health, people must have income sufficient to provide adequate food and shelter. It is indeed difficult to separate the social and economic components from health care, and in many national and state/provincial governments, the functions of social welfare and health have been brought together in one department. In the United States, for example, the Department of Health and Human Services administers both the national health and the national social welfare programs, as does the Department of National Health and Welfare in Canada.

The provision of adequate health measures is viewed as an essential component of a country's overall social policies. In the United States and in Canada (and in many other countries too), we believe that society has a responsibility to look after its older people who have reached the age of retirement and may be unable to care for themselves financially. The assumption of this responsibility is a social policy to which both countries subscribe. The policy is evidenced in our social (income) security programs that ensure a basic minimum income for all senior citizens and in programs that provide health services for older people through public monies.

EXPLICIT AND IMPLICIT HEALTH POLICIES

The health programs for senior citizens illustrate national health policies that have been adopted in our countries. A policy is an administration decision that is used to guide and determine a plan of action.

At every level of government, national, state/provincial, and municipal, health programs are based on certain policies that the prevailing government either initiated on its own or endorsed from a previous governmental policy. When policies are proclaimed in written statements, they are called "explicit" policies. It is not uncommon for a newly elected government, for example, to make a formal statement of the health policies it intends to follow during its term of office; indeed, these may have been planks in its election campaign, which are then made into explicit policy commitments after election. The following statements, taken from a speech made by one health minister in outlining his government's Ten Year Health Plan, are examples of explicit policy statements:

(development of) a Maternal Health Programme which would cover 75 per cent of the population

and

decentralization and regionalization of the health services and the establishment of Community Health Advisory Boards made up of the people and the nursing personnel in the particular community.[2]

Health policies, once adopted, are frequently incorporated into legislation. In the United States, the issue of national health insurance has been debated for many years, but no consensus has been reached on overall policy. In Canada, a policy of universal prepaid medical and hospital insurance has been incorporated into national health insurance laws.

Sometimes, health policies are not explicitly expressed in formal statements, nor incorporated into legislation, but they may be inferred from the programs that are carried out by the department of government responsible for health. In this case, they are called "implicit" policies. An example here might be the policy of a municipal government to protect all children, insofar as possible, from the communicable diseases to which they are particularly vulnerable and for which there are known immunizations. Although the policy may not be explicitly stated, it would be demonstrated in citywide preschool and school immunization programs carried out by the municipal department of health.

HEALTH CARE FOR ALL: A MAJOR POLICY ISSUE

A major policy issue concerning most countries of the world is how to ensure that the services needed to promote and maintain health, to prevent disease, and to treat illness, as well as the rehabilitative services needed to restore the sick to an active functioning role in society, are made available to all persons in the country.

The importance attached to this concern is evidenced by the increasingly large sums of money being spent annually on health care, and by the rapidly growing number of people engaged in providing health care services. During the 1970s, national health expenditures more than doubled in the United States, reaching $192.4 billion in 1978. This amount averages out to a health bill of $863 per person per year. Health care expenditures in the United States in 1970 represented 7.6 per cent of the Gross National Product; in 1978, 9.1 per cent.[3]

In Canada, national health expenditures rose from $6 billion in 1970 to over $16 billion in 1978 (or $688.77 per capita). Total health expenditures as a percentage of the Gross National Product remained fairly steady at around 7 per cent during these years.[4]

The allocation of health monies by type of expenditure (United States figures) is shown in the figure above.

The increased expenditure on health care has been accompanied by a marked increase in the number of people who provide health care services. Reports indicate that the number of people employed in the health field has been increasing at more than twice the rate of the number of employed persons in the total economy. It has been said that the "health care industry" now encompasses a combined manpower force larger than that of any other industry. In 1978, it was estimated that there were 6.7 million persons employed in health-related occupations in the United States, an increase of nearly 60 per cent over 1970 figures. More than half of these people worked in hospitals.[3] In Canada, with a population roughly one tenth that of the United States, over half a million people are engaged in the provision of health services.

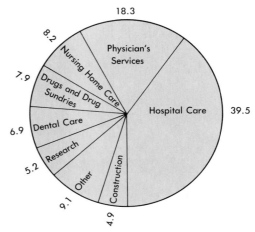

Types of health expenditures, fiscal year 1978. (Source: *Health United States 1979*. Hyattsville, Maryland, U.S. Department of Health, Education and Welfare Publication No. (PHS) 80–1232. Public Health Service. Health Resources Administration, National Center for Health Statistics, p. 238.)

INCREASED DEMAND FOR HEALTH SERVICES

The basic reason for the increased health expenditures and, also, the growing number of people engaged in providing health services, has been an increase in the demand for health care. A number of factors have contributed to this increased demand, including changes in the size and structure of the population, a growing public recognition of the value of health care, and increased awareness of social needs in regard to health care, government subsidies for the construction of health facilities, and enlargement of the scope of health services through increased knowledge and improved technology in the biomedical field.

Both the United States and Canada experienced tremendous spurts of growth in the third quarter of this century. Canada's population increased from an estimated 11.5 million in 1941 to almost 23 million in 1976. Similarly, the population of the United States increased from 132 million in 1940 to 215 million in 1976. Through the 1950's and 1960's and into the early 1970's, health services were being expanded as rapidly as possible, as we struggled to keep up with the increased demands put on our health care system by the rapid population explosion.

The rates of population increase have slowed considerably in both countries during the past decade, owing mainly to the record low fertility rates of the 1970's. Our primary concern now is the change in composition of the population, which is putting additional pressures on our health care system.

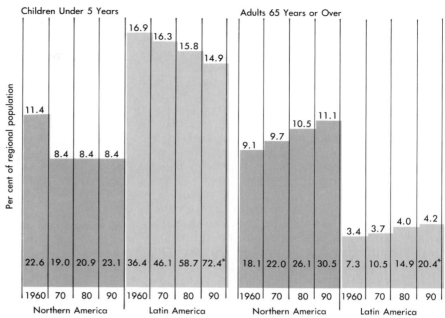

Population in two age groups—children under 5 years, adults 65 or over—in Northern America and Latin America, 1960–1990. (Source: *Health Conditions in the Americas 1973–1976*. Washington D.C., Pan American Health Organization. Pan American Sanitary Bureau, Regional Office of the World Health Organization, 1978, p. 9.)

The three population groups usually requiring the most health services in a country are its youngest and its oldest citizens, and women in the childbearing years. As we can see in the figures above and below, the populations of both South and Central America contain a large proportion of women and children, with a relatively small percentage of people over 65 years old. In North America, however, we have had an unprecedented increase in recent years in the number of older people in the population. Those over 65 now constitute approximately 10.5 per cent of the total population—a phenomenon that

Britain and the Scandinavian countries are well used to, but one that we have not had to cope with before in North America.[5]

The total number of people over the age of 65 years in the United States in 1977 was estimated at 23.5 million.[3] By the year 2000, it is expected that this figure will reach approximately 31.8 million. In Canada, it is anticipated that the number of senior citizens will grow from an estimated 2 million in 1976 to approximately 3.4 million by the year 2001.[6] Older people have more health needs than people in the middle years of the health spectrum. Because of their

Number of women 15–49 years of age in the regions of the Americas, 1950–2000. (Source: *Health Conditions in the Americas 1973–1976*. Washington, D.C., Pan American Health Organization. Pan American Sanitary Bureau, Regional Office of the World Health Organization, 1978, p. 10.)

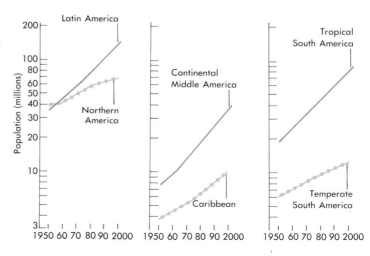

longer lifespan, they tend to suffer from more chronic and degenerative diseases. The needs for hospital, nursing home, home care, and other services to care for our senior citizens have put a strain on existing services and increased the demand for both facilities and personnel. There has been a major expansion in both the numbers and capacities of nursing homes to care for the sick among our aged population. This has meant additional requirements for trained workers in general and a heightened demand for professional nurses in particular to carry the major responsibility for supervising care in these homes.

Increasingly, too, it is being recognized that the provision of health promotion, health maintenance, and home care services for older people in the community can help to reduce the numbers needing to be cared for in hospitals and other institutional facilities. Many innovative programs are being tried, with nurses becoming increasingly involved in the development and implementation of health clinics, health counseling, visiting nurse services, and the like for our senior citizens.

Although the number of children has been decreasing in proportion to the total population in recent years in both the United States and Canada (because of the low fertility rates), there were still an estimated 20.9 million children under 5 years of age in North America in 1980—a sizeable number when one considers their health care needs. Children need a great deal of health supervision to promote their optimal growth and development and to protect them against the numerous diseases to which they are particularly vulnerable, in addition to the curative and restorative services required when they are sick. Much of the preventive and health promotional care is provided by physicians, nurses, and other workers in child health clinics. In both the United States and Canada, community health nurses and specially prepared nurse practitioners are taking increasing responsibility for supervising the health care of children.[5]

We mentioned in Chapter 4 that better health care for women during the maternity cycle is felt to have been a major factor in the remarkable decline in maternal mortality in North America over the past 50 years—thus contributing significantly to lengthening the lifespan for women in our society. We are still working hard to try to ensure that *all* women receive competent health care early in pregnancy, and maternal and child health programs form a large part of most community health programs. Nurses have traditionally carried much of the responsibility for maternity care. In most countries of the world the nurse/midwife is a familiar and highly respected figure in both rural and urban communities. In

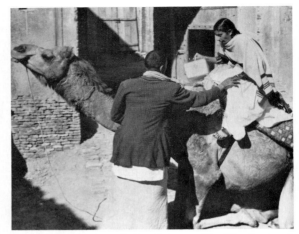

Midwife Shakuntla of the Primary Health Center in Toshan, Punjab State, India, alights from her camel after visiting patients in rural Punjab. (Source: UNICEF. Courtesy Canadian Nurses Association, Helen K. Mussallem Library.)

North America, there has been a strong movement in recent years to re-establish midwifery as a major specialty for nurses, and a growing number of nurses are becoming qualified in this field.

Although the number of women in the childbearing years is proportionately smaller in the United States and Canada than in South and Central America, they still constitute a very sizeable group. The children of the postwar baby boom are now in the young adult years, creating a major bulge in the population at that point. It is these people who are now producing the children and, although they are not having as many as their parents did, and many of the women are having them later, still the needs for maternal and child health services are there and continue to grow.

Another major factor contributing to the increased demand for health services has been a growing public awareness of the value of health care. Health is no longer considered a privilege, but a right. People have been made aware through educational programs in the schools and through radio, television, newspapers, and popular magazines of the importance of maintaining their health and the value of seeking professional help promptly in the event of suspected illness.

Then, too, an increased awareness by the public of social needs has led to more extensive governmental involvement in health care and to an expansion of health care programs to cover all segments of the population, rich and poor. There has been a rapid expansion of private prepaid health insurance in the United States and increased outlays on both Medicare and Medicaid, the two federal programs that pay for care for persons over 65 and the poor, respectively. In Canada, all provinces participate in a system of government-sponsored health insurance that covers almost 100 per cent of the population. Subsidies by government for the construction of hospitals, clinics, and health centers in both the United States and Canada have also contributed to the rapid growth in demand for both health care services and workers.

Although in the United States a total surplus of physicians is expected by 1990, the supply is not distributed according to need and there are still many parts of the country where there are shortages of physicians and other highly trained professional people to care for the health needs of the population. This is particularly true of rural and isolated areas, but it is also true of low-income neighborhoods in our big cities. Many nurses are discovering challenging careers as community or family nurse practitioners in underserviced areas.

Last, but by no means least, on the list of factors contributing to the increased demand for health services has been the explosion of scientific knowledge that has characterized the latter half of this century. More complex surgery, the development of complicated machines for the diagnosis and treatment of disease, and radical changes in therapy have intensified the need for people with highly specialized skills in the health care field. An ever increasing number of workers are engaged in research to promote still better methods of preventing and treating disease and newer and better ways of delivering health care services.

THE ESCALATING COSTS OF HEALTH CARE

Considerable concern has been expressed in both the United States and Canada over the rapidly escalating costs of health care. In Canada, the annual rate of cost escalation has been between 12 and 16 per cent in recent years;[7] in the United States, the average rate of change in national health expenditures has been around 12 to 13 per cent during the past decade.[3] In both countries, these rates are far in excess of the rate of economic growth. Many people feel that if left unchecked, health care costs may soon be beyond the capacity of society to finance them.[7]

While population growth and factors such as increased utilization of services and quality changes account for a large proportion of the increased expenditures on health care, price increases accounted for approximately half of the total increase. These price increases have been mainly in the increased cost of physician services and in increased hospital costs.[8]

Pressures created by the increased demand for health care services and the escalating costs of providing these services have forced a re-examination of our health care resources. Despite the huge sums of money being spent on health care and the growing numbers of people engaged in the health field, gaps and deficiencies in our present system of health care delivery have been pointed out in numerous studies and reports. If we are to provide adequate health services to all of our citizens at a price they can afford to pay, we must utilize our resources as efficiently and effectively as possible.

At the present time, there is considerable turmoil in the field of health care. Existing arrangements for providing health services are being critically examined, and new approaches to the delivery of health care are being tried in many parts of the country.

HEALTH CARE SYSTEMS

The set of arrangements for the provision of health care in a country is usually referred to as its "health care system." Systems vary considerably from one country to another, both in the extent of responsibility assumed by government for the provision of health care and in the administrative control of services. At one extreme is the completely free enterprise system, in which all services are bought and paid for by the consumer on an open market basis, in accordance with his perceived needs and his ability to pay. At the other extreme is the completely socialized system in which the government assumes full responsibility for the health care of all its citizens. In some countries the system is centrally controlled, that is, all services are administered by one central agency; in others, a multiplicity of agencies provide services. Between the extremes are a wide variety of systems. The American and the Canadian health care systems both lie between the extremes. Although they differ in the extent of government sponsorship of programs, in both countries a wide variety of agencies provide services. The types of agencies providing services are similar in the two countries.

HEALTH CARE IN THE UNITED STATES AND IN CANADA

It is principally in the financing of personal health care services that differences currently exist in the American and the Canadian health care systems. Personal health care expenditures are usually taken to include spending for services provided by hospitals and related institutions, services rendered by physicians, dentists, and other health practitioners, nursing services, drugs and drug sundries, eyeglasses, appliances such as artificial limbs and supplies and equipment used in health care.

In the United States at the present time, personal health care is paid for in a variety of ways. Government-sponsored programs include Medicare and Medicaid for senior citizens and the medically indigent, respectively. A large proportion of the remainder of the population is covered for personal health care expenses through private insurance plans. Many employers help people to meet the costs of personal health care through employer-employee cost-shared insurance plans or, in some instances, through the direct provision of health services for their workers as, for example, in a company hospital. Philanthropic (charitable) organizations also finance health services, particularly for specific groups in the population, such as the Shriners' hospitals for children, and the charitable clinics and hospitals run for the poor. Finally, there is the direct payment method of financing, whereby the individual pays for services directly out of his own pocket.

An increasingly large proportion of personal health care in the United States is being financed through public monies. In 1950, it was estimated that only one fifth of the nation's expenditures for personal health care was paid for by the government. By 1978, nearly 38.7 per cent of these expenses were covered by government-sponsored programs, chiefly Medicare and Medicaid. There has also been a considerable increase in the amount paid for by private health insurance plans—from 8.5 per cent in 1950 to 27 per cent in 1978. It is estimated that approximately three quarters of the American public now have some form of health insurance that covers major hospital and medical-surgical expenses. The out-of-pocket expenses borne by the individual consumer have decreased proportionately with the increase in public financing of health care and the expansion of private insurance plans.[3]

In Canada, the major portion of personal health care expenditures is taken care of for the consumer of health services through a system of universal prepaid health insurance. The costs are borne almost entirely by the federal and provincial governments and indirectly by the consumer. The federal government's share of the costs is derived from general tax revenues. The provinces raise their share in different ways. Some finance the program entirely out of general tax monies. Others require the individual to pay a premium. In provinces where a premium is required, it is waived for people who would have difficulty in paying it, such as senior citizens and people on low incomes, and it is waived or reduced for students.

The range of services covered by the government-sponsored program varies from one province to another. All provincial plans must provide basic hospital and medical care services. Some include additional benefits, such as pharmaceutical services, foot care services, and eye

Distribution of personal health care expenditures, by source of funds, selected fiscal years 1950–1978. (Source: Health United States 1979. Hyattsville, Maryland, U.S. Department of Health, Education, and Welfare Publication No. (PHS) 80–1232. Public Health Service. Health Resources Administration, National Center for Health Statistics, p. 251.)

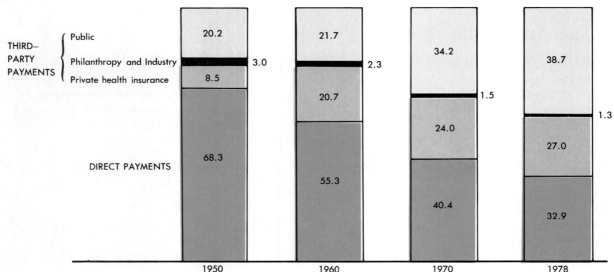

care services. A number of people supplement the government program with private insurance plans to cover additional expenses they might incur, such as the costs for private or semiprivate accommodations in a hospital, or else to provide income security in the event of illness. In addition, industrial and commercial firms frequently offer supplementary benefits, such as dental insurance, to their employees on an employer-employee cost-shared basis. As in the United States, industrial firms also share in the financing of health clinics and hospitals in some instances.[9]

THE SPECTRUM OF HEALTH CARE SERVICES IN THE COMMUNITY

People seek the help of health services for many reasons. The new mother may take her infant to the physician's office or to a "well-baby" clinic to make sure that he is developing normally, to obtain advice on caring for him in order to promote his optimal growth and development, and to receive immunizations to protect him from disease. Some people go to their physicians for periodic health checkups, not because they are ill, but to be reassured that they are well. Most people, however, do not seek the help of health professionals unless they are worried about their health. The majority of these people receive diagnostic services and are treated in physicians' offices, in clinics, or in outpatient departments of hospitals. Many who are ill, however, need to be hospitalized. They may later require rehabilitation services in specialized agencies. People with chronic or prolonged illnesses often need to be cared for in nursing homes or other extended care facilities over a long period of time.

The spectrum of health services in a community ranges from health promotion and protection services, through primary care facilities, to inpatient services and home care for the sick and rehabilitation services for those who require them. A wide variety of agencies provide these services, and many agencies combine a number of them. Hospitals, for example, often have outpatient services for the detection and treatment of illness, as well as inpatient services for the acutely ill and home care programs for the convalescent. A city health department may work in combination with a visiting nurse service to provide nursing care in the home. Nurses work in all phases of the health care spectrum and are employed in every type of health agency.

THE PROVIDERS OF HEALTH CARE

In both the United States and Canada, health care services are provided by a wide variety of

health agencies and health professionals. We will discuss these in regard to their roles in the provision of services in the various areas of the health care spectrum. It may be helpful, however, for the student to keep in mind the major headings under which the providers of health care may be categorized. These include:

1. Government agencies
2. Private, non–profit-making agencies
3. Private, profit-making (or proprietary) agencies
4. Private practitioners.

AGENCIES PROVIDING HEALTH PROMOTION AND HEALTH PROTECTION SERVICES

The nurse's role in the promotion of health and the prevention of disease is an expanding one. At the present time, most nurses whose work is primarily concerned with these aspects of health care are employed in official or voluntary agencies, and more and more nurses are being employed to develop and carry out health teaching programs in agencies like the Health Maintenance Organizations. Official agencies are agencies of the government; voluntary agencies are supported by contributions from people within the community and are operated as private, non–profit-making agencies. The specific services provided by official and voluntary agencies in any community depend to a large extent

In some rural and remote areas, the public health nurse is the chief source of health care. Here, the nurse and a native community health worker set off from a northern outpost nursing station to make their rounds.

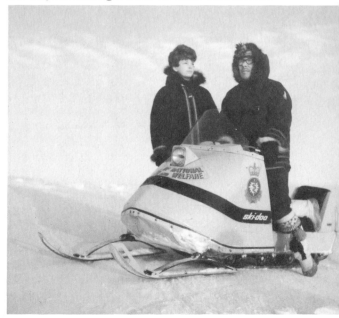

on the apparent needs of the people. In some communities, most health services may be provided through private physicians and private agencies; in others, official health agencies may offer more extensive programs.

Official Agencies

Official health agencies have been established at the local, state/provincial, and federal levels. At all levels, these agencies are concerned with the prevention of illness and the promotion of health. They often provide services of a curative and rehabilitative nature as well.

The local government agency is usually a city or a county health department, although other branches of a local government may also provide health services as, for example, the welfare department of the school board. The health department of a city or a county usually develops its own health program, based on the needs of the people in the community and the resources available to meet these needs. The general community program usually includes preventive measures, such as communicable disease control, the control of pollution, the safeguarding of water, milk, and other food supplies, and the maintenance of cleanliness of public beaches and swimming pools. Health education is also a large part of the program of most local community agencies.

Many official agencies at the local level provide a number of specialized health services in addition to the general community program. These frequently include maternal and child care services; immunization clinics; and often diagnostic, treatment, and rehabilitative services, particularly for people in low income groups. The school health program usually consists of health supervision of the students and counselling and consultative services for teachers and parents, as well as the supervision of environmental sanitation. School nurses may also participate in classroom teaching activities that relate to health matters.

The local government may also be responsible for the operation of hospitals and related facilities for the care of the sick. These are discussed later in this chapter under inpatient services.

State and provincial health departments, for the most part, assume leadership and advisory roles to local health agencies, but they may also provide direct services such as the operation of laboratories, the licensure of individuals and agencies, the dissemination of information, and the provision of financial assistance. In some states and provinces, community health agencies serving centers outside the large metropolitan areas may be organized directly by the state department of health. State governments also operate hospitals, particularly tuberculosis hospitals and psychiatric facilities. Community mental health clinics may be directly operated by a state or provincial agency, as, for example, are mental hospitals, schools for the mentally retarded, and other related psychiatric facilities.

Federal health agencies are concerned with promoting the general health of the nation. In both the United States and Canada, health is primarily the responsibility of the individual states or provinces. National health policies are therefore initiated at the federal level, but are implemented by the states. The federal government contributes a large share of the monies required to carry out various health programs at the state and community levels, as, for example, the Medicare and Medicaid programs in the United States and the National Health Insurance programs in Canada. The federal government, through its numerous agencies, provides advisory and consultative services for local and state health agencies. Another federal responsibility is the maintenance of a national information service about health matters. Federal agencies, for example, collect vital statistics and statistics relative to the prevalence of disease, health facilities, and health manpower. The federal government's role in research in all aspects of health care is also highly significant.

At the direct services level, the federal government is concerned with the control of interstate hazards such as pollution, with the control of communicable disease, and with the setting of standards for food and drug control. The federal government is also directly responsible for the provision of health care services to certain segments of the population such as armed services personnel and their families, war veterans, and the members of the native Indian and Inuit populations.

Voluntary Agencies

Voluntary agencies are established by the people in a community in response to a particular need that is felt in that community. They are usually supported by donations, and the services they provide serve to supplement or augment the functions performed by official agencies. Voluntary agencies usually provide services of a specific nature. They may be concerned with the preventive, curative, and rehabilitative aspects of one disease, as for example, heart disease, tuberculosis, diabetes, or arthritis. Some agencies confine their attention to a particular segment of the population, such as handicapped children or the mentally retarded. A number of voluntary groups are presently concerned with environmental programs such as pollution control. The visiting nurse agencies that provide care for the sick in the home are organized in many communities by voluntary associations. Voluntary agencies may develop at a strictly local level or at a state level, or they may be national in scope. In the United States, most visiting nurse services are locally organized; in Canada, on the other hand, the major visiting nurse service is the Victorian Order of Nurses, which is a national organization.

PRIMARY CARE SERVICES

Although many health professionals tend to think of the hospital as the principal place where sick people receive care, in actual fact it has been estimated that approximately 95 per cent of this care is given outside of hospitals. Most of the health service that people receive is provided in physicians' offices, in clinics, or in other community agencies. The term "primary care" is used to designate the initial health care given, that is, the point at which an individual enters the health care system.

The area of primary care has been singled out as one of the most pressing problems in the health field today. A shortage of physicians, particularly in rural areas and in low income neighborhoods in urban centers, has been given as one of the principal reasons for the inadequacy of primary care services. Many hospitals have found their emergency wards overtaxed with nonemergency health problems, because people have been coming to them for care that was not available elsewhere. Because of this problem, a number of alternative methods of providing needed health services are being tried. The principal providers of primary care services in the community at the present time are private physicians, the clinics operated by community health agencies, the outpatient departments of hospitals, the Health Maintenance Organizations (HMOs), Neighborhood and Community Health Centers, and "free" or storefront clinics.

Private Physicians' Services

A large number of nurses are employed in physicians' offices. They may work with one physician who is in "solo" practice or with a group of physicians. Although the majority of physicians in the United States and Canada are still in individual practice, group practice is becoming more common. In this type of practice, several physicians may work together to provide more comprehensive care for individuals and families. For example, there may be one or two

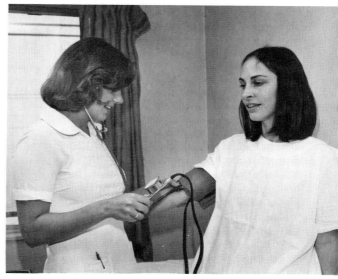

Many nurses who work in physicians' offices now undertake the initial assessment of patients.

family practitioners in the group, an obstetrician, a pediatrician, and a surgeon. Frequently, there is also a psychiatrist, and there may be other specialists as well. Some group practices are small; others are quite extensive. In a large group practice, several nurses may be employed as well as other supportive personnel.

The nurse's role in a "solo" physician's office or in a group practice setting varies. The traditional "office nurse" role included receiving patients in the office, making appointments and referrals for the patient, and assisting the physician with physical examinations and treatments. Increasingly, however, nurses are assuming a much more independent and expanded role in working with physicians in community practice. Many nurses these days undertake the initial assessment of patients, including history-taking and physical examination. They frequently do a considerable amount of health counselling, advising people and helping them to promote and maintain their health. Some nurses working as associates to physicians make home or hospital visits; some carry a caseload of patients, consulting with the physician about their care and referring to him (or her) those problems that he (or she) alone is qualified to handle.

Health Maintenance Organizations

Health Maintenance Organizations (HMOs) have been developing in increasing numbers in the United States in recent years. Their development was greatly encouraged by passage of the 1972 Social Security Amendments, which facilitated the use of HMOs by Medicare and Medicaid recipients, and the Health Maintenance Organization Act of 1973, which spelled out guidelines for HMOs seeking to be federally qualified.

The HMO is essentially a form of prepaid group practice. It provides a comprehensive range of services on a fixed contract basis, which is paid for in advance by people enrolling in the organization. The emphasis in the HMOs is on health promotion and the prevention of illness. The range of services provided by HMOs covers both preventive and curative care and includes physician services, health counselling, inpatient and outpatient hospital services, and diagnostic and therapeutic services, including home care. Many nurses are employed in HMOs, where they often work as associates to the physicians in an expanding role such as that described previously.

Clinic and Outpatient Services

The term "clinic" may be applied to a group practice of private physicians such as that just described or may be used to designate the services provided by a community agency for care and treatment of the sick on an ambulatory basis. In ambulatory care, the patient remains at home but comes into the agency for care and treatment. When community agencies operate clinic services, these usually are provided free of charge to the patient, or a nominal charge may be made. Outpatient services, also of an ambulatory nature, are provided by many hospitals. Again, these may be offered on a charitable basis, or the patient may pay a small fee. In the clinics and outpatient departments, diagnostic and treatment services are provided and often rehabilitative services as well. The nurse working in a clinic or outpatient service is frequently responsible for the day-to-day management of the clinic, and she assists the physicians with physical examinations and with treatments. She may also perform laboratory tests. The nurse is often involved in health teaching activities in the clinic and in health counselling for individuals and families.

Neighborhood Health Centers

Another development in the area of primary health services for the people in a community has been the establishment of Neighborhood Health Centers. Originally these centers were set up by the Office of Economic Opportunity in the United States to provide health care services in poverty and ghetto areas. The centers provide comprehensive health services (exclusive of inpatient services) for the residents of a given community in their own neighborhood. They employ a clinic type of approach but are concerned with both health and social problems. They frequently utilize people who live in the community as adjunctive health workers.

Community Health Centers

The Community Health Centers that have been developing in Canada are similar in concept to the Neighborhood Health Centers in the United States. They are not, however, intended for any specific segment of the population, such as the poor, but rather for the use of all residents in a community. Community participation is encouraged on the advisory boards of the centers, which are usually government agencies, and a comprehensive range of services is offered, including social as well as health services.

"Free Clinics"

The so-called free, or storefront, clinics that developed in both the United States and Canada in the 1960's and 1970's offer another example of innovation in the field of primary health care. These clinics have been set up in poverty or ghetto neighborhoods to provide health services for people who, because of an inability to pay, or a reluctance to use traditional agencies, were not receiving the care they needed. They offer a readily accessible care, usually 24 hours a day, on a free or minimal charge basis in a setting that is as devoid of "red tape" as possible. The clinics have been staffed for the most part by health professionals, young doctors, nurses, and social workers (often students), or retired professionals, who work on a voluntary basis to provide needed health care. Although there are many problems associated with this type of agency, as, for example, the legal implications of who does what, the provision of personalized, accessible, and nonjudgmental care with a minimum of bureaucratic structure appears to be meeting an otherwise unmet need in many communities.

Emergency Services

We have become increasingly conscious in the past few years of the need for highly skilled personnel to deal with medical emergency situ-

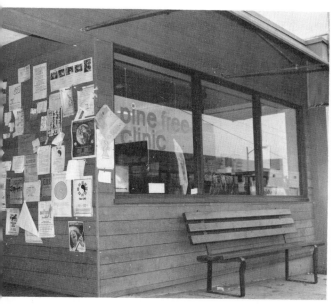

"Free clinics" offer easily accessible primary care to many who would otherwise not obtain needed health services.

ations in the community. Most large hospitals, and many small community ones, have well-staffed, well-equipped emergency rooms that are open 24 hours a day. The patient, however, does not usually wait to have his heart attack in the emergency unit—it may occur while he is shopping in a crowded plaza, driving on a busy highway, or even shoveling snow in his front yard. Accidents and sudden attacks of illness may occur at any time and in any place. The first few minutes of care an individual receives are often crucial to his survival and subsequent recovery.

In many communities, the fire department operates ambulance services and provides emergency care. Sometimes, ambulances are owned and operated by private firms that have a contract with the community to provide services. Occasionally, a hospital provides transportation (via ambulance) as part of its emergency services. In most parts of the United States, and in many parts of Canada, ambulance drivers are being equipped with basic training as Emergency Medical Technicians to enable them to carry out first aid competently. This training includes techniques of cardiopulmonary resuscitation (CPR) and other basic emergency treatment for people who have been injured or have suffered an acute attack of illness. The fire and police departments in a community usually like to have all of their regular forces trained in basic first aid and CPR so that they can render basic life support care if necessary. Often, the depart-

ments like to have some personnel with advanced training in emergency skills as well.

In many communities, the Red Cross has a disaster team of emergency workers who will assist in the event of a major accident or calamity. The community may also have a Civil Defense unit that is prepared to coordinate services in an emergency. The Red Cross and Civil Defense workers are usually volunteers who turn out when their services are needed. The nurse should become familiar with the emergency services available in her community and the agencies providing these services.

AGENCIES PROVIDING INPATIENT SERVICES FOR THE CARE OF THE SICK

The majority of registered nurses in both the United States and Canada are employed in hospitals or related institutions that provide inpatient services for the care of the sick. In addition, a large proportion of the clinical experience of nursing students takes place in hospitals. The nurse should therefore be familiar with the functions of hospitals, the kinds of hospitals and related institutions in her community, and the various departments within a hospital.

The Hospital

The hospital is an institution whose chief purpose is the care of sick and injured people. Hospitals are the centers in which a wide range of specialized functions are brought to bear on health problems. People who are acutely ill generally come to a hospital to avail themselves of the services of the professional people and the facilities necessary for their care.

Hospitals, like other community health agencies, perform curative, preventive, and rehabilitative functions, and are also involved in two additional areas of commitment: research and education. The emphasis placed upon any of the three areas varies with the agency. Generally, the policies of agencies in this regard are determined by the following factors:

1. The cultural, religious, and social groups within the community
2. The nature of the health problems of the patients admitted to the hospital
3. The availability of medical and related personnel
4. The specific needs of the particular community and the facilities that are already available

5. The money available to provide these facilities

6. The existence of nearby institutions, for example, a university

7. The size of the community that the hospital serves.

Hospital policies are usually set by the hospital board of directors. Although the membership varies from hospital to hospital, the board usually consists of people representative of the community served by the hospital. There is usually also one or more representatives of the medical department on the board and, in hospitals operated or financed by government agencies, a member representative of government interests. The hospital administrator usually attends board meetings and frequently serves as secretary to the board. In some hospitals, the director of nursing also attends board meetings, on either a regular or an occasional basis; in others, she does not. Sometimes she is a full-fledged member of the board.

In performing its basic function, the care of the sick and injured, the hospital usually renders emergency care as well as diagnostic, therapeutic, and rehabilitative services. Many hospitals also provide facilities for research so that members of the health disciplines avail themselves of the clinical resources of the hospital. Education, the third function of most hospitals, includes the in-service education of institutional personnel and programs for medical students, nursing students, laboratory technicians, dietetic interns, and a variety of other students in the health disciplines.

Kinds of Hospitals. There are many kinds of hospitals; they can be described according to their size, ownership, control, services, or the length of stay of the patients. Usually a hospital is described in terms of its available beds. The small community might have a hospital of 10 beds; a large metropolitan area might have one of 2000 beds. Often, smaller hospitals offer limited services, but they may have an arrangement with larger hospitals for the prompt transfer of patients in need of specialized facilities.

Hospitals may be owned or controlled by the government, by private groups, or by a single individual. Government ownership of hospitals may be at the federal, state, or local level. Often these institutions are governed jointly by representatives of the government and representatives of the community in which the hospital is situated. This arrangement is usually true of the county or municipal hospital. Private groups also own hospitals; for example, it is not unusual for religious organizations to have their own health institutions. An individual or a group of individuals may also operate a hospital or clinic. Physicians in particular often own and operate their own hospitals.

The services offered are another way of describing a hospital. Thus, a hospital may be a general hospital; that is, one that offers a diversity of services, such as surgery, medicine, psychiatry, obstetrics, and pediatrics. Or it may be a special hospital, admitting only patients of one sex, people with a particular type of illness or children of a specific age group. In years past, psychiatric hospitals were the most obvious special hospitals, and often they were situated in rural areas. Today, however, there is a trend to incorporate a psychiatric nursing unit into the general hospital rather than isolate the mentally ill from the community. There has also been a considerable expansion of psychiatric outpatient facilities that enable people to carry on their normal activities while receiving care on an ambulatory basis.

The length of stay of the patient is also a basis upon which to classify an institution. Generally speaking, there are acute care hospitals, extended care hospitals, and day care hospitals. The acute care hospital has restrictions upon the length of stay of patients; some permit patients to stay 30 days at the maximum, after which they are transferred to extended care facilities. The extended care hospital, as its name implies, is for long-term patients. Often its accent is upon the retraining and rehabilitating of patients over a period of months. Nursing homes also provide long-term care for the sick who require nursing services over an extended period of time.

The day care hospital is a relatively new addition to hospital services. Originally intended for psychiatric patients, it now offers services to patients with various other illnesses. The patient stays at the hospital during the day and returns to his home at night. This arrangement has the obvious advantage of lowering hospital expenses and also maintains the home orientation of the patient. Many hospitals also operate outpatient surgery units for people requiring minor operations who do not need to be hospitalized for more than a few hours.

Standards for the quality of service in the hospital have been established by the Joint Commission on Accreditation of Hospitals. Instituted in 1952, the commission is composed of representatives of the American College of Surgeons, the American College of Physicians, the American Hospital Association, and the American Medical Association. The commission can accredit a hospital, provisionally accredit it, or not accredit it at all. A similar commission accredits hospitals in Canada.

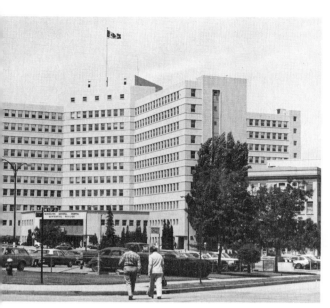

The hospital provides a center where a wide variety of specialized functions are available to combat health problems.

The Departments Within the Hospital. The many services available within the hospital can be classified as direct or indirect with respect to the patient. These services can be divided into three groups: patient care services, institutional services, and financial services. The services correspond roughly with the departments of the hospital.

Usually, however, the number of separate departments in a hospital is dependent upon its size. The larger the hospital, the greater is the number of departments. The patient is usually aware of the medical department, the x-ray department, and the nursing department. He may be less aware of the maintenance department and the purchasing department, yet their services are also important to his comfort and welfare. The following departments are commonly found in the average hospital.

The Medical Department. The medical department includes the members of the medical staff who are responsible for the care of the patients. Often this department designates a board whose members keep watch on the quality of medical care given by the physicians attending the patients.

The Nursing Department. The nursing department includes registered nurses, practical nurses, nursing orderlies, and nurse's aides. These people usually give direct care to the patients under the guidance of the head of the department and according to the policies of the

hospital administration. The head of the nursing department is usually the director of nursing; she may have an assistant director as well as supervisors and head nurses to carry out administrative duties.

If a hospital has a school of nursing, it may be included within the department of nursing. However, a school of nursing can affiliate with a hospital and yet be a separate entity financially and administratively.

The Dietary Department. The dietary department includes dietitians as well as cooks, kitchen workers, and persons who deliver trays to patients. The chief responsibility of this department is to supply food to the patients, and sometimes to the staff of the hospital. This responsibility usually includes the preparation of therapeutic diets for many patients.

The Laboratory Department. The function of the laboratory department is to perform laboratory tests ordered by the physician. These tests include blood serology and chemistry tests, urinalyses, bacteriological tests, and analyses of specimens for pathological diagnosis. The laboratory technologist collects some specimens; the nursing staff is responsible for the collection of others.

The X-Ray Department. One of the obvious functions of the x-ray department is to take x-rays of patients as ordered by medical practitioners. In addition to the x-ray technologists who work in the department, many hospitals employ radiologists, physicians who are specialists in interpreting x-rays and can aid other physicians in their diagnostic work. The use of x-ray equipment, radium, and the like for therapeutic purposes is also an important function of many x-ray departments.

The Maintenance Department. The services provided by the maintenance department vary from hospital to hospital. The department often performs carpentry, plumbing, and electrical services, as well as cleaning, heating, and possibly laundry services.

The Pharmacy Department. The pharmacy department provides pharmaceutical supplies that are ordered by physicians for their patients. The pharmacist prepares some of the medications himself, while others are purchased commercially and are dispensed to the nursing units.

The Business Department. This department is responsible for the financial business of the hospital. It prepares the patient's hospital bills, administers the hospital payroll, and is involved in budget preparation and general hospital business.

The Central Supply Department. The central supply department of the hospital is usually responsible for the cleaning, the sterilizing, and often the delivery of equipment used in the institution. It may also be responsible for the purchasing of supplies if the hospital has no purchasing department. In some hospitals, the central supply department is included in the nursing department.

The Personnel Department. This department is responsible for hiring personnel and for job placement within the hospital. Some nursing departments assume the responsibilities for hiring nurses, whereas at other hospitals this task is handled entirely by the personnel department.

The Social Service Department. Many hospitals have a separate department to provide welfare services for the patients. Among the concerns of the social worker are family finances and nursing home placement. Usually she maintains liaison between the hospital and other welfare agencies in the community.

Other Departments. Large hospitals may have many other departments. There may be separate departments for electrocardiography, physical therapy, public relations, and hairdressing. The services that hospitals supply vary considerably; however, no matter how many departments there may be, they have a common goal: to help meet the needs of the hospital patient and his family.

HOME CARE SERVICES

Home care programs may be operated by a health agency that also provides other types of care, by one that has been separately incorporated to provide home care, or by a combination of agencies. Sometimes it is an official agency, such as a city, provincial, or state health department, that administers the program. The home care programs may utilize their own nursing staff or they may contract with another agency, such as a voluntary visiting nurse service, to provide the direct care. Many hospitals and agencies, like the HMOs, are also incorporating home care into their services.

Although nursing care is the most frequently used service in home care programs, physical therapy, occupational therapy, and other specialized rehabilitative services may also be included. Often homemaker and social services are part of the total program.

EXTENDED CARE SERVICES

A growing number of registered nurses and licensed practical nurses work in agencies whose primary purpose is the care of people with long-term illness. The majority of residents in these agencies are older people who require varying amounts of nursing care. With the rapidly growing numbers of older people in our society, there has been a great proliferation in both the number and types of extended care facilities. Included in this category are personal care homes, nursing homes, extended care units in hospitals, and hospitals solely for the care of long-term patients. The improvement of standards in long-term care is a current concern. Whereas many formerly operated with a minimal number of professionally qualified staff, regulations requiring adequate numbers of qualified nursing personnel are now being enforced. There has consequently been a considerably increased demand for registered nurses and licensed practical nurses to work in these agencies. The emphasis in extended care agencies is changing, too, from a custodial type of care to one stressing the restoration of the individual to his optimal level of functioning, physically, mentally, and socially. Nurses specializing in the care of the long-term patient find the work rewarding and challenging. It demands a high

Outdoor recreational areas are important for people requiring long-term care.

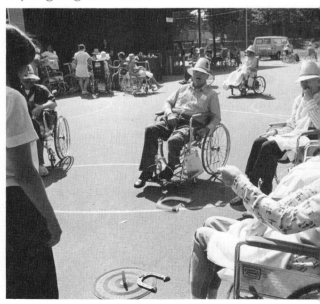

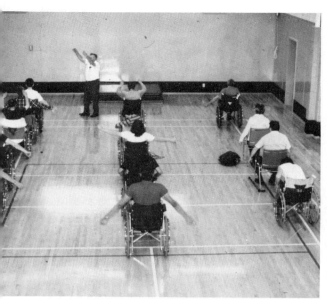

Rehabilitation centers usually have a gymnasium where patients learn corrective or preventive exercises individually or in groups.

level of nursing skill and, while perhaps not as dramatic as nursing in the acute care setting, offers considerable satisfaction.

HOSPICES

A new type of health agency that is being seen in increasing numbers across the United States and Canada is the hospice. Its purpose is to provide care for dying patients, while enabling them to live as normally as possible with as much freedom from pain as possible. The hospice is both a philosophy of care and an agency for inpatient and home care services. Care is provided so that the dying person can be maintained in his home as long as feasible, with health professionals providing the assistance and support required by the patient and his family. When he can no longer be maintained at home, the individual is transferred to the inpatient facilities—or, he may move in and out as his condition warrants.[10]

REHABILITATION SERVICES

Rehabilitation is the restoration of an individual who has been ill, from whatever cause, to the most complete level of social, physical, and mental functioning that is possible for him. The concept of rehabilitation should permeate all health care, and should be a factor in the therapeutic plan of care for each patient. Rehabilita-

tion does not commence when the patient is over the acute phase of an illness; nor is it the responsibility solely of specialized agencies. It begins with the patient's admission to whatever agency he comes to for the care and treatment of an illness; his restoration to an active, functioning role in society, insofar as this is possible, should be the aim of all who care for him.

In the past, the major health problems in our society were the acute infectious illnesses, which were usually of short duration; the patient either recovered quickly or succumbed to the infection and died. Today, with the increasing prevalence of the chronic and degenerative diseases, and the vast numbers of people suffering permanent injuries as a result of accidents, there is a growing need for long-term restorative services, and considerably more emphasis is being placed on rehabilitation.

For many people injured in accidents or crippled with degenerative disorders, restoration to their optimal level of functioning is a lengthy process that may take years of encouragement and require specialized care. Frequently these people need the help of members of a variety of health disciplines—physicians, nurses, therapists, clergymen, and social workers, among others—to assist in their rehabilitation. Often, they require facilities that are not usually provided in acute care hospitals, such as gymnasiums, swimming pools, and outdoor recreational areas, as well as nursing units especially adapted to facilitate increasing independence in the activities of daily living.

In response to the growing need for these types of services, specialized agencies have developed whose primary purpose is rehabilitation. Rehabilitation programs in independent centers in the community and as part of the programs of other health agencies and institutions offer comprehensive service to the disabled. A rehabilitation unit coordinates the efforts of many disciplines in order to plan an approach designed to meet individual needs. Generally, each patient follows an individual plan of therapy during his rehabilitation. The rehabilitation team meets regularly to discuss the patient's progress and revise the plan to meet his changing needs. In addition to the specialized agencies in the community, many acute care hospitals now have a rehabilitation unit to which the patient can be transferred when he is ready. At this time, the rehabilitation team assumes the major responsibility for his therapy.

Most people require physical and occupational therapy in order to restore maximum physical function. Learning to walk and regaining the use of various skeletal muscles are important aspects of therapy. Most rehabilitation

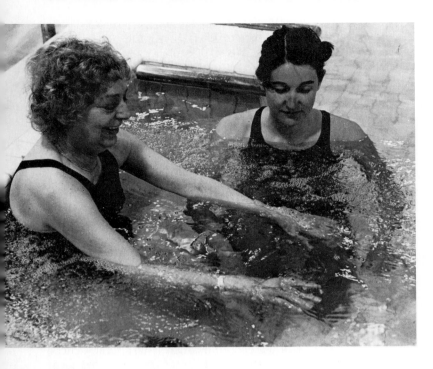

Swimming pools are often used in physical therapy. Water helps to support the patient's weight, making movement easier during recuperation.

centers provide gymnasium facilities for corrective and preventive exercises for patients. Such exercises are conducted by a physical therapist both on an individual basis and in classes. Workshops where patients relearn skill in utilizing muscles through using them in arts and crafts are also an important part of most rehabilitation agencies. These workshops are staffed by occupational therapists.

Relearning the activities that are necessary for daily living is most important to patients. To dress oneself, to prepare meals, and so on, represent areas of independence in which the handicapped person can maintain his self-respect. Rehabilitation programs teach the patient to carry out these activities for himself, often providing him with specially constructed tools, such as a fork with an enlarged handle, which a person with a partially paralyzed hand can grasp more easily.

Some patients require vocational education before they can obtain employment that is compatible with their limitations. Vocational counsellors can advise patients about fields in which they are likely to succeed and about the employment opportunities in these fields.

The psychologist and the psychiatrist are also important members of the rehabilitation team. Their professional help is often required to help patients cope with the psychological stresses accompanying illness and disability. Moreover, since rehabilitation services can be fully effective only when the patient is motivated to help himself and to cooperate in his plan of therapy,

the guidance of the psychologist and the psychiatrist is often necessary to the success of the program.

Before a patient in an inpatient facility is ready for discharge, he is visited by a member of a community health agency who assists him and his family in making arrangements for his return home. For example, if a patient cannot climb stairs, it may be necessary to change his sleeping arrangements in his home. Many community agencies provide nursing and rehabilitative services within the home. Encouragement and instruction carried on after discharge from a hospital help a person to continue to progress.

The Nurse's Role in Rehabilitation

Nurses play a key role in rehabilitation, both in the acute care setting and in the specialized rehabilitation agency. When the patient is acutely ill, good nursing care supports the patient's own resources in all areas of functioning and helps prevent the development of complications that can delay or prevent full recovery. To illustrate this point, most people who are acutely ill—with a heart attack, a stroke, a fracture, or any other type of illness—are placed on bed rest. The patient's position in bed is important to maintain good body alignment and to prevent the development of deformities in joints, such as the wrist or the ankle, which the patient may not be able to move himself. Good skin care and frequent changes of position are essential to prevent the development of pressure sores that can take months to heal. Muscles that are not being used need to be exercised within the patient's level of tolerance, or they soon become weak and require considerable restorative treatment to regain their normal strength. The nursing care plan for every patient must take into consideration not only the immediate problems with which the patient needs help, but also the potential problems that can arise if good preventive care is not given.

Then, too, in both the acute care setting and in the specialized rehabilitation unit, nursing is the one constant in a variety of services that are needed to restore people to their optimal level of health. Nursing is *there*, on a 24 hours a day, 7 days a week basis, whereas other health workers come and go, spending varying amounts of time with the patient. It is frequently up to the nurse, then, to ensure that all aspects of the rehabilitation plan for the patient are carried through, and that there is continuity and consistency in the approach used by all members of staff.

Because of her day-to-day contact with patients, the nurse is often the first person to recognize or become aware of many of the patient's needs. Patients often talk easily to a nurse whom they have come to know and who has helped them in the acute phase of their illnesses. Her observations, her understanding, and her knowledge, therefore, can be valuable assets to the rehabilitation team.

Another important responsibility of the nurse is to encourage and support the patient during the period of rehabilitation. Progress is not always steady; there are sometimes plateaus, and during these periods patients feel discouraged. An understanding nurse can help people through these periods of discouragement by reassuring them about their progress. In so doing, the nurse reinforces and supports the teaching of other members of the rehabilitation team.

Patients frequently find it necessary to relearn many skills of living. The nurse's role is vitally important in ensuring that all who care for him are aware of the patient's needs and support him in his relearning activities. She also helps him to plan his day's activities so that practice and learning sessions are well spaced in order to avoid fatigue.

Above all, the nurse is frequently responsible for coordinating the patient's care. Since she has contact with the various members of the rehabilitation team, the patient's family, and the patient, it is often the nurse who is in the best position to schedule the activities of the patient and to help interpret his needs to the various members of the team.

THE INTEGRATION OF HEALTH CARE SERVICES

Despite the increasing numbers and types of agencies providing health services, it has become evident that there are still many deficiencies in the system and, at the same time, much duplication of effort. A person may go to one physician for treatment of a gastric disorder, to another for examination of his eyes, to the hospital emergency unit for a cut hand, and to a public health clinic for immunization for his children, and may call in the visiting nurse service to give weekly liver injections to his aged aunt who is living with the family. Still, he may wonder to whom he should go with many of his health problems. The frustrations and delays in getting to the appropriate agency in our confusing health care maze result in many problems being left untreated, and referrals to agencies that could help are often not made.

Attempts are being made throughout the country to bring some order to the health care system. There is a major move toward the integration of services in order to eliminate some of the gaps and deficiencies of the present system and the duplication of services. Hospitals are becoming "hospitals without walls." In small communities, many hospitals have become community health centers and offer a wide variety of services in addition to their traditional care of the bedridden sick. The local physician, for example, may have his office there, as may the community health nurse and the social worker. A community mental health center may also be housed in the same hospital building. Many city hospitals are providing a wide range of services these days also. Some offer home care services for the follow-up of discharged patients, and many have expanded their outpatient departments to provide more ambulatory care. A number also provide health promotion and health maintenance programs, such as prenatal and well-baby clinics, for people in the neighboring area. The development of multipurpose clinics and health centers with links to hospitals and other community agencies (such as a visiting nurse service) is another example of an attempt to provide comprehensive and coordinated services to people.

At the state or provincial level, there is a move toward the regionalization of services, that is, bringing all services in a geographical region under one administrative umbrella in order to ensure that all aspects of health care are covered and also to avoid duplication of services. In a regionalized plan, for example, one hospital might be designated as the center for care and treatment of people requiring highly sophisticated (and expensive) medical care. People needing heart surgery, for example, would be sent to this hospital, where the necessary equipment would be centralized.

This movement toward the integration of health services means that nurses must become more versatile. Many feel that tomorrow's nurse will need to be able to function with equal ease in the hospital or the community setting.

ADMISSION OF AN INDIVIDUAL TO A HEALTH AGENCY

Most people are anxious when they go to a health agency for the first time. Even if they are going for a routine checkup, there is always the nagging worry that something may be wrong. Minor irritations suddenly become magnified, and a person can imagine all sorts of horrible diseases that he may have. For example, the small rash on his arm may be the first sign of cancer—he had better remember to ask the doctor about that. Having to enter a hospital is especially traumatic for most people, and the transfer, if one is made, to an extended care facility frequently carries with it thoughts of being relegated to the "never going to get better" category. The admission of a patient to any type of health agency is therefore always a critical point in his care.

The patient is, as we have said, usually apprehensive, and the attitude and behavior of the nurses and other agency personnel concerned with his admission can do much to make him feel more comfortable. A sincere welcome and genuine interest in the patient help to reassure him that he is a person of worth and dignity. Many health agencies, particularly large ones, have been criticized for their impersonality. Much of the criticism stems from the fact that the agencies are busy places and the personnel are often rushed. But it does not take extra time to be kind or to convey to the patient that he is welcome.

Although each agency has its own admitting procedure, there are some commonalities that the nurse will find in all agencies. We have concentrated here on the admission of a patient to a hospital, because much of the experience a student will have is in a hospital setting, but it is important to remember that the principles are the same, regardless of the type of health agency to which the patient is being admitted.

When a patient comes to a hospital, he usually goes initially to the admitting office. Here he answers the questions of the admitting clerk or admitting nurse about his financial status, his age, his address, his next of kin, and his usual employment. Most hospitals supply an admission sheet for this purpose.

Often the patient's initial impression of a hospital is formed in the admitting department. Thus, the appearance of the area and the kind of reception provided by the staff are of utmost importance. If a patient is acutely ill, however, he may be admitted to the emergency department of the hospital. In this case it is often a member of the family of the patient who gives the needed information to the admitting clerk. Most hospitals ask patients to sign a consent form during the admitting procedure. This form usually gives the hospital staff permission to perform diagnostic and treatment procedures considered necessary during the patient's stay. In recent years there has been considerable controversy about the validity of consent obtained by having the patient sign a routine form on admission. Many agencies have revised their forms and their method of obtaining consent to ensure that the patient is well informed about the procedures to which he is giving his consent (see Chapter 7).

After the patient has given the requested information to the receptionist in the admitting department, he is usually shown to a nursing unit. When the patient arrives at the nursing unit, a sincere welcome is again important in helping to ease the adjustment to his new environment. The patient should be greeted by name. His family or friends who have accompanied him to the hospital should also be made welcome. The patient's room or his bed unit should be ready for him so that he feels expected and welcome. The nurse can help the patient by showing him where showers and bathrooms are located, also telephones and other facilities, and by explaining various routines such as mealtimes and visiting hours. Many hospitals have prepared patient information booklets, which are helpful in this regard.

It is important, too, to introduce the patient to the nursing personnel who will be caring for him, and to give him an explanation of their responsibilities. If he is in a room with other people, the patient will find it helpful to have an introduction to those who share the accommodation.

The nurse should also find out if the patient has any particular needs or desires that would make his stay in the hospital more comfortable. Some patients, because of their religious or cultural backgrounds, have specific dietary requests, and the dietitian should be informed about these. The nurse should also find out from the patient if he has any allergies and if he has

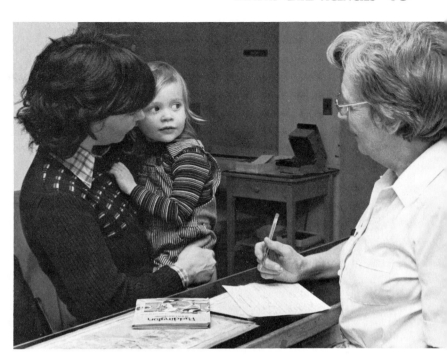

Even a very young patient may form an initial impression of a health agency in the admitting office.

been on any medications at home, such as steroids. These observations should be noted on the patient's record and reported to the attending physician.

Once the initial orientation to the hospital has been completed, the patient is usually examined by the hospital physician. This examination includes a medical history, a physical examination, and routine screening tests. In most hospitals, all newly admitted patients have a urinalysis and a hemoglobin or hematocrit test. Many hospitals require a chest x-ray and a blood serology test for syphilis as part of the admission routine. Tests for pulmonary function and also tests for blood sugar are performed routinely for all newly admitted patients in some hospitals.

During her contact with the patient, the nurse's initial observations are of particular importance in identifying problems with which the patient needs help. The initial observations are an important part of the nursing assessment and provide a basis for the nursing care plan for the patient (see Chapter 8).

Basic Principles for the Care of the Patient Admitted to a Health Agency

Much has been written about the psychological effect of the admission procedure on the patient. Hospitals have been especially criticized for the impersonal manner in which this procedure is frequently carried out, and the depersonalization the individual feels as a result of the routines many hospitals have considered essential. From the patient's point of view, he is first asked a lot of personal questions—to which he is expected to give answers to a stranger. Then, he is given a number and "tagged" with an armband. He is taken to a nursing unit that is usually also designated with a number, not a name, and assigned to a room or a bed, likewise numbered. Once there, he is stripped of all of his clothes and most of his valuables that help to identify him as a person. A procession of strangers then begins to arrive at his bedside—to ask more personal questions and perform various examinations on his body. Sometimes, these people do not even introduce themselves, and the patient is left to guess who they are by the uniform they are wearing. If the patient is assigned to a room in which there are other patients, he often has to make their acquaintance himself.

The nurse can do a great deal to dispel the impression of agency impersonality and minimize the patient's feelings of depersonalization. The following basic principles are helpful as guides to action for the nurse in admitting a new patient.

The Unknown Produces Fear. When people enter a hospital, they encounter a new environment and a new set of behavioral norms. Their security is threatened. They are often not sure what is expected of them, nor what to expect. A number of items that should be included in the new patient's orientation were mentioned on page 64. Most patients recognize their need to become familiar with the customs and the policies of the hospital. In fact, the patients themselves often provide the new patient with information about the hospital and nursing unit personnel, anticipating his need for information and allaying his fears by explanations.

Illness Can Be a New Experience. People need to have an understanding of their illness and an opportunity to come to terms with their new situation. Most people want to know what is wrong with them. The nurse can help by giving all the information she can about his condition to both the patient and the worried family or friends who accompanied him to the hospital. If the nurse is unable to furnish a sufficient amount of information to answer the patient's questions herself and allay his and his family's anxiety, she has a responsibility to relay the questions to someone who can. The patient should be told in advance about the various examinations and procedures that are going to be performed and given an explanation of why they are being done.

Patterns of Response Are Learned. A person may fear a situation not because of the situation itself but because of conditioning through previous learning. Thus, a patient may have had a badly administered injection at some time and react with more than the usual amount of apprehension when he sees the nurse advancing toward him with a syringe and needle in hand. The nurse's confidence in her own ability to give an injection competently, based on sufficient practice in the skill, will help her to reassure the patient and allay his fears. It is helpful for the nurse to find out from the patient about previous experiences he may have had with hospitals and with health personnel, and his feelings about these experiences. With this information, she is better able to anticipate his needs and reactions.

Maintaining Personal Identity Is Important. A person's name, clothes, and valuables frequently serve as symbols of his identity. They also represent security to many people, since they serve as a link with the understood and the familiar. The nurse can help a patient to maintain his identity by making a point of calling him by name and by encouraging him to use his own clothes and personal possessions whenever it is feasible to do so.

Subgroups Within a Culture Tend to Develop their Own Norms of Behavior. During the course of her career the nurse will meet a wide variety of people, often with ethnic and socio-economic backgrounds that differ from her own. It is important to remember that someone's behavior is not necessarily wrong just because it is different from our own. As long as a pattern of behavior does not jeopardize a person's health, he should be permitted to maintain it. An elderly Chinese gentleman may wish to keep a large thermos of tea at his bedside and, as long as he is not on restricted fluids (or there are no other contraindications), there is probably no reason why he should not be permitted to do so.

Specific Admitting Measures

Two nursing care measures that are concerned specifically with the admission of a patient to a hospital are the care of his clothes and the care of his valuables.

Care of the Patient's Clothes. Each agency will have its own policies regarding the care of patient's clothes. Most hospitals and other inpatient facilities have bedside lockers or closets in which the patient can keep his clothes. Often, the patient's family are asked to take those that he does not need home with them. The patient is usually asked to sign a form stating that he assumes responsibility for all belongings kept at his bedside.

Some agencies maintain a central clothes storage area. If clothes are to be sent there for safekeeping, it is usually necessary to list each article on an agency form designed for that purpose. Occasionally, a patient's clothes are infested with vermin. Most hospitals have facilities for sterilizing such clothes before they are returned to the patient.

Care of the Patient's Valuables. If a patient is unconscious, very ill, or otherwise incompetent when he comes to the hospital, his valuables are often sent to the cashier's office for safekeeping. The valuables of the patient usually include his money, jewelry, personal papers, and any other personal effects of value. Valuables that the patient usually wants to keep at his bedside include eyeglasses or contact lenses and dentures. If a patient is lucid and rational upon his admission to the hospital, he usually signs a statement in which he assumes responsibility for the valuables that he keeps at his bedside. Patients are often encouraged to ask their relatives to take home articles of great value rather than risk their theft or damage. Many hospitals routinely provide facilities for the safe storage of valuables.

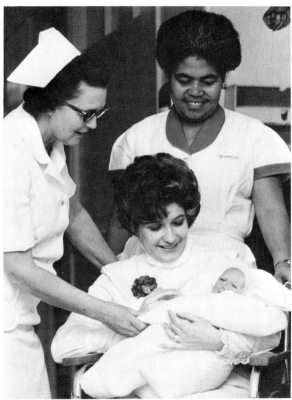

Discharge from a health agency may give rise to feelings both of joy and of some degree of anxiety.

DISCHARGE FROM A HEALTH AGENCY

Preparation for discharge should begin with the patient's admission to the hospital. The patient should be given every opportunity to gain increasing independence during his stay in an inpatient facility.

Hospitals provide a protective environment for their patients, and the world outside often becomes remote, threatening, and somewhat awesome to them. Thus, at discharge, the joy of being united with one's family and being restored to a state of good health are often mixed with fear and anxiety about the future.

Patients are genuinely concerned about their discharge. They wonder about how they will be able to manage, about being a burden to their families, and about their ability to contribute as a functioning member of the family and the community.

Many patients are anxious about changes they are going to have to make in their lifestyle because of physical limitations imposed by an illness: A newly diagnosed diabetic, for example, may have to rearrange his daily routine to accommodate testing his urine for sugar and acetone before meals. A patient will not be able to resume his regular exercise pattern for a while if he has had surgery.

Some of the common needs of patients are:

1. The need to accept the limitations imposed by illness
2. The need to learn to function effectively within these limitations
3. The need to be accepted as a member of the family and the community.
4. The need to learn specific skills and possess specific knowledge pertinent to healthful living.

Patients are usually discharged from the hospital, or other health agency, when they no longer require the services it offers. Should a patient require the services of another agency, the referral is made prior to his discharge. The patient may require home care services, for example, or he may need to be transferred from an acute care hospital to an extended care facility such as a nursing home. Sometimes, a community agency providing services in the home will maintain a liaison nurse within the hospital to facilitate the referral process. Or, a hospital may employ a nurse whose chief responsibility is to make arrangements for and coordinate the services needed by patients on discharge. In any case, the arrangements should be made well in advance of the patient's discharge to ensure the smooth transfer of care from one agency to another.

Occasionally, however, a patient leaves a hospital against the advice of the doctor. In such instances, most hospitals require the patient to sign a form that relieves the hospital and the physician of responsibility for any subsequent ill effects. If a person refuses to sign this release, the hospital administrator and physician are informed directly.

In a hospital, the business office must also be notified in order to prepare the patient's financial record so that the patient or his family can make the final business arrangements on the day of discharge.

On the day of discharge, the nurse assists the patient with his clothes and personal valuables. She also checks with the patient about any last minute questions he may have about his aftercare. New learning material should not be given to the patient just before he leaves the hospital, because patients find it difficult to remember instructions at this time. Moreover, last minute teaching never replaces a teaching plan that has extended over the time of the patient's stay in the hospital. Any final details are written down: for example, the date and time of his appointment with the physician.

When a patient leaves the hospital, he is escorted to the door of the hospital. Some hospitals have a policy that all patients are discharged in a wheelchair. In this way a patient does not overtax his strength while leaving the nursing unit.

In summary, the nurse has certain responsibilities in a patient's discharge from an agency.

1. Checking that the physician has signed the order for discharge
2. Helping the patient, as he requires, with his transportation, clothing, and personal effects
3. Clarifying any questions that the patient might have about aftercare
4. Notifying the business office and other related services in advance of the patient's discharge
5. Arranging the necessary referrals
6. Escorting the patient to the door of the hospital upon discharge.

An important part of any discharge procedure from a hospital is the entering of discharge notes on the patient's record. It is general practice to include in the nurse's notes the general condition of the patient, the time of discharge, and any particular circumstances relevant to his discharge.

STUDY SITUATION

The Parent-Teachers' Association of one of the schools in your district has asked you to talk to them about the health agencies in their community. In preparing your talk, you need to answer the following questions:

1. Has the local government (municipal or county government, for example) outlined specific health policies that effect agencies in the community? Are there pertinent state (provincial) or federal policies that apply?

2. What agencies provide health protection and health promotion services in your community?

3. What primary care services are available in the community? Which agencies provide emergency services?

4. What hospitals are located in the community? What services do they provide?

5. Are home care services available? Through what agencies?

6. Are extended care facilities available? If so, where are they located?

7. What services are available for rehabilitation in the community?

SUGGESTED READINGS

A New Perspective on the Health of Canadians. A Working Document. Ottawa, Department of National Health and Welfare, 1974.

Abalos, D. T.: Strategies of Change in the Health Delivery System. Nursing Forum, 17(3):284–316, 1978.

Aiken, L. H.: Nursing Priorities for the 1980's: Hospitals and Nursing Homes. American Journal of Nursing, 81(2):324–330, February, 1981.

Brown, M. C.: The Health Care Crisis in Historical Perspective. Canadian Journal of Public Health, 70:300–306, September-October, 1979.

Chopoorian, T., et al.: Nursing and Health Care Delivery . . . Health Planning and Resources Development Act. American Journal of Nursing, 76(12):1988–1991. December, 1976.

Curtin, L. L.: Is There a Right to Health Care? American Journal of Nursing, 80(3):462–465, March, 1980.

Dorsey, J. L.: The Health Maintenance Organization Act of 1973 (P.L. 93–222) and Prepaid Group Practice Plans. Medical Care, 13:1–9, January, 1975.

Health United States 1979. Hyattsville, Maryland, U.S. Department of Health, Education and Welfare Publication No. (PHS) 80–1232. Public Health Services. Health Resources Administration, National Center for Health Statistics.

Johnston, M.: Ambulatory health care in the 80's. American Journal of Nursing, 80(1):76–79, January, 1980.

Kennedy, E. M.: The Congress and National Health Policy. American Journal of Public Health, 68:241-244, March, 1978.

Martin, A.: Hospice Nursing: Walking a Fine Line. Nursing 81, 11(2):81, February, 1981.

Schueler, A.: Utilization Review for Medicare. Does It Open a New Gap in Services? American Journal of Nursing, 77(7):1155–1159, July, 1977.

REFERENCES

1. Doronzynski, A.: *Doctors and Healers*. Ottawa, Canada, International Development Research Centre, 1975, p. 5.
2. 10 Year Health Plan Outlined, *Guyana Sunday Chronicle*, June 20, 1976.
3. *Health United States 1979*. Hyattsville, Maryland, U.S. Department of Health, Education and Welfare Publication No. (PHS) 80–1232. Public Health Services. Health Resources Administration, National Center for Health Statistics.
4. *National Health Expenditures in Canada 1970–1978*. Provisional issue. Health Information Division, Information Systems Directorate, Policy, Planning and Information Branch, Department of National Health and Welfare, August 1980.
5. *Health Conditions in the Americas 1973–1976*. Washington, D. C., Pan American Health Organization. Pan American Sanitary Bureau, Regional Office of the World Health Organization, 1978.
6. *Population Projections for Canada and the Provinces 1976–2001*. From Statistics Canada.
7. *A New Perspective on the Health of Canadians*. A Working Document. Ottawa, Department of National Health and Welfare, 1974.
8. *Health United States 1975*. Rockville, Maryland. U. S. Department of Health, Education and Welfare Publication No. (HRA) 76–1232. Public Health Services. Health Resources Administration, National Center for Health Statistics.
9. *The Standard Department Letter of Explanation on the Canadian Health System*. Prepared in the Department of National Health and Welfare, Ottawa, 1978.
10. Walborn, K. A.: A Nursing Model for the Hospice: Primary and Self-Care Nursing. *Nursing Clinics of North America*, 15(1):205–217, March, 1980.

6

The Nurse Should Be Able to:

- List the major fields in which nurses are currently employed
- Distinguish between members of the nursing team on the basis of their preparation and major responsibilities
- List other members of the health team with whom the nurse comes in frequent contact
- Describe the principal functions of these team members
- Explain the nurse's role in relation to its:
    care aspects
    curative aspects
    protective aspects
    teaching aspects
    coordinating aspects
    patient advocate aspects
- Differentiate between independent, dependent, and interdependent nursing functions
- Describe the role of the nurse practitioner
- Describe the role of the clinical nursing specialist
- Explain the concept of primary nursing in a hospital setting
- Explain what is meant by total care nursing and by modular nursing

NURSING PRACTICE

CHAPTER 6

INTRODUCTION

As each decade passes, nursing seems to become increasingly sensitive to health care needs, increasingly creative in meeting these needs, and more objective in analyzing its professional efforts and goals.[1]

Nursing is a dynamic profession and its practice is constantly changing. It is one of the helping professions, with a long and honorable tradition of service to humanity. Although we tend to date the emergence of modern nursing from the era of Florence Nightingale in the latter half of the last century, we should not forget that we owe much of our nursing heritage, and indeed much of the high regard in which the nursing profession is held in our countries, to the work of the nursing sisters who followed early in the wake of the first French colonists to the "New World." The Hotel Dieu Hospital of Quebec, for example, was established in 1639 by the Nursing Sisters of Dieppe in response to the request of the early colonists for help in ministering to the needs of the sick among both the new settlers and the native Indian population. Later, but still early in the development of the New World, the Order of Grey Nuns in 1738 organized district nursing services to assist in providing health care for residents of the rapidly growing community of Montreal. The work of the early French nursing sisters won them the respect and affection of settlers and Indians alike.[2]

Throughout our relatively short history in this part of the world, nurses have played an important role in bringing needed health services to the people, a role that has been continuously reshaped by the changing needs of our society. In the preceding few chapters, we have discussed some of the changes in health care needs that are affecting the current practice of nursing. Among these are the change in social thinking that has led us to view health as the right of every individual, with the resultant expansion of health services to ensure that right; a decided change of focus that is occurring, from a health care system that has been primarily illness-oriented to one stressing health promotion and the prevention of illness; a trend away from institutionalized and toward community-based services; and the integration of services.

These changes are having a profound effect on the practice of nursing. Nurses are being challenged to assume new roles, to work in new and different health care settings, and to accept increasing responsibility in the provision of comprehensive health care. In discussing nursing practice as it currently exists, it is well to remember that the utilization of nurses in an expanded role (which we will discuss later in the chapter) is already a national trend, and may well be the accepted practice role for all nurses in the not-too-distant future.

NURSES AND THEIR CURRENT FIELDS OF PRACTICE

Nurses constitute the largest single group of workers in the health field in both the United States and Canada. In 1977, there were an estimated 1,011,000 nurses registered and actively practicing in the United States,[3] and 143,388 in Canada.[4] These figures, representing professional nurses alone, constitute over one fifth (in Canada, almost one fourth) the total number of persons employed in health care. When we add to these numbers the licensed practical nurses and the nursing aides, orderlies, and attendants, nursing personnel account for roughly one in every two workers in the health field. To a large extent, then, the quality of our health care is dependent on the quality of the nursing component of that care.

The number of professional nurses has risen sharply in both the United States and Canada over the past few decades, both in absolute numbers and in proportion to the population. The United States and Canada are both in a very favorable position with regard to their nursing resources vis-a-vis other countries of the Amer-

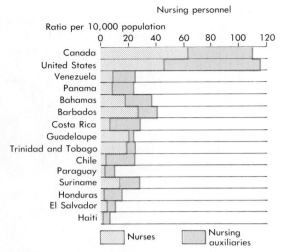

Nursing personnel per 10,000 population in countries of the Americas, 1975 or 1976. (Source: *Health Conditions in the Americas 1973–1976*. Washington, D.C., Pan American Health Organization. Pan American Sanitary Bureau, Regional Office of the World Health Organization, 1978, p. 124.)

Nursing is predominantly a women's profession in most countries of the world. The number of men in nursing has been increasing in both the United States and Canada in recent years; however, men still account for less than 2 per cent of the total number of registered nurses in both countries. Not too many years ago, the majority of nurses were young, unmarried women; today, more than two thirds of all employed registered nurses are married, and their average age is now just under 40 years in the United States and 35 years in Canada. These last figures would tend to indicate that nurses, like women in other professions, are today engaging in longer careers. This trend has been borne out in a number of studies that have been done on the career patterns of nurses.

At the present time, the overwhelming majority of professional nurses are employed in hospitals, nursing homes, and other inpatient facilities for the care of the sick. Relatively few (approximately 8.8 per cent in the United States and 6.9 per cent in Canada, according to the latest figures available) are currently employed in the community health field. As discussed previously, however, there is a great deal of evidence to suggest that in the future more health care will be provided in the community, as, for example, in community health centers, clinics, and other types of health agencies offer-

icas. Whereas our ratios of nursing personnel to population give us more than 100 registered nurses and auxiliary nursing personnel per 10,000 population, some countries in the region have less than 10.

Percentage of registered nurses in various fields of employment in the United States and Canada. (Sources: American Statistics: *Second Report to the Congress, March 15, 1979* (Revised), Nurse Training Act of 1975. Health Manpower References. Hyattsville, Maryland, U.S. Department of Health, Education and Welfare. Division of Nursing. DHEW Publication No. (HRA) 79–45, 1979. Canadian Statistics: *Nursing in Canada*. Canadian Nursing Statistics, 1978. Statistics Canada Health Division, Health Manpower Section, Ottawa, 1980.)

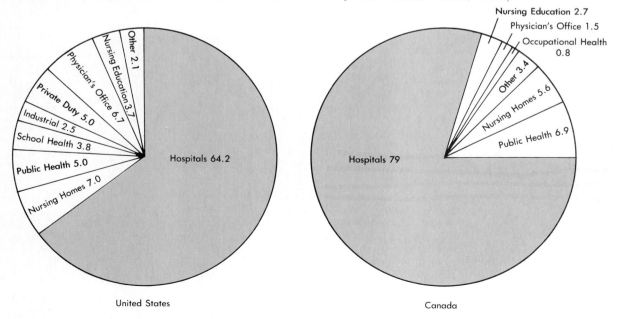

ing ambulatory and home care services for people. The majority of nurses working in the field of "public health" currently are employed in governmental and voluntary agencies, as discussed in Chapter 5.

A growing number of nurses are also being employed in the field of occupational health. Many nurses today are working in factories, in industrial plants, in department stores, and, in fact, in virtually any place where large numbers of people are employed. An important aspect of their work is participating in safety programs to protect the health of people in their work environment. Occupational health nurses are also often responsible for rendering emergency care to people who are injured or become ill on the job, as well as for providing health counseling and other health promotion and health protection services for employees.

Another field that is attracting an increasing number of nurses is nursing education. With the rapid expansion of nursing schools that has taken place in the past decade in order to prepare the large numbers of nurses needed for our health services, more and more nurses are being recruited into this field; yet, we never seem to have enough nursing teachers. Nursing education is a field that has been perennially short of qualified people.

We have mentioned earlier the nurses who work in association with physicians in solo or group practice in the community. This is also a major field of nursing practice. We can anticipate that an increasing number of nurses will be employed in physicians' offices in the future, as more nurses become prepared to function in an expanded role in both general and specialized practice.

One field that has declined in recent years is private duty nursing. Many acutely ill patients still require nursing care on a one nurse–one patient basis; but, increasingly, the type of care required for these patients demands highly skilled technical competence, and this care is usually provided by the nursing staff of a hospital's intensive care units. As the demand for the traditional type of private duty nurses has decreased, however, an increasing number of enterprising nurses are establishing themselves in private practice as independent nurse practitioners.

THE NURSE AS A MEMBER OF THE HEALTH CARE TEAM

Regardless of where the nurse practices today, even if she has "hung up her shingle" and is engaged in independent practice, she functions as a member of the health care team. The provision of comprehensive and continuous care to people requires the services of a number of different categories of health workers. The health team of today is composed of a variety of personnel representing professional disciplines concerned with the health and welfare of people.

In addition to the traditional health professions of medicine, nursing, dentistry, and pharmacy, a number of other, highly specialized positions in health care have developed. Many of the people in these specialties provide direct care services to patients that are complementary to medical and nursing care, such as the physical therapists and the occupational therapists. Some are technologists whose occupations have evolved because of the need for people with specific skills in handling the complex machinery used in the care of patients, such as the respiratory technologists and the renal dialysis (artificial kidney) technicians. Several of the newer groups have emerged as a result of the delegation of certain functions by the major professionals. These include the "physician's assistant" group, licensed practical or vocational nurses (called nursing assistants in some provinces in Canada), dental hygienists, dental nurses, dental assistants, and pharmacy assistants.

Increasing awareness of the contribution that each discipline can make to health care has led to increased responsibility being given to those in the allied health disciplines. The provision of health care today requires a multidisciplinary team approach.

In some instances, the team may consist of only three members—the physician, the nurse, and the patient; in others, there may be a dozen or more health professionals involved in the care of one individual, a family, or a community. Each member of the team possesses knowledge and skills unique to his discipline, and each contributes his special expertise to the care of the patient. There are also many areas of shared knowledge and skills. Students who have all or part of their educational program in the health sciences division of a community college, or in a university health sciences center, may find themselves sharing common core courses with the students in several other health disciplines. Most of the health professions require that their practitioners have a good foundation in the biophysical and the social sciences, and, frequently, students from several health sciences programs take classes together in such subjects as anatomy, physiology, microbiology, psychology, and sociology.

Many skills are also shared among various members of the health team. Communications skills, for example, are needed by all health professionals, not only by those who work directly with patients. The nursing student and the medical student must both learn to give injections and to start intravenous infusions. The nurse must also learn to perform many of the common laboratory tests that are a part of the laboratory technologist's repertoire of skills.

The essence of the team concept is that all members work cooperatively with the patient, whether an individual, a family, or a community. Together, they are able to make a concerted effort toward their common goal of attaining the highest level of health possible for that patient.

The Nursing Team

The nursing team is a component part of the overall health team. Essentially, the nursing team consists of registered nurses, licensed practical nurses (designated as licensed vocational nurses in some states and as nursing assistants in some provinces in Canada), and nurse's aides or attendants.

The preparation of the registered nurse takes place in three different types of educational programs in the United States: the 3-year diploma school of nursing in a hospital; the 2-year associate degree program in a community or junior college; and the 4-year baccalaureate program in colleges and universities that grant Bachelor of Science degrees in nursing. In 1981 there were 1,403 nursing programs in the United States preparing students for RN licensure: 385 baccalaureate programs, 707 associate degree programs, and 311 diploma schools. Approximately 76,000 students graduated from such programs in the school year 1978–1979.[5] Many professional nurses undertake additional academic preparation in masters' and doctoral level programs in universities.

The responsibilities of the various members of the nursing team vary according to the policies of the agency in which they are employed. In general, however, the registered nurse is responsible for coordinating and supervising the work of other members of the nursing team. She also carries out nursing care herself, which we will discuss in detail in a later section of this chapter.

The licensed practical nurse, who has usually had a 1-year educational program in a community college or in a vocational school, may perform standardized nursing procedures and treatments, working under the direction of a registered nurse.

The nurse's aide is frequently trained on the job, or in a course of a few weeks' duration. The nature of the tasks assigned to the nurse's aide varies considerably from one agency to another. In some agencies, nurse's aides perform tasks that are essentially housekeeping in nature, while in others they assist with the care of patients.

Other nursing attendants, designated by a variety of names (such as personal care attendant), may be employed to assist with such care as helping patients with their meals, helping them to dress and undress, and assisting them with personal hygiene. These attendants are usually given a short course of instruction by the agency that employs them.

Members of the Medical Team

Patients are admitted to a health agency in most instances under the care of their own private physician or a physician on the staff of the agency to whom they have been assigned. The physician is usually responsible for directing the diagnostic and therapeutic plan of care for the patient. Most teaching hospitals and their related community agencies also have interns and resident physicians. Interns are recent graduates of medical school who have a planned program of clinical experience on the various services of these agencies in order to complete requirements for licensure as practicing physicians. Residents are qualified medical practitioners who are preparing for practice in a medical specialty. In some parts of the country, the internship year is no longer a basic requirement and may instead count toward specialization. If the agency is affiliated with a medical school, there will also be medical students receiving clinical instruction and experience in the various units of the agency.

Another member of the medical team in the United States (and in a number of other countries) is the physician's assistant. Designated by various titles in various parts of the country, such as Medex, Primex, or simply Physician's Assistant, he or she is usually employed by a physician and performs, under the supervision of the physician, many tasks traditionally considered a part of medical practice. These tasks may include taking the medical history and undertaking the initial physical examination of a patient, assisting in primary care, and monitoring the progress of people under the care of the physician. Many physician's assistants work in rural areas with physicians in solo practice, where they help to extend the range of medical coverage in areas where there is a scarcity of doctors. Many are former army corpsmen, some

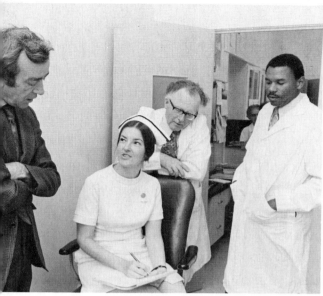

The nurse has frequent contact with various members of the medical team, such as the patient's private physician, the podiatrist, and the resident pictured here.

are nurses, and others enter the educational programs for preparation as physician's assistants without previous experience in the health field. The course of studies, which is usually offered in a university setting in conjunction with a medical school, ranges from 1 to 5 years in length, depending on the individual's previous training and experience in the health field.

Members of the Health Team Concerned Primarily with Health Promotion

With the trend toward the emphasis on health, as opposed to sickness-oriented care, the nurse should be aware of those in other disciplines who are working in the field of health promotion.

The *health educator*, for example, is a relatively new member of the health team. He or she (many health educators are women) is primarily responsible for the development of health education programs in the community. A large part of his or her work lies in community development—that is, in working with people in a community, assisting them in identifying their health needs, and in taking steps to improve health conditions in the community as well as the health status of the people who live there. The nurse will find the health educator an excellent resource person in her own work in health promotion. The health educator has usually had a university course of studies at the

baccalaureate or higher degree level to prepare him for his work.

Also in the field of health promotion, the *recreation specialist* is increasingly being considered a member of the health team. His or her (again, many are women) responsibilities include the development of recreation, sports, and physical fitness programs in the community. The recreation specialist is usually a graduate of a baccalaureate program in physical education (or recreation).

The *family nutritionist* is rapidly becoming a familiar staff member in many community health agencies. The special area of expertise for this member is food and its relationship to health. He or she advises people about good dietary habits, counsels them about their nutrition problems, and undertakes nutrition education programs for people in the community. The nutritionist has usually had a 4- to 5-year program of studies in a university, followed by a year of internship in various health agencies.

The nutritionist who works in a hospital or other institutional setting is called a *dietitian*. The dietitian is usually responsible for planning meal service for patients and staff, supervising other workers in the preparation of food, and counseling patients about their nutritional problems.

Members of the Health Team Concerned Primarily with Environmental Health

In working in the community, the nurse will also meet a number of workers whose primary concern is the improvement, control, and management of man's environment. The term "environmentalist" is increasingly being used in the United States, and "environmental technologist" in Canada, to refer to workers in this field.

The *sanitarian* (U.S.) and the *public health inspector* (Canada and some other countries) are traditional workers in this field. The responsibilities of these workers are principally the elimination or control of "nuisances," that is, factors in the environment that may endanger health (such as excessive noise, offensive odors, and the like); ensuring the safety of water, milk, and food supplies; ensuring that garbage and sewage disposal is properly carried out; enforcing public health laws with regard to sanitation; and assisting in control of communicable diseases. The sanitarian in the United States usually has a baccalaureate degree in the biological, physical, or sanitary sciences; in Canada, programs for the preparation of public health inspectors are usually offered in institutes of technology or in community colleges.

A large number of workers are emerging in this field of environmental health. Some are primarily concerned with the control of pollution, for example. Another worker in this field is the *industrial hygienist*, whose main concern is the detection and control of hazards in the work environment.

Other Members of the Health Team

It is difficult to separate into discrete categories by area of primary interest all of the workers in the health field today. Like the nurse, many other health professionals have functions that include assisting people in all areas of the health care spectrum. Some of the other workers with whom the nurse will come in frequent contact are the social worker, the pharmacist, the physical therapist, the occupational therapist, the respiratory technologist, the medical laboratory technologist, and the radiology technologist.

The *social worker* assists in evaluating the psychosocial situation of the patient and helps people with their social problems. She (or he) usually has extensive knowledge of community agencies and frequently makes arrangements for the patient to be cared for by the appropriate agency, as, for example, to receive home care services and/or "Meals on Wheels," or to be admitted or transferred to a nursing home. The majority of social workers hold a bachelor's or master's degree in social work; many community colleges are now offering courses for the preparation of assistant social workers.

The *pharmacist* is an individual whose primary area of responsibility is the preparation and dispensing of drugs and other chemical substances used in the detection, prevention, and treatment of illness. The neighborhood "druggist" is a familiar person to many students. Because drug therapy is an important part of the treatment of many illnesses, most hospitals and other health agencies in the community usually employ a staff of pharmacists. The pharmacist is an excellent source of information for nurses on the nature of medications ordered for patients—their composition, mode of action, method of administration, dosage, and possible side-effects. Most pharmacists in North America receive their preparation in a 4-year course of studies at a university; a number of community colleges are developing courses for pharmacy assistants. In many countries of the world, new programs to prepare pharmacists (to replace the old apprentice type of training) are being located in community colleges and technological institutes as well as universities.

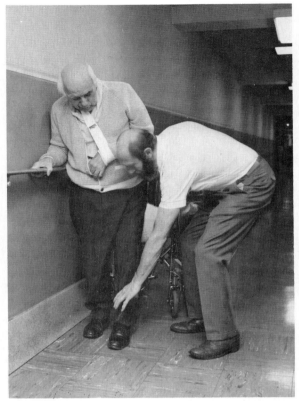

The physical therapist frequently helps patients with the difficult task of learning to walk again.

The *physical therapist* has specialized preparation in physical therapy in a 3- to 4-year program of studies, usually in a university setting. He assists in assessing the patient's functional ability, strength, and mobility; carries out therapeutic treatments, particularly those dealing with the musculoskeletal system; and teaches families and patients exercises and other measures that can contribute to the patient's recovery and rehabilitation.

Closely allied to the physical therapist are two other occupational groups, the *remedial gymnast*, whose speciality is rehabilitation through exercise, and the *kinesiologist*, who is a specialist in human movement and human performance. Kinesiology is offered in baccalaureate programs, usually of 4 years duration, in a university setting. Remedial gymnasts are often trained by people who have specialized in kinesiology; theirs is usually a certificate or diploma program at the community college or technological institute level.

The *occupational therapist* has a preparation similar to the physical therapist; many individuals, in fact, hold a combined degree (or certificate) in physical and occupational therapy. The occupational therapist, however, is primarily concerned with the restoration of bodily functions through specific tasks or skills, rather than exercises and treatments. Occupational therapists frequently play a large role in rehabilitation by helping people to develop new skills or to relearn skills lessened or lost through illness.

The *respiratory technologist* (therapist) is an expert in diagnostic procedures and therapeutic measures used in the care of patients with respiratory problems. He is skilled in handling oxygen therapy equipment, for example. Programs in respiratory technology are usually 2 to 3 years in duration and are offered in community colleges or other types of post-secondary educational institutions.

A large variety of clinical laboratory technologists also assist in patient care in both the institutional and the ambulatory care setting. The student has already probably come in contact with the *medical technologist* (medical laboratory technologist), for example, when she went to the laboratory to have blood and other tests done in connection with her physical examination prior to entry to her school of nursing. The medical technologist is responsible for collecting many of the specimens needed for laboratory tests; he or she treats and analyzes these specimens and advises physicians and nurses on the results of these tests. The technologist is also helpful in advising nurses on the nature of tests and the specific procedure for carrying these out if the nurse is to do this task. In the United States, clinical laboratory technologists are usually required to have a baccalaureate

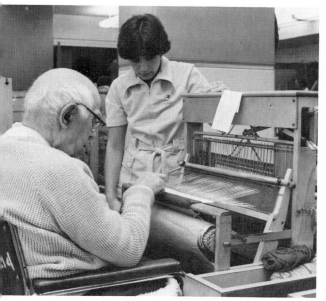

The occupational therapist helps patients with the restoration of function through specific tasks or skills.

degree in medical technology, chemistry, or a biological science. In Canada, courses in medical laboratory technology are offered in community colleges and technological institutes, and are generally 2 to 3 years in duration.

Most nursing students will have also met the *radiologic technologist* (x-ray technologist), again probably in connection with their pre-entry physical examination, since most schools of nursing require candidates to have a chest x-ray done, and it is the radiologic technologist who usually performs this task. He or she is specifically prepared to perform diagnostic and therapeutic measures involving the use of radiant energy. The radiologic technologist's preparation is usually a 2- to 3-year program of combined academic work and clinical experience. The programs are usually conducted by hospitals or post-secondary educational institutions, such as a community college or technological institute, with hospital affiliation.

Members of the Health Team Primarily Concerned with Emergency Services

Personnel in agencies providing emergency medical services require training that ranges from basic first aid to professional level training in emergency care. The basic first aid course offered by the American Red Cross is a 9-hour multimedia, or 16-hour regular course in first aid and lifesaving. An advanced first aid course, usually of 50 to 60 hours, provides advanced skill training. In Canada, the St. John's Ambulance Society offers a 16-hour basic first aid course. An advanced level course is also offered in some provinces. Virtually all health professionals and others working in the clinical field today are required to become certified in cardiopulmonary resuscitation (CPR). As student nurses, you will probably take the 6-hour CPR training as part of your introductory nursing course. The CPR course is often put on by local branches of the American or Canadian Heart Association, and is also a regular offering of inservice educational programs in most health agencies today.

In Canada, people working as first aid personnel in industry (in industrial plants, canneries, logging operations, mining operations, and the like) are usually required to have an Industrial First Aid Certificate. The program leading to this certificate consists of a 50-hour course which may be given in a concentrated 2-week period, or extended over a period of several weeks. A "survival first aid" course of 8 hours may be given to first aid attendants in work settings where the services of an industrial first aid attendant are not warranted (when there are a small number of employees, for example, or when the probability of accidents requiring additional skills is minimal). In the United States, first aid personnel working in industry are usually required to have either First Responder or Emergency Medical Techinician training.

A 40-hour *First Responder* course is frequently incorporated into the basic training program of policemen and firemen, who, by the nature of their work, are often first on the scene in an emergency situation. The First Responder course combines advanced first aid and CPR training. This course is often required for Civil Defense volunteer workers, and is also available to others whose work would benefit from such training.

We mentioned in Chapter 5 that, in many cities and towns in the United States, the fire department is responsible for ambulance services. Personnel manning ambulances (whether they are fire officers or others) are now being trained as *Emergency Medical Technicians.* The EMT-A (A for ambulance) program is an 81-hour course in basic life support skills and leads to certification by a national registry in the United States. A more advanced, 5-month course in advanced life support training and skills (EMT-II training) is taken by people functioning as *paramedics.* The EMT-A program and the paramedic program are offered in many community colleges across the country.

Nurses and physicians working in emergency services also need to have specialized training to be able to react quickly and without hesitation to competently carry out the care that is required. Emergency or trauma medicine has become a recognized specialty in the medical field. For nurses, a variety of continuing education courses are now being offered to assist those working in emergency units. The courses may be given on an inservice basis in a health agency, or offered as part of a continuing education program for nurses by an educational institution, or other agency.

All emergency workers need to have their skills refreshed regularly. Most agencies granting certificates require that individuals be recertified annually.

THE UNIQUE ROLE OF THE NURSE

With the sometimes bewildering array of other workers in the health field, and the many changes that are taking place in health care today, the beginning student may well wonder just what it is that nurses do. Many of the nurse's traditional tasks have been delegated to other workers. Nurses have been relieved of most of the housekeeping chores that formerly occupied much of their time. Ward clerks and unit managers in many health agencies have taken over many of the clerical duties that nurses used to do. Auxiliary nursing personnel often look after a good deal of the patient's personal care and are now doing a number of treatments that were once carried out only by professional nurses.

The International Council of Nurses has stated that "the fundamental responsibility of the nurse is fourfold: to promote health, to prevent illness, to restore health, and to alleviate suffering."[6]

In carrying out their responsibilities, nurses assist individuals, families, and communities in the promotion of health and the prevention of illness; they minister to the needs of the sick, helping them to the fullest restoration of health compatible with their illness, or providing comfort and support in the event of incurable disease. In so doing, nurses work in close coordination with a growing number of other health disciplines to provide health services for people.

The scope of the professional nurse's practice, as outlined in this description of her role, implies a much broader spectrum of activities than is represented by the traditional image of the nurse as the ministering angel who soothed the patient's fevered brow, changed his linen, and dressed his wounds. The nurse still performs many of these activities, but today she is a skilled person who carries out a multiplicity of complex functions. She cares for the patient and about the patient. She participates in the detection and treatment of illness. She protects the patient from harmful factors that could endanger his health. She is an advisor and a teacher on health matters. She is expected to coordinate the activities of other members of the nursing team and to work with a variety of people in other disciplines as a cooperating member of the health team. She also acts as a spokesman, or advocate, for the patient.

The Care Aspects

From its earliest inception, nursing has had a nurturing quality, and this quality is best evidenced in the care aspects of the nurse's role. In caring for the patient, the nurse assists him in carrying out those activities that he would normally do for himself if he were able. Much of nursing action is concerned with the daily living of the patient. Helping him to meet his needs for water, food, rest, and sleep and helping him to maintain normal body functioning are primary concerns of the nurse in caring for the

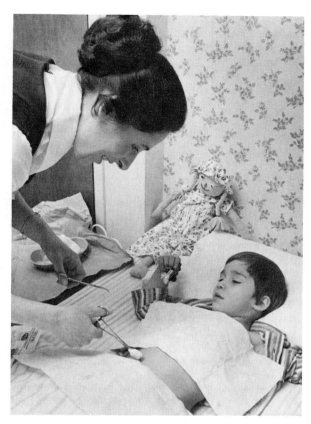

Nurses carry out many measures that are part of the patient's therapeutic plan of care.

The nurse's initial assessment of a patient, along with that made by other members of the health team, contributes to the identification of his health problems (see Chapter 8). The nurse is often responsible for carrying out many of the diagnostic tests that help to establish the exact nature of these problems. Although the diagnostic and therapeutic plans for an individual patient are usually the responsibility of the physician, nursing observations of the patient's condition and assessment of the need for medical or nursing intervention contribute significantly to the development of these plans.

Nurses also carry out a good many of the therapeutic measures that are part of the plan of care for each patient. The administration of medications and the carrying out of treatments are illustrative of some of the therapeutic measures undertaken by nurses. The nurse's skill in carrying out these measures—for example, in giving an intramuscular injection or in operating complicated monitoring equiment—is essential. In innumerable instances, the nurse must use her own judgment in initiating therapeutic action when she feels it is needed. For example, many medication orders are written "to be given as needed" (p.r.n.), and the nurse administers these when, in her judgment, the patient requires them.

The nurse also participates in evaluating the effectiveness of therapeutic measures. Nurses usually have more frequent contact with patients than do other members of the health team, and the immediacy of the nurse's presence (particularly in the hospital situation) provides her with a unique opportunity to observe the patient's reactions to therapy. These observations are of inestimable value in appraising the patient's total plan of care and modifying it as needed.

patient. Part of the caring function is the provision of comfort and support to the patient and his family. Here, the nurse is concerned not only with the patient's physical comfort but also with assisting him to cope with his health problems and the stress and anxiety that accompany even slight deviations from health. In all of these activities the nurse works with the patient, helping him to regain his independence as rapidly as possible and as much as he is able within the limitations imposed by illness.

In caring *for* the patient, the nurse also cares *about him.* Many patients perceive the caregiver, that is, the one who actually gives him his bed bath or backrub, as the person who really cares about him. Carrying out nursing activities with compassion, with empathetic understanding, and with respect for the patient as an individual of worth and dignity is caring about the patient.

The Curative Aspects

Many of the nurse's activities involve participation in the detection and treatment of illness.

The Protective Aspects

An important aspect of nursing care is assisting the patient to take those measures that will protect him from adverse influences in the environment and protecting and supporting his physiological defense capabilities. When the patient is unable to do this for himself, it is the nurse's responsibility to see that all protective measures are taken for his safety. In working in a community setting, the nurse must be alert to environmental factors that may endanger health and take steps to see that, insofar as possible, her patients' homes and the neighborhoods in which they live are conducive to healthy living. She also encourages people in the development of good health habits, such as eating a balanced diet, developing and maintaining good hygiene practices, getting a sufficient amount of rest, and relaxation—all of which help to reduce the individual's vulnerability to illness. She also encourages people to have all of the advised immunizations to further increase their resistance to specific diseases.

When an individual is ill, his protective capabilities and his resistance to other diseases are usually diminished. He may not be in a position to protect himself from environmental hazards and he is particularly vulnerable to infection. It then becomes the nurse's responsibility to see that the environment of the sick room is free from harmful (or potentially harmful) factors, and that all measures are taken to prevent the spread of infection.

The Teaching Aspects

Many of the teaching activities of the nurse have already been mentioned in the preceding section. Nurses both act as advisors to people on health matters—which is in essence teaching on a one-to-one basis—and engage in more formal teaching activities. Teaching functions are a very important part of nursing care. They may involve such diverse activities as advising new mothers on the care and feeding of babies, teaching hygiene measures to protect against illness, advising a patient about his diet, teaching deep-breathing exercises to patients before surgery to prevent postoperative complications, or helping a patient to cope with the activities of daily living when he has been handicapped by illness.

The nurse is also frequently involved in helping the patient to carry out activities that have been prescribed or in supervising him while he is doing them. For example, the visiting nurse may go into a patient's home to help him carry out exercises to strengthen his abdominal and leg muscles in preparation for learning to walk again. The nurse also helps the patient and his family to plan for his home care or to work through health problems and develop a plan for overcoming them.

The Coordinating Aspects

The delegation of many routine tasks to auxiliary personnel has freed the nurse for more specialized work, but it has also added to her responsibilities for the administration and coordination of the activities of others. The nurse plans and supervises the care given by such auxiliary nursing personnel as the licensed practical nurse, the nursing orderly, and the nurse's aide. In addition, she consults with other professional workers regarding the care given to the patient. She consults with the physician about his plan of therapy. She may need to talk with the dietitian about the foods the patient likes that are permissible on his diet; with the physical therapist about his exercise program; with the social worker and the community agency about plans for his home care. The nurse sees that appointments for the patient's laboratory tests and x-ray examinations are made and kept. If he is in the hospital, she makes sure that the housekeeping staff has cleaned his room and that the aide has brought him drinking water. In most health agencies that have inpatient facilities, nursing is the only service that is provided on a 24 hour a day, 7 day a week basis. Other workers come and go, usually during the daytime hours and not on weekends. It is the nurse, then, who establishes a plan for the patient's care and serves as the coordinator for all activities concerned with it. In this, she works coop-

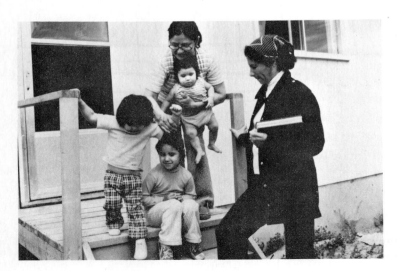

Meeting with a family at their home provides the nurse with an opportunity to learn more about the family's health needs and to give advice on matters of health.

eratively with the patient and his physician, with the patient's family, and with the other members of the health care team.

The Patient Advocate Aspects

As the health care system has become more complex, with a number of different agencies and an increasing variety of workers concerned with different aspects of the patient's care, the need for someone who can speak on the patient's behalf and intercede in his interest has become essential. This speaking for the patient and interceding on his behalf is an important aspect of nursing care.

The multitude of workers who do things for and to the patient, particularly in a hospital, seems never-ending. Some patients have reported that as many as 50 employees were in and out of their rooms in one day while they were in hospital. The patient needs some one person to whom he can relate in a meaningful way, and who can act as his spokesman with other members of the health team.

In the community setting, people often do not know about (or if they do know, have difficulty in contacting) the appropriate agency to help them with their health problems. The nurse, with her knowledge of the services offered by various community agencies, and by virtue of her professional contacts in these agencies, can facilitate the process of getting the patient to the appropriate people who can help him.

INDEPENDENT, DEPENDENT, AND INTERDEPENDENT NURSING FUNCTIONS

The terms "independent," "dependent," and "interdependent" are frequently used in connection with nursing functions. These terms refer to the extent of independent decision-making the nurse exercises in initiating and carrying out nursing activities. When a nurse makes a decision that certain actions should be taken in the care of a patient, and either takes that action herself or delegates this responsibility to another member of the nursing team, she is performing an *independent* nursing function. The nurse may decide, for example, on assessing the condition of a patient's mouth, that he needs special mouth care that he is unable to do himself. She develops a plan for seeing that this care is given; for instance, she may write a directive on the nursing care plan to the effect that the patient is to have special mouth care every 4 hours. She then undertakes this care herself, or delegates it to another member of the nursing team.

The nurse also carries out some of her responsibilities under the legal orders, or under the direction or supervision, of another health professional. The physician, for example, may order a medication for a patient. The decision that the individual should receive the medication is made by the physician. In giving the medication to the patient, the nurse is carrying out a *dependent* nursing function.

In other instances, decisions regarding the actions to be taken by nurses may be made jointly by two or more members of the health team. At a team conference concerned with the rehabilitation of a patient, for example, the nurse, the physician, the physical therapist, and perhaps other members of the team may together decide on a course of action to increase the patient's independence in the activities of daily living. Each member of the team may have specific responsibilities in this regard. The physician might order that the patient be up twice a day to sit in a chair. The physical therapist might start the patient on an exercise program to increase his muscle tone in limbs that have not been used while he was in bed. The nurse may include in her plan of care directives to other members of the nursing team to encourage the patient to feed and dress himself and to take increasing responsibility for his own hygiene. In carrying out these activities, the nurse functions *interdependently*, that is, on the basis of decisions made in consultation with other health personnel.

EXPANDED ROLES FOR NURSES

The distinctions between independent, dependent, and interdependent nursing functions are not always as clear-cut as the previous examples would indicate. Traditionally, the independent functions of the nurse have been principally in the care aspects of nursing and, to a certain extent, in the protective and teaching aspects. In all aspects of her role today, the scope of the nurse's independent functions, wherein she makes decisions and implements action on her own, is rapidly being expanded. Two examples of new nursing roles in which expansion of the nurse's realm of independent functioning are evident are the nurse practitioner role and the clinical specialist role.

The Nurse Practitioner

The nurse practitioner role is seen as an extension of the present nursing role, through the development and more effective utilization of the nurse's unique skills in the provision of health care and through the assumption by the nurse of certain tasks that have traditionally been considered a part of medical practice. Although there was initially some controversy over use of the term "nurse practitioner" (mainly on the basis that any nurse who is practicing nursing might be deemed to be a nurse practitioner), it appears to have gained fairly common acceptance now, not only in the United States and Canada but on a worldwide basis. The California Nurses' Association Glossary of Terms provides this definition:

Nurse practitioners are registered nurses with additional skills in physical diagnosis, psychosocial assessment, and management of health-illness needs in primary care: who have been prepared in formalized programs affiliated with institutions of higher learning. The extended role of the nurse practitioner integrates health maintenance, disease prevention, physical diagnosis, and treatment of common episodic and chronic problems in primary care with equal emphasis on health teaching and disease management.[7]

Inherent in all descriptions of the role of the nurse practitioner is the premise that the nurse exercises more independent judgment than has been permitted herefore.

The nurse practitioner may be a generalist, that is, a family nurse practitioner, or a specialist, as, for example, a pediatric nurse practitioner. Those specializing in maternal health usually become certified to practice midwifery. As we mentioned earlier, midwifery is a rapidly

Many nurses employed in official and voluntary community health agencies are being given an opportunity to extend their scope of independent functioning.

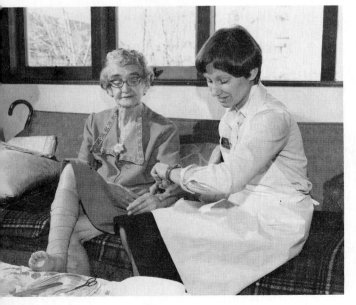

growing field for nurses in the United States, although its practice is still not permitted in Canada.

It has been demonstrated that the nurse practitioner can function effectively in a variety of settings—in Health Maintenance Organizations, clinics, health centers, schools, industry, home care settings, and physicians' offices, as well as in acute care settings. The nurse practitioner works in a colleague relationship with the physician. She may practice in a remote, rural area where she has minimal contact with medical personnel, she may work for a community health agency or in industry, or she may work side by side with a physician, or a group of physicians, in an urban setting. She may provide care independently to some patients, and may work closely with a physician in the joint management of other patients' problems.[8]

The concept of the nurse practitioner is not really new. Many nurses working in rural and isolated areas in the United States and in Canada have been practicing in such an expanded role for a good many years, as have nurses in many other countries. Well-known examples that might be cited to illustrate this point are the Frontier Nurses of Kentucky, the Northern Nurses in Canada, the "Sick Nurse Dispensers" in the hinterlands of Guyana, the public health nurses in the outback in Australia, and also the nurses attached to the famous "Flying Doctor Service" in that country. What is new in the concept of the nurse practitioner is that nurses are now being given an opportunity to practice in this role in urban communities as well as in isolated areas, and in settings where their scope of independent functioning has previously been limited, as, for example, in official and voluntary community health agencies, in physicians' offices, in occupational health settings, and in the emergency departments of hospitals. Nurses are now being prepared to undertake this role through formal university-based educational programs. In other words, the role is being legitimized. An ever-increasing number of nurse practitioners are being prepared in post-basic programs for registered nurses in universities across the country. A number of university schools of nursing are also including preparation for the nurse practitioner role in their basic baccalaureate programs. The number of nurses working as primary care nurse practitioners has increased rapidly since the first educational program—one to prepare pediatric nurse practitioners—was started at the University of Colorado in 1965. In 1972, there were a reported 1,398 nurse practitioners in the United States. Estimates for 1980 were over 18,000, with this number expected to more than double by the year 1990.[9]

The Clinical Nursing Specialist

The clinical nursing specialist is a nurse who has expanded her nursing knowledge and skills in one particular branch of nursing. The term was coined by Frances Reiter in the early 1940's to describe the nurse who has achieved a high level of competence in her nursing practice, that is, as she saw it, in giving direct care to patients. Such a nurse would have increased her range of functions in regard to care, cure, and counseling (as Reiter described the nurse's functions); she would have a broad knowledge base from which to operate; and she would be able to provide a more extensive scope of services than nurses had previously given.[10] At the time that Reiter first outlined this concept, there was little opportunity for the nurse to increase her clinical competence except through experience in the field and through the preparation offered in a few hospital postgraduate courses of short duration. Career advancement, both academically and job-wise, was achieved by means of additional preparation (or demonstrated ability) in administration or teaching. Clinical competence was not rewarded—a complaint that has been noticed in other fields too, such as education, where the excellent teachers, it seems, must become administrators in order to advance their careers.

Although the clinical nursing specialist does not necessarily have to have an academic degree (a good many nurses have achieved clinical excellence by experience and self-instruction), the development of university programs at the master's degree level for preparation in a clinical specialty has advanced the concept considerably. The advent of the nurse practitioner programs has also furthered the idea, and in the United States in particular the role of the clinical nursing specialist is rapidly becoming one with the role of the specialized nurse practitioner.

The clinical nursing specialist may work in a hospital setting or in ambulatory care in the community. In the institutional setting, at the present time, her responsibilities vary, depending on the agency in which she is working. The role is still relatively new, and many clinical nursing specialists have had to develop their own "job descriptions" as they worked and could see how they best fit into the existing nursing service structure of the agency. They often give direct care to patients, particularly those with multiple problems (or one problem that is especially difficult to resolve). They also function as a role model for other nurses, and provide consultative and advisory services for nursing personnel who are working in the specialist's particular area of expertise. Many health agencies have replaced the traditional nursing supervisor, whose functions were mainly administrative, with clinical nursing specialists who can provide more clinical guidance for nursing personnel.

In the ambulatory care setting, the clinical nursing specialist functions in much the same manner as that described for the family nurse practitioner, except that her area of practice is limited to a clinical specialty. Thus, the clinical nursing specialist in an ambulatory care setting might, for example, be a pediatric nurse practitioner, a nurse midwife, or a medical, a surgical, or a psychiatric nurse practitioner.

PRIMARY NURSING AND OTHER PRACTICE MODES IN THE HOSPITAL SETTING

The number of nurses working as clinical nursing specialists and as nurse practitioners is still relatively small. The vast majority of nurses at the present time are employed as "staff nurses" in a hospital setting. We have said that in this capacity, the registered nurse frequently acts as the leader of a nursing team, which may comprise a variety of nursing personnel. The team is usually responsible for the care of a group of patients. If the team is large, the number of patients, too, is likely to be quite large, and the nurse is often busy with the coordination of care and supervision of other members of the team.

Nurses, frustrated with duties and responsibilities that have taken them away from the bedside, have sought alternatives to team nursing that would get them back to the patient, who is their primary concern. One method of allocating nursing responsibility that provides the nurse with an opportunity for more direct patient care is that of *primary nursing*. In primary nursing, each patient is assigned, on admission, to a specific nurse. This nurse is responsible for the patient's care throughout his hospital stay. She becomes "his" nurse, in other words. The primary nurse plans for her patient's needs over the 24-hour period and gives direct care when she is on duty. Through the use of nursing care plans, conferences, referrals, and collaboration with other nurses, she supervises and guides the patient's care when she is not on duty. The primary nurse sees the patient with the physician when he makes his rounds, confers with him about the patient's care, and confers with other health team members, such as the physical therapist, who may be involved in his care. The usual "caseload" for a nurse is three to four patients, although she may assist with the care of patients assigned to other nurses.

Another method of assigning nursing responsibility that involves the nurse in direct patient care is called *total care, or case assignment*. The nurse is assigned a group of patients for whom she is responsible during the 8 (or 12) hours that she is on duty. She assesses her patients' needs and plans, implements, and evaluates their care. This method is often used to provide students with experience in the clinical area. It is also used frequently for nursing assignments in intensive care units.

Still another method is *modular, or district*, nursing. In this method, the nurse is assigned a group of patients, usually eight to twelve, whose beds (or rooms) are close together in one geographic area of the nursing unit. The nurse may have the same group of patients over a period of time, or she may not. Often other nursing personnel, such as a licensed practical nurse, are also assigned to the module, so that it becomes, in effect, a small team approach to nursing care.

Sometimes primary nursing is used in conjunction with total care or with modular nursing. That is to say, one can have total care nursing and also use a primary nursing approach. The essence of primary nursing is that the nurse is responsible, and accountable, for her patients on a 24-hour basis, not just during the time she is on duty. Also, assignment of patient responsibility by geographic location of patient units is one way of determining a caseload for primary nursing. Another way is to assign patients on the basis of the nurse's particular talents and skills in caring for patients with certain problems. For example, one nurse may have strong skills in the area of patient teaching, and particularly like teaching new diabetics. Another might like, and be good at, handling the complex machinery used in the postoperative care of some patients. The charge nurse would take these factors into consideration in assigning patients to her nursing staff.

Nurses who have worked in settings where these alternatives to team nursing are being tried appear to find them very satisfying. They are able to get back to the bedside, to provide direct care to patients, and to individualize that care in a way that more closely approximates the way they have been taught to nurse patients.

STUDY SITUATION

You are a staff nurse on a surgical ward in a large city hospital. The head nurse has assigned you a new patient, Mrs. Majorie Jones, who was admitted last night with acute pain in her upper abdomen, nausea, and vomiting. From her patient record you learn that Mrs. Jones is 35 years old, is 5'2" (157 cm.) tall, weighs 147 pounds (67 kg.), and has had no serious illnesses previously. Her husband is an executive in a large national firm and they have three children, aged 12, 10, and 7 years. You note that she is allergic to penicillin and subject to hay fever. Her physician has left orders for bed rest, clear fluid diet, medication p.r.n. for pain, and instructions for x-ray examination and laboratory tests. His tentative diagnosis is cholecystitis (inflammation of the gallbladder).

You go down to talk with Mrs. Jones and find her sitting up in bed, smoking a cigarette. She tells you that she is hungry—they did not give her anything to eat for breakfast. She wants to know what they are going to do to her and if she will have to have surgery. She is anxious about her family, since they have recently moved to this city and have no relatives here. She says she hopes this doctor can do something about her weight problem. She is a compulsive eater and has tried several diets, but can never stay with them. She states that she smokes about a pack of cigarettes a day to keep from eating. She does not have any interests outside the home. Now that the children are in school all day, she reads a lot, watches television, and usually takes a daily nap after lunch.

1. As Mrs. Jones' primary nurse, what would your responsibilities include?

2. Discuss the nursing care of Mrs. Jones under the following heading: care aspects, curative aspects, protective aspects, teaching aspects, coordinating aspects, patient advocate aspects.

3. Name members of the health team currently involved in Mrs. Jones' care.

4. Identify other members of the health team who might be able to help in the resolution of Mrs. Jones' health problems.

SUGGESTED READINGS

Bakke, K.: Primary Nursing: Perceptions of a Staff Nurse. *American Journal of Nursing,* 74:(8):1432–1438, August, 1974.

Blust, L. C.: School Nurse Practitioner in a High School. *American Journal of Nursing,* 78(9):1532–1533, September, 1978.

Ciske, K.L.: Accountability—The Essence of Primary Nursing. *American Journal of Nursing,* 79(5):890–894, May, 1979.

Douglas, C., et al.: How Could We Help Betty? *The Canadian Nurse,* 77(1):30–31, January, 1981.

Engelke, M. K.: Nursing in Ambulatory Settings: A Head Nurse's Perspective. *American Journal of Nursing,* 80(10):1813–1815, October, 1980.

Ford, L. C.: A Nurse for All Settings: The Nurse Practitioner. *Nursing Outlook,* 27:516–521, August, 1979.

Graydon, J., et al.: Outpost Nursing in Northern Newfoundland. *The Canadian Nurse,* 73(8)34–37, August, 1977.

Harris, J.: On Becoming a Public Health Nurse. *The Canadian Nurse,* 77(1):27–28, January, 1981.

Hegyvary, S. T.: Symposium on Primary Nursing. *Nursing Clinics of North America,* 12(2): 185–186 (Foreword), June, 1977.

Hess, M. P.: Hospital Nursing As a Family Nurse Practitioner. *Nursing 80,* 10(1):12–14, January, 1980.

Hymovich, D. P.: How Children, Mothers and Nurses View Primary and Team Nursing. *American Journal of Nursing,* 80(11):2041–2045, November, 1980.

Joel, M.: Adult Nurse Practitioner: One of the Most Satisfying Nursing Roles. *Nursing 79,* 9(1):17–19, January, 1979.

Kowalchuk, B.: A Challenge in Office Nursing. *The Canadian Nurse,* 75(8):48–49, September, 1979.

Manthey, M.: If You Are Instituting Primary Nursing. *American Journal of Nursing,* 78(3):426, March, 1978.

McTavish, M.: The Nurse Practitioner: An Idea Whose Time Has Come. *The Canadian Nurse,* 75(8):41–44, September, 1979.

Moses, E., and Roth, A. Nursepower: What Do Statistics Reveal about the Nation's Nurses? *American Journal of Nursing,* 79(10):1745–1756, October, 1979.

Pesznecker, B. L., et al.: Family Nurse Practitioners in Primary Care: A Study of Practice and Patients. *American Journal of Public Health,* 68:977–980, October, 1978.

Ramaekers, M.: A Lesson in Courage. *The Canadian Nurse,* 77(1):28–30, January, 1981.

Roberts, L. E.: Primary Nursing: Do Patients Like it? Are Nurses Satisfied? Does It Cost More? *The Canadian Nurse,* 76(11):20–23, December, 1980.

Rushowick, B.: That's Me, a Prairie Public Health Nurse. *The Canadian Nurse,* 77(1):25–27, January, 1981.

Williams, C. A.: Community Health Nursing—What Is It? *Nursing Outlook,* 25:250–254, April, 1977.

REFERENCES

1. McGivern, D.: Baccalaureate Preparation of the Nurse Practitioner. *Nursing Outlook, 22:*94, February, 1974.

2. Gibbon, J. M., and Mathewson, M. S.: *Three Centuries of Canadian Nursing.* Toronto, The Macmillan Company of Canada Limited, 1947, pp. 1–8.

3. *Second Report to the Congress, March 15, 1979* (Revised), Nurse Training Act of 1975. Health Manpower References. Hyattsville, Maryland. U.S. Department of Health, Education and Welfare. Division of Nursing. DHEW Publication No. (HRA) 79–45, 1979.

4. *Nursing in Canada.* Canadian Nursing Statistics, 1978. Statistics Canada Health Division, Health Manpower Section, Ottawa, 1980.

5. State Approved Schools of Nursing—R. N. NLN Publication 19–1853, 1981.

6. Ethical Concepts Applied to Nursing 1973. *ICN News Release,* No. 6, September, 1975.

7. *Standard of Care: Glossary of Terms.* California Nurses' Association, 1974.

8. *Joint Statement on Family Nurse Practitioners in Primary Care.* California Joint Practice Commission, 1975.

9. *Health United States 1979.* Hyattsville, Maryland. U.S. Department of Health, Education and Welfare. Public Health Service. DHEW Publication No. (PHS) 80–1232, 1980.

10. Reiter F.: The Nurse-Clinician. *American Journal of Nursing,* 66:274–280, February, 1966.

7

The Nurse Should Be Able to:

- Outline the role and functions of her national and international professional associations and national student association
- Discuss implications for nursing practice of the International and the American Nurses' Association Codes of Nursing Ethics
- Differentiate among licensure, registration, and certification
- Discuss mandatory continuing education requirements for licensure and registration
- Discuss the need for a legal definition of nursing practice
- Compare the functions of the registered nurse and the practical nurse
- Discuss the legal status of the nurse
- Discuss consumer rights in the health care system
- Outline methods of quality assurance in nursing
- Discuss the meaning of the term "informed consent"
- Define the following legal terms: tort, crime, negligence, malpractice, assault, battery, defamation of character, slander, libel, false imprisonment, and invasion of privacy
- Give examples of common types of incidents involving nurses that may lead to legal suits in which negligence is a factor
- List guidelines helpful to nurses in maintaining the confidentiality of patients
- Discuss the nurse's responsibility if she is present at the scene of an accident
- Explain the legal implications of witnessing a will
- Discuss the legal, moral, and religious considerations of abortion
- Explain the implications for nursing practice of laws controlling narcotic and other harmful drugs

THE LEGAL AND ETHICAL BASIS OF NURSING PRACTICE

CHAPTER 7

INTRODUCTION

People place a great deal of trust in health professionals. It therefore seems reasonable for individuals to expect that the people who provide health care are qualified to practice their profession and that they will be assured of safe and competent care in their hands. It also seems reasonable to assume that their basic rights as human beings will be respected by all who care for them.

Although nurses are not responsible for all aspects of health care, they have a responsibility to ensure that, insofar as the nursing component is concerned, the patient is assured of safe and competent care and that his fundamental rights, such as the right to courtesy, to privacy, and to information on his condition, will be safeguarded during the process of care.

Most of the developed countries of the world have laws that regulate the practice of health professionals; these laws are intended to protect the public from unqualified practitioners. In some cases, the laws also define the scope of professional practice—that is, they specify the functions that the qualified practitioner may undertake. In many instances, however, the law is vague in this respect, particularly in regard to the practice of nursing and medicine. Often it has been the professional associations that have undertaken to define the role and functions of the practitioner, based on currently accepted patterns of practice.

In most countries of the "free" world, an individual's basic human rights are protected, either in the constitution of the country or in its legally enacted laws. The consumers' bills of rights developed in both the United States and Canada have sought to further clarify an individual's basic rights as these are applicable to health care. Safeguarding the patient's rights is also an important aspect of the ethical codes adopted by each of the major health professions. These codes extend beyond the legal basis for practice and into the realm of social values to which members of the particular profession are committed.

The professional associations have also become increasingly concerned with the need to develop standards to ensure that patients will receive safe and competent care. Both the American and the Canadian Nurses' Associations, for example, have been developing statements regarding standards that must be maintained in various fields of nursing practice in order to assure the consumer of good quality nursing care.

The nurse should be familiar with the International Code of Nursing Ethics and other such codes, which describe social responsibilities considered important in nursing practice. She should also be familiar with the laws in her state or province concerning the provision of health care to the public, and particularly with the acts that control the practice of nursing. She should be aware of her functions and responsibilities, both as defined by law and as delineated by her professional nursing associations. It is important, also, for the nurse to be familiar with the various charters that have been developed to outline consumers' rights in the health care system, and she should be aware of how the law protects the patient in this regard. She should also be cognizant of her own legal status both as a student and as a graduate nurse.

PROFESSIONAL NURSING ASSOCIATIONS

Professional nursing associations in the United States, in Canada, and in other countries, as well as the International Council of Nurses, have been instrumental in developing and promoting a sound legal and ethical basis for nursing practice. We will be referring time and again throughout this chapter to statements made by the professional associations. It would seem important, then, for the beginning student of nursing to know a little about these organizations.

The International Council of Nurses is a nonpolitical, self-governing organization, with headquarters in Geneva, Switzerland. It was founded in 1899 as a federation of national nurses' associations. The ICN meets once every 4 years and provides an opportunity for nurses from all member associations, now including 84 countries, to meet to share common interests and discuss common problems. The stated functions of the ICN are:

1. To assist national nurses' associations to improve the standards of nursing and the competence of nurses;
2. to promote the development of strong national nurses' associations;
3. to serve as the authoritative voice for nursing internationally;
4. to assist the national nurses' associations to improve the status of nurses.[1]

Each member association has one representative (usually its current president) on the Council of National Representatives, which is the highest governing body of the ICN. The Council meets once a year. An elected president, three vice presidents, and 11 other members make up the ICN Board of Directors, which conducts the business of the organization on an ongoing basis. The *International Nursing Review* is the official journal of the ICN.

In the United States, the American Nurses' Association was founded in 1896 and was a charter member of the International Council of Nurses. The ANA now has over 200,000 members. Its purposes, as stated in its bylaws, are:

1. To foster high standards of nursing practice;
2. to promote the professional educational advancement of nurses;
3. to promote the welfare of nurses so all people may have better care.[1]

The Canadian Nurses' Association had its origins in a joint American/Canadian association called the American Society of Superintendents of Training Schools, which was concerned over the need to improve educational programs for student nurses. This group was established in 1894 and worked closely together for a number of years until 1908, when it divided to form the Canadian Nurses' Association and the National League for Nursing Education (in the United States). The latter subsequently became the National League for Nursing, with a broadened scope that includes the improvement of nursing services as well as nursing education. The CNA, whose membership now exceeds 127,000, also retained its interest in the improvement of nursing education but broadened its scope, too, as befitted a national nursing association. Its objectives are stated as follows:

All associations of professional nurses in Canada strive to promote health and to seek conditions conducive to the best possible patient care. To achieve this, the Canadian Nurses' Association is continuously concerned with:
— quality and quantity of nurses available to the health team;
— standards of preparation and performance of professional nurses;
— social and economic welfare of nurses;
— advancement of knowledge, techniques and competence within the profession;
— promotion of understanding, unity and good professional citizenship among its members;
— representing and speaking for the organized nursing profession, both nationally and internationally.[2]

Both the American Nurses' Association and the Canadian Nurses' Association are tri-level organizations, that is, they are composed of national, state/provincial, and district associations. The American Nurses' Association has 53 constituent (state association) members, including one in each of the 50 states, the District of Columbia, Guam, and the Virgin Islands. In Canada, 10 provincial associations, plus the Association of Nurses of the Northwest Territories, together make up the Canadian Nurses' Association. In both the United States and Canada, with the exception of the smallest jurisdictions (such as Guam), the state or provincial associations are subdivided into district nursing associations, which provide all members with the opportunity to participate in the affairs of their professional association.

In both the United States and Canada, the national nursing associations represent nurses and serve as the official voice of nursing in relations with allied national and international organizations, governmental bodies, and the public. The state and provincial associations function similarly within their jurisdictions.

The American Nurses' Association and the Canadian Nurses' Association both publish monthly professional journals, the *American Journal of Nursing* and *The Canadian Nurse*, respectively. These journals serve as the principal resource for nurses in regard to national and international affairs affecting nursing. Both journals also help to keep nurses up-to-date with new developments in nursing through articles of a clinical nature. The ANA also publishes a monthly newspaper called *The American Nurse,* which is distributed to all members. It contains news about issues in nursing and in health care that are of interest to nurses.

In both Canada and the United States, student nurses' associations have been formed. The National Student Nurses' Association, Inc. (NSNA) is the national association for undergraduate students in the United States; the Canadian Student Nurses' Association (CSNA) is its counterpart in Canada. Both associations are concerned with fostering high standards of nursing education to promote the highest quality of nursing care. A particular concern of the NSNA at the present time is the recruitment of members of racial minority groups (and men) into programs preparing registered nurses. In 1975, the NSNA adopted the Student Bill of Rights and Grievance Procedures for the purpose of guaranteeing students' rights and assisting the establishment of grievance procedures in schools of nursing. The NSNA publishes a magazine, *Imprint,* which is put out four times a year and distributed to all members.

At least one provincial nursing association, the Registered Nurses' Association of British Columbia, permits undergraduates enrolled in RN programs to hold "student membership" in the Association for a nominal fee. Student members may participate in chapter and provincial activities, may serve on committees, and may represent chapters as voting delegates to annual and special meetings.

The National Federation of Licensed Practical Nurses Inc. and the Canadian Association of Practical Nurses are national organizations analogous to the ANA and the CNA. The purposes of the NFLPN are stated as being:

—to speak, act and establish policy for its members on the local, state and national level, in all areas where their welfare may be affected;

—to establish educational programs for its members . . . ;

—to seek the betterment of all LPNs as an integral part of the health care team; and

—to assure the public that optimum standards of personal nursing care are observed.[1]

The Federation maintains a liaison committee with both the American Nurses' Association and the National League for Nursing. It also publishes a monthly journal entitled *Nursing Care.* Student nurses in practical nursing programs do not have a separate student association, but may belong to the NFLPN as affiliate members and may attend meetings.

CODES OF NURSING ETHICS

Every profession is based on a code of ethics that commits its members to certain social values that are above the selfish ones of income, power, and prestige. At its Congress in 1973, the International Council of Nurses adopted a code of nursing ethics that focuses on the nurse's responsibilities in regard to people, to society, to practice, to co-workers, and to the nursing profession. Following is a statement of the Code in its entirety.

Code for Nurses—Ethical Concepts Applied to Nursing

The fundamental responsibility of the nurse is fourfold: to promote health, to prevent illness, to restore health, and to alleviate suffering. The need for nursing is universal. Inherent in nursing is respect for life, dignity, and the rights of man. It is unrestricted by considerations of nationality, race, creed, colour, age, sex, politics, or social status. Nurses render health services to the individual, the family, and the community and coordinate their services with those of related groups.

Nurses and People. The nurse's primary responsibility is to those people who require nursing care.

The nurse, in providing care, promotes an environment in which the values, customs, and spiritual beliefs of the individual are respected.

The nurse holds in confidence personal information and uses judgment in sharing this information.

Nursing and Society. The nurse shares with other citizens the responsibility for initiating and supporting action to meet the health and social needs of the public.

Nurses and Practice. The nurse carries personal responsibility for nursing practice and for maintaining competence through continual learning.

The nurse maintains the highest standards of nursing care possible within the reality of a specific situation.

The nurse uses judgment in relation to individual competence when accepting and delegating responsibility.

The nurse when acting in a professional capacity should at all times maintain standards of personal conduct which reflect credit upon the profession.

Nurses and Co-Workers. The nurse sustains a cooperative relationship with co-workers in nursing and other fields.

The nurse takes appropriate action to safeguard the individual when his care is endangered by a co-worker or another person.

Nurses and the Profession. The nurse plays the

major role in determining and implementing desirable standards of nursing practice and nursing education.

The nurse is active in developing a core of professional knowledge.

The nurse, acting through the professional organization, participates in establishing and maintaining equitable social and economic working conditions in nursing.[3]

American Nurses' Association Code for Nurses

The American Nurses' Association first developed its code of nursing ethics in 1950. This code has been amended twice since then to reflect the changing concerns of nurses in practice. The most recent version was adopted in 1976. Its guidelines for ethical conduct reflect the increasing autonomy of the nursing profession, its broader practice base, its concern with maintaining the quality of nursing care, and the assumption by nurses of increasingly broad social responsibility in the community. The code is reprinted below.

1. The nurse provides services with respect for human dignity and the uniqueness of the client unrestricted by considerations of social or economic status, personal attributes, or the nature of health problems.
2. The nurse safeguards the client's right to privacy by judiciously protecting information of a confidential nature.
3. The nurse acts to safeguard the client and the public when health care and safety are affected by the incompetent, unethical, or illegal practice of any person.
4. The nurse assumes responsibility and accountability for individual nursing judgments and actions.
5. The nurse maintains competence in nursing.
6. The nurse exercises informed judgment and uses individual competence and qualifications as criteria in seeking consultation, accepting responsibilities, and delegating nursing activities to others.
7. The nurse participates in activities that contribute to the ongoing development of the profession's body of knowledge.
8. The nurse participates in the profession's efforts to implement and improve standards of nursing.
9. The nurse participates in the profession's efforts to establish and maintain conditions of employment conducive to high quality nursing care.
10. The nurse participates in the profession's effort to protect the public from misinformation and misrepresentation and to maintain the integrity of nursing.
11. The nurse collaborates with members of the health professions and other citizens in promoting community and national efforts to meet the health needs of the public.[4]

The Canadian Nurses' Association endorsed the ICN Code for Nurses in 1973. The Associa-

tion has also developed a statement on an ethical basis for nursing in Canada which was approved by the Board of Directors in 1980 but is currently under revision.

Ethics and Nursing Research

One area of practice that has been of considerable concern to nurses from an ethical point of view is research that involves human beings as subjects. Both the American and the Canadian Nurses' Association have developed position papers regarding this matter. The CNA paper, "Ethics of Nursing Research," in its preamble, states that:

Respect for the value of human life, for the worth and dignity of human beings, and their rights to knowledge, privacy and self-determination must underlie research practices in nursing as in other health disciplines. The legitimacy of involving human subjects in nursing research must be assessed within the context of these values. The right of the subject to informed consent, confidentiality, positive risk value, and competence of the investigator must be assured.[5]

The American Nurses' Association has two position papers on research, one dealing with the rights of nurses in conducting research, and the other concerning the rights of patients participating in research studies. The latter is similar in content to the CNA paper, stating that:

The relationship of trust between patient and nurse has always been an essential element of the professional code of ethics. In research, the relationship of trust between subject and investigator requires that the investigator assume special obligations to safeguard the subject in several ways. The subject needs to be assured that his rights will not be violated without his voluntary and informed consent. Secondly, the investigator guarantees that no risk, discomfort, invasion of privacy, or threat to personal dignity beyond that initially stated in describing the subject's role in the study will be imposed without further permission being obtained. Finally, the subject is assured that if he does not wish to participate in the study, he will neither be subjected to harrassment nor will the quality of his care be influenced by this decision.[6]

NURSING PRACTICE ACTS

The laws in both the United States and Canada derive from two main sources: the statutes passed by lawmaking bodies, such as Congress or Parliament, and the decisions of the courts. The latter are collectively known as common law. The law is a reflection of public opinion and of civic and social movements within a community. The law therefore is not static; rather, it is constantly changing. Changes in the statutes and the decisions of the courts in cases involving nursing reflect changes in public thinking about the development of nursing.

In recent years, there has been an increasing awareness by nurses and by the public of the need to standardize the laws concerning the practice of both the professional and the practical nurse. The authority to control nursing, together with various other professions and occupations concerned with health and welfare, has been vested in the states (or, in Canada, in the provinces). Thus, each state and province has enacted its own laws to control the practice of nursing. These laws are generally termed "nursing practice acts," although the exact title of the statute varies in the different jurisdictions. Because each state and province has set up its own law, it is understandable that the statutes vary somewhat. Nevertheless, the purpose of these laws is the same—that is, to protect the health of the public through the establishment of minimum standards, which a qualified practitioner must meet in order to practice as a nurse.[7]

Licensure and Registration

The responsibility for administering the nursing practice act has been delegated to a board of nursing in each of the 50 states and in Washington, D.C., Puerto Rico, Guam, and the Virgin Islands. Sometimes the board functions as a separate government entity; sometimes it is part of a department within the state government structure, as, for example, a department of health or a department of licenses. The responsibilities of state boards of nursing include the tasks of examination of candidates for the profession, licensure of qualified candidates, discipline of nurses who violate the law or ethical principles pertaining to nursing, and establishment of standards for, and accreditation of, basic nursing education programs.

In Canada, with the exception of Ontario and Quebec, provincial governments have delegated administration of the nursing acts to the professional nursing association. In Ontario the responsibility rests with a College of Nurses, which is separate from the nursing association. The College undertakes the same types of tasks as those carried out by the state boards of nursing in the United States. In the Province of Quebec, the provincial government, in its Health Disciplines Act of 1975, established an Order of Nurses, which is charged with similar responsibilities.

In the United States, nurses are issued a license by the state board of nursing. A license is a permit granted by a government agency to an individual to engage in the practice of a profession and to use a particular title. Basically, the purpose of licensure is to protect the public from unqualified practitioners. The individual must meet certain requirements laid down by the licensing board (and also pay a fee) in order to receive a license in a particular field of endeavor. The state boards of nursing issue licenses to registered nurses who have successfully completed a course of studies in a school of nursing accredited by the state board and have passed the national qualifying examinations with a score that is acceptable to the board. Acceptable passing scores may vary in different states. A state board may also grant a license to a nurse who holds an active practicing license in another state, through a process of endorsement, without the candidate having to rewrite examinations, providing she has attained a passing score on the national examinations that is equal to, or above, that considered acceptable in the state in which she wishes to practice. Nurses returning to active practice after being out of nursing for a while may be granted licensure by reinstatement (in the state in which they were originally licensed). Nursing is changing so rapidly at the present time, however, that many people feel that any nurse who has been out of the work force for 5 years or more should update her knowledge and skills before resuming active practice. Increasingly, state boards are requiring nurses who have not practiced for a number of years to take a refresher course before engaging in active practice again.

In Canada, nurses are not licensed except in the province of Quebec. They are, however, registered by their provincial nursing association and by the College of Nurses of Ontario.* The term "registration" means the listing of an individual's name on the official roster of a governmental or nongovernmental agency. Nurses who are registered are permitted to use the title "Registered Nurse"; nurses who have failed to register are not permitted to do so. In order to be registered, the nurse must have completed a basic course of nursing studies in a program approved by the registering body, and have passed the national qualifying examinations with an acceptable grade. As with state boards of nursing in the United States, provincial registering bodies vary in the score they consider an acceptable passing grade. Nurses from other provinces in Canada may be granted

*Nurses in the United States are also registered but must, in addition, be granted a license to practice.

registration by endorsement, as may nurses from other countries, providing their qualifications meet the criteria established by the provincial registering body. As in the various states of the United States, nurses wishing to return to practice after an interval of absence from the professional working force may have their registration reinstated. Again, provincial agencies are beginning to demand that the nurse take a refresher course to update her knowledge and skills if too many years have elapsed since she was last in active practice.

Both licensure and registration must be renewed on an annual basis (in some states every 2 years) in order to be valid. A nurse's license (or, in Canada, registration) may be *revoked* if, in the opinion of the disciplinary committee of the licensing or registering body, it is not safe to permit her to practice nursing. The three principal reasons for revoking a license are professional misconduct, incompetence, and negligence.

In the past few years, there have been a considerable number of changes in licensing/registration regulations in the United States and Canada. In the United States at present, only Indiana, Texas, and the District of Columbia do not have a *mandatory* licensing regulation for Registered Nurses, that is, a rule requiring the nurse to hold a current, valid license as a Registered Nurse in the state in which she is employed in order to be able to practice. In Canada, most of the provincial registered nursing acts are permissive in nature, that is, the nurse may or may not register, depending on whether she wishes to have the privileges that accompany registration. These privileges are, in general, that she may designate herself as a registered nurse and that she may place the initials "R.N" after her name. There is a strong movement under way in Canada to make registration compulsory in all provinces.

In addition to the laws controlling professional nurses, all states now have mandatory licensing acts for practical nurses, except California, Wisconsin, Indiana, and Texas, along with the District of Columbia. The exceptions have permissive licensing acts for LPNs. In Canada, all provinces but Newfoundland have practical nursing laws. Practical nurses are granted licensure by provincial government agencies.

Continuing Education Requirements

The rapidity with which new knowledge and technology are becoming available in nursing has created problems in keeping the practitioner up-to-date with the latest developments in her field.

As of November 1982, 16 states had, or soon would have, continuing education requirements for renewal of nursing licensure. In these states it is necessary for a nurse to show that she has had a specified number of contact hours in continuing education in order to renew her license to practice as a nurse in the state. In 11 states, the requirement applies to all R.N.'s; in the other five, it applies only to Nurse Practitioners.[8]

In Canada, although there has been considerable discussion about mandatory continuing education as a requirement for continued practice, no province to date has incorporated it into its registration renewal process.

Certification

The American Nurses' Association has a program of certification for nurses specializing in particular fields of practice. In order to be certified as a specialist, the nurse must demonstrate by examination that her knowledge of the field is current and she must show evidence of excellence in practice. The certification program provides a mechanism for ensuring the quality of practitioners' competence at a level higher than simple licensure.[9]

Certification programs are currently offered in:
1. Adult and Family Nurse Practitioner
2. School Nurse Practitioner
3. Gerontological Nursing (nursing of older people)
4. Nursing of the Child/Adolescent with Acute or Chronic Illness or Disabling Condition
5. Pediatric Nurse Practitioner
6. Medical Surgical Nurse
7. Clinical Specialist in Medical Surgical Nursing
8. Psychiatric and Mental Health Nurse
9. Clinical Specialist in Psychiatric and Mental Health Nursing—Adult or Child and Adolescent
10. Nursing Administration
11. Nursing Administration Advanced[9]

In addition to the ANA Certification Program, other agencies also certify practitioners in specialized fields as, for example, Nurse Anesthetists, who are certified by the American Association of Nurse Anesthetists.

AREAS OF NURSING FUNCTION

Nursing practice, as we have already noted, is constantly changing in response to societal needs. Guidance on what constitutes nursing practice has come principally from two sources, the nursing practice acts and the statements of the professional nursing associations. Because of the interdependent nature of nursing and medical practice, it has become quite common too for joint statements to be made by nursing and medical associations on functions nurses may undertake. The opinions of state and provincial attorneys generally provide some additional assistance from the legal point of view, although these opinions are usually offered in response to requests from governmental agencies and pertain for the most part to specific situations.[10]

The Law and Nursing Functions

In the past few years, there have been an unprecedented number of changes in nursing practice acts in the United States and in Canada, as nurses have felt the need to have imbedded in the law a more precise definition of nursing practice and a clearer description of their role and functions than previous statutes contained. Most nursing (and medical) practice acts in the past were written in broad, general terms. The general nature of the wording permitted both disciplines to enlarge the scope of their practice without the need for changes in the law each time and, also, made possible the orderly transfer of many procedural functions from medicine to nursing without recourse to the law. Not too many years ago, for example, only physicians were permitted to start intravenous infusions, yet today this is an accepted nursing procedure.

One of the principal reasons for the need for a more precise definition of nursing practice has been the development and rapid proliferation of expanded roles for nurses, as described in Chapter 6. In some aspects of expanded role practice, as, for example, when a nurse practitioner initiates treatment on her own, the question of the legality of her actions has arisen. Another reason for the need felt by the nursing profession for clearly identified roles and functions for nurses has been the increasing concern by governments for legislation pertaining to all health manpower and government suggestions for changes in existing statutes.

In the United States, the nursing practice acts in all but 11 states now contain a definition of the practice of nursing. Although the definitions vary in wording from state to state, many contain similar provisions. The Washington State Nurse Practice Act provides an example of current definitions of nursing practice.

Section 3, Section 4,

The practice of nursing means the performance of acts requiring substantial specialized knowledge, judgment and skill based upon the principles of biological, physiological, behavioral and sociological sciences in either:

1. The observation, assessment, diagnosis, care or counsel, and health teaching of the ill, injured or infirm, or in the maintenance of health or prevention of illness of others.

2. The performance of such additional acts requiring education and training and which are recognized jointly by the medical and nursing professions as proper to be performed by nurses licensed under this chapter and which shall be authorized by the board of nursing through its rules and regulations.

3. The administration, supervision, delegation and evaluation of nursing practice: PROVIDED, HOWEVER, that nothing herein shall affect the authority of any hospital, hospital district, medical clinic or office, concerning its administration and supervision.

4. The teaching of nursing.

5. The executing of medical regimen as prescribed by a licensed physician, osteopathic physician, dentist, or chiropodist.[11]

Statements by Professional Nursing Associations

Statements issued by both national and state or provincial nursing associations have also helped to define the scope of nursing practice. In 1954, the American Nurses' Association published a "Statement of Functions" of the professional nurse. This was followed in 1955 by a definition of nursing practice. In 1970, the ANA suggested, in a memo to Executive Directors of State Nurses' Associations, a new section to its definition of nursing, this section encompassing new areas of responsibility for nurses engaged in expanded role practice. These statements by the ANA have provided a model for development of the definitions of nursing and identification of areas of nursing practice contained in many of the state nursing acts, such as the Washington State statute.

In addition to the statements made by national nursing associations, most of the state boards of nursing and the provincial nursing associations have issued guidelines from time to time regarding the additional functions that may be performed by nurses when these are delegated by a physician. Increasingly common, also, have been joint statements issued by various professional groups, such as state nursing, medical, and sometimes hospital associations regarding the transfer of specific procedural functions from physicians to nurses. Although statements made by professional associations lack the authority of legally enacted laws, they are generally persuasive in that they reflect prevailing custom.[10]

Professional Versus Practical Nursing Functions

Creighton considers that "the essential difference between the registered professional nurse and the practical nurse is that by professional education and training and more refined skills, the registered professional nurse is obliged to evaluate and interpret facts in order to decide necessary action that may be required."[9]

Creighton has summarized the areas of the professional nurse as being:

1. Supervision of a total, comprehensive nursing care plan for the patient;
2. observation, interpretation and evaluation of the patient's symptoms and needs (mental and physical);
3. accurate recording and reporting of facts and evaluation of patient care;
4. carrying out nursing procedures and techniques, especially those that require judgment, modification or calculation, based on technical information;
5. supervision of auxiliary help (practical nurses, student nurses, other health workers) who give patient care;
6. giving health guidance and participating in health education;
7. carrying out the legal orders of physicians for medications and treatments.[9]

One would infer from this that the professional nurse's practice encompasses more independent nursing functions, whereas the practical nurse performs more dependent ones, and this is borne out in the statements regarding their functions.

The National Federation of Licensed Practical Nurses has issued a statement outlining the role, functions, and vocational responsibilities of the practical/vocational nurse as follows:

An LP/VN through education and clinical experience has acquired the necessary knowledge, skill and judgment to provide nursing care at the direction of a registered nurse, a licensed physician, or a licensed dentist. Through continuing education, the LP/VN prepares to assume progressively more complex nursing responsibilities.

Functions

The LP/VN

1. Participates in the planning, implementation, and evaluation of nursing care, and teaches the maintenance of health and prevention of disease.
2. Observes and reports to the appropriate person significant symptoms, reactions, and changes in the condition of the patient, and records pertinent information.
3. Performs and/or assists in nursing functions such as:
   a) the administration of medications as prescribed.
   b) therapeutic and diagnostic procedures.
   c) procedures requiring the use of medical/surgical aseptic technique.
4. Assists with the rehabilitation of the patient and family according to the patient care plan:
   a) provides support for emotional needs.
   b) teaches appropriate self-care.
   c) advocates use of community resources.
5. Assists in performing nursing services in specialized units, with appropriate preparation.
6. Assumes responsibilities as a charge nurse under direction, with appropriate preparation.

Vocational Responsibilities

The LP/VN

1. Practices nursing according to state law.
2. Performs those nursing functions for which he/she has been prepared.
3. Seeks further growth through educational opportunities.
4. Participates in nursing organizations.

Closing Statement

The LP/VN should be an example of dignity and grace and maintain a spiritual approach to all nursing care.[12]

THE LEGAL STATUS OF THE NURSE

The nurse in her practice can be classed as either an independent contractor or an employee. Private duty nurses, that is, nurses who are engaged by the patient to perform nursing service, come under the category of independent contractors. Nurse practitioners who are working independently in the community (not in the employ of a community agency) would also be considered independent contractors. Nurses who work in hospitals or clinics, in public health agencies, in industry, or for private physicians are considered employees. The distinction is a matter of control. On private duty or in independent community practice, the nurse works on her own; in the hospital, she works under the direction of the employing institution.

Student nurses, when assigned for clinical experience to a hospital or other health agency, are usually considered as employees, since they are subject to the control of clinical instructors, head nurses, and physicians.[9] In a school of nursing controlled by a hospital, students are generally held to be employees of the hospital insofar as they perform services for the hospital and are supervised by its staff. Students in collegiate or other independent schools of nursing may, however, be entirely under the supervision of the faculty of their school while in the practice area. Creighton considers that in these instances "the student would not seem to be an employee of the hospital, but might be held as an employee of the college."[9]

It is helpful for the student to remember that even though she may be considered an employee, she is still responsible for her own actions. Anyone who gives nursing care, whether student or graduate, assumes certain duties, and it is expected that these will be carried out with "reasonable prudence" under the circumstances. "Reasonable prudence" is taken to mean that the individual acts with the care that any reasonable person with his or her knowledge, training, and experience would take.

The reason for the importance of determining the status of the nurse is that, under the law, not only is an individual liable for his own actions but also his employer is liable under the rule of respondeat superior (Let the master answer). Thus, if a nurse is negligent and a patient is harmed, both the nurse and her employer can be sued by the patient.

In some states, charitable institutions and government hospitals, such as municipal or county hospitals, are exempt from the rule of respondeat superior and may not be sued; however, the employee of such an institution who performs a negligent act may still be sued. The law is somewhat different in various states in this regard.

Nor is the nurse absolved of responsibility for her actions simply because she is carrying out the orders of a physician. The law states that the nurse must understand the cause and effect of the treatment that she undertakes. If she carries out an order that she knows is wrong, she is guilty of negligence. At all times the patient's safety must be paramount.

If the nurse undertakes work that she knows is beyond the scope of her professional training—for example, if she performs some action or treatment that is defined as being within the province of medical practice—she may again be considered negligent or guilty of malpractice.[13]

CONSUMERS' RIGHTS IN THE HEALTH CARE SYSTEM

The art of healing has, from ancient times, been imbued with an aura of mystery, and magical powers have been attributed to those who practice the healing arts. Even modern practitioners of "scientific Western medicine"—doctors, nurses, and other health professionals—have, until fairly recently, tended to perpetuate the feeling that the average lay person could not possibly understand the complex workings of the human body and does not have the knowledge and experience to judge what treatment is best for himself. Through the use of technical jargon that is incomprehensible to anyone outside the health field, and in many other subtle (and some not-so-subtle) ways, health professionals usually managed to convey to the patient that he really should not question what was being done for him but simply trust in the experts to cure him of his ills.

There is no doubt that trust is still a very important ingredient in the relationship between health professional and client, but today's patient is viewed as an active member of the health team rather than a passive recipient of care. No longer is it felt that the doctor or the nurse, or any other health professional, has a "divine right" to knowledge that is too far above their heads to be understood by average citizens. The average citizen of today is much more knowledgeable about the complicated mechanisms of the human body, and the things that can go wrong with it, than his parents or grandparents were. He learns from the popular media about the latest advances in medical treatment and surgical procedures. He also feels that he has a right to question the treatment he is being given, to have a say in this treatment, and to be kept informed of his progress.

There has been an active and growing consumer movement in the health field in recent years. Increasing public awareness of health issues, increased knowledge about health and illness, and the rising costs to the consumer of health services are three major factors that have contributed to this movement. Additionally, the fact that people have become more conscious of their rights generally—as women, as native people, as members of minority ethnic groups, and so forth—has had repercussions in the health field. Consumer bills of rights have been developed and widely publicized, in the United States by the American Hospital Association and in Canada by the National Consumers' Association.

Consumer Rights in Health Care

I Right to be informed
  1 — about preventive health care including education on nutrition, birth control, drug use, appropriate exercise
  2 — about the health care system, including the extent of government insurance coverage for services, supplementary insurance plans, and referral system to auxiliary health and social facilities and services in the community

3 — about the individual's own diagnosis and specific treatment program, including prescribed surgery and medication, options, effects and side effects

4 — about the specific costs of procedures, services and professional fees undertaken on behalf of the individual consumer

II Right to be respected as the individual with the major responsibility for his own health care
— right that confidentiality of his health records be maintained
— right to refuse experimentation, undue painful prolongation of his life or participation in teaching programs
— right of adult to refuse treatment, right to die with dignity

III Right to participate in decision making affecting his health
— through consumer representation at each level of government in planning and evaluating the system of health services, the types and qualities of service and the conditions under which health services are delivered
— with the health professionals and personnel involved in his direct health care

IV Right to equal access to health care (health education, prevention, treatment and rehabilitation) regardless of the individual's economic status, sex, age, creed, ethnic origin and location
— right to acess to adequately qualified health personnel
— right to a second medical opinion
— right to prompt response in emergencies[14]

Bill of Rights for Patients

In the interest of "more effective patient care and greater satisfaction for the patient, his physician, and the hospital organization," the American Hospital Association has adopted a "Patient's Bill of Rights" as a national policy statement and distributed it to its member hospitals throughout the country. Intended to "give the consumer something to go by," the 12 rights, in summary, are:

1. The patient has the right to considerate and respectful care.

2. The patient has the right to obtain from his physician complete current information concerning his diagnosis, treatment, and prognosis in terms the patient can be reasonably expected to understand.

3. The patient has the right to receive from his physician information necessary to give informed consent prior to the start of any procedure and/or treatment.

4. The patient has the right to refuse treatment to the extent permitted by law, and to be informed of the medical consequences of his action.

5. The patient has the right to every consideration of his privacy concerning his own medical care program.

6. The patient has the right to expect that all communications and records pertaining to his care should be treated as confidential.

7. The patient has the right to expect that within its capacity a hospital must make reasonable response to the request of a patient for services.

8. The patient has the right to obtain information as to any relationship of his hospital to other health care and education institutions insofar as his care is concerned.

9. The patient has the right to be advised if the hospital proposes to engage in or perform human experimentation affecting his care or treatment.

10. The patient has the right to expect reasonable continuity of care.

11. The patient has the right to examine and receive an explanation of his bill regardless of source of payment.

12. The patient has the right to know what hospital rules and regulations apply to his conduct as a patient.[15]

More recently, charters on the rights of members of special groups have been developed and made public. For example, declarations on the rights of the mentally retarded and those of disabled persons were adopted by the General Assembly of the United Nations in 1971 and 1975 respectively; the Dying Person's Bill of Rights was developed in 1975 at a workshop in Lansing, Michigan, on care of the terminally ill; and the Pregnant Patient's Bill of Rights was published by the International Childbirth Education Association in 1975.

While these charters do not have the force of legally enacted statutes, they have been influential in raising the consciousness of consumers of health services so that they feel freer to express their dissatisfactions with the health care system and are less reluctant to demand their rights. The charters have also increased the awareness of health care workers of the fundamental rights of patients as human beings and as citizens.

ACCOUNTABILITY, SAFETY TO PRACTICE, AND QUALITY ASSURANCE

One of the most pressing concerns of individual nurses and of professional nursing associations at present is to ensure that patients receive safe and competent nursing care regardless of the setting or the circumstances under which that care is given. Health professionals have long been concerned about the need to maintain high standards of practice. However, the growing rise of consumerism in the health field and the generally increased sophistication of the public in relation to health care matters have put additional emphasis on the accountability of health professionals to the public they serve. Then, too, our elected representatives in government are becoming increasingly concerned about the quality of health care, since more and more of that care is being paid for by public funds. They too are demanding that the work of health professionals be monitored to ensure that high quality standards are maintained.

We are hearing a lot these days about accountability, about safety to practice, and about quality assurance. As beginning students, you are probably wondering what these terms mean exactly, and how they affect you. The term "accountability" means basically that a person is answerable (or accepts responsibility) for his own actions. The health professional must be able to "account" for the care he gives, to tell precisely what he did and why he did it. The term was initially used in the business world, but has now taken on a much broader meaning that includes social values. Individual practitioners and health care institutions are being held accountable for both what they do and what they have said they will do, as well as for the process by which it is done.[16]

"Safety to practice" means simply what it says. The nursing profession, along with other health professions, makes sure that beginning practitioners have the knowledge and skills necessary to practice their profession competently and without harming the people to whom they render care. Ensuring that the practitioner remains "safe to practice" is a matter that has become of increasing concern to the health professions. It used to be that once a physician, nurse, or dentist had completed his basic educational program and passed his qualifying examinations, his name would be inscribed on a permanent roster and he could practice throughout his lifetime—providing, of course, that he did not commit some flagrant offense that caused him to have his license or registration revoked. The rapidity with which health care is changing, however, and the increasing stress on accountability have made it imperative that the professions develop mechanisms to ensure that practitioners remain competent and "safe to practice" throughout their professional careers.

"Quality assurance," another term borrowed from the business world, refers to a program designed to try to ensure that health care provided to patients is consistently of good quality.

In any situation in which health workers are providing services for the public, the quality of care the patient receives is dependent on a number of variables. Four of the principal elements that can vary and affect care are: (1) the providers, that is, the people who give the care—the nurses, physicians, and all others who contribute to patient care; (2) the standards that are maintained in the agency providing care; (3) the environment, or setting, in which the care is given; and (4) the recipient of care, that is, the patient himself. In attempting to ensure that patients receive good nursing care at all times, the nursing profession has given a great deal of consideration to each of these four variables and has developed a number of mechanisms to try to ensure that the practice of nursing is consistently safe and of good quality.

The Providers of Care

We have already mentioned several ways in which the nursing profession tries to ensure that its practitioners are competent and safe to practice. Perhaps it is time, however, to pull all of these together with others that we have not discussed so far.

1. Accreditation/Approval of Basic Nursing Education Programs. Minimum standards for basic nursing education programs have been established in each state of the United States and in each province in Canada. All programs preparing candidates for licensure or registration are carefully monitored by the state boards of nursing (or a designated body) in the U.S. and by the provincial nursing associations (or the College of Nurses in Ontario or the Order of Nurses in Quebec) in Canada. State accreditation or provincial approval is granted to schools of nursing meeting the minimum criteria.

Another type of accreditation of schools of nursing is that done by the National League for Nursing. This accreditation is concerned with optimum, rather than minimum, standards. In other words, accreditation by the NLN certifies that an educational program has not only met minimum standards, but is considered "good" by national standards.

2. National Qualifying Examinations. The National Council of State Boards of Nursing and the Canadian Nurses' Association provide national testing services in their respective countries, which may be used by state and provincial licensing and registering bodies for the examination of candidates for the nursing profession. The Canadian set of examinations is available in both French and English, the two official languages of Canada.

3. Licensing/Registration. The licensing/registration mechanism is the basic safeguard protecting the public from unsafe practitioners and assuring employers that the individual has met certain standards established by the licensing/registering body as minimum requirements for entry to practice.

4. Disciplinary Bodies. All professional nurse licensing/registering agencies in the United States and Canada have established disciplinary bodies that monitor the practice of nurses to whom they have granted licensure or registration. Depending on the severity of a nurse's transgression, the disciplinary body may reprimand the individual, suspend the individual's license or registration for a time, or revoke the license or registration completely.

5. Mandatory Continuing Education. The rapid expansion of knowledge in the health field means that all practitioners need to update their knowledge and skills on a continuing basis throughout their professional careers. A number of states (14 in 1980) require that a nurse present evidence of having attended a specified number of continuing education classes (contact hours) in order to be able to renew her license each year. Several other states, and some provinces in Canada, are currently considering this step.

6. Certification. Certification provides yet another mechanism for ensuring the competence of practitioners—at a level higher than licensure. The ANA now has a certification program for each of 11 specialty areas of nursing practice. The Canadian Nurses' Association is currently contemplating establishment of a certification program for nurses who have achieved excellence in practice in specialized fields of nursing.

7. Assessment of Clinical Competence. A number of mechanisms have been developed that attempt to judge a nurse's competence in clinical practice. The traditional method has been through a *supervisor's rating* of the nurse's performance in the work setting. Although numerous types of performance rating scales have been tried in efforts to make these as objective as possible, it is difficult to eliminate the subjective bias from an assessment of one person's work by another.

Peer review is a method of assessing the quality of care provided by a practitioner through a review of her work by a group of her peers. Methods used in this review may include looking at care plans written by the nurse and patient records she has completed, gathering evaluations from patients cared for by the nurse and from professional co-workers, and reviewing evidence of attendance at continuing education programs.

A *nursing audit* is a method of evaluating nursing care through a review of patient records which document the care given. It may be used for evaluating a single nurse's clinical performance, or for assessing the quality of care on a given nursing unit or in an agency. (See Chapter 12 for further details.)

The *problem-oriented medical record (POMR)* has been hailed as an excellent means of evaluating the quality of care given by practitioners since it requires a detailed analysis of the individual patient's problems, a statement of the reasoning behind actions the practitioner takes, and precise documentation of those actions and their results. (See Chapter 12 for further details.)

Standards of Care

In assessing the quality of care provided by individual health practitioners or by health agencies, it is essential to have objective criteria by which to judge whether the care given is "good," "adequate," or "unsafe." The American Nurses' Association has developed a set of *Standards of Nursing Practice* which are often used in evaluating an individual's nurse's clinical practice. In addition to the basic set of standards that are applicable in any nursing situation, the Association has developed standards of practice for medical-surgical, maternal-child, geriatric, psychiatric, and community health nursing. The basic (generic) standards are listed below. Copies of these standards and the ones for specific areas may be obtained from the American Nurses' Association for a nominal fee.

Standard I: The collection of data about the health status of the client/patient is systematic and continuous. The data are accessible, communicated, and recorded.

Standard II: Nursing diagnoses are derived from the health status data.

Standard III: The plan of nursing care includes goals derived from the nursing diagnoses.

Standard IV: The plan of nursing care includes priorities and the prescribed nursing approaches or measures to achieve the goals derived from the diagnoses.

Standard V: Nursing actions provide for client/patient participation in health promotion, maintenance and restoration.

Standard VI: Nursing actions assist the client/patient to maximize his health capabilities.

Standard VII: The client's/patient's progress or lack

of progress toward goal achievement is determined by the client/patient and the nurse.

Standard VIII: The client's/patient's progress or lack of progress toward goal achievement directs reassessment, reordering of priorities, new goal setting, and revision of the plan of nursing care.[17]

In addition to the standards for practice developed by the professional nursing associations, individual health agencies have been attempting to determine standards that nurses in their agency consider important in the care of patients. This work has resulted in the development of standard nursing care plans for the care of patients with particular health problems, as, for example, patients who have had a cerebrovascular accident (stroke), who are unconscious, or who are undergoing different types of surgery. We will be discussing this topic at greater length in connection with the nursing process in Unit 2. The important point here is that these standard plans provide guidelines for nurses to assess, through reviewing documented records of patient care, whether everything that should have been done in the way of nursing care for a patient with a particular health problem was indeed done.

The Practice Setting

In order for nurses to give good care to patients, the environment in which they work must be such as to permit, and encourage, good nursing care. When we were talking about the environment as one of the major factors affecting health (in Chapter 3), we discussed both the physical and the social environment, and their effects on an individual's health. Similarly, in considering the environment in which nursing is practiced, one must take into account both the material things necessary to provide care and the social environment of the agency that encourages or discourages the maintenance of high standards of nursing care.

Individual nurses and their professional nursing organizations have become increasingly concerned about such matters as ensuring that nurses have a safe environment in which to practice, that they have sufficient equipment in good working order to work with, that nursing units are adequately staffed with competent personnel, and that nurses are not required to work in areas for which they are not prepared, or in situations that conflict with their ethical, moral, or professional beliefs.

In this regard, two statements on the professional rights of nurses, which have been developed and widely publicized, are appropriate.

One is a summary of nurses' rights by Fagin, a nurse researcher who has done a considerable amount of study in this area. Her statement of rights includes:

1. The right to find dignity in self-expression and self-enhancement through the use of our special abilities and educational background.
2. The right to recognition for our contribution through the provision of an environment for its practice, and proper, professional economic rewards.
3. The right to a work environment which will minimize physical and emotional stress and health risks.
4. The right to control what is professional practice within the limits of the law.
5. The right to set standards for excellence in nursing.
6. The right to participate in policy making affecting nursing.
7. The right to social and political action on behalf of nursing and health care.[18]

The second statement is a resolution prepared by the Michigan State Nurses' Association, which reads:

Resolved, that the nurse practitioner has the responsibility to inform employers, present and prospective, of her educational preparation, experience, clinical competencies, and those clinical beliefs which would affect her practice, and be it,

Resolved, that the nurse practitioner has the responsibility to alter, adjust to or withdraw from situations which are in conflict with her preparation, competencies and beliefs, and be it,

Resolved, that the employer shall provide the resources through which health services are made available to the recipient, and be it,

Resolved, that the nurse practitioner has the right and responsibility to collaborate with her/his employer to create an environment which promotes and assures the delivery of optimal health services, and be it further,

Resolved, that the nurse has the right to expect that her/his employer will respect her/his competencies, values and individual differences as they relate to her/his practice.[18]

The Patient

The fourth variable in any health care situation is the patient himself. Because patients are human beings, in all their infinite variety, this is probably the least predictable element in the situation—and the most difficult to provide with adequate safeguards. The best prepared practitioner working in an agency with the highest standards and under the best possible conditions of work can still not guarantee the patient's response to care. The elderly woman whose mouth needs attention may spit the mouthwash the nurse has given her all over the bed. A "helpful" patient may lend his salt shaker to a neighbor who is supposed to be on a salt-free diet.

Earlier in the chapter we discussed the patient's rights in the health care system. If a person has certain rights, it follows that he also has certain responsibilities. According to one legal authority who has done considerable study in the area of nursing and the law, the patient has a responsibility to act as any reasonable patient would under similar circumstances. According to Rozovsky, the patient has four duties:

1. The duty of honest disclosure, that is, the patient has a responsibility to tell those who are caring for him everything that is pertinent to the health condition for which he is seeking their help.
2. The duty to cooperate during actual treatment. The patient has a right, of course, to refuse treatment (providing he is a mature adult and in his right mind). If, however, he has consented to undergo treatment, he has an obligation to cooperate with those people who are carrying it out.
3. The duty to follow instructions.
4. The duty of returning for further treatment, as directed.[19]

Rozovsky suggests that there are some things that nurses and other health personnel can do that make it easier for the patient to carry out his responsibilities to himself. These include:

1. Asking the patient specific and direct questions to obtain the information needed for diagnosis and treatment.
2. Informing the patient of what he is to do and what he is not to do (and recording this information). It is often helpful, in this regard, to give the patient written instructions in addition to telling him what to do.
3. Telling the patient specifically why he needs to be seen again, when he is to return and where he is to report when he comes back.[19]

LEGAL ISSUES OF INTEREST TO THE NURSE

Torts and Crimes

In addition to understanding her responsibilities as a professional nurse, the nurse should be aware of the types of legal proceedings in which she may become involved either as a witness or as a defendant. Generally speaking, there are two types of court actions in which a nurse can be involved. The first is called a tort. A tort is a legal wrong committed by one person against the person or property of another. The injured party may sue for damages and, if the

suit is successful, he is usually awarded money to be paid by the other party. Sometimes this is spoken of as a civil suit, as opposed to a criminal action.

A crime is also a legal wrong but, in general, it refers to a wrong committed against the public and punishable by the state. The punishment for a crime is either a fine or imprisonment. In a criminal action, the case is designated in the form The People versus Mary Jones; in a tort, the form used is John Doe versus James Jones, or Mary Doe versus the Blank Hospital. Acts such as murder, manslaughter, and robbery are considered criminal, whereas negligence and malpractice are usually torts.

Negligence and Malpractice

It has already been noted that each individual is responsible for his own actions and that a nurse can be held liable for her own negligent actions. Negligence on the part of nurses has been defined by the courts as "the failure to exercise that degree of skill, care, and diligence exercised by professional nurses in light of the present state of nursing science in comparable situations."[10] As a general rule, nursing negligence usually means failure by the nurse to take the appropriate action to protect the safety of the patient.[10] Negligence may involve either doing something that ought not to be done or failing to do something that ought to be done. Thus, if the nurse does not carry out a physician's order correctly, as, for example, if she gives a wrong medication, she may be considered negligent. Similarly, failure to put up side rails on the bed of a confused patient could also be considered negligence on the nurse's part.

Malpractice has been defined as "any professional misconduct, unreasonable lack of skill or fidelity in professional or judiciary duties, evil practice, or illegal or immoral conduct."[10] The term "malpractice" is virtually synonymous with professional negligence. Any individual, professional or nonprofessional, may be sued for negligence; when the negligence is on the part of a professional person, it is deemed malpractice. Some courts have held that the term "malpractice" should be used only in connection with the professions of medicine and law.[10] The term is, however, being more widely applied to other professional groups, including nurses.

It should be noted that, although the term is most frequently used in connection with cases involving negligence, malpractice may include other claims against a professional person, as, for example, breach of contract.

Common Acts of Negligence. Professional nurses may be called upon to testify in a legal proceeding in regard to some matter pertaining to their work. The most common types of incidents leading to legal proceedings involving a patient and a nurse are those in which negligence is a factor. Some of the more common of such acts of negligence that have resulted in suits for damages are:

Overlooked Sponges. In any operative procedure care must be taken that no sponges are left inside the patient. Counting sponges is a nursing responsibility in most instances, and the nurse may be held liable if she fails to make a count when it has been ordered or if she makes an error in her count. Many hospitals now require that instruments and needles also be counted both before and after surgery.

Burns. Hot water bottles, heating pads, inhalators, steam radiators, enemas, douches, and sitz baths are all items that can cause a patient to be burned. The nurse may be held responsible if she has neglected to take the usual safety precautions, such as taking the temperature of the water used in a solution administered to a patient or keeping articles that might burn the patient out of his reach.

Falls. Another common type of accident that may result in injury to the patient and subsequently a suit for damages is falling from bed. The usual safety precautions include the use of side rails and other restraints. Most health agencies have rules regarding the use of side rails for the beds of postoperative patients and patients under sedation. Many extend this ruling to include the beds of all irrational patients, patients over 70 years of age, and children under a certain age. It should be remembered that, if side rails are used on a patient's bed to protect him from falling, both rails should be put up. All too often, one sees the bed against the wall, with one side up but no railing on the side nearest the wall. This is a dangerous practice because the patient can push the bed out from the wall and easily fall.

Wrong Medicine, Wrong Dosage, Wrong Patient, Wrong Concentration. Another common area in which negligence occurs is in giving medications. Labels can be misread or may not be read at all. The nurse may fail to identify the patient correctly and consequently give a medication to the wrong person. Numerous errors are made in giving medicines. With the tremendous increase in the number of medications ordered for patients and the numerous trademarks commonly used for the various drugs, safety precautions assume greater importance in ensuring that the right patient gets the right drug in the proper concentration at the right time and in the proper manner.

Defects in Apparatus or Supplies. Patients can be injured by the use of defective equipment. The nurse is not held responsible if the patient is injured as a result of a hidden defect, but if she uses equipment or supplies that she knows to be faulty, she may be held liable. The use of unsterile gauze for a surgical dressing could be an example of this.

Abandonment. Instances in which patients have been left unattended and have injured themselves as a result have led to suits for negligence. For example, if the nurse leaves a baby on a table and the baby falls while she is absent, she can be held negligent.

Loss of or Damage to a Patient's Property. The nurse is held liable if a patient's property is lost when it has been entrusted to her care. Most hospitals now try to safeguard against suits for lost articles by asking the patient to sign a statement to the effect that he is responsible for items he retains in his possession while he is in the hospital. Nevertheless, there are still many instances in which the care of a patient's property becomes of necessity the nurse's responsibility. For example, when the patient goes to the operating room for surgery, his valuables are placed in safekeeping. The property of the unconscious or irrational patient is also to be safeguarded. Perhaps the most commonly lost items are dentures, although diamond rings, watches, and money also seem to disappear quite frequently.

Other Negligent Acts. The above is by no means an exhaustive list of all the acts of negligence which have resulted in suits for damages. In her book *Law Every Nurse Should Know*, Creighton discusses a number of others in which nurses have been involved, including the administration of injections, the administration of blood by nurses, failure to communicate important information, failure to exercise reasonable judgment, errors due to family assistance in patient care, infections, cardiac arrest, elopement (patient leaving the agency without notifying anyone), and pronouncing the patient dead.[9]

Incident Reports

The nurse has a moral and legal responsibility to report to the health agency any accidents, losses, or unusual occurrences. Most health agencies have special forms for this purpose. Filling out this report should not be interpreted as a punishment. The primary purpose is to ensure that there is a record of the details of the incident and the subsequent action taken, in the event that legal proceedings are instituted. Incident reports are also useful as a source of information in research to improve the quality of care and the effectiveness of policies.

Good Samaritan Laws

The majority of states (and some provinces) have enacted legislation designed to protect the professional practitioner from malpractice suits arising from care given to the injured at the scene of an accident or other emergency. Some of these statutes cover physicians only; others, all practitioners of the healing arts. These laws are usually referred to as "Good Samaritan" laws and are intended to encourage qualified people to give aid in an emergency. In general, these laws protect the individual who renders emergency care from civil liability for this care, unless he, or she, is guilty of gross negligence or extreme malpractice in giving the care.

In some states, there is specific legislation to the effect that no one may leave the scene of an automobile accident without first giving aid to those injured in the accident. In Vermont, a person is required to give first aid in any emergency; if he does not he can be criminally charged.[9] The Ontario Highway Traffic Act also places an obligation on people directly or indirectly involved in an accident to render assistance to those who have been injured. In the absence of such a law, there is no legal compulsion for the nurse, or anyone else for that matter, to give assistance in an emergency. If aid is given voluntarily, the person giving the aid is under an obligation to give the best care possible under the circumstances, commensurate with his knowledge, training, and experience. Most medical practice acts contain a waiver to the effect that, in an emergency, a volunteer who is not medically qualified may perform procedures to "save life or limb" that ordinarily lie within the scope of medical practice. In doing so, the volunteer is not considered guilty of practicing medicine without a license.

If a nurse is present at the scene of an accident, or finds herself in an emergency situation and feels morally obligated to give assistance, she should first of all ascertain that she is the best-qualified person there to give aid. She should also make sure that a state of emergency truly exists. The nurse should then render the care that is necessary and transfer the patient as soon as possible to a medically qualified practitioner for continued treatment. In such a situation, the nurse is expected to act as any other nurse of equal training and experience would act under the same or similar circumstances.[20]

Assault and Battery

In some instances, nurses have been involved in legal proceedings as a result of a charge of assault and battery by a patient. Assault refers to attempts or threats to do bodily harm to another. Battery is "the unlawful beating of another or the carrying out of threatened physical harm."[9]

Assault and battery are considered criminal offenses as well as torts. Nurses have sometimes been involved in suits for assault and battery because of the use of restraints on patients. It is important to remember that, except in emergencies, restraints should not be used unless they are ordered by the physician. At all times, undue force is to be avoided in handling patients. The law protects every individual against bodily harm by another person and also against any form of assault due to interference with his person. Therefore a person cannot take a blood sample from a patient without his consent. Nor may a person be operated on for any condition unless he has given his consent to the procedure and understands the significance of the procedure. Autopsy without the consent of relatives may be considered assault and battery.

Informed Consent

One of the most fundamental rights of patients is the right to consent to treatment. It is, indeed, a well established principle of law that "an adult of sound mind has the right to decide what shall or shall not be done to his body."[9] The fact that health professionals feel that certain treatment is desirable for a person does not give them the right to go ahead with that treatment without the consent of the patient, except in an emergency. In an emergency when treatment is a matter of life and death and the patient is unable to give permission, consent may be implied.

In the past few years a number of lawsuits have centered on the issue of a patient's lack of consent to treatment. Although suits of this nature usually involve physicians or health agencies, the nurse may be called upon as a witness, for example, to attest to the patient's mental condition at the time he gave his consent to treatment. The nurse is also frequently asked to obtain the patient's signature on a consent form. She should be aware of the implications of her actions from a legal, ethical, and moral point of view.

In order for a patient's consent to be valid, the patient must be of such an age and mental capacity that he is capable of deciding for himself whether or not he wishes to have the proposed treatment. In order to make that decision, the patient must be given sufficient information in language that he understands so that he can give his informed consent. Informed consent is taken to mean that the patient has been given:

1. An explanation of the condition
2. A fair explanation of the procedures to be used and the expected consequences
3. A description of alternative treatments or procedures
4. A description of the benefits to be expected (not assured)
5. An offer to answer the patient's inquiries
6. An understanding that the patient is not being coerced to agree and may withdraw if he changes his mind[21]

It is the physician's direct responsibility to inform patients about medical or surgical treatment, and this is not a responsibility that can be delegated. The nurse may, however, present the form granting permission for treatment to the patient for his signature. Sometimes, the nurse is asked to sign as a witness to the patient's signature. In doing so, the nurse is simply verifying the identity of the patient—her signature does not require the nurse to determine whether the patient has had sufficient information to make a rational decision.

The ethical and moral implications of witnessing a patient's signature on a consent form are, however, different from the legal implications. Professional nursing associations have been concerned about the nurse's ethical and moral responsibilities in such situations, and some have issued guidelines for nursing action in the form of policy statements. The Registered Nurses' Association of British Columbia, for example, in a "Policy Statement on Informed Consent" states that:

Nurses responsible for obtaining a patient's signature on a consent form have the additional responsibility to:

1. assess and document the patient's understanding of the nature, purpose, inherent risks and alternatives of her/his treatment;
2. inform the physician and/or the appropriate agency representative if there is reason to believe the patient has any misunderstanding regarding the nature, purpose, inherent risks, or alternatives of her/his treatment;
3. inform the physician and/or the appropriate agency representative if there is reason to believe the patient signed the consent while under age, or under sedation or other medication that might affect his/her mental ability and judgment.[22]

In most hospitals, the patient is requested to sign, on admission, a standard form granting permission for treatment and operative procedures deemed necessary while he is under the care of the agency. In addition, a separate consent form is often used to obtain the patient's permission for specific aspects of care. If a special form is used prior to surgery, the signature should be obtained before the patient is sedated, since consent obtained while the patient is under sedation can be questioned. Consent must be voluntary and the individual giving it must be rational. In the case of mentally incompetent persons, it is necessary to obtain the consent of the patient's legal guardian.

In the case of children, either parent may give permission for treatments and operative procedures. The age when individuals are no longer considered minors and can give their own consent to medical treatment varies in different jurisdictions, from 14 years of age (in the province of Quebec) to 21 years in some states and provinces. A teen-ager who no longer lives at home and is self-supporting is considered an "emancipated minor" and, as such, able to give consent for medical treatment. A "mature minor" is one who has demonstrated that he has the intelligence, understanding, and independence to make his own decisions in regard to the acceptance or rejection of medical treatment. In the case of treatment for venereal disease, the courts have usually upheld the principle of confidentiality between physician and client, ruling that the physician is not under obligation to obtain permission from parents to treat a teenage patient.

Many hospitals are in the process of revising both their procedures for obtaining consent from patients and the forms that are used. The nurse should familiarize herself with those that are being used in the agency in which she is having clinical experience (or will be working). Sample forms from one hospital, a general consent form and one used for specific operations or other special procedures, are shown on pages 104–105.

GENERAL CONSENT

I hereby authorise any member of the medical or nursing staff of the Ottawa General Hospital to carry out medical examinations, tests and treatments on _____
(Insert "myself" or name of patient)
while a patient in the hospital.

Date: _____   Signature: _____

Witness: _____   _____
(Relationship to patient)

Note: If the patient is unable to sign by reason of mental or physical disability, this consent is to be signed by his spouse, parent or one of his next of kin.
If the patient is unmarried and under **sixteen** years of age, this consent is to be signed by his parent or guardian.

AUTORISATION GÉNÉRALE

Je soussigné(e) autorise, par la présente, les médecins autorisés et le personnel infirmier de l'Hôpital Général d'Ottawa à effectuer les examens médicaux, analyses et traitements qu'ils jugeront nécessaires, sur _____
(Inscrire "moi-même" ou le nom du malade)
durant mon séjour à l'hôpital.

Date: _____   Signature: _____

Témoin: _____   _____
(Lien de parenté)

N.B.: Si le malade ne peut signer en raison d'une incapacité mentale ou physique, cette autorisation devra être signée par son époux(se) ou un parent responsable.
Si le malade est célibataire et n'a pas **seize** ans, cette autorisation doit être signée par son père, sa mère ou son tuteur.

REFUSAL OF TREATMENT

I hereby agree to assume all responsibility for whatever might happen to _____
who is leaving the Ottawa General Hospital against the advice of the attending Physicians or Surgeons.

Date: _____   Signed: _____

Witness: _____   Relation to patient: _____

REFUS DE TRAITEMENT

Je, soussigné reconnais avoir été averti des risques encourus par le départ de _____
patient de l'Hôpital Général d'Ottawa, quittant l'hôpital malgré l'avis des Médecins et dégage entièrement la responsabilité de l'hôpital et des Médecins pour ce qui peut en advenir.

Date: _____   Signé: _____

Témoin: _____   Parenté: _____

A general consent form for medical examinations, tests, and treatments. Forms printed in all languages commonly used in an area allow the patient to exercise his right to give or withhold his informed consent to medical care. (Courtesy of the Ottawa General Hospital.)

False Imprisonment

An individual who is unjustifiably detained, or confined against his will and without a legal warrant for his detention, may bring a charge of false imprisonment against the individual or the agency that has detained him.[9] Most instances in which nurses have been involved in court proceedings on charges of false imprisonment have been in relation to mental patients. United States and Canadian law does provide for the detention without a warrant of a person who is mentally disturbed and who may hurt himself or others, or destroy property, and also for the confinement of persons with communicable diseases, which present a danger to society. However, this covers only the length of time required to obtain legal authority for the person's restraint.[9]

A person cannot be prevented from leaving a health agency if he is of sound mind, even if it is advisable that he stay for additional care. If the patient insists on leaving, most agencies require that he sign a form stating that he will not hold the agency responsible for any harm resulting from his leaving.

The use of force to hold someone against his will, or even the threat of forcible restraint made in order to detain a person, is considered assault and/or battery. The nurse must therefore exercise caution in the use of restraints, as we have noted above.

Invasion of Privacy

Under both American and Canadian law, every individual has the right to withhold both himself and his property from public scrutiny. The right does not hold, however, if the individual has given consent for exposure; nor is there a tort when the person is a public figure or does

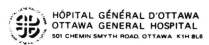

HÔPITAL GÉNÉRAL D'OTTAWA
OTTAWA GENERAL HOSPITAL
501 CHEMIN SMYTH ROAD, OTTAWA K1H 8L6

Consent to Operation

or

Special Procedure

I hereby authorise Dr._____ ("the doctor") and such other medical practitioners and other assistants as he may select or approve to perform or assist in performing on _____ at the Ottawa General
                                      (insert "myself" or name of patient)
Hospital the following operation or special procedure:

The doctor has given me an explanation of and I understand the nature of this operation or procedure, the risk involved and its probable effects.

I authorise the doctor to take whatever measures he considers necessary or desirable in addition to or different from the operation or procedure initially contemplated in the event that any condition is discovered in the course of the operation or procedure that was not previously apparent.

I consent to the administration of anaesthesia and to the use of such anaesthetics as may be deemed advisable.

I consent to the disposal by the Hospital authorities of any tissues or organs removed in the course of the operation or procedure.

Date:_____

_____   _____
(Witness)   (Signature)

                                        _____
                                        (Relationship to patient)

Note: If the patient is unable to sign by reason of mental or physical disability,
         this consent is to be signed by his spouse, parent or one of his next of kin.

         If the patient is unmarried and under SIXTEEN years of age, this consent is
         to be signed by his parent or guardian.

44-03(10/80) cat:410670

A consent form for operations or other special procedures. (Courtesy of the Ottawa General Hospital.)

acts of public interest.[9] A common instance in which the nurse must guard against invasion of a person's right to privacy is in the taking and use of photographs of patients. Consent must be obtained if these are to be used in any way not connected with the patient's medical treatment. Care must be taken by nurses also to avoid the exposure of patients to roommates, visitors, or others during the process of nursing care or when the patient is being transported from one area to another in the health agency.

The right to privacy extends also to information about the patient. The patient's record contains confidential information; it should not be left where it might be read by unauthorized persons. In using information from patients' records (or information she has obtained from the patient) for case studies or other types of classroom work, the student should be careful not to reveal the patient's identity; nor should information about a patient be discussed carelessly with people who are not entitled to that information. The nurse should always be discreet in giving out information about patients. People have become increasingly aware of their right to privacy as a result of national publicity about prominent cases of wiretapping and subsequent legislation to safeguard the individual's rights in this regard. The use of tape recorders and Dictaphones without the patient's knowledge and consent could undoubtedly be taken as an invasion of privacy and should be avoided by the nurse.

Defamation of Character

Another area of the law of which the nurse should be aware is that of suits arising from defamation of character. The term "defamation of character" means that a person's reputation is damaged by written or spoken words that tend to lower his esteem in the eyes of other people. If written, as in a letter to a third party, or depicted in a cartoon that causes the person to be the subject of ridicule or contempt, the term "libel" is used to describe the action.[9] "Slander" is the term used for defamation of character through spoken words, as, for example, if one speaks badly of someone in conversation with another person. The nurse should always be careful not to discuss patients except with others who are concerned with their care. Not every mention of a patient is slander or libel, of course; these terms are used only when there is a threat to the individual's reputation. For example, most courts consider it defamatory to let other people know that an unmarried woman is preg-

nant, or that a patient has venereal disease. To state that a patient had a broken leg would not ordinarily be considered defamatory. If, however, one added that the broken leg resulted because the patient was intoxicated and fell down the stairs, this might be considered to be defamation of character.

The Nurse and Confidential Information

The International Code of Nursing Ethics and the Code of Ethics of the American Nurses' Association both specifically state that the nurse has a responsibility to hold in confidence all matters of a personal nature entrusted to her. Legally, the betrayal of a patient's confidence is covered under the area of professional misconduct, and a nurse found guilty of such action may be disciplined by her professional organization.[9]

Whether confidential information entrusted to the nurse by the patient is considered to be a privileged communication and therefore inadmissible as evidence in court proceedings has not been definitely settled. A few states have enacted statutes that specifically state that the nurse-patient relationship is a privileged one, and therefore confidential information given to the nurse cannot be used in proceedings. In instances in which the doctor-patient communication is considered privileged, the ruling has been held to extend to nurses when they are acting as agents of the physician. In Canada, the rule of privilege for confidential information is not absolute. Although the nurse and the physician should not disclose confidential information entrusted to them, they may be directed to do so if this is justified by public policy or if the law requires reporting of the matter.[9] In the United States, a witness cannot be required to give evidence that would tend to incriminate him, whereas in Canada the law requires that a witness answer all questions that are relevant whether or not the answer tends to incriminate him. He can, however, invoke the protection of the Canada Evidence Act in certain cases.

Some guidelines suggested by Creighton in regard to the maintenance of confidentiality by nurses are helpful to keep in mind, from both an ethical and a legal point of view:

1. Think before you speak.
2. Close doors when giving reports.
3. Refrain from shop talk in public places.
4. Avoid repeating what you hear about patients from other staff members.
5. Keep confidential any information noted in the patient's chart.

6. Do not repeat a patient's diagnosis to others.
7. Do not discuss patients with other patients.[9]

Abortions

An abortion is the premature termination of a pregnancy. It may occur spontaneously, in which case it is usually called a miscarriage, or it may be induced by medical or surgical means. Until fairly recently, in both the United States and Canada, the intentional termination of a pregnancy for reasons other than preserving the life of the mother was considered a criminal offense. In 1973, however, a new abortion ruling was established when the U.S. Supreme Court found that a Texas state law banning all abortions except those to save the mother's life was in violation of a woman's right to privacy in making an abortion decision. This ruling paved the way for the legalization of abortions. Guidelines issued by the Court made the procedure a matter between a woman and her physician during the first trimester, with the protection and preservation of the mother's health the primary consideration during the second trimester, and protection of the unborn infant's life—but not at the expense of the mother's life and health—of prime importance during the third trimester. Although the ruling is federal in scope, individual states have the power to regulate such matters as by whom abortions shall be performed and where they may be done.

In Canada, although abortion has not yet been removed from the Criminal Code, therapeutic abortions, for the protection and preservation of the mother's health, are permitted. These may be carried out only in accredited or approved hospitals and only by physicians licensed in the province in which the abortion is performed. The procedure must be approved by an abortion committee of the hospital. Neither hospitals nor individual physicians are forced to perform abortions if they do not wish to do so.

Abortion is an issue about which people often have very strong feelings. Public opinion, as reflected in the law, is much more liberal about abortion than it was previously. Still, a great many people oppose abortion because of moral, ethical, or religious beliefs against taking the life of an unborn child. The Roman Catholic Church, for example, stands firmly against abortion, as do the Greek Orthodox Church and the Church of Jehovah's Witnesses. Some Mennonite sects also oppose abortion. Other people object on ethical or moral grounds because of their own convictions.

The professional nursing associations have been concerned about the need for nurses to participate in abortions or sterilizations when they hold strong moral, ethical, or religious beliefs against these procedures. The Nurses' Association of the American College of Obstetricians and Gynecologists has issued a statement specifying that nurses have the right to refuse to assist in such procedures. As noted earlier in this chapter, this was a major point in the Michigan State Nurses' Association Resolution on nurses' rights.

Wills

Nurses are often asked to witness a will for a patient. A will is a declaration of an individual's wishes regarding what is to be done with his property after his death. The individual making the will is called the testator. A will must ordinarily be in writing and must be signed by the testator. The law usually requires the signature of two or three competent witnesses in addition. An individual who may expect to benefit from a will should not act as a witness to the signing of that will. The family and close friends of a patient are naturally reluctant, then, to be witnesses, and the nurse is frequently called upon to act in this capacity since she is a disinterested party. The nurse should not agree to act as a witness, however, if she is a minor. Minors, that is, persons under the legal age as defined by the law of the particular state or province, are not usually acceptable as witnesses.

In most jurisdictions, all witnesses are required to be present at the same time and to sign the will in the presence of the person making it. The witness should see the testator sign the will before signing it himself. If, however, the will has already been signed, the witness should either ask the testator to sign again or to declare that this is his will and he has signed it. In affixing his signature to a will, the witness indicates either that he has seen the person sign the document or that the testator has declared to him that he has signed it, and that the testator was competent to sign.[20] It is not necessary for the witness to know the contents of the will, nor in most jurisdictions is it necessary for the witness to be told that the document is a will.

For a will to be valid, the person making it must be capable of understanding what he is doing. If the patient dies and the validity of the will is questioned, a nurse may be called upon to testify in court concerning the mental capacity of the individual at the time the will was made, whether or not she acted as a witness to the will. If the nurse is aware that a patient has made a will while in the hospital, it is a good practice for her to note on the patient's record the fact that a will was made, the date and time that it was signed, and the nurse's observations regarding the mental state of the patient at the time the will was made.

Controlled Substances Legislation

Another area of the law in which the nurse is involved is the control and administration of narcotics and other potentially harmful drugs. In the United States, there are both federal and state laws controlling narcotics and certain other drugs. The principal federal law is the Comprehensive Drug Abuse Prevention and Control Act, commonly known as the Controlled Substances Act. This Act was passed in 1970 and replaced virtually all pre-existing federal laws dealing with narcotics, stimulants, depressants, and hallucinogens (drugs that alter perception, such as LSD and hashish). The Federal Food, Drug, and Cosmetic Act is concerned with the control of non-narcotic drugs, such as the barbiturates and hypnotic drugs. In addition to the federal laws, almost all the states have their own laws further regulating harmful drugs.[9]

In Canada the control of narcotic drugs is under federal jurisdiction, the pertinent legislation being the Narcotic Control Act and the Narcotic Control Regulations. This legislation, which was enacted in 1961, controls the use of opium, coca leaves (and their salts and derivatives), and a number of other drugs classified as narcotics, including cannabis. Certain other drugs, for example the barbiturates, have been designated as "controlled drugs." Regulations regarding these drugs are included in the Food and Drugs Act and Regulations of Canada (1961).

A list of the "controlled drugs" appears in Schedule G of the Food and Drugs Act.[9]

Under both American and Canadian law, only certain persons are authorized to prescribe and dispense narcotics and other controlled drugs. These persons include physicians, dentists, and veterinarians, but not nurses. The nurse is considered to be acting as an agent of the physician when she administers controlled drugs. Nurses functioning as nurse practitioners in areas with few doctors usually prescribe and dispense medications (including controlled drugs) under "standing orders" from the physician, who is providing medical supervision, albeit on a remote basis. It is unlawful for the nurse to have narcotic drugs in her possession. The attempt to obtain narcotic drugs by fraud or deceit is a violation of the law. Penalties for violation include fine or imprisonment or both. The nurse must be careful when handling narcotics to see that they have been ordered in writing by a duly licensed physician and that careful records are kept of their use.

Malpractice Insurance

Because of the increase in the number of malpractice suits in general, and against nurses in particular, many authorities now recommend that each nurse carry her own malpractice insurance to cover the cost of lawyers' fees and possible damages. The American Nurses' Association and several of the provincial nursing associations in Canada have made malpractice insurance available to their members at a reasonable cost.

Many nurses have the mistaken belief that, because they are employees, their employer will carry the burden of responsibility for their negligent actions. This is not so; the nurse can be sued as an individual.

STUDY SITUATION

As you are driving along a lonely country highway late one evening on your way home from a party, you and your escort notice skid marks on the pavement and a car overturned in the ditch at the side of the road. A young man, his clothes muddy and torn, waves his arms frantically to get you to stop. You think you hear a woman's voice moaning somewhere.

1. What would you do?

2. What are your legal responsibilities if you stop and find that the woman is badly injured? Your ethical and moral responsibilities?

3. Is there a Good Samaritan law in your state/province?

4. What protection do you have against possible charges of negligence or malpractice if you render first aid in this situation?

SUGGESTED READINGS

Besch, L. B.: Informed Consent: A Patient's Right. *Nursing Outlook*, 27:32–35, January, 1979.

Curtin, L. L.: Is There a Right to Health Care? *American Journal of Nursing*, 80(3):462–465, March, 1980.

Doll, A.: What to Do after an Incident. *Nursing 80*, 10(1):15–19, January, 1980.

Flynn, B. C., et al.: Quality Assurance in Community Health Nursing. *Nursing Outlook*, 27:650–653, October, 1979.

Hemelt, M. D., and Mackert, M. E.: A Nursing 79 Handbook. Your Legal Guide to Nursing Practice.
Part 1: *Nursing 79*, 9(10):57–64, October, 1979.
Part 2: *Nursing 79*, 9(11):56–64, November, 1979.
Part 3: *Nursing 79*, 9(12):49–56, December, 1979.
Part 4: *Nursing 80*, 10(1):57–64, January, 1980.

Kohnke, M. F.: The Nurse as Advocate. *American Journal of Nursing*, 80(11):2038–2042, November, 1980.

Mancini, M.: Nursing, Minors and the Law. *American Journal of Nursing*, 78(1):124+, January, 1978.

Moser, D., and Cox, J. M.: Perspectives: Resolving an Ethical Dilemma. *Nursing 80*, 10(5):39–43, May, 1980.

O'Sullivan, A. L.: Privileged Communication. *American Journal of Nursing*, 80(5):947–950, May, 1980.

Schmidt, M. S.: Why a Separate Organization for State Boards? *American Journal of Nursing*, 80(4):725–726, April, 1980.

Sklar, C.: You and the Law. Regular series of articles in *The Canadian Nurse*. For additional material on topics covered in this chapter, see:
The Patient's Choice vs. the Nurse's Judgment. 74(4):11–12, April, 1978.
Unwarranted Disclosure. 74(5):6–8, May, 1978.
Can You Afford to Be a Good Samaritan? 74(6):15–17, June, 1978.
Minors in the Health Care System. 74(9):18–20, September, 1978.
Error of Judgment: Is It Always Negligence? 75(3):14–16, March, 1979.
Patient's Advocate—A New Role for the Nurse. 75(6):39–41, June, 1979.
Hands That Care: Are They Safe? 75(9):10–11, October, 1979.
Sinners or Saints? The Legal Perspective.
Part 1: 75(10):14–16, November, 1979.
Part 2: 75(11):16–21, December, 1979.
The Extension of Hospital Liability. 76(2):8–11, 48, February, 1980.
Consent. 76(3):14–16, 52, March, 1980.
Was the Patient Informed? 76(6):18, June, 1980.
The Responsibility of the Patient. 76(7):14, July, 1980.
Student Nurses and the Law. 76(9):7–11, October, 1980.
Nurse, You Did This to Me! It's Your Fault. 76(10):10–12, November, 1980.

Smith, S. J., and Davis, A. J.: Ethical Dilemmas: Conflicts among Rights, Duties, Obligations. *American Journal of Nursing*, 80(8):1463–1466, August, 1980.

REFERENCES

1. American Nurses' Association: *Facts About Nursing 1976–77*. Kansas City, Mo., American Nurses' Association, 1978.
2. Canadian Nurses' Association: *1980 The Canadian Nurses' Association is . . . .* Ottawa, Canadian Nurses' Association, 1980.
3. International Council of Nurses: *Code For Nurses*. Geneva, Switzerland, International Council of Nurses, 1973.
4. *Code for Nurses with Interpretive Statements*. Kansas City, Missouri, American Nurses' Association, 1976.
5. Canadian Nurses' Association: Ethics of Nursing Research. *The Canadian Nurse*, 68(9):23–25, 1972.
6. *Human Rights Guidelines for Nurses in Clinical and Other Research*. Kansas City, Missouri, American Nurses' Association, 1975.
7. American Nurses' Association: *Principles of Legislation Relating to Nursing Practice* (revised). New York, American Nurses' Association, January, 1958.
8. CE Now Required for Licensure in 16 states. *American Journal of Nursing*. 82(11):1668–1675, November, 1982.
9. Creighton, H.: *Law Every Nurse Should Know*. 4th edition. Philadelphia, W. B. Saunders Company, 1981.
10. Anderson, B. J.: Orderly Transfer of Procedural Responsibilities from Medical to Nursing Practice. *Nursing Clinics of North America*, 5:313, June, 1970.
11. State of Washington, Law Regulating the Practice of Nursing, Ch.133, Laws of 1973.
12. *Declaration of Functions of the Licensed Practical/Vocational Nurse*. Revised. New York, National Association for Practical Nurse Education and Service, Inc., 1976.
13. Gray, K. G.: Law and Nursing. *The Canadian Nurse*, 60:546, June, 1964.
14. Consumer Rights in Health Care. *Canadian Consumer*, 41, April 1974.
15. Bill of Rights for Patients. *Nursing Outlook*, 21:82, February 1973. Adopted by American Hospitals Association as a national policy statement and distributed nationally to all member hospitals.
16. Credentialling in Nursing: A New Approach. Report of the Committee for the Study of Credentialling in Nursing: *AJN* 79(4):674–683, April 1979.
17. American Nurses' Association: *Standards of Nursing Practice*. Kansas City, Mo., American Nurses' Association, 1973.
18. Fagin, C. M.: Nurses Rights. *AJN* 75(1):82–84, January, 1975.
19. Rozovsky, L.: The Patient's Duty to Himself. *Dimensions of Health Services*. 56:27–28, December, 1979.
20. Sarner, H.: *The Nurse and The Law*. Philadelphia, W. B. Saunders Company, 1968.
21. Kelly, L. Y.: The Patient's Right to Know. *Nursing Outlook*, 24:28, January, 1976.
22. *Policy Statement of Informed Consent*. Registered Nurses' Association of British Columbia, April, 1980.

THE NURSING PROCESS

2 UNIT

8

The Nurse Should Be Able to:

- Define the term nursing process
- Explain the circular nature of the four basic steps in the process
- Lists types of information needed to plan nursing care
- Identify sources of information available to the nurse
- Describe content usually included in a nursing history
- Explain the functional abilities approach in the nurse's clinical appraisal of a patient
- Demonstrate beginning skill in:
  — collecting baseline data about a patient
  — analyzing data
  — synthesizing information from all sources
  — identifying and stating nursing problems
  — arranging a problem list in order of priorities
  — identifying relevant principles to assist in planning care
  — developing goals in terms of expected patient outcomes
  — developing a nursing care plan for one patient
- Discuss the use of flowsheets and other forms as aids in planning and implementing nursing care
- Discuss methods of evaluating the effectiveness of nursing intervention

THE NURSING PROCESS

INTRODUCTION

Nursing care may range from the simple act of cleansing and putting a bandage on the child's cut finger to the highly complex measures involved in caring for a patient in the intensive care unit of a hospital, or in helping a family with multiple problems to meet their health needs in a community setting. The process of nursing is the same, however, whether the nursing care given is a basic first aid measure or a sequence of complicated nursing activities.

The term "nursing process" designates the series of steps the nurse takes in planning and giving nursing care. Described by a number of authors as application of the problem-solving, or scientific, approach to nursing practice, the process provides a logical framework on which to base nursing care. Moreover, a terminology is evolving that can be readily understood by all nursing personnel as well as by other members of the health team.

The essential elements of the process are that it is planned, it is patient-centered, it is problem-oriented, and it is goal-directed. The term "patient" is used here to denote the recipient of care and can mean an individual, a family, or a community. Four basic steps are involved in the process:

1. Assessment
2. Planning
3. Implementation
4. Evaluation

The focus of this text is on the care of the individual, since the fundamental basis of nursing practice is the one-to-one relationship of the nurse and the patient. In this chapter, then, we will discuss the nursing process in relation to the individual patient. It should be noted, however, that the nursing process applies whether the patient is an individual, a family, or a community.

The steps in the process follow logically one after the other. As a basis for making decisions about actions that she will take, the nurse must first assess the need for action. This assessment involves the gathering of all pertinent information, the analysis of the information, the synthesis of information from all sources, and the identification of problems that the nurse, by her actions, can help to resolve. Once problems are identified, expected outcomes are established and a plan of action developed to help the patient to attain these objectives. The next step is to implement the plan of action—that is, to carry out the specified measures (nursing interventions) outlined in the plan. The final step is to evaluate the results of the action taken, or, in other words, to determine if the expected outcomes have been attained. The last step may result in new information that leads to modification in the problem list, changes in the plan of action, or a restatement of expected outcomes. Thus, the process becomes a circular one that involves a continuing dynamic set of activities on the nurse's part.

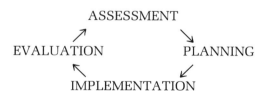

Diagram of the nursing process

ASSESSMENT

In the past, much of nursing care was based on the nurse's intuitive assessment, which was often the result of her previous experience in similar situations. An experienced nurse could—and still can, for that matter—walk into a home to visit a new mother and baby and, within a few minutes, assess the situation and identify several problems. Although the baby seems to be thriving well, 2-year-old Mark has a cold that has persisted too long, and the mother is in dire need of rest and is anxious and worried about how she is handling the baby. An experienced nurse in a hospital setting can enter the patient's room and immediately sense that he is uncomfortable, that his position needs changing, that he is having difficulty in breathing, and that he is worried and apprehensive. But nurses, even experienced nurses, have often found it difficult to explain how they arrived at their assessments.[1]

The development of a systematic method of nursing assessment and identification of the necessary tools to undertake it have only recently evolved. Today many health agencies use forms that they have developed to assist the nurse in her assessment and to provide a written record of the information she obtains. Although the format used and the specific items recorded vary in different agencies, they have a common purpose in that they help to guide the nurse in making a systematic appraisal of all relevant factors. The assessment is undertaken in an orderly manner; the nurse knows what to look for and there is less danger that important factors will be overlooked.

Systematic nursing assessment involves four sets of activities on the nurse's part: the collection of information, the analysis of that information, the synthesis of information from all sources, and the identification of problems.

The Collection of Information

The systematic collection of information for a specific purpose is called "data gathering," and one uses the information collected to develop a "data base," which can be analyzed in a number of different ways, depending on the purpose for which the information was collected in the first place. In order to develop a solid data base for the planning and implementation of nursing care, the nurse needs to know (1) the purpose for which she is collecting information, (2) what information is needed, (3) what sources can be used to obtain data, (4) how these sources can be tapped, and (5) how to organize and utilize the information collected.

Purpose. The objective of the nurse in collecting information about a patient is to identify areas in which nursing intervention is required. The information gathered in the initial assessment enables the nurse to make a beginning plan of care for the patient. Information gathered by the nurse, however, may identify problems that require the intervention of other members of the health team, such as the physician, the social worker, or the physical therapist. The initial data collected by all members of the team provide a baseline for assessing an individual's health status, for identifying existing and potential health problems, and for developing a combined plan of action to assist the patient.

Information Needed by the Nurse. Virginia Henderson, in her well-known and often-quoted definition of nursing, has stated, "The unique function of the nurse is to assist the individual, sick or well, in the performance of those activities contributing to health or its recovery (or to peaceful death) that he would perform unaided if he had the necessary strength, will, or knowledge."[2]

We might rephrase this to say that the nursing care of an individual is primarily concerned with assisting him to cope with the activities of living in such a way as to promote his optimal level of functioning or, in the case of incurable disease, to cope with terminal illness.

In order to identify areas in which the individual requires nursing assistance to be able to cope with either of the above, the nurse needs to have information that will tell her:

1. Something about the individual as a person
2. His usual abilities (or lack of abilities) in coping with the activities of living
3. The nature of any health problems that are interfering with his abilities to cope
4. His current status in regard to these abilities
5. The physician's plan of care for the individual

Some of this information the nurse collects herself; some she gathers from other sources.

Sources. The first, or "primary," source of information is always the patient. Other sources, termed "secondary sources," include other people, such as family members or "significant others" with whom the individual has a close relationship. In the case of a child or an unconscious or irrational patient, much of the information the nurse needs to know must be obtained from someone other than the patient.

The patient's health record is also a valuable source of data for the nurse, and today an increasing number of health team members contribute to it. If a record has already been stated, or if old records are on file, the nurse should review these, if possible, prior to setting out to gather information herself. This review helps to avoid duplication in gathering information and also gives the nurse the benefit of data gathered by others. The physician, for example, is usually responsible for taking the patient's medical history, for identifying medical problems the patient has, and for developing diagnostic and therapeutic plans for the individual, if such are warranted. The results of the physician's findings and the medical plan of care are incorporated into the patient's record. In order to develop her plan of care for the patient, the nurse must be aware of the nature of the patient's medical problems and of the physician's plan of care.

Other members of the health team also contribute to the nurse's understanding of the patient and his health status. Observations and interpretations may be communicated by the social worker, the nutritionist (dietitian), the physical therapist, or the occupational therapist, to name only a few, through written notes on a patient's record, in consultations with the nurse, or in conferences and other meetings of various members of the health team. Nor should the nurse overlook the importance, as sources of information, of the reports on x-ray findings and the results of laboratory tests performed on the patient. These reports are usually attached to the patient's record.

If the individual has a known medical problem, the nurse will probably want to increase her knowledge about it by reading available literature on the subject in the library and by reviewing notes she may have from classes that will contribute to her understanding of this particular patient's problem.

Methods. The basic methods used by nurses to gather information about an individual patient are the interview (talking with the patient), observation and examination, consultation (with other members of the health team), and review of records and other written material.

Essentially there are two types of information that the nurse gathers through interviewing the patient and through her observations and examination. One is information of a relatively "constant" nature that is not expected to change during the period of care. For example, the fact that an individual wears dentures or that he is right-handed would be considered data of a constant nature. This type of information is usually collected by talking with the individual, that is, through an interview. The second type of information the nurse collects is concerned with the current status of the patient; this may be expected to change and such facts are therefore called "variable" data. A person's temperature, for example, may change from day to day and even during the course of one day. Temperature recordings from individual patients, then, would be considered variable data. Variable data are obtained through the nurse's observations and/or examination of the patient.

Specific tools have been developed to assist the nurse in gathering the information she needs to collect in interviewing and in observing the patient. Most health agencies now use a "nursing history" form to provide a written record of the information about a patient that the nurse gathers by interview. A number of agencies now use in addition a "clinical appraisal guide" (or an initial patient progress record) to record baseline information the nurse has gathered in her observations/examination of the patient's current functioning abilities.

The forms shown on pages 117 to 119 were developed during a project on nursing information systems sponsored by the Division of Nursing, U.S. Department of Health, Education, and Welfare.[3] The first form (p. 117), used in connection with the nursing history, is intended for gathering basic patient data of a constant nature, which can be obtained by interviewing the patient. The second form (p. 156), used in discussing the nurse's clinical appraisal of a patient, is for collecting baseline and reassessment data on factors that may vary in the patient's health/illness status. This particular form was developed for use with hospitalized patients. It is intended that these and other forms developed during the project be used with a manual of instructions that provides the nurse with guidelines for completing them.

The Nursing History. The nursing history provides a guide for systematically obtaining information which can help the nurse to (1) plan and modify her care to suit the individual patient's preferences and usual living patterns, and (2) establish a baseline from which to evaluate the results of nursing action.

The history is taken as soon after the patient's admission to the agency as is feasible, preferably by the nurse who has primary responsibility for planning the patient's care. The technique for obtaining the history is a structured interview—that is, the nurse controls and directs the interview for the purpose of gathering specific information.

The information gathered includes items that nurses in a particular agency have found helpful in assessing patients' needs and in planning care for the majority of patients.[4] Among the items frequently included are: events leading up to the patient's admission to the health agency, basic social data about the patient, basic physiological data (verbal information that can be obtained by interview), the person's usual patterns of daily living, environmental factors that may affect his health, the individual's understanding of his health and illness status, and the patient's concerns and his expectations of the care he will receive in the agency.[4] Not all nursing histories include all of these items. Some of the data (all of which is helpful to the nurse) may be obtained from other sources, as for example, the basic physiological data may be gathered by a physician during initial examination of the patient.

Events Leading Up to the Patient's Admission. In order to know how she can help the individual, the nurse needs to be aware of the reasons for his admission to the health agency. In an ambulatory care setting, the individual may have come for any one of a number of reasons. He may want assistance in promoting his physical fitness or in protecting himself from illness, or he may be worried and anxious about his health. He may or may not have a health problem. The person who has been admitted to the hospital has a recognized problem and has come for diagnosis or treatment or both. The patient used here to illustrate the nursing process was admitted to a large city hospital following transfer from another agency. He had been injured in a car accident and suffered compression fractures of three vertebrae. Details of events leading to his admission are recorded on page 117.

Basic Social Data. The basic social data gathered about an individual usually includes biographical information (or vital statistics), and information about the person's educational level and his employment status. Often included are items about his interests, hobbies, and community affiliations.

Vital statistics about an individual help to give the nurse some idea of what this patient is like. The name sometimes helps to identify ethnic origin, as does information about birthplace and citizenship. The person's address can give some indication of the type of neighborhood in which he lives. Information can be elicited about whether there are relatives who might be helpful, and whether they live nearby or far away. Knowledge of the language a person speaks is essential for communicating with him. Age, sex, and employment status are important in understanding a person's perceptions of his health and illness status. For example, a woman of 40 who is admitted to the hospital for termination of her first pregnancy may be expected to react quite differently from the 30-year-old woman who is in the hospital for a therapeutic abortion and already has four children. A singer who is to have even a minor operation on his throat may be extremely anxious about the results of the surgery and its effects on his career. Knowing the individual's marital status and next of kin assists in the identification of significant family members and helps the nurse to assess the potential support of family and friends.

Knowledge of the individual's educational

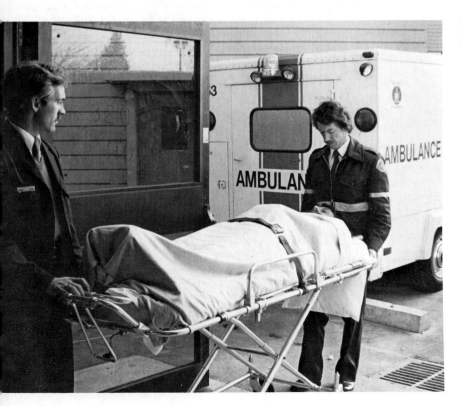

Paul Jordan arriving at the emergency ward by ambulance.

HOSPITAL _North West General_

NURSING ASSESSMENT: BASIC PATIENT INFORMATION

ADMISSION TIME _1600 HRS._ DATE: _16/9/82_

Sept. 16, 82
Jordan Paul
2465 Washington Ave. Shore City
234-7566
Smith James 1600   Surg. R.C.
Same
9-16-82   PATIENT'S IDENTIFICATION

1. GENERAL ADMISSION INFORMATION

MODE:	ACCOMPANIED BY:	SOURCE OF DATA:
walking ☐	family ☐	patient ☑
wheelchair ☐	friend ☑	family ☐
stretcher ☑	no one ☐	_____ other

PRIMARY LANGUAGE: (If not English) _____

DIFFICULTY WITH ENGLISH IN RELATION TO:

comments: _____

speaking ☐

understanding ☐

2. PRESENT ILLNESS

Instructions: Check first box for single term or first double term, check second box for second term

Reason for present admission _CAR ACCIDENT - COMPRESSION FRACTURE 3 VERTEBRAE_

Primary signs/symptoms:

blurring/double vision	fatigue/weakness	pain ☑
chills/fever	heart burn/indigestion	pruritis
cough	incontinence	voiding difficulty ☑
		weight loss/gain
cyanosis	injury/trauma ☑☑	L.M.P. _____
diarrhea/constipation	insomnia	Date
		Site of
dysphasia	jaundice	{ discharge _____
S.O.B./dyspnea	loss of appetite	{ bleeding _____
edema/swelling	nausea/emesis	

DURATION: _7_ hrs.; _____ days; _____ weeks; _____ mos.; _____ yrs.

LOCATION: _D11, D12, L1_

SEVERITY: _POSSIBLE NERVE DAMAGE   PAIN VERY SEVERE_

comments: _TRANSFERRED FROM NORTHCOAST HOSPITAL - BY PLANE X-RAYS WITH PATIENT_

3. PREVIOUS HOSPITALIZATION(S)

NONE ☐   NUMBER _1_   LAST ADMISSION   reason and date _MOTORCYCLE ACCIDENT 1972_

PREVIOUS ADMISSION in this hospital: No ☐ Yes: ☑ reason/date _AS ABOVE_

FEELINGS ABOUT NURSING CARE   strongly positive ☐   positive ☑   neutral ☐

negative ☐   strongly negative ☐   Why liked/disliked? _RECEIVED GOOD CARE_

comments:

4. ALLERGIES

NONE KNOWN ☑

	DRUGS	FOOD	OTHER
1.	_____	_____	_____
2.	_____	_____	_____
3.	_____	_____	_____
4.	_____	_____	_____

comments:

5. MEDICATION(S) HISTORY

MEDICATION(S) TAKEN ROUTINELY: None ☑

	name or reason	freq.	last dose
1.	_____	_____	_____
2.	_____	_____	_____
3.	_____	_____	_____

comments:

DRUG(S) WITH PATIENT?   No ☑

sent home:	1 2 3
given to staff:	1 2 3
with patient:	1 2 3
_____	1 2 3
other	(circle)

HOSPITAL _____

NURSING ASSESSMENT: BASIC PATIENT INFORMATION

PATIENT'S IDENTIFICATION _____

6. CHRONIC HEALTH PROBLEMS

None known ☑

(a) Diabetes ☐
(b) Heart Disease ☐
(c) Emphysema ☐

(d) Hypertension ☐
(e) Arthritis ☐
(f) Ulcer ☐

(g) Epilepsy ☐
(h) Amputation ☐
(i) _____ other

RESTRICTED ACTIVITIES (specify) _____

POSSIBLY HAD T.B. AGE 12 YRS. ANNUAL CHEST X-RAYS

Comments:

7. RESPONSE TO ILLNESS(ES)

to indicate which disease(s) the information pertains (Sect.6), place the letter(s) of disease(s) in the box(es) following statement(s). Place a check mark to indicate which information pertains to present illness.

PERCEPTIONS OF SIGNS/SYMPTOMS:

denies presence of ☐
preoccupied with ☑
has misconceptions ☐
inadequate information ☐
other _____

Unable to evaluate ☐ ☐ ☐   comments: _____

PERCEPTIONS OF PROGNOSIS:

complete recovery ☐
partial recovery ☐
to die ☐
doesn't know ☑
no change ☐

8. SUPPORTIVE AIDS

PROSTHESES:

DENTURES
upper ☐
lower ☐
partial ☐

rt lt
leg ☐
arm ☐
breast ☐
eye ☐
other _____

DOMINANT HAND:

Right ☑
Left ☐

AIDS TO MOBILITY:

crutches ☐
cane ☐
walker ☐
brace ☐
wheelchair ☐
other _____

comments: _____

9. ELIMINATION

USUAL DEFECATION FREQUENCY

OD: (am)/pm   QOD: am/pm
(circle)

impacted ☐
other _____
date of last BM *SEPT. 16, 1982*

Colostomy ☐
ileostomy ☐
_____
duration _____
No self care ☐

AIDS USED AT HOME (name & frequency)

dietary _____
laxative _____
suppository _____
enema _____

URINATION:

frequency ☐
urgency ☐
nocturia _____
no. of times

INCONTINENCE:

total ☐
stress ☐

Comments: _____
_____
_____
_____

FORM 0001

HOSPITAL *NORTH WEST GENERAL*

NURSING ASSESSMENT: BASIC PATIENT INFORMATION

PATIENT'S IDENTIFICATION

10. SENSORY STATUS

VISION: rt lt
- uncorrected ☐☐
- severely impaired ☐☐
- blind ☐☐

Uses Aid(s): _____ (type)

Does not have glasses ☑

HEARING: rt lt
- severe loss ☐☐
- deaf ☐☐
- wears Aid ☐☐

_____ (type)

Does **not** have hearing aid ☑

TASTE:
- loss of taste ☐
- distorted ☐
- circle: dec./inc. ☐

comments: _____

SMELL:
- loss of smell ☐
- distorted ☐
- dec./inc. ☐

SPEECH:
- Slurring ☐
- Stuttering ☐
- Dysphasia ☐
- Other _____

COMMUNICATION:
- Unable to speak ☐
- Unable to write ☐
- Sign language ☐
- Reads lips ☐

SENSE OF FEELING:
circle: dec (inc) sensitivity to:
- Pressure ☑
- Heat ☐
- Cold ☐

Locate *SACRAL AREA*
comments: *BRUISED, TENDER*

11. NUTRITION

HEIGHT *177.8 cm. (5'10")*
WEIGHT *61.4 kg (135 lb.)*

USUAL APPETITE:
- anorectic ☐
- voracious ☑

SPECIAL DIET AT HOME:
- diabetic ☐
- low salt ☐
- bland ☐
- soft ☐

other _____

RESPONSE TO DIET:
- Lack of understanding ☐
- Strong dislike ☐

other _____

comments: _____

12. USUAL REST AND SLEEP PATTERNS

SLEEPING PATTERNS:
usual hours of sleep: (circle)

from *11* ~~a.m.~~ / p.m. to *5* a.m. / ~~p.m.~~

insomnia ☐ Daily naps ☑

comments: _____

AIDS USED TO SLEEP (name & frequency):
- position in bed _____
- extra pillows _____
- medication _____
- food _____
- other _____

13. SOCIAL HISTORY

WORK
OCCUPATION *FISHERMAN*
SHIFT evening ☐ night ☐
- Head of Household ☑
- Homemaker ☐
- Retired ☐
- Dependent ☐

comments: *SELF-EMPLOYED COMMERCIAL FISHERMAN*

INTERESTS/HOBBY
- radio ☐
- T.V. ☐
- reading ☐
- needlework ☐
- crafts ☐
- puzzles ☐
- other *PLAYS GUITAR*

HOUSING
patient lives with:
- no one ☐
- family ☐
- friend ☑
- other _____

comments: _____

- nursing home ☐
- institution ☐
- single dwelling ☐
- multiple dwelling ☑
- walk-up ☐
- Floor *GROUND*
- Bed & Bath on separate floor ☐
- Bath shared with other tenants ☐
- other _____

14. VISITORS

NO VISITORS ANTICIPATED ☐

RESTRICTIONS DESIRED
- family only ☐
- no visitors ☐
- other _____

comments: _____

level is helpful both in adjusting the nurse's use of language for communicating with him and in assessing his ability to comprehend information about his health/illness status. Knowledge of his interests, hobbies, and community affiliations also helps to give the nurse insight into the person as an individual and some understanding of his inner resources.

An example of the basic social data is given below.

NAME: Paul Jordan
SEX: Male
MARITAL STATUS: Single
BIRTHDATE: October 2, 1951
RELIGION: Roman Catholic
BIRTHPLACE: Philadelphia, Pennsylvania
CITIZENSHIP: U.S.
ADDRESS: 2465 Washington Avenue, Shore City
LANGUAGE: English
EDUCATION: 2 years university
EMPLOYMENT STATUS: Self-employed commercial fisherman. Works April–October, 7 days/week. Fishing trips average 8–10 days out; 1–3 days ashore. Hours: 0400–2300 during season.
INTERESTS: Plays guitar; skiing, hiking, camping
COMMUNITY AFFILIATIONS: None

Basic Physiological Data. The amount of basic physiological data included in the nursing history depends on the policy of the health agency. In some agencies much of this type of data may be obtained during the initial physical examination of the patient. If this is the case, the information would not be duplicated in the nursing history. In many agencies, however, the nurse gathers basic physiological data about the individual in the course of taking the nursing history.

The type of information that is helpful for the nurse to have about the patient's physiological status includes a general body description, which takes into account such constant factors as: height and weight (often both the "usual" weight and the present weight are noted), the individual's dominant hand, prostheses (artificial parts such as a limb, dentures, and the like), amputations the individual may have had, visual or auditory impairments of long standing, the person's ability to communicate, and his mobility status. Observations about the individual's current status in regard to these items are often noted as well as past history. In addition, chronic health problems the individual may have, as well as known allergies, are often noted. Many nursing histories also include information about medications the person is currently taking, and some include the person's immunization record.

This type of information helps to provide baseline data on which to assess the individual's current health status. It is also useful in the identification of nursing problems and in the establishment of realistic goals for nursing care.

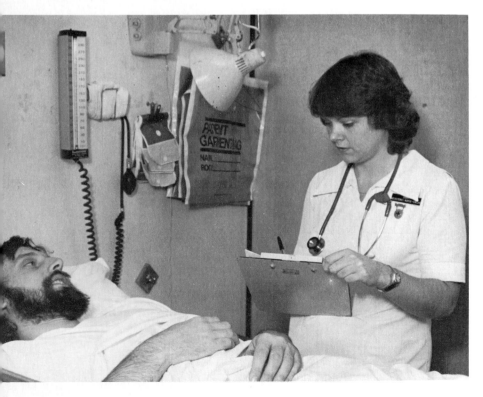

Nurse taking Paul Jordan's history on arrival in the emergency ward.

Let us add the basic physiological data to our information about Mr. Jordan.

HEIGHT: 177.8 cm. (5 ft. 10 in.)
WEIGHT: 61.4 kg. (135 lb.)
DOMINANT HAND: Right
VISION ⎫
HEARING ⎬ Normal
COMMUNICATION: No problem
HEALTH HISTORY: No known allergies
  Possibly had tuberculosis when approximately 12 years
  No prostheses
  No medications
  Immunization: Had all recommended childhood ones
  Other: Has chest x-rays once/year
MOBILITY STATUS: Normally no problem
  Present mobility limited by injury
  Confined to bed rest
  Cannot lift arms above head because of pain

Usual Patterns of Daily Living. Most nurses have found it helpful in planning care for an individual to have information about his usual habits of daily living. Information generally collected includes habits in regard to rest and sleep, eating, elimination, and hygiene practices. Habits relating to smoking and alcohol consumption are increasingly being included as a part of the nursing history.

The person's usual time for going to bed, the number of hours he sleeps, and the aids he may use to get to sleep are particularly helpful if the person is ill and needs to be cared for in an inpatient facility. The individual's usual appetite and normal diet are important in assessing nutritional status, in identifying problems with regard to nutrition, and in planning this essential element of his care. If the person has been on a special diet at home, the nurse needs to be aware of this fact and also of his response to it. Does he understand this diet? Is he adhering to it? These are among the questions that should be asked. With regard to elimination, the usual time and frequency of defecation are noted, as well as aids the person uses regularly, such as foods or fluids that the person feels are helpful in maintaining regularity. If the individual is in the habit of taking laxatives regularly or using suppositories or enemas to aid in elimination, it is helpful to have this information.

The nurse also needs information about the person's usual pattern of urination and any problems he has, such as frequency, urgency, or having to get up at night to void. Habits with regard to hygiene are also important to note. Particularly if the patient is ill, it is helpful for the nurse to know if he prefers a tub bath or a shower, for example, and the time of day he usually takes it.

The type of information gathered about usual habits of daily living is useful not only in planning care, but also in detecting existing and potential problems. It also provides a base for assessing the individual's present functional abilities.

Let us add the information about Mr. Jordan's usual patterns of daily living to the data we already have.

USUAL REST AND SLEEP PATTERNS: During fishing season, 5 to 6 hours a night and approximately 1 to 2 hours during day.
  No aids, no medications. Sleeps soundly.
NUTRITION: Three meals/day plus snacks when available. Healthy appetite. Well balanced meals: meat, potatoes, vegetables, fruits, and milk.
ELIMINATION: Daily bowel movement after breakfast. No problems, no laxatives.
  No problems with urinary elimination.
  Never has to get up at night.
HYGIENE: On shore—daily shower and washes hair. On boat—daily wash and wash with disinfectant after cleaning fish (hands and face)
SMOKING: One to two packs a day since age 16
ALCOHOL: Socially with other fishermen and when on shore
  Not a heavy drinker

Environmental Factors. Among the environmental factors that affect a person's health are his family, where he lives, and where he works. The amount of detail included about these factors in the nursing history is a matter of agency policy. Usually much more information is gathered in a community health agency than in a hospital about a person's family, his living accommodations, and the neighborhood in which he lives. If the individual is living with other family members, it is helpful to have basic social data about them and information about their health history and present health status.

In planning and adjusting care for the patient at home, or discharge care for the person who has been hospitalized, it is important to have information about the person's living accommodations. For example, if the bathroom is located on a different floor from the sleeping area, this may pose a problem for the person who becomes short of breath on climbing stairs. With older people, especially, it is important for the nurse to be aware of the location of shopping areas and other facilities in relation to the home. Knowledge of this type can be very helpful in identifying existing and potential problems, as well as in planning realistic care for people.

Knowing the environment in which a person works is important too. Again, it is helpful not only in identifying problems, but also in planning for the rehabilitation of the individual if he has a health problem.

Let us suppose that the community health nurse has made a visit to Mr. Jordan's home and work environment and has gathered the following information:

RESIDENCE: 2465 Washington Avenue, Shore City
NEIGHBORHOOD DESCRIPTION: Urban residential. Mainly apartments and multi-family dwellings
PROBLEMS: Noisy—on a main thoroughfare. Near beach. Good parks nearby.
LIVING ACCOMMODATIONS: Ground floor apartment (one bedroom)
  Safety hazards: Old building—fire potential
FAMILY MEMBERS: Family in Philadelphia (parents, 2 sisters, 5 brothers)
SIGNIFICANT OTHERS: Lives with fishing partner, Joe Smith aged 21 years. Girl friend in city.
WORK ENVIRONMENT: Fishing boat cabin clean but difficult to maintain; area where fish are cleaned is rinsed constantly by seawater during cleaning process and thoroughly scrubbed after each catch has been cleaned

The Individual's Perceptions of His Health and Illness Status.

In planning care for an individual, it is essential for the nurse to be aware of how the patient regards his health and illness status. People vary considerably in the way they view health and illness, as we discussed in Chapter 3. Although many people today are highly sophisticated in their knowledge of health matters, it is not uncommon to find mistakenly held views about the causes of illness and the significance of signs and symptoms. Then, too, illness is caused by a multiplicity of factors; it is helpful to know what the patient thinks is causing his health problem.

People vary in their reactions to illness, as we also discussed in Chapter 3. Some people become very angry; some react by denying that it exists; some people can talk of nothing else but their signs and symptoms. Usually, if a person has been injured, or admitted to a health agency for emergency treatment of any kind, his physical well-being is the most important thing on his mind and he is naturally going to be preoccupied with his condition. Some people may realize the implications of their signs and symptoms; others may be totally unrealistic about these or about their *prognosis*, that is, the expected outcome of their health problem. People often have some knowledge about the state of their health, but it may not be enough for them to be able to cope with a major health problem.

Knowing how a person views his current health and illness status enables the nurse to identify discrepancies between his perceptions and factual findings. This type of information is helpful in identifying his learning needs and also in anticipating the amount of support the patient may need in accepting his health problem, if he has one, and its implications. For example, the person who has a stomach ulcer may need help in accepting the limitations imposed on his diet, particularly if he has had only a mild attack and is not convinced that there is anything seriously wrong with him.

Let us see how Mr. Jordan views his current health problem and what his anxieties are. Following are the nurse's notes in this regard:

Mr. Jordan is in great pain. He knows that he has broken his back. He does not know how bad it is and is worried and anxious about whether he will have to have surgery. He guesses he's "going to be laid up for a long time." He is also anxious about his clothes and money, which have been lost during the transfer from North Coast Hospital.

Expectations of Care.

An indication of the patient's expectations regarding his care, i.e., what he expects to happen to him and the care he anticipates from nursing personnel, helps the nurse to understand how much explanation the patient will require and may help to clarify some of his reactions to the care he receives. Asking the patients about these matters in itself indicates interest and helps to establish a trusting relationship between nurse and patient.

People usually have preconceived ideas of what they may expect from a health agency. These expectations are conditioned by their own previous experiences with the agency, if they had any, and the accounts of care received by relatives and friends, as well as by information they have picked up from other sources, such as newspapers, books, and magazines, or radio and television programs.

Their expectations may or may not be realistic. In any case, it is helpful for the nurse to know just what these are.

Let us see what Mr. Jordan expects of his care.

Mr. Jordan says he will be happy if they can just relieve his pain and fix his back. He was in the hospital 4 years ago following a motorcycle accident in which he suffered a head injury. He was released after observation because there was no apparent fracture or brain damage. He says he has positive feelings about the nursing care and the treatment he received at that time.

The Patient's Concerns.

An indication of the things about which the patient is concerned is important for the nurse both in planning care and in establishing a trusting relationship with the patient. Knowing about the things that are worrying him helps to identify some sources of anxiety and provides the nurse with some guidance on what she can do to help the patient. The woman who is worried about how her husband and children are managing while she is in the hospital might be relieved by having a telephone at her bedside so she could call home, or the nurse might ask the social worker to see the patient, with a view to making arrangements for "homemaker" services while the mother is in the hospital.

An indication of what is important to the individual helps the nurse to attend to the small details that mean so much to patients. A woman patient may request the nurse to telephone her husband to bring in a clean nightgown and her make-up, for example. This may seem an unimportant detail to the nurse who is busy with medications and treatments, but it is important to the patient in contributing to her sense of well-being. Attention to such requests helps the patient to feel more secure and comfortable in a strange environment; it also helps maintain the patient's feelings of self-worth.

Asking the patient about his concerns in itself helps to make him feel that he is being treated as an individual—that someone cares. In following through and doing something about his concerns, the nurse helps to establish a feeling of trust between herself and the patient, which is essential in any nurse-patient relationship.

Here are Mr. Jordan's expressed concerns:

Mr. Jordan was primarily concerned with his excruciating pain. He wants to know if he has to have surgery and whether he will be OK. He is concerned about his clothes and money, which were lost in transit.

The Clinical Appraisal. In her assessment of the patient's problems and his needs for nursing care, the nurse must have a good basis of information about the present state of his physical and mental health. Some of the information needed is obtained by interview. During the course of taking the nursing history, as we mentioned earlier, the nurse gathers basic physiological data about the patient and data about his usual patterns of daily living. Any deviations from the patient's normal—such as a recent sudden loss of weight or changes in bowel habits—will probably have been noted. But some information must be gathered by observations the nurse makes herself.

To be systematic, the nurse's observations must follow a logical and orderly plan. In recent years, a considerable amount of research has been undertaken and numerous articles and reports have appeared in the nursing literature on the development of systematic methodology for nursing observations. Most of the study reports and articles have included examples of forms (such as the nursing assessment forms shown in this chapter) and manuals that provide guidelines for the nurse in making observations. Although the format and specific items recorded vary in different agencies, there is a growing consensus on general content areas to be included in the initial appraisal of an individual patient. These content areas, for the most part, follow the functional abilities approach to nursing assessment outlined originally by R. Faye McCain in 1965 and described by her as "an orderly, precise method of collecting information about the physiological, psychological and social behavior of a patient."[1]

McCain identified 13 functional areas in which the individual's abilities should be assessed: "the patient's social, mental, emotional, body temperature, respiratory, circulatory, nutritional, elimination and reproductive status; state of rest and comfort; state of skin and appendages; sensory perception and motor ability."[1] It is essential that both abilities and disabilities be noted so that the nurse can identify both the individual's strengths and his weaknesses in all functional areas.

The concept of functional assessment provides a logical framework on which the student can begin to develop skills in observation of an individual patient. A detailed discussion of the kinds of observations the nurse makes in her initial assessment of the current status of a patient's functional abilities is included in Chapter 9. Meanwhile, we will include here the observations noted by the nurse who admitted Paul Jordan to the nursing unit. These are shown on the following pages, on the forms headed "Nursing Assessment: Patient Progress."

Problem Identification

Analysis of Information. Once the nurse has gathered information about the patient through taking the nursing history and through her observations, her next step is to analyze that information. The question is, what does it all mean?

In order to critically examine the data she has collected, the nurse will find it helpful to group the information by categories. This helps to put it into some sort of logical order and to develop a structure, or framework, which not only makes the mass of data she has collected more meaningful, but also makes it much easier to manage. If her observations have been made on a basis of functional areas, for example, this already gives the nurse a framework on which to analyze the data logically and systematically.

When the data are organized (or grouped), the next step is to look at them from the point of view of significant deviations from the normal. What is unusual in the findings about this patient? In what way does the status of his functional abilities differ from normal functioning? How important are the deviations from normal that the nurse has found in this patient? In this analysis, the nurse is aided by: (1) her knowledge of normal functioning, derived from courses in the basic biophysical and social sciences; (2) her understanding of normal and abnormal factors that may affect functioning in a particular area; and (3) her awareness of common problems, signs, and symptoms that accompany various health problems.

At the beginning of her nursing program, the student will not, of course, have an extensive knowledge base from which to draw. She can, however, identify many deviations from the normal and can relate these to the knowledge she does have. As her knowledge increases and her clinical experience grows, she will be able to assess the significance of her findings more readily and with a greater depth of understanding. At all times, however, it is important that the nurse communicate her findings and interpret them honestly at the level of her understanding.

In taking the nursing history, the nurse has noted the patient's usual functional abilities and has gained some information about him as an individual. In her clinical appraisal, she has made observations about his current status in regard to his functional abilities and has noted deviations from the normal. By comparing data from her observations with data from the history, she is able to note any changes that have occurred between the person's usual functioning and his present abilities. Now she separates the abnormal findings from those that appear to be normal and assesses the importance of these in relation to his current health status. A person may have a long-standing abnormality which may or may not be significant in the present situation. For example, the patient may have had an amputation of one of his little fingers a number of years ago. This is a deviation from the normal, but probably is not significant if he is in the hospital to have surgery for removal of his appendix. On the other hand, the fact that a person has been confined to a wheelchair for years is significant in planning his care.

In Mr. Jordan's case, the nurse will note deviations from the normal in regard to his rest and comfort status (he is in pain), to his mobility status (he cannot walk or lift his arms above his head, and movement aggravates the pain), to his elimination status (voiding is difficult), to his nutritional status (his weight is below normal for his height), to the status of his skin and appendages (he has several large bruised areas on his lower back). All of these findings would appear to be significant.

Synthesis of Information. When the nurse has analyzed the information she has collected and identified significant findings she has made, she then relates it to information she has obtained from other sources. From the admission notes she has learned that Mr. Jordan was in a car accident and suffered compression fractures of three vertebrae. She has noted the location of the injury, vertebrae T11, T12, and L1. The nature and location of the injury have been confirmed in the report of the x-rays taken on admission to this hospital. The laboratory reports of blood tests and urinalysis (telephoned to the ward) show normal findings. From the physician's notes, she learns that he has ruled out surgery at this time, that he suspects there may be internal injuries, and there is a possibility of nerve damage.

The physician's orders include:

Bed rest
Fracture board
Bed flat—pt. to maintain back-lying position, may turn on side for care
2 pillows under head—1 supporting shoulders
1 pillow under knees
NPO 48 hr
Dextrose—Saline 5% 1500 ml/d × 2
Vital signs q4h—48 hr
Intake and output
Demerol—100 mg IM q4h p.r.n. for pain

By putting this information together with the data she has collected, the nurse can begin to think about some of the things that will be important in Mr. Jordan's care. He is having severe pain—it will be important to relieve that. She will have to be careful in helping him to move—he will probably need instructions on "log rolling" in turning and in maintaining his position as the doctor has ordered. NPO (nothing by mouth)—this might be a problem, since Mr. Jordan normally has a voracious appetite. Watching the vital signs—that will help determine presence of internal injuries. Watching intake and output—that's to watch for signs of damage to the nerves innervating the bladder, also for possible internal injuries.

The nurse is ready now to begin organizing her initial impressions and identifying specific problems that require nursing intervention.

Problem Identification. A nursing problem is any condition or situation in which the patient needs the nurse's help. The term "nursing diagnosis" is increasingly being used to describe the statement of a problem the patient has that the nurse can help to resolve through her actions. A series of national conferences has been

ACCEPTED NURSING DIAGNOSES

Anxiety
Body Fluids
Bowel Elimination, Alteration in
Cardiac Output, Alteration in
Comfort, Alterations in
Consciousness, Altered Levels of
Coping Patterns, Maladaptive (Individual)
Coping, Ineffective Family
Digestion, Impairment of
Family Process, Inadequate
Fear
Fluid Volume Deficit
Grieving
Home Maintenance Management, Impaired
Injury, Potential for
Knowledge, Lack of (Specify)
Manipulation
Mobility, Impairment of
Noncompliance (Specify)
Nutritional Alteration
Parenting, Alterations in
Respiratory Dysfunction
Role Disturbance
Self-Care Activities, Alterations in
Self-Concept, Alterations in
Sensory-Perceptual Alteration
Sexuality, Alteration in Patterns of
Skin Integrity, Impairment of
Sleep-Rest Activity, Dysrhythm of
Spirituality, Matters of
Social Isolation
Suffocation, Potential for
Thought Processes, Impaired
Tissue Perfusion, Chronic Abnormal
Trauma, Potential for
Urinary Elimination, Impairment of
Verbal Communication, Impairment of

Identified by the National Group on Classification of Nursing Diagnoses at Conferences on Nursing Diagnosis, St. Louis, Missouri, 1973, 1975, 1978.

Source: Price, M. R.: Nursing Diagnosis: Making a Concept Come Alive. *The American Journal of Nursing,* 80(4):668–671, April, 1980.

held in the United States to try to develop a systematic method for classifying nursing diagnoses. From these deliberations, a list of accepted nursing diagnoses is currently evolving. Those identified by the National Group on Classification of Nursing Diagnoses as of 1982 are listed above.

Nurses are frequently confused about *needs* versus *problems.* To illustrate the difference, the following example may be helpful. The patient is having difficulty in breathing and requires oxygen therapy. The *problem* is the difficulty in breathing. The *need* is for oxygen therapy. The problem identifies the difficulty the person is having. The need spells out the type of intervention that the nurse feels would resolve the problem. There may be several possible alternatives, so the nurse has to decide which intervention is most appropriate for that problem. Changing the patient's position, for example, might relieve the difficulty in breathing; giving medication might be another possibility.

In order to plan nursing care and decide on the intervention that is most suitable for the situation, it is necessary first to identify the problems the patient is having. These may be either actual or potential problems. *Actual problems* are those that, in the nurse's opinion, are causing the patient difficulty at the present time. For example, Mr. Jordan has an actual problem with pain (to select one problem). *Potential problems* are those that may arise because of the nature of the patient's health problem or because of the diagnostic or therapeutic plan of care. Mr. Jordan, for example, is not allowed out of bed, and he is restricted to a certain position in bed. He is thin and there is a potential problem of skin breakdown, particularly over bony prominences, such as the lower part of his back, his heels, and his elbows.

Problems should be identified systematically. Again, using the functional abilities approach helps the nurse to systematically check where the patient needs help with either actual or potential problems. In stating problems, the most important thing is that the nurse communicate the intent of her message so that it can be understood by others. Wherever possible, the nurse should state the cause of the problem as she understands it.

If we review the information we have about Mr. Jordan by functional area, we can identify several problems, some actual and some potential, with which he needs the nurse's help. Following each problem, there is a statement that gives some of the nurse's thinking in relation to that problem:[5]

Social Status: No actual problem: potential problem of feelings of isolation because family is in the East.

> *Analysis:* Mr. Jordan has mentioned his family. Would like them to be notified of his accident. His friends in the city are all working.

Mental Status: (1) Restlessness due to pain.

> *Analysis:* Pain relieved by medication, restlessness more noticeable as time approaches for medication.

(2) Potential problem of disorientation and drowsiness due to medication for pain.

> *Analysis:* Patient will probably be kept sedated while pain is severe to ensure his safety from further injury.

Emotional Status: (1) Anxiety due to uncertainty about physician's plan of care and prognosis.

Analysis: Physician has decided against surgery "at this time." Patient unsure as to just what this means.

(2) Anxiety over loss of clothes and money.

Analysis: Patient admitted first to North Coast Hospital. Transferred by plane, then by ambulance. Money and valuables could have been left in any one of three places.

Temperature Status
Respiratory Status } No actual problems
Circulatory Status

Potential problems due to possibility of internal injuries.

Analysis: Vital signs may change quickly if there is internal bleeding. Physician has ordered monitoring of vital signs q4h, or more often if changes are noted or if observations warrant it.

Nutritional Status: (1) Hunger, due to NPO.

Analysis: Patient says he is hungry. Aware that he can have nothing to eat or drink for 48 hours; aware of reason for order. Normally has a big appetite.

(2) Potential problem of maintaining nutritional status if NPO is continued.

Elimination Status: (1) Difficulty in voiding, possibly due to nerve damage.

Analysis: Injury to vertebrae T11, T12, and L1 could have caused damage to nerves leading to bladder. There could also be a possibility of damage to kidneys as a result of trauma suffered in accident.

(2) Potential problem of constipation due to bed rest and lack of solid food intake.

Analysis: Immobility and lack of sufficient food and fluids may cause constipation. Possibility of nerve damage may also cause interference with intestinal elimination.

(3) Potential anxiety about finances due to anticipated lengthy convalescence and possible need to change his line of work.

Analysis: People with the sort of back injury Mr. Jordan has usually require a long time to recover. He will probably be unable to work for several months. He may not even then be able to return to fishing as a career.

State of Rest and Comfort: (1) Severe pain in lower back due to injury, aggravated by movement.

Analysis: Pain relieved by medication. Pain causes restlessness, and increased movement when restless increases pain.

(2) Sensitivity to touch in area of injury and bruised area due to damaged tissues.

Analysis: Sensitivity confirmed by patient's facial expression and involuntary exclamations when back is touched.

State of Skin and Appendages: (1) Bruises in sacral area due to trauma.

Analysis: Area very sensitive to touch, as noted above.

(2) Potential problem of pressure areas developing over bony prominences because of bed rest and limited movement.

Analysis: Patient is thin; this will increase possibility of pressure areas developing. Restlessness increases rubbing of skin surfaces on bedclothes.

(3) Inability to maintain own hygiene due to limited mobility.

Analysis: Patient unable to raise arm to upper part of head; can reach mouth; unable to reach below thighs without pain. Cannot comb hair; hair is long and curly.

(4) Potential problem of poor oral health due to NPO.

Analysis: Patient says that his mouth feels dry. Teeth and gums in good condition at present.

Reproductive Status: No actual problems.

Motor Status: Limited mobility due to pain and restrictions on position.

Analysis: Patient is careful about moving; restricts movement because of pain. Physician has left specific instructions about position. Patient can turn on side for bed-making and back care. Patient will need assistance with exercises to maintain muscular strength and tone, and to prevent contractures if on extended bed rest.

Priority Setting. Once problems are identified, they are placed in order of importance. It is not possible to attend to all problems at the same time, nor is it possible to help the patient with all of his problems all of the time. It is necessary, then, to decide which problems the nurse can assist the patient in resolving and which of these should be attended to first.

In establishing priorities to assist in planning nursing intervention, a helpful guide is Maslow's hierarchy of human needs, which was introduced in Chapter 2 and will be described in detail in Chapter 13. To review these briefly, the basic human needs, in order of priority according to Kalish's model, are:

1. Physiological needs
2. The need for knowledge
3. The need for safety and security
4. The need for love and belonging

5. The need for esteem and self-worth
6. The need for self-actualization

It may not be possible, even under the most favorable circumstances, for the nurse to help the patient to meet all of his needs. Through her awareness of basic human needs, however, she can direct her actions toward helping the patient to resolve problems that interfere with his ability to meet those needs that are essential to his well-being or to his recovery.

In Mr. Jordan's case, the nurse's problem list might be arranged in order of priority as given below. Note that the statements of problems have been shortened in some cases for ease of communication.

1. Pain, due to injury, aggravated by movement
2. (a) Limited mobility because of pain and prescribed position
   (b) Potential problem of loss of muscle tone
   (c) Potential problem of contractures of ankle joints
3. Sensitivity to touch in lower back area due to site of injury and bruised tissues
4. Potential deviations in vital signs because of possible internal injuries
5. Difficulty in voiding, possibly due to nerve damage or internal injuries
6. Anxiety because of uncertainty about physician's plan of care and prognosis
7. Anxiety due to loss of clothes and money
8. (a) Hunger due to NPO
   (b) Potential problem of maintaining nutritional status if NPO is continued
9. Decreased mental alertness due to sedation for pain
   (a) May fall from bed
   (b) May burn self or set fire to bed while smoking
10. Potential problem of maintaining good oral health status due to NPO
11. Potential pressure areas over bony prominences, sacral area, elbows, and heels (see No. 2)
12. Potential problem of constipation due to bed rest and NPO
13. (a) Inability to look after own hygiene (see No. 2)
    (b) Potential problem of poor status of skin and appendages (see No. 13a)
14. Potential problem of feelings of isolation because family is far away and friends are working
15. Potential problem of anxiety about finances due to anticipated lengthy convalescence and possible need to change occupation

The student will note that this ordering does not follow exactly the priority listing of Maslow's hierarchy of human needs. The nurse uses her judgment in allocating priorities; the hierarchy only provides a base from which to start. The concerns that were causing Mr. Jordan anxiety were very important to him and the nurse felt they should be attended to as quickly as possible. Hence, his anxiety problems were given high priority. Also, the patient was smoking frequently; his safety was a matter of immediate concern.

When problems are resolved, they may be crossed off on the nurse's problem list, or they may be left on and the date of resolution recorded. Policies in this regard vary from one agency to another. (See Chapter 12 for discussion on resolved problems when the problem-oriented medical record is used.) The statement of problems that have changed is modified. For example, constipation may become an actual problem rather than a potential one; this would necessitate a change in the problem statement. New problems that emerge are added to the list.

PLANNING

Planning is the second major step in the nursing process. It involves determining what the nurse can do to help the patient and selecting appropriate nursing interventions to accomplish this.

It has been said, and rightly so, that nurses have always planned the care of their patients. In the past, however, planning often was a mental process on the nurse's part, with minimal guidance in the form of written material developed to assist others in their care of the patient when that particular nurse was not on duty.

Taking time to sit down and write out a plan of care helps the nurse to organize her mental activities: to think through what she hopes to accomplish by nursing care; to take into account potential problems as well as those that are actually present; to review the possibilities of alternative nursing interventions; and to develop a plan of care that can be followed through by all nursing personnel concerned with the patient. A written plan of care helps to ensure continuity and completeness of care—that everyone is using the same approach with the patient, and that nothing is left to the uncertainties of human memory.

Planning is a continuous process. The patient's problems change. Some are quickly resolved; some seemingly minor problems suddenly become acute; new ones arise. Sometimes a nursing intervention does not succeed in accomplishing its purpose and alternative approaches must be explored. The planning of nursing care, then, is constantly under revision.

Professional nursing care is based on principles, rather than the application of routine or standard techniques. The body of scientific knowledge that is the foundation of nursing is constantly enlarging; techniques and routines of care are continuously being revised because new information has emerged. The nurse cannot depend on a learned repertoire of skills and procedures to carry her through a lifetime career; skills and techniques soon become obsolete. She must instead base her practice on relatively unchanging principles to guide her in modifying techniques she has learned or in acquiring new skills and techniques.

Many situations the nurse will encounter are unique. She may have never met this set of circumstances before. Indeed, because every person is a unique individual, nursing care must be adapted to suit each patient's particular needs. In order to help the patient in resolving his problems, the nurse must draw on principles rather than rely on rule-of-thumb techniques or standard procedures.

Planning involves basically two sets of activities on the nurse's part: setting goals for the patient to attain and developing a plan of action to achieve these goals. Before the student sets out to undertake these activities, however, she will find it helpful to identify relevant principles applicable to the set of problems her patient has.

Identifying Relevant Principles

Nursing is an applied science. The theoretical basis of nursing draws from many areas, including the biophysical sciences, the medical sciences, pharmacology, nutrition, and the social sciences. The principles applied in nursing practice may be derived from any of these areas.

People's interpretations of the word "principle" vary, but it is used here to mean essentially one of four things: a concept, a scientific fact, a law of science, or a generally accepted theory.[6] Principles are used as guides in determining appropriate nursing action. For example, the holistic concept of man as an integrated being who functions as a whole (discussed in Chapter 2) leads the nurse to consider his social and psychological needs as well as his physical needs when planning care and deciding on specific nursing interventions.

Scientific facts derived from anatomy and physiology guide the nurse in many of her actions. The normal ranges for measurements of body processes, such as those for temperature, pulse, respirations, and blood pressure, are scientific facts that alert the nurse to take action when she observes deviations from the normal in her patients. From the physical sciences, the student will learn in body mechanics that pulling or sliding an object requires less effort than lifting it, since lifting necessitates moving against the force of gravity (see Chapter 23). We have just used the theory of a hierarchy of human needs (drawn from psychology) as a guide in setting priorities for nursing actions for solving patient problems.

Taking the case of Mr. Jordan, some principles applicable in his care would include:

1. The bony vertebral column protects and supports the spinal cord *(anatomy and physiology)*.

There is not much space between the spinal cord and the bony structure supporting and protecting it. Injured vertebrae that are out of alignment or broken may press on or actually damage the cord and the roots of nerves innervating the part of the body below the site of the injury. Therefore, the injured vertebrae must be immobilized until the broken pieces of bone knit together sufficiently to maintain their normal structure and placement. This means that the physician's orders regarding Mr. Jordan's positioning must be followed exactly. Thus, in turning Mr. Jordan, when the nurse is changing the bed linen, it is important that his trunk be maintained in good alignment at all times. Later, when Mr. Jordan is allowed out of bed, he will have to learn to do such activities as getting up, walking, and picking things up without bending his back.

This principle is probably *the* most important one for the nurse to remember in caring for Mr. Jordan. His fractured vertebrae are, after all, the reason for his hospitalization.

2. The loss of blood volume causes a decrease in systemic blood pressure *(anatomy and physiology)*.

When a person is bleeding heavily at any point in the circulatory system, his blood volume drops and his blood pressure is lowered. When this happens, the heart greatly increases its activity in an attempt to increase its output and maintain the amount of circulating blood; blood is withdrawn from surface areas and shunted to vital organs; the skin becomes cold (and clammy); temperature drops (to lessen demands for oxygen transported by the blood); and respirations become rapid and deep (to supply more oxygen for the body).

The physician suspects that Mr. Jordan may have internal injuries as a result of the trauma his body suffered in the accident. There is therefore a possibility of internal bleeding. Vital signs

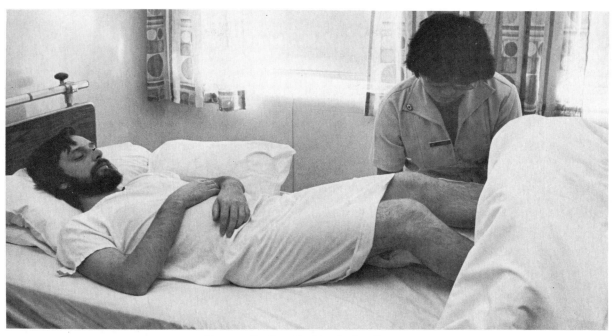

Nurse adjusting Paul Jordan's pillows.

are monitored to watch for: decreased blood pressure, increased and/or irregular pulse, subnormal temperature, and rapid and deep respirations.

3. Adequate elimination of wastes is essential for efficient body functioning (anatomy and physiology).

Mr. Jordan is having difficulty voiding and the physician suspects that there may have been damage to the nerves innervating the urinary system. Monitoring of intake and output is therefore essential. This principle is also applicable in regard to intestinal elimination.

4. Demerol depresses the central nervous system (pharmacology).

The physician has ordered Demerol for the relief of Mr. Jordan's pain. From pharmacology, the nurse knows that this drug causes drowsiness and dulling of mental faculties. It may also cause a person to experience a feeling of happy well-being (euphoria); Mr. Jordan described it as a feeling of "floating." The person may not be fully alert to his surroundings and his safety must be protected.

5. All body cells require adequate amounts of essential nutrients (nutrition).

The physician has ordered NPO for 48 hours, and has prescribed intravenous feedings. If the NPO order is extended, maintaining adequate nutrition will be a problem.

6. The intact skin is the body's first line of defense against infection (microbiology).

Because of his injury, Mr. Jordan is more vulnerable to infection than he normally would be. It is important therefore to maintain skin integrity and prevent the development of pressure areas.

7. Friction is caused by the rubbing together of two irregular surfaces (physics).

The rubbing of the skin surfaces on bed sheets causes friction. The irregularities between the skin surfaces and the bedclothes can be minimized by keeping the sheets smooth and by separating the surfaces as, for example, by using a lubricant to coat the surface of the skin.

8. The need for knowledge is a basic human need, ranked by some theorists as second only to physiological needs (psychology).

Mr. Jordan is very worried because of his lack of information about his therapy (is he going to have to have surgery?) and also about his prognosis. He is also worried about the loss of his clothes and valuables. Therefore, it is important that the nurse take action to see that he receives information about these matters.

9. One of the functions of the family is to support its members in times of crisis (sociology).

Mr. Jordan has asked that his family be notified of his accident. It is important that the nurse take steps to see that this is done.

Determining Expected Outcomes

The identification of patient problems leads to the development of goals or expected out-

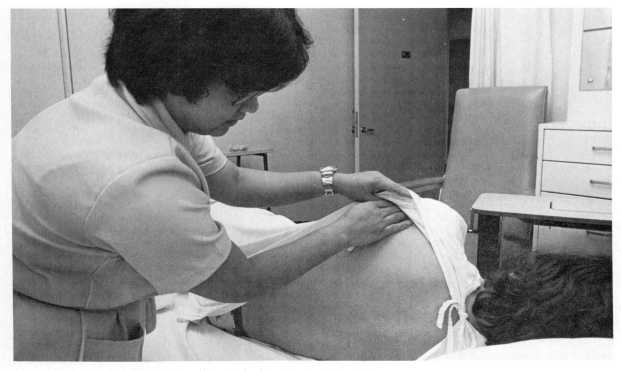

Nurse examining Paul Jordan's back for pressure sores.

comes to be attained by the patient with the assistance of nursing action. These goals should be realistic and attainable both in terms of the potentialities of the patient and the ability of the nurse to help him to meet them. For example, to set as a goal that the patient regain normal motor functioning may be completely unrealistic for a patient who has been partially paralyzed by a stroke, but the patient may be able to achieve independence in feeding and dressing himself, and these are goals that the nurse can help him to achieve.

Goals are stated in terms of expected patient outcomes, rather than nursing activities. Nursing intervention is then planned to help the patient to achieve these. The *expected outcomes* describe the behavior the patient is expected to attain. For example, "The patient dresses himself each morning without help" might be one goal for the partially paralyzed patient. The statement of a goal usually includes: (1) the healthy response, or desired patient behavior (dresses himself); (2) the conditions, if any, under which it is to occur (without help); and (3) a criterion of performance, or standard for judging the performance (in this case, each morning). Some agencies ask that a target date be included (for example, by April 10, the patient should be dressing himself without help every morning).

The expected outcomes, or goals, should always describe behavior that is observable and measurable. In this case, the nurse can actually observe the patient while he is dressing and can note whether he is able to do it himself, and how well he dresses himself on his own. The goals, too, should be developed in conjunction with the patient if at all possible. If Mr. "X" does not want to dress himself, or was not involved in deciding that this was a goal for him to achieve, he is not likely to put forth maximum effort to achieve it.

Long-range goals such as "The patient will regain optimal motor functioning" are important, but in planning specific nursing intervention for one patient, it is helpful to have goals that are worded more specifically. Another objective for the partially paralyzed patient might be, "The patient maintains his right arm and leg [if these are the affected ones] in good anatomical position at all times." Goals worded in terms of expected behavioral outcomes help to communicate to other personnel, to the patient, and to his family just what is to be attained.[7] They also provide scope for prescribing definitive nursing intervention, such as the use of a footboard and pillows to support the arm and leg, and the use of a roll in the patient's hand to maintain flexion of the fingers, in the case of the objective just stated. Stating the expected outcomes also provides the means for evaluating the patient's progress and the effects of nursing action.

THE NURSING PROCESS 131

Some agencies advocate the use of deadlines, or intervals, for checking on the progress the patient has made in relation to the expected outcomes. Thus, in the case of the goal stated above, the patient would be checked at regular intervals (e.g., q4h) to ensure that his right arm and leg were being maintained in good position. One would expect that the nurse caring for the patient would, in the course of giving other care, check the positioning, but a designated deadline draws attention to this aspect of care, and ensures that it is not neglected or forgotten.

In Mr. Jordan's case, one expected outcome in relation to his problem of pain might be that he is quiet and comfortable at all times as evidenced by his relaxed facial expression, his decreased restlessness, and his statements that his pain is lessened.

Expected outcomes in regard to Mr. Jordan's other problems are shown in the nursing care plan prepared for him (see pp. 132–133).

There have been a number of articles and books in the nursing literature about the writing of behavioral objectives. Some of these are included in the list of suggested readings at the end of this chapter. For additional help, the nurse is directed to Mager's book, *Preparing Instructional Objectives*.[8] This book, which is considered a classic in the field, was originally intended for teachers, but nurses will also find it useful.

Developing a Plan of Action

Once objectives have been established in relation to the identified problems, the next step is to determine those nursing interventions which will best help the patient to attain the expected outcomes. This involves the exploration of possible courses of action and a decision to try one approach. In assessing the merits of different courses of action, the nurse is guided by her knowledge of the biophysical and the social sciences, her understanding of the patient's health problem and of the physician's plan of care, and her knowledge about the individual patient as a person.

In deciding on a course of action in relation to any one specific problem, the nurse has basically three options: she may decide (1) that no action is necessary (or possible); (2) that nursing intervention can resolve the problem; or (3) that the problem should be referred to another member of the health team.

In Mr. Jordan's case, his hunger may be the one thing the nurse can do nothing about until the order for nothing by mouth is terminated. There are, however, a number of other problems that require nursing intervention. Pain is, of course, one of these. The patient's anxiety about the therapeutic plan of care for him, and his prognosis, would need to be referred to the physician.

The types of nursing intervention possible should be reviewed systematically. The nurse may find it helpful here to think in terms of the various aspects of nursing discussed in Chapter 6. For example, does the problem require intervention in regard to the care aspects of nursing, the curative aspects, the protective aspects, the teaching aspects, the coordinating aspects, or the patient advocate aspects?

In Mr. Jordan's case, he requires a number of interventions in regard to care, since he is unable to do many things himself. He will need help with hygiene, to list just one. In regard to the curative aspects, it is essential that he maintain the prescribed position in bed. He will require instruction (teaching aspect) in regard to maintaining the prescribed position in bed and in regard to turning. The protective aspects of Mr. Jordan's care include preventing the development of pressure areas. With regard to coordinating aspects, this may involve asking the social worker to help with locating Mr. Jordan's clothes and valuables. The nurse will act as a patient advocate when she requests the physician to discuss Mr. Jordan's plan of care with him and also his prognosis. These examples give just one possible intervention for Mr. Jordan in each of the six aspects of nursing; the nurse will note others in the plan of care for him.

Nursing interventions may also be categorized on the basis of whether they are preventive in nature, palliative (as, for example, to relieve suffering), restorative, or rehabilitative. The nurse will find it helpful to review the patient's problems under the headings used in this categorization of nursing interventions in planning her care of a patient.

In assessing the relative merits of different nursing interventions, the nurse uses her judgment to decide on the best alternative to use for this particular patient, at this particular time. For example, medications for pain are usually ordered q4h p.r.n. This is generally interpreted to mean that the medication may be repeated after an interval of 4 hours; it may be delayed longer than the 4 hours; or it may not be given at all if, in the nurse's judgment, the patient does not require it. There are several alternatives to giving medications to relieve pain. Sometimes altering the patient's position, straightening out the bedclothes and rearranging the pillows, giving a back massage, or talking with the patient may relieve his pain. (The subject of pain is discussed in Chapter 21.) In Mr. Jordan's case,

NURSING CARE PLAN — MR. PAUL JORDAN

Patient Problems	Expected Outcomes	Nursing Directions
1. Pain due to injury, aggravated by movement	1. Quiet and comfortable at all times. Calm facial expression, decreased restlessness, statements indicating that pain is lessened or absent	1. Medication for pain q4h. Give before pain too severe
2A. Limited mobility due to pain and prescribed position	2A. (a) Maintains prescribed position at all times except when on side for care	2A. (a) Prescribed position on back/bed flat: 2 pillows under head 1 pillow supporting shoulders 1 pillow under knees Verify that pt. understands prescribed position
	(b) Keeps trunk in good alignment at all times when turning on side	(b) May turn on side for back care, linen change. Pt. can help with turning Teach "log-rolling" technique for turning; repeat p.r.n.
	(c) When allowed out of bed, maintains trunk in good alignment at all times when sitting, standing, walking	(c) Discuss long-range plans with pt.'s M.D.
2B. Potential problem of loss of strength and tone in unused muscles	2B. Prevent	2B. Same as 2A (c)
2C. Potential problem of contractures in ankle joints	2C. Prevent	2C. Apply footboard and cradle to bed
3. Sensitivity to touch in lower back area due to site of injury, bruised tissues	3. Absences of sudden involuntary movements and verbal expressions of pain or facial grimaces when given care	3. Use gentle movements, extreme care when giving back massage, assisting pt. with bath, or giving other care Avoid pressure on vertebral column, also bruised area
4. Potential deviations in vital signs because of possibility of internal injuries	4. Normal vital signs	4. Monitor v.s. q4h Report deviations from normal Observe: (a) Rate, volume, quality of pulse (b) B.P., watching for marked or sudden change (c) Rate and depth of respirations (d) Temperature (e) Color and temperature of skin
5. Difficulty in voiding, owing to possible nerve damage or internal injuries	5. Normal urinary output	5. (a) Intake and output q shift (b) Observe output: 1. Amount 2. Color 3. Blood in urine (c) Report promptly if no output >8 hr. or output under 200 cc. q shift
6. Anxiety due to uncertainty about M.D.'s plan of care, prognosis	6. Relieved by information as evidenced by verbal statements and relaxed facial expression	6. Ask M.D. to explain his plans and discuss prognosis with pt.

NURSING CARE PLAN — MR. PAUL JORDAN (*Continued*)

Patient Problems	Expected Outcomes	Nursing Directions
7. Anxiety due to loss of clothes and valuables	7. Relieved by information that belongings have been found, as evidenced by verbal statements of pt.	7. Request social worker to come in as soon as possible
8. Possible decreased mental alertness due to medication for pain (a) May fall from bed (b) May burn self when smoking or set bed on fire	8. (a) Prevent (b) Prevent	8. (a) 1. Apply siderails to bed 2. Keep siderails up at all times (b) Delegate someone to stay with pt. when smoking q shift
9A. Dry mouth due to NPO	9A. Moist lips and tongue; moist mucous membranes in oral cavity at all times	9A. Oral hygiene q4h and p.r.n. Offer chewing gum p.r.n. Check with M.D. about ice chips to suck Offer lip moisturizer q4h p.r.n.
9B. Potential problem of dry mucous membranes in oral cavity, lips dry and cracking (see #9A)	9B. Prevent, as evidenced by #9A	9B. As in #9A
9C. Potential problem of maintaining nutritional status due to NPO	9C. Prevent	9C. 5% D/S I.V. t.i.d. × 2 (see medication order) Check with M.D. about d/c
10. Potential pressure areas over bony prominences: sacral area, heels, elbows (due to #2)	10. Prevent, as evidenced by good condition of skin, absence of redness and abrasions	10. (a) Gentle massage of back and areas mentioned q4h Use hospital lotion Be careful when massaging back (see 1.b) Pt. can be on side for back massage (note instructions above) (b) Apply lubricant to elbows, heels
11. Potential problem of constipation due to NPO and bed rest	11. Normal bowel movement q1-2 days	11. Note B.M. record q shift Check with pt. daily in a.m. Report deviation from normal Observe stools for signs of blood (see #5)
12. (a) Inability to look after own hygiene	12. (a) Maintains good hygiene at all times	12. (a) Assist pt. with bed bath daily Pt. can clean teeth himself—needs help to hold kidney basin Comb hair daily after bath and p.r.n. Pt. can clean and cut fingernails Clean and cut toenails p.r.n.
(b) Potential problem of poor status of skin and appendages	(b) Prevent. Skin clean and in good condition at all times; hair untangled at all times; nails clean, in good condition	(b) As in #12(a)
13. Potential feelings of isolation (family far away, friends working)	13. Prevent, as evidenced by patient's verbal statements	13. Request a friend to phone family in East Encourage friends to visit when not working
14. Potential problem of anxiety over finances due to anticipated lengthy convalescence and possibility of having to change occupation	14. Prevent, as evidenced by patient's verbal statements following discussions with social worker	14. Alert social worker to potential problem (see #7)

he is having severe pain and it is important that the medication for pain be given sufficiently early to keep him comfortable and relaxed at all times while the pain is so severe. Restlessness caused by mounting pain could cause further injury to his damaged vertebrae.

Writing a Nursing Care Plan. To facilitate the implementation of nursing action, many agencies have developed a system of nursing care plans. The nursing care plan is just what one would expect it to be: the plan of care for the patient. It usually includes a statement of the patient's problems, the expected outcomes that have been established, and the specific nursing measures that are to be used in caring for the patient. The care plan is developed as soon after the patient's admission as sufficient data are available on which to base a plan. It is developed by the nurse who has primary responsibility for the patient's care; or, in some agencies, it is developed jointly by the nursing team responsible for caring for the patient.

Because the patient's problems may change from day to day when he is acutely ill, the nursing care plan for the sick person is constantly under revision. Care plans for patients in ambulatory care settings, and for those in extended care facilities, also need frequent revision but usually not as often as those for patients in acute care settings.

In some agencies, the nursing action to be taken is written in terms of nursing orders, which are prescribed and followed through in much the same way as doctors' orders. In other agencies, the term "nursing approach," "nursing actions," or "nursing directions" may be used to identify the specific nursing interventions to be used in the care of the patient.

The nursing care plan is a means of communicating in writing, to other nursing personnel and to other members of the health team, the patient's problems, the expected outcomes of nursing care, and the specific nursing action to be taken in the care of the patient. In many agencies, the care plans are incorporated into the patient's record; in some, they form part of a Kardex report. Sometimes a separate notebook is kept for nursing care plans.

A nursing care plan for Mr. Jordan is shown on pages 132–133.

Standard Care Plans. Because nurses have found that most patients with similar types of conditions have many problems in common, a number of agencies have developed standard care plans for use with patients who have a particular type of condition. There might be a standard care plan for all medical patients, for example, supplemented by a plan for all patients who have suffered a stroke. There might be another standard care plan for all surgical patients, supplemented by one for patients who are having one particular type of surgical intervention. It should be noted that space is always left on these standard care plans for unusual problems that a patient has—problems that are not anticipated and are unique to this patient.

IMPLEMENTATION

Once nursing care plans have been developed, the next step is to put them into action. The nursing directions (or nursing approach or orders) must be sufficiently detailed and sufficiently specific to enable all nursing personnel to carry them out in the same manner and at the designated times.

In some agencies, the nursing care plans are supplemented by a record that lists the nursing directions (taken from the care plan) and provides spaces for the nurse to tick as each intervention is carried out. This type of record acts as a checklist for the nurse responsible for the patient's care on each shift so she may quickly see what is to be done. It is also easy to see at a glance if any intervention was omitted.

Another type of form, similar in purpose to the one described above, is the flowsheet. When one specific intervention or a group of related interventions are to be done on a regular basis (as, for example, daily, or at more frequent intervals), it is helpful to have a special form that details the intervention specifically and documents the results of that intervention. See Chapter 12 for more details.

In implementing nursing action, the nurse may give direct care to a patient or engage in indirect activities that contribute to his care. She may give the patient a bath, administer his medications, or supervise others in doing these things for him. Nursing care includes a wide variety of specific nursing interventions. As the student progresses through her educational program, she will learn a good many types of interventions; she will continue to do so throughout her nursing career. Specific nursing interventions in Mr. Jordan's care have been identified in the plan of care prepared for him.

EVALUATION

Throughout her care, the nurse constantly evaluates the progress the patient has made toward reaching the pre-established goals. Evaluation is the process of determining the extent to which objectives have been attained. It implies measurement against predetermined standards. If the expected outcome of nursing care has been carefully thought through and the standards have been clearly stated, the nurse can compare the patient's attainments with these standards. For example, in Mr. Jordan's case, one expected outcome for his problem of limited mobility has been stated as "maintains prescribed position at all times, except when necessary to turn on side for care." The physician has been very explicit in describing the prescribed position. In evaluating the patient's attainment of the expected outcome, the nurse checks through the points enumerated regarding the position. Is Mr. Jordan's bed flat? Is he on his back? Does he have two pillows under his head? Is one supporting his shoulders? Does he have a pillow under his knees? Is he maintaining this position at all times, except when it is necessary to turn on his side for a back rub or for the bed linen to be changed?

In evaluating the effectiveness of nursing action, it is important to have definite criteria in mind. These criteria should be observable and they should be measurable. Then progress can be noted and, if a particular nursing approach does not appear to be effective, an alternative course of action can be tried. The attainment of certain goals may mean that the patient is ready for more far-reaching ones. The patient who has learned to dress himself, for example, may be ready to learn other activities of daily living.

Stating criteria in question form helps the nurse to be objective and to look for specific indications that expected outcomes have been met. Questions are not always written down, but the beginning nurse may find it easier to develop the habit of asking herself the questions implicit in the nursing goals for the patient if she does put them onto paper.

The effectiveness of nursing care is evaluated by the nurse through her observations of the patient. Is his paralyzed arm in good anatomical position, or is the hand in a dependent position? It is also necessary to ask the patient if nursing intervention has been effective. Is he more comfortable? Is he free from pain?

In addition to evaluating the effectiveness of nursing action in relation to the patient's attainment of the expected outcomes, the nurse examines critically the soundness of the plan that was developed. Did she have enough information? Did she take all relevant factors into consideration in assessing the data she had? Did she omit any problems for which nursing care could have helped this patient? Were the priorities she established indeed the most important things to be taken care of? Was her plan a logical outgrowth of the problems she identified? Did she take into consideration unique factors in regard to this patient? Was her plan consistent with the physician's plan of therapy? Were the expected outcomes logical and attainable, in view of the patients' problems? Were the nursing directions clearly stated? Was the plan successful? Were there factors that interfered with its success? Factors that contributed to its success? Is the plan current and up-to-date? Have some of the problems been resolved? Have any new ones emerged?

As was stated at the beginning of the chapter, the nursing process is a circular one. Evaluation means a reassessment and a gathering of additional new information. On the basis of her reassessment, the nurse may identify new problems, modify her plan of care, or decide to try alternative interventions for ones that were unsuccessful.

To complete the story on Mr. Jordan: his clothes and valuables were found; they had been left in the plane and the air charter company returned them (one problem resolved). He was taken off NPO after 48 hours (another problem resolved) and progressed through a normal convalescence. His nursing care plan needed to be revised several times.

SUMMARY

The nursing process provides a methodology for a systematic approach to nursing care. The four basic steps in the process (assessment, planning, implementation, and evaluation) follow one another in logical, sequential order. Nursing is primarily concerned with assisting an individual to cope with the daily activities of living in such a way as to promote his optimal level of health, or to cope with the exigencies of terminal illness, if such be the case. In order to help the individual, the nurse needs to know something about him as a person, his usual coping abilities, anything that is interfering with these, and his present status in relation to these abilities. She also needs to know the plans his physician has for his care if the individual has a recognized health problem.

The nurse gathers the information she needs from several sources. Some of it she collects herself through the nursing history and through her observations of the patient; some comes from the individual's family, his friends, or significant others. She also utilizes data collected by other health professionals and she makes use of records, reports, and other forms of written material to extend her data base about the patient.

She analyzes the information she has gathered

from all sources in order to identify problems that can be resolved by nursing actions, and to set priorities for action.

She uses relevant scientific principles gained from her studies to guide her in establishing objectives that define the expected outcomes of nursing action in terms of the patient's behavior and in developing a plan for nursing interventions that will enable the patient to attain these objectives.

Continuous reassessment takes place during the process of implementing the plan of care as new information is gathered and the patient's progress in attaining the expected outcomes is evaluated. Implicit in this reassessment is the need for constant revision of nursing care plans as new problems emerge, some are resolved, and some change. Priorities may need to be reordered, objectives modified or new ones established, and decisions made regarding appropriate nursing interventions in the light of new information, changes that have occurred in the patient's condition, and the success or failure of interventions that have been tried.

STUDY SITUATION

In conjunction with your instructor, select one patient who has recently been admitted to the nursing unit on which you are having clinical experience:

1. Review the nursing history and initial clinical appraisal done on this patient.

2. Review other data that have been collected that you feel would be helpful in planning his nursing care.

3. State nursing problems you can identify.

4. Arrange these problems in a list according to priorities as you see them.

5. Identify principles relevant to this patient's care.

6. State the expected outcomes of nursing care in relation to each of the problems you have listed.

7. Compare your problem statement list and statements of expected outcomes of care with those on the nursing care plan prepared by unit staff. Did you identify the same problems? Did you miss any? Identify different ones not listed? Use similar wording in stating problems? Did you rank priorities in the same order? If not, why do you think it was different? Were your goal statements similar?

8. Review the nursing directions included in the nursing care plan, and flowsheets or other forms prepared to facilitate care. Relate these directions to the patient's problems and to principles underlying care.

9. Describe how you would evaluate the effectiveness of the nursing care plan.

SUGGESTED READINGS

Catanzaro, M.: MS: Nursing Care. *American Journal of Nursing,* 80(2):286–291, February, 1980.

Gordon, M., Sweeney, M. A., and McKeehan, K.: Nursing Diagnosis. Looking at its use in the clinical area. *American Journal of Nursing,* 80(4):672–674, April, 1980.

Gray, J. W., and Aldred, H.: Care Plans in Long-term Facilities. *American Journal of Nursing,* 80(11):2054–2057, November, 1980.

Lewis, L.: *Planning Patient Care.* 2nd Edition. Iowa, Brown Co., 1976.

Little, D. E., and Carnevali, D. L.: *Nursing Care Planning.* 2nd Edition. Philadelphia, J. B. Lippincott Co., 1976.

Marriner, A.: *The Nursing Process, A Scientific Approach to Nursing Care.* St. Louis, C. V. Mosby, 1975.

Price, M. R.: Nursing Diagnosis: Making a Concept Come Alive. *American Journal of Nursing,* 80(4):668–671, April, 1980.

Robinson, J. (ed.): *Documenting Patient Care Responsibility.* Horsham, Pa., Intermed Communications, 1978. (Nursing 78 Skillbook Series.)

Silverhorn, A.: Nursing Care Plans: A Vital Tool. *The Canadian Nurse,* 75(3):36–41, March, 1979.

Vasey, E. K.: Writing Your Patient's Care Plan . . . . Efficiently. *Nursing 79,* 9(4):67–71, April, 1979.

Wells, T. J.: Clinical Nursing: Curiouser and Curiouser. *American Journal of Nursing,* 79(10):1757–1760, October, 1979.

REFERENCES

1. McCain, R. F.: Nursing by Assessment—Not Intuition. *American Journal of Nursing*, 65:82–84, April, 1965.
2. Henderson V.: *The Nature of Nursing: A Definition and Its Implications for Practice, Research and Education*. New York, Macmillan Company, 1966.
3. Taylor, D. B., and Johnson, O. H.: Systematic Nursing Assessment: A Step Toward Automation. DHEW publication No. (HRA) 74–17. Washington, D.C., U.S. Government Printing Office, 1974.
4. Pearlman, E.: *Manual for the Use of the Nursing History Tool*. Gainesville, Fla., University of Florida College of Nursing, 1971.
5. Mayers, M. G.: *A Systematic Approach to the Nursing Care Plan*. New York, Appleton-Century-Crofts, 1972.
6. Nordmark, M. T., and Rohweder, A. W.: *Scientific Foundations of Nursing*. 3rd edition. Philadelphia, J. B. Lippincott, 1975.
7. Registered Nurses Association of British Columbia: *Manual of Information for the Preparation and Utilization of Nursing Care Plans*. Vancouver, British Columbia.
8. Mager, R. F.: *Preparing Instructional Objectives*. Palo Alto, Cal., Fearon Publishers, 1962.

9

The Nurse Should Be Able to:

- Describe methods and techniques of observation used in the clinical assessment of a patient
- Demonstrate skill in taking a patient's temperature (oral, rectal, and axillary)
- Demonstrate skill in taking a pulse
- Demonstrate skill in observing respirations
- Demonstrate skill in taking blood pressure
- Demonstrate beginning skill in observing deviations from the normal in a patient's functional abilities
- Outline responsibilities of the nurse in assisting with the physical examination of a patient
- Describe common positions patients are asked to assume for examination or treatment, i.e., supine, Sims's, knee-chest
- Outline nursing responsibilities in assisting with laboratory tests
- Explain the use of common diagnostic tools such as roentgenography (x-ray, fluoroscopy, CAT scan), nuclear medicine studies, ultrasound scans, thermography, and electrodiagnostic examinations (EEG, ECG, EMG)
- Outline guidelines for assisting with tests and examinations before, during, and after the procedure

CLINICAL ASSESSMENT SKILLS

CHAPTER 9

INTRODUCTION

Nurses today take increasing responsibility for both the initial and the ongoing assessment of patients in the health care system. Not too long ago, only physicians were allowed to take a blood pressure. Today, nurses in many areas have the responsibility for assessment. For example, specially trained nurses in maternal and child health often undertake the first critical examination of the newborn. Community health nurses and pediatric nurse practitioners are responsible for ongoing health assessment of infants and children, while more and more nurses involved in school health programs carry out the pre-school health examination of children.

We could continue with many more examples of nurses who are taking increasing responsibility for clinical assessment—of adults as well as children. We mentioned several when discussing nurse practitioners and clinical nursing specialists in Chapter 6. The important point is that assessment is an integral part of every nurse's daily practice. The nurse begins to develop her assessment skills early in her educational program and continues to expand them during her nursing studies and throughout her professional career. These skills begin with the ability to make intelligent observations.

Intelligent observations are based on the nurse's knowledge of the biomedical, physical, and social sciences. As the nurse's knowledge increases through education and experience, she develops increasing skill in observing significant factors in the patient's appearance, behavior, and physical and social environment. She learns what to look for in making observations, and how to differentiate the normal from the abnormal. Skill in observing requires a knowledge of what is normal, the ability to identify and de-

scribe deviations from the normal, and the capacity to assess the significance of these deviations.

We have chosen here to use the functional abilities approach for the development of beginning skills in clinical assessment. The observations described in this chapter do not require extensive skills in physical examination. They depend rather on acquisition of basic skills such as taking temperature, pulse, respirations, and blood pressure, and utilization by the student of her awareness of the structure and functioning of her own body to detect readily observable deviations from the normal in regard to an individual's functional abilities.

As we progress through this textbook in our discussions of the nurse's role in helping people to meet their basic needs in order to promote their optimal health, we will enlarge on the assessment of specific functional abilities. For example, assessing an individual's nutritional status will be described in greater detail in the chapter on nutritional needs, assessing respiratory status in the chapter on oxygen needs. In schools of nursing where preparation for an expanded role is incorporated into the basic curriculum, the student will learn additional skills in physical examination. Nurses who do not gain these extended skills in their basic program may learn them in any of the numerous continuing education courses on physical assessment that are available in many colleges and universities.

Besides making observations for her own nursing assessment, the nurse often assists in carrying out procedures that are part of the medical assessment of a patient's health status. She is usually responsible for preparing patients, both mentally and physically, for the various diagnostic tests and procedures that they undergo and often collects the specimens for different laboratory tests. She carries out many of the tests and procedures herself, either as dependent functions on orders from the physician or, more and more often today, as independent functions on her own initiative.

We have included in this chapter, then, information of a general nature about the more common measures used in the detection of illness. More detailed information about diagnostic tests and examinations used in the assessment of various body systems is included where pertinent in the chapters on specific needs.

OBSERVATION TECHNIQUES AND VALIDATION

Some authorities call any information that the nurse acquires about an individual observations. The term is used here, however, to denote the information the nurse obtains about the patient through the use of her senses of *sight, hearing, smell,* and *touch.* The nurse *looks* at a child's face, for example, to inspect the rash on his cheek; she *listens* to the wheezing breath sounds of the asthmatic; she *smells* the fruity breath odor of children with high fevers; she *touches* a painful ankle to see how much swelling there is.

Visual examination for the detection of abnormalities is called *inspection*. The observations are detailed and focused on a particular area of the body. *Palpation is the method of examining by using one's fingers*. Size, texture, temperature, swelling, and hardness are qualities noted by palpation. *Auscultation* is the listening for sounds within the body. Direct auscultation, with the ear placed on the body, is seldom used; instruments to amplify the sounds are used instead, the most common example being the stethoscope. *Percussion* is the tapping of various parts of the body and listening to the sound that ensues. It may be done directly, as in striking the chest wall with a fingertip, or by laying one finger on a body surface and striking it with another.

The nurse's physical senses are augmented by tools such as the *clinical thermometer,* the *sphygmomanometer* (instrument used for measuring blood pressure) and the *stethoscope* (mentioned above), which have been developed to obtain measurements indicative of the functioning of various body processes. In addition to these commonly used tools, a wide variety of instruments and machines are used to assist in the observation and measurement of vital body processes. The student will see, and later will probably use, cardiac monitoring machines, for example, in emergency rooms and in the intensive and coronary care units of most hospitals.

Observations reported by the nurse include both *objective findings, that is, what the nurse observes, and the patient's subjective observations*. To use an example, the nurse may observe that an individual is not moving his right arm; this is an *objective* observation made by the nurse. The individual may say, "My right arm is very painful." This is a *subjective* observation on the patient's part.

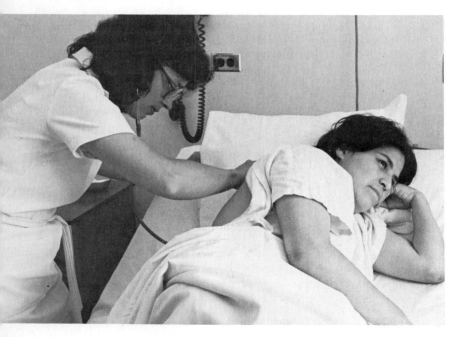

Ongoing assessment is an integral part of nursing care.

The Validation of Observations

Information the nurse obtains from talking with the patient and from her observations should always be validated by checking with the patient as to whether the impressions she has gained are in line with his perceptions.

THE VITAL SIGNS

Temperature, pulse, and respirations have traditionally been referred to as the *vital*, or *cardinal*, signs of life. Together with blood pressure and heart beat, they indicate basic physiological functioning, specifically in the functional areas of temperature status, circulatory status, and respiratory status. In making observations about an individual's current functional abilities, the nurse frequently starts with the vital signs.

In assessing vital signs, it is important to remember that each individual has his own *circadian (diurnal) rhythm*, or a 24-hour biological time clock, that regulates the daily events in his life. The rhythm is evident in biological functioning such as body temperature, sleep, and blood pressure, and the nurse will note differences in the vital signs of her patients at different times of the day. Normally, a person's temperature, for example, is lowest in the early morning hours and highest in the late afternoon or early evening. Blood pressure, in most individuals, is also highest after the individual has been active for a good part of the day.

Although temperature, pulse, respirations, and blood pressure readings vary from individual to individual and at different times of the day in the same individual, there is a range that is generally considered to be normal for each of these signs. Normal ranges for individuals in different age groups are included in each of the following sections on temperature, pulse, respirations, and blood pressure.

Because of the variable nature of vital sign measurements—from one individual to another, and within the same individual at different times of the day and in various states of health and illness—it is important to establish a data base for each patient as soon after admission to a health agency as possible. A series of readings, undertaken systematically and in a consistent manner (preferably by the nurse who is caring for the patient), helps to determine what is normal for that particular individual, to identify deviations from the normal and to pick up trends in the early stages. For example, if a patient's temperature is usually around 97.0° F (36.1° C) before breakfast but, one morning, you find it to be 99.5° F (37.5° C) and, by noon, it is 100.4° F

(38° C), you would suspect that he is developing a fever, even though all temperature readings fall within the 'normal' range.

It is important, too, to interpret vital sign readings in relation to other information you have about a patient. In Mr. Jordan's case (Chapter 8), vital signs are being monitored closely for the first 48 hours after admission to watch for indications of internal injury. A sudden drop in his blood pressure, an increase in pulse rate (or irregularity of rhythm or weakness of the pulse), or a lowered body temperature, with or without rapid and deep respirations, would alert the nurse to the possibility of internal bleeding and should be reported promptly to the physicians in charge of Mr. Jordan's case.

Temperature

The surface temperature of the body fluctuates with the temperature of the surroundings. In a cool room, for example, exposed skin surfaces soon feel cold and are cold to the touch. The internal, or core, temperature of the body, on the other hand, is precisely regulated and maintained within a very narrow range. It is this internal temperature which is usually measured as an indicator of a person's temperature status. Under normal conditions it does not vary more than a degree or so from the mean, or average, for that person. Variances greater than that are usually indicative of disturbed functioning of the body's heat regulating system.

The temperature regulating system is one of the principal homeostatic mechanisms whereby the internal climate of the body is maintained at an optimal level for functioning. The center for controlling the internal temperature of the body is located in the hypothalamus, in the lower portion of the brain. In health this center maintains a fairly precise balance between heat production and heat loss. Heat is continually being produced in the body as a byproduct of metabolism. It is also constantly being lost through *evaporation* (perspiration from the skin); *radiation* (the transfer of heat in the form of electromagnetic waves), e.g., from the body to cooler objects in the environment; *conduction* (the transfer of heat from a warmer to a cooler substance by direct contact), e.g., from the body to the surrounding air; and *convection* (movement of air), as currents around the body carry away heat that has been conducted to the air from the body surface. The factors affecting heat production and the processes by which heat is lost from the body are described in more detail in Chapter 19.

The *body temperature*, as measured by a clinical thermometer, reflects the balance between heat production and heat loss. It usually varies slightly during the course of a 24-hour period in any one individual, being lowest during the early morning hours before a person wakens and highest in the evening. The cycle may be reversed in persons who work at night and sleep during the day. Many people who are ill have an elevated temperature; it is often one of the first observable indications of disturbed body function. In addition, a temperature below normal may be indicative of illness.

Factors other than disease processes, however, can affect body temperature. The activity of the individual can make some difference, with the active person usually having a higher temperature than the sedentary person. Exercise can cause a marked, but temporary, elevation in body temperature. Age also affects temperature; the infant and the aged often have a body temperature of 0.6° C (1° F) higher than the young adult. Emotions and anxiety can increase the basal metabolic rate of an individual and thereby elevate temperature.

The normal range for body temperature in most adults is considered to be between 36.1° C and 38.0° C (97° F and 100.4° F) when taken orally. The rectal temperature is expected to be approximately 0.6° C (1° F) higher and the axillary temperature, 0.6° C (1° F) lower. Pyrexia and fever are two terms used to refer to an elevated temperature. The term hypothermia refers to a temperature that is below normal.

Procedures for Taking Temperature. Body temperature is usually measured with a clinical thermometer, which is an elongated glass tube calibrated in degrees Celsius (centigrade) or degrees Fahrenheit. Within the tube is a column of mercury, which expands in response to the heat of the body. The scale on the thermometer generally starts at about 33° C (91.5° F) and terminates at 44° C (111° F). The conversion between the Fahrenheit and Celsius scales is shown in the table above. Calibrations beyond this scale are considered unnecessary, because temperatures above and below these limits rarely occur.

In addition to the standard clinical thermometer, a number of other devices are also used to measure body temperature. Disposable thermometers are available. Also commercially marketed is a temperature-sensitive tape that can be used in the home (it is also used in some health agencies) for infants and small children. The tape is usually applied to the child's abdomen and will change color if the temperature is above or below normal. If deviations are noted, the temperature should be taken with a standard

FAHRENHEIT AND CELSIUS (CENTIGRADE) SCALES IN MESUREMENT OF BODY TEMPERATURE

Fahrenheit	Celsius
93.2	34.0
95.0	35.0
96.8	36.0
97.7	36.5
98.6	37.0
99.5	37.5
100.4	38.0
101.3	38.5
102.2	39.0
103.1	39.5
104.0	40.0
105.8	41.0
107.6	42.0
109.4	43.0
111.2	44.0

In order to convert Fahrenheit to Celsius, subtract 32 from the Fahrenheit reading and multiply by the fraction 5/9; thus $C = 5/9 \ (F - 32)$. To convert Celsius to Fahrenheit, multiply the Celsius reading by 9/5 and add 32; thus $F = 9/5 \ C + 32$.

thermometer to obtain a more accurate measurement.

Electronic thermometers are also widely used today. With these, it is possible both to get an accurate temperature reading in a few seconds and to monitor temperature over a period of time. The electronic thermometer consists of a monitor that registers the temperature on a dial and an attached probe for insertion into a body cavity. When it is considered important to maintain a constant surveillance of the body temperature, an alarm attached to the probe may be set to alert the person watching the monitor when the patient's temperature deviates from within a set range. Different types of probes are used with the electronic thermometer, depending on the purpose for which it is being used. For example, sometimes it is considered important to monitor a small infant's temperature. For this procedure, a small, flexible vinyl probe might be inserted into the infant's esophagus. An attachable surface probe would be used for assessing skin temperature.

The most common site for obtaining a measure of internal body temperature is the mouth (per os). The small blood vessels on the underside of the tongue lie close to the surface. When the thermometer is placed under the tongue (in the sublingual pocket) and the mouth is closed, it is possible to obtain a reasonably accurate estimate of the body's internal temperature. If the patient has been smoking, or has just had a hot or a cold drink, it is best to wait at least 15 minutes before taking an oral temperature. The thermometer is wiped off, shaken down, and placed

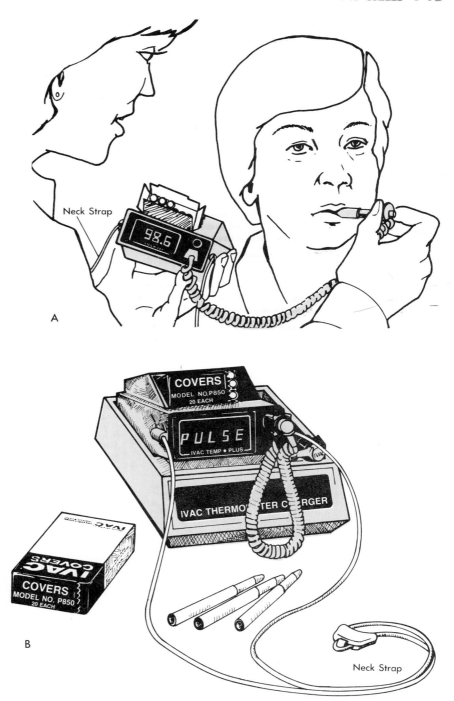

A

B

Electronic thermometers provide quick, accurate temperature readings in both Fahrenheit and Celsius degrees and can be used for monitoring temperature over a period of time.

sublingually (under the tongue) for 7 to 10 minutes. The patient is instructed to hold the thermometer between his lips and avoid biting it. After the thermometer is removed and the temperature noted, the thermometer is wiped off, shaken down, rinsed under cold running water and dried. In wiping a thermometer, a rotating or twisting motion is used. The thermometer is wiped starting from the tip and working down-ward to the mercury bulb, that is, from clean to dirty.

The conventional clinical thermometer is usually kept in a small vial containing a disinfectant. Various kinds of disinfectants are used to soak the thermometers; the synthetic phenols, isopropyl alcohol (70 per cent), and tincture of Zephiran (1:1000) are all considered suitable. Because thermometers are soaked in a disinfectant when not in use, they need to be washed or wiped off carefully before they are given to patients. The method of disinfecting thermometers varies in different agencies. However, the same basic steps are usually followed: wiping off the thermometer to remove mucus and secretions, shaking down the mercury, rinsing in cold water, drying, and soaking in a disinfecting agent.

It is frequently necessary to take a patient's temperature via the *rectum*. Traditionally, the temperature of infants has been taken rectally, but this practice has been questioned by researchers.[3] This method is indicated for adults when it is considered either unsafe or inaccurate to take the temperature by mouth, as when a patient is unconscious or irrational. It is customary in many agencies for a rectal temperature to be taken when a person is receiving oxygen therapy, when he has a Levin tube in place, or when he has had oral or nasal surgery. The rectal method should not be used for people with diseases of the rectum, those with diarrhea, or those who have had rectal surgery. The patient lies on his side for this measure. After the thermometer is wiped off and shaken down, it is lubricated with petrolatum or other lubricant. This facilitates the insertion of the thermometer into the rectum and lessens the danger of irritating the mucous membrane. The thermometer is inserted from 1 to 2 inches and held in place for at least 2½ minutes. When it is removed, the temperature is noted, and the thermometer is wiped, washed in cold soapy water, and gently shaken down before being returned to its container. It is important to removal all fecal material and to wash the thermometer in cold or lukewarm water, since organic materials interfere with disinfection. The use of cool water prevents the coagulation of protein material. Hot water is never used because it may damage the thermometer.

• Rectal and oral thermometers are sometimes differentiated by the color of the bulb. Oral bulbs are often silver and rectal bulbs are blue. In addition, some rectal thermometers are more rounded at the ends, although many thermometers may be used for taking either rectal or oral temperatures.

Taking an axillary temperature is safer than taking an oral temperature for irrational or mentally disturbed patients. Axillary temperature readings are also safe and accurate for infants in a controlled environment. The thermometer is treated in the same manner as the oral thermometer. For adults, the axilla is dried before the thermometer is inserted, because moisture conducts heat. The thermometer is placed between the inner surface of the patient's arm and the

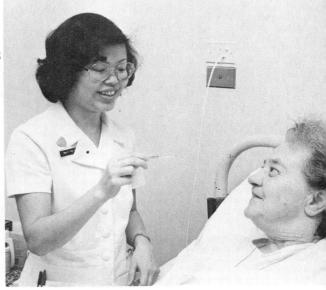

An elevated temperature is often one of the first indications of disturbed body functioning.

side while his arm is held across his chest. The thermometer is left in place for at least 10 minutes; then it is removed and the temperature is noted. The nurse can expect the axillary temperature to be approximately 0.6° C (1° F) lower than the oral temperature.

A temperature reading taken in the *esophagus* is considered to be a more accurate reflection of the internal or core temperature of the body than that taken at any other site. It is difficult to obtain, however, and is only used when precise measurements are required as, for example, in premature infants, or in adults who are receiving a type of therapy that involves lowering of the body temperature (hypothermia). The esophageal temperature is usually a little more than one half of a Fahrenheit degree, or 0.3° C, higher than that taken by the oral route.

Sometimes it is important to assess the tem-

In order to obtain an axillary temperature the thermometer is placed in the patient's axilla, and then his arm is placed across his chest.

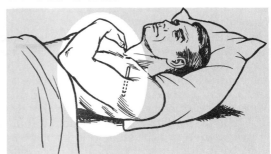

perature of the *skin surface*, as, for example, in patients who have had a skin transplant. A general assessment may be done by using the fingers to palpate the area. It is suggested that the backs of the fingers be used for this procedure, because the nerve endings are more sensitive to subtle temperature changes there than on the pads of the fingers. If more accurate measurements are needed, it is better to use a clinical thermometer, for example, an electronic thermometer with a surface probe.

Pulse

Pulse is the throbbing of an artery as it is felt over a bony prominence. When the left ventricle of the heart contracts, blood surges through the systemic arteries. This wave of blood is felt as the pulse.

At rest the heart is required to pump only 4 to 6 liters of blood per minute. This volume is increased as much as five times during exercise. Normally each ventricle pumps 70 ml. of blood with each contraction, although wide variations in the amount are compatible with life. This volume of output is reflected in the pulsations that can be felt where arteries pass over bones.

When taking a pulse, the rate, rhythm, size (volume), and tension (elasticity) of the pulse are noted. The *rate* of the pulse is the number of beats per minute. Deviations from the normal frequently are seen in illness. In addition, a number of factors other than disease processes also affect the pulse rate. Pulse rate varies according to age, sex, size, and physical and emotional activity, for example. The pulse rate decreases as a child grows and continues to decrease until extreme old age. Men generally have a slower pulse rate than women. Exercise increases the rate of cardiac contractions, and when a person is experiencing strong emotions, such as anxiety, fear, or anger, the heart usually beats faster also (see Chapter 29). A pulse rate between 60 and 80 beats per minute is usually considered normal for most adults. The normal range and average of pulse rates for children from birth to 18 years is shown in the table above. If the pulse rate is greatly accelerated (for example, over 100 beats per minute), the condition is referred to as *tachycardia*. A very slow pulse rate (under 60 beats per minute) is called *bradycardia*.

The *rhythm* of the pulse refers to the pattern of the beats. In health the rhythm is *regular*; that is, the time between beats is essentially the same. The pulse is *irregular* when the beats follow each other at irregular intervals.

The *size*, or amplitude, of a pulse wave reflects

NORMAL PULSE AND RESPIRATORY RATES FOR SPECIFIC AGES*

Age	Pulse (Beats per Minute)	Average Pulse
Newborn	70–170	120
2 years	80–130	110
4 years	80–120	100
6 years	75–115	100
8 years	70–110	90
10 years	70–110	90
12 years	70–110	85
14 years	65–105	85
16 years	60–100	85
18 years	50–90	80

*These are averages and vary with the sex of the child. From Tackett, J. J. M., and Hunsberger, M.: *Family-Centered Care of Children and Adolescents*. Philadelphia, W. B. Saunders Company, 1981.

the *volume* of blood pushed against the wall of the artery in the ventricular contraction. A *weak* pulse lacks a feeling of fullness and a definite beat; it may feel thready. When a pulse cannot be felt or heart, it is said to the *imperceptible*. A *bounding* pulse is one in which the volume reaches a higher level than normal, then disappears quickly.

The *tension* (elasticity) of the pulse refers to the compressibility of the arterial wall. If the pulse is obliterated by slight pressure, that is a pulse of low tension. A pulse that is obliterated only by relatively great pressure is a pulse of high pressure. The words "*soft*" and "*hard*" are used to describe pulse tension. Some health agencies prefer to use a numerical scale to assess the quality of the pulse. One such scale, with measurements from 0 to +4, describes the numerical measurements as follows:

0—Pulse is imperceptible (not palpable)
+1—Pulse is thready, weak and difficult to palpate—may fade in and out and is easily obliterated with pressure
+2—Pulse is difficult to palpate, may be obliterated by pressure—but stronger than +1
+3—Pulse is easily palpable, does not fade in and out, is not easily obliterated with pressure (considered to have normal volume)
+4—Pulse is strong, bounding, or hyperactive, easily palpable and not obliterated with pressure.[1]

Procedure for Taking the Pulse. Pulse is assessed by palpation, and there are numerous sites on the body at which a pulse may be obtained. When a person is lying on his back, one can normally observe pulsations from the carotid artery and, also, from the jugular vein. The carotid pulse shows as a brisk, localized throbbing; the jugular pulse is slow and undulating. In emergency situations, the carotid pulse is convenient to palpate to assess cardiac functioning. Care must be taken, though, to make sure that one does not inadvertently cut off, or seriously slow down, carotid circulation. Palpation should be done high in the neck, to avoid undue pressure on the carotid sinus, which is located just above the bifurcation of the artery into its external and internal branches. Excessive pressure on the artery is to be avoided and only one carotid artery should be palpated at a time.

In non-emergency situations, for assessment of a person's circulatory status, the peripheral pulses located in the head and the extremities are commonly used. Of these, the radial and the brachial pulses are the ones most frequently used by nurses. The radial site is used to assess the pulse, and the brachial site is used in taking the blood pressure. Other peripheral sites may be used for pulse assessment if the radial pulse is obscured, or if there is a need to test the circulation of blood to a specific area. The temporal, femoral, and dorsalis pedis pulses are three that are used most often.

The *radial pulse* is located on the inner aspect of the wrist on the thumb side where the radial

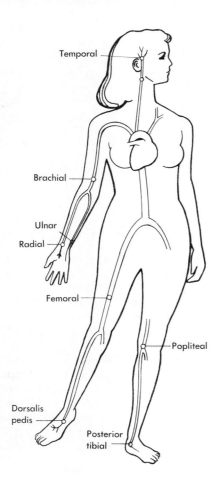

Temporal

Brachial

Ulnar

Radial

Femoral

Popliteal

Dorsalis pedis

Posterior tibial

artery passes over the radius. With slight pressure, the artery may be held against the radius so that the pulsations of blood may be felt. The *brachial pulse* is located on the anterior surface of the arm, just below the elbow, where the brachial artery passes over the ulna. The *temporal pulse* is felt anterior to the ear at the mandibular joint, where the temporal artery passes over the temporal bone. It can also be felt at the temple, that is, to the side of the eyebrow just in front of the hairline. The *femoral pulse* may be taken at the point in the middle of the groin where the femoral artery passes over the pelvic bone. The *dorsalis pedis pulse* (usually taken to assess circulation in the foot) can be felt on the dorsum of the foot in a line between the first and second toes, just above the longitudinal arch.

Other peripheral pulses that are sometimes used include the *ulnar*, which is on the opposite side of the wrist to the radial, the *posterior tibialis*, on the inner aspect of the ankle, and the *popliteal* pulse, which can be felt on the inner aspect of the back of the knee.

When the nurse takes the patient's pulse, she places her second, third, and fourth fingers lightly on the skin at the place where the artery passes over the underlying bone. The thumb is not used because the nurse might feel the pulsations of the radial artery of her own thumb. Usually, counting the rate for 30 seconds and then multiplying by two gives an accurate record of beats per minute. Some people prefer to count the rate for 15 seconds and multiply by four. If the pulse is irregular in any way it is counted apically for a full minute.

Generally the patient should lie or sit quietly so that his pulse rate can be compared with previous observations. Exercise and anxiety accelerate the pulse rate to an extent that it does not reflect the normal rate at rest.

Apical Beat. It is often necessary to determine the rate of the apical beat of the heart. The apical beat is the beat of the heart as felt at its apex. The apex is considered to be the point of maximal impulse. The apical beat can usually be heard in the fifth intercostal space, 2 to 3 inches to the left of the sternum, just below the left nipple. By listening with the stethoscope in this area, the point of maximal sound can usually be found.

To determine the apical beat, the bell of the stethoscope is placed over the apex of the heart and the beats are counted for a full minute. A heart beat is heard as "lubb-dubb." The "lubb" represents the closure of the atrioventricular or tricuspid and mitral valves; it occurs at the onset of systole. The "dubb" represents the closure of the semilunar (aortic and pulmonic) valves at the end of systole. The rhythm of the heart beat can also be noted and recorded in the patient's chart.

An *apical-radial* pulse is ascertained by two nurses. One nurse counts the patient's radial pulse at the same time that the second nurse counts the apical beats of the heart with the same watch. Each is counted for a full minute. In health, the apical and radial rates are the same, but in illness they sometimes differ, as when some apical beats are not transmitted to the radial artery. The difference between the apical rate and the radial rate is the *pulse deficit*.

Respirations

Respiration is a term used to cover both the exchange of oxygen and carbon dioxide that takes place in the lungs, and the exchange of these gases that takes place in the tissues (between the blood and body cells). The former is technically called *external* respiration, the latter *internal* (or *tissue*) respiration. When we are assessing respiration as one of the vital signs of body functioning, it is the external process we are measuring.

There are two principal movements involved in this respiration, *inspiration (inhalation)*, the act of breathing in, and *expiration (exhalation)*, the act of breathing out. The process is controlled primarily by the respiratory center in the medulla oblongata. This center is influenced by several factors, including chemical changes in the body (e.g., a high carbon dioxide level, which stimulates respiration), alterations in blood pressure (e.g., increased blood pressure, which inhibits respirations), and stimuli arising from the muscles (as, for example, exercise, which increases respiration). A more detailed discussion of the factors affecting respiration will be found in Chapter 18.

Respirations controlled in this manner are automatic. Their rate and depth are regulated within a range that meets the metabolic needs of the body for oxygen. Any activity that necessitates increased oxygen supply will result in more rapid and usually deeper respirations. It should be noted, however, that the rate and depth of respirations are to a certain extent under voluntary control. A person can take deep breaths or shallow breaths, or breathe more quickly or slowly, within the limitations imposed by the body's needs for oxygen.

Procedure for Observing Respirations. It is important to observe a person's respirations unobtrusively. It is often done after taking the pulse,

while the nurse has her fingers on the wrist. If a person is aware that his respirations are being observed, he usually finds it difficult to maintain his normal breathing pattern. In assessing respirations, they are observed for rate, depth, rhythm, and character. One counts the rate, watches the chest movements, and listens for breath sounds.

In calculating the respiratory *rate*, you count the respirations as you would the pulse, that is, count for 30 seconds and multiply by 2. If the respirations are irregular, they should always be counted for a full minute. Either the inspirations or the expirations are counted, but not both. Sometimes it is impossible to see a person's chest movements or hear his breathing. By placing a hand on the patient's chest, you can often feel the movements of the chest and count these. The average normal respiratory rate for infants is 34 to 40 per minute; for children, 24 to 32 per minute at 2 years, slowing down gradually to 20 to 26 at 10 years; in adults it is 14 to 20 per minute.[2] An abnormal increase in the respiratory rate is called *tachypnea (polypnea)*, and an abnormal decrease is technically referred to as *bradypnea*. Normal breathing, which is effortless, regular, and noiseless, is called *eupnea*. An absence of breathing is termed *apnea*.

The *depth* of respirations refers to the amount of air inhaled and exhaled with each breath movement. It is observed by watching the chest movements. Normal respirations result in deep and even movements of the chest. In *shallow* respirations, the rise and fall of the chest and abdomen are minimal. If the respirations are shallow and rapid, the person is said to be *short of breath*. The term *air hunger* is frequently used to describe respirations that are abnormally deep and accompanied by an increased respiratory rate.

The *rhythm* of respirations refers to the regularity of inspirations and expirations. Normal respirations follow one another evenly, with little variation in the length of the pauses between inspiration and expiration. *Symmetry* refers to the synchronous movements of each side of the chest. You may observe *asymmetrical* breathing in some individuals.

The *character* of respirations refers to digressions from normal, effortless breathing. *Labored breathing*, for example, involves active participation of accessory inspiratory and expiratory muscles. In normal breathing the principal muscles concerned are the diaphragm and, to a lesser extent, the external and internal intercostal muscles. If, for any reason, respiration becomes difficult, all the muscles attached to the thoracic cage are brought into play. These include the major and minor pectoral muscles, the sternomastoid, the scalene, and the subclavius. Difficulty in breathing accompanied by whistling sounds is called *wheezing*. If bubbling sounds can be heard in air cells (alveoli) or bronchial tubes, the term *rales* is used. Another descriptive term that is commonly used for noisy breathing is *stertorous* respirations.

Coughing is a means by which a person clears his respiratory tract of secretions and foreign material. A cough is almost always abnormal and should always be noted. The individual may tell you that the cough has come on suddenly (*acute cough*) or that he has had it for a long time (*chronic cough*). By listening to the person cough, you can usually ascribe certain qualities. Common descriptive terms include *hacking* (frequent short cough), and *paroxysmal* (sudden, periodic attack of coughing). A cough may be termed *dry* or *nonproductive* if the individual does not bring up any *sputum* (secretions from the bronchi or lungs) with the cough. If the person does bring up sputum (the cough is *productive*), you will need to describe the appearance of these secretions since sputum varies in character. It may appear *watery* (thin and colorless), *frothy* (having the appearance of being light and aerated, containing bubbles), or *viscous* (containing a thick, tenacious mucoid exudate). Sputum may also be described according to color; it may be *green, yellow, blood-tinged*, or *gray*. Sometimes sputum has a distinctive odor—it may have an offensive (*foul*) smell, for example, or sometimes a *sweetish* smell. In recording observations about sputum, you should also indicate the amount: *scant* (small amount), *moderate*, or *copious* (large amount). Often a 24-hour specimen of sputum is collected to obtain a more accurate estimate of volume.

Blood Pressure

Blood pressure refers to the pressure of the blood within the arteries of the body. When the left ventricle of the heart contracts, blood is forced out into the aorta and travels through the large arteries to the smaller arteries, arterioles, and capillaries. The pulsations extend from the heart through the arteries and disappear in the arterioles. The *systolic pressure* is the arterial pressure at the height of the pulsations; it is normally 120 mm. of mercury in a young adult. The *diastolic pressure* is the arterial pressure at the lowest level of the pulsation, that is, during ventricular relaxation. It is normally 80 to 90 mm. of mercury. The difference between the systolic and diastolic pressure is the *pulse pressure*.

A number of variables affect the arterial blood pressure. It is dependent on the *force* of the ventricular contractions of the heart and on the amount of blood ejected from the heart with each ventricular contraction (cardiac output). The force of the contractions depends on the pumping action of the heart. The greater the

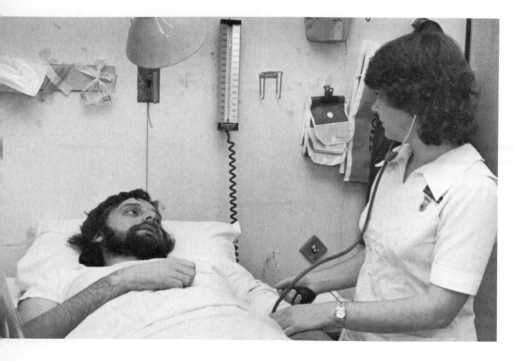

The nurse checks Paul Jordan's blood pressure as she monitors his vital signs.

strength of the pumping action, the more blood is ejected with each contraction.

The amount of cardiac output is also affected by the total *volume of blood* circulating in the body. A decrease in blood volume, such as occurs in hemorrhaging, will result in a lowered blood pressure. Changes in the *elasticity* of the muscular walls of the blood vessels also affect the blood pressure. Aging, for example, decreases the elasticity of muscular tissue, and an older person's blood pressure is usually higher than a younger person's. Blood pressure is also affected by the *viscosity* (thickness) of the blood, which is dependent on the number of red blood cells and on the amount of plasma protein it contains. Viscosity may be altered by disturbances of fluid balance. Another factor which affects the blood pressure is the *resistance of the peripheral vessels* (peripheral resistance). Normally, the pressure in the large blood vessels is high, and the pressure in the smaller vessels (the arterioles and capillaries) is low. Blood, as any other liquid, tends to flow from areas of high pressure to areas of low pressure. Factors that decrease the lumen of the blood vessels affect the smaller vessels proportionately more than the larger ones, and increase the amount of pressure required to pump the blood through them. Any constriction of the vessels, e.g., as when deposits occur on the lining of the vessels, increases the peripheral resistance and, therefore, the blood pressure.

An individual's blood pressure varies from hour to hour and from day to day. It falls during sleep and may be strikingly elevated by strong emotions, such as fear and anger, and by exercise. When a person is lying down, his blood pressure is lower than when he is sitting or standing. Also, the pressure may differ in the two arms of the same patient. Therefore, before taking the blood pressure for a comparison value, the nurse should check (a) the time of day, (b) the arm used, and (c) the position the patient was in for previous readings. The upper limits of normal blood pressures (over the brachial artery) as determined by the American

Standard blood pressure monitoring kit.

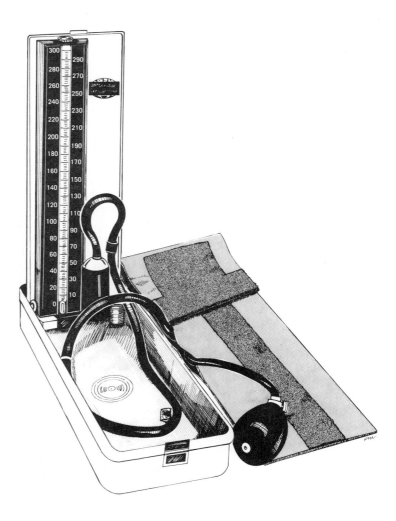

Heart Association for individuals of different ages are as follows:

✓	Infants	90/60 mm. Hg
	3–6 years	110/70
	7–10 years	120/80
	11–15 years	130/80
	15–20 years	130/85
	20–40 years	140/90
	40–60 years	160/95
	60–75 years	170/95
	75 years and older	180/100

An abnormal elevation of blood pressure is referred to as *hypertension*. *Hypotension* refers to abnormally low blood pressure. Hypertension has become so prevalent that the World Health Organization calls it "a widespread epidemic." In the United States, it is estimated that some 23 million people have high blood pressure. With governments and health professional organizations now engaged in a massive public and professional educational program to promote early detection and treatment, it is important that the nurse gain proficiency in the skill of taking blood pressures accurately at an early stage in her career.

Procedure for Taking the Blood Pressure. The equipment for taking the blood pressure usually includes a blood pressure cuff, a stethoscope, and a sphygmomanometer. The most common site used is the upper arm, although it is sometimes necessary to take a blood pressure reading on the thigh. The cuffs come in various sizes to fit infants, children, and adults; sizes for the thigh as well as the arm are available. For best accuracy, the cuff should be approximately 20 per cent wider than the diameter of the extremity on which it is being used. Thus, if you have a very obese patient, it may be necessary to use a thigh cuff rather than an adult arm size one. Mercury, aneroid, and electronic sphygmomanometers are available commercially. The aneroid instruments are the smaller, more compact ones usually used in hospitals and other health agencies. Mercury sphygmomanometers, which are less compact, are frequently used in physicians' offices, where they are often mounted on the wall above an examining table. The electronic sphygmomanometers have a microphone and a transducer built into the cuff; hence, one does not need to use a stethoscope to listen to the sound of the blood pulsating through the artery as one does with the other types of sphygmomanometers.

In taking the blood pressure, the cuff is wrapped smoothly and firmly around the pa-

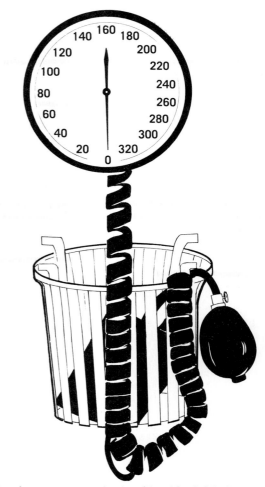

Blood pressure monitoring kit with dial indicator that can be mounted on a wall.

tient's upper arm so that the lower border of the cuff is 2.5 cm. (1 in.) above the antecubital space. The disc of the stethoscope is placed over the site of the brachial pulse and the cuff is pumped to 30 mm. of mercury above the pressure at which the pulsation in the brachial artery disappears. (The pulsation disappears when no sounds can be heard through the stethoscope.) This means that the artery is collapsed by the pressure of the cuff and no blood is flowing through it. The pressure is then gradually released and, when the blood slips through the artery, sounds are heard in the stethoscope. At the same time, the manometer is watched closely. The reading when the first sounds are heard is the *systolic pressure*.

With the continual lowering of the pressure in the cuff, the sounds continue to be heard as the artery alternately collapses and fills. Eventually the sounds diminish in intensity as the

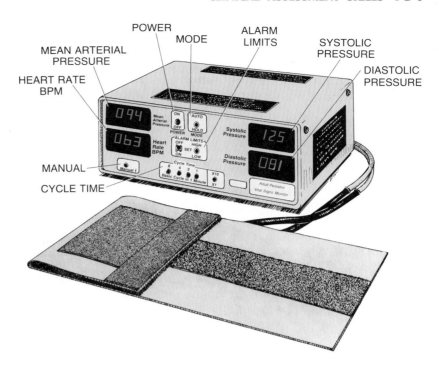

Electronic blood pressure kit with digital readout and pulse meter.

artery no longer collapses; weakened beats are usually heard for a few seconds and then disappear altogether. The onset of muffling (point at which the sounds change) is used by many clinicians as the index of *diastolic pressure,* although some prefer to use the point at which the sounds disappear entirely. In some agencies, both points are recorded.

It usually takes practice to learn to distinguish the systolic and diastolic points of pressure with ease and accuracy, and in some patients they are very difficult to discern. Care should be taken, however, to avoid repumping the sphygmomanometer repeatedly within a short space of time.

In using an electronic sphygmomanometer, the cuff is inflated to the desired pressure (as is done with the mercury sphygmomanometer). Then, the pressure is released and the needle on the gauge allowed to fall. The appearance of a flashing light and a "bleeping" sound indicates the systolic pressure, its disappearance the dias-

The blood pressure cuff is wrapped evenly around the upper arm so that the lower edge is 2.5 cm. (1 inch) above the antecubital space. The arm is positioned so that the cuff is at the level of the heart.

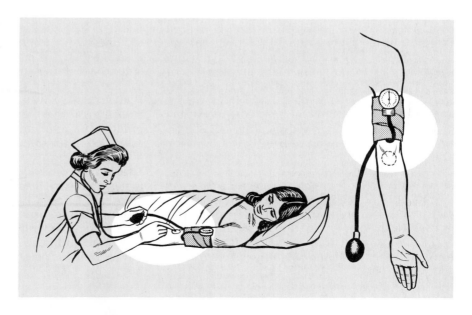

tolic. The electronic instruments help to give a more accurate reading, since they eliminate the human error possible when one has to interpret sounds and coordinate hand and eye movements at the same time. They are very sensitive instruments, however, and should not be used with restless patients.[2]

FUNCTIONAL ABILITIES

Nutritional Status

In assessing an individual's nutritional status, the nurse may have information about his *height*, his *usual weight*, and his *present weight* from the nursing history. It is customary practice in most health agencies to take height and weight measurements on all newly admitted patients, and this is usually a nursing responsibility. Many agencies use a combination height and weight measuring scale. The patient is asked to remove his shoes and to stand on the scales. It is a good hygienic measure to use a fresh paper towel on the scales for each patient. The nurse usually measures the person's height first (with his back to the measuring scale), and then his weight. If the patient is too ill, the height and weight measurements might not be taken on admission. A portable set of scales that can be wheeled to the bedside is used if it is important to monitor the weight of a patient confined to bed. An individual's height and weight may be compared with the average for his age, sex, and type of body frame to aid in assessment of his nutritional status. Tables showing desirable weights for individuals of different ages are included in Chapter 14.

In addition to noting the patient's height and weight, the nurse also observes his general appearance—does he look *obese, plump, average* in build, *thin,* or *emaciated*? She should also be aware of the individual's usual eating habits. Does he usually have a small, average, or big appetite? The nurse should also know about special diets he has been following as well as any dietary restrictions he observes for cultural or religious reasons or because of allergies. Observations can be made regarding the individual's *present response to food* and eating. Normally people enjoy food, although they do not always eat enough of the proper nutrients. Abnormalities that should be noted in the person's ability to eat or in his response to food include: *nausea* (a queasy feeling in the stomach); *anorexia* (loss of appetite); refusal to eat; difficulty in swallowing; *distention* (enlargement of the abdomen due to internal pressure of gas or liquid); or *distorted tastes*. The nurse should

also note if the patient has any difficulty in swallowing (dysphagia). The nurse notes the amount of food or fluids that the individual takes. If he takes only small amounts of food or fluids, this too should be noted.

Elimination Status

Constant data collected about an individual's elimination status are usually included in the nursing history (see page 121). In assessing the individual's current elimination status, the nurse makes observations about the following:

Emesis. Emesis is the vomiting of contents of the gastrointestinal tract through the mouth. Vomiting is always an abnormal condition. The nurse should make observations about the *amount* (it should be measured or approximated) and the *contents* of the emesis. Common terms used to describe the latter include: *bloody* (containing red blood); *liquid* (primarily liquid in consistency); *undigested food* (recognizable particles of food); and *bile* (a thick, viscid fluid varying in color from yellow to brown or green, and having a bitter taste).

Bowel Status. Significant observations about current bowel status include the date and time of the individual's last bowel movement, the color of the stools, and the frequency of bowel movements. Normal stool is brown, soft, and formed. Abnormal findings should be noted, such as *clay-colored* stools; *tarry* stools (black or blackish-brown viscous semi-liquid or liquid stools). Common problems with bowel functioning that the individual may report are *diarrhea* (frequent bowel movements; stools of more or less fluid consistency); *constipation* (infrequent passage of feces or difficult defecation; stools are unduly hard and dry); and *flatulence* (gas in the digestive tract). When the individual is unable to control the movement of his bowels, he is said to have *involuntary bowel* movements (incontinence). The term *impacted* bowel refers to a condition in which there is an accumulation of feces in the rectum pressed firmly together so as to be immovable.

Urinary Status. Normal urine is clear and straw colored. Observations should include its color, clarity, and amount. Common terms used to describe abnormalities are: *cloudy, dark orange, pink, red, frothy,* or *containing sediment.* Common problems in urinary functioning that the individual may report include: *frequency* (urinating at short intervals); *urgency* (the need to void suddenly, with an inability to retain,

diplopia - double vision

urine without acute distress); *burning* (a scalding sensation on voiding); *dribbling* (an intermittent flow of urine). A person is said to be *incontinent* of urine when he is unable to control urination.

Sensory Perception

The abilities to see, to hear, to feel, to taste, and to smell are vitally important in coping with the daily activities of living. In making observations relating to an individual's sensory perception, the nurse is concerned with the integrity of the anatomical structures needed for functioning in these areas: the eyes, the ears, the nose, the mouth and throat, and the skin, as well as their disturbances in functioning per se. Deviations from the individual's normal abilities, as indicated in the constant data collected about that person, should be noted in all sensory areas.

Vision. In assessing current visual status, the nurse makes observations about the condition of the eyes, the eyelids, and the pupils, as well as asking the person about visual disturbances he may be experiencing. When observing the individual's eyes, the nurse should look first at the condition of the eyelids. They may be *reddened* and look irritated, or they may appear *swollen* (puffy enlargement). The individual may complain of *itching* or *burning* of the eyes or lids; frequent rubbing of the eyes is often indicative of this feeling. The nurse should also look for *tearing* or *exudate* from the eyes. In addition, she should ask the individual if he has any visual disturbances such as *blurring* (seeing objects as vague or lacking in outline), or *diplopia* (double vision, seeing two objects when there is only one). In noting comments about the eyes the nurse should record which eye is affected—right, left, or both.

The nurse also observes the pupils of the eyes. The average normal pupil is 4 to 5 mm. in diameter. If the pupils are excessively large, they are said to be *dilated*; very small pupils are termed *pinpoint*. It is often important also to observe the reaction of the pupils to light. Normally an individual's pupils contract when exposed to a strong light. A flashing light directed at the eyes is used to observe this reaction. The nurse should note if both pupils react at the same time (consensually), as well as watch the separate reactions.

Hearing. The average individual can hear a normal conversation from a distance of approximately 15 feet. Hearing is one of the senses that become less acute as one grows older. Men lose the ability to hear high sounds first (women's voices, for example), whereas women find the low tones more difficult to hear as they grow older. Long-standing deficits in hearing are included in the constant data collected about an individual.

The nurse observes the condition of the ears. Normally, these are clean and free from discharge. Abnormalities that should be noted include the presence of *cerumen* (earwax), a sticky substance, usually brownish in color, and any discharge coming from the ear. These may be described as *watery* secretions, *purulent* (yellowish), or *bloody* (usually red in color). The amount of discharge should be noted as scant, moderate, or copious. The nurse always records which ear is affected (right, left, or both).

The nurse also asks if the individual has noticed any disturbances in hearing, such as a buzzing or ringing in the ears *(tinnitus)*, or any dizziness or *loss of balance.*

Smell. The nose is not only instrumental in the ability to smell, but it is also an important part of a person's respiratory apparatus. Common abnormalities include *nasal discharge* (secretions from the nose), or bleeding *(nosebleed)*. Disturbances in the sense of smell, such as an *absence of this sense*, or *distorted odors* (odors usually considered agreeable are unpleasant, and vice versa), should also be noted.

Taste. The condition of a person's mouth and throat is important not only to his sense of taste

The nurse observes the condition of the patient's mouth and throat in her clinical appraisal.

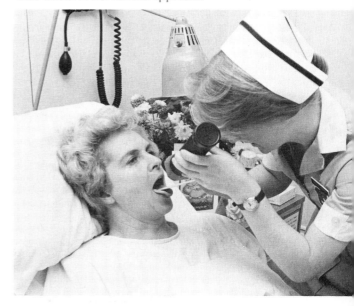

but also to his ability to take food and fluids, thereby affecting his nutritional status. Pertinent observations include noting if the mouth looks dry. A *dry mouth* is evidenced by a lack of saliva, and often one can see fine cracks in the surface of the lips or mucous membrane lining of the oral cavity. A mouth that is *not clean* has a collection of mucus and food particles around the teeth and gums or adhering to the mucous membranes. Sometimes the oral cavity appears *red* and inflamed. Any *bleeding* in the mouth should be noted; it usually occurs in the gums around the teeth.

The nurse also observes the condition of the tongue. The term *coated tongue* is used to describe the presence of a thick, furry covering, which may be variously colored. The mouth may also have a *foul odor*. Another abnormality to look for is *lesions* in the mouth, such as sores or fever blisters. The nurse notes whether the individual's teeth are in good condition. *Dental caries* (decayed teeth) may be observed. If the individual wears dentures, the nurse should note this fact and also their condition. A person without teeth is said to be *edentulous*.

Disturbances in taste that the individual may describe include a *bad taste* in the mouth, an *absence of taste*, or *distorted taste* (misinterpretation of tastes). Or he may report that he has an *increased acuteness* of this sense or, conversely, *decreased ability* to distinguish tastes. When looking at the mouth, the nurse should observe the throat; it may appear *reddened* or *swollen*, and the individual may complain of a *sore throat*.

Touch and Feeling. Touch and feeling are subjective experiences, and the nurse must rely on the individual's observations regarding deviations from the normal in this sensory area. Disturbances in feeling, such as *numbness, prickling*, or *tingling*, are most commonly noted in the extremities or in the facial area. Sometimes there is a *heightened sensitivity* to touch (pressure), heat, or cold, or, conversely, a *decreased sensitivity*.

The Skin and Its Appendages. The intact skin provides a protective covering for the body. Normal, healthy skin is clear (free from blemishes), intact (unbroken), warm to the touch, and has a·characteristic color, depending on the person's ethnic background and inherited complexion tones. Although each individual's skin coloring varies to a certain extent, the nurse may observe common abnormalities such as *flushing* (redness of the skin, particularly noticeable in the face and neck), *pallor* (lack of color), cy-

anosis (bluish or grayish cast to the skin, particularly noticeable in the lips, earlobes, and nailbeds), and *jaundice* (yellow color of the skin or whites of the eyes).

The nurse should also look for blemishes and breaks in the skin. Common blemishes include *rashes* (eruption of the skin, usually reddish in color); *bruises* (superficial discolorations due to hemorrhage into the tissues from ruptured vessels); *reddened areas* (diffuse red discoloration); *weeping areas* (oozing a watery secretion); *dry, itching areas* (rough and scaly skin which the individual has a desire to scratch); and *mottled areas* (marked with blotches of different shades of color). *Scabs* (crust of a sore, wound, ulcer, or pustule) and *lesions* (open areas or breaks in the skin surface) should be noted, as well as scars on the body or incisions from surgical operations. The presence of *lumps* under the skin (abnormal masses that perform no physiological function) should also be observed. Both the location (specific area of the body on which the blemish or lesion appears) and its size should be recorded.

Other observations that the nurse may make about the skin are the presence of excessive perspiration, which may be seen on the forehead, upper lip, palms of the hands and/or soles of the feet, in the axillary area, or covering the entire body. If the entire body is bathed with perspiration, the term *diaphoresis* is used. The nurse may also notice abnormalities in the temperature of the skin. For example, it may feel *hot* (abnormally warm) or *cold* (abnormally cool) to the touch.

Motor Status

A normal individual can sit, stand, walk, and perform a great number of movements, provided that the bones and muscles, circulation, and nerve supply are intact. Limitations in mobility due to chronic health problems, as, for example, paralysis, weakness, or difficulty in movement of one or more limbs (or parts of limbs), should be included in the constant data collected about the individual. Nursing observations to gather variable data pertaining to present motor status usually focus on the integrity and functioning ability of the extremities. Abnormalities to which the nurse should be alert in the extremities include disturbances in circulation or sensory perception, limitation of movement, and abnormal muscular movements.

An important observation which the nurse should make relative to circulation is the *presence or absence of distal* (peripheral) *pulses*— that is, whether a pulse can or cannot be ob-

pallor - lack of color
cyanosis - blue/gray
diaphoresis - perspiration all-over

CLINICAL ASSESSMENT SKILLS 155

tained by compressing the arteries at the points farthest from the heart in any of the extremities (see page 146). Other pertinent observations include the presence of *swelling* (abnormal localized enlargement) or *edema* (an excessive amount of tissue fluid) in any part or all of an extremity. Sensory disturbances that the individual may tell the nurse about include *paresthesia*, that is, an abnormal sensation without objective cause, such as *numbness, prickling*, or *tingling*, or a *heightened sensitivity* (to pressure, heat, or cold) in any part, or all of one or more limbs.

The nurse should also observe the limbs for deficiencies in range of motion of a part or of the whole extremity (see Chapter 23, pp. 493–496). *Weakness* (that is, a lack of strength in any area) should be noted, especially a marked decrease in the ability to grasp an object *(weak hand grip)*.

Abnormal muscular movements include: *contractures,* a permanent contracture of a muscle due to spasm or paralysis; *tremors,* a quivering or involuntary convulsive muscular contraction; and *muscle spasms,* involuntary convulsive muscular contractions. *Missing limbs,* or parts of a limb, absent as a result of a birth defect, trauma, or surgery, should be noted if not already reported in the constant data.

The nurse includes observations relating to the individual's response to activity. Some common terms that people use to describe abnormal responses to activity are: feelings of *dizziness,* a whirling sensation in the head that gives the affected person a tendency to fall; *faintness,* a feeling of weakness; *fatigue,* a feeling of tiredness or weariness; and *shortness of breath,* slow, rapid respirations on exertion. It should be noted that these observations are predominantly subjective. The nurse must ask the individual if he has noticed any of these symptoms in response to normal activities, such as walking, climbing stairs, and the like.

The individual's mobility should also be determined. Aids to mobility required at the present time, such as crutches, a cane, a walker, a wheelchair, or persons to assist the individual, are noted. If restrictions have been placed on his activities because of a current illness (such as bed rest or bathroom privileges only), these are included also.

State of Rest and Comfort

The individual's usual patterns of rest and sleep are noted in the constant data collected about him. Problems that the person is currently experiencing should be noted in the variable data, e.g., insomnia or excessive drowsiness. The nurse notes the presence of any pain, since it is one of the most common causes of disturbances in rest and sleep. Pain is, of course, a subjective experience, and the nurse must rely on the patient's observations of the pain he feels. She records the exact location of the pain, if the patient is able to tell her, and also its nature. People use a variety of expressions to describe pain that they are experiencing. Common terms which the individual may use include; *sharp,* (acute or cutting); *aching* (dull, generalized, persistent); *cramp-like* (severe paroxysmal type); *throbbing* (pulsating); *constant* (continuous, unchanging); *intermittent* (coming and going at intervals). The nurse also notes whether the pain reacts to therapy—whether the severity or intensity of the pain is, or is not, appreciably alleviated by the ministrations of the nurse or by the medication or treatment specified.

intermittent - coming + going

Reproductive Status

Age, sex, and marital status are vital statistics about the individual that are noted in the constant data. Other information about reproductive status that is collected in the nursing or medical history of a female patient includes data about usual menstrual pattern, and, if applicable, the age of menopause and of menarche, the number of pregnancies and of live births, the number and ages of children, and information about contraceptive methods used.

Variable data about an individual's reproductive status include the data of last menstrual period (if female) and the presence of any discharge from the genitals (both sexes). If the patient reports, or the nurse observes, discharges from the vagina or penis, it is important to note the color and amount of the discharge. Common types of discharge include *bloody, white,* or *yellow* discharges. An intermittent bloody discharge is termed "*spotting.*" If a discharge has a *foul odor,* this also should be noted.

Mental Status

Normally, during his waking hours, a person is alert and responsive. In appraising the mental status of an individual, the nurse should observe his movements. If he is slow or sluggish in moving, or appears to suffer from abnormal drowsiness, he is said to be *lethargic.* If he appears bewildered and perplexed, and/or makes inappropriate answers to questions, the

Text continued on page 160

NURSING ASSESSMENT: PATIENT PROGRESS

HOSPITAL   NORTH WEST GENERAL

SEPT. 16, 82

JORDAN PAUL
2465 WASHINGTON AVE SHORE CITY
SMITH JAMES   234-7566
SAME
             1600   SURG.   R.C.
9-16-82 PATIENT INFORMATION

DATE	9/16		
HOSPITAL/P.O. DAY	1		
TIME	1800		

DATE	9/16		
HOSPITAL/P.O. DAY	1		
TIME	1800		

1. VITAL SIGNS

BLOOD PRESSURE	Systolic	120		
	Diastolic	60		
TEMPERATURE (O) R A (circle)		37		
PULSE/min.	radial	80		
	apical			

PULSE/min.				
	irregular	☐	☐	☐
	bounding	✓	☐	☐
	weak	☐	☐	☐
	imperceptible	☐	☐	☐
	other	☐	☐	☐

RESPIRATIONS/min.		16		
	non-rhythmic	☐	☐	☐
	labored	☐	☐	☐
	rales	☐	☐	☐
	wheezing	☐	☐	☐
	shallow	☐	☐	☐
	short of breath	☐	☐	☐
	other	☐	☐	☐

2. RESPIRATORY AIDS   none ✓ ☐ ☐

OXYGEN	flow	l/min.	l/min.	l/min.
	nasal	☐	☐	☐
	mask	☐	☐	☐
	tent	☐	☐	☐
	trach collar	☐	☐	☐

TRACHEOSTOMY				
	cuffed	☐	☐	☐
	not cuffed	☐	☐	☐
	mist	☐	☐	☐
	suctioned	☐	☐	☐

VENTILATOR				
	rate/min.			
	controlled	☐	☐	☐
	assisted	☐	☐	☐
	other			

*AMOUNT/SEVERITY = 1 small/occasionally
2 moderate/frequently
3 copious/most of the time

3. EENT

R=right L=left				
	blurring	☐	☐	☐
	diplopia	☐	☐	☐

PUPILS				
	dilated	☐	☐	☐
	unequal	☐	☐	☐
	pinpoint	☐	☐	☐
	do not react to light	☐	☐	☐

	tinnitus	☐	☐	☐
	nasal discharge	☐	☐	☐
	nosebleed	☐	☐	☐
	throat irritation	☐	☐	☐
	other	☐	☐	☐

MOUTH				
	dry	✓	☐	☐
	not clean	☐	☐	☐
	coated tongue	☐	☐	☐
	reddened	☐	☐	☐
	bleeding	☐	☐	☐
	foul odor	☐	☐	☐

4. COUGH*

	acute	☐	☐	☐
	chronic	☐	☐	☐
	hacking	☐	☐	☐
	non-productive	☐	☐	☐

SPUTUM				
	green	☐	☐	☐
	yellow	☐	☐	☐
	blood-tinged	☐	☐	☐
	gray	☐	☐	☐
	viscous	☐	☐	☐
	not deep-breathing	☐	☐	☐
	other	☐	☐	☐

5. POSITION IN BED

PRESCRIBED POSITION				
	legs elevated	☐	☐	☐
	side only	☐	☐	☐
	semi-Fowlers	☐	☐	☐
	Trendelenberg	☐	☐	☐
	other BED FLAT	✓ -	☐	☐

NURSING ASSESSMENT: PATIENT PROGRESS

HOSPITAL *NORTH WEST GENERAL*

DATE	9/16		
HOSPITAL/P.O. DAY	1		
TIME	1800		

DATE	9/16		
HOSPITAL/P.O. DAY	1		
TIME	1800		

6. SKIN*

flushed	☐	☐	☐
pale	✓	☐	☐
cyanotic	☐	☐	☐
jaundiced	☐	☐	☐
perspiration	☐	☐	☐

LOCATION

rash	☐	☐	☐
bruise	✓	☐	☐
reddened	☐	☐	☐
weeping	☐	☐	☐
dry/itching	☐	☐	☐
mottled	☐	☐	☐

LOCATION *SACRAL AREA*

size/cm (approx.) _____

depth/cm (approx.) _____

other *SEVERAL BRUISED AREAS* ☐ ☐ ☐

7. EXTREMITIES*

R=right
L=left
B=both
A=arm
D=leg

NO distal pulses	☐	☐	☐
paresthesia	☐	☐	☐
limited movement	✓	☐	☐
paralyzed	☐	☐	☐
swelling	☐	☐	☐
edema	☐	☐	☐
weakness	☐	☐	☐
hand grip weak	☐	☐	☐
contractures	☐	☐	☐
muscles spasms	☐	☐	☐
tremors	☐	☐	☐
missing	☐	☐	☐
other _____	☐	☐	☐

8. GENITALS*

L.M.P. DATE ___/___/___

DISCHARGE white	☐	☐	☐
yellow	☐	☐	☐
spotting	☐	☐	☐
foul odor	☐	☐	☐
other _____	☐	☐	☐

9. RESPONSE TO FOOD/EATING

WEIGHT			
nausea	☐	☐	☐
anorexia	☐	☐	☐
refuses to eat	☐	☐	☐
distention	☐	☐	☐
diff. swallowing	☐	☐	☐
distorted taste	☐	☐	☐

SPECIAL DIET _____

SMALL INTAKE OF: fluids	☐	☐	☐
food	☐	☐	☐
other *NPO*	☐		

10. ELIMINATION*

EMESIS	bile	☐	☐	☐
	undigested food	☐	☐	☐
	bloody	☐	☐	☐
	liquids	☐	☐	☐
	other	☐	☐	☐

BOWEL	bowel movement	☐	☐	☐
	constipated	☐	☐	☐
	diarrhea	☐	☐	☐
	involuntary	☐	☐	☐
	impacted	☐	☐	☐

URINARY	cloudy	☐	☐	☐
	dark orange	☐	☐	☐
	pink	☐	☐	☐
	red	☐	☐	☐
	bladder distended	☐	☐	☐
	scanty amount	✓	☐	☐
	not voiding	☐	☐	☐
	dysuria	✓	☐	☐
	incontinent	☐	☐	☐
	frequency	☐	☐	☐
	urgency	☐	☐	☐
	other _____	☐		

*AMOUNT/SEVERITY = 1 small/occasionally
2 moderate/frequently
3 copious/most of the time

NURSING ASSESSMENT: PATIENT PROGRESS

SEPT, 16, 82

HOSPITAL *NORTH WEST GENERAL*

JORDAN PAUL
2465 WASHINGTON AVE SHORE CITY
SMITH JAMES   234·7566
SAME   1600   SURG.   R.C.
9 - 16 - 82   PATIENT INFORMATION

DATE	9/16		
(HOSPITAL)/P.O. DAY	1		
TIME	1800		

DATE	9/16		
(HOSPITAL) P.O. DAY	1		
TIME	1800		

11. WOUND*

inflamed			
hematoma			
gaping			
DRAINAGE serous			
sero-sanguineous			
sanguineous			
muco-purulent			
bile			
fecal matter			
urine			
_____ odor			
other _____			

12. CAST/TRACTION*

describe/locate _____

DRAINAGE sanguineous			
sero-sanguineous			
purulent			
odor			
pale			
cyanotic			
cold			
swelling			
other _____			

13. DRAINAGE TUBES*

A. N/G	B. Foley	C. H'vac	Use letters/tubes opposite
D.	E.	F.	related term(s).

not patent			
suction			
gravity			
irrigated			
cloudy			
pink			
red			
dark amber			
clots			
viscous			
other _____			

*AMOUNT/SEVERITY = 1 small/occasionally
2 moderate/frequently
3 copious/most of the time

14. ACTIVITY LEVEL

bed only	✓		
dangles only			
chair only			
BRP only			
room only			
one level only			
ambulates			
other _____			

15. AIDS TO MOBILITY

crutches			
cane			
walker			
brace			
wheelchair			
person(s)			
other _____			

16. RESPONSE TO ACTIVITY*

dizziness			
faint	✓		
fatigued			
short of breath			
other _____			

17. PAIN*

R=right
L=left
B=both

incisional			
chest			
abdominal			
lower back	3		
calf of leg			
head			
sharp	3		
aching			
cramp-like			
throbbing			
constant	✓		
intermittent			
not relieved by therapy			
other _____			

NURSING ASSESSMENT: PATIENT PROGRESS

HOSPITAL *NORTH WEST GENERAL*

DATE	9/16		
(HOSPITAL)/P.O. DAY	1		
TIME	1800		

DATE	9/16		
(HOSPITAL)/P.O. DAY	1		
TIME	1800		

18. MENTAL STATUS*

lethargic			
confused			
disoriented			
inattentive	1		
forgetful			
unresponsive			
other _____			

19. SPEECH COMMUNICATION*

reticent			
evasive			
verbose			
stuttering			
slurring			
unable to speak			
other _____			

20. OBSERVED BEHAVIOR*

restless	2		
crying			
withdrawn			
underactive			
combative			
abusive			
noisy			
other _____			

21. SOCIAL RESPONSE*

wants to be alone	1		
doesn't want to be alone			
UPSET BY: family			
visitor(s)			
roommate(s)			
staff			
other _____			

*AMOUNT/SEVERITY = 1 small/occasionally
2 moderate/frequently
3 copious/most of the time

FORM 0002

22. FEELINGS EXPRESSED BY PATIENT*

depression			
nervousness	2		
anger			
fear			
wants to die			
undersired changes due to illness			
other _____			

23. PERCEPTIONS OF ILLNESS* - PATIENT

misconceptions			
inadequate information			
refuses to talk about illness			
preoccupied with illness	3		
denial			
other _____			

24. PERCEPTIONS OF PROGNOSIS* - PATIENT

complete recovery			
no change			
to die			
doesn't know	✔		
partial recovery			
other _____			

25. COMMENTS

Pt. in severe pain
Wants to know if he's going
to have surgery, will he be o.k.
Worried about clothes and
money lost in transit

26. SIGNATURES

Instructions:
sign your name
under column of
date you recorded.

(1.) *J. Smith* R.N.

(2.) _____ R.N.

(3.) _____ R.N.

term *confused* is commonly used to describe his mental state. The *disoriented* individual perceives himself and/or his environment incorrectly in relation to time, place or person. He may not know who he is (or recognize familiar people), where he is, or what day it is. A person is said to be *inattentive* when he is unable to focus his mind on an idea or on some aspect of his surroundings or on reality. The term *forgetful* is used when a person has a temporary loss of memory, e.g., he cannot remember what you asked him a few minutes ago, or whether he has eaten lunch. When the individual makes no response to sensory stimulation, meaning that he does not answer or obey simple commands such as, "Please raise your hand," or he does not turn his head away from a bright light or react to touch, he is said to be *unresponsive*.

Emotional Status

✓People are not happy all the time. Most people experience a range of emotions in their day-to-day lives. These emotions are communicated to other people both by what the individual says and by his actions. In assessing an individual's emotional status, the nurse needs to identify both the individual's feelings as he expresses them in words and his observable behavior. These feelings include: *depression* (a feeling of sadness or melancholy); *nervousness* (easily excited, irritated, jumpy, uneasy, or disturbed); *anger* (strong feelings of displeasure or antagonism); and *fear* (unpleasant emotion caused by anticipation or awareness). The person may say that he *wants to die*. He may have feelings of *anxiety* concerning possible ill effects from his present state of health, or from surgery.

Some common types of observable *behavior* include: *restless* (continually moving the body or parts of the body); *crying* (weeping or lamenting); *withdrawn* (socially detached and unresponsive); *underactive* (not moving about as much as is desirable); *combative* (physically striking or attempting to strike others); *abusive* (harshly attacking others verbally); and *noisy* (talking loudly, shouting, or banging objects).

Social Status

People normally are gregarious; they enjoy the company of other people. The ability to make contact and to exchange communication with other members of the human race not only makes life more interesting and enjoyable, but is essential to daily living. People convey messages to other people by speaking, by writing, and through their behavior. Deviations from the normal in regard to an individual's social status may be observed through his speech, writing, and behavior.

Verbal Communication. Normally a person has the ability to carry on a conversation with another person and to respond to questions in such a way that his meaning is clear. This, of course, assumes that there are no language problems. Two common abnormalities of speech that the nurse can identify by listening to a person talking are *stuttering* (stumbling and spasmodic repetition of the same syllable), and *slurring* (sliding or slipping over word sounds that would normally be heard). A person who is unable to make his meaning clear (provided everyone is speaking the same language) is said to be *incoherent*. When an individual who previously was able to speak normally is unable to speak at all, the term *aphasia* (or aphasic) is used. *Dysphasia* is a general term used to refer to difficulties in speaking.

In observing an individual's speech, the nurse should note his willingness to communicate. He may, for example, be *reticent* (inclined to be silent and uncommunicative); evasive (avoids answering people directly); or *verbose* (extremely talkative). If the individual is unable to write, this fact should be noted.

Social Response. People respond to other people in an infinite variety of ways. Behavior that is normal for one individual may be abnormal for another. If the individual is ill, however, the nurse should note his response to the presence of others.

It is important to note, for example, if the individual wants to be alone (to have minimal or no contact with *anyone*) or does not want to be left alone, but desires or needs constant companionship. The nurse should also record her observations if the patient becomes *upset by contact* with his family, friends, staff, visitors, or roommates.

EXAMINATIONS AND DIAGNOSTIC TESTS

In her assessment, preparatory to developing a plan of care for a particular patient, the nurse makes use of data collected by other members of the health team. A comprehensive health assessment today usually includes a large number of tests and examinations requiring the talents of many different types of health workers.

The first step in the assessment is usually a complete physical examination, performed by a physician or by a nurse practitioner. In conjunction with the examination, laboratory tests are usually ordered, and x-rays and other special examinations may be scheduled. The gamut of specialized tests and procedures used in the detection of illness today includes not only the standard x-ray with which most of us are familiar but also its sophisticated offspring, the CAT scan, as well as the ultrasonic scan, nuclear medicine studies, electrodiagnostic studies, thermography, cardiopulmonary laboratory examinations, and tissue biopsies. The neuropsychiatric field also has a number of specialized tests to help in assessing an individual's mental status.

Examinations and diagnostic tests create a good ideal of anxiety in most people. Of primary importance to anyone undergoing them is what the results will mean in terms of prognosis (medical opinion of the final outcome of a health problem) and treatment. Some of the questions that run through a person's mind are: Will the results indicate that I have an incurable disease? Will I be a cripple? Do I have to have surgery? These questions often preoccupy a person even if he is just going to have a routine chest x-ray or blood test. People also want to know the reasons for the tests, and when they will be able to have the results.

Under present rules of ethical practice, the nurse does not give the patient the results of examinations or tests. This is the responsibility of the attending physician. The nurse can, however, provide the patient with emotional support before, during, and after many procedures. She provides this support by confirming and explaining what the physician has said about the "whys" of the test or examination and by giving the patient information he feels he needs. She explains how the procedure is to be carried out, in terms the patient can understand, and answers his questions to the best of her ability. The patient often feels a need to help in the procedure, and the nurse can assist him by explaining what he can do before, during, and after the test to facilitate the examination. She can also communicate to the patient her understanding of his anxiety and his need to have confidence in the measures that are being taken for his care. If she feels that the patient does not understand what is being done, she has an important responsibility as a patient advocate to communicate this to the physician. The nurse also has an important coordinating function in regard to diagnostic tests and examinations. She assists in the scheduling of many of these, car-

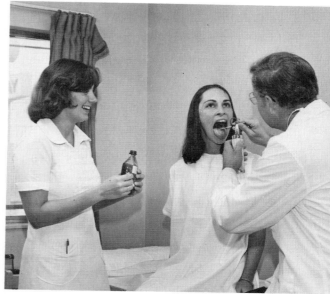

The nurse participates in carrying out many of the tests and examinations used in the detection of illness.

ries out some herself, and assists other members of the health team in carrying out many others.

The Physical Examination

The nurse is very often asked to assist the physician, or a nurse practitioner, in carrying out the physical examination of a patient. A complete examination usually consists of a health history, the examination itself, and special tests. The health history includes both the personal and medical history of the patient. The examiner will want to know about the patient's present problems as well as previous illnesses. Information is also gathered about the family history, since many diseases tend to recur in families, and some are inherited. The personal history usually includes the patient's social, religious, educational, and economic backgrounds, as well as his feelings of achievement and frustration. Habits of nutrition, sleeping patterns, bowel habits, and, for women, the menstrual history are usually included. Also noted are lifestyle patterns, such as smoking and drinking habits, regularity of exercise, and the like.

The physical examination generally proceeds from the head to the feet of the patient, with the findings being described in some detail. The examiner usually requires the following equipment; a scale with a height measuring rod, to take height and weight measurements; a clinical thermometer, stethoscope, blood pressure cuff, and sphygmomanometer, to assess vital signs; an otoscope for examining the ears and the nose; a tuning fork to assess hearing; an ophthalmoscope for examining the eyes; and an eye chart (e.g., Snellen chart) to assess vision; tongue blades, a laryngeal mirror, and a head mirror to examine the mouth and throat; a percussion hammer to test reflexes; a tape measure to measure such things as the circumference of a baby's head; and a vaginal speculum, if an internal examination is to be performed on a female patient. Usually these instruments are kept in the examining room in an ambulatory care setting, such as a physician's office or a clinic, or in the nursing unit of an inpatient facility. In addition to the instruments, the examiner will need supplies such as cotton balls and cotton applicators, lubricant, rubber gloves (sterile or clean), and containers or slides for specimens.

The responsibilities of the nurse who is assisting usually involve gathering the necessary equipment and supplies, preparing the examining room or patient's unit, and helping both the examiner and the patient with the physical examination. Most patients need some explanation about the examination—what is to be done and why. The patient will need to remove most or all of his clothing, and may need help in putting on the gown provided; the gown may be removed during parts of the examination. It is important to ensure the patient's privacy and also to make sure that he is not cold. If the patient lies on a bed for the examination, a light blanket may be put over him.

The nurse does not always stay throughout the entire physical examination, although many agencies today, and also many physicians, request that a female nurse be present during the examination if the patient is female and the examiner male. The reason for this is twofold: it contributes to the psychological comfort of the patient and also provides legal protection for the examiner. The nurse should also consider the patient's age, mental alertness, balance, and cooperativeness in judging whether she needs to stay with the patient throughout the examination.

● The physical examination usually includes the taking of vital signs, observation of the general physical and emotional status of the patient, and a general inspection of posture, skin, head, eyes, ears, nose, mouth, throat, neck (including the thyroid gland and lymph nodes), chest and lungs, heart, breasts, abdomen, genitalia, extremities, back and spine, nervous system, and rectum.

● During the examination the nurse is usually responsible for draping the patient as appropriate for comfort and modesty, and helping him, as needed, to assume the best position to facilitate the examination.

If the patient is ambulatory, a general inspection is often done with the patient standing; that is, one assesses posture and general appearance and notices abnormalities. Alternatively, it is done with the patient lying on his back (supine position). Most examiners prefer to have the patient sitting up for examination of the head and neck and the chest and lungs (back and front). The supine position is the usual choice for examination of the breasts, heart, and abdomen. The examiner may also look at the extremities when the patient is lying down but will often want to do a further examination with the patient sitting and, also, standing. For examination of the rectum, a male patient may be asked to bend over the examining table. For a bed patient, or a female patient, Sims's position or a knee-chest position may be used. Sims's position is also known as the semi-prone or three-quarter prone position. It is a position that is frequently used for people who are unconscious and is described in detail in Chapter 20.

In the knee-chest position, the patient kneels with the buttocks upward. It is important that the patient who assumes this position be adequately draped. Many health agencies have special rectal drapes that completely cover the buttocks of a patient except for a circular cutout over the anus. The patient will generally need additional covering for his shoulders and a pillow for his head.

If the health agency does not have special drapes, the nurse can improvise with a cotton drawsheet. The drawsheet is placed across the patient so that the lower edge just covers the buttocks. The corners are tucked around the medial aspect of the patient's thighs. By raising the fold of the sheet, the anal area is exposed.

During this procedure, the examiner needs a rectal glove, lubricant, and kidney basin. He (or she) inserts his lubricated gloved finger into the patient's rectum, palpating for abnormalities such as hemorrhoids and fissures.

The *lithotomy position* is used chiefly for examinations and operations involving the reproductive and urinary tracts for both sexes. In this position the patient lies on his back with a small pillow for his head. His hips are flexed and slightly abducted and his knees are also flexed. The patient needs support for his feet if he is to maintain this position for more than a few minutes. The stirrups provide a means for supporting the feet.

Because this position is also embarrassing for

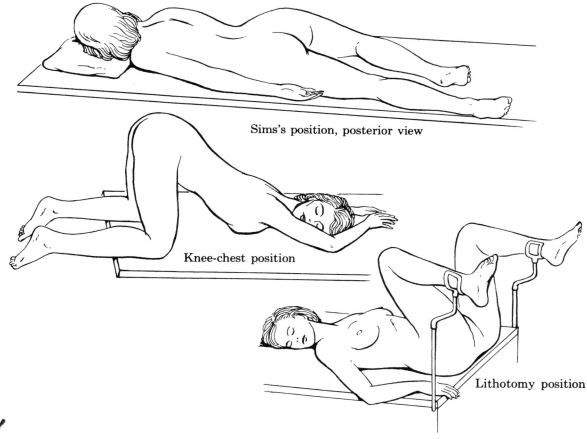

Sims's position, posterior view

Knee-chest position

Lithotomy position

Various positions used in examination or treatment. From *Dorland's Illustrated Medical Dictionary.* 26th ed. Philadelphia, W. B. Saunders Company, 1981.

most patients, it is important that adequate drapes be provided. One way of draping the patient is to place a drawsheet across the patient so that the lower border is 10 cm. (4 in.) below the symphysis pubis. Then each of the lower corners of the drawsheet are brought to the medial aspect of the patient's thighs and tucked around the patient's legs. When the upper fold of the drawsheet is lifted the patient's perineum is exposed. The nurse should also provide the patient with a covering for the upper part of the body. Another method is to place a bath blanket diagonally over the patient. The opposite corners (at each side of the patient) are wrapped around the legs and anchored at the feet. The lower corner can be drawn back and tucked under the top layer of the bath blanket to expose the perineum.

For a vaginal examination the examiner requires rubber gloves, lubricant, a vaginal speculum, a kidney basin, and a good light. This equipment is sterilized after use in order to prevent the transmission of infection. The phy-

sician may also want a tongue blade and a microscopic slide in order to take a sample of the cervical secretions, which are then sent to the laboratory for examination for abnormal cells. This is called a Papanicolaou smear.

Laboratory Tests

In conjunction with a physical examination, various laboratory tests are usually ordered. These generally include blood tests and a urinalysis in the initial assessment of an individual's health status, or a periodic health checkup. In the blood work, the tests commonly ordered include white blood cell count (WBC) and differential, hematocrit (Hct), a red blood cell morphology and platelet examination, and a hemoglobin estimate. In many places where laboratory data systems are computerized, it is now common practice to order a battery of tests, instead of ordering them singly. One such battery, the SMA-12, includes 12 separate analyses on one sample of blood and provides an assessment of nutritional status, liver and kidney function, tissue injury, and parathyroid function. In a routine urinalysis, the urine is tested for pH, specific gravity, albumin, and sugar, and a microscopic examination is done (see Chapter 15). If abnormalities are found in the blood tests or urinalysis, further laboratory investigation or other special tests are undertaken.

Frequently, the nurse is responsible for collecting specimens from patients. These may include specimens of blood, urine, sputum, and drainage from wounds. For these tests, patients usually need explanations as to what they can do to help. Most patients like to be able to assist, and often the success of a test is dependent upon the patient's willingness to provide a specimen or perform some activity at a particular time. When the nurse collects specimens, her functions include:

1. Explaining the procedure to the patient and gaining his cooperation
2. Collecting the right amount of specimen at the correct time
3. Placing the specimen in the correct container
4. Labeling the container accurately (this usually includes the patient's full name and registration number, the date, the physician's name, and if in a hospital, the number of the nursing unit)
5. Completing the laboratory requisition (this specifies what tests are to be carried out and gives pertinent data about the patient)
6. Recording anything unusual about the appearance of the specimen

Various specimens are sent for microbiological examination in the laboratory. Specimens of a patient's secretions, excretions, and any exudates are frequently examined in order to isolate and identify an infecting organism. A secretion is a product produced by a gland (for example, bile); an excretion is a substance excreted or discharged by the body (for example, urine). An exudate is an inflammatory fluid, such as pus, that is discharged from an infected area of the body.

For most specimens, a sterile container is required, and precautions must be taken to avoid contaminating the specimen with organisms in the environment. A smear or culture may be needed. If a specimen is required for a smear, clean (preferably new) slides and a sterile, cotton-tipped applicator are needed. The specimen is gathered with the applicator, which is rolled over the center of the slide. The smear is covered with another glass slide. The slides are appropriately labeled and sent to the laboratory.

For cultures, the specimen is placed in a sterile container. Urine, blood, ascitic fluid, and the like are usually put in sterile test tubes. For cultures of specimens of wound discharge, many agencies furnish sterile test tubes that are equipped with sterile applicators suspended from the cork that seals the tube. When the cork is removed the applicator is removed with it. The applicator tip is touched to the area of discharge and then returned carefully to the sterile container.

Sputum specimens are collected in wide-necked sterile containers or on Petri dishes. Sputum is collected early in the morning, when the patient is most able to cough up sputum from his lungs.

When stools are sent for culture, it is seldom necessary to send the entire specimen. Normally a sterile applicator dipped in the feces is sufficient. If the feces are to be examined for amebae, the specimen is sent to the laboratory while it is warm and it is examined within 30 minutes after it is obtained. Only a small quantity (approximately 3 ml.) of feces is needed for this examination.

It may be necessary to test a culture for differentiation and sensitivity. *Differentiation* is accomplished by means of Gram's stain, which divides bacteria into two classes: gram-negative organisms stain red; gram-positive organisms stain purple. *Sensitivity* refers to the effect of specific antibiotics upon bacteria. The organisms are streaked on nutrient plates, various antibiotics are then added to the plates, and the plates are placed in an incubator. The areas where the growth of the bacteria is inhibited indicate the particular antibiotics to which the bacteria are sensitive.

X-rays

Radiation is a highly publicized and emotionally charged word these days, and many people are afraid that having any kind of an x-ray will harm them. Excessive radiation is most certainly dangerous, and special precautions are taken to ensure that people who work in x-ray departments or in places where radiation therapy is used (such as in a cancer clinic) are not being exposed to excessive amounts. You may have noticed the monitors that workers in the x-ray department wear on their uniforms. These monitors, which look something like metal pencils, are carefully checked on a regular basis to make sure that the worker has not had a dangerous level of radiation exposure. The amount a person receives during diagnostic tests, however, is minimal. A person does not receive enough radiation to destroy tissue unless this is being done therapeutically, as, for example, for treatment of a tumor.

X-rays today are used in diagnosis and therapy on virtually every system of the body. In diagnosis, their purpose is to assist in the visualization of internal structures of the body, so that pictures of these structures can be put on film. X-rays, which are also called *roentgen rays*, are electromagnetic radiations, or energy waves, of short wave length.

When x-rays are passed through the body, denser structures, such as bone tissue, absorb more of the rays and, hence, register heavier shadows on the photographic film. Less dense structures, such as soft organs (like the stomach), permit the rays to pass through them more easily. These structures register lighter shadows on the film. It is the contrast between light and dark shadows (because of the differing density of tissues and, hence, the differing amount of rays they absorb) that enables the person reading the x-ray to find abnormalities.

In order to visualize softer structures within the body, such as the gastrointestinal tract, a substance (called a contrast medium) is often used to make the structures radiopaque so that they will show on photographic film. The contrast media usually used are either metallic salts or gases. Barium sulfate, for example, is the contrast medium used for the gastrointestinal tract. If the upper part of the tract (the esophagus, stomach, and duodenum) is to be visualized, the patient drinks the barium solution; to allow visualization of the lower part (colon and rectum), the barium is given as an enema. For x-rays of the ventricles of the brain, oxygen is injected into the spinal canal. Organic soluble iodides are used to visualize the gallbladder, urinary tract, and blood vessels.

The ordinary diagnostic x-ray is like a still photograph and provides a permanent record. Sometimes, however, it is desirable to observe body organs or systems in motion, as for example, the filling and emptying of the stomach. Then, *fluoroscopy* is used. In this procedure, x-rays are passed through the body and images of the moving internal structures are projected onto a fluorescent screen. Again, a contrast medium may be used to aid in the assessment.

The CAT scan (also known as CT and as CAT) is another form of x-ray. The initials stand for *computerized axial tomography*. In this procedure, x-rays are passed through the body in the region of the structure to be "scanned." A 180° sweep of the structure, at 3 or 4 different planes, is used. The x-rays are fed into a computer, which records the "absorption potential" of different tissues at varying planes within the structure. The computer prints out a visual representation of these. Photographs are also taken of the image on the screen. Usually these are in black and white, although color photography is also possible.

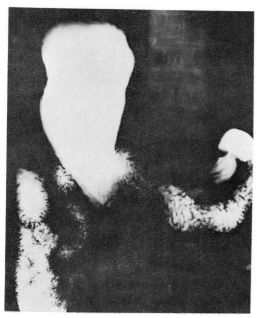

An x-ray showing barium sulfate filling the stomach and the first portion of the small bowel.

Nuclear Medicine Studies

Radioactive isotopes, which are also known as *radionuclides* or *radiopharmaceuticals*, are another form of radiation that is used in both diagnosis and treatment. These substances give off radioactivity in known, predictable quantities as they decay, and they can thus be traced in the body by a monitor that picks up radioactivity. Certain radioactive substances have a particular affinity for specific parts of the body; for example, radioactive iodine taken orally (it is usually given in a drink) will find its way to the thyroid gland, where it tends to accumulate. Given in large doses, it will destroy tissue in much the same way as radiation therapy using x-rays. In smaller doses (called tracer doses) it can be used to identify abnormalities in the thyroid gland. The radioactivity given off by the iodine as it decays can be picked up by a scanner (much like a form of Geiger counter) and the emissions transformed into electrical impulses, which can then be counted. Or, a camera, called a gamma camera, may be used to take photographs of the accumulation and distribution of the radioactive iodine in the body. It is possible, using radioactive substances, to detect abnormalities or malignant tumors in such tissues as the brain, bone, lungs, liver, kidneys, spleen, pericardium, and thyroid.

Electrodiagnosis

Various organs of the body, including the heart, the brain, the stomach, the muscles, and the skin, constantly emit electrical impulses as they function. These impulses can be picked up on a machine and transformed (transduced) into a set of tracings that provides a graphic representation of the impulses. The tracings are then "read," or interpreted, by an expert to assess the functioning of the particular organ. In this way, graphic representations can be made of the electrical impulses emitted by the heart (*electrocardiogram*, also called an ECG or EKG), brain (*electroencephalogram*, or EEG), and muscles (*electromyogram*, or EMG).

Ultrasonic Scan

Auscultation, the listening for sounds within the body, is one of the basic methods of observation we discussed at the beginning of this chapter. The *ultrasonic scan* is a diagnostic tool that utilizes this basic methodology. Sound waves of too high a frequency to be heard by the human ear are directed at the organ or structure of the body that is to be assessed. The vibrations that come back are transformed (transduced) into tracings, called *oscilloscope tracings*, which can be read to detect pathological changes in tissues of the muscles and joints, the brain, or the heart. Ultrasonic scans are used with increasing frequency to assess fetal development.

Thermography

Thermography is the assessment of the temperature of various body areas for the purpose of detecting underlying pathological processes. It is basically a technique using self-emanating infrared radiation to portray surface temperatures of the body photographically. It is frequently used in the detection of tumors of the breast, for example, and may also be used in assessment of blood vessels and inflammatory processes.

Tissue Biopsies

Sometimes it is considered important to examine a sample of living tissue from a particular structure of the body. Usually this is done to look for either abnormal cells that may indicate the presence of a tumor or structural changes indicative of an infectious process. The procedure for obtaining a specimen of tissue from the body is called a *biopsy*. The specimen is sent to a pathology laboratory for microscopic examination. There are basically three ways that a tissue biopsy may be obtained: (1) by use of a needle for puncture or aspiration; (2) by endoscopy; and (3) by surgical excision.

A sample of bone marrow may be obtained by inserting a hollow needle through the surface tissue of the body and into the marrow cavity of a bone. A small amount of the marrow is aspirated to obtain the specimen. The sternum is the most common site for this procedure, although the iliac crest, the posterior superior ilium, and the spine are also used.

Endoscopy is the examination of body cavities and openings through the use of specially designed instruments that enable the examiner to observe tissues more clearly. The instruments are called scopes and usually come equipped with a small light at the inserting end and, often, a small mirror to make visualization easier. If a tissue sample is wanted, a narrow instrument is inserted through the scope to pick up cells for the biopsy.

For obtaining a sample of tissues that are imbedded in a body structure as, for example, from a lump in the breast, it may be necessary to use surgical excision to get specimen cells for laboratory examination.

Cardiopulmonary Laboratory Tests

A large number of tests and examinations have been developed to aid in the assessment of functioning of the heart and lungs—so many that there are now specialized laboratories devoted to this diagnostic area. The electrocardiogram mentioned above is a procedure commonly ordered as part of a complete physical examination for all patients over the age of 40 years. In addition, various x-ray techniques may be used to visualize the size, positioning, and functioning of the heart, lungs, and blood vessels. A number of specialized tests may also be done, such as the stress tolerance test and treadmill test that assess cardiac functioning, and the pulmonary function tests that measure lung volumes, capacities, and flow rates. We will be discussing the more commonly used diagnostic tests for cardiopulmonary functioning in Chapter 18.

Tests of Mental Functioning

In some cases, particularly when it is considered important to establish a psychiatric diagnosis, specialized psychological tests may be used. These include the objective type of tests, such as the intelligence tests with which most of us are familiar, the vocational interest and aptitude tests, and the personality tests (for example, the Minnesota Multiphasic Personality Inventory). These may be supplemented by projective tests, such as Draw-a-Person, the Rorschach ink blot test, or the thematic apperception test. The latter two call for the individual to interpret different shapes of ink blots and pictures of people in different situations, respectively. The projective tests are said to reflect a person's fantasies and his modes of adaptation. They are always administered and evaluated by a skilled psychologist.

GUIDELINES FOR ASSISTING WITH TESTS AND EXAMINATIONS

Before the procedure:

1. Prepare the patient
   a. Explain the procedure, what exactly is to be done and why it is being done, in terms the patient can understand
   b. Explain how the patient can help with the examination
   c. Provide the patient with a gown and assist him in getting into it, if necessary
   d. Provide privacy for the patient to dress and undress and to wait for the examination
   e. Help the patient to assume the position required for the examination
   f. Drape the patient for his comfort and to facilitate the examination

2. Prepare the equipment
   a. Obtain all the equipment needed for the examination
   b. Maintain the sterility of the equipment before and during the examination, as necessary
   c. Obtain the containers needed for specimens and label these with the patient's name, the examiner's name, and the date

3. Prepare the examining room
   a. Close the windows and eliminate drafts
   b. Ensure privacy
   c. Place equipment so that it is convenient for the examiner
   d. Provide a chair for the examiner when this is indicated

During the procedure:

1. Provide emotional support for the patient

2. Provide physical support for the patient as needed, for example, when he is maintaining a position

3. Assist the examiner with equipment as necessary

4. Observe the patient for his reactions to the examination

After the procedure:

1. Carry out measures for the patient's comfort, e.g., cleaning lubricant off the skin or drying areas that may have been dampened

2. Observe the patient closely for any untoward reactions

3. Send labeled specimens to the laboratory

4. Clean and dispose of equipment as necessary

5. Enter details of the examination on the patient's record, such as date, time, exactly what was done, and whether and for what purpose specimens were sent to the laboratory

STUDY SITUATION

With the help of your instructor, select one patient in the clinical area where you are having experience:

1. Review data already accumulated on the patient's record, paying particular attention to the admitting data (name, age, sex, and other vital statistics, plus reason for admission), the nursing history, and the medical history.

2. Undertake a clinical assessment of the patient's functional abilities, including:

   — temperature, pulse, and respirations
   — blood pressure
   — nutritional status
   — elimination status (emesis, bowel status, urinary status)
   — sensory perception (vision, hearing, smell, taste, and touch)
   — motor status
   — state of rest and comfort
   — reproductive status
   — mental status
   — emotional status
   — social status (verbal communication and social response)

3. Identify deviations from the normal that you observed in the patient's functional abilities.

4. How important are these deviations in terms of planning nursing care for this patient?

5. What diagnostic tests and examinations have been ordered for this patient? Was a complete physical examination done? What laboratory tests were ordered? Roentgenography? Other? Why were they ordered? Are the results back on any of these yet? Do they show deviations from normal? What are the implications in terms of nursing care?

SUGGESTED READINGS

Alder, J.: Patient Assessment: Pulses. *American Journal of Nursing,* 79(1):115–132, January, 1979.

Assessing Vital Functions Accurately. Nursing Skillbooks Series. Horsham, Pa., Intermed Communications, Inc., 1977.

Assessing Your Patients. Nursing Photobook Series. Horsham, Pa., Intermed Communications, Inc., 1980.

Dossey, B.: Perfecting Your Skills for Systematic Patient Assessment. *Nursing 79,* 9(2):42–45, February, 1979.

Farrell, J.: The Human Side of Assessment. *Nursing 80,* 10(4):74–75, April, 1980.

Meissner, J. E.: A Simple Guide for Assessing Oral Health. *Nursing 80,* 10(4):24–25, April, 1980.

Pepler, C. J.: Your Fingers on the Pulse: Evaluating What You Feel. *Nursing 80,* 10(11):32–39, November, 1980.

Reynolds, J. I., and Logsdon, J. B.: Assessing Your Patient's Mental Status. *Nursing 79,* 9(8):26–33, August, 1979.

Schweiger, J. L., et al.: Oral Assessment: How to Do It. *American Journal of Nursing,* 80(4):654–657, April, 1980.

Thomas, S.: Pulse, Respirations and Blood Pressure. *Nursing Mirror,* May 10, 1979.

REFERENCES

1. Alder, J.: Patient Assessment: Pulses. *American Journal of Nursing,* 79(1):115–132, January, 1979.
2. Thomas, S.: Pulse, Respirations and Blood Pressure. *Nursing Mirror,* May 10, 1979.
3. Eoff, M. J., and Joyce, B.: Temperature Measurements in Children. *American Journal of Nursing,* 81(3):1010–1011, 1981.

10

The Nurse Should Be Able to:

- List five basic characteristics of a helping relationship
- Describe three major phases in the nurse-patient relationship
- Outline the process of contracting with a patient
- Explain the SMCR model of the communication process
- Give examples of factors that can interfere with elements of the communication process
- List factors the nurse should consider when she wants to convey a message
- Discuss characteristics of language to be considered by the nurse in communications with patients
- Give examples of various ways by which people communicate nonverbally
- Discuss ways of fostering an open climate for nurse/patient communications
- Develop beginning skills in listening to patients
- Discuss the interview as a tool in nurse/patient communications
- Give examples of various media used for information exchange between members of the health team

COMMUNICATION SKILLS

CHAPTER 10

INTRODUCTION

The fundamental core of nursing is the relationship that is established between the nurse and the patient. This is a professional relationship, based on trust and mutual respect. An individual who comes to a health agency is there because he needs help in relation to his health; the nurse and other health professionals are there to provide the help he needs. In order to develop a relationship whereby she can help the patient, the nurse must develop skills in communicating, since, without communication, no relationship is possible.

Communication is the process by which one person conveys thoughts, feelings, and ideas to another. It is a tool that provides a means for one person to understand another, to accept and be accepted, to convey and receive information, to give and accept directions, to teach and to learn. The nurse communicates with the patient and the patient with her. Communication is always a two-way process. The nurse also communicates with the patient's family and friends, with visitors to the agency, with other members of the health team and other personnel, and with a host of other people during the course of a day. She should, then, know something about the process of communication.

THE NURSE-PATIENT RELATIONSHIP

Nursing is one of the helping professions. Nurses, in their work, help other people—to promote and maintain their optimal health, to prevent them from becoming ill, to restore them to health following an episode of illness, or to cope with the exigencies of chronic or terminal illness. The relationship that is established between nurse and patient is a helping relationship. This relationship is the basis of nursing practice, and it is woven into the fabric of every interaction that occurs between nurse and patient.

In the health field, the helping relationship is often referred to as a therapeutic relationship, because it is a key element enabling the health professional to administer care to the patient. The helping relationship is not, of course, unique to nursing or to the health field. It is an integral part of the practice of law, medicine, the ministry, and all of the other helping professions. The type of help a clergyman, a doctor, or a lawyer provides is different from that provided by the nurse, but the relationship is essentially the same.

Several characteristics of the helping relationship have been identified by different authors. One essential element is empathy, which is the ability to recognize and understand another person's feelings in a given situation. Empathy means trying to imagine yourself in the other person's place and looking at things from his point of view. For example, a child brought to a hospital from the hinterlands in Surinam for removal of a growth in his neck was found sleeping on the floor underneath his hospital crib instead of in it. His actions were understandable (you could feel empathy for him) when you realized that he had probably never seen a crib before in his life. Most likely, his sleeping cot had been a hammock slung beside those of his brothers and sisters in the sleeping room of his home in the jungle village. Unfortunately, the hospital was not equipped with hammocks. To use a more commonplace example, the removal of a mole from a woman's face may seem like a minor surgical procedure when you compare it with open heart surgery, but, to the person who is having it done, there are all sorts of frightening possibilities. The doctor said it was probably just a harmless little growth, but he was going to send it to the laboratory just to make sure. What if it turns out to be cancer? Will it grow back? Do moles spread? Thoughts such as these may be running through the patient's head. It is always helpful to try to think of the implications of any procedure from the point of view of the person who is having it done. What if it were happening to you? How would you feel?

Another commonly cited characteristic of the helping relationship is mutual *respect*. You respect the patient as a person of worth and dignity, and you observe the social courtesies that indicate respect. You call the person by the name and title he prefers. Many older people do not like to be addressed by their first name, particularly by a younger person, but prefer the Mr. or Mrs. title with their surname. It is, therefore, always a good idea to ask the person how he would like to be addressed. In Oriental cultures, age is highly respected and deference is shown in many ways. A younger person asks permission of an older person to sit down, or to speak. In some cultures, a young girl is expected to keep her eyes cast down and not look directly into the face of an elder when speaking to him. Western societies, too, have polite and courteous ways of addressing people and of asking them to do something—ways that show respect for the other person. You ask permission to take up the patient's time for an interview, for example; you introduce yourself by name and explain what you are doing. You also respect the autonomy and independence of the individual. It is, after all, his body that is being treated, and he has a right to participate in decisions regarding what shall be done with it.

The nurse also needs to have the respect of the patient if the relationship is to be effective. Your nursing education qualifies you to help others in regard to health matters, and these qualifications engender respect from others who have not had this professional training. Competence in carrying out the nursing measures that need to be done, whether it is teaching preoperative exercises, putting on a dressing, or taking a blood pressure, reinforces the inherent respect for the professional felt by the lay person. Then, too, respect for oneself, as evidenced in such things as personal grooming, good posture, and a manner that conveys confidence in your own abilities also helps. It is important to know what you are doing and how to do it, in other words.

Both empathy and mutual respect contribute to fostering a *climate of trust*, which is a very basic element in the helping relationship. The patient must be able to trust the nurse as a person who is concerned first and foremost with his welfare before he can accept her help wholeheartedly. He has to be sure that she will not betray his confidence before he feels free to discuss personal matters or express his feelings. He has to be sure in his own mind that she is competent in her basic nursing skills before he can trust her to carry out more complex measures such as inserting an intravenous needle into his arm. The nurse, too, must trust the patient to carry out his responsibilities in regard to his health care. Trust usually develops slowly as one gets to know the other person. It is built up of small things, such as remembering to make the phone call the patient asked you to make, and reporting back to him, of being honest and giving only reliable information, and, again, of competence in your nursing care.

Genuineness, or *authenticity*, is another characteristic of the helping relationship that is helpful in creating a climate of trust. Spontaneity of response, a lack of defensiveness on the nurse's part and absence of a superior ("I know better than you do") attitude all contribute to genuineness. There has to be a certain amount of openess on both sides. The patient will probably want to know something about you as a person, and, as someone who is going to help him, you have to be prepared to disclose some of your feelings and values. Most patients, however, are much more interested in themselves and their own problems than in anyone else, and these are the real focus of the relationship.

The nurse and the patient are both primarily concerned with the reasons the patient has sought help. There is then, a *specificity of purpose to the relationship*. The nurse's goal is to help the patient to meet his health needs. She accomplishes this through utilizing the nursing process to assess his needs, to identify his immediate problems, and to work with him to resolve these problems.

People who have undertaken studies of the nurse-patient relationship have identified three major phases in the relationship. There is first of all an *introductory, or orientation,* phase, when nurse and patient get to know and trust each other, then a *working phase*, and, finally, a *termination phase*. Some authors subdivide these phases, and some identify them as more than three, but since the components coincide, we will discuss them under the three major headings.

I.W.T.

Orientation

This is the phase when nurse and patient get to know and begin to trust each other. Under normal circumstances, they start off as strangers. The nurse, however, usually has the advantage of having some information about the patient before she meets him. If you are assigned a patient in the clinical area, for example, you can obtain a good deal of information about him from the patient's record, and you will probably have a verbal report about him from the charge nurse (or the nurse who has been looking after him) before you meet the patient.

The nurse takes the initiative in the relationship that is being established. It is up to her to set the tone for the encounter (or series of encounters), and she takes the lead in establishing guidelines for the working relationship. Both nurse and patient are identified by name and roles are clarified during this introductory phase. Both the nurse and the patient come with preconceived ideas about the nature of the relationship. The patient may have been conditioned by television or motion pictures to have certain beliefs about hospitals and nurses. He may have heard comments about the agency he has selected from friends or relatives. He may have had previous experiences in the health care system that influence his expectations of the care he will receive. The nurse will have her previous experiences in the clinical area and the teaching she has received in the classroom as a basis for her expectations. The two sets of expectations may not coincide, and it is well in this orientation phase to come to an agreement on the nature of the working relationship between the two parties. The patient, for example, may expect the nurse to do everything for him while he lies in bed "getting better." The nurse, on the other hand, may hold the philosophy that promoting as much self-care as the patient is capable of doing is the best medicine. It is a good idea, as we mentioned in Chapter 8, to find out the patient's expectations of care and to discuss with him what is expected of him in this situation, as well as what he can expect from you as his nurse.

An orientation to the nursing unit, or to the health agency if it is an ambulatory care facility, is usually part of the introductory phase. It is important that the patient be introduced to the persons who will be participating in his care and that their roles be explained to him. Taking the nursing history is often a part of this phase and is sometimes the first opportunity the nurse has to get to know the patient. During this phase of the relationship there is often a good deal of testing, as both parties attempt to find out about each other and as trust begins to be established.

Working Phase

The working phase of the nurse-patient relationship begins when the nurse has gathered all of her data and is beginning to draw up a tentative plan of care for the patient. Increased emphasis on accountability and responsibility for both providers and consumers of health services has led to the premise that both are equal partners in the process of health care. It is this premise that guides the nurse in her working relationship with the patient. The nurse and the patient share in developing mutually agreable goals, and both have a definite role to play in achieving these. There is a division of responsibility, and it is well to clarify at the beginning of the working phase who will be responsible for which aspects of care.

A relatively new concept is that of establishing a contract with the patient. The contract may simply be a verbal agreement, as for example, "I will teach you how to do the deep breathing exercises before surgery, but I expect you to practice them four times a day on your own." Or, the contract may be a written statement that is signed by all parties concerned. (A family member or significant other person may be involved, and there may be more than one nurse or other health care provider.)

Zangari and Duffy have identified seven steps in the process of contracting, and these provide good guidelines for nurses wishing to initiate the process:

1. The nurse collects her data base information
2. The nurse and the patient discuss each other's expectations (in regard to the end results of care)
3. Together they set up mutually agreeable short-term and long-term goals
4. A contract is established stating how responsibilities toward achievement of each goal will be divided
5. The nurse coordinates the contract with other staff members providing care and with the patient's family
6. The nurse and the patient evaluate progress towards the stated goals
7. If the the goals need modification, a new contract is negotiated. If the goals have been met or the patient has been discharged, the contract is terminated[1]

The authors stress the importance of making the contract very specific to ensure that the terms of the agreement are clearly understood by all concerned. It should contain not only specific daily activities but also the variables of the activity. For instance, in the verbal contract described above, the nurse would specify the number of times she would help the patient with deep-breathing exercises and the times of the day the patient should practice before surgery. It is likely that more than one nurse is involved in the patient's care; therefore, they would all need to be agreeable to the arrangements if the contract is to be fulfilled. The patient's primary physician should also be involved in the contract design. Depending on the nature of the activity, the physician's orders may need to be included and, in any case, the contract must be consistent with the overall plan of care for the patient.

The nurse has an important motivating role during the working phase of the nurse-patient relationship, in addition to her responsibilities in carrying out specific nursing care measures. She encourages the patient to take increasing responsibility for his own care as he is able, and she helps him to keep working towards the goals they have established together. A review of progress made each day and honest praise for accomplishment of the various tasks that are his responsibility help to keep the patient motivated. Family and friends, who often are as concerned about his health as the patient, can also provide support in motivating him to work toward the established goals.

Termination Phase

The nurse-patient relationship terminates when the patient is discharged from the agency or the nurse leaves for another assignment or for vacation, or for any other reasons ceases to provide care for the patient. Sometimes the relationship is of short duration, as, for example, when the nurse has had the responsibility of caring for the patient for one shift only. For the nurse working in an acute care setting, the relationships are usually short, extending over a few days or a few weeks. In long-term care facilities, in which the patients are often residents, the nurse may work with one group of patients for several months. The community health nurse may have patients she works with over a period of years. Whatever the length of the relationship, there is an inevitable sense of loss when the relationship is terminated. This feeling is more acute, of course, the longer the relationship has been.

It is helpful during the termination phase to review with the patient the accomplishments that have been made, or progress toward the previously established goals. It helps to assuage the feelings of loss if the goals have been met and the patient no longer needs the nurse's care. There is a great deal of satisfaction in seeing the patient recovered from a bout of illness and able to take responsibility for his own health once more, or to see a child grow to adulthood after having successfully passed the health hazards of infancy and childhood with the help of your guidance to the mother. Patients, too, have a feeling of accomplishment if goals have been achieved or if there has been definite progress toward them with the nurse's help. Sometimes, it is necessary to hand over the care of your patient to another person. In these situations it is always helpful if you can introduce the patient

to the person who will be caring for him next. The patient may be transferred to another agency. In this case, he needs to be prepared for the transfer. Reviewing his progress to date and giving him information about the agency he is going to help to make the transfer easier. If the patient, for example, is being moved from an acute care hospital to an extended care unit, he will appreciate knowing where the agency is located, the type of accommodation he will have, and something about the care he can expect. If a member of the family can visit the facility, this is helpful. In many larger hospitals, a nurse is employed as discharge coordinator and can assist in facilitating the transfer.

THE PROCESS OF COMMUNICATION

Communication involves both the sending and the receiving of a message. If the message is not received, no communication has taken place.

Because communication is such as essential component of most people's work, as well as a basic social process, it has received a great deal of study. Numerous models have been developed to illustrate the process. The Source, Message, Channel, Receiver (SMCR) model[2] of the communication process (shown below) is one that illustrates the process simply, contains all the basic elements, and is easily understood.

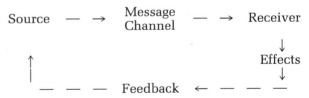

The essential elements in this process are:

1. A source (sender)—someone who wishes to send a message to another person
2. A message—the thought, feeling, or idea that the sender wishes to convey
3. A channel—the means by which the message is conveyed
4. A receiver—the person for whom the message is intended

Let us consider an example. The nurse in a doctor's office wishes Mr. Brown to go into the examining room and tells him so. The *source* is the nurse. The *message* is "Please go to the examining room." The *channel* is the spoken word. The intended *receiver* of the message is Mr. Brown. The desired effect on the receiver is that he gets up from the chair on which he has been sitting and proceeds to the examining room. If he does, the nurse will know that he received the message. If he does not, she will assume that the message was not received. The *effects* on the receiver provide the sender with *feedback*, since they enable the person who has sent the message to know if it was received or not. If it was not, communication has not taken place and the sender should try again.

FACTORS AFFECTING COMMUNICATION

Effective communication means that the message the sender intended to convey reached the intended receiver, was received by him, and was interpreted correctly, and that the receiver was able to respond in some meaningful way to indicate that he received the message. Difficulties can occur anywhere along the way in the communication process.

The Source (Sender)

The sender may have a problem in putting his message into a form that can be communicated. This is called coding the message. Some people are very skilled at translating their message into drawings (as, for example, cartoonists), into painting, or into music. Most of us, however, communicate with words, both in speech and in writing, and with nonverbal behavior, such as facial expression, gestures, body postures, and touch. A person can sometimes communicate quite eloquently using nonverbal means, but, in order to convey many of the messages he wants to send, he needs to be able to attach symbolic meanings (in the form of words) to both living creatures and inanimate objects. He must also be able to arrange these symbols to form messages that can be understood by others, and he must be able to send his message clearly.

Consider the person who is in a foreign country, for example, and is unable to speak the language. He can get along to a certain extent by pointing, using gestures, and pantomiming, but, when it comes to asking directions or ordering a meal, he may be unable to attach the right symbols to get his meaning across. He will then probably encounter difficulties. A person who has suffered brain damage and is unable to speak, or cannot put his thoughts into verbal expressions that can be understood by others, has similar problems. Difficulties in making vocal sounds also interfere with the ability to communicate.

Someone who has lost the use of his voice must depend on written forms of communication, gestures, and other ways of expressing himself nonverbally in order to convey messages.

An individual's physical well-being and his emotional state also affect his ability to communicate. A person who is ill may find trying to communicate just too much of an effort, or his thought processes may not function well enough for him to put together a coherent message. A person's emotional state can make communication easier, may hinder his ability to express himself, or may put a stop to his communicating at all. When a person is at ease emotionally and feels comfortable with another person, he usually finds it much easier to talk and express himself. Nervousness and anxiety often interfere with a person's ability to put together a clear message and send it. The nervous applicant at a job interview, for example, frequently finds it difficult to say what he wants to say in the way it should be said, and comes out of the interview feeling that he has said all the wrong things.

All types of emotions can affect one's ability to communicate. A person can be so overwhelmed with happiness that he cannot find the words to express himself adequately. He can also be so angry that no suitable way of expressing his anger comes to him, or too frightened to say or do anything. In these cases, however, the person usually conveys his feelings in nonverbal ways. The look on a person's face can tell you that he is happy. The clenched fist, the pounding on the table, or the slamming of a door can convey anger as eloquently as words. The eyes and the taut facial expression often tell you that a person is frightened.

The Message

The message itself may not be clear. Some people have a problem in getting the message they want to send clear in their own minds. Often, however, a person knows what he wants to communicate, but the way it comes out is not at all what he intended. Sometimes two conflicting messages are being sent simultaneously. For example, the nurse may say to a patient, "I am glad that you came, even if it is late," but the impatient tapping of her foot, or surreptitious glances at her watch, may convey an entirely different meaning to the patient. Noise or other distractions can also interfere with a message exchange. The child who is watching a television program may not hear his mother calling him to come to bed.

In order to convey the meaning intended by the sender, the message must be sent in a form the intended received can understand. If Mr. Brown does not speak English, the communication process breaks down, unless the nurse is able to put her message into a language he does understand, or can convey the intent of her message by nonverbal means. Even with someone who does speak the same language as the nurse, the words must be in terminology that the patient can understand, or again the message is unclear. If the intent of the message is not completely and explicitly stated, as, for example, if directions on how to get to the examining room are not included for the person who is unfamiliar with the physical layout of the office, the message is not complete.

The Channel

The channel chosen for sending a message must be appropriate. Basically, there are three main channels by which we communicate with other people: oral (speech), written, and nonverbal communication.

For oral communication, we have a number of tools at our disposal: talking directly with a person in a face-to-face meeting, recording messages on tape, telephoning, or communicating by radio or television. All are media for the spoken word. There are also many forms of written communication: notes, letters, interoffice memos, records and forms, newpapers, books, and magazines all convey messages in written form. But we also convey messages nonverbally. It has often been said that a person communicates his true feelings more in his actions and his mannerisms than he does in words. A whole area of study in recent years has been on "body language"—that is, the interpretation of messages people send through their facial expressions, gestures, postures, ways of walking, and so forth.

Then, too, pictures and diagrams are often useful as an adjunct to, or in place of, words. Consider the use of diagrams, slides, and films in your own educational program, for example. You can listen to a description and read the directions on how to make a bed and probably learn to do it adequately. But it is much easier when you can see a filmstrip or follow an illustrated manual.

The important point, here is that the medium chosen must be appropriate for the message and must make the intent of the message clear to the intended receiver. Touch can sometimes convey more sympathetic understanding than words to someone who has suffered a loss. Direct face-to-face talking is often a more effective means of communication than telephoning, or writing a message. Some people have difficulty expressing themselves orally and can put their thoughts and feelings down on paper easier. When there is a long list of instructions for someone to follow, it is usually better if these are written down and supplemented with oral clarification as needed. At times the individual just needs time to think about the message, and thus, the written format serves as a future reference.

The Receiver

Problems in communication can also occur at the receiving end of the process. The message may reach someone other than the intended receiver. If Mr. Jones gets up and moves in the direction of the examining room while Mr. Brown continues to sit in his chair, the nurse knows that the wrong person received the message. An individual who is hard of hearing may have difficulty receiving spoken messages, unless he wears a hearing aid, or unless the message is given loudly enough and clearly enough for him to receive it. A person who cannot read or write is unable to receive communications sent in written form. The intended receiver must not only receive the message but also be able to interpret it.

A large number of physical and psychosocial factors can affect a person's ability to understand communications. Age, for example, must be taken into consideration. A child often will not understand messages that are directed to him by an adult, either because the child's language skills have not developed sufficiently for him to be able to symbolize in the same terms as the adult, or because his intellectual development has not reached a level where he can comprehend the idea the adult is trying to convey. The integrity of the anatomical structures and physiological processes involved in interpreting messages must also be intact. When a person's mental faculties have been impaired by brain damage, or his ability to use his mental faculties is lessened by drowsiness, by alterations in his level of consciousness, or by alcohol or drugs, for example, his ability to receive and interpret messages is decreased.

A person's emotional state may also interfere with both his ability to receive messages and and his ability to interpet them. The frightened individual attends only to those messages that concern the object of his fear. He may not receive messages about anything else, or he may misinterpret messages sent by people who are trying to help him. The patient who is afraid that the injection he is about to receive will be painful may perceive the nurse's smile as sadistic rather than reassuring. Most people are at least a little bit afraid of injections; some people have a real phobia about them.

It has often been said that people hear only

what they want to hear. Receiving and interpreting messages is an active process. A person who is told that he has inoperable cancer may not hear the message because he has "turned off" the sound of the doctor's voice. Nurses and other health professionals often do not receive messages sent by patients, simply because they are not attentive to what the person is trying to tell them.

Then again, because each person is a unique individual, who has his own personality traits, background of life experiences, and set of values, each person may interpret a message differently. He will interpret it according to the way he *perceives* it. Therefore, the meaning he atttaches to a message may be completely different from the one intended by the sender. The nurse may take the arm of an older person as he walks along the hall. The gesture by the nurse may be intended to convey her warmth of feeling for the older person, but he may interpret it as, "She thinks I can't walk by myself." He then sees it as a threat to his independence and brushes her hand aside.

Words, of course, do not have the same meaning for everyone. The meanings attached to symbols we use in our language differ, depending on the context in which the words were learned. In some countries, the examining room in a doctor's office is known as the doctor's surgery. Telling someone who is not used to this terminology to go to the doctor's surgery, then, might conjure up visions of a major operation about to take place, whereas the doctor may just want to put a simple dressing on the patient's injured hand.

Messages are received and interpreted on both an intellectual and an emotional level. Mr. Brown may be afraid to go into the examining room, particularly if the nurse calls it a "surgery," because of what he thinks may happen to him there, and he may not respond to the nurse's message. Or, he may react with hostility toward the nurse, perhaps because he did not like the tone of her voice, or the way she addressed him. He responds to the attitude that is conveyed nonverbally at the same time as the nurse's spoken words. He may think, "If that's the way she is going to treat me, I'm not going to do anything she wants me to do." This type of situation arises frequently with children, who will often do anything for someone they like and trust, but nothing for the person who has failed to win their confidence.

Source credibility is important, though, with adults too. That is to say, a person must believe that the other person is telling him the truth and that the person is a reliable source of information. In order to promote effective communica-tion, the nurse must foster an atmosphere in which the patient feels that he is safe, that he is accepted as a person, and that he can trust the nurse.

THR NURSE AS SENDER IN THE COMMUNICATION PROCESS

There is an old rhyme that goes, "I have six honest serving men who taught me all I know. Their names are Who and What and When, and Where and Why and How."

In thinking about communication and how to get a message conveyed to an intended receiver so that the message is received and correctly interpreted, the nurse may find it helpful to ask herself the six questions contained in the rhyme. We will start with the what, since the first thing to do is to get the message clear in your own mind before you decide how to send it.

What is to Be Communicated?

Is it directions, such as how to get somewhere or how to do something?

Is it information, such as explaining to a patient what is going to happen to him when he goes down to the x-ray department for a series of tests?

It is an attitude, such as a feeling of warmth and acceptance?

Who is the Intended Receiver?

What is this person like as an individual?
What is his background?
What is likely to be his point of view?

Why is This Message to Be Communicated?

Does the patient need to know something, in order to become oriented to the agency?

Does he need help to overcome his fear of surgery?

Does he need this message for his safety? To increase his independence?

How Should It Be Communicated?

Should I talk to the person, should I give him information (or directions) in writing, or would nonverbal communication be best for this particular message?

Where Should the Communication Take Place?

In the patient's room, in the nursing station, in a classroom outside the nursing unit?

When Should It Be Communicated?

Is the person receptive to the message?
Does he need the message now?
Should it be delayed?

The nurse will probably think of many more questions that could be asked, but, if she remembers the six basic ones, it will help her to keep in mind some of the fundamental elements of the communication process when she is in the position of being the sender in the process.

THE SPOKEN WORD AS A MEDIUM OF COMMUNICATION

In sending a message to anyone, either in speech or in writing, the language chosen for the message should be simple and clear. Some people have a tendency to overcommunicate. The message gets lost somewhere among the explanations, embellishments, or general extra wordage that the sender feels he should include. Some people undercommunicate, so that the message is incomplete, and the receiver has to ask for further clarification. If a person has something important to communicate, the message should be sent in the simplest language and with as few words as possible (but as many as are necessary to get the meaning across), if he wants to be sure his message will be interpreted correctly.

Then there is the choice of words. Although many people in our health-oriented society are quite knowledgeable about health matters, such as the causes and treatment of illness, they often do not understand the technical terms that health workers use. Each line of work has its own jargon—that is, technical terms that are used in that particular field but are not in common use outside the field. Health professionals have their own language and use a good many technical terms that are readily understood by other health workers but are incomprehensible to the average layman. The terminology that nurses learn in order to be able to communicate effectively with other health professionals is often not understood by patients. Effective communication with others depends on the use of a common language. It is important, then, that nurses talk to patients in terms that they can understand. The nurse must assess the patient's language level and use appropriate words to express her meaning clearly.

For example, the nurse might ask and environmental health technician or a medical officer of health. "What measures are taken for vector control?" and expect a satisfactory answer. If an average homeowner were asked the same question, he or she probably wound not know what the nurse was talking about. On the other hand, if she were to say, "Do you have screens on the doors and windows to keep out insects?" The person would probably be able to understand the question more clearly.

Health workers commonly use technical terms to refer to vital bodily functions. The words "void" and "defecate," for example, are used for urination and defecation, but terms like "pass water," "pee," and "bowel movement" are probably more readily understood by most people. In working with children, it is important to find out the particular terms that they have been taught.

NONVERBAL COMMUNICATION

Feelings and attitudes are conveyed not only in the words a person says, but also in his nonverbal behavior. Nurses should be aware that their facial expression, tone of voice, gestures, and posture all convey in subtle ways their regard and feeling for another person. At the same time, the nurse should be aware that clues about the patient's feelings, attitudes, and often his physical condition can be picked up through observations of his nonverbal behavior.

Facial expression is perhaps the most common way in which feelings are expressed by people nonverbally. One conveys feelings of happiness, fear, surprise, anger, disgust (contempt), and sadness by using the facial muscles. Facial expressions speak a universal language. In cross-cultural experiments, psychologists have found remarkable agreement in people from different countries in interpreting emotions expressed in photographs. Both literate and illiterate cultures have been tested, with remarkably similar results.[3]

Patients are very quick to note the expression on a nurse's face and to relate it to their own needs and anxieties. Conversely, the nurse can learn a great deal about people from their facial expressions. For example, the patient in pain has a typical facial grimace; the face of the fearful patient looks anxious; the worried patient usually wears a frown.

Human beings, as opposed to the lower animals, can use the muscles around their eyes and

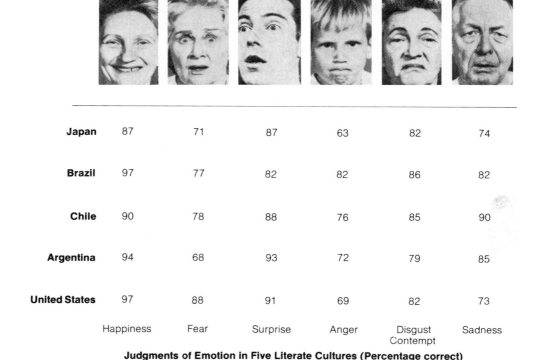

	Happiness	Fear	Surprise	Anger	Disgust Contempt	Sadness
Japan	87	71	87	63	82	74
Brazil	97	77	82	82	86	82
Chile	90	78	88	76	85	90
Argentina	94	68	93	72	79	85
United States	97	88	91	69	82	73

Judgments of Emotion in Five Literate Cultures (Percentage correct)

(From Ekman, P.: Facial Muscles Talk Every Language. Psychology Today, 9:36, September 1975.)

mouths to express their feelings. Actors on the stage are aware of the impact of facial expression and learn to control their muscles to such an extent that the audience is able to tell, merely by looking at their faces, the emotions they wish to convey. Perhaps the nurse does not need as much skill in facial expression as the actor, but she does need to be able to control nonverbal expressions of dislike, hostility, and disgust. She can begin to accomplish this by examining her own motivations and feelings.

Body posture is also a means of communicating. An erect, upright posture usually indicates that a person has a feeling of self-esteem and a considerable degree of inner poise. Sadness, depression, or a low regard for oneself usually makes a person stoop or slouch. It is not uncommon, for example, to see a severely depressed person sitting slumped over in a chair or shuffling along with his head down and shoulders rounded.

Grooming also conveys meaning. A neat, well-groomed look indicates that a person takes pride in his appearance. The attitude of the patient towards his grooming is often indicative of his state of well-being. Very ill people often do not have the strength or the desire to keep up their grooming. The request of a female patient for a mirror and her cosmetics has often been noted as an indication that she is feeling better.

People are often unaware of the gestures they use, but gestures play an important role in conveying thoughts and feelings. The welcoming gesture as you ask a person to sit down helps to put him at ease. A hurried manner with quick

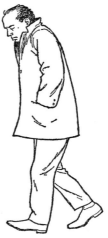

The dejected walker. (Reprinted from Nierenberg, G. I., and Calero, H. H.: How to Read a Person Like a Book. New York, Hawthorn Books, 1971.)

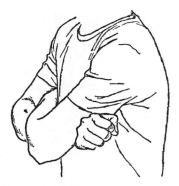

Tension indicated by the folded arms and clenched fists. (Reprinted from Nierenberg, G. I., and Calero, H. H.: How to Read a Person Like a Book. New York, Hawthorn Books, 1971.)

gestures on the part of the nurse evokes a feeling that the nurse does not have much time and, as a result, the patient becomes reluctant to ask questions or to confide his fears and worries. Significant, too, are the patient's gestures. Lowered eyes or an averted glance usually indicates a wish to avoid communication on a topic. A person who sits with his arms folded and his body occupying as little space as possible is often tense.

A wide variety of subtle meanings are conveyed by the *intonation of one's voice*. There is an adage that it is not so much what you say as how you say it. Small children in particular respond much more to the tone of a person's voice than to his words. Adult patients, however, are also sensitive to coldness or warmth as conveyed in the tone of the nurse's voice.

A person's tone of voice is often indicative of his feelings of well-being. An anxious person frequently has difficulty in expressing himself, as we have noted. A person who is ill usually speaks more slowly and in a lower tone than usual. With excitement, the voice often rises and is more highly pitched. A myriad of feelings may be expressed simply by changing the intonation of one's voice as, for example, in saying "Good morning." People are seldom aware of how their voice sounds to others. Listening to a tape recording of one's voice is often useful in helping to hear oneself as others do.

CREATING A CLIMATE FOR PATIENTS TO COMMUNICATE FREELY

In order to foster an atmosphere of openness in which the individual feels free to communicate, the nurse must convey a feeling of warmth and acceptance.

Warmth implies a genuine liking for people; *acceptance*, the ability to understand another person's point of view and to respect the right of each individual to be different. Acceptance means being nonjudgmental. This is not an easy task. Each person brings to his or her own work conscious and unconscious attitudes, biases, and prejudices that reflect his or her own social background and the learning and life experiences he or she has had. And, everyone tends to evaluate other people and events in the light of his or her own experiences. A member of one of the helping professions, however, must learn to understand other people in the light of *their* backgrounds and experiences. Learning to be nonjudgmental is a conscious undertaking for most people. It is helpful for the nurse to first become aware of her own attitudes, biases, and prejudices and to understand how they were acquired. Attitudes, biases, and prejudices are all learned; they can all therefore, be unlearned or, at least, modified by additional learning and life experiences. Taking courses in psychology can help the nurse to gain an increased understanding of her own self and also greater insight into individual differences and the factors motivating behavior. Courses in sociology and anthropology help in developing an appreciation of cultural and social influences on behavior. Working with people from other cultures and from different social backgrounds, and getting to know them as individuals, also helps to change attitudes previously held, consciously or unconsciously.

Giving Information

Communication is always a two way process and, in order to keep the communication channels open, the nurse must contribute too. She is an important source of information for the patient, as we have noted before. She should always answer the patient's questions, both those he has verbalized and his unspoken ones. Her answers should be specific, with as much information as she can provide and in terms that the patient can readily understand. The patient, for example, may say to the nurse, "The doctor said he was sending in a referral for a neurologist to investigate this ringing in the ears I've been having. What, exactly, did he mean?" The nurse might answer, "He has asked Dr. Smith to come in and check you over. He thinks the problem may be related to the nerves that are involved in hearing. Dr. Smith is one of our top-flight specialists in this field. He'll probably be in to see you later this morning." Or, the patient may say, "I hear they are going to operate on me tomorrow. I wish I knew what time." The nurse might say, "I have just seen the schedule for tomorrow's surgery. Your operation is down for 8 a.m." Or, if she doesn't have the information, she might say, "I don't know just yet. They make up the schedule in the afternoon and we usually have it by 3 p.m. As soon as it comes, I will let you know.''

LEARNING TO LISTEN

In any nurse-patient communication, the patient's problems, interests, feelings, and activities are the primary focus. In order to help the patient, the nurse must learn to listen. Most people will communicate quite readily if they have an attentive listener who is not going to impose his or her own values on them, nor proffer unwanted advice. The techniques of being a good listener can be learned. Many such techniques, developed in the behavioral sciences, are now being taught to students in the health professions. Although most beginners tend to feel a little self-conscious using them, the techniques soon become a habitual way of responding, particularly if the rationale for their use is understood, and practice is gained in using them.

One of the first things to learn is to listen attentively. To the patient, this conveys that someone is interested in him as a person and is willing to devote time and energy to hearing what he has to say.

The nurse's posture is important in conveying to the patient that she is listening attentively. Much nurse-patient communication occurs during the process of giving care, and the nurse, particularly in a hospital setting, is usually standing as she works. For an interview (such as taking the nursing history), a discussion of problems the patient has, negotiating a contract, or the like, it is always better if the nurse can sit and talk with the patient. You do not want the patient to think you are in a hurry. Sitting down to talk implies a more relaxed manner than standing. Getting out from behind a desk and sitting in a comfortable chair (with the patient also in a comfortable chair) helps to create a more relaxed atmosphere for both the nurse and the patient in a community health setting. It also helps in saying to the patient that you and he are equal partners in this relationship. Preferably nurse and patient should be on the same level so that good eye contact can be maintained. It should be remembered, however, that in some ethnic cultures, it is considered disrespectful to look another person directly in the eyes. In the American Indian culture, for example, it is felt that this is tantamount to looking into a person's soul.[4]

The nurse should sit facing the patient directly—this helps to indicate a willingness to listen. Neither arms nor legs should be crossed, as these actions tend to portray a defensive posture and what you are striving for is a nondefensive posture to foster openness in the relationship. It helps to lean slightly forward, toward the patient, as you talk. You will probably find that you do this automatically—most people do in conversational situations.

You need to watch, too, the distance you are from the patient. Each of us likes to have a certain amount of space around us. It is a natural protective instinct, and we feel threatened when other people intrude upon it. If you are in a crowded elevator, for example, and a number of people get off at one floor, you will almost automatically move to put more space between you and the next person. The amount of room a person likes as his personal body space varies, depending on personal idiosyncrasies, on cultural mores, on how a person feels at the time, and on the intimacy of the situation. Many North American Indians, for example, do not like to be touched (except in intimate family situations) because they feel that their personal body space is being violated. In some other ethnic groups, such as the Italian, there is often much hugging and kissing even among people who do not know each other very well. Some people when they are ill do not want anyone near them. You may have felt that way on occasion yourself— you just don't want anyone to touch you or come close to you.

Studies have been done on the distances most commonly used for various types of social interaction.[5, 6] A knowledge of these ranges is useful in judging the space to keep between you and the patient in different situations, so that you both feel comfortable.

For intimate interaction 3 to 18 inches (7.5 to 45 cm.) is the average range. This distance is used for confidential information-a whisper can be heard by most people. It is also used in nonverbal communication, such as putting an arm around the shoulder to comfort someone or cuddling an infant. For personal interaction, when you are discussing personal matters, the range is from approximately one and a half to 4 feet (0.4 to 1.2 meters). At this distance, a soft voice can be heard by the person with normal hearing but people at a farther distance cannot overhear the conversation. This is the distance to maintain when you are discussing personal matters with the patient. You should be near enough to shake the person's hand or touch his shoulder. Distances from 4 to 12 feet (1.2 to 3.7 meters) are used for most social interactions (as in small group discussions). The normal speaking voice is used, but it is important to remember that it can be heard by others within the range. This distance is suited to discussions on nonpersonal matters. In public interactions, such as teaching in a classroom or giving a talk to a fairly large group of people (more than 10 to 12), the distance may be beyond 12 feet (3.7 meters). One has to be careful in these situations to speak in a loud, clear voice and enunciate your words clearly. Twenty to 24 feet (6.0 to 7.4 meters) is usually as far as the average person can project his voice indoors without the use of a microphone, although he may be able to do so up to 100 feet (30 meters) outdoors.

Many of the measures nurses use in caring for patients necessitate being in the intimate range of interaction. People often feel uncomfortable at this distance with someone they do not know well, and they may react with a reflex withdrawal. The nurse should, whenever possible, alert the person beforehand as to what she is going to do.

Listening attentively is an active process. The person must have the nurse's undivided attention. Some people feel that the nurse should not take notes when she is talking to a patient to obtain information; others, however, feel that taking notes does not hinder the communication process. Certainly, if a lot of information is needed from the patient, it is difficult to remember everything that has been said without the benefit of notes. It may be reassuring too for the patient to know that details of the things he likes and does not like, and his particular concerns, for example, have been noted and will not be forgotten. Attentive listening is also indicated by the responses the nurse makes.

Responses That Help

Minimal Responders. Sometimes just a word or a nod of the head is sufficient to give the patient the feeling that the nurse is interested in what he is saying and would like him to continue. Words or utterances such as "Mmm . . . ," "Yes," "I understand," and so forth, have been termed "minimal responders" and are frequently used, although the nurse may find other words that she feels more comfortable in using.

Silence. Sometimes it is best not to say anything, particularly if you feel that the patient has something he wants to add to his last statement. Most of us feel uncomfortable when conversation lapses and, if a pause lasts too long, we want to rush in to fill the vacuum. Often, however, people need to think about what they are going to say and, given a little time, will continue with their train of thought. Or, they may decide that they don't want to pursue the subject any further and will introduce a new topic. One should not press, or give the appearance of prying into another person's private affairs. Some people just do not want to talk

about personal matters, and the nurse should respect their wishes in this regard. People brought up in the traditional Japanese culture, for example, usually do not like to talk out their emotional problems. Sometimes, just sitting quietly with the patient or walking with him down the corridor is enough to let him know that you understand his feelings.

Touch. Touch is a very important form of nonverbal communication for nurses. We use our hands in so many of our nursing measures. Touching the patient's hand or shoulder or holding the sobbing child can convey empathy. There is often no need for words. Touch is something that has to be used with discretion, however, because, as we have already mentioned, people of some cultures find touch distressing. For some, it is an outright taboo. According to one study most Israeli patients do not like to be touched too much when they are sick, nor do adult Puerto Rican patients.[7]

Reflecting Feelings. Another way of indicating interest and attention is through the reflection of feelings the person has expressed. People sometimes express their feelings directly in words, as, for example, "I was so angry that I . . . ." Sometimes they describe their actions, and it is through this description that the nurse is able to identify the person's feelings. For instance, if the person says, "I can't stand it any longer, so I banged on the door," he is obviously expressing feelings of frustration and probably feelings of anger and hostility toward whoever was on the other side of the door. The nurse may also pick up clues about the patient's feelings from his nonverbal behavior, as discussed earlier in this chapter. The nurse might respond in words that acknowledge the feelings as, for example, by saying, "I understand that you were angry [or annoyed, or hurt]" or "You were upset by . . . . [whatever it was he was describing]," or "I can see that this bothers you." Although it is sometimes useful to use the patient's own words in response, it is more important to reflect his feelings. Repeating the individual's words can make the nurse's response sound mechanical, as if she were parroting a learned response.

Repeating Key Words or Phrases. At times, though, it is helpful to repeat key words or phrases that the person has used, particularly if he has expressed a number of thoughts at one time. To use an example, a person might say, "Nothing seems to have gone right since I had that operation a year ago. I can't seem to work the way I used to. I haven't been able to go to the lodge either and I miss that. You know, the lodge folks are a mighty nice group of fellows."

Here it might be useful for the nurse to pick up the key phrase "since I had that operation a year ago," rather than responding to the lodge item. Repeating a key word or phrase helps to keep the conversation focused on important issues rather than irrelevant items.

Using Open-ended Questions or Statements. If the nurse wishes to obtain more information about a specific point, it is often helpful to repeat a key word or phrase in a question or statement that gives the person an opportunity to say more. The nurse might say, "You said that you had an operation a year ago" (repeating the key phrase). "Perhaps you could tell me more about it." Or, she might simply say, as a question, "You had an operation a year ago?" Sometimes the nurse can use an open-ended statement or question, such as "You were going to say . . ." or "Would you like to tell me more about it?"

Asking for Clarification. Sometimes it is difficult to identify feelings or to understand the meaning of a person's words. The nurse may then want to ask for clarification. Phrases such as, "You mean that you were angry?" or "Am I right in thinking that you felt guilty [or depressed, or sad]?" are examples of responses the nurse could make to verify her impressions. Asking for clarification also helps to indicate to the patient that the nurse is trying to understand his point of view.

Exploring Alternatives. Sometimes the nurse can help an individual to explore possibilities in regard to resolving problems he has identified. She may be aware of factors in the situation that he has not mentioned, or she may help him to think about things he might want to take into consideration in working through his solution to these problems. She may then want to mention these factors in her responses to his statements or questions. She should be careful, however, not to give her own opinions on what he should do, but rather to help him consider all factors and possible alternatives in the situation.

Responses That Hinder

Reassurance. Responses that hinder the flow of conversation can be made if the nurse is not thinking about the impact of her words. One of the most common ways of cutting off communication is the use of reassurance. We want to make the patient feel better—therefore, we say things like, "Don't worry, everything is going to be all right," "Everybody feels like that," or "We haven't lost a patient yet" (from a simple or routine procedure). Comments such as these may be said with the intention of reassurance, but they may convey to the patient that the nurse is denying he has a problem.

The patient isn't really interested in how "everybody else" feels. He is interested in his own feelings and problems. Procedures that are routine and simple to the nurse are new and problematic to the patient.

Social Cliches. Closely allied to reassurance are the social clichés that seem to come almost automatically to our lips if we are not thinking too much about what we are saying. Expressions like, "You'll feel better after a good night's sleep," "Your doctor knows what is best for you," and "Everything will work out in time" are examples of common clichés, that is, pat answers that are trite and have lost their meaningfulness through overusage. They tend to convey to the patient that you weren't really listening to what he was saying. You probably were thinking of something else and answered automatically.

Hostility. People who are anxious frequently react with anger and hostility to those around them. Nurses and other health workers often bear the brunt of this anger from patients and their families, and it is difficult not to be hostile in return. A hostile response made by a nurse, such as, "You shouldn't say things like that," can humiliate the individual and, most certainly, will hinder the progress of the nurse/patient relationship.

Imposing Values. The nurse should be careful not to impose her own values on the patient. "You shouldn't have done that," or "If I were you, I would have done this or that," are examples of evaluative responses that are best avoided.

Giving Advice. Giving advice implies to the other person that you know better than they do what they should do. If your advice is being requested on matters pertaining to the patient's health, this is an area in which you are expected to have more knowledge, and advice may be acceptable. Advising people on matters other than health is generally not acceptable. For example, statements such as, "I think I would tell your sister to stop bothering you," or "If I were you, I'd sell all those stocks and bonds and buy real estate" are likely to cut off communication. Most people don't want advice, unless they specifically ask for it. Even if they ask for your opinion, it is wise to refrain from giving advice in areas in which you are not an acknowledged expert. Even when it is a matter of health, it is preferable to help the patient to explore alternatives, so he can make his own decisions, rather than giving cut and dried answers.

Probing. We have already mentioned that the nurse should avoid the appearance of probing into another person's private life. Questions such as, "Why do you feel this way?" or "Why did you do that?" or statements like "Tell me more about your relationship with your sister" are probing responses. Often, the person himself may not know the answer to the why, or if he does, may resent someone asking him. It puts him in an uncomfortable position when he has to explain his actions. Silence is often preferable to asking direct questions, particularly if an individual appears to feel deeply about something.

Belittling. Belittling the feelings or actions of another person engenders resentment. Saying things like, "Other people don't seem to feel this way" conveys to the patient that there must be something wrong with him if he is reacting in this fashion. Or, telling the patient about other people's accomplishments or their problems that are greater than his make him feel small and insignificant. If a post-partum patient says, "My stitches hurt" and the nurse answers, "You have to expect a little pain. My sister told me she couldn't sit down for a week after she had her baby," the patient is not likely to confide further in the nurse.

Rejection. The nurse can cut off communication, consciously or unconsciously, by rejecting the patient's feelings, thoughts, or actions. Statements such as, "You shouldn't feel like that," "I don't want to hear about it," or "How could anyone do that?" give the impression to the other person that his thoughts, feelings, or actions are unworthy. He is likely, then, to avoid talking further about that subject, and may be hesitant to bring up other matters. Rejection can be communicated also by nonverbal means. Turning away from a person, averting your eyes, and subconsciously backing away can all indicate rejection.

A Case in Point

The following example shows how the nurse can affect the patient's well-being through communication.

Mr. Angelo Niccolini is a 64-year-old widower who was admitted to the hospital suffering from difficulty in breathing and pain in his chest, left arm, and back. Mr. Niccolini emigrated from Italy 50 years ago and, although he is fluent in English, he prefers to speak only Italian at home.

He lives with his daughter and son-in-law and their four teenage children in a predominantly Italian neighborhood. He is a baker, head of the family business, which he runs with his three sons, who live in the same neighborhood. Mr. Niccolini's working day is usually from 0400 to 1800 hours, 6 days a week. He smokes about a pack of cigarettes a day. He enjoys food and is consequently overweight. He drinks what he considers a moderate amount of wine every day. He has never been hospitalized before and appears very anxious about being separated from his family.

Mr. Niccolini is sitting up in bed playing solitaire and muttering to himself when the nurse walks in.

N.: Good morning, Mr. Niccolini. How are you feeling this morning?

Mr. N.: What's good about it? I feel fine. Why can't I go home? I just sit here all day. Why can't I have a cigarette and some decent food? How can you expect me to eat these meals? Now, what I would like is some good pasta, some decent bread, and a little wine. I can't even taste the food you give me here.

N.: You seem to be upset this morning, Mr. Niccolini.
   (reflecting feeling)
   You say you want to go home?
   (picking up key words)

Mr. N.: Yes, I want to go home. Nobody's doing anything for me here. They just take my temperature and my blood pressure now and then, and expect me to lie around like this. I have better things to do with my time.

N.: What sort of things do you feel you have to do, Mr. Niccolini?
   (asking for clarification)

Mr. N.: Well, who's looking after the bakery, for example? They need me there.

N.: Don't your sons work in the bakery with you?
   (asking for clarification)

Mr. N.: Yes, yes, my sons. But they all have their own jobs to do—who's going to make the bread? I always make it myself every morning. They need me.

N.: I'm sure they do need you, Mr. Niccolini. Is someone making the bread now while you are in the hospital?

(accepting the patient's feelings and helping him to explore situation)

Mr. N.: Yes, my oldest boy. But he has his jobs to do too. And who will mind the counter when everyone is busy?

N.: You mind the counter as well as make the bread?
(picking up key phrase)

Mr. N.: My daughter does most of the time, but I help out when things get busy. Luigi comes in and helps on the weekends.

N.: Luigi?
(asking for clarification)

Mr. N.: He's my oldest grandson. He seems to like the bakery or maybe he just likes the money he earns.

N.: Could Luigi come in and help after school?
(helping the patient to explore)

Mr. N.: That might be an idea. Luigi is 17 now and should now be taking more responsibility. I'll call my daughter and see about it.

When the nurse comes back a little later, Mr. Niccolini seems a little more cheerful.

N.: Well, Mr. Niccolini, do you feel better now that you've talked with your daughter?
(showing interest in patient)

Mr. N.: Yes, I do, but I just remembered something.

N.: What's that, Mr. Niccolini?
(encouraging patient to elaborate)

Mr. N.: I'm supposed to give a speech at the baker's association meeting next week. I've never missed a meeting. I guess that's how I became president. Now I won't be able to go on the day I'm supposed to give my speech.

N.: Do the members of the association know you are in the hospital?
(picking up key words and helping patient to explore the situation)

Mr. N.: No. But my sons will tell them at the meeting tonight. Two meetings in a row I'm going to miss.

N.: Would you like to talk with one of the other members? The vice president perhaps?
(helping patient to explore the possibilities to resolve problem)

Mr. N.: Yes, I would, but not until tomorrow. Otherwise, they might decide to let someone else give my speech, and I want to give it myself.

INTERVIEWING

The interview has been defined as a "talk with a purpose." It is a basic tool of communication that is used a great deal by health workers, although its use is not, of course, limited to the health field. Most nursing students will have had experience with interviews. If they have applied for a summer or full-time job, for example, they probably had an interview with their prospective employer. Prior to entering most schools of nursing, students are interviewed by a member of the school faculty as part of the admission procedure.

In the health field, the interview is used for a number of different purposes, and by most health professionals. The physician may interview an individual to obtain a medical history, to use a common example, or to assess the results of therapy.

Social workers use interviewing extensively in their work, as, for example, in discussing financial problems with a patient. The nutritionist may interview someone to find out his food preferences or to counsel a person about his special dietary needs. The psychologist uses the interview mainly as a therapeutic tool, as in helping a person to resolve his emotional problems.

Nurses, in their practice, may use interviewing for any or all of the purposes exemplified above—for gathering information or for verifying it, for assessing the results of nursing care, in counseling people about health matters, in planning with individuals about their care, and as a therapeutic tool.

When planning an interview, the nurse takes into account not only its purpose, but also the time and the setting for the interview. She should be familiar with some of the basic techniques of interviewing, such as those used in beginning and ending an interview, and in eliciting specific information. As with other skills, interviewing requires practice. One should not expect to become an expert overnight, or in one easy lesson. The material presented here is intended simply as an introduction to the subject. Many textbooks and articles have been written

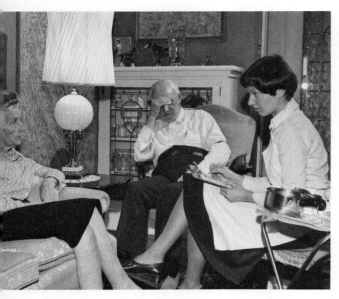

The nurse frequently uses the interview to gather information from a patient.

on interviewing, and the nurse will probably want to supplement the material presented here with additional readings from the list of references suggested at the end of the chapter.

Setting the Time and Place for the Interview

An adequate amount of time should be set aside for the interview, the length depending on the purpose and nature of the interview. Judgment must be exercised on both the length of time allotted for the interview and the time at which it takes place. If a person is seriously ill and many new and frightening things are happening to him, or if he has just been admitted to the hospital and is having numerous tests and examinations, it may be best to delay an interview until the immediate crisis is over. Again, if the person appears to be becoming fatigued, it is wise to terminate an interview and complete the session at another time. Interviews should be scheduled for a time when both the patient and the nurse are free from other commitments. They should not conflict with appointments the patient has for x-rays, laboratory tests, treatments, or visiting hours. Nor should the nurse feel hurried or rushed because she has other things to do. In short, one strives for a relaxed, unhurried atmosphere.

It is always best to have a quiet and private room in which to interview an individual. This is, however, not always possible in our busy and often crowded health agencies. It is important, though, that the person being interviewed feel that he has the undivided attention of the nurse and that his confidentiality is being respected.

A corner of a lounge or of an office can be used, or the curtains can be pulled around the patient's bed if he is in the hospital and not in a private room.

Beginning an Interview

An interview is essentially a conversation between two people—often, as when the patient has just been admitted to the agency and the nurse has not met him before, between two strangers. The nurse, as the interviewer, has a responsibility to put the other person at ease. For the beginning student, who is perhaps a bit apprehensive about interviewing someone, it is helpful to remember that the patient, too, is probably anxious. Most people who seek the help of health professionals by coming to a health agency are either ill or in some way concerned about their health. Even those who are well and attending a health maintenance clinic usually have some minor worries. They are all, therefore, at least a little anxious. It helps if the nurse observes the common courtesies of greeting people by name, offering them a seat (in an ambulatory setting), or asking their permission to sit down and talk (if the person is in an inpatient facility). The nurse should also introduce herself by name. These courtesies convey a feeling of respect for the person who is being interviewed and help to put him at ease. The common ritual also helps the nurse to feel more comfortable.

The nurse should also state the purpose of the interview and the approximate amount of time it will take. This information helps to set the climate for the interview. The patient feels more comfortable when he knows what to expect and why the nurse is interviewing him. The nurse might say, for example, that the purpose is to learn something about the person so that his care can be planned to suit his individual needs and preferences if it is an initial assessment interview. Or she may say she would like to talk with him about plans for his going home.

Eliciting Specific Information

Although the nurse often has specific information that she wants to obtain from the individual during the interview, it should not be conducted as a question and answer session. It may be a structured interview in the sense that the nurse controls and directs the conversation, as when the nurse gathers information in her assessment interview, but the individual should feel free to discuss his feelings and concerns and the things that are important to him. Most people will give all the information needed, and more, if an open climate is created.

In this regard the section in this chapter on creating a climate in which the patient feels free to communicate and on learning to listen will be helpful.

When there is specific information that the nurse would like to obtain, some direct questions will have to be asked. In such cases it is probably a good idea to start with the person's immediate concerns, that is, his feelings and perceptions in regard to whatever the interview is about, without interjecting too many questions in the beginning. If the nurse does not do this, there is a possibility that important factors may be missed. It is usually considered best, in asking questions, to start from the general and then proceed to the specific details. Also, people usually respond much better to impersonal questions at first. The nurse should leave the more personal ones until the patient has had a chance to get to know the nurse a little during the course of the interview. In our computer-age society, most people are used to filling in forms and answering questions about their name, age, education, and place of employment. These are relatively impersonal items. An individual's likes and dislikes and his feelings are more personal. These should be left until after the general questions have been answered.

Ending an Interview

When the purpose of the interview has been accomplished, the nurse should take some time to ask the patient if he has any questions, or if there are other things that he is concerned about that were not discussed. Patients often feel that the nurse is busy and they are sometimes reluctant to take up her time. But taking a few minutes to listen to the patient's concerns often saves the nurse time in the long run, since the patient is less apt to make frequent requests later if he is reassured that someone is concerned about him as a person.

In terminating an interview, it is again helpful to observe the social amenities. Thanking the person for his time, saying that you will see him again, and assuring him that he can call on you if he is concerned about anything are all ways of conveying to the patient that he is a person worthy of respect.

COMMUNICATING WITH OTHER MEMBERS OF THE HEALTH TEAM

Nurses very seldom work in complete isolation. Even in a remote nursing station where she may be the sole provider of health care for a community, the nurse almost always has at least radio contact with a base hospital where she can communicate with other members of the health team. Very few nurses work in isolated rural settings, of course. More usually, the nurse is employed in a busy, urban health agency where there are large numbers of nurses and a variety of other health personnel.

Communication with other members of the health team is an important part of the nurse's work. It is essential to facilitate the process of patient care. Information gathered by all team members provides the basis for planning comprehensive care for the patient. Sharing information helps to avoid duplication of effort in gathering data and also enables each team member to benefit from the information others have collected. Communication is essential too in the planning of patient care so that everyone shares the same goals for the patient; in that way, care is coordinated and people are not working at cross-purposes.

The actual implementation of health care today is also very much a team effort. The provision of comprehensive care requires the skills and talents of many different categories of workers. The physician and the nurse have always worked closely together in many aspects of patient care and continue to do so. With the number of specialized workers in the health field today, however, it is more than ever essential that all coordinate their efforts in caring for patients. There must be adequate, effective communication channels for the achievement of this coordination.

Communication between members of the health team takes place in many ways. A great deal of information is exchanged informally, through face-to-face meetings and telephone conversations. But there are also more formal channels, both oral and written, that help to facilitate the exchange of information.

The patient's record is one very important tool that helps to keep all team members up-to-date on the latest information that has been gathered about a patient and the most recent developments regarding his progress. Patient records will be discussed in Chapter 12, so we will not go into them further at this point. Other commonly used communication media that the nurse will utilize frequently are reports, both oral and written, consultations, conferences, referrals, and patient rounds.

Reports

Reporting of information to other members of the health team is essential if they are to be briefed on events that have taken place (or are likely to take place), be told of developments that have occurred in regard to patients' progress, and be alerted to things to watch for in the care of specific patients. Reports may be given either orally or in writing. At the end of each shift, members of the nursing team usually report orally to the team leader on the progress of each patient they cared for during that shift. The team leader, in turn, reports to the head nurse, who uses this information to prepare her change-of-shift report for the nurses who are coming on duty.

The change-of-shift report is usually a fairly formal report, in which the nurse completing her tour of duty "hands over" the care of patients on the unit to those who will be responsible for their care on the next shift. At this time, the progress of each patient on the unit is reviewed, and the nurse who is leaving briefs the newly arrived staff on treatments or other activities that are still in progress, and on events that are likely to occur on the next shift. She may, for example, say that Dr. X is coming in to take out Mr. Smith's sutures this evening, or that the Admitting Department has called to say we are receiving a new patient, giving as many details as she has received herself.

As part of the change-of-shift report, the head nurse often makes rounds with the nurses coming on duty, and they exchange information about each patient in the process. Many agencies are now using tape recorders or Dictaphones to make the change of shift report less cumbersome. Each nurse who has been responsible for the care of a group of patients can dictate the report on her patients. Nurses coming on duty then need to receive only a minimal report from the head nurse going off duty and can obtain direct information about each patient from the nurse who cared for him during the previous tour of duty. The head nurse also reports to her supervisor about the patients on the unit. This is often a written report, supplemented by an oral report as needed.

In addition to patient care reports, most health agencies have a large number of other reports and forms that nurses utilize. These vary from agency to agency and the nurse must familiarize herself with those used in the agency in which she is working. There are usually forms for requesting laboratory, x-ray and other types of diagnostic tests, forms for recording the administration of narcotics and other controlled drugs (a count has to be kept of these), forms for ordering drugs and other supplies, and a good many others. We have already mentioned the accident (incident) report, which is completed whenever an unusual occurrence takes place (Chapter 7).

Consultations

The nurse often feels the need to consult with another health practitioner about the care of her patients. She usually consults informally with her team leader, or with the head nurse, or with both. She also consults with the physician about the patient's plan of care and progress. If there is a clinical nursing specialist available, the nurse may want to consult with her about the patient's plan of care, or about unusual problems the patient has. She consults with the physical therapist frequently and with the nutritionist and the social worker—in fact, with all who may be involved with the patient's care.

Physicians consult with other physicians; they frequently call in specialists to see the patient and give opinions regarding diagnostic or therapeutic measures for that patient. The nurse will note the requests for specialist consultations and the specialist's report on the patient's record.

Conferences

Members of the nursing team usually meet daily in a team conference to exchange information about their patients and to review and revise their care plans. Increasingly common too are team conferences, at which various members of the health team meet to review their findings about a patient, to develop a combined plan of care or to review the patient's progress. Until very recently team conferences have been used most frequently in rehabilitation settings, in community health agencies, in psychiatric settings, and in agencies providing long-term care for people who are ill. However, they are becoming more common in all types of health care settings.

Referrals

Referrals are basically of two types, those requesting the services of another department within an agency in the care of a patient, and those referring a patient to another agency for care. In a multiservice ambulatory health care agency, such as a Health Maintenance Organization (HMO), a Community Health Center (CHC), or the Outpatient Department of a hospital, patients are frequently referred from one service to another for specialized care. A patient might be referred to the dental or eye clinic, for example, or to the nutritionist or social worker from a generalized service. In a hospital setting, a referral might be made to such departments as social service, physiotherapy, or inhalation therapy (respiratory technology) for their specialized services for the patient. Patients may also be referred from one agency to another. An HMO or CHC might refer an individual to a hospital if he needs inpatient care (he would be admitted under the care of his attending physician) or a hospital might refer a patient to an HMO or

CHC. If a patient is being discharged from the hospital and requires home care services, a referral would be made to the appropriate agency. Referrals may be made by a community health nurse (or a school nurse) for individuals to receive care from any number of agencies in the community.

A referral system is important to assure continuity of care. It is essential that the agency to which the patient is being referred have sufficient information to assure that continuity. Most agencies have referral forms on which summary information about a patient is written; it is often the nurse who is responsible for completing these forms, although policies vary. In a hospital, the patient's record would be available to the member of the department being called in to see a patient; therefore, the referral is usually simply a request for services.

Patient Rounds

Another means of communicating information about patients is through patient rounds. We have already mentioned one type, when nurses make the rounds on a nursing unit during the change of shift report. The nurse usually makes rounds with the physician when he visits his patients on a hospital nursing unit. A considerable amount of information is exchanged at this time, as opinions are shared regarding the patient's progress and plans are discussed for his care. Often, nursing rounds are made by the head nurse on a unit with her supervisor, with the clinical nursing specialist, or with staff nurses on the unit. Teaching rounds are also made for the benefit of students; both medical and nursing schools use patient rounds as learning experiences for students.

STUDY SITUATION

With the help of your instructor, select a patient in the clinical area in which you are gaining experience. Arrange a time for you to visit the patient for the purpose of taking a nursing history, using the agency's form. By utilizing some of the techniques outlined in the section on learning to listen, see what you can find out about this patient as a person.

SUGGESTED READINGS

Almore, M. G.: Dyadic Communication. *American Journal of Nursing*, 79(6):1076–1078, June, 1979.

Cohn, L.: Barriers and Values in the Nurse/Client Relationship. *ARN Journal*, 3:3–8, November-December, 1978.

Crews, N. E.: Developing Empathy for Effective Communication. *AORN Journal*, 30:536+, September, 1979.

Fire, M., et al.: A Smile and Eye Contact May Insult Someone. *Journal of Nursing Education*, 15:14–17, September, 1976.

Knight, I.: Communication Methods. Part 3. *Nursing Times*, 73:11–12, June 23, 1977.

Long, R.: A Tale of Two Cultures . . . Asian Lady. Arab Lady. Nursing Times 73:1215–1216, August 4, 1977.

Poole, K.: Breaking the Ice. Nursing 81, 11(2):31–32, February, 1981.

Presley, S. R.: When It Came to Communicating without Words . . . Cyrus Was an Expert. *Nursing 80*, 10(10):18, 1980.

Schneggenberger, C.: History-Taking Skills: How Do You Rate? *Nursing 79*, 9:97–101, March, 1979.

Shubin, S.: Nursing Patients from Other Cultures. *Nursing 80*, 10(6):26–29, 1980.

Veninga, R.: Are You a Successful Communicator? *The Canadian Nurse*, 74(3):4–7, November, 1978.

Yearwood-Grazette, H. S.: An Anatomy of Communication. *Nursing Times*, 74:1672–1679, October 12, 1978.

REFERENCES

1. Zangari, M.-E., and Duffy, P.: Contracting with Patients in Day to Day Practice. *American Journal of Nursing*, 80:451–455, March, 1980.
2. Rogers, E. M., and Rogers, A.: *Communication in Organizations*. New York, The Free Press, 1976.
3. Ekman, P.: Face Muscles Talk Every Language. *Psychology Today*, 9:35, September, 1975.
4. Primeaux, M.: Caring for the American Indian Patient. *American Journal of Nursing*, 77(1):91–94, January, 1977.
5. Hall, E. T.: *The Hidden Dimension*. Garden City, N.Y., Doubleday and Co., 1969.
6. Hall, E. T.: *The Silent Language*. Garden City, N.Y., Doubleday and Co., 1959.
7. Shubin, S.: Nursing Patients from Other Cultures. *Nursing 80*, 10(6):26–29, June, 1980.

11

The Nurse Should Be Able to:

- Discuss the importance of the teaching aspects of her role
- List the principles of learning that are relevant to teaching patients
- Give an example from her own learning experiences to illustrate each of these principles
- Explain how each of the following may affect the process of teaching-learning: characteristics of the learner, characteristics of the teacher, the social climate, and the nature of the material to be learned
- Name the basic types of learning tasks
- Describe teaching strategies suitable for each type of task
- Discuss the goal of patient learning as a basis for identifying learning tasks
- Formulate specific objectives for patient learning
- Discuss points to consider in planning and organizing a teaching session, conducting a teaching session, and selecting the time and place for teaching
- Describe methods for the evaluation of patient learning suitable for different types of learning tasks

TEACHING AND LEARNING SKILLS

CHAPTER 11

INTRODUCTION

An important part of nursing is helping the patient to learn the things he needs to know, or to be able to do, in order to promote his optimal well-being. In Chapter 6, we identified teaching as one of the major roles of the nurse. The teaching aspects of nursing are receiving a great deal of emphasis these days, for several reasons. Many of the major health problems in Western societies today are directly or indirectly attributable to life style factors. We discussed this matter in Chapter 4. Overeating, insufficient exercise, smoking, overindulgence in alcohol, excessive speed on the highway, and the stresses of urban living were among the factors we mentioned. Tackling the problems resulting from these (such as obesity, hypertension, heart dis-

ease, respiratory problems, alcoholism, accidents, and mental illness) all involve a large educational component. People must be motivated to change their lifestyles and helped to learn, and adopt, alternatives, if these problems are to be lessened.

Then, too, it is increasingly being acknowledged that people have a responsibility to protect and promote their own health. If they are to assume this responsibility, they have to learn measures that will enable them to do so. Indeed, the emphasis today on patients' rights in the health care system has led to consumer demands that health professionals share their knowledge and skills. The consumer wants to be given the necessary information and taught the requisite skills to look after his own health insofar as he is able. Failure on the part of health profession-

Being taught the proper technique for walking on crutches can allow a patient to function independently while recovering from an injury.

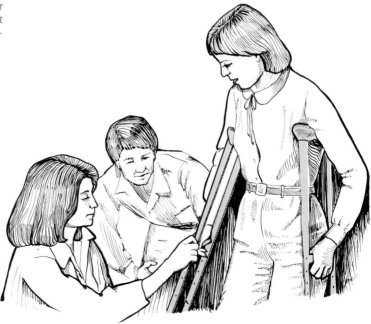

191

als to teach the patient adequately may, in fact, be construed as negligence.

Nurses are playing a key role in educating patients. The nurse is regarded by the public as a person knowledgeable about health matters; her opinion is respected and her advice is sought by people on matters that concern them about their health. By now, you have probably found that your friends and your family—and other people too—are beginning to ask you questions about health matters, even though you are just at the beginning of your nursing program. A comment you will hear frequently throughout your lifetime is, "You should know—after all, you are a nurse." You cannot possibly expect to be able to teach everybody all that they want or need to know about their health at this stage of your career, nor even after you have completed your nursing course. But you can help them to learn what they want to learn.

Every individual, whatever the state of his health, has learning needs in relation to health matters. The person who is active and in good health may need to learn more about nutrition in order to control his weight, or he may want to embark on a regular exercise program to improve his physical well-being. Most people want to know how to protect their health. Parents are usually particularly anxious to learn measures they can take to protect their children from the disorders to which youngsters are particularly vulnerable, as well as steps they can take to promote their child's optimal growth and development.

Most people who become ill have learning needs relative to their new situation. They usually want knowledge about tests and examinations, about their disease process, and, if they have been hospitalized, about their environment. Some people must learn ways of planning for the future, regaining their health, or coping with physical, psychological, and sociological stresses.

Nurses and other health personnel should always keep in mind the ultimate goal of restoring the sick individual to an active, functioning role in society insofar as this is possible. The individual and his family must be assisted from the onset of an illness, and throughout its duration, to engage in activities that will help him achieve the highest level of well-being that is possible for him. To use an example, the person who has had a stroke needs to be encouraged to maintain independent bladder and bowel functioning and given the opportunity to do so, or, if necessary, to regain independence in this area as quickly as possible if it has been lost temporarily during a period of unconsciousness. Nurses all too often accept incontinence as an inevitable result of illness, particularly in older people—yet it need not be so. Rehabilitation is a learning process that should not be left until an episode of acute illness is over.

Patients with terminal illnesses, and their families, also have learning needs. They may need to learn measures to control pain, for example. Lifestyles may need to be altered to accommodate the person with an illness. If the patient remains at home, a bed may need to be moved to a downstairs room, close to a bathroom and to a kitchen, to make care easier. The family may need to learn home nursing skills, such as giving the person a shampoo in bed or making a bed with the person in it.

Helping the individual to learn new skills or to relearn old ones should be a fundamental part of care for all patients.

In order to fulfill her teaching responsibilities, the nurse must know something about the learning process, be able to identify the patient's learning needs, and be able to select appropriate methods and techniques to facilitate the learning process. She should also be able to evaluate the effectiveness of the patient's learning.

THE LEARNING PROCESS

Learning is an active process that continues from birth to death. Throughout his lifetime, an individual is constantly learning as he gains information, develops skills, and applies these in adjusting to new life situations. Learning takes place basically in one of two ways: either informally, through the ordinary activities of living, or formally, through a series of selected learning experiences designed to achieve specific goals.

People learn a great deal about health and illness through informal means. In the family environment, for example, parents usually teach children basic hygiene measures, such as washing their hands before meals and using a tissue to blow their nose. Children also learn measures to protect their health as, for example, "Don't go outside without your coat on—you'll catch cold" or "Wear your rubber boots—you don't want to get your feet wet and take a chill." Care during illness is also a part of childhood learning experiences in the home. The child is put to bed when he has a fever. The parent has certain remedies for a cold, and these are passed on to the child through informal teaching methods. Dietary habits too are learned in the home. The learning that occurs in the family is often supplemented by informal talks with people in the health field, such as the family doctor or a nurse who lives in the community. Other means, such as reading articles in the newspapers about health matters, or the health columns written by medical experts that are a feature in many newspaper and popular magazines, also contribute to a person's informal learning about health matters. Similarly, people learn a great deal about health and illness from radio and television.

People who are sick and need the help of health professionals often learn much about their health problems and how to care for themselves informally through the actual experience of being ill. However, there has been a substantial amount of evidence to indicate that many patients' learning needs are not met through informal channels. One of the most frequent complaints of patients is that they do not receive enough information. This concern has been voiced in the statements of Patients' Bill of Rights (see Chapter 7). Yet it has been shown that the better informed the patient is about his condition, the more effective is his therapy. The value of good teaching in contributing to the sick person's recovery and his rehabilitation has been well documented. Adequate preoperative instruction has been shown to be a factor in the prevention of many postoperative discomforts, such as pain and vomiting, and a contributing factor in early recovery from surgery. Good teaching programs for diabetic patients and for cardiac patients, to cite two examples, are accepted as important aspects of the care of patients with these health problems. Other examples of people whose sole responsibility is to teach patients about their disease include the diabetic teaching team and the "ostomy nurse."

Many ambulatory agencies employ a nurse full time to develop and carry out a program for teaching patients. An HMO, for example, may have a nurse on staff whose responsibilities include teaching prenatal and postpartum classes, weight-control classes (which might include an exercise program), and classes for patients with other kinds of specific health problems.

An "ostomy nurse" teaches patients who have had operations like colostomies and ileostomies how to care for themselves. A colostomy is an artificial opening (stoma) created in the large intestine and brought to the surface of the abdomen for the purpose of evacuating the bowel. An ileostomy is a similar opening in the small intestine.

How Learning Takes Place

Learning causes changes in the learner's thought processes, actions, or attitudes. Evidence of these changes can, for the most part, be observed in the learner's behavior. If your anatomy and physiology instructor asks you to learn the names and functions of the cranial nerves, for example, he or she can observe whether learning has taken place by asking you to list the cranial nerves and explain their functions. Your nursing fundamentals teacher can observe your actions in making a bed and judge whether the requisite amount of learning has taken place to consider that you have mastered the skill. Attitudinal scales have been developed to assess the amount of change that has taken place in a person's opinions or feelings as a result of a learning experience. For example, a scale could be used to assess changes in your attitude toward working with old people after you have had experience in an extended care unit or in a nursing home.

The internal process of learning—what actually goes on inside the learner—does not, however, lend itself to direct observation. One cannot peer into a person's brain to see what is actually taking place. We are perhaps closer to understanding the phenomenon of learning motor skills (the psychomotor area of learning) as a result of research into the physiology of muscular activity. We know, for instance, that complex movements such as those learned in skill development involve the establishment of a series of connections in the neural pathways enervating muscle action. In gaining knowledge (the cognitive area of learning) and in acquiring attitudes (the affective areas) there is still a great deal of mystery as to what actually takes place.

Theories have been postulated by a number of educators over the past century to explain the phenomenon of learning. Most theories have been based on studies that have measured the ease with which learning took place (how much was learned? how long did it take?), the extent of learning retention (how much was retained? for how long?), and observations of changes in the thinking patterns of children as they develop. From these theories, a set of principles, in the nature of generally accepted facts about the learning process, has evolved. Several of these principles are relevant to patient learning. (You will find that they apply in your own learning, too.)

Principles of Learning

1. *Learning is more effective when it is in response to a felt need on the part of the learner.* It is amazing how much learning takes place the evening before a class quiz — when you know that you are going to need the material the next day. And there is no greater stimulus to learning

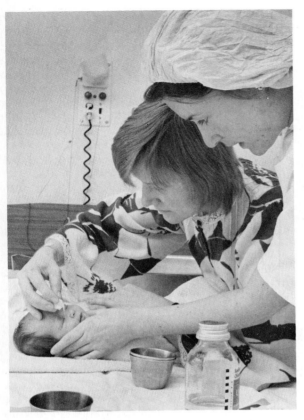

This mother is learning to bathe her new baby by doing it herself under the nurse's supervision.

subject to learn as much as you can before the teaching session. The patient too has to feel a real need to learn for optimum learning to take place. The new mother about to go home from the hospital with her first baby is usually eager to learn all she can about caring for the infant before she leaves the hospital. She is, most likely, going to have to feed, change, bathe, comfort, and soothe that infant by herself when she gets home. On the other hand, the person who has had a colostomy may be reluctant to learn to care for it himself. Changing a colostomy dressing is not a pleasant procedure—there are offensive odors and, as long as the nurse changes the dressing, the patient may be able to view the opening into the intestine as something detached from himself. Reality sets in when he does the dressing himself, and he may want to put that off awhile. (Some people, of course, feel embarrassed at having the nurse do the procedure and are anxious to do it themselves.)

2. *Active participation on the part of the learner is essential if learning is to take place.* Learning takes place in the learner, and he must be actively involved in the process. Telling the patient what to do or handing him a set of written instructions will not ensure that he will follow these instructions on his own. The use of discussions in which the patient takes an active part, problem-solving by the patient, and actual practice in performing procedures and handling equipment are much more effective than straight "telling," in which the activity is almost all on the nurse's part. It is helpful, in this regard, to make use of as many of the senses as are applicable in your teaching—that is, hearing, sight, smell, touch, and taste.

than having to teach someone else. If you have been asked to take part in a diabetic teaching program, for example, you will probably find yourself delving into all the books and journals you can find in the library with material on the

PRINCIPLES RELEVANT TO TEACHING PATIENTS

1. **Learning is more effective when it is in response to a felt need on the part of the learner.**
2. **Active participation on the part of the learner is essential if learning is to take place.**
3. **Much learning takes place through the mechanism of association.**
4. **Learning is facilitated when the learner achieves a reward as a result of his behavior.**
5. **Learning is made easier when the learner understands the fundamental concepts on which material to be learned is based.**
6. **Learning is made easier when the learner can see the material to be learned as part of an overall whole.**
7. **Learning is made easier when the material to be learned is related to what the learner already knows.**
8. **Learning is made easier when the material to be learned is meaningful to the learner.**
9. **Learning is retained longer when it is put into immediate use.**
10. **Learning must be reinforced to be retained.**

3. *Much learning takes place through the mechanism of association.* We associate the name with a person and we learn his name. You learn medical terminology by associating the new words with terms you already know. A child who is given an injection by the nurse may associate pain from the injection with the person who gave it, and cry on seeing the nurse on subsequent visits to the health clinic. She has learned to expect pain from that person. (The learned fear may, however, be extinguished if it is not reinforced by subsequent painful encounters with the nurse.

4. *Learning is facilitated when the learner achieves a reward as a result of his behavior.* We all learn best when our efforts are rewarded. The good grade on an examination paper, or praise from your instructor in the clinical situation, motivates you to keep up your studies and practice your skills. Innumerable studies have shown that reward is a much more effective stimulus to learning than punishment. We tend to avoid situations that cause us pain or embarrassment or from which we do not gain a feeling of satisfaction. The reward may be *extrinsic* (from an outside source), such as the good grade on your paper or praise from your teacher. Many physicians keep a supply of small toys or lollipops on hand to reward children for good behavior during an examination or treatment. Telling the child that he has been a good boy, or girl, is also a form of extrinsic reward. The use of rewards helps to build up pleasant associations with visits to the clinic. Rewards may also be *intrinsic* (from the inside), such as the feeling of satisfaction you get from doing something well or learning something new. In teaching a patient, you can help him in his learning by giving him honest praise and encouragement. The patient who is learning to walk again, for example, finds each step a challenge. The nurse's helpful encouragement enables the patient to take pride in his accomplishment (for example, that he has walked farther today than he did yesterday). There is, if you like, both the extrinsic reward of the nurse's praise and the intrinsic reward of the satisfaction he feels on accomplishing this feat.

5. *Learning is made easier when the learner understands the fundamental concepts on which the material to be learned is based.* As in the matter of communications, some people have a tendency to include too many details when they are teaching. The most important message—the main point they are trying to get across—often gets lost in a mass of extra detail. It is important to get the basics clear in your own mind, and to emphasize these in teaching others. For example, if you are teaching sterile technique to someone who is going to have to give himself injections at home, one of the most important points is to teach the person to avoid contaminating the syringe and needle. *Therefore* the package is opened (or the syringe and needle are lifted out of the container used for sterilizing) in a certain way, the needle is fitted onto the syringe in a certain manner, the top of the bottle is swabbed with an antiseptic solution, and so on. The patient will find it much easier to learn, and to remember, if the nurse begins by emphasizing the main point, and relates each step in the procedure to this principle, than if she starts off with "now, the first thing you do is this . . . and the next is . . ." Principles are basic concepts that can be used effectively in helping people to learn complex material.

6. *Learning is made easier when the learner can see the material to be learned as part of an overall whole.* The matter of relevance is involved in this principle. We all want to be able to see where things fit into the total scheme of things, and we look for the pattern, or total configuration. If something does not fit, it seems irrelevant and we think, "Why bother learning it?" Students in professionally oriented programs, such as nursing, are almost always concerned about the relevance of material they are asked to learn. There is so much material they feel they really need to learn that they question material that they do not see as being relevant; they learn it with reluctance, if at all. In teaching patients, it is always helpful at the beginning of a teaching program or teaching session to go over the total program—to give a brief synopsis that enables the person to see how the component parts combine to make a unified whole.

7. *Learning is made easier when material to be learned is related to what the learner already knows.* We build up chains of associated knowledge in learning theoretical material, and chains of motor responses in learning skills. Therefore, it is important in teaching new material, or a new skill, to build on what the person already knows or is able to do. Learning to make an anesthetic bed for the patient returning from the operating room, for example, is much easier to learn once you have mastered the skills of making an ordinary bed. Similarly, the woman who has made jams and jellies, or put up fruit in jars at home, will find it easier to learn how to sterilize a syringe and needle, or bottles for an infant's feedings, if the nurse relates these activities to the preparation of jars for canning. The new learning, then, is an extension of what the person already knows and is learned more readily.

8. *Learning is facilitated when the material to be learned is meaningful to the learner.* One

can of course learn nonsense syllables, and many experiments have been conducted to see how fast people can learn material that has no meaning. In nursing, however, we are more concerned with the patient's application of his knowledge than with his ability to recite facts and figures. A nurse can tell the patient that he needs so many grams each of carbohydrates, fats, and proteins in his daily diet, but unless the patient knows the foods that contain these elements and the size of a portion that constitutes so many grams, he is not likely to put the knowledge to use. It is important also to use terms that the patient can understand. The use of technical terminology should be avoided and simple words used wherever possible. It is particularly important to explain fundamental concepts in simple terms so that the individual grasps the meaning readily. You do not want the main point to get lost in a fog of words the person does not understand.

9. *Learning is retained longer when it is put into immediate use.* Material you learn in class, for example, about caring for a patient with fractured vertebrae, is retained better and longer if you are able to care for a patient with that condition during your next clinical experience. For the same reason, if the experience is delayed, you will probably find that you have forgotten a lot of what you learned in class.

10. *Learning must be reinforced to be retained.* This is the basic reason for repetition in learning. We forget knowledge that we have not used or reviewed for a period of time. Skills that are not used tend to become rusty. The quizzes your teacher gives you in class reinforce your learning by helping you to review material that you have learned. Practice sessions for your nursing skills also help to reinforce the original learning (and improve efficiency in performing the skill). Similarly, in teaching a patient, questioning him about material he has previously learned and providing for sufficient practice of skills are important ways of reinforcing his learning. Rewards also serve as reinforcers of behavior.

THE TEACHING PROCESS

Teaching and learning are reciprocal processes. The teacher's role is to assist the learner to acquire the knowledge, skills, and attitudes that he needs to learn. Teaching facilitates the learning process. It is not a matter of imparting information, of giving someone the ability to do something, or of changing his opinions or feelings. The behavioral changes all have to take place in the learner, and the teacher can only guide and direct the learning process, so that it takes place more easily and more effectively. There is an old adage in the education field that, if the student hasn't learned, the teacher hasn't taught, and this saying sums up the reciprocal nature of teaching and learning.

Teaching Styles

Basically, the style a teacher uses—his way of conducting classes and guiding other learning experiences—is his style in assuming a leadership role with his students. At one end of the continuum is the *autocratic* style, in which decisions are all made by the teacher, and there is little or no opportunity for the student to have a voice in the goals to be achieved or the nature of the learning experience, or to take some responsibility for its direction. An extreme example of the autocratic style of teaching is the nurse who tells the patient, "These are the things you need to know," and proceeds to give a nonstop talk on his eye condition, or whatever his health problem happens to be. This type of teaching implies that the nurse knows better than the patient what he needs to know, and this usually engenders resentment. At the other end of the continuum is the *laissez-faire* style of teaching, in which decisions about what is to be learned and how it is to be learned are left entirely up to the students. While this style may be effective with a group of well-motivated and well-educated adults, it is all too easy for a group to be sidetracked and to deviate from its original goals. The middle style is the *democratic* style, in which the learner participates in establishing goals, assumes some responsibility for the conduct of the learning session, and feels free to participate in decisions regarding the direction of the experience. This style has been shown to be the most effective in facilitating learning. However, the styles are on a continuum; some people tend to be more autocratic in their teaching, and some more laissez-faire. It is always wise, however, to strive for a middle-of-the-road, democratic approach in teaching patients.

FACTORS AFFECTING TEACHING AND LEARNING

A number of factors affect the reciprocal processes of teaching and learning. The most important variables in these processes are the characteristics of the learner, the characteristics of the teacher, the nature of the material to be learned, and the social climate of the situation in which teaching and learning take place.

Characteristics of the Learner

In developing a teaching program for one patient, or for a group of patients, it is important to know something about the learner or learners. *Age,* for example, is a factor that affects both learning and the teaching done to facilitate learning. Young children do not think in abstract terms. For them, things need to be concrete—involving something they can see, do, feel, touch, taste, or smell, or something they have experienced. They usually have fertile imaginations, but their imagery is based on past experiences they have had. If imaginary situations are used in teaching, then, they need to be based on experiences familiar to the child, such as going to the store, playing with friends, helping Mommy or Daddy, and the like. Adults are usually more goal-oriented in their learning than children are and more selective in what they learn. The adult learner usually wants to see the relevance to his own situation of material to be learned. As people get older, their reaction time decreases, and the older person generally needs more time to learn new material than a young person. It is better if the older person can be allowed to learn at his own pace.

The individual's *communication skills* need to be taken into account also. Both hearing and vision become less acute with advancing age. You will probably find that you have to talk a little louder than you normally would, enunciate your words more clearly, and perhaps provide written material in larger print if you are teaching a group of senior citizens. Language is often a considerable barrier to teaching and learning. The teacher and the learner have to be talking a common language. If the patient speaks only a language that is foreign to you, you can use nonverbal communication to a certain extent—gestures for directions, pantomiming some actions, diagrams, or printed material in the person's language. When there are complicated instructions, or complex material to be learned, an interpreter is needed. Often, a family member or friend accompanying the patient can interpret for him. Many agencies whose clientele includes people of different ethnic origins have phrase books that are helpful or staff members who speak one or more of the languages commonly used by patients. Even if the language is common, the words must be understandable to the patient. You have to consider the vocabulary used by the patient. You would use different terms in teaching adults and children, for example. You would probably expect a college graduate to understand terms that a person with less education would not. However, many people without a college degree have extended their formal education through reading, attendance at continuing education classes, or life experience and have gained an extensive vocabulary. One should never make the mistake of "talking down" to a person just because he has not had much formal education.

Then, too, the cultural background of the patient is important. Customs and mores vary from one ethnic group to another, from one part of the country to another, and from one socioeconomic group to another. New mothers in a hospital in northern India, for example, scoffed at the nurse's demonstration of bathing a baby. When asked why they laughed, they said they could bathe six babies in the time it took the nurse to bathe one. On further questioning, they said they would not use a basin, soap, and a washcloth as the nurse did. They would sit on the mud floor of a one-room home and, holding the baby between their ankles with one hand, pour water from a jug over him with the other, letting the water flow off the baby into an open drain in the floor. The nurse did a little research with a community health nurse and, in the next round of classes, demonstrated a "safe" method for the procedure the mothers had described. She also showed them the basin method (sitting on a mat on the floor). This time the teaching was accepted with no scoffing. It should be pointed out that the nurse was from the same region as the mothers, but from a different socioeconomic group.

In teaching patients, the *state of a person's health* must be considered. The person who is ill usually has a shorter attention span than when he is well. Teaching sessions need to be short, then, and gauged to the person's ability to participate. One should not attempt to teach the patient any more than he needs to know for his own safety when he is seriously ill. Hence, one teaches deep-breathing exercises preoperatively, when the patient is feeling relatively well, rather than postoperatively, when he may be in considerable pain, possibly not as alert as he normally would be owing to effects of the anesthetic used during surgery or to medication, and generally not feeling well.

It is important, too, to find out what the patient already knows about his health status and/or his health problems. People today are much more knowledgeable about health matters in general and their own health problems in particular than were patients of 20 years ago. Medical information is much more readily available to the average layman in newspapers, popular magazines, movies, television, and public school programs. The patient may, in fact, sometimes know much more than the nurse about his particular health problem, and she will have to do some extra studying in order to help him extend his knowledge and skills. However, the nurse should never assume that, because the patient is well-educated and perhaps even a health professional, he knows everything he wants or needs to know about tests and procedures, or wants to know about his health and health problems. It is always wise to ask the person both what he knows and what he wants to know.

The individual's motivation for learning is also vitally important. As we discussed when talking about the principles of learning, to be most effective, learning must be in response to a felt need.

The person who has participated in a hypertension screening clinic, in a shopping mall perhaps, and been told that his blood pressure is a little elevated is much more motivated to learn about hypertension and what he can do to bring his blood pressure down than is the person whose reading was normal or the obese individual who walked on by the clinic without stopping (unless, of course, that individual was already under treatment). The confirmed smoker may not be motivated to learn techniques for breaking the nicotine habit until he has a sore throat that will not go away or he finds he is having trouble breathing. For some people, it is only when they see noticeable changes in their health that they really feel the need to stop. The alcoholic, too, has to really want to stop drinking before he can be helped to learn another lifestyle.

Characteristics of the Teacher

The teacher is, of course, a key figure in the process of teaching and learning. We can all think of memorable teachers we have had who influenced us more than others, from whom we feel we learned the most and, with their guidance, most easily. Perhaps reading the following section will help you to remember particular attributes of these teachers who helped you in your learning and to remember them when you are in the role of teacher yourself.

A good *knowledge of the subject matter* is basic. If you are going to teach a group of overweight individuals—or even one individual—how to control their diet to lose weight, you will need to have a good knowledge of foods and the nutrients they contain, as well as their caloric content. You should be familiar with the Food Guides put out by the federal government in both the United States and Canada. You should also know the number of calories expended during various types of activity, such as swimming, jogging, resting, and so forth. In fact, you will want to be prepared to answer any questions that might arise. It is a good idea to try when you are planning a teaching session to think of questions people might ask. If, during the actual teaching session, you find you do not have the answer to someone's question, you can say, "I don't know, but I will find out and give you the answer tomorrow [or next session]." If you feel competent in your mastery of the subject matter on other points, you will feel more comfortable in saying this. Even the best of teachers cannot be expected to know everything.

When you are teaching skills, you must be sure of your own mastery of these before you attempt to teach someone else. It is always helpful to practice the skill beforehand, even if you think you know it well, just to refresh your memory. You might enlist the help of one of your classmates to observe, so you can have the point of view of someone watching you perform the procedure.

Knowledge of the subject matter is, however, not enough to guarantee effective teaching. The teacher also has to have *skill in using teaching strategies* to put the material across effectively. We will discuss strategies commonly used in teaching patients later in the chapter. A knowledge of the various methods that can be used will help you to select the one best suited to meet a particular patient's needs. Skill in using the different strategies will come with practice, as is true of any other skill. A wide range of teaching aids, including models, charts, diagrams, films, filmstrips, and tapes on a wide variety of health topics are available to help you in your teaching. You will need to become skilled in handling the various types of audiovisual equipment to use them successfully.

The teacher must also have skill in assessing the learner's needs and in planning and organizing the material to be taught. In thinking of teaching the patient, the fundamental questions are: What is the patient going to have to do? What does he therefore need to learn? We will discuss these questions in detail later in this chapter. When the material to be learned has been identified, the teacher needs *planning and organizing skills*. How much material should be included? Can it all be taught in one session, or are several sessions needed? What should be presented first? Are there things that need to be taught before something else can be learned? Where should the teaching be done? Do I need to prepare the place beforehand? What materials do I need? Are there teaching aids I can use? These are some of the questions to ask yourself when you are planning and organizing a teaching program. (Who said that teachers have an easy job?)

The Social Climate

The person who is teaching also needs good *interpersonal skills* to be able to foster a climate that is conducive to learning. A person cannot learn easily if he feels threatened. Most patients view the nurse as an authority figure and it is important to dispel any threats the patient may feel. In this regard, material in Chapter 10 on creating an open climate for communication is relevant in the process of teaching and learning. In teaching, both on a one-to-one basis and in groups, it is important that you have an atmosphere in which each person feels free to participate and the communication channels remain open. When you are teaching a group of patients, you will find that there is interaction not only between you as teacher and the learners but also among the learners. People feel more comfortable in a group when they know who the other members are and why they are there. It is helpful at the beginning of a teaching session to have everyone introduce themselves and, perhaps, tell a little about their background and why they are there attending the program. The authority aspects inherent in the nurse's role are lessened if the nurse can sit as a member of the group, rather than stand at the front of the room behind a lectern. A more relaxed, informal atmosphere is promoted if everyone can sit around a table. In many situations, however, this is not feasible. If the group is large or if the nurse needs to use aids such as flip-charts or a blackboard, she should stand where everyone can see her and she can see everyone in the class. It is important that the nurse and the learners feel comfortable and at ease, and that everyone is within sight and hearing range.

Nature of the Material

Basically, there are four different types of learning tasks: those that involve the acquisition of knowledge, those that involve the development of skills, those that involve attitudinal changes, and those that involve the application of these. During your educational program, you will acquire a considerable amount of knowledge through the classes you attend, the reading you do, the projects you undertake, and the assignments you are asked to do, as well as from your experience in the clinical area. You will also develop a repertoire of nursing skills.

In the course of your program, you will probably change your attitude about a good many things. For example, you may overcome a fear of the operating room once you have had experience there; you are likely to develop more tolerance toward people who are from a different background than your own. You may even begin to enjoy getting up in the early morning hours to be on duty by 7 a.m. It is during your clinical experiences that you learn to apply your knowledge and skills, and you put the attitudes you have acquired into practice in the real-life situations that constitute nursing.

In teaching patients, you will find that many of your patients' learning needs come under the heading of knowledge to be gained. As we have stated before, this is the need most frequently expressed by patients. People want to know what is happening to them, what the test or examination is all about (and the results as quickly as possible), and what they can do to become more physically fit, to hasten their recovery, or to meet whatever goal led them to seek help from the health agency.

Many times, the patient needs to learn new skills. Mr. Jordan, our patient from Chapter 8, needed to learn the skill of log-rolling for turning himself in bed, to use just one example. We have already cited a number of other instances of patients having to learn new skills, such as the diabetic who has to learn to test his urine for sugar and acetone and the new mother who needs to learn the skill of bathing a small infant.

Often, before other learning can occur, attitudinal changes need to take place. The person has to recognize the need to take his medications on time and appreciate the significance of skipping a dose. If the individual feels that the material to be learned is not important or relevant to him, he is likely to adopt an attitude of "Why bother?" Attitudes are also very important in the application of learning.

The nurse's primary concern in teaching patients is that the individual use his knowledge and skills in day-to-day living. This application involves the integration of knowledge, skills, and attitudes and their use in the activities the person usually engages in, or wants to or needs to engage in, in his everyday living. A person may learn all about nutrients and calories, for example, and may develop skill in planning meals that contain nutritious but low-calorie foods, but he is not likely to lose weight—which was the purpose of the learning—unless he actually carries through with his planned menu at home and does not deviate by adding additional snacks or increasing quantities.

TEACHING STRATEGIES

The nature of the learning task helps you to determine the methods used in teaching. Various strategies are particularly suitable for each type of learning task.

For Acquiring Knowledge

For an individual to gain knowledge, the information must be made available to him in one form or another. It may be presented in the form of a lecture, or short talk, for example, or during the course of a conversation. Conversation is suitable when you are dealing with one patient, or a very small group (two to four patients). For most groups, the *lecture* or *talk* is usually more appropriate. A straight lecture, or uninterrupted talk, however, does not involve much activity on the part of the learner, except through his sense of hearing, and it depends on the ability to listen attentively. If you are giving a talk, it is wise to remember that the attention span of the average adult is only about 20 minutes. It is less for children and for old people, and usually less when the person is ill. One should vary the techniques used in teaching, then, and intersperse talking with other techniques such as looking at diagrams, or other visual aids, and with discussion.

Discussion, which involves participation on the part of the patient, facilitates the retention of learning. In conversation and in group discussions, however, the participants have to have some knowledge of the subject at hand in order to discuss it intelligibly. There also needs to be some structure to the session, i.e., someone guiding and directing it, for it to be effective. The combination of a short talk followed by discussion is often a good way of structuring a teaching session.

Illustrating a talk with diagrams or stick pictures on a blackboard, flip-chart, or just a piece of paper, will often help you to get points across that are difficult to grasp through words alone. If you think of trying to give someone directions on how to get some place in a strange city, it is much easier for the person to follow the directions if you draw a small map. Models are also useful adjuncts to teaching. Models of various portions of food, for example, are often used in teaching people to estimate the size of a portion that weighs a certain number of ounces or grams.

Information can also be presented through the use of *audiovisual materials*. Many films, filmstrips, slides, and tapes have been developed on common health problems to help in teaching patients.

If you are using audiovisual aids in your teaching, you will need to review these ahead of time, so that you can assess their suitability and relevance to the class and, also, so that you are familiar with the content. The actual presentation should be introduced with an explanation of the purpose in viewing it and the point to watch for during the presentation. Opportunity should be provided for discussion during or after the presentation to clarify a point or to emphasize basic concepts or key points that are illustrated.

Written materials are also available on a number of different health topics. Your local health department and agencies concerned with specific health problems, such as the national Heart Associations, will probably have pamphlets on smoking, nutrition, exercise, hypertension, heart disease, and a great many other topics that will be useful to you in teaching patients. The health agency in which you are having clinical experience may have developed handouts for teaching patients with particular problems. Handouts are very useful to supplement teaching by other means. The person can have something to take home with him, or keep at his bedside, to read and review at his leisure, as well as something to refer to at a later date if he wishes.

Storytelling is a useful technique to present information to children. Again, situations used in the story are best if they are based on things familiar to the child, either through his own experience in doing them or through other ways such as reading about them or watching programs on television. A number of illustrated children's books are available on the market to help children prepare for a hospital experience, and cartoons and comic strips have been developed to help children learn about health topics such as nutrition, brushing their teeth, and other hygiene measures.

For Developing Motor Skills

In order to develop skill in carrying out a procedure, a person must actually go through the movements of doing it and practice these movements until he develops proficiency in them. A person who is learning to give himself

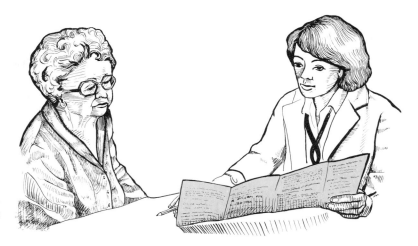

The use of written materials often facilitates discussion of health problems between the nurse and the patient.

an injection of insulin, for example, has to go through the motions of sterilizing the syringe and needle (or unwrapping the package), assembling the equipment, disinfecting the top of the insulin container, drawing up the correct amount, selecting an injection site, cleansing it, and giving himself the injection. A complicated series of sequenced movements is involved in the skill. Appropriate methods for learning various skills are used extensively in nursing education programs, and you are probably already familiar with the demonstration (or lecture-demonstration), the return demonstration, and skill practice.

In demonstrating a specific skill, the nurse should wherever possible use the type of equipment the patient will be using at home. Is the patient going to use disposable syringes, for example, or glass ones that will need to be sterilized?

Many health agencies have standard trays of home care equipment consisting of common household items. The nurse can use these to advantage in demonstrating many nursing measures to patients.

In giving a demonstration, you should first of all explain what you are going to do and why it is to be done in this way. (Referring to basic principles or concepts is helpful in this regard.) You should always be sure that the patient can

In teaching two diabetic children how to take blood samples from their fingers, the nurse uses written materials as well as the same kind of equipment the patients themselves will use.

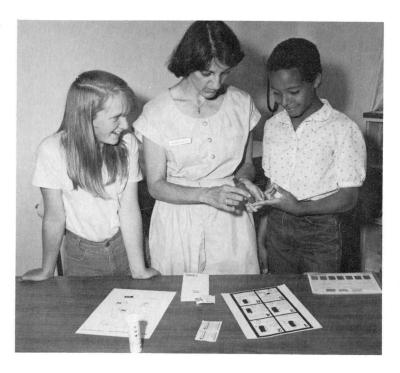

see exactly what you are doing. For example, the patient should be able to see the numbers on the syringe when he is learning to draw up a liquid. An overview of the procedure is given first; then the procedure is broken down into steps. Key points are stressed while you are demonstrating. The material that is being taught can often be related to something that is familiar to the patient, so that the learning can be transferred from the familiar to a new area. We used the illustration earlier of the woman who is familiar with canning procedures finding it easier to learn to sterilize equipment when similarities in the procedures are pointed out to her.

Audiovisual materials can be used advantageously in teaching many skills. A short film, filmstrip, or videocassette can help the learner to visualize the procedure and can often be used as a substitute for an actual demonstration by the teacher. A written outline of the procedure, with diagrams illustrating key points, is also helpful, particularly if there are several steps involved in the procedure. These provide a set of directions to which the learner can refer when he is returning the demonstration or practicing on his own.

The patient should have an opportunity to perform the procedure in a return demonstration soon after the nurse has demonstrated it—preferably immediately afterward. It is helpful to guide and direct the person through the various steps when he is returning your demonstration, so that he performs them correctly and in the right sequence. In learning a skill, accuracy is more important than speed in the beginning. Efficiency and speed will come with practice. Sufficient practice sessions should be arranged so that the patient feels competent before he is on his own.

For Attitudinal Changes

Learning experiences to help people change their attitude about something are, perhaps, the most difficult to structure. Attitudes often develop over a long period of time many we acquire almost subconsciously from other people around us. A person's attitude towards the importance of having regular meals, for example, is usually acquired in the home through early childhood experience. Attitudes can be changed, however, through a variety of teaching strategies. To use an example, through an intensive educational program over the past few years on the part of government and private health associations, we are changing from a nation of armchair athletes to one where millions of people consider a regular exercise program an essential part of their lives. We have changed our attitude, then, about exercise. We have also changed attitude toward smoking. A generation ago, learning to smoke was almost a part of the initiation into nursing training. Today, very few nursing students smoke. The proportion of smokers in the general population has declined substantially. The strategies used to bring about these changes have included a massive propaganda campaign that has utilized every available form of mass communication, including radio and television programs, newspaper articles, and the wide distribution of pamphlets and other written materials, the development of physical fitness testing centers, and the holding of clinics and workshops on common health problems across the country.

A person's attitude toward the material to be learned will affect whether or not he actually puts his learning into practice. The person has to recognize the need to take his medications on time, and appreciate the effect of skipping a dose, if he is to maintain a regular schedule of taking them. If the material learned does not seem important or relevant to him, he is not likely to apply it.

Often, attitudinal changes come about with increased knowledge. If a hypertensive person understands the effects of obesity on blood pressure, for example, he is more likely to recognize the importance of losing weight and more likely to participate in a weight-reduction program. An awareness of the potential problems of high blood pressure, such as heart disease, a stroke, or kidney failure, will help him to realize the importance of keeping to his treatment regimen.

In helping a person to change his attitude and apply his knowledge and skills, it is important to remember two of the basic principles of learning: Learning is more effective when it is in response to a felt need on the part of the learner, and learning is made easier when the learner achieves a reward as a result of his behavior. In changing attitudes, then, it is important to know something about the individual's needs and priorities. What things are important to him? What are the things that give him satisfaction—from which he achieves a feeling of reward?

THE APPLICATION OF LEARNING

We stated that the nurse's primary concern is that the patient apply the knowledge and use the skills he has learned. Having the information, and being able to perform the skills in his day-to-day living, is not enough; he must learn to apply these. To learn to apply his knowledge and skills, the learner must be actively involved.

The *problem-solving* method has been suggested by educators as a very appropriate method for learning to apply knowledge. This method is useful in teaching patients. The steps in problem-solving include: (1) identification of the problem, or the perception of a felt learning need by the patient (this involves gathering information and pinpointing what the problem is); (2) suggesting possible solutions; (3) selection of one solution to be tried; (4) putting the solution into action; and (5) evaluating the results of this action, reconsidering, and possibly trying other solutions.[1]

The nurse's role becomes one of supportive assistant. She helps the patient to identify his problem, gather information, and assess the relative merits of various possible solutions. She may help him to select and try one course of action, and assists him in evaluating this action.

For example, a patient may have been told by his physician that he should stay on a salt-free diet. The nutritionist, or dietitian, has talked to the patient and instructed him regarding foods that are low in salt, and the patient appears to accept the idea of salt substitutes to flavor his food. He seems worried about being able to stay on the diet at home. The nurse may help him to identify the problem by gathering information and helping to pinpoint the difficulty. The patient and his wife are elderly and they live alone. His wife does the cooking. He is afraid that it is going to give her extra work to cook his meals without salt. The nurse helps him to work through possible solutions. Has he talked to his wife about this? In this example, it would seem that the wife, who does the cooking, should be consulted in solving the problem. Together the patient and his wife might examine possible solutions. The patient's food may be cooked separately, in which case there will be two meals to prepare and two sets of pots and pans to wash. Or, food for both may be cooked together without salt, the wife adding salt to hers later. Many people find food tasteless when salt is not added during the cooking, and the wife may not like her food cooked this way. Both alternatives should be explored and a decision reached. The couple may decide to try cooking meals for both together without salt. If this solution does not work, then they can try the alternative.

There are many examples that could be cited of situations in which problem-solving seems the logical method for helping patients to understand their disease processes and make realistic plans to care for themselves. Often the patient's family needs to be included, since many problems related to health and illness involve adjustments in family living. The family frequently provides excellent assistance in developing and carrying out plans for the patient's care at home.

The *case study* is another method that is often used in helping people to apply knowledge. The case study involves the description of a person with the particular problem the patient has, and a series of questions or points to consider in a discussion. Situations the person might encounter in real life may be described and the individuals asked to tell what they would do. The use of an imaginary person is often helpful in that it is less threatening to the individual concerned. It is a strategy that is often useful in helping to bring about attitudinal changes. People often feel freer to express their feelings and opinions about an imaginary person than about themselves.

Role-play is another useful strategy in helping people to apply knowledge and skills. Again, an imaginary situation is used. People in a weight-reduction program, for example, might be asked to think of going to the market and selecting foods to feed themselves and their families. The situation might then be acted out by participants in the class. This strategy is also helpful in encouraging people to express feelings and attitudes or to work through difficult situations. It is most effective when it is relatively unstructured, and the participants are permitted to develop the situation as they go along. Not everyone feels comfortable with role-play, however, and it is time-consuming.

Children usually love role-playing, and this is a strategy that can be used very effectively with them. Not only is it a good way to help them acquire new information, as, for example, with the nurse in the role of teacher, storekeeper, TV character, or other suitable figure. Role-playing can also be used for demonstrations, return demonstrations, and practice sessions in learning new skills. It can also be very effective in helping children to put into practice material that they have learned in a simulated situation that is close to real-life situations they may encounter.

Behavior modification is a strategy that is frequently used in helping people to facilitate the use of new behaviors that are desirable in lieu of ones that are undesirable. Originally used in mental institutions to bring about changes in the behavior of mentally retarded individuals, it is now being utilized in many situations where lifestyle patterns need to be changed. The process involves the substitution of healthy habits (or behaviors) for unhealthy ones. The desirable behavior has to be learned first. The technique is used in many programs designed to help people to stop smoking, for example, or to stop overeating. It is also used in helping children to 'unlearn' behavior that is undesirable, such as bullying, or fighting with other children, and to

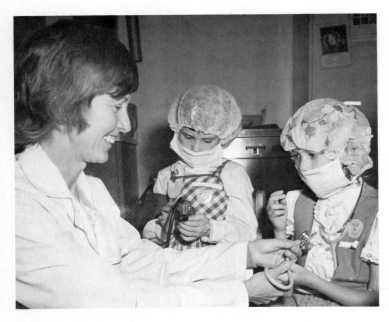

Role-playing can help young patients understand the medical treatment they are going to receive.

substitute desirable behavior, such as playing cooperatively, helping smaller children, and the like. Behavior modification is based on rewarding the desirable behavior and extinguishing the undesirable through a lack of reinforcement. The child is rewarded for good behavior with praise, stars on a chart, or other suitable tangible rewards. The undesirable behavior is ignored and is extinguished because it is not reinforced. Sometimes an aversive response to the undesirable behavior, such as separating the child from a group temporarily when he is disrupting it, may be used in combination with rewards for good behavior. One of the methods used for helping people to stop smoking uses this technique. The person is encouraged to smoke continuously for a period of time until he gets to the point where he cannot stand the sight or smell of cigarettes. His pleasure in smoking is replaced by distaste. A similar method has been used in some instances in treating alcoholics. A substance to induce vomiting is put into alcoholic drinks the person consumes, so that every time he takes a drink, he vomits. The theory involves substitution of an unpleasant response to alcohol consumption in place of the pleasurable effect it had for the individual.

INCORPORATION OF TEACHING IN NURSING CARE

Teaching, we have said, should be included in the nursing care of every patient. The teaching aspects of care, then, need to be incorporated into the steps of the nursing process as you work through these in providing care. This involves:

1. Assessing the patient's learning needs
2. Developing a teaching plan
3. Implementing the plan
4. Evaluating the learning that has taken place

Assessing the Patient's Learning Needs

In assessing learning needs, the basic question is, what is it that the person needs (or would like) to be able to do? This is the *goal* (or overall performance objective) to be achieved through learning. It is important to clarify the goal with the individual who is to do the learning, to be sure that you, as teacher, and he, as learner, are both headed in the same direction, i.e., toward the same goal. The following illustration is a situation you may well encounter. One of your neighbors is having coffee with you. She says she has been hearing a lot about health and physical fitness, and she would like your help, as a person knowledgeable about health matters, in getting started on a program "to put her into better shape," as she puts it. Here, you think, is a chance for some informal health teaching. Before you embark on trying to teach her everything you know about health and physical fitness, however, it would be well to find out exactly what she wants you to help her with—getting started on an exercise program, losing weight (she doesn't look as if she needs that one), learning to handle stress, or all three. She says she is careful to eat a well-balanced diet and, so far, has been able to cope with stress pretty well. What she really wants your help with is incorporating a regular exercise schedule into her lifestyle to improve her overall physical fitness. Once the goal has been definitely established, then you can proceed with helping her.

In following through on the various steps involved in assessing learning needs, developing a plan to meet these needs, implementing the plan, and evaluating the learning that has taken place, let us take an illustration that involves teaching a small group in a slightly more formal situation. We will use as our example teaching a skill you have already learned (in Chapter 9).

Let us suppose that, as one of your learning experiences in developing teaching skills, your instructor has arranged for the class to participate in teaching. You and two of your classmates will be teaching the procedures for taking vital signs (temperature, pulse, and respirations) to a group enrolled in a home nursing course at the local community center. There are eight people in the group. They are all women, mainly middle-aged, although one is over 65. The reason most of them have given for taking the course is that they expect to have to take care of aging parents, or to look after grandchildren when they are ill. The woman who is over 65 will be looking after her husband when he comes home from the hospital following recovery from a heart attack. The educational level of the women varies from 9 years of formal schooling to a baccalaureate degree in history. Your responsibility is to teach the group how to take temper-

atures. You clarify with your instructor just exactly what is to be included. The goal is that the group learn how to obtain an accurate temperature reading on both adults and children, using the types of thermometers commonly available for home use. In this situation, the goal has been made clear. Often, as in our example above, you will find that before you can teach, it is necessary to clarify with the individual precisely what it is he wants to be able to do at the end of the learning experience.

Once you have a clearly stated goal, the next step is to identify the learning tasks involved in achieving it. They include the knowledge, skills, and attitudes the learner needs to gain. The questions in this case, then, are: What does the person need to know in order to take an accurate temperature reading on adults and children (knowledge component), what does he need to be able to do (skill component), and what attitudes is it desirable for him to have?

It is helpful to list the learning needs under the headings of knowledge, skills, and attitudes, as in the table shown below, so that you do not overlook any in planning your teaching.

Developing a Teaching Plan

When you have identified the learning tasks (or needs), the next step is planning for the teaching. Planning involves determining expected outcomes for each of the learning tasks, selecting appropriate strategies and teaching

LEARNING NEEDS FOR TAKING TEMPERATURES

Goal	Knowledge Components	Skill Components	Attitude Components
To be able to obtain an accurate temperature reading on children and adults	Normal ranges of body temperature Equivalents of Fahrenheit and Celsius temperatures Factors affecting body temperature Dangerous levels of temperature Sites for taking temperature Indications for using each site Types of thermometers commonly used Temperature-sensitive tapes Time required for accurate reading. Temperature variations due to site Assessment of temperature reading Methods of cleansing and storing thermometers	Preparing thermometer for use Shaking down mercury in thermometer Inserting and removing thermometer Reading thermometer Cleansing thermometer Applying temperature-sensitive tapes Reading temperature indicated on tape	Appreciation of need for care in handling thermometers Appreciation of need for precautionary measures in inserting, removing thermometer Appreciation of need to leave thermometer in place for an adequate length of time

PLAN FOR TEACHING THE PROCEDURE OF TAKING TEMPERATURES

Learning Task (Need)	Expected Outcome	Possible Strategies to Use	Possible Aids to Use
Normal ranges of body temperature	States normal ranges of body temperature for infants, children, and adults	Present material in short talk	Write on blackboard, flip-chart, or overhead projector May be included in handout
Factors affecting body temperature	Explains how age, time of day, activity, emotions, and illness can affect temperature	Allow for discussion, questions from and to participants	
Dangerous levels of temperature	States temperatures that would be considered dangerously high or low in infants, children, and adults	As above	Write on blackboard, flip-chart, or overhead projector
Sites for taking temperature	Names sites usually used for taking body temperature	Present material in short talk	Write on blackboard, flip-chart, or overhead projector Use filmstrip if available May be included in handout
Indications for use of each site	Describes situations in which oral, rectal, and axillary sites are appropriate	Present material, allow for discussion, questions	As above
Temperature variations due to site	States expected differences in readings of temperature taken at oral, rectal, and axillary sites	Present material	As above
Types of thermometers commonly used	Differentiates between thermometers used for oral and those used for oral or rectal, and ones used for only rectal readings	Demonstate with explanation Allow participants to handle	Use actual thermometers May supplement with diagrams
Appreciation of need for care in handling thermometers	Takes adequate precautions to prevent breakage in shaking, inserting, removing and reading thermometer	Explain in talk, demonstrate	As above

aids, and developing a plan for the teaching session(s). It is always helpful, in doing your planning, to keep in mind the principles of learning discussed earlier in this chapter.

Determining Expected Outcomes. The first step in planning teaching is to determine the outcomes you expect for each of the learning tasks. The outcomes should be stated specifically and in behavioral terms. For example, under the heading Knowledge Components, for the component of normal ranges of body temperature, an expected outcome might be stated as: "(Individual should be able to) state the normal ranges of body temperature for infants, children and adults." An example from the skill component list, shaking down mercury in thermometer, might be stated as: "(Individual should be able to) shake mercury in thermometer

down to 95° F (35° C)." And, from the list of attitudinal components, appreciation of need for taking care in handling thermometers, might be stated as: Takes adequate precautions in shaking down, inserting, removing, cleansing, and storing thermometer to prevent breakage. Other behavioral outcomes expected for the learning tasks we have identified are shown above in the Plan for Teaching the Procedure of Taking Temperatures.

Group and Ordering Expected Outcomes. When expected outcomes have been determined for each learning task, they need to be organized into groups. For example, you would probably teach all content dealing with normal ranges of temperature and factors affecting temperature as a unified whole. Similarly you would probably teach the sites for taking temperatures, temper-

PLAN FOR TEACHING THE PROCEDURE OF TAKING TEMPERATURES *(Continued)*

Learning Task (Need)	Expected Outcome	Possible Strategies to Use	Possible Aids to Use
Temperature sensitive tapes	States indications for use and limitations of temperature sensitive tape	Show samples Explain uses, limitations	Show samples of ones commercially available
Preparing thermometer for use	Cleanses thermometer before use Lubricates, if for rectal use	Demonstration, return demonstration, practice	Use participants for demonstration mannikins for rectal temperature and infants
Shaking down mercury in thermometer	Shakes down mercury in thermometer to 95°F (35°C)		
Inserting and removing thermometer	Inserts and removes thermometer safely in mouth, axilla, rectum		
Reading thermometer	Reads thermometer accurately		May use diagrams to assist
Applying and reading temperature sensitive tapes	Applies temperature sensitive tape to infant or child	Demonstration	
Reading temperture indicated by tape	Interprets color change of tape or markings correctly		May use color chart to show differences, or diagram if markings must be read
Appreciation of need to leave thermometer in for an adequate length of time	Leaves thermometer in place adequate time for oral, rectal, and axillary temperatures	Explain need, tell participants time considered adequate	
Appreciation of the need for precautionary measures in inserting and removing thermometers	Takes adequate precautions when taking temperature by oral, rectal, or axillary route	Explain precautions, and demonstrate	
Methods of cleansing and storing thermometers	Uses safe methods of cleansing and storing thermometers	Demonstrate with explanation	Case for thermometer Small container for keeping thermometer, for sick person at home

ature variations due to site used, and indications for using each site together, as shown in the teaching plan. Then, they need to be arranged in sequential order. This involves the matter of establishing priorities. What is most important to be achieved first—because of its critical nature (for the learner's or other people's safety)? What is necessary to learn before other behaviors can be learned? Do any of the tasks (or outcomes) involve something the person may find frightening? (It is usually wise not to try to tackle these first.) What are the key, or most important, behaviors you want to be sure to have the person learn? What would be a logical order for teaching to be done? These are some of the questions you might ask yourself. In the illustrations we have used, the person would need to know the normal ranges of body temperature for infants, children, and adults before he could state whether a temperature reading might be considered to be normal, elevated, or below normal. Safety precau-

tions in taking temperature via the various sites would need to be learned before the person demonstrates taking a temperature by that route, especially if live models are used. You rearrange your list of expected outcomes, putting things together that belong together, and listing them in sequential order. We have grouped and put in a sequential order the expected outcomes for teaching the procedure of taking temperatures, and these are shown in the overall plan.

At this point it is a good idea to find out whether any of the expected outcomes you have listed have already been covered or will be covered in future classes, or whether the learners already know how to do them. If so, they can be omitted from your list for teaching. The next step is to identify suitable learning experiences so that the learners can achieve the desired outcomes. You will need to select the appropriate strategies, such as lecture or short talk, discussion, demonstration, return demonstration, or others we have discussed. You should also identify teaching aids that could be helpful, such as filmstrips, diagrams, handouts, and the like.

The teaching plan may be brief, including simply the expected outcomes and the method you are going to use in teaching. Or, you may want to include, also, the content in brief or key points or both. Many agencies have developed teaching plans for patients with specific problems, and you may want to look at plans described in some of the current nursing journals.

Each person who teaches will develop his own style of lesson plan. The important thing to remember is that the plan is to help you to keep in mind the expected outcomes (your reasons for teaching) and to serve as a reminder of what you were going to do. It is your guide, in other words.

Implementing the Plan

Selecting the Time and Place for Teaching. In our illustration, the time and the place for the class will have already been determined for you. When you are teaching one patient, or a group of patients, in an inpatient facility or a community agency, you will need to consider both when and where you are going to do the teaching.

All teaching, if it is to be worthwhile, takes time. Some of the nurse's teaching may be done informally, during the process of talking with the patient, but when specific material is to be taught, a definite plan should be developed and sufficient time should be allocated. A time that is suitable for both the patient and the nurse— when neither feels rushed and the patient is not overly tired—should be selected. The choice of time varies, depending upon the patient's activities and the nurse's schedule. In an ambulatory care setting, there may be definite times allocated when classes are scheduled for people with common concerns as, for example, the prospective parenthood classes run by some agencies, or classes for people with diabetes or other specific health problems. There may also be regularly scheduled classes in an inpatient facility to accommodate people with similar problems. Often, however, the teaching needs to be done on an individual basis. For people in inpatient facilities, the period in the morning after treatment and care have been completed, or the early afternoon, frequently can be used to advantage for teaching. For the sick, teaching periods are kept relatively short because most people, during illness, have a decreased attention span and generally do not feel well, and the nurse must be careful not to try to cover too much in any one session.

The place for teaching in a hospital is most often at the patient's bedside, although some health agencies have separate rooms for consultations with a health worker. It is important that privacy be provided in learning situations that involve personal matters.

Wherever possible, one nurse should initiate and carry through the teaching plan. Patients usually prefer to have the same person teaching them, and the nurse can develop a more effective relationship with the patient if she carries through the complete teaching plan. It also helps to provide for continuity if only one nurse is involved. If this not feasible, however, a team approach in which each nurse is responsible for one aspect of teaching can be used quite effectively.

Preparing for the Teaching Session. The place where the teaching session is to take place may need to be prepared ahead of time. You will need to prepare the content you are going to teach. You will have to decide how much content to include that is appropriate to the goals of the learners and relevant to their needs. You would not include as much theoretical content in teaching people enrolled in a home nursing course to take temperatures, for example, as you have had in your classes. The best criterion for selecting content is what is important and what can be covered in the time allotted. You may want to do some research or extra studying so you are sure of the subject matter and review your skills to be sure of your mastery of these.

The place where the teaching is to be done may need to be prepared ahead of time. It is always a good idea to check that everything you need is there in the room. You may want to use a blackboard, flip-chart, or audiovisual aids. You want to make sure there are enough chairs, and a place to put your notes, materials, and equipment. Equipment you are planning to use, such as a slide or film projector, should be checked to make sure it is in working order. You should gather all your materials you plan to use ahead of time, and have your diagrams prepared if you are going to use them. Whenever possible, it is helpful to go through the entire session in a "dry run," by yourself or with another person. A classmate or family member can be helpful in this regard.

Conducting the Teaching Session. In conducting a teaching session, whether for one patient, or a group of patients, it is important that the expected outcomes are made clear to the learners at the beginning of the session, in your introduction. The session should then proceed logically from one point to the next. It is important that the learners understand one step, or point, before you go on to the next. Feedback techniques, such as asking the person (or group) if everything is clear to them or if they have any questions, are useful in helping you to decide whether you should go on with the next point. Asking the person to restate in his own words what he has just heard is another useful technique. It is always a good idea, too, to watch for signs of disinterest or irritability that may indicate that the person is not ready to go on to new material. In concluding the session, it is a good idea to emphasize key points that you made. At the end of the session, the learners should be left with a clear idea of what it was all about.

Evaluating the Learning That Has Taken Place

Evaluation is the assessment of how far along the road toward attainment of the pre-established goals the learner has come. If the objectives have been stated specifically in terms of what the learner is expected to be able to do at the end of the teaching program, the task of evaluating the effectiveness of his learning is relatively simple. If, for example, one objective for learning is that the patient should select foods that are low in fat content for his meals, then the extent of his learning would be evaluated through his reporting of the foods he has eaten, or the nurse's observations of the foods he selects.

Methods of evaluating learning will vary with each of the four types of learning task. If the task has been one of acquiring information—for example, learning the danger signals to watch for in patients with a diabetic condition—questioning the patient is a good method of finding out the extent of his knowledge. Can he list the danger signals? Does he understand their significance? Does he know what to do about them?

The acquisition of skills can be assessed by observing the patient's ability to carry out the specific procedures. Can he give himself a hypodermic injection or do his own dressing? Does he know how to prepare the equipment, handle it, and maintain good technique while doing it? Questioning the patient while he is performing the procedure helps to ascertain whether he understands the principles involved (or the "why's" of doing things a certain way). In assessing attitudes it is important to look at whether a person applies his knowledge and skills and the way he applies them. For example, is he careful in measuring the exact amount of insulin in the syringe? Does he take his medications regularly and on time?

In assessing the application of knowledge and skills, observing what the patient does in a given situation is the best way of measuring this type of learning. In the example of the patient on a fat-free diet just cited, the nurse must either rely on the patient's accurate reporting of what he has eaten or actually observe the foods he eats. Many times evaluation of the application of knowledge can be done only by observing the patient in his home situation. This emphasizes the importance of follow-up visits in the home. Indeed, one of the most important responsibilities of the community health nurse is teaching the patient and helping him to apply his knowledge in day-to-day living.

APPLYING YOUR OWN LEARNING IN THE CLINICAL SETTING

The goal of your educational program is that you use the knowledge, skills, and attitudes you acquire during the course of the program in your subsequent nursing practice. Your learning experiences in the clinical area are designed to help you in applying what you have learned in the classroom and the laboratory. To this end, you will probably have clinical experience in a variety of patient care settings—in an acute care agency, probably in an extended care facility or nursing home, and in various community health agencies. In these experiences, you will be assisted and guided by your clinical instructors and also by staff of the agency. The following suggestions are intended to provide you with some practical methods for getting the most out of your clinical experiences. These are particularly relevant to experience in inpatient facilities—where a large portion of your clinical time will be spent, and where the majority of graduate nurses work.

1. Always be punctual for clinical assignments. Few things feel worse (or are more annoying to people who are waiting for you) than being late before you get started. The day starts early in most inpatient health agencies, and it is up to you to arrange your personal life so that you arrive at the right place, dressed in the approved attire and looking neat and well-groomed (professional), ready to start work at the appointed hour.

2. Become familiar with the physical layout of the unit. You will probably have an orientation tour of the unit, but it is hard to remember where everything is—particularly if you have clinical experience in a number of different agencies. Do not hesitate to ask if you are not sure where the linen cupboard is or where supplies are kept if you have forgotten. It will save

you considerable time if you don't have to search on your own.

3. Make sure you know the names of key personnel on the unit, such as the head nurse, the team leader (or nurse responsible for patients you will be caring for), and other staff with whom you will be working. It is always helpful to write the names down.

4. Find out all you can about the patient, or patients, to whom you will be giving care, before you start your care. Your instructor will probably give you a brief rundown, and you may have sat in on the change of shift report, but you will want to supplement this with by looking at the patient's record and the Kardex (if it is used on the unit). In some programs, students are expected to go to the nursing unit the evening before clinical practice to prepare for the next day's assignment. If this is the case in your program, it is wise to go when the unit is not too busy. The early evening hours are a good time in many units. Don't forget to introduce yourself to the nurse in charge of the unit, explain why you are there, and ask permission to look at charts and other records. You will probably need identification if the person does not know you. In many situations, however, it is not practical or feasible for students to go to the unit in advance of clinical practice. Your instructor may give you time at the beginning of the clinical practice period to review charts and plan your activities, or you may have to incorporate these activities into your own plan.

5. Make sure you know exactly what you are supposed to do in your assignment. Uncertainties frequently arise even if you think you know. Are you supposed to help with serving meals and gathering up meal trays, for example, or is this done by staff from the food service department? Are you expected to take your patient's temperature, pulse, and respirations as part of morning care, or is this task assigned to one staff member? Are you supposed to fill the humidifier at the patient's bedside, or is this done by a respiratory technologist? Should you empty a drainage bag, or, if it is full, alert the team leader to this fact? Do you throw the contents away? Most of these things will probably have been explained to you by your instructor (or team leader whose patients you are caring for), but routines vary from one agency to another. Or, you may not remember exactly what was said. Don't hesitate to ask!

6. Take the initiative in getting as much experience as you can. If there are procedures you have not been supervised in doing, and they are available on the unit, ask if you can do them. Your instructor cannot remember everything that everyone has done, particularly if she has several students to supervise. She will check with her group, to make sure all procedures included in the objectives for the assignment have been done, but there may have been something that has been left over from an earlier assignment. There may not have been opportunity for you to have had the experience. Some procedures that you will be expected to do as a graduate are not done very frequently any more—catheterization is one example. You have to take a certain amount of responsibility for your own learning. Or a treatment may be being performed on the unit that you would like to see. Again, ask your instructor if it can be arranged that you can watch it.

7. About asking—always be courteous. You will get a better response if you are polite and respectful when you are asking questions, asking for assistance, or requesting the opportunity to do something. Address the person by name, phrase your request in good English, and do not forget to thank the person for his or her assistance. Try not to interrupt when people are busy unless the matter is urgent, such as if you need help with a patient right away. The patient's safety is paramount in any situation.

8. Learn to organize your activities so that you usually complete your assignments on time. In nursing, there are always unexpected things happening—the patient's physician may come to see him when you are in the midst of giving the patient a bed (blanket) bath, the operating room schedule may have been rearranged and you find that the time your patient is scheduled to go to surgery has been advanced. It is not always possible to stick to the plan you have made, but you should have a plan. It is a good idea to list all the things you are going to have to do during the clinical practice period, and arrange them in the order in which you will be doing them. If you have just one patient to care for, things are less complicated and reasonably straightforward. You will need to put into your plan the times when you must do certain activities, such as giving a medication or helping a patient to ambulate. Allow time for other activities to be completed, so you can do these on time.

If you have two or more patients to care for, you will need a little more organizing skill. At this point, we will introduce you to a technique that is borrowed from administration courses. It is called the 'critical path' technique. In fact, you will find that you use the basic methodology of this technique in coordinating all of your morning activities to get yourself to class or to the clinical area on time. The idea is that you have a given starting time, a given finishing time, and a certain number of things to do

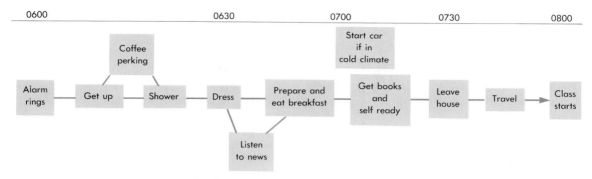

Critical path for organizing morning routine.

between these times. For example, if you need to be in class by 8 a.m., you have to set your alarm clock for 6 a.m. to have time to get up, get washed (or have a shower), get dressed, listen to the early morning news, have breakfast, get your books and other things ready to take with you, start your car (or get out the exact change for the bus), and allow sufficient time to get wherever you are going. You have probably found that you can do some things at the same time as others. You can listen to the news while getting dressed, for example. Or you may have the coffee perking or breakfast cooking while you take a shower. Some things need to be done before others. You have to get washed or have a shower before getting dressed. Most people have their morning activities down to a science—some to split-second thing. Others just never seem able to get themselves organized.

In applying the same methodology to organizing care for two or more patients, as with one patient, it is helpful to list all the activities you need to do for each patient. Note the time when specific tasks need to be done, such as giving medications, taking vital signs, and carrying out treatments. These are the critical points in your overall plan. Estimate the amount of time needed to do the various activities. It is always wise to allow a little extra time, so that you do not feel rushed, and to allow for the unexpected. Identify priorities for the activities you have to do. A good general rule is to look after the sickest patient first, but other considerations may also determine your priorities. For example, if you know from experience that Mrs. J.'s bed is usually a mess, you may feel she needs to be attended as soon as possible after breakfast. Or, if Mr. S. goes down for occupational therapy every morning at 9:30, he needs to be given morning care, be dressed, and be up in his wheelchair ready to go by that time. Some activities many need to be done before others, such as taking a patient's temperature, pulse, and respiration before you start your care, helping the patient with a bath before he gets up for the first of his scheduled walks down the corridor.

In any case, you make up a tentative time schedule for getting everything done. You may be able to do some things simultaneously, such as getting Mrs. J started with her bed bath while Mr. Y is sitting up in a chair. It is a good idea, especially when you are starting out, to write

Critical path for planning care of patients.

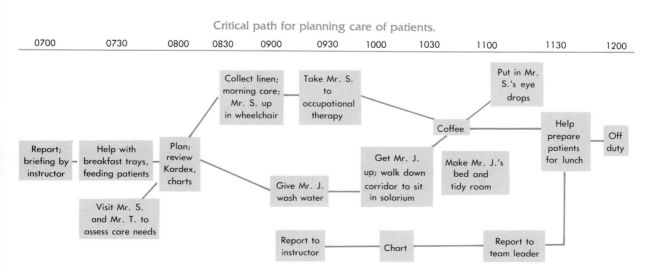

out your time schedule and keep it handy in your pocket while you are working. When you are busy, you may forget things, and it is wise to check your schedule when you have finished one activity, to remind yourself of what you should be doing next. In the days when student nurses wore aprons, the inside hem of the apron often served as a memo pad (with the writing in pencil) for students. Today, most agencies provide a form for nurses to use in planning and organizing their activities.

You may find that you have to rearrange your time schedule if an activity takes longer than you anticipated, or if priorities change, as when one of your patients vomits and you need to change the bed right away.

9. Get help when you need it. Many times, nurses will try to do things themselves when they really should have help, such as lifting a heavy person up in bed. Remember that your health is at stake, as well as the patient's, because you may injure yourself performing these tasks alone. You will learn techniques for lifting and moving patients. Use them. Some of them, such as placing a semi-helpless patient in a wheelchair, require two or more people to be done properly. Be sure you wait until you have assistance before undertaking these tasks.

If you are not sure how Mr. J.'s sling is supposed to go on—you may have never seen that kind before—be sure you get someone who knows the proper method to help you with it.

Whom do you ask for assistance? Your instructor is a good person to ask when you are doing procedures you are not sure of. Even if you have been supervised in it once, you may have not developed sufficient skill that you feel comfortable in doing it yourself. Or, an agency may have equipment that is different from the equipment with which you have had previous experience. Your team leader, or person responsible for your patients, is another good source of assistance, as are other team members.

10. If you are concerned about a patient who seems to be having difficulty, get help at once. Reasons for summoning help may include that the patient is bleeding, has difficulty breathing, is in severe pain, displays sudden erratic behavior, has an ashen color, falls out of bed, or fails to respond to sound, light, or touch. A stopped IV or equipment failure may also indicate a need to summon help. Pressing the call bell in the patient's room is the best way to get help. Only if this fails to bring help, and if you think the patient can be left safely, should you leave the room to get help. Remember that the patient's safety is the most important consideration.

11. If you make an error, such as giving the wrong medication or putting drops in the wrong eye, tell someone at once. Again, it is the patient's safety that is most important. Fill in an incident report with exact details of what happened.

12. Be sure to follow basic health rules yourself. Be sure to eat a good breakfast. Nursing sick people is hard work. If you don't eat breakfast, you can hardly wait for coffee break, and it becomes the most important part of the morning. Also, your breath may be offensive if you don't eat and you are in close contact with your patients. Make sure you engage in a regular schedule of exercise. You really need to be in top physical condition to accomplish all the activities involved in the hard physical work of lifting and moving patients, making beds, and being on your feet for several hours at a time. (You will be glad to be able to sit down and do your charting at the end of the morning.) Be sure to maintain a balance of work and recreation.

13. Enjoy the rewards of helping people. That is what you came into nursing for, after all. Even if your contribution is small, you will enjoy the feeling of at least doing something to make a patient feel more comfortable. This is mainly where the rewards come from in nursing. People are the most interesting creatures on this earth, and you will find yourself enriched by the wide variety of interesting people you meet in the course of your work.

14. Avoid coffee room chatter about patients or discussing your patient's personal affairs with your classmates, family, or friends. You may be excited over something you have done on the ward and want to tell everybody about it when you see them at coffee break or lunch in the agency cafeteria. Remember, however, that most agency cafeterias are open to patients and to visitors as well as to staff. The unthinking remark that Mrs. X really doesn't look as if she is going to make it, or Mr. B is an awful complainer, or the like may be overheard by Mrs. X's daughter or Mr. B's wife. Snatches of coffee-time conversations among nurses (or other health professionals) can be very disturbing to patients, relatives, and other visitors.

SUMMARY

Meeting the patient's learning needs is a primary responsibility of nurses. The topic deserves much more extensive coverage than it has been possible to give in this short chapter. Like the subject of communication, the nurse's role in teaching patients merits a book on its own. The nurse is therefore directed to the books and articles included in the Suggested Readings for more thorough coverage of this topic.

GUIDE TO EVALUATING YOUR TEACHING OF PATIENTS

The following questions will help you in evaluating how you conduct a teaching session with one patient or a group of patients. The questions are organized under the headings that correspond to characteristics of the teacher that we discussed as affecting teaching and learning, although not in the order we discussed them.

Planning Skills

1. Did you have a written plan?

2. Did you state the objectives for the session clearly and specifically, in behavioral terms?

3. Were the objectives attainable in the time available for the session?

4. Was the content you included relevant to the patients' needs?

5. Was it appropriate in terms of what the persons already knew or were able to do?

6. Did you include appropriate material and strategies?

Organizing Skills

1. Were the time and place for the teaching adequate? Appropriate?

2. Did you make sure the place for teaching was ready?

3. Did you have all your equipment and supplies ready before the session?

4. Did you make sure that all participants had a clear, unobstructed view of equipment and materials used?

5. Did you make the objectives clear to participants at the beginning of the session?

6. Did you develop the lesson logically and sequentially?

7. Did you stop to see if the participants understood and were clear on one point before you proceeded to the next?

8. Did you emphasize key points in your conclusion?

9. At the end of the session, did the participants have a clear idea as to what it was all about?

Skill in Using Teaching Strategies

1. Do you feel the strategies you used were effective in gaining and holding the attention of participants?

2. Do you feel they were appropriate for the content of the session?

3. Did you use teaching aids effectively (blackboard, diagrams, audiovisuals)?

4. Was the language you used clear and precise? Was it appropriate for the participants?

5. Did you explain any technical terms you used?

6. Did you project your voice clearly so that everyone could hear you?

7. Do you think the participants found the session interesting?

8. Were the patients attentive?

9. Did the patients participate in the session?

10. Did you use appropriate techniques to evaluate the extent of the patients' learning?

Mastery of Subject Matter

1. Was subject matter correct in terms of current theory and practice?

2. Did you explain basic concepts clearly and simply?

3. Did you explain to the patients how this session related to the total program? How it was related to their needs?

4. Did you use approved technique in demonstrating a skill?

5. Do you feel you answered the patients' questions appropriately?

STUDY SITUATION

Jimmy Smith, who is 8 years old, has an infected cut on his thigh. He is at home and his physician has asked you as the community health nurse to visit his home and teach his mother how to apply hot compresses to the cut. Jimmy's mother is Spanish and speaks very little English.

1. What factors would you consider before initiating any teaching?

2. What methods would best be used for teaching in this situation?

3. What factors might inhibit learning?

4. What aids could you use to facilitate learning?

5. How could you evaluate the learning of the patient and his mother?

SUGGESTED READINGS

Banning, J.: A Personal Commitment to Fitness Results in Healthier Clients. *The Canadian Nurse,* 76(5):38–41, May, 1980.

Freedman, C.: *Teaching Patients,* San Diego, Courseware, Inc., 1978.

Gross, S., and Algrim, C.: Teaching Young Patients and Their Families—about Home Peritoneal Dialysis. *Nursing 80.* 10(12):72–73, December, 1980.

Guinee, K.: *Teaching and Learning in Nursing.* New York, Macmillan, 1978.

Guinee, K.: *The Process of Patient Teaching in Nursing.* 3rd ed. St. Louis. C. V. Mosby, 1976.

Hallburg, J. C: The Teaching of Aged Adults. *Journal of Gerontological Nursing,* 2(3):3–19, May-June, 1976.

Huckstadt, A. A.: Work Study: A Bridge to Practice. *American Journal of Nursing,* 81(4):726–727, April, 1981.

Kornguth, M. L.: Nursing Management. *In* When Your Patient Has a Weight Problem. *American Journal of Nursing,* 81(3):553–554, March, 1981.

Langford, R. W.: Teen-agers and Obesity. *In* When Your Patient Has a Weight Problem. *American Journal of Nursing,* 81(3):556–559, March, 1981.

Loustau, A., and Blair, B. J.: A Key to Compliance—Systematic Teaching to Help Hypertensive Patients Follow Through on Treatment. *Nursing 81,* 11(2):84–87, February, 1981.

McCreary, C. S., and Watson, J.: Pickwickian Syndrome. *In* When Your Patient Has a Weight Problem. *American Journal of Nursing,* 81(3):555, March, 1981.

Overeaters Anonymous—A Self-Help Group. *In* When Your Patient Has a Weight Problem. *American Journal of Nursing,* 81(3):560–563, March, 1981.

Pelczynski, L., and Reilly, A.: Helping Your Diabetic Patients Help Themselves. A Plan for Inpatient Education. *Nursing 81,* 11(5):76–81, May, 1981.

Pierce, P.M.: Intelligence and Learning in the Aged. *Journal of Gerontological Nursing,* 6(5): May, 1980.

Ross, M. Nursing the Well Elderly. The Health Resource. *The Canadian Nurse,* 77(5):50–55, May, 1981.

Sivesind, D.: A Teaching Program for the Elderly on Developmental Tasks. *Journal of Gerontological Nursing,* 6(11):659–662, November, 1980.

Talarico, D.: Four Basic Steps to Successful Patient

Teaching. *The Canadian Nurse, 74*(5):22–24, May, 1978.

Tymkiw, G.: Obesity: A Challenge for Patient Teaching. *The Canadian Nurse, 74*(11):42–44, November, 1978.

White, J. H., and Schroeder, M. A.: Nursing Assessment. *In* When Your Patient Has a Weight Problem. *American Journal of Nursing, 81*(3):549–553, March, 1981.

Whitehouse, R.: Forms That Facilitate Patient Teaching. *American Journal of Nursing,* (7):1227–1229, July, 1979.

REFERENCE

1. Collins, R. D.: Problem Solving a Tool for Patients, Too. *American Journal of Nursing, 68*:1483–1485, July, 1968.

12

The Nurse Should Be Able to:

- Explain the principal purpose of the patient's record
- List types of information that are kept on this record
- Describe ways in which the record is used
- Discuss the nursing audit as a means of monitoring the quality of care
- Describe the following parts of the traditional patient's record, including the type of information contained on it and nursing responsibilities in regard to it:
    1. Fact sheet
    2. Doctor's order sheet
    3. History sheet
- Outline pertinent data that should be included in the nurse's notes for each of the six categories of information recorded
- List information included in the data base of the POMR
- Write a patient profile based on the data collected in the nursing history
- Discuss the use of the problem list as an index to the patient's record
- Write narrative notes using the SOAP format
- Discuss the initial plans portion of the POMR as a source of information for the nurse
- Name four guiding points to keep in mind when recording

RECORDING SKILLS

CHAPTER 12

INTRODUCTION

Recording is the communication in writing of essential facts in order to maintain a continuous history of events over a period of time. Reporting is the communication of information to another individual (or group of individuals) and may be either written or oral. A number of different records and report forms are kept by various health agencies, and the nurse will find that these vary from one agency to another. All types of health agencies maintain a patient's record or chart, however. The form of the record formerly depended on the type of agency—that is, hospitals used one type of patient record, public health agencies another, and extended care institutions yet another.

The introduction of the system called Problem-Oriented Medical Records has, however, caused a revolution in the recording practices of many agencies. Since the POMR, as it is usually abbreviated, can be utilized equally effectively in all types of agencies, it is doing much to bring about greater uniformity in health records. In fact, the day may be coming when each individual carries a list of his health problems and record of therapy with him and presents it to whatever health practitioner or agency he has engaged to undertake his health care.[1]

Not all agencies have yet adopted the problem-oriented system of records, however, and the nurse may work in a hospital or other agency in which the traditional type of patient record is used. We will, therefore, describe briefly both systems of recording. There are, of course, some similarities in both systems; the purpose of the patient's record remains the same, and there are some general rules for recording that are applicable in both systems.

THE PURPOSE OF THE PATIENT'S RECORD

A person's record or chart is a written record of his health history, his health problem(s), the preventive, promotional, diagnostic, and therapeutic measures used to assist him in meeting his health needs, and his response to these measures while he is a patient in the agency. In other words, it is a record of the events that took place during the period of time he was receiving care in a particular agency.

Hospitals and other types of health agencies are required to keep records by state or provincial laws and by regulatory agencies such as those concerned with accreditation. A variety of records are kept by health agencies in addition to patient records. For example, there are financial records, records of births, details of communicable diseases, and records relevant to legislation regulating narcotics. The nurse is concerned chiefly with the patient's health care record, which contains information regarding his nursing care as well as the care he has received from the physician and other members of the health team.

The chief purpose of the patient's record is to provide a written record of data that have been gathered about the patient. Thus, it serves as a means of communication among those whose professional talents are directed towards his care. This concise compilation of data serves as the basis upon which the physician plans his diagnostic and therapeutic regimen for the patient and the nurse plans her care. Physicians other than the one primarily responsible for the patient's care (such as specialists—e.g., the radiologist, the pathologist, and other consultants called in by the attending physician) contribute information to the patient's record, as do a variety of other members of the health team. The patient's record, as we have already noted, is a valuable source of information for the nurse in the development of her plan of care for the patient.

The patient's record is a legal document and is admissible as evidence in court. Some jurisdictions, in recognition of the confidentiality of communications between the patient and his physician, have ruled that information gathered in such a setting is inadmissible in court if the patient objects. Although the record is the property of the health agency, it is generally felt nowadays that the patient has a right to the information contained on his record.[2] The current emphasis on the patient's rights has strengthened this viewpoint, although in many agencies it is still not considered right or proper for the patient to read his own record. Some people contend, however, that if the patient is to be considered an equal partner on the health team, it is essential not only that he have access to the information on his record, but that he also check the accuracy of it. The nurse will have to be guided by the policy of the agency in which she is working in regard to the matter of whether the patient does or does not see his chart.

With the increasing stress on the accountability of all health professionals to the people they serve, the function of the patient's record as a means of documenting the care he has received has become very important. The POMR is very helpful in this regard in that all members of the health team must, in this type of recording system, not only state the care the patient has received but also give their reasons for that care. The patient's progress is systematically noted, so that it is easy to review the record to make sure that all the things that should have been done for the patient have, in fact, been done. Thus, the record provides a means of checking on the quality of care that the patient has received.

Patients' records also provide material for research. Many disciplines in the health field avail themselves of this source of information in a diversity of research programs—for example, to show trends in the utilization of the services of a community health agency. The records maintained by health agencies are also a source of statistical information used by governments in the compilation of information about the health status of people and health conditions in the municipality, state or province, or country (see Chapter 4). Statistical information, such as the number of births, deaths, or hospital admissions in a health agency, also serves as a basis for making plans for the future and anticipating the health needs of people in a given area. Some of the statistics are required by law; for example, the record of births must be filed with a government agency.

Another use of the patient's record is in the education of students in the health disciplines. The record provides learners with a comprehensive picture of the patient, his problems, and the care planned for him. Nursing students, medical students, interns, residents, and students in virtually all of the health disciplines

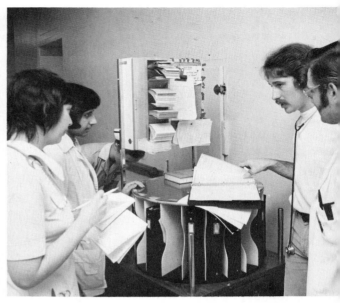

The patient's record is a valuable source of information for all members of the health team.

utilize patient records as reference sources. The records enable them to see the application of theory in a practical situation.

Nursing Audit

The *nursing audit* consists of a review of patient records to evaluate the quality of nursing care as documented in the record. It may be *retrospective*, that is, looking back at the care received by patients who have been discharged, or *concurrent*, looking at care that is currently being given. In either case, it is looking to see if nursing care meets established standards. The process of care, as documented in the record, is compared with criteria for good nursing care as determined by members of the nursing profession.

A nursing audit may be undertaken to evaluate either the quality of care given by individual nurses or the care provided by the entire agency. In either case, it is individual patient records that are reviewed. A nursing audit committee within the agency is responsible for determining the standards of care to be met. If the agency's quality of nursing care is being evaluated, an outside committee would be established. Representatives on this committee might include members of the state or provincial nurses' association and other nursing organizations, nurses from an accrediting agency, and, possibly, nurses employed by a government agency. Because these audits are done by members of the same professional group, the procedure is often referred to as *peer review*.

Criteria for evaluation are established through such aspects of care as the data base; the identification of problems; the expected outcomes of care; the selection of nursing interventions; and the degree to which the plan of care was carried out, as evidenced by the nurse's notations on the patient's record. In measuring the quality of the process of care, one asks: "Was everything done that should have been done?" In evaluating the outcomes of care, one asks: "What were the results of care in terms of changes in the patient's health status?" So far, auditing procedures for judging the quality of care have been developed to a greater extent than those for evaluating the outcomes of care.

Another mechanism for establishing quality assurance in nursing care is the development of *standards* for nursing service, which outline criteria in respect to the structure of services provided. Are the facilities, equipment, and personnel adequate to permit nurses to give good, high-quality nursing care? The ANA has developed standards with respect to both nursing care and nursing services, and the CNA is currently in the process of developing similar standards.

MEDICAL TERMINOLOGY

The nurse may find it helpful at this point to have a knowledge of some of the terminology used by physicians (and others) in their notations on the patient's record.

Pathology refers to the disease process itself; it is generally classified as either organic or functional. *Organic pathology* refers to diseases that can be identified physically—a tumor or a communicable disease, for example. *Functional pathology* refers to diseases that have no apparent physical basis; emotional disturbances frequently come under this heading. With the intensive research that is being conducted at the present time, the line between organic pathology and functional pathology has become less distinct and their frequent interrelatedness is recognized. The term *psychosomatic* illness is used to refer to the connection between emotional factors and organic illness, as, for example, between anxiety and a peptic ulcer.

A *medical diagnosis* is the physician's opinion of the nature of the disease. *Prognosis* means the medical opinion as to the final outcome of the disease process. A prognosis can be described as negative, positive, or uncertain, and as good, poor, or fair.

A *symptom* is evidence that there is a disease process or disturbance in body function. *Subjec-*

tive symptoms are those symptoms that can be perceived only by the patient. For example, the patient is really the only person who can describe his pain. Through her observation of the patient's facial expression or his body position, the nurse may interpret that a patient has, or does not have, pain, but only the patient himself can actually describe this symptom. An *objective symptom* is one that can be observed and described by others. A flushed face, a swollen ankle, and rapid respirations can all be observed and described objectively. Subjective and objective symptoms are, in fact, the same things as the subjective and objective observations we noted in Chapter 9.

A *sign* is an objective symptom that is detected through special examination. For example, fever is detected by the clinical thermometer, an abnormal heart beat by the stethoscope.

Prefixes and suffixes commonly used in medical terms are listed in the Appendix.

THE TRADITIONAL PATIENT RECORD

The traditional patient record still used in many health agencies generally has the following components:

1. An admission sheet
2. A face sheet
3. A doctor's order sheet
4. A history sheet
5. Nurses' notes
6. Other reports and records, such as reports of laboratory and x-ray findings, preoperative anesthetic record and surgical reports, and the results of other diagnostic and therapeutic measures the patient has.

The traditional patient record is sometimes referred to as a source-oriented record (as opposed to the problem-oriented record). Material in it is organized in sections, with each section being compiled by a different source. For example, there is a separate nursing section, a separate section for laboratory reports, and so forth.

The Admission Sheet

Most agencies have an admission sheet upon which are recorded basic biographical and some social data about the patient. This sheet is generally completed upon admission to an agency and then sent to the nurse or to the nursing unit to become a part of the patient's chart. Admission sheets contain accurate information which the nurse can transcribe to other records when necessary. The material on this sheet, like all the material in the chart, is confidential, to be disclosed only to professional people.

Often admission sheets record a unit number for the patient. This number serves as one means of identification and, also, as a basis for cataloging medical records. The information on the admission sheet generally includes:

1. Patient's full name, including maiden name
2. Address
3. Classification number
4. Nursing unit or agency
5. Date and hour of admission
6. Date of birth
7. Name of physician
8. Details of financial responsibility
9. Sex and marital status
10. Nearest relative
11. Occupation and employer
12. Diagnosis
13. Previous admission or previous call
14. Religion

The Face Sheet

The face sheet is the front sheet of a chart; it has a number of uses. Frequently it is used to record allergies, but it may also be used to record the history at discharge, in which case it is completed by the physician at the end of the patient's care.

The nurse's responsibilities are generally minimal with respect to the face sheet. Usually the headings and the notation of a patient's allergies are recorded when a patient is admitted to the agency.

The Doctors' Order Sheet

The doctors' order sheet is a written record of the orders given by the physician for the patient's treatment. The sheet may be kept with the patient's chart. However, in some hospitals it is kept in a central book on the nursing unit.

Doctors' order sheets are checked regularly by the nursing staff for new orders. Frequently a nursing unit has a method of flagging a patient's chart to indicate that a new order has been written. When the nurse has noted an order and put it into effect, she indicates this in the prescribed manner on the order sheet.

In some hospitals, when the physician orders a medication that is not kept on the nursing unit, he writes his order on a prescription pad as well as on the chart, so that the order can be sent to the pharmacy and a record kept on the nursing unit.

When the physician telephones an order to the nursing staff, the nurse so indicates on the order sheet. She also enters the name of the doctor, the time of the order, and her own signature. Doctors are usually asked to countersign their telephone orders within 24 to 48 hours.

The History Sheet

The history sheet is a record of the personal and medical history of the patient; it is filled in by the attending physician. Frequently the doctor also outlines the therapeutic regimen for the patient and makes notes on the medical progress of the patient after each visit.

The history sheet can be a valuable reference for the nurse in making her nursing care plan for the patient. It provides information about the patient's present medical condition, previous illnesses, family history, and current medical therapy.

The Nurses' Notes

The nurses' notes in a patient's chart can serve as a record of the medical and related therapies, including nursing, and the responses of the patient to these ministrations. In some agencies only nurses record these notes, whereas in others auxiliary nursing staff, which includes orderlies and nursing aides, also record their care and observations of patients.

Generally the nurses' notes serve to record and convey six categories of information:

1. Therapeutic measures carried out by various members of the health team
2. Measures ordered by the physician and carried out by nursing personnel
3. Nursing measures that are not ordered by the physician but that the nurse carries out to meet the specific needs of a patient
4. Behavior and other observations of the patient that are considered to be pertinent to his general health
5. Specific responses of the patient to therapy and care
6. In many agencies a record of the teaching the patient has received is also kept in the nurses' notes

In many situations the nurses' notes serve as a record of the therapeutic measures that are carried out by various members of the health team. For example, when the physician changes a dressing on a patient's wound, it is recorded by the nurse in these notes. She includes not only the name of the doctor performing the

SPEEDISET   MOORE BUSINESS FORMS LTD.

RIVERSIDE HOSPITAL OF OTTAWA

PHYSICIAN'S ORDERS

ATTENDING PHYSICIAN _Dr. L S White_

ALLERGIC TO _____

NOV 4 82

SMITH   MARY   SP 1246
2321 MARKET ST OTT 234-7566 600
JONES   RICHARD   HUS
SAME
23.10.82   2PM F 23 M SURG RC

420   1

DATE	TIME	ORDERS	EXECUTED
Sept 4/82	2 pm	DAT	Noted
		Up as desired	Noted
		APC ∘ C 30 mg tab ī q4h prn for headache	T
		Seconal 100 mg qhs prn	T
TOK		Consult ī Dr. Brown regarding headaches	Notified 3 pm
		Hgb, Hct, WBC, Diff on admission	DONE
		AC blood sugar in a.m.	Req
		Large chest x-ray in a.m.	Req
		Valium 5 mg TID pc & qhs	T ordered
		Dr. White	

NURSE SHALL CLOSE OFF ORDER
SHEET IF NO PHARMACY COPY.

IMPORTANT: NURSE SHALL USE COPY BENEATH AS
PHARMACY REQUISITION.
EACH ORDER MUST BE SIGNED

PHYSICIAN'S ORDER

FORM #2 - 8208

FORM #2 - 8208

PHARMACY COPY A

A sample physician's order sheet. (Courtesy of the Riverside Hospital of Ottawa.)

procedure but also relevant details such as the appearance of the wound, the amount and nature of any discharge, the application of a medication, and the removal of sutures. In some agencies, the nurse also records visits by the doctor and other members of the health team, such as the physical therapist and dietitian. This type of charting serves chiefly as a record of care and therapy and therefore as a communication tool for all members of the health team.

Nurses also record measures that are prescribed by the physician and for which the nurse has the primary responsibility. For example, the nurse records the administration of medications ordered by the physician and the time they were given. She also notes any unusual difficulties she encountered in administering the medication or unusual reactions observed in the patient. If a patient refuses to take a medication that has been prescribed, this fact is noted, together with the patient's stated reason for refusal if possible.

The third type of recording comprises the nursing measures that are independent nursing functions. These are the measures not ordered by the physician, but rather those the nurse judges to be necessary for the patient's care.

The nurses' notes also serve as a record of behavior observed in the patient that the nurse considers pertinent to his health problems or that constitutes a problem in itself. Behavior in this sense includes not only body action but emotional tone, verbal communication, and physiological reactions. In this type of recording, objective observations are made and then recorded, the description being as complete and concise as possible. In describing verbal communication that reflects emotional tone, the nurse uses direct quotations rather than a paraphrase.

Often, the lack of a bodily reaction can be significant, and this information should also be recorded. For example, the lack of shortness of breath in a patient who sits in a chair after spending 4 weeks in bed can be significant in determining the ability of the patient to tolerate increased activity.

The fifth area of charting is the specific response of the patient to therapeutic and nursing care measures. This includes the effect of an analgesic on pain, of a sponge bath on a fever, and of the application of cold to a swollen joint. In recording such reactions, the nurse records the perceptions of the patient and objective observations, such as a reduction in temperature or in the swelling of a joint. When the patient's perceptions are recorded, this fact should be made clear in the record. For example, the nurse may write, "The patient says . . ." Often, the words "The patient" are omitted, since it is inferred that the notation refers to the patient. The abbreviation c/o, for "complaining of" is frequently used, as in "c/o pain in left shoulder."

It is important to note accurately the date and time that a patient receives a treatment or a medication. Time is often denoted by the use of a.m. or p.m., although most agencies use the 24-hour clock to avoid ambiguity. Each entry in the nurses' notes is accompanied by the legal signature of the person who does the recording.

THE PROBLEM-ORIENTED MEDICAL RECORD

The POMR is simply a method of documenting the problem-oriented approach to patient care. Adoption of this system of recording in more and more health agencies reflects the increasing use of the problem-oriented approach by all members of the health team in all aspects of patient care.

The student who has understood the problem-oriented approach to nursing care used in the nursing process and is able to apply this in the clinical situation should have no difficulty in understanding the POMR nor in learning to record in the format prescribed. We have deliberately introduced some of the terminology that has developed in regard to the POMR in Chapter 8 in order to acquaint the student with the language used. We have also discussed some of the forms used in the POMR because they serve a dual purpose of assisting in the planning and implementation of nursing care and in the documentation of care.

Components of the POMR

The problem-oriented medical record has four components:

1. A data base
2. A problem list
3. Initial plans or orders
4. Progress notes

The Data Base. The data base contains the information that is considered necessary for the development of a comprehensive plan of care for the patient. It is a "defined" data base in that there usually are specific instructions on what information is to be gathered. Questionnaires have been developed and are used by most agencies to ensure that the needed data are gathered. What is included depends on the type of patient with whom the record is being used. For example, if the record is intended for use with patients who have one particular health problem such as hypertension, the information gathered will probably concentrate on factors particularly relevant to this condition.

The data base usually includes:

1. Information about the patient's chief complaint, or reason for admission to the health agency
2. A description of his present health status and a systems review
3. The patient's medical history and family history
4. A patient profile

5. Findings from the initial physical examination.

6. Baseline laboratory data and x-ray findings

7. The nursing history

Most of this information is gathered by the physician and the nurse in their initial assessments of the patient. If special data have been requested to be gathered by other members of the health team, this information is also included in the data base.

The nurse who took the nursing history is usually responsible for preparing the patient profile. The profile is intended to give members of the health team working with the patient a "thumbnail sketch" of this person as an individual. The information contained in the profile varies somewhat from one agency to another. Generally, however, it includes some of the basic social data the nurse has collected about the individual, pertinent information about his lifestyle and personal habits that may be significant in his care, any physical disabilities that he has, his ability to communicate, and the availability of family or significant others. The following patient, for example, has been referred to a rehabilitation center from an acute care hospital.

Mrs. Doe is 72 years old and was admitted to the Center on referral from _____ Hospital. She has right hemiparesis and aphasia due to left cerebral accident on 5/5/71. Historian is husband, aged 83 years, a retired civil servant on limited income. He is attentive and protective towards his wife; seems interested in learning about her care. States his goal is to assist his wife to return home and have some pleasure in life. They are proud of their four well-educated children, three sons and one daughter, all of whom live a major distance from them. Mr. and Mrs. Doe have a modern, two-bedroom, one-floor house in _____ (city) _____ (state). Mr. Doe plans to rent an apartment near the Center so he can visit his wife daily.[3]

The patient profile is usually affixed to the front of the patient's chart. In many agencies, the nurse also includes the profile as part of her admission notes on the chart.

The Problem List. Problems are identified from the data base of information collected about the patient. If the data base is incomplete, this becomes the first problem on the list. The patient's physician is responsible for developing the initial problem list. The nurse and other members of the health team contribute to its development.

The identified problems are listed in order of priority; each problem is dated and assigned a number. The problem list becomes an index for the rest of the patient's record and is placed at the beginning of the record. All subsequent notations made are referred to the numbered problems. Problems that are resolved are identified with the date of their resolution.

The problem list is kept current and up-to-date by the dating of resolved problems, new statements of those that have changed, and the addition of new problems that have arisen since the original list was compiled. Erasures usually are not permitted. If new information causes a change in the index, the new problem (with a different number) is added to the list, and reference is made to the previous number.

As we stated earlier, a problem has been defined as anything with which the patient requires help. The statement of the problem may be a diagnosis, a symptom, or a finding. Psychosocial, economic, and demographic problems (such as excessive smoking or eating) are included, as well as physical ones.

An example of a numbered patient problem list is shown on page 224.

Problems are identified as either active or inactive. Active problems are those the patient has now and inactive ones are those he had previously. The inactive ones are usually shown in a separate column and usually are not numbered. An arrow is often placed after an active problem that requires resolution. When it is resolved, the date of resolution may be written along the line of the arrow, or in a separate column.

Potential problems—those that are suggested by findings but have not yet developed into actual problems, such as an initial occurrence of vomiting—are not included in the problem list but are written up in the progress notes. If they do turn out to be actual active problems, they are then added to the active problem list.

Initial Plans or Orders. The initial plans for the patient's care are made relative to each problem on the active list. The plans are numbered to correspond with the number of the problem. The plan for each problem contains three parts: the diagnostic measures, therapeutic measures, and a plan for patient education. The doctors' order sheet is an extension of these plans. Orders are written, again being numbered to correspond with the number of the problem to which the order relates.

This system makes it much easier for the nurse to understand the reasoning behind the physician's diagnostic and therapeutic regimens for the patient and also the doctor's orders for medications and treatments. It also provides her with a better basis for planning nursing care. She is able to anticipate some of the patient's reactions and is guided in her observations in knowing better what to look for and what is important in her assessments of the patient. Knowing what the physician has planned in the way of patient

	PROBLEMS:	Originator's Initials	Physician	Active	Inactive
1	Left CVA	M.S.	J.B.	6/10/71	
2	Aphasia			6/10	
3	Ulcer Over Sacrum			6/10	
4	Urinary Incontinence			6/10	
5	Bowel Incontinence			6/10	6/23/71
6	Decreased Ambulation			6/10	
7	Decreased Activities of Daily Living			6/10	
8	Discharge Planning	M.S.		6/10	
9	Subluxation Rt. Shoulder		J.B.	6/11	

Problem list on patient Jane Doe. (From Rosemarian Berni and Clyde Nicholson: *Nursing Clinics of North America,* 9:266, 1974.)

education and what information he or she has told (or is going to tell) the patient is of considerable assistance to the nurse in planning her teaching program for the patient.

INITIAL PLANS

PATIENT: Jane Doe
(DATE, TIME)

#1 Lt. CVA
   a. Passive range of motion to Rt. U.E. with positioning.
   b. PROM. to Lt. L.E. to tolerance.
   c. Padded foot board.
   d. Confer with physiatrist.
   e. Teach patient and husband the exercises.
#2 *Aphasia due to #1*
   a. Record extent of language deficit.
   b. Use very short sentences or phrases.
   c. Test response to communication in pantomime only.
   d. Maintain frequent sensory input.
   e. Omit distractions when trying to communicate.
   f. Plan constant daily routine. Write schedule on patient's bulletin board for team information.
   g. Confer with speech pathologist.[3]

Progress Notes. The progress notes provide a record of the progress made by the patient toward the resolution of his problems, as one would anticipate from the name of this compo-

nent of the record. Therefore, notations made by the physician, the nurse, and other team members, laboratory and x-ray reports, the record of surgical intervention and of other diagnostic and therapeutic measures all form part of the progress notes. More strictly, however, the term "progress notes" is usually taken to refer to three parts of the overall record of progress: narrative notes, flow sheets, and the discharge summary.

Narrative Notes. These are the notations made by the physician, the nurse, and other members of the health team relative to the patient's problems. The narrative notes are numbered according to the problem to which they refer; they are dated; and the person making the notation affixes his signature and title at the bottom end of his notation. A specific format has been developed for the writing of narrative notes; it is usually referred to as the SOAP format because it contains subjective observations, objective observations, assessments, and plans.

The *subjective notation* is the problem (or sign or symptom) as the patient perceives and expresses it. It is not the observer's interpretation of what he or she thought the patient meant. The patient's own words should be used, rather than an interpretation of what the observer thinks the person meant. If the patient is unable to communicate his thoughts or feelings, or does not do so, this section of the notation is left blank.

The *objective notation* is what the observer sees, hears, or feels, or it includes observations made through the senses of seeing, hearing, touching and smelling, or with the aid of various tools, such as the thermometer, the stethoscope, and so forth (as described in Chapter 9). Laboratory and x-ray findings, and the findings from other diagnostic and therapeutic measures, are also included in the objective notation.

Assessments are the observer's impressions, interpretations, and conclusions drawn from the subjective and objective observations. All persons making notations are urged to state their assessments honestly, that is, at their level of skill and understanding of the situation. This is quite a change from the days not so long past when nurses were told not to write any impression or interpretations on the patient's chart, but to confine their comments to factual data.

The *plan* communicates the specific action the observer intends to take to work toward the

resolution of this particular problem. As in the initial plans, the observer is encouraged to think in terms of diagnostic, therapeutic, and teaching actions.

#5 *Bowel Incontinence* (date, time)[3]
  S: Husband reports enemas given about every three days. Last accident—yesterday. Pt. "used to go to the bathroom right after breakfast."
  O: Rectal sphincter tone present. Very soft stool on rectal glove. Rectum empty.
  A: Loss of normal bowel function due to too many enemas.
  P: 1. Evaluate bowel function for possible initiation of structured bowel program. Start daily record on flowsheet.
     2. Omit enemas.
     3. Order bedside commode and commode cushion.

Mary Smith, R.N.

Flowsheets. The purpose of the flowsheet is to show in graphic form interventions or observations in respect to one particular problem.

Flowsheet for recording bowel program. (From Rosemarian Berni and Clyde Nicholson: *Nursing Clinics of North America, 9*:269, June 1974.)

Date	Start Related *Meal* Breakfast	Suppository Time	Toileting Time	Rectal Massage Time	B.M. Time	Description: Amount, Color, Consistency	Place
6/10/71	---	---	---	---	7 PM	Smearing, brown	Bed
6/11/71	7:15 AM	---	7:45 AM	---	10 AM	Smearing, brown	Bed
6/12/71	7:15 AM	7:45 AM	8:00 AM	8:15 AM	Noon	Smearing, brown	W.C.
6/13/71	7:15	7:45 AM	8:00	8:15 AM	8:20 AM	Small, brown, hard	Commode
6/14/71	7:15	7:45	8:00	8:15	8:30 AM	Moderate, brown, hard	Commode
6/14 PM	---	---	---	---	9:00 PM	Smearing	Bed
6/15/71	7:15	7:45	8:00	8:15	8:20 AM	Large, brown, formed	Commode
6/16/71	7:15	7:45	8:00	8:15 AM	8:20 AM	Moderate, brown, formed	Commode
6/17/71	7:15	7:45	8:00	D.C.	8:15 AM	Small, brown, formed	Commode
6/18/71	7:15	7:45	8:00	---	8:15 AM	Moderate, brown, formed	B.R.
6/19/71	7:15	7:45	8:00	---	8:20 AM	Small, brown, formed	B.R.
6/20/71	7:15	D.C.	8:00	---	8:20 AM	Moderate, brown, formed	B.R.
6/21/71	7:15	---	8:00	---	8:15 AM	Moderate, brown, formed	B.R.
6/22/71	7:15	---	8:00	---	8:20 AM	Small, brown, formed	B.R.
6/23/71	7:15	---	8:00	---	8:05 AM	Moderate, brown, formed	B.R.

Flowsheets are usually developed for use for a designated period of time. They may cover a week or a 24-hour period. The TPR form used in most hospitals is an example of a flowsheet that is used to record vital signs for a week at a time. When it is necessary to monitor vital signs more frequently than every 4 hours, as allowed for on the usual TPR form, a separate flowsheet would be used. The minute-to-minute monitoring of vital signs of patients in the intensive care unit of a hospital serves as an appropriate example.

Flowsheets are helpful in ensuring continuity of care in that each nurse caring for the patient knows exactly what is to be done and when it is to be done. She can also note quickly the results of previous nursing interventions and assess the patient's progress in relation to the expected outcome. The flowsheet also serves to document the care that has been given. Notations made on it are not repeated on the narrative notes.

An example of a flowsheet developed for a patient on a bowel retraining program is shown on page 225. This particular flowsheet covers a 15-day period.

The Discharge Summary. The physician in charge of the patient's care is usually responsible for writing the discharge summary when an individual leaves the agency. With the increasingly widespread use of the POMR system in community agencies, such as a visiting nurse agency, it is often the nurse who prepares the discharge summary. The summary follows the format used elsewhere in the record—that is, notes are made concerning the progress attained in regard to each of the problems identified on the problem list. Again, the discharge notes are numbered by problem.

GUIDES TO CHARTING

The nurse may work in an agency in which the problem-oriented system of patient records has been implemented, or in one in which a traditional type of patient record is used. In either case, she will find that every agency has specific policies regarding charting on the patient's record.

Each nurse should be aware of the regulations for the agency for which she works. The following guides, however, will help a nurse in her recording, no matter what the particular policy happens to be.

Accuracy

The nurse records all factors accurately and truthfully. The omission of a recording is as inaccurate as an incorrect recording. Time is recorded accurately in the notations the nurse makes; all treatments and medications are recorded immediately after their administration, never before. Observations are specific and accurate; for example, the pain of a patient is described in detail as to type, exact location, duration, and any precipitating factors and accompanying signs and symptoms.

Because the chart is a legal document, most agencies do not permit the use of erasures when an error is made in recording. Each institution has its own method of correcting mistakes. Often the error is crossed out, and the word "error" is added and initialed by the writer. The correct information is then inserted immediately following the error.

Headings on the chart sheets are entered accurately. Many health agencies use Addressograph plates, which print data about the patient directly on the sheet. An Addressograph plate usually prints the patient's name, date of admission, nursing unit (if applicable), agency unit number (some agencies have a classification system in which each patient has a number), and the name of the attending physician. The Addressograph has the advantage of recording this information quickly and accurately.

Brevity

All recording is concise and complete. Vagueness is to be avoided. Extra words such as "patient" can usually be eliminated from charting because it is obvious that it is the patient about whom the nurse is recording.

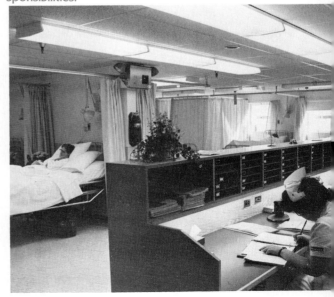

Charting is an important part of the nurse's daily responsibilities.

Legibility

Most agencies permit either printing or script on a patient's chart, provided that the script is legible. Ink is used because pencil does not provide a permanent record.

In making entries on the patient's record, the nurse is required to sign her name following her notations. Her signature includes her first initial and full last name. In most health agencies the nurse is also required to record her status, for example, R.N. or, for a student nurse, S.N.

Format

There is usually a standard format for recording, which ensures consistency and facility of communication. For example, all medications and treatments might be recorded on separate flowsheets (or in one column of the nurse's notes if the traditional type of record is used).

Most agencies use blue or black ink for all charting, but occasionally red ink is used for night charting (2400 to 0700 hours).

COMMONLY USED TERMS AND ABBREVIATIONS

It is an important part of charting that only correct spelling and acceptable abbreviations be used. Some hospitals provide a list of abbreviations that are acceptable; others accept the commonly used abbreviations. The list below illustrates only a small portion of abbreviations in use. The student is advised to refer to medical terminology books and dictionaries that specialize in this type of material. She should also become familiar with the abbreviations that are accepted in the agency in which she is having clinical experience.

abd.	abdomen
a.m.	morning
amb.	ambulatory, walking
amt.	amount
approx.	approximately (about)
ax.	axillary (armpit)
B.M.	bowel movement
B.P.	blood pressure
B.R.P.	bathroom privileges
C	Celsius (Centigrade)
c̄	with
ca	cancer
CBC	complete blood count
cc	cubic centimeters
C.D.	communicable disease
CHF	congestive heart failure
c/o	complains of
COPD	chronic obstructive pulmonary disease

CVA	cerebrovascular accident
DC	discontinue
dist.	distilled
ECG (EKG)	electrocardiogram
E.R.	emergency room
exam	examination
F	Fahrenheit
G.I.	gastrointestinal
G.U.	genitourinary
gr.īss̄.	1½ grains
gr.x̄	10 grains
h(hr.)	hour
hi-cal	high calorie
hi-vit	high vitamin
H_2O	water
h.s.	bedtime
I and O	intake and output
I.M.	intramuscular
invol.	involuntary
irrig.	irrigate
I.V.	intravenous
kg.	kilogram (weight)
lab.	laboratory
L.L.E.	left lower extremity
L.L.Q.	left lower quadrant
L.U.E.	left upper extremity
L.U.Q.	left upper quadrant
mid.	middle
min.	minute
ml.	milliliter
no. (#)	number
noc.	night
NPO	nothing by mouth
O_2	oxygen
O.B.	obstetrics
O.O.B.	out of bed
O.R.	operating room
o.d.	right eye
o.s.	left eye
o.u.	each eye
p.	pulse
Ped(s).	pediatrics
per	by or through
p.o.	per os (by mouth)
p.r.n.	when necessary
Psych.	psychology (psychiatry)
pt.	patient
P.T.	physical therapist
q.	every
r (resp.)	respirations
RBC	red blood cell
R.L.E.	right lower extremity
R.L.Q.	right lower quadrant
R.U.E.	right upper extremity
R.U.Q.	right upper quadrant
s̄.	without
S.C.	subcutaneous
sp. gr.	specific gravity
stat	at once
staph	staphylococcus (microorganism)

TL	team leader	×	times
TPR	temperature, pulse, respiration	>	greater than
V.D.	venereal disease	<	less than
via	by way of	↑	increase(d)
WBC	white blood cell	↓	decrease(d)
wt	weight		

STUDY SITUATION

Mrs. J. Rossten is a patient who has undergone abdominal surgery. She has been on the nursing unit three days postoperatively. Her orders from the physician include dressing changes once a day as necessary and Demerol, 100 mg. I. M. p.r.n., for pain.

Her dressing is soaked through with reddish brown fluid and she complains of pain. As her nurse you give her 100 mg. of Demerol and change her dressing.

The following questions should be answered for recording on:

a. A problem-oriented medical record

b. A traditional patient record.

1. Where should you check for Mrs. Rossten's orders?

2. Give a sample of the charting for the Demerol, including what should be recorded about the patient.

3. What should be included in recording the dressing change? Give an example.

4. Where are these data recorded?

5. How would a change in the physician's orders be indicated to nursing personnel?

SUGGESTED READINGS

Atwood, J., and S. R. Yarnall (eds.): Symposium on the Problem-Oriented Record. Nursing Clinics of North America, 8:2, June 1974.

Eggland, E. T.: Charting: How and Why to Document Your Care Daily . . . and Fully. Nursing '80, 10(2):38–43, February, 1980.

Hanna, K. K.: Nursing Audit at a Community Hospital. Nursing Outlook, 24:33–37, January, 1976.

Lindeman, C. A.: Measuring Quality of Nursing Care. Part 2. Journal of Nursing Administration, 6:16–19, September, 1976.

Mezzanotte, E. J.: Getting It Together for End-of-Shift Report. Nursing '76, 6(2):21–22, April, 1976.

Phaneuf, M. C.: The Nursing Audit: Profile for Excellence. New York, Appleton-Century-Crofts, 1972.

Sultan, S.: Nursing Audit. What's It All About? Canadian Nurse, 76(5): 33–35, May, 1980.

Thompson, A. B., and Wilson, A. M.: Quantity First, Then Quality: A Hospital Looks at Cost-effective Staff Utilization. Canadian Nurse, 77(5):22–26, May, 1981.

Vaughn-Wrobel, W. C.: The Problem-Oriented System in Nursing: A Workbook. St. Louis, C. V. Mosby Co., 1976.

Weinstein, E. L.: Developing a Measure of the Quality of Nursing Care. Part I. Journal of Nursing Administration, 6:1–3, July-August 1976.

Will, M. B.: Referral: A Process, Not a Form. Nursing '77 7(12):44–45, December, 1977.

Woody, M., and Mallinson, M.: The Problem-Oriented System for Patient-Centered Care. American Journal of Nursing, 73:1168–1175, July, 1975.

REFERENCES

1. Woody, M., and Mallinson, M.: The Problem-Oriented System for Patient-Centered Care. American Journal of Nursing, 73:1168–1175, July, 1975.

2. Berni, R., and Readey, H.: Problem-Oriented Medical Record Implementation. St. Louis, C. V. Mosby Company, 1974.

3. Berni, R., and Nicholson, C.: The POR as a Tool in Rehabilitation and Patient Teaching. Nursing Clinics of North America, 9:267, June, 1974.

MEETING
BASIC NEEDS

3
UNIT

13

The Nurse Should Be Able to:

- Discuss the nature of Maslow's hierarchy of needs
- Discuss Kalish's adaptation of Maslow's hierarchy of needs
- Discuss Freud's Psychosexual Development Theory
- Describe the four stages of Piaget's Theory of Cognitive Development
- Explain Kohlberg's Theory of Moral Development
- List the stages and conflicts in each stage of Erikson's Theory of Psychosocial Development
- Discuss the different Passages of Adulthood described by Sheehy
- Describe growth and development inside the womb
- Discuss needs requiring special attention during pregnancy and factors affecting needs
- Describe the development of an individual through the various stages of the life cycle from birth to old age
- Identify factors affecting basic needs during each stage of the life cycle

MEETING BASIC NEEDS THROUGHOUT THE LIFE CYCLE

INTRODUCTION

In Unit 1, we discussed some of the basic concepts that underlie our current beliefs about health and illness. One of the concepts we talked about briefly in Chapter 2 was Maslow's theory of a hierarchy of human needs. Maslow, as you will recall, suggested that everyone has certain basic needs that must be fulfilled if an individual is to attain an optimal level of well-being. These needs, he felt, are common to all human beings and include:

1. Physiological needs, such as the need for air, for water, for food, for elimination, and the like
2. Safety and security needs
3. Needs for love and belonging
4. Esteem needs
5. Needs for self-actualization

Much of nursing is concerned with helping people to meet their basic needs when they are unable to do so by themselves because they are ill or because they lack the necessary knowledge, skill, or motivation. This part of nursing is embodied in the *caring* aspects of the nursing role and includes basic nursing measures that are applicable in the care of patients of all ages, regardless of their medical diagnosis. The concept of basic needs is the framework for Unit 3. In the chapters that comprise this unit, you will learn to apply the nursing process in the care of patients who, for one reason or another, are unable to fulfill their basic needs.

It is generally agreed that people have the same basic needs throughout the life span. However, the nature of these needs and their relative importance to an individual's well-being vary, with a person's age and his stage of physical and psychosocial development being important variables affecting these needs. A growing child's nutritional needs are different, for example, from those of a middle-aged adult; the child needs more protein, for instance, to build bones and muscle tissue. Both the very young and the very old have increased safety needs.

The very young have not yet learned to be aware of danger, and so need the help of others to protect them from harm. The elderly have bones that are more fragile and break more easily than those of younger people. Their sensory faculties are also usually not as efficient in alerting the individual to dangers in the environment. Therefore, they are more likely to trip and fall over a stool in their path, for example, and suffer a broken wrist or ankle as a result.

In this chapter, which serves as an introduction to Unit 3, we will explore the nature of man's basic needs. We will also look at some of the theories of growth and development that contribute to our understanding of differences in basic needs, and their relative importance, at various stages in the life cycle. Finally we will try to put it all together in a discussion of changes that occur as an individual grows and develops throughout his life, and the needs requiring particular attention at each stage.

THE NATURE OF THE BASIC NEEDS

The basic needs identified by Maslow were listed at the beginning of this chapter. Maslow believed that there is a certain prioritization to these needs—hence, his concept of a hierarchy. According to Maslow, the more fundamental needs must be satisfied first before a person can proceed to seek satisfaction for needs of a higher order.

Physiological needs, of course, take precedence over all others because they are essential for survival. These include the need for water, for food, for air, for elimination, for rest and sleep, for temperature maintenance, and for the avoidance of pain. When a person is starving, life revolves around the need to obtain food. Similarly, a person deprived of water for a long period of time is concerned above all else with relieving his thirst. The fulfillment of certain needs is so essential that if there is interference with attainment of them, immediate action must be taken to save the person's life. If there is interference with breathing, for example, and a person's air supply is cut off, prompt measures must be initiated to restore adequate respiration or the person will die within a matter of minutes. The relief of pain is also a priority item. If pain is severe, a person cannot rest, he cannot sleep, and he can think of nothing else until he obtains relief from it.

Next in order of priority, according to Maslow, are the *safety and security needs.* These include such fundamental components as adequate shelter from the elements and protection from harmful factors in the environment. But a person must also *feel* that he is secure and protected from both real and imagined dangers. People usually feel more secure when they are in familiar surroundings, with accustomed routines, with people they can trust, with things about them that they know. Conversely, they feel threatened when they are in strange places, when their *usual pattern* of living is disturbed, or when they are among strangers or have no familiar objects around them. Often, inanimate objects assume a symbolism that represents safety and security for an individual. Linus's blanket (in Charles Schulz's cartoon "Peanuts"), which he carries everywhere with him, has become a symbol of security that is recognized by most North Americans. Almost all children have a toy, or other object, that has become important to them; they often like to take their favorite Teddy bear, car, blanket, or pillow with them wherever they go. The familiar object helps to give them a feeling of security when they are in strange surroundings or unfamiliar situations. Many adults, too, have their lucky charms, talismans, or other objects that they feel give them special protection against harm. Maslow has suggested that many of our religious rituals, our superstitions, and our traditions have their origins in this basic need for safety and security.

Maslow placed the *needs for love and belonging* as next most important. There is little question that these are very basic needs indeed.

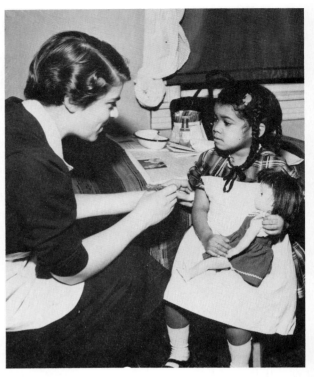

Most children have a favorite toy that provides them with a feeling of security when they are in strange surroundings or unfamiliar situations. This little girl has Dolly ready for her injection when the nurse has finished with hers.

Infants deprived of love and affection just do not thrive, even if all of their physiological and safety needs are met. But adults, too, need love and affection. They need to have people who are close to them to share their joys and sorrows, their anxieties, and their doubts. People who do not have close ties with other people often have pets—a cat, a dog, or a canary, for example—on whom they lavish all the love and affection they do not have the opportunity to share with other people.

Next in the hierarchy Maslow put the *esteem needs.* A person has to feel that he is worthwhile as a human being—that is, he must have self-esteem—and he must also feel that he is considered a person of worth and dignity by his family and by other people. Maslow has suggested that many of the problems of people in our impersonalized society, particularly in big cities, are due to failure to satisfy the two basic needs of love/belonging and esteem. If people do not have these needs satisfied, they come to have a low regard for themselves, and feelings of inadequacy, frustration, alienation, and hopelessness result.[1]

Finally, in Maslow's hierarchy, are the *needs for self-actualization.* These include the need to attain one's highest potential and achieve one's ambitions in life. Maslow included here also the need for knowledge and the aesthetic needs, that is, the need for something beautiful in one's life.

Subsequent theorists have suggested modifications to Maslow's hierarchy. Richard Kalish, for example, believed that the need for knowledge, as exemplified by man's curiosity, is a more fundamental need than Maslow depicted in his hierarchy. He placed it second, after physiological needs, and included in this category sex, activity, exploration, and novelty.[2] Again, to use an example drawn from childhood, infants who do not have sufficient opportunity to explore their surroundings and to manipulate objects, or who are kept in a monotonous environment, do not attain their optimal development physiologically, emotionally or socially. Older children and adults will often forget about safety and security in a desire to obtain stimulation or, sometimes, just to satisfy their curiosity.

The sex drive is also, of course, very fundamental and very strong, since it is essential for the survival of the species. However, it is a drive that can be sublimated; that is, it can be channeled into other forms of activity, such as a career. Or, its gratification can be delayed. It may sometimes be delayed indefinitely, as, for example, in the case of people in some religious orders who take vows of chastity.

In using the concept of basic human needs as a framework for Unit 3, we have essentially followed Kalish's adaptation of Maslow's hierarchy. We have, therefore, started with a section on physiological needs, and followed this with one on activity needs. Safety and protection needs logically accompany activity of any sort, so the chapters covering these needs are third. We have concluded with a section on love,

security, and self-esteem needs. You will note that we have deviated somewhat from the Kalish model, in incorporating sexual needs as a component of the love, security, and self-esteem needs rather than including it with activity needs. This is our own personal bias. We have also not developed a separate chapter on self-actualization needs, because we feel that a discussion of these needs more rightly belongs in a senior text on psychiatric nursing or one on rehabilitation nursing.

THEORIES ABOUT GROWTH AND DEVELOPMENT

In Maslow's hierarchy (and others subsequently developed) the individual is seen as constantly striving to fulfill his basic needs. As one set of needs is gratified, others of a higher order emerge and become more powerful. A person who seemingly has all his needs fulfilled still looks for something further. He may develop his aesthetic needs and hunt for rare art objects, for example, or he may seek to increase his knowledge and become a scholarly authority on a particular subject.

The concept that is presented in Maslow's theory, then, is not of man as a static entity, trying simply to maintain his equilibrium in a changing world, but of man as a developing being, constantly reaching out for things beyond his immediate grasp. This concept embodies the idea of continuous growth and development of the human organism, which begins at the moment of birth and continues until death.

The study of human development has received a great deal of attention in recent years from educators and social scientists, as well as from people in the health field. Our knowledge

Maslow's hierarchy of needs, as adapted by Kalish. (From Kalish, R. A.: *The Psychology of Human Behavior*. Belmont, California, Wadsworth Publishing Company, 1966).

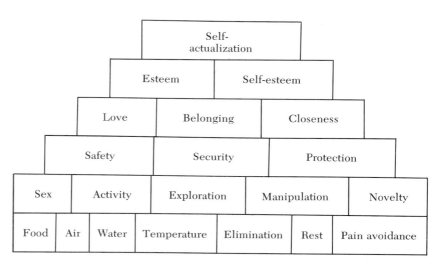

of physical growth and development has increased tremendously with advances in scientific technology that permit us to measure, with a great deal of accuracy, the changes occurring in most body tissues and processes throughout the life span. Our understanding of man's social and psychological development, however, has to be derived from studies of observable behavior. Since the range of possible human behaviors is enormous, a wide variety of theories have been developed, each stressing one or more aspects of development.

Freud and Psychosocial Development

One of the pioneers in the field of personality development was Sigmund Freud. His theory of psychosexual development shocked the scientific and lay community of the early 1900's and still evokes controversy whenever it is discussed. According to Freud, each individual must progress through five stages from infancy through puberty, and it is the quality of his experiences in each stage that determines his adult personality. Deprivation, or overindulgence, of the individual's needs in any one of the stages may cause him to become "fixated" at that stage. The five stages identified by Freud were:

1. Oral Stage (birth to 18 months). Freud believed that during this stage, the infant derives his greatest sensual satisfaction through his mouth. Behavioral traits that may develop as a result of too little or too much oral satisfaction in infancy, he felt, included aggression, a preoccupation with food or drink, cigarette smoking, and nailbiting.

2. Anal Stage (18 months to 3 years). Freud felt that the toddler's greatest pleasure comes from moving his bowels. The management of toilet training during this stage is therefore crucial to one's development. If this training is not handled correctly, the individual may show behavioral characteristics as an adult that include hoarding, an obsession with cleanliness, or the reverse, that is, slothfulness. If training is too rigid, Freud felt, the parent might even stifle the child's creativity.

3. Oedipal Stage (3 to 6 years). During this stage, it was felt that the child identifies with and derives sensual satisfaction from the parent of the opposite sex, and views the parent of the same sex as a rival. Behavioral traits that Freud felt may develop from overindulgence or deprivation at this stage include competitiveness, seductiveness, and a preoccupation with older partners.

4. Latent Stage (6 to 11 years). The child at this stage identifies with the parent of the same sex, and learns to assume the appropriate social role. Behavioral characteristics that Freud believed were formed at this stage include the development of a conscience as well as the seeds for later rebellion if this stage is not handled properly by parents.

5. Genital Stage (11 to 14 years). Freud believed that the adolescent derived his most pleasurable experiences through his genital organs. Personality traits felt to result from mishandling of this stage include a tendency to rationalization and a preoccupation with sex.

The terms coined by Freud are still widely used, although most people feel that his theory of psychosexual development is too restrictive, focusing as it does on only one aspect of growth and development.

Piaget and Intellect Development

Looking at growth and development from a different perspective, Jean Piaget formulated a theory of cognitive, or intellectual, development based on four sequential stages. Subsequent studies have confirmed that although the rate of development may vary, children do indeed seem to progress through the stages of intellectual development in a sequence such as Piaget outlined. These stages are briefly described below:

Sensorimotor Stage (birth to 2 years). During this stage the infant is concerned mainly with actions and sensations that affect him directly. He begins to relate to outside events, at first tentatively, then actively experimenting with his environment. He develops *object permanence* (knowledge that an object exists even though it is not visible to him). At birth, the infant's response range is basically limited to reflex actions. By the age of two he is capable of thinking through a problem before taking action.

Preoperational Stage (2 to 7 years). At this stage a child's thinking is still *egocentric*, that is, concerned mainly with himself. He believes that everyone sees the world as he does. Language becomes an important vehicle of communication. Piaget has divided this stage into two distinct periods:

Preconceptual Period (2 to 4 years). The child at this point is not yet capable of reason, although he is able to form general concepts. He may call all soft, stuffed toys "bear," for example, or he may use a facecloth (with which he has just wiped his face) to polish the furniture.

Perceptual (Intuitive) Period (4 to 7 years).

Children at this stage are capable of reason, yet it is not a logical, adult form of thinking. They can only concentrate on one aspect of an object or idea at a time. For example, if a child at this stage of development saw you put an equal number of candies in each of two jars, one tall and narrow, the other short and stout, he would think there were more candies in the tall narrow jar because the level of candies was higher.

Concrete Operational Stage (7 to 11 years).

During this stage, the child's reasoning becomes logical but is limited to his own experiences. He is now able to understand concepts and to concentrate on more than one aspect of an object or idea. For example, if you asked a 7-year-old child to describe a coin, he could probably tell you that it is round, that it is shiny, and that it is a form of money. At this point the child acquires the ability to reverse his thinking, learning the relationship of cause and effect.

Formal Operational Stage (11 to 16 years).

During this stage the individual acquires the ability to develop abstract concepts for himself. His thinking is oriented towards problem-solving and transcends concrete experience; that is, he no longer has to experience things before he can understand them. Science fiction has a great appeal for persons at this stage.

Piaget's Theory of Cognitive Development is currently well accepted, although some feel that it is incomplete because Piaget believed that the highest level of cognitive development is reached by the end of adolescence. Subsequent studies indicate that an individual does not reach his full mental capacity until about age 25, and that he continues to learn throughout his life span. Another criticism of Piaget's theory is that he does not give enough consideration to the effects of environmental factors on intellectual development.

Kohlberg and Moral Development

On a different theme, Lawrence Kohlberg has presented a theory of moral development, defining three stages that, like Piaget's, are inflexibly sequential, but are attained at varying rates. According to Kohlberg, the individual's progression through these stages occurs as conflict is encountered, often through interaction with a person at a higher stage. Progression through

these stages is not necessarily age-related; in fact, it may be more dependent on socioeconomic status. According to one study, more middle-class adolescent boys reached stages 2 and 3 than did their lower class peers.[3] Kohlberg's stages are defined as follows:

1. Preconventional Stage. During this stage the individual's main concern is with himself. He is occupied only with satisfying his own needs, without regard to others. An individual in this stage will obey an authority figure, although only to avoid punishment.

2. Conventional Stage. During this stage the individual is concerned mainly with pleasing others and maintaining order. He shows great respect for rules and socially accepted authority figures, such as policemen.

3. Autonomous Stage. During this stage an individual's morality is based on personal conscience, dictated by the desire to avoid self-condemnation. The individual shows a profound respect for human dignity and life. He is able to think abstractly and to take another's point of view.

Erikson and Psychosocial Development

Erik Erikson formulated a theory of psychosocial development that, like Kohlberg's theory of moral development, is based on conflicts. According to Erikson's theory, however, a person encounters the conflicts within himself. Although, ideally, the individual resolves each conflict as it is encountered, failure to do so does not mean that he will forever be burdened with it. It is possible to resolve the conflict at a later stage. According to Erikson, there are a number of developmental tasks, related to the principal conflict, that an individual must complete at each stage.

Resolution of the conflicts during the stages of infancy through the preschool years is largely dependent on the parents. During middle childhood and the adolescent years this responsibility is shared with the child's teachers. Beginning in adolescence and continuing through the adult years, the individual assumes responsibility for his own development. A brief outline of Erikson's stages of development, including the principal conflict and some related developmental tasks, is given below.

Infancy (birth to 18 months). *Principal Conflict: Trust vs. Mistrust.* During this stage the infant develops either a basic trust or mistrust of others, depending on the relationship he de-

velops with his mother (or other principal caregiver) and the quality of care he receives.

Tasks: Mother and infant adjust to each other. Infant learns to take solid foods, to walk, and to talk.

Early Childhood (18 months to 3 years). *Principal Conflict: Autonomy vs. Shame.* During this stage the child either develops a sense of pride in his independence and new accomplishments or he develops feelings of shame and doubt concerning his abilities to deal with other people and the world.

Tasks: The child seeks independence in his actions, learns to control elimination, learns to communicate through language, and learns to differentiate between right and wrong.

The Preschool Years (3 to 6 years). *Principal Conflict: Initiative vs. Guilt.* In this stage the child learns to initiate activities, and it is the response he receives to these activities that determines whether his sense of initiative will remain intact or whether he will feel a sense of guilt for his actions.

Tasks: The child establishes relations with his peers, begins to form concepts based on reality, refines his motor control, and learns a social role based on gender identification.

Middle Childhood (6 to 11 years). *Principal Conflict: Industry vs. Inferiority.* During this stage the child divides his time between home and school. A negative response received at home to his new sense of industry can be neutralized by a positive response at school, or vice versa. If the child encounters consistent failure or discouragement, however, he will experience feelings of inferiority.

Tasks: The child learns autonomy, refines his coordination, learns cooperation and self-control, develops social skills, learns to view the world objectively, and forms values.

Adolescence (11 to 18 years). *Principal Conflict: Identity vs. Role Confusion.* During this stage the adolescent ideally develops a positive and stable sense of identity, or self-image, in relation to his past and future. Lacking this, he will experience a sense of confusion with regard to his social role.

Tasks: The adolescent accepts his changed physique, seeks and achieves independence from adults, forms close peer relations, defines his social role, and reasons logically.

Early Adulthood (18 to 35 years). *Principal Conflict: Intimacy vs. Isolation.* During this stage the individual establishes close relationships with others of the same and opposite sex. If the individual is not close to anyone, he will experience feelings of isolation.

Tasks: The individual decides on a career path, chooses a marriage partner, raises children, and assumes social responsibilities.

The Middle Years (35 to 65 years). *Principal Conflict: Generativity vs. Self-absorption.* Generativity means being concerned with the future of society and the world in general. A person lacking in this quality is overly concerned with himself.

Tasks: The individual adjusts to physical and physiological changes, accepts the needs of his children and of his aging parents, and attains his career and social goals.

The Later Years (65 plus). *Principal Conflict: Integrity vs. Despair.* During this stage most adults take stock of their lives and their accomplishments. If they are content with what they have done, they experience what is called "integrity," or a sense of "wholeness." A person who is dissatisfied with his life, who wishes he could do it over again, yet knows that it is impossible, succumbs to despair.

Tasks: The individual accepts the aging process, adjusts to retirement, and adjusts to the death of his spouse and friends.

Sheehy and the Passages of Adulthood

Erikson was one of the earliest of the developmentalists to go beyond the realms of childhood and incorporate changes occurring during adulthood into his life cycle theory of growth and development. His work has subsequently been extended by others in the field. Notable among those who followed Erikson is Gail Sheehy, who has contributed much to our understanding of the nature of the inner changes taking place as a person passes through the various turning points of adulthood.[4] Sheehy preferred to call these turning points "passages," rather than crises, because people so often think of a crisis as something bad. The passages, Sheehy felt, are very normal, as well as being highly predictable. Although the individual experiences a period of instability as he passes each turning point, it is not necessarily a "bad" experience. Rather, it is an essential factor in his growth and development as a person.

In her research, Sheehy found that, although men and women both reported going through the same passages in adult life, they did not necessarily do so at the same ages, or in the same sequence. A woman who has spent her young adult years at home raising a family, for example, may be just entering the labor force at the age of 40. On the other hand, a man who has been the bread-winner of the family since his early 20's may feel that he has reached just about the peak of his career at age 40 and be looking for something else to round out and enrich his life.

Early Adulthood. Sheehy divides the early adult period (from 18 to 35 years) into four stages, or passages:

1. Pulling Up Roots (after age 18). In our North American society, an individual usually begins to sever dependence on his family sometime in his late teens or early 20's. Most young people like to move out of the family home about this age and establish a social and sexual role based on peer relationships (rather than on family expectations). This is the time when the individual makes decisions regarding a career and takes steps to prepare himself for the one of his choice. It is also a time when countless hours are often spent in serious consideration of social and moral issues as the young adult seeks to develop his own personal philosophy of life.

2. The Trying Twenties. During the 20's decade, the individual actively sets about achieving his goals. For the man, the choice is usually clear-cut—this is the time to get started on a career. At this point, the young adult is ready for an intimate relationship, usually with a person of the opposite sex. However, joined with the urge to settle down is an equally strong desire to experience as much of life as possible. Many young people like to travel or experiment with different jobs before settling down. For the man, settling down usually involves seriously embarking on a career. A young woman, however, has options. She may opt for marriage and babies in her 20's to fulfill her nurturing role, or she too may decide to get started on a career and defer children and/or marriage until later. When a person is in his 20's, there seems to be a lot of time ahead to do all the things he wants to do in life. Everything seems possible, and the individual is convinced he is invincible—that he is not going to get hurt if he drives his car at 100 miles per hour down the freeway or climbs the highest mountain in the Andes.

3. Catch-30 (approaching age 30). As the individual approaches the age of 30, he usually feels a need to reassess and change many aspects of his life. Often he finds his present lifestyle restricting—he is caught in a bind, and he wants to free himself. He discovers that the decisions made previously are not necessarily irrevocable. A large number of divorces take place around age 30. Many men change jobs or career paths at this time. Women who are childless often decide to have a baby (before they are too old, is the usual rationale). Those who have spent the 20's engrossed in their nurturing role may suddenly feel they have been missing something and decide to resume their education or career.

4. Rooting and Extending (to age 35). During the first half of the 30's, most individuals settle down in earnest and begin to put out roots in the community. This seems to be an instinctive action that is coupled with all-out efforts to achieve success in a career. The early 30's is usually a stable age when responsibilities are taken seriously. This is the time when many couples are buying homes, raising a family, and making a place for themselves in the community. The single 30's also seem to crave stability. They want their own "nest," and become serious about achieving their career goals.

Later Adulthood. Erikson grouped together the years from age 35 to age 65, calling them the "middle years." Sheehy, however, divides these years into two distinct "passages." The period from age 35 to 45 she calls the "Deadline Decade." It is a crossroads, a time when the individual must come to terms with himself and set a life course before time runs out. Daniel Levinson has coined the term "BOOM" (becoming one's own man) to describe this maturational crisis. According to Sheehy, women often feel this push around age 35, and men feel it around age 40.

"Renewal or Resignation" is the term Sheehy uses to describe life after age 45. If the individual has responded to the urge to reorganize his life during the preceding decade, he will experience a feeling of happiness or renewal during the remainder of his life. If he has simply continued on in the same course he set earlier, he will experience a feeling of stagnation, becoming resigned to the idea that now it is too late to change. For men, the late middle years are often a period when they become actively involved in community organizations. They are on planning committees for the local community, for example, the board of the community center, their union executive, church council, or other board, or they may become active in a service club, such as the Rotary, Lions, Kiwanis, or the like. Many women pursue like activities at this age, but many others go back to school or get a full-time job once the children are grown up. Some women today experience a new sense of freedom when they are in the 40's, with household responsibilities minimized and opportunities for a career outside the home opening up new horizons for them. Sheehy presents a much more optimistic picture of adulthood than the strictly physical point of view that everything is downhill after the age of 25, or even Erikson's rather depressing premise that the later years are filled with compromise and adjustment to lessening abilities. Sheehy, indeed, paints with vivid clarity an exciting portrait of continued growth and development throughout the adult years as an individual enlarges his experiences and enriches his personality. Unfortunately, she did not explore the period from 65 years onward, when many individuals report enjoying a new freedom and a renewed zest for life that they had not anticipated.

GROWTH AND DEVELOPMENT INSIDE THE WOMB

There is a great deal of controversy, particularly in regard to.the debate over abortion, as to whether the fetus is legally a human being. However, for the purposes of this discussion, we will take it that human life begins at conception when the male sperm unites with the female ovum (or ova) during its journey down the fallopian tube. *Gestation* is the term used to describe the development of new life that takes place in the womb between conception and birth. This development normally takes 9 months and can be divided into three stages.

Germinal Stage (Fertilization to 2 Weeks)

During this stage, the cells of the fertilized ovum, now called a *zygote*, multiply rapidly and the new cell mass moves down the fallopian tube and into the uterus. Approximately 2 weeks after fertilization the zygote attaches itself to the uterine wall.

Embryonic Stage (2 to 8 Weeks)

After the zygote has attached itself to the uterine wall, the cells continue to multiply, forming three distinct layers. The *ectoderm*, or outer layer, will later form the nervous system and sense organs; the *mesoderm*, or middle layer, becomes the skeletal, muscular, and circulatory systems; the *endoderm*, or inner layer, becomes the digestive system.

It is during the embryonic stage, also, that the amniotic sac and the placenta are formed. The *amniotic sac* is a protective membrane filled with fluid that surrounds the developing embryo, providing warmth, moisture, and relative freedom of movement. The *placenta* is an organ that attaches to the uterine wall and to the fetus by means of the *umbilical cord*. Through the umbilical cord, the unborn child receives nourishment and oxygenated blood and disposes of wastes. The placenta also serves as a barrier protecting the developing child from potentially harmful agents.

By 8 weeks gestation, the embryo is recognizably human, with distinct arms, legs, fingers, and toes, although the head comprises about half its length. It is only about 1 inch long, but already its systems are beginning to function.

Fetal Stage (8 Weeks to Birth)

The most striking change that occurs during the fetal stage is the dramatic increase in size from approximately 1 to 1½ inches to an average length of 18 to 20 inches at birth. The systems that began to form in the embryonic stage increase in complexity and maturity. The fetus begins to move by the third month, although this is not usually felt by the mother until the fourth or fifth month when its actions become more vigorous. By the sixth month, the eyelids open and the fetus begins to take amniotic fluid into its lungs as a rudimentary form of breathing.

The greatest brain development occurs during the last few months of the fetal stage. Until the seventh month, the fetus is virtually incapable of living outside the womb owing to the immaturity of its nervous system.

The 7-month fetus is neurologically mature enough to survive in the extrauterine world in a controlled environment. It can breathe, although the lungs are not fully developed until approximately 36 weeks gestation, or just before birth in a full-term infant. Also, the fetus at 7 months has not accumulated the layers of fat so noticeable in a full-term baby, which protect him from temperature changes and enable him to go without nourishment for the first day or two after birth.

The eighth and ninth months of fetal development are devoted primarily to maturation of the lungs and nervous system and to the accumulation of fat, as mentioned above. Toward the end of the ninth month, activity often diminishes as the fetus becomes cramped for space. Shortly before the onset of labor the fetus becomes "engaged" in the pelvic cavity, normally with its head down, in preparation for birth.

During its period of development inside the womb the fetus is totally dependent on the mother to satisfy its basic needs. She provides nutrients, oxygen, warmth, and protection and disposes of fetal wastes. Although the placenta provides some protection from harmful agents, many others pass through the placental barrier to the fetus. As the fetus is very vulnerable to infection and the effects of noxious stimuli, particularly in its early developmental stages, the mother must take care to protect her unborn child from such dangers. Studies have suggested that maternal emotions affect the developing fetus, too, and can have long-range effects on personality. To date, the results of such studies have been inconclusive, largely owing to the difficulty of collecting data over a period of several years, and of separating out other influences that may affect a person's psychological make-up.

PREGNANCY

Although pregnancy, as a chronological event, occurs traditionally during the stage of early adulthood, we feel that it belongs more logically in a discussion on fetal development. While the unborn child grows and develops inside the womb of the mother, many other changes are occurring that affect the pregnant woman herself. The duration of an average pregnancy is 38 weeks from conception, or 40 weeks from the last menstrual period, divided into trimesters of 3 months each.

First Trimester

A woman's first indication that she is pregnant may be the cessation of menses, or swollen and tender breasts. Or, she may feel generally "out of sorts." During the first trimester of pregnancy there is a marked increase in the production of hormones, particularly estrogen and progesterone. These hormonal changes account for many of the early signs of pregnancy. As mentioned above, the woman usually (but not always) misses a menstrual period. She may feel tired and her breasts may swell, tingle, and feel tender as the milk glands prepare to produce milk. She may experience nausea and vomiting, especially first thing in the morning (usually called morning sickness).

The pelvic structure begins to widen to accommodate the growing uterus. During pregnancy, the uterus will increase its weight from approximately 60 grams (pre-pregnant weight) to approximately 1100 grams at full term. Many women feel the need to urinate more frequently owing to pressure of the uterus on the bladder as well as to hormonal changes. The increase in

PREGNANCY

Needs Requiring Particular Attention	Factors Related to These Needs
Nutrition	Growth of new tissue, requiring additional nourishment
	Fetus nourished at expense of mother
Elimination	Hormonal changes affecting kidney function and digestion
	Expansion of uterus in pelvis and into abdominal cavity
Circulation	Increase in total fluid volume
	Increased body mass
Comfort, rest, and sleep	Weight gain, increasing body bulk
	Altered body proportions, making some resting positions difficult
Pain avoidance	Medications may cross placenta and have harmful effects on the fetus
Movement and exercise	Awkwardness due to
	(1) Weight gain, (2) increase in fluid volume, (3) shift in center of gravity, affecting balance, and (4) relaxing of ligaments
	Slowing down of body processes
Protection and safety	Dependence of fetus' well-being on mother
	Shift in center of gravity, affecting balance
Hygiene	Hormonal changes affecting skin texture and secretions
Infection control	Placenta only a partial barrier to harmful agents
Love, security, and self-esteem	Possibility that strong emotions may affect the fetus
Sexuality	Note: There are conflicting beliefs regarding possible harm to the fetus from intercourse
	Altered body proportions
	New role of "mother"

progesterone has a relaxing effect on smooth muscle, which causes bowel irregularity and, in many cases, constipation.

The degree to which these changes are felt depends on the individual—on her physiological make-up and on her emotional response to her pregnancy. While one woman may experience nausea every day for the first trimester, another may simply feel tired, while yet another may feel no different from the way she felt before she became pregnant. Then, too, no two pregnancies are exactly alike, as any woman with more than one child will tell you.

Second Trimester

During the fourth to the sixth month of pregnancy, the future mother usually experiences a feeling of overall well-being. Her body has adjusted to the hormonal changes and she has more energy. She can feel the baby move, which usually has a positive effect. Many women take on a "radiant glow" at this time.

By the fourth month, weight gain is usually evident. There is a thickening of the waist as the uterus expands and rises out of the pelvis. The amount of body fluid increases by approximately 7 liters, about 3 liters of which is increased blood volume. The cervix softens and is closed by a mucous plug. The breasts, including the nipples, enlarge and may begin to produce colostrum (a thin, yellowish substance rich in maternal antibodies). The nipples may become darker, and a vertical line of dark pigment, called the *linea nigra*, appears between the pubic area and the navel. Some women develop *stretch marks* (reddish streaks) on their breasts and abdomen.

Third Trimester

During the third trimester, the future mother again often experiences fatigue and a new feeling of heaviness. A general relaxation of all body ligaments occurs in late pregnancy, and the continually enlarging uterus pushes her center of gravity backward. The enlarged uterus is responsible for much of the discomfort the woman feels at this time. It may press on the lungs or the diaphragm or both, causing shortness of breath; on the bladder, causing urinary frequency; or on the stomach, causing indigestion.

Approximately 1 month before birth the baby "drops" as its head settles into the pelvic cavity. This makes the mother generally more comfortable, although the uterus may now be pressing on the bowel, causing constipation. During this stage *Braxton-Hicks contractions,* that is, tightening of the uterine muscles in preparation for labor, often occur.

The loss of the mucous plug (often called a "show") and the appearance of amniotic fluid are generally good indications that labor is imminent. *Labor* is the process by which the baby

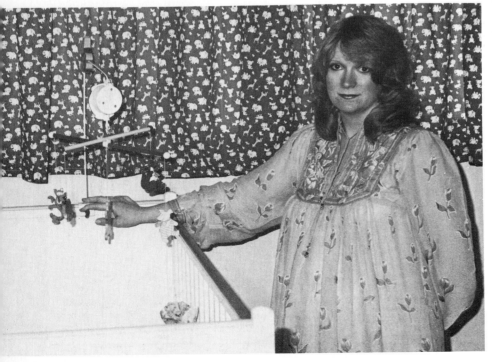

The future mother contemplates the arrival of her baby as she prepares the baby's room.

is expelled from the uterus. It consists of a series of strong contractions, and can be divided into three stages.

During *first stage labor* the cervix shortens, and becomes thinner (*effacement*) and opens (*dilation*) to allow the baby to pass through. *Second stage* labor begins as the baby's head "crowns" or becomes visible, and ends with the birth of the infant. During *third stage* labor the placenta is expelled.

During pregnancy and labor many women sense a diminution of their self-image, a loss of respect on the part of others for their needs and wishes. All too often, especially during labor, the pregnant woman's wishes have been over-ruled or ignored in favor of the convenience of hospital personnel. It should be remembered that while the health and safe delivery of the infant are important, so are the needs and wishes of the parents.

INFANCY (Birth to 18 Months)

The first sight of a newborn baby comes as a shock to most of us. Expecting to see a plump, rosy-cheeked, bright-eyed infant (as often depicted on television), we are instead presented with a squalling bundle with reddish or blue-tinged wrinkled skin, a puffy face, a flat nose, and, often, a misshapen head. He is covered with a creamy white substance called *vernix*, which protected his skin in the womb and eased his passage through the birth canal. He may also be covered with *lanugo*, a thick downy hair, and he may be splattered with blood. Upon closer

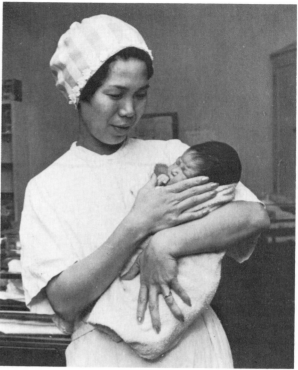

Nurse with newborn. (From the Canadian Nurse *75*(10):30, November, 1979. Courtesy Canadian Nurses Association, Helen K. Mussallem Library.)

inspection you may notice that his skin is peeling in some places or he may be bruised from a forceps delivery. As if that weren't enough, his legs may be bowed and his toes bent in odd ways from his cramped position in the womb.

✔ INFANCY

Needs Requiring Particular Attention	Factors Related to These Needs
Nutrition	Immaturity of gastrointestinal system
	Rapid growth of all body tissues, requiring increased nutrition
	Appearance of teeth
Elimination	Immaturity of gastrointestinal system
	Immaturity of neuromuscular structures necessary for control
Temperature regulation	Immaturity of temperature regulation system
Comfort, rest, and sleep	Rapid growth, requiring increased rest and sleep
Sensory stimulation	Quality of environment
	Mobility status
Movement and exercise	Neuromuscular development
	Opportunity for exploration of environment
Protection and safety	Lack of experience to perceive danger
	Inability to protect self
Hygiene	Vulnerability to infection
	Sensitivity of skin
Infection control	Maternal antibodies in young infants—prolonged by breast-feeding
	Immunization schedule
Security and self-esteem	Mother-infant adjustment or primary importance
Love and belonging	Mother-infant "bonding" important
	Quality of care, extent of cuddling, affection important

At birth the infant must make immediate adjustments in order to survive. Accustomed to having his needs met automatically in the womb, he is now forced to rely on his own systems to satisfy many of his basic needs, such as nutrition, elimination, oxygen, and circulation. Newborns typically fall into a deep sleep shortly after birth, and this sleep can last up to 12 hours. During the first few months of life in this world, they spend most of their time sleeping or resting.

The first 18 months of life are a period of rapid growth. By the end of their first year, most infants have tripled their birth weight and increased their length again by half. Normally born without teeth, they begin teething around 5 or 6 months. Most infants have 6 to 8 teeth by 1 year and 4 to 6 more by 18 months. Babies have a relatively immature gastrointestinal system at birth. For the first few months they can handle only breast milk or formula; anything else passes through them without being absorbed. By 18 months, however, the gastrointestinal system has matured to the point at which toddlers can handle most adult foods.

Newborns and young infants generally have

Age	Anatomic Progression	Motor Skill

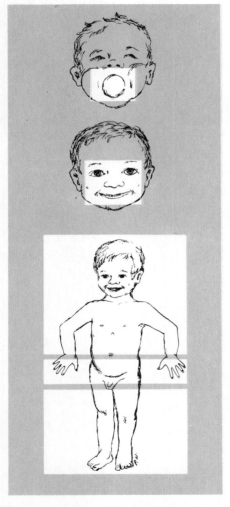

Mnemonic for motor development. (From Sells, C. J.: Infancy—The First Two Years. *In* Smith, D. W., Bierman, E. L., and Robinson, N. M. (eds.): *The Biologic Ages of Man.* 2nd ed. Philadelphia, W. B. Saunders Company, 1978, p. 113.

Age	Motor Skill
Birth (full term)	Suck, breathe, and swallow in a coordinated fashion*
3 Months	Directed vision — reaching for objects with eyes
6 Months	Sit with head erect when hips are supported; reach for objects, though grasp of them is immature
9 Months	Sit unaided indefinitely; grasp, using opposition of thumb and fingers (pincer grasp)**
12 Months	Walk unaided

*This motor skill can be better appreciated if compared to the necessity of passing a feeding tube into the stomach of an infant born at 28 rather than 38 weeks of gestation.
**Sitting unaided indefinitely is but one of the skills children acquire with control over movement at the hips. Creeping (moving on hands and knees); getting from a prone into a sitting position and back to prone—all of these become a part of the child's activities about this age.

very sensitive skin. It breaks down easily, providing an ideal site for bacteria and other organisms to grow. Skin rashes on the face and especially in the diaper area are common. Young babies are also very sensitive to even mild fluctuations in temperature, as their temperature regulating system is immature and does not adapt quickly. They do not shiver; instead their metabolic rate increases when they are cold.

Infants receive some protection from disease during their first 2 to 3 months through their mother's antibodies that remain in their system. It is possible to prolong this immunity through breastfeeding, as breast milk is high in maternal antibodies. In the United States and in Canada, the recommended immunizations are usually begun when the infant is 2 or 3 months old and are continued throughout his childhood years (See Chapter 25).

The newborn has very little motor control; most of his movements are reflexes, that is, automatic responses to stimuli. He will withdraw from a pinprick, turn toward a sound, grasp your fingers or startle at a loud noise. When his cheek is stroked he will turn his head in that direction and begin sucking movements. This reflex is called rooting. Many of the reflexes present at birth disappear as the infant achieves control over his actions. He progresses from simple movements, such as watching his mother move around a room, to complex skills within a relatively short time. By 18 months, an infant is capable of negotiating stairs, for example, or turning the pages in a favorite book. Development of motor skills appears to progress in a head to foot, central to peripheral direction.[5] By 12 months most infants have learned to walk, and by 18 months they are running and climbing.

In the area of communication, the infant progresses from just crying to smiling in a few short weeks. Soon he begins to vocalize. By 1 year, most infants have two or three words with many meanings; at 18 months they may have an "understandable" vocabulary of about a dozen words. An infant can understand his own name by about 8 months, and by 1 year he knows and can say the names of those close to him. He is capable of understanding more than he can say and enjoys being read to, although his attention span is very short.

Erikson identified the principal conflict of this stage as "Trust vs. Mistrust." Perhaps the most important task during infancy is the adjustment that mother and child must make to each other. The bonding, or attachment, that occurs between parent and newborn is important in creating a sense of security in the infant. When the mother cares for her infant in a loving and consistent manner, meeting his needs as they arise, the infant develops a sense of trust in others. This sense of trust also appears to be a motivational force. Studies have shown that in institutions such as orphanages, where there is not always sufficient staff to deal with each infant's needs as they arise and on an individual basis, the infants are generally anxious and display little curiosity about their environment. This passivity has the effect of slowing their rate of development.

EARLY CHILDHOOD (18 Months to 3 Years)

During the early childhood stage, the child continues to grow, although not quite so rapidly as during infancy. The proportions of his body begin to change—his head does not appear quite so large, and his limbs begin to lengthen in relation to his trunk. The body systems continue to mature, and mental functions increase in complexity. For example, between 18 and 24 months, most children have the neuromuscular capacity for sphincter control; that is, they are capable of controlling elimination. This is the time when most patients initiate "toilet training."

Language plays an important role for children at this stage. They are learning to make their wants and needs understood by others. By 2 years, the average child has a vocabulary of 50 to 100 words; by the age of 3 he is capable of forming complex sentences to express his ideas.

The child's motor coordination improves greatly during this stage. He can hold a crayon to draw, and he can manipulate buttons to put on and take off his clothes. There is a new sense of mobility as he learns to ride a tricycle or push himself in his wagon.

Small wonder, then, with all his new abilities, that the child seeks to employ them. This stage is often referred to as the "Terrible Two's" as the charming and compliant child of one is transformed into a veritable monster. At this stage he seems to be "on the go" all day. His new abilities, combined with an insatiable curiosity about his world, turn him into a little dynamo, busily exploring everything within his reach. He wants to do things himself, without his parents' help, and he can be very vocal when expressing his disapproval of their interference. Unfortunately, children of this age have little concept of danger, and even less understanding of cause and effect. It is often necessary to curtail their activities for their own protection.

Erikson identified the principal conflict of this stage as "Autonomy vs. Shame." The child is actively seeking independence, yet he also needs approval for his actions. It is important, then, in

EARLY CHILDHOOD

Needs Requiring Particular Attention	Factors Related to These Needs
Nutrition	Continued growth and maturation of systems
Elimination	Proportional fluid constituency of body is great compared with that in adults
	Achievement of control of elimination
Sensory stimulation	Increased mobility and improved motor control, making exploration further afield possible
	Developing sense of autonomy
	Independence of movement
Movement and exercise	Increasing neuromuscular maturation
	Improved motor control
	Development of motor skills
Protection and safety	Developing independence
	Insatiable curiosity
	Improved motor control
	Inability to understand danger
Hygiene	Parental teaching
	Toilet training
Infection control	Increased contact with other children
	Immunization schedules
Security and self-esteem	Developing sense of autonomy
	Home atmosphere
Love and belonging	Quality of parent-child interactions
	Stability of relationships with parents, siblings
	Development of trust
Sexuality	Gender identification
	Relationships with parents and siblings important

setting limits, to help the child to understand the distinction between right and wrong, without discouraging him in his activities.

Before age 3, children take little notice of one another. They will play side by side, (*parallel play*), but there is little interaction. Around age 3, however, children begin to have more contact with others their age, and they learn to play together as a sense of cooperation emerges. The primary influence on a child of this stage, however, is still his immediate family. He learns mainly through observation and imitation of his parents and siblings. The home atmosphere has a profound effect on a child's image of himself.

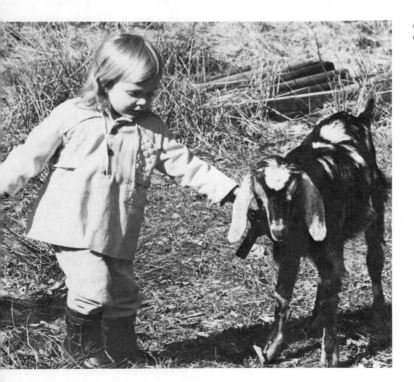

All the world is new to the toddler who enjoys her explorations.

THE PRESCHOOL YEARS

Needs Requiring Particular Attention	Factors Related to These Needs
Nutrition	Continued growth and maturation of systems
Elimination	Functional maturity of systems
Sensory stimulation	Maturation of vision
	Improved muscle control making exploration easier
Movement and exercise	Improved neuromuscular control
	Developing motor skills
Protection and safety	Lack of awareness of danger
	Expanding horizons
Infection control	Increasing contact with others
	Development of active immunity to infection
	Immunization schedule for communicable diseases
	Nutritional status affects vulnerability to infection
Sexuality	Gender identity with parent of same sex
Love and belonging	Home environment
	Development of initiative
	Parents' and siblings' attitudes toward child
Security	Development of initiative
	Support and guidance from parents
	Stability of home
	Accustomed routines
Self-esteem	Interaction with peers
	Family atmosphere

THE PRESCHOOL YEARS (3 to 6 Years)

During the preschool years, the child's rate of growth begins to slow down, although he will continue to gain 2 to 3 inches a year until he reaches puberty. In appearance, his proportions resemble more closely those of an adult. His bones become harder and his muscle control and coordination improve noticeably. In general, boys of this age have better large muscle control and may enjoy such sports as soccer or baseball. Girls usually have better fine motor coordination and may be more interested in crafts such as painting or sewing.

By the age of 3, most children have all their primary teeth. Their body systems have reached functional maturity. For example, they can handle adult foods, and they are capable of controlling their elimination and taking care of their various toilet needs. Although infants are capable of seeing at birth, full visual maturity does not occur until about age 5.

Children develop active immunity through exposure to disease. From the time they start playing with other children on a regular basis, at preschool or kindergarten, for example, they seem to catch whatever is going around, be it a cold, the flu, or a disease such as measles, mumps, or chicken pox. Immunization programs, usually begun in infancy, continue throughout the childhood years. Although inoculations do not guarantee that a child will not succumb to a particular disease, they usually mean a less severe attack and a quicker recovery. The preschool stage is a time when children begin to actively socialize with each other, as

mentioned above. Many children attend preschool or nursery school at age 3 or 4, and almost all school systems now incorporate a kindergarten class for 5-year-olds. The child's world expands beyond his home and family, although the family is still a major influence on his development. During this stage, the child begins to identify with the parent of the same sex, learning a social role based largely on imitation of this parent. He practices these newfound social skills during play with his peers; the differences between the sexes become apparent.

Language continues to play a major role throughout this stage. It is a means by which the child can capture the attention of others and assert himself. As his horizons broaden and he is capable of doing more and more for himself every day, the child wants to tell people about it. Sometimes children of 3 and 4, especially, just can't seem to stop talking. They have fertile imaginations and often get reality and fantasy mixed up. Children at this stage are highly impressionable; that is, they will take to heart what others, particularly adults, tell them. It is important to recognize, in talking with young children, that they are not always capable of detecting teasing or sarcasm.

According to Erikson, the principal conflict of this stage is "Initiative vs. Guilt." A child's delight as he explores the world and discovers his own emerging capabilities is truly wonderful to see. He is so proud of his accomplishments. However, not all his endeavors may fall into the category of "acceptable behavior," and often it may be necessary to redirect his energies. Chil-

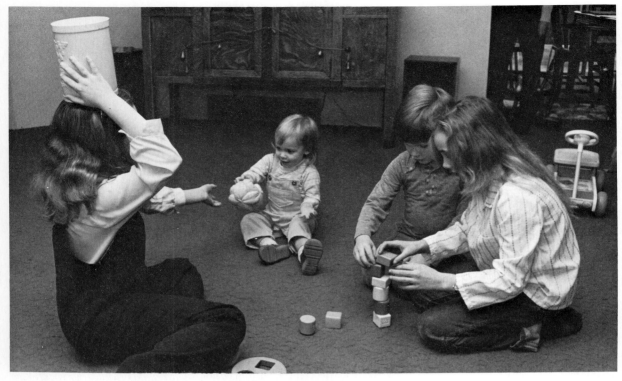

Preschoolers often enjoy playing with older siblings.

dren of this age are mainly motivated by a sense of discovery, and it is important to discourage unacceptable behavior without discouraging initiative or making the child feel guilty.

MIDDLE CHILDHOOD (6 to 11 Years)

During middle childhood, the child's growth continues at a slow and steady rate. Boys are generally heavier and taller than girls of the same age. The child's body proportions now resemble those of an adult. There is further maturation of the body's systems and brain development is virtually complete by puberty. Neuromuscular coordination is further refined, and team sports become a major activity for children of this age. As they continue to develop their active immunity, school age children are prone to the various "childhood diseases." Im-

MIDDLE CHILDHOOD

Needs Requiring Particular Attention	Factors Related to These Needs
Nutrition	Continued growth and maturation of systems
Movement and exercise	Further refinement of neuromuscular control
Protection and safety	Understanding of relationship of cause and effect
Infection control	Increased contact with others (school and extracurricular)
	Development of active immunity
	Immunization schedule
	Nutritional status
Sexuality	Adoption of social role based on sex
Self-esteem	Establishment of independence
	Home atmosphere and school atmosphere
	Relations with peers, adults outside home
	Success in endeavors
Security	Parental support
	Teachers' support
Love and belonging	Stability of home environment
	Continuity of school environment
	Routines and schedules
Sexuality	Development of social role based on gender
	Role model (parent or parent-substitute of same sex)

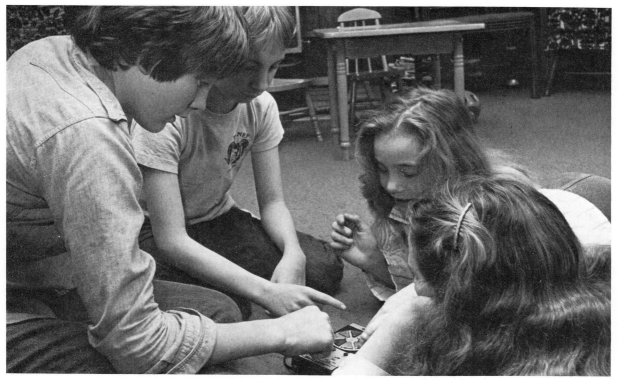

Playing an electronic game in this high technology world.

munization schedules generally continue throughout this stage.

In the schoolroom and through participation in team activities, the child develops an attitude of cooperation and self-control. His thinking and actions are no longer so completely self-centered as he learns that not everyone shares his viewpoint. He begins to think about things that do not necessarily affect him directly and to express his thoughts and feelings about himself and others. He learns that there is a relationship between cause and effect.

The period of middle childhood is a critical one in terms of psychosocial development. This is when the child firmly establishes his sense of independence and defines his social role. According to Erikson, the principal conflict of middle childhood is "Industry vs. Inferiority." The child is on a quest of discovery throughout both his inner and outer selves. He asks many questions, seeking to understand every aspect of the world. He may want to know where he came from, for example, or who made the world. He might enjoy taking things apart to see what makes them work. (He may not be so successful in putting things back together again, though.)

If the child is encouraged to try new things and taught to learn from his mistakes, he will develop a positive image of himself and his capabilities. If, on the other hand, he is continually discouraged in his endeavors through failure of his ideas or negative comments from others, he will soon feel incapable of anything worthwhile, assuming what is commonly called an "inferiority complex." Success in any endeavor, no matter how small, is necessary for an individual to feel good about himself.

As mentioned above, the child during this stage establishes his independence from his family. He spends a large part of his day now away from home. As well as attending school, he may also participate in such community activities as Scouts or team sports. Although the home and family remain a primary factor in his development, other adults and his peers are beginning to play an important role in his life, too.

ADOLESCENCE (11 to 18 years)

Much has been written about the "turbulent" adolescent years. The notion that adolescence is an unsettling (or unsettled) period in one's life, however, seems to be peculiar to the modern Western world. In Samoa, for example, where adult roles are clearly defined, the transition from childhood to adulthood is gradual and serene.[6] Even in our own Western society less than a century ago, children gradually assumed adult responsibilities at home and then apprenticed at an early age in a vocation that, as often as not, was chosen for them. Perhaps these days

ADOLESCENCE

Needs Requiring Particular Attention	Factors Related to These Needs
Nutrition	Growth spurt
	Maturation of systems
Oxygen	Rapid increase in vital capacity of lungs
Movement and exercise	Change in body proportions
Protection and safety	Risk-taking behavior
Hygiene	Excessive sebum production
	Attainment of puberty
Infection control	Sexual experimentation
Sexuality	Maturation of reproductive system
	Establishment of social role
Self-esteem	Physical appearance
	Peer relations
	Attainment of independence
	Establishment of identity

there are just too many options open to the adolescent.

Adolescence has been defined as "the period of psychobiologic maturation during which the secondary physical growth spurt is completed and sexual maturity and the ability to reproduce are achieved."[5] It is a stage involving many changes for the individual. As mentioned above, there is a growth spurt during adolescence, including an increase in both height and weight. Girls usually attain their maximum height earlier, but boys are generally taller. Also, there is a rapid increase in the vital capacity of the lungs during adolescence, greater in boys than in girls.

Body proportions change—girls develop breasts and hips, and boys' shoulders become broader. Other physical changes are apparent as the reproductive system matures. There is an increased production of the hormones *testosterone* in males and *estrogen* in females, which are primarily responsible for the appearance of the secondary sex characteristics. (See Chapter 28.) *Puberty* is marked by *menarche* (the onset of the menstrual cycle) in girls, and by the production of sperm in boys. The increased production of hormones also results in the secretion of excess amounts of *sebum*, a thick, oily substance that can plug the hair follicles, often resulting in skin eruptions called *acne*.

Most adolescents enjoy general good health, having already established immunity to most contagious diseases. The principal infections suffered by adolescents these days are sex-related. In the past 25 years, over half the cases of gonorrhea reported in the United States have involved persons between the ages of 15 and 24.[5]

As the adolescent takes on the appearance of an adult he wants to be treated as one also. He can be very critical of his parents, partly because he is dependent on them, partly because he feels that they do not understand him. This is a

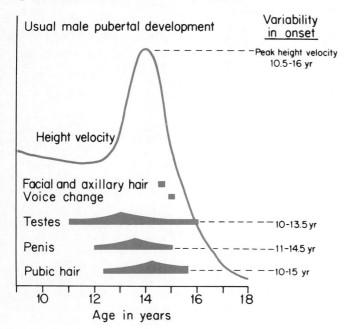

Diagram of sequence of events at adolescence in males. (From Hammar, S. L.: Adolescence. *In* Smith, D. W., Bierman, E. L., and Robinson, N. M.: *The Biologic Ages of Man.* 2nd ed. Philadelphia, W. B. Saunders Company, 1978, p. 172. Adapted from Hammar S. L.: Adolescence. *In* Kelley, V. C. (ed.): Brenneman's Practice of Pediatrics. Hagerstown, Maryland, Harper & Row, Publishers, Inc., Vol. 1, Chapter 6, 1970.)

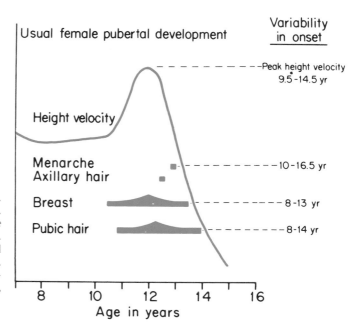

Usual female pubertal development

Variability in onset

Peak height velocity 9.5-14.5 yr

Height velocity

Menarche
Axillary hair — 10-16.5 yr

Breast — 8-13 yr

Pubic hair — 8-14 yr

Age in years

Sequence of events at adolescence in females. (From Hammar, S. L.: Adolescence. *In* Smith, D. W., Bierman, E. L., and Robinson, N. M. (eds.): *The Biologic Ages of Man.* 2nd ed. Philadelphia, W. B. Saunders Company, 1978, p. 173. Adapted from Hammar, S. L.: Adolescence. *In* Kelley, V. C. (ed.): Brenneman's Practice of Pediatrics. Hagerstown, Maryland, Harper & Row, Publishers, Inc., Vol. 1, Chapter 6, 1970.)

common complaint of adolescents. As they seek independence, they also desire parental guidance and approval—contrary to popular belief.

Communication with parents is difficult at this stage, and so the adolescent turns to his peers. The importance of peer relations during adolescence cannot be overemphasized. The peer group provides the individual with a sense of belonging. Conformity is the order of the day, as no one wants to be "different." Peer pressure is an important influence on an adolescent, affecting all aspects of his life. For example, the attitude of the group usually decides the degree to which an individual will engage in sexual experimentation, the leisure activities in which he will participate, how long, or short, he will

Appearance and peer approval are important to adolescents.

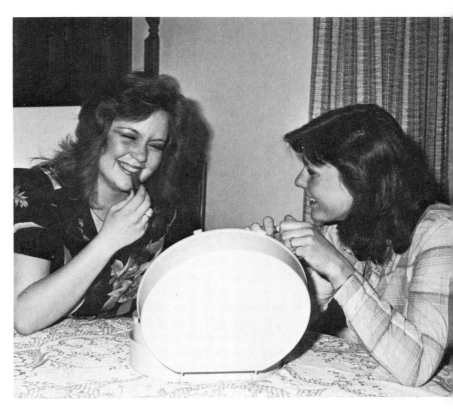

wear his hair, and what style of clothes he will buy. Adolescents are particularly concerned with their physical appearance, often spending literally hours in front of a mirror (as any parent of a teenager knows).

Adolescence is characterized by experimentation as the individual seeks to gain knowledge about himself and about the world around him. During this stage many adolescents engage in risk-taking behavior, often pushing themselves and each other to test their limits. For example, they may drive at high speeds, experiment with drugs or alcohol, or engage in sex without taking precautions against pregnancy. Experimentation with their new-found sexuality is a major concern of most adolescents, both boys and girls, although boys have the stronger sex drive at this stage of development.

Adolescents also experiment with their own self-image, trying on various roles in an effort to establish a true sense of self. For example, a parent may watch his teen-age son drive off with his friends in a great roar on his motorcycle one moment, and yet later in the same day, he may find this same son strumming his guitar and singing quiet folk songs. Erikson has defined the principal conflict of this stage as "Identity vs. Role Confusion." The individual who does not have the opportunity to try on different roles may ultimately be unable to settle on one identity. This leads to role confusion and can disrupt one's relationships with others.

In the area of intellectual development, the adolescent differs from younger children in his ability to think and reason in a logical manner. Also, he is capable of understanding and forming abstract thoughts. Values acquired in childhood are questioned and new ones formed. The adolescent is often critical of the stage of the world in general, and actively seeks to change it. He strives for perfection, yet often gets carried away by his emotions.

EARLY ADULTHOOD (18 to 35 years)

As they enter adulthood, most people have reached their physical maturity and their body systems are functioning at their optimum level. Sensory and intellectual perception and muscular strength are at their peak.

Young adults comprise the healthiest segment of our population. They rarely succumb to contagious diseases, and when they do, their illness is generally brief and without complications. As with adolescents, however, the major causes of infection are sexually transmitted diseases. Gonorrhea, nongonococcal urethritis and vaginitis, venereal warts, trichomoniasis, and genital herpes have reached epidemic proportions in the young adult age group.[5] owing largely, it is felt, to the general relaxing of sexual mores in our society.

There is a tendency, among young adults, to view themselves as indestructible and as having limitless physical capabilities. The notion that "It can't happen to me" is very prevalent among this age group. Consequently, as with adolescents, there is much risk-taking. High-risk activities may also provide a release for the individual from the many stresses he encounters at this stage of his life.

Initiation to adulthood involves many major decisions. For the first time, probably, the individual needs to make a plan and set goals for the future. He must decide whether to continue

EARLY ADULTHOOD

Needs Requiring Particular Attention	Factors Related to These Needs
Nutrition	Continued growth and development in early adult years
	Establishment of own dietary habits (early training and habits formed in childhood important here)
	Time and work pressures
Movement and exercise	More sedentary lifestyle
	Development of own lifestyle
	Gradual decline in physical performance from peak fitness
Protection and safety	Feelings of indestructibility
	Risk-taking behavior common
Infection control	Strength of sexual drive
	Choice of sexual partners
Sexuality	Self-image
	Ability to establish close relationships
	Choosing a marriage partner
Security and self-esteem	Decline in physical performance
	Relationships with others
	Ability to make major decisions
Love and belonging	Ability to form close ties with others

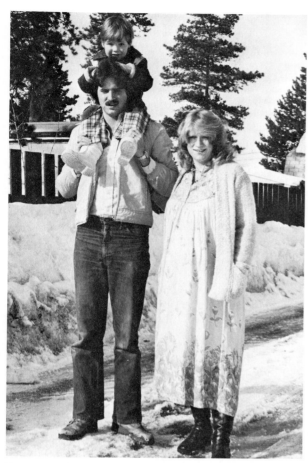

Young adults take on new responsibilities, including raising a family.

ance of which he was capable just a short year or two ago. If he is unwilling to accept these new physical limitations in his activities, he may push himself to succeed, causing more harm than good in most cases. If he does accept them, he may feel that he has compromised his image of himself.

According to Erikson, the principal conflict of this stage is "Intimacy vs. Isolation." The individual needs to establish a close relationship with one or more persons with whom he can share his innermost thoughts and feelings, and who will accept him as he is. Many individuals achieve such closeness only with their marriage partner. Others may have several good friends on whom they can rely for emotional support. A person who has no one to share his intimate thoughts experiences a feeling of profound loneliness or isolation. He may feel worthless, lacking in positive qualities. An individual's relationships with others during this stage—that is, family and, especially, friends—are important in the development of his self-esteem. He looks to them for advice and support as he seeks to establish his own personal lifestyle.

THE MIDDLE YEARS (35 to 65 Years)

During the first decade of this period (Sheehy's "Deadline Decade"), the physical changes accompanying the aging process may be almost imperceptible. Individuals who have participated in a regular exercise program, maintained good nutritional habits, and had a generally healthy lifestyle throughout their young adult years often look, feel, and are remarkably fit in their late 30's and early 40's. Many young adults, however, are too busy—climbing the corporate ladder, raising children, or just earning a living—to look after their health. They are often, then, suddenly brought up short by the realization that the odd gray hair is beginning to show, the waistline has thickened, or wrinkles have suddenly appeared around the eyes or mouth. A person may notice a decrease in the perception of taste and smell, or find that he needs to wear glasses for the first time in his life. Sometimes, the change in health status is more serious. For example, there has been an alarming incidence of heart attacks among men around the age of 40. As part of the general reassessment of one's lifestyle that is done sometime between the ages of 35 and 45 years, health is usually an important consideration. An increasing number of people of this age group are joining fitness programs as they begin to realize that their health is not indestructible and that it is time to take action to safeguard it.

with his education, or find a job immediately after completing school; whether he will remain in his parents' home or move out. There are also the questions of whether to settle down, choose a marriage partner, and have children.

The numerous major decisions an individual must face can make this stage of his life an extremely stressful one. Often a person literally leaves his home, family, and friends as he moves to a different city to pursue his education or a career goal. Or, he may be unable to make a definitive career choice. He may want to travel, yet feel pressured by his family and friends to settle down and get married. A major factor contributing to the stress an individual experiences at this stage in his life is his own conviction that the decisions he makes at this time, once made, are irrevocable. He wants to be sure to make the right decision now.

Another cause of stress for the individual in the later years of this stage may be the realization that his physical performance is diminishing. He can no longer match the strength and endur-

THE MIDDLE YEARS

Needs Requiring Particular Attention	Factors Related to These Years
Nutrition	More sedentary lifestyle
Sensory stimulation	Greater intensity of stimulation required
Movement and exercise	Decline in physical performance
	Awareness of preventive value of regular exercise program
	Availability of programs
Hygiene	Decrease in skin integrity
Sexuality	Elimination of fear of pregnancy for women
	Decrease in fertility
	Self-image
	Attainment of career and social goals
Self-esteem	Attainment of career and social goals
	Decline in fertility and sexual function
Security	Visual signs of aging process
	Mid-life crisis
Love and belonging	Decline in sexual function
	Teen-aged children
	Aging parents

The physical changes of the aging ·process inevitably catch up with people in the late middle years. The "change of life" usually begins when the person is in his early to mid-40's. Generally, this means the *menopause*, or end of the childbearing years, for women. The onset and duration of menopause varies with each individual. It may start and end abruptly, or it may be a gradual process. There is a decrease in the production of estrogen, causing the ovaries to cease releasing ova. Other changes directly related to decreased estrogen production are "hot flashes," a thinning of the vaginal linings, and urinary dysfunction.[6]

Some women experience other symptoms such as fatigue, dizziness, or nervousness, for example, which, although not directly attributable to estrogen reduction, may result from a combination of factors at this stage in a woman's life. We do not seem to be hearing so much about the dreaded female menopause these days, however. Many women, indeed, look forward to the cessation of menstruation as a blessed end to an inconvenience, and view the last child's leaving home as an opportunity to assert their individuality and seek their own fulfillment. Perhaps the new lease on life being experienced by so many women as they go back to school or work in their late 30's (and on through the 40's and 50's) has taken the sting out of nature's withdrawal of the ability to reproduce.

There has been much written lately, however, about the "male menopause." Although men do not lose their ability to reproduce, they do experience a decrease in the production of testosterone, which reduces fertility and the ability to achieve orgasm. Impotence can also be a problem. In our youth-oriented North American society, many men seem to have difficulty accepting the "change of life" process. They may feel the need to compensate by wearing loud clothes, driving flashy sports cars, and seeking involvement with younger people—particularly of the opposite sex. It is not uncommon for a man in this age group to abandon his wife of many years, and all he has worked hard to achieve, for a new life with a younger woman.

This woman, in her middle years, had decided to return to college now that her children are grown.

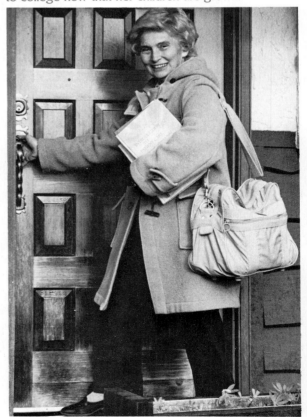

THE LATER YEARS

Needs Requiring Particular Attention	Factors Related to These Needs
Nutrition	Fixed or diminished income
	Reduced caloric intake
	Oral problems
	Loneliness, depression
Elimination	More sedentary lifestyle
	Loss of muscle tone
	Poor eating habits
Circulation	Slowed heart rate
	Fatty deposits around heart
	Chronic conditions
Oxygen	Decrease in vital capacity of lungs
	Chronic conditions
Temperature regulation	Diminished adaptation to extremes of heat and cold
Comfort, rest, and sleep	Loss of skin integrity
Pain avoidance	Reduced sensitivity to pain
Sensory stimulation	Diminished perception in all areas
Movement and exercise	Loss of muscle tone, mass
	Loss of cartilage
	Limited range of motion
	Slower coordination
Protection and safety	Loss of cartilage
	Bones more fragile
	Presence of osteoporosis
	Slower reflexes
	Diminished sensory perception
Hygiene	Loss of skin integrity
	Loss of teeth
	Dentures, gum disease
Infection control	Loss of skin integrity
	Decreased isoimmunity
	Immunosuppressive drugs
	Chronic conditions
Sexuality	Privacy
	Past sexual patterns
Self-esteem	Financial status
	Leisure, social activities
	Dependency status
	Attitudes of family, others
Security	Financial, social status
	Dependency status
	Death of spouse, friends
	Attitudes of family, others
Needs related to terminal illness	Death of spouse, friends
	Inevitability of own death

There are also other adjustments associated with the middle years. Often, an individual finds himself, at this stage, caught in the middle of three generations. While coping with the problems of teen-aged children and adjusting to their eventual independence, the individual is often faced with the realization that his own parents are getting old. They may now need his help and support with their physical, emotional, or financial problems.

In spite of the many changes and adjustments one experiences, the late middle years are often referred to as the "prime of life." It can be a time of general good health and relative stability, when the individual attains the goals he has set for himself. This is often the most productive period in a person's life. Through his various life experiences, the individual has achieved a measure of self-assurance and will feel satisfied as he reaches the peak of his career and earning power and attains his most influential role in society. As the children grow up and leave home, many married couples find that they have more time to devote to leisure activities and more time for each other. Many women report having a renewed interest in and considerably more enjoyment from sex at this time of their lives than at any other.

THE LATER YEARS (Age 65 Plus)

The final stage in an individual's development has been called the "golden age." It is a time when the individual no longer has to strive to achieve—when he can relax and enjoy the fruits

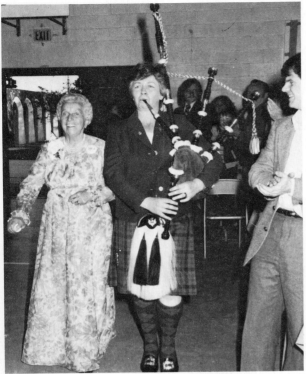

Mrs. Julia Hemphill being "piped in" to her 90th birthday party.

ical needs, then, assume a great deal of importance for people in their later years.

Protection and safety needs are also increased. There is a diminishing of sensory perception with aging, so that an individual is not so alert to danger. There is also a lessened physical ability to cope with it. The reflexes are not as fast as they were, for example, and coordination is not as good. Thus, the person's reaction to dangerous situations is slower and less effective. Combined with these changes is an increased fragility of the bones. This is due to a loss of cartilage (which in many parts of the body provides a cushion to protect bony structures) and, also, a loss of calcareous material from the bones. The elderly are, therefore, more likely to suffer a fracture when they fall than a younger person would. Healing is also slower, largely because circulation is not as efficient, and the elderly do not bounce back from an illness as rapidly as younger adults do.

In the psychosocial realm, the later years are marked by many lifestyle changes. Retirement, for men especially, involves a major adjustment. Most companies in the United States and Canada require that their employees retire by age 70. Even though it is expected, many people find retirement a traumatic experience. Often, it means a reduced income, a loss of self-esteem (one no longer feels useful) and diminished social status. (Ours is, unfortunately, not a culture in which old age is revered for its wisdom.) It may also mean dependence on one's family or others, or on the state for financial, physical, or emotional assistance. Increasingly, however, companies are helping their employees to prepare for retirement. Those who have prepared for their withdrawal from the work force can find it a very rewarding period. In an article on "Pre-Retirement Counseling," Diekelman has suggested that there are six areas an individual should consider as he plans for his later years: income, activities, living arrangements, role change, health, and legal matters.[7]

Income affects many aspects of a person's life—the food he eats, the activities in which he participates, and his self-esteem, to name a few. Most people contribute to pension or retirement plans during their working years in order to supplement the state-provided pension. In most communities in the United States and Canada, senior citizens also benefit from a number of financial concessions such as reduced fares for bus, train, and ferry transportation, special rates for admission to movies, concerts, sports events, and other entertainment, and reduced tuition fees at colleges and universities. Often, tuition fees are waived completely for senior citizens.

of his labor. In the United States and in Canada, we believe that the state has a responsibility to care for its older people, who have already made their contribution to society. Through our social security program, older people are assured of an income sufficient to meet their basic needs, at least minimally (although the size of the check always seems to lag behind the increases in inflation). Senior citizens are also provided with health care, largely at government expense.

The latter is important because a person's health typically diminishes as he gets older. This is characterized by a general decline in the functioning of all body systems. The body, in this respect, is rather like a motor that begins to show the effects of long usage. Various body parts start to wear out (luckily, an increasing number of them can be replaced these days) and the different systems are unable to tolerate the wear and tear they did when a person was younger. An individual may have to be a little more selective in the food he eats, for example, or pay the penalty of indigestion. Like a vintage model car, the older person's body needs gentle handling, and preventive maintenance to ensure that all systems are kept functioning as well as possible, for as long as possible. The physiolog-

Financial considerations such as these help people to stretch a fixed income and also enable them to participate in a great many activities they would otherwise not be able to afford. The secret of a happy old age, according to many in that age bracket, is to keep active, and certainly there is no dearth of activities for people over 65 these days.

Living arrangements are also an important consideration for older people. It is important that they can retain their independence as long as they are physically capable of doing so. An increasing number of services are helping people to remain in their own homes, such as "meals on wheels," homemaker services, "good neighbor" programs, and the like. In New Zealand, even laundry services are provided for older people who find this job too much of a chore. Inevitably, however, the stairs become too much to climb, the house becomes too much to keep up, or illness strikes, and the older person is no longer able to manage alone. Many people, at this stage, decide to go into a smaller house or an apartment, or they may move in with relatives. A wide variety of alternative housing arrangements for senior citizens have developed in recent years, including the very expensive, privately developed "retirement communities" complete with golf course, swimming pool, and

other amenities, the publicly financed low-rent apartment complexes, the housing projects sponsored by church groups and service clubs, and boarding and personal care homes both private and state-run. Regardless of the type of accommodation, however, the move is always a difficult one for the older individual. It is less painful if the individual can retain an essence of privacy and if steps are taken to ensure that he is always treated with dignity and respect.

One of the major adjustments for the older person is the reversal of roles that takes place with one's children, as the individual becomes more dependent on them. Another role change that many elderly must face is that of being widowed. The sense of loss experienced by an elderly person at the death of a spouse is often overwhelming. Although the support of family and friends can be a great comfort, the surviving spouse may never recover from his despair. Many who have become widowed do, however, recover and remarry, and indeed weddings in senior citizen communities are becoming quite common.

As a person ages, he must accept not only the death of those close to him, but his own death as well. In preparation for this eventuality, many individuals make out a will (see Chapter 7). Often, the older person is able to discuss the

Many elderly people who cannot look after themselves are in extended care facilities. Here, the residents are celebrating the birthday of an elderly lady.

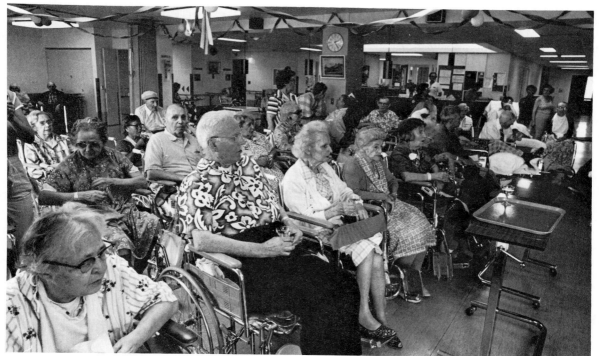

disposal of his worldly assets with relative equanimity, but his family become upset at the thought of the parent's death. Many older individuals like to have a "squaring up" of their accounts—to get all their affairs in order. Often, too, there is a renewed interest in religion as one gets older. The individual's spiritual counselor can usually provide much solace and support. Counseling in matters related to death and dying has been developed in recent years largely as a result of work done by Elisabeth Kübler-Ross in this field. This matter will be further discussed in Chapter 30. As science continues to extend the time we mortals spend on this earth, we are becoming wiser about how to enrich the later years. In your clinical experiences on the medical-surgical wards of acute care hospitals, in nursing homes and extended care units, and in your work in community agencies, you will undoubtedly meet many 90-year-olds and even 100-year-olds. If you take the time to talk with some of your older patients, you will find that a rapidly growing number of people continue to lead full, active, and interesting lives long after the traditional retirement age of 65 years.

SUGGESTED READINGS

Bee, H.: *The Developing Child.* 2nd Edition. New York, Harper and Row, 1978.

Bower, T. G. R.: *A Primer of Infant Development.* San Francisco, Freeman, 1977.

Bromley, D.: *The Psychology of Human Ageing.* Baltimore, Penguin, 1975.

Butler, R. N.: *Why Survive?* New York, Harper and Row, 1975.

Caplan, F.: *The First Twelve Months of Life.* New York, Grosset and Dunlap, 1973.

Caplan, F., and Caplan, T.: *The Second Twelve Months of Life.* New York, Grosset and Dunlap, 1977.

Combs, K. L.: Preventive Care in the Elderly. *American Journal of Nursing,* 78(8):1339–1341, August, 1978.

Diekelmann, N.: Staying Well While Growing Old. Pre-retirement Counseling. Part 2. *American Journal of Nursing,* 78:(8):1337–1338, August, 1978.

Diekelmann, N.: The Young Adult. The Choice is Health or Illness. *American Journal of Nursing,* 76(8):1272–1277, August, 1976.

Dresen, S. E.: Autonomy: A Continuing Developmental Task. *American Journal of Nursing,* 78(8):1344–1346, August, 1978.

Flanagan, G. L.: *The First Nine Months of Life.* New York, Simon and Schuster, 1962.

Green, M.: Adolescent Health Care. *Children Today,* 8:8–11, September-October, 1979.

Hogstel, M. O.: How Do the Elderly View Their World? *American Journal of Nursing,* 78(8):1335–1336, August, 1978.

Hunt, B., and Hunt, J.: *Prime Time.* New York, Stein and Day, 1974.

Inhelder, B., and Piaget, J.: *The Growth of Logical Thinking from Childhood to Adolescence.* New York, Basic Books, 1958.

Klaus, M. H., and Kennell, J. H.: *Maternal-Infant Bonding.* St. Louis, C. V. Mosby Company, 1976.

Kohen-Ruz, R.: *The Child from 9–13.* London, Aldine-Atherton, 1971.

Lantz, J.: Aging: Birth of an Individual. *Journal of Gerontological Nursing,* 3(4):32-36, July-August, 1977.

LeShan, E.: *The Wonderful Crisis of Middle Age.* New York, Warner, 1973.

Lipsitz, J. S.: Adolescent Development. *Children Today,* 8:2–7, September-October, 1979.

Munsinger, H.: *Fundamentals of Child Development.* 2nd ed. New York, Holt, Rinehart and Winston, 1975.

Papalia, D. E., and Olds, S. W.: *Human Development.* New York, McGraw-Hill Book Company, 1978.

Quinn, J. L., and Ryan, N. E.: Assessment of the Older Adult: A "Holistic" Approach. *Journal of Gerontological Nursing,* 5(2):13–18, March-April, 1979.

Seidl, A. H., and Altshuler, A.: Interventions for Adolescents Who Are Chronically Ill. *Children Today,* 8:16–19, November-December, 1979.

Sheehy, G.: *Passages, Predictable Crises of Adult Life.* New York, Dutton, 1976.

Smith, D. W., Bierman, E. L., and Robinson, N. M., (eds.): *The Biologic Ages of Man.* 2nd ed. Philadelphia, W. B. Saunders Company, 1978.

Tichy, A. M., and Malasanos, L. J.: Physiological Parameters of Aging, Part II. *Journal of Gerontological Nursing,* 5(2):38–41, March-April, 1979.

Troll, L. E.: *Early and Middle Adulthood: The Best Is Yet to Be—Maybe.* Monterey, Cal., Brooks/Cole, 1975.

White, B. L.: *The First Three Years of Life.* Englewood Cliffs, N. J., Prentice-Hall, 1976.

Wuerger, M. K., The Young Adult. Stepping into Parenthood. *American Journal of Nursing,* 76:(8):1283–1285, August, 1976.

REFERENCES

1. Bourne, L. E., Jr., and Ekstrand, B. R.: *Psychology: Its Principles and Meanings.* 3rd ed. New York, Holt, Rinehart and Winston, 1979.

2. Kalish, R. A.: *The Psychology of Human Behavior.* Belmont, California, Wadsworth Publishing Company, 1966.

3. Munsinger, H.: *Fundamentals of Child Development*. 2nd ed. New York, Holt, Rinehart and Winston, 1975.
4. Sheehy, G.: *Passages. Predictable Crises of Adult Life*. New York, Dutton, 1976.
5. Smith, D. W., Bierman, E. L., and Robinson, N. M. (eds.): *The Biologic Ages of Man*. 2nd ed. Philadelphia, W. B. Saunders Company, 1978.
6. Papalia, D. E., and Olds, S. W.: *Human Development*. New York, McGraw-Hill, 1978.
7. Diekelmann, N.: Staying Well While Getting Old. Pre-retirement Counseling. Part 2. *American Journal of Nursing*, 78(8):1337–1338, August, 1978.

14

The Nurse Should Be Able to:

- Discuss the role of food in meeting basic human needs
- Outline nutrient and energy requirements in health
- Discuss variations in nutritional needs throughout the life cycle
- Identify factors affecting the nutritional status of an individual
- Assess his nutritional status
- Identify common nutritional problems
- Identify situations requiring immediate intervention in the care of patients with nutritional problems
- Apply relevant principles in planning and implementing nursing interventions in patients
  a. to promote optimal nutritional status
  b. to prevent potential nutritional problems
  c. to restore optimal nutritional status in patients with nutritional problems
- Evaluate the effectiveness of nursing intervention

NUTRITIONAL NEEDS

CHAPTER 14

INTRODUCTION

Food and the partaking of meals have a significance in human society that goes far beyond the provision of nourishment for the body. In addition to fulfilling a basic physiological need, food may also help to satisfy one or more of an individual's many other needs. It has long been recognized, for example, that food is closely related to feelings of security. This is not merely the presence or absence of food in sufficient quantity to satisfy hunger, but the availability of specific foods. For many people, milk is a basic security food; for others, it may be meat, potatoes, rice, or some other familiar food that helps most to foster feelings of security. When a person is ill, it is sometimes necessary to deprive him of certain foods. If any of these foods hold strong security meanings for him, it is understandable that the individual may feel threatened by its absence from his diet.

Food is often used to promote a feeling of social acceptance. Sitting down to eat with another person, even if the food that is taken is simply a cup of coffee, conveys to the person that you consider him your equal. Offering someone a cup of tea or coffee, our "ritual of hospitality," can do much to foster an atmosphere of warmth and friendliness that is often difficult to attain in other ways. In some hospitals, nurses use a "coffee-get-together" with new mothers to provide a relaxed and informal setting in which to teach about the care of their infants.

Then, too, some foods are used for their prestige value, to enhance feelings of self-esteem. In many cultures, bread is a prestige food. For many years, steak and roast beef were considered prestige foods in North America. Now that the world has become a "global village," however, and we have been introduced to the delights of cooking from other countries, we tend to want our steak in the form of "Chateaubriand," and our fowl as "duck à l'orange" or "Tandouri" chicken. Steak or roast beef may no longer be the most expensive item on the menu. It may be flying fish imported from Barbados, or Arctic char from Alaska or Northern Canada. Food may also be used to express creativity. Many women and men enjoy using their creative talents to prepare gourmet meals to please their families and friends.

The partaking of food in one form or another plays an important role in many religious ceremonies. One has only to think of the Christian ceremony of Communion to be aware of the significance of food in this regard. At Communion, one partakes of bread, which symbolizes the flesh of Christ, and of wine, which symbolizes His blood. In some religions, as for example in Judaism and in Islam, the preparation of food is in itself a ritual. There are also many food taboos associated with specific doctrines of other religions. The devout Muslim will not eat pork, for example, nor the Hindu, beef.

Food is, in fact, interwined with the traditions, superstitions, and prejudices of virtually every culture. The Easter ham in our country and the Devali* gift of sweets in India are but two examples of the incorporation of food into traditional customs. To spill salt is considered by many people to be bad luck—a common example of a superstition involving food. Most of us have prejudices against certain foods; yet these foods may be eaten with great enjoyment by others. Few North Americans would have eaten snails 15 years ago; today they are often included

---

*Devali, the "Festival of Lights," is a major religious festival in India.

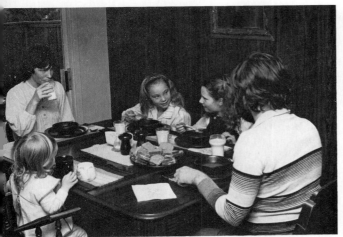

Being together for meals can help to strengthen family ties.

on the appetizer list in expensive restaurants. The fruit bat is considered a delicacy in Guam, but few "state-side" Americans relish it.

Mealtime, in most parts of the world, is a significant aspect of family life. In many cultures, eating is considered a private affair, to be shared and enjoyed only with one's family or intimate friends. Meals often play an important role in reaffirming solidarity within the family group. In most North American homes, the mother likes to have all members of the family present for the evening meal. The traditional gathering of a family for Thanksgiving or Christmas dinner serves to strengthen ties within the extended family unit. Meals, too, may provide a time when family roles are defined and clarified, as when father (or mother, in many single parent families) sits at the head of the table, a tangible symbol of the role as head of the family.

In our culture, we usually like to think of mealtime as a pleasant time—a period of relaxation, when we can enjoy the company of others and engage in social conversation. Health agencies today are doing much to make mealtimes more pleasant for patients. Food is arranged attractively on trays; there is usually a menu from which the patient may select the foods that he likes; and many hospitals now have small dining areas next to the nursing units, where patients who are able may gather to eat their meals.

As well as having psychological, social, and cultural significance in our daily lives, food is vitally important to our physical well-being. Because all cells in the body require adequate nourishment for optimal functioning, all systems of the body may be affected by nutritional problems. The synergism between poor nutritional status and infections was discussed in Chapter 4. The direct effect of malnutrition on brain tissue is currently receiving considerable study. Listlessness and poor concentration resulting in poor performance in school children are frequently linked to poor nutrition. Some researchers believe that hyperactive children are helped by alterations in diet.

Many skin and gastrointestinal problems are directly attributable to poor dietary habits. Nutrition is certainly a factor in a person's strength and endurance, as athletes prove.

Nutrition is so vital to all aspects of health that nurses should be well versed in helping people to develop and maintain good dietary habits.

NUTRITIONAL NEEDS IN HEALTH

A person cannot exist for long without taking some form of nourishment. Food is the fuel with which we run our human bodies. It is necessary for the growth and maintenance of bones and other tissues, and for the regulation of all body processes. In order for a person to function at his optimal level, he must consume adequate amounts of foods containing the nutrients essential to human life. A nutrient is defined as any chemical substance found in foods that functions in one or more of the three ways mentioned above. The amount that is adequate varies from one individual to another, depending on age, sex, current physical status, lifestyle, physical environment, and many other factors. The essential nutrients are carbohydrates, proteins, fats, vitamins, minerals, and water.

Essential Nutrients

Carbohydrates. *Carbohydrates* are composed of carbon, hydrogen, and oxygen and are used by the body primarily as a source of energy. They are the most common nutrients in the majority of diets because of their availability. Carbohydrates are found in most plants and fruit sugars, and in natural starches. The cellulose in plants is an important ingredient for digestion. Excess carbohydrates consumed are stored in the liver in the form of glycogen or changed into fat.

Fats. *Fats* are also composed of carbon, hydrogen, and oxygen, but in different ratios than in carbohydrates. They are also primarily a source of energy to the body, and because they contain less oxygen, they release their energy more quickly and in greater quantity than do carbohydrates. Fats are found in nature in animals and in plant seeds. The most common sources of fats in our diets are butter, margarine, nuts, eggs, and oils used for cooking and in salad dressings (for example, corn, peanut, olive, and soybean oils). It is thought that the saturated fats (e.g., butter, meat fats) are a contributing factor in high blood pressure, arteriosclerosis, and other circulatory diseases.

Proteins. Like carbohydrates and fats, proteins are composed of carbon, hydrogen, and oxygen, but with the added element of nitrogen. Most proteins also contain sulfur and some contain other minerals as well. The primary functions of proteins in the human body are the release of energy and the building and repair of body tissues. Protein is found in nature in animals and plants. The most common sources in our diets are dairy products, meat, fish, eggs, legumes (such as peas and beans), nuts, and seeds.

Vitamins

Vitamins are a natural component of most foods. They are necessary for the growth, maintenance, and repair of body tissues and for the regulation of body processes. Since the body is unable to manufacture vitamins, they must be obtained from foods we eat. Vitamins are designated as A, B, C, D, E, and K and are classified into two main groups, the fat-soluble and water-soluble vitamins.

The fat-soluble vitamins (A, D, E, and K) are transported throughout the body in fats.

● Vitamin A, often considered the most important vitamin, is essential for growth and maintenance of tissues, for proper development of bones and teeth, and for good vision. It is found in yellow and green fruits and vegetables, egg yolk, butterfat, and liver.

Vitamin D promotes the growth of teeth and bones. Called the "sunshine vitamin," it is most commonly obtained through sunlight and in enriched foods. Other sources of vitamin D are fish liver oils, egg yolk, and butterfat. Many foods on the market today are "fortified" by the addition of vitamin D, as, for example D–fortified milk, infant formula preparations, and margarines.

Vitamin E is important for normal creatine excretion and for the prevention of blood disorders. Taking large quantities of this vitamin has become something of a fad—it is thought by some to enhance sexual powers, prevent tissue scarring, and increase sensory perception, among other things. However, these claims are not clinically proven. An excellent source of Vitamin E is wheat germ oil; other common dietary sources are whole grains, salad and cooking oils, liver, and fruits and vegetables.

Vitamin K is necessary for blood coagulation. It can be found in liver, egg yolk, green leafy vegetables, and soybean oil.

The water-soluble vitamins (the B complex and C) use water as their vehicle. For this reason, foods containing these vitamins are most effective when eaten raw, since cooking tends to remove the vitamins.

Particularly important for the formation and maintenance of healthy blood are pyridoxine (vitamin B_6), vitamin B_{12}, and folic acid. The vitamins thiamine (vitamin B_1), riboflavin (vitamin B_2), and niacin are especially needed for normal growth and development and a healthy nervous system and, together with vitamin B_6 and pantothenic acid, for promoting and maintaining a healthy appetite and good digestion.

Vitamin C is essential for the building and maintenance of teeth, bones and joints, muscles, gums, and connective tissues. It also functions to protect the body from infection and promotes wound healing. Common sources of vitamin C are citrus fruits, tomatoes, and green leafy vegetables.

Minerals. Minerals are necessary to the body in the building and maintenance of bones, teeth, and the various body systems. The main essential minerals are considered to be calcium, iron, phosphorus, and magnesium. Other minerals, called trace minerals, are equally essential, but are needed in much smaller amounts. Some of these other minerals required by the body are copper, iodine, manganese, zinc, and fluorine.

Calcium is important for the proper formation of teeth and bones, for muscle tone and nerve transmissions, and for the coagulation of blood. The main sources of calcium in most diets are milk and other dairy products, but calcium is also found in dark green leafy vegetables, eggs, meat, and cereals.

Phosphorus aids in the formation and strengthening of bones. It can be obtained from dairy products, meat, fish, poultry, nuts, whole grains, and legumes.

Magnesium is an important factor in regulation of the body's temperature, nerve conduction, and muscle contractions. Commonly dietary sources of magnesium are green leafy vegetables, nuts, whole grains, and beans.

Iron is important for building hemoglobin in red blood cells, and preventing nutritional anemia. The best sources are liver, red meats, and egg yolk, but it is also found in lentils, green leafy vegetables, whole grain and enriched cereals, flours, bread and pastas.

Water. Water is the single most important nutrient in the human body. It is a component of most foods, both liquid and solid. Water is a vehicle of absorption for most nutrients in the body and is present in all body excretions and secretions. Approximately 60 to 70 per cent of the adult body is composed of water. Because water is so important in the regulation and maintenance of all body tissues and processes, it will be discussed in more detail in Chapter 17.

Energy Requirements

Dietary requirements are generally considered in terms of both specific nutrients and energy requirements. The body's needs for energy are usually expressed in calories (a term taken from the physical sciences), which measure heat units. A *calorie* is the amount of heat required to raise the temperature of one gram of water by one degree Celsius. The calorie used in nutrition is often written as kcal (for kilocalorie) to indicate that it represents 1000 of the calories used in the physical sciences.

The body's requirements for energy vary considerably from one individual to another, depending principally on age, sex, body frame, amount and kind of daily activity, and the secretions of endocrine glands.

Basal Metabolic Rate.   In discussing energy requirements, it is helpful to start with the *basal metabolic rate*, which represents the energy requirements of the body at rest—the amount required for the internal work of the body. A person's basal metabolic rate is influenced by body size, age, sex, and the secretions of endocrine glands, principally the thyroid gland. It is higher in children and adolescents than in adults, the normal pattern showing an increase during the first few months of life, followed by a fairly rapid initial, then gradual, decrease through childhood and adolescence, with a still slower decline with advancing age in adults.

The Effect of Activity.   To the basal metabolic requirements are added the energy needs to carry out our daily activities. It is primarily the work of body muscles that demands the energy. Mental activity consumes very little, because the brain is always active in any case and is therefore accounted for in the basal metabolic rate. Since it is muscular work that creates the need for additional energy, over and above the basal metabolic needs, it stands to reason that the heavier the workload, the more energy is required (and, hence, the more caloric intake is needed).

A great deal of research has been done, both to estimate the number of calories expended in the course of different activities and to work out average energy expenditures of people in different age groups.

Common activities in which people engage have been categorized into levels according to the amount of energy expended in carrying them out. A commonly used categorization includes five levels:[1]

1. Maintenance activities: sitting most of the day, with about 2 hours of moving or standing
2. Light activity: typing, teaching, shop work, laboratory work, some walking but no strenuous exercise
3. Moderate activity: walking, housework, gardening, carpentry, light industry, little sitting
4. Strenuous activity: unskilled labor, forestry work, skating, outdoor games, dancing; little sitting
5. Very strenuous activity: tennis, swimming, basketball, football, running, lumbering; little sitting

People whose work involves sitting most of the day and who do not engage in additional exercise require approximately 1.5 times their basal metabolic needs. Housewives, carpenters, and those others whose work is considered moderate activity, expend energy at 1.6 times their basal rate. Those engaged in strenuous activity, such as construction workers, use 1.7 times the energy they would at rest. Football players, lumberjacks, and others whose occupations are in the very strenuous activity category expend energy at twice their basal rate.

One has to realize that these are only approximations. The vigor with which a person works and the amount of time per day he spends at the activities vary considerably from one individual to another. You would not expend as much energy in dancing a slow waltz, for example, as a fast square dance. You might play a leisurely game of tennis for an hour two or three times a week, but your energy expenditures per hour would not be as great as the professional who puts full effort into every point. There is also a wide variety of energy expenditure involved in the specific jobs that might be found in any given line of work. A person living alone in a small apartment usually would not expend as much energy in housework as one who has to clean an eight-room house and cook for a large family. A cabinet maker whose work involves small detail would not expend as much energy as a carpenter building houses.

The Effect of Climate.   Contrary to popular belief, the body's nutrient and energy requirements do not vary considerably with changes in climate. There may, however, be a small amount of additional energy expenditure by people who live and work in cold climates. Certainly, a person feels hungrier in the cold, brisk air of autumn than in the hot, humid days of summer.

ENERGY EXPENDITURE BY A 150-POUND PERSON IN VARIOUS ACTIVITIES

Type of Activity	Kilocalories per Hour
Rest and light activity	50–200
Lying down or sleeping	80
Driving an automobile	120
Standing	140
Moderate activity	200–350
Walking (2½ mph)	210
Gardening	220
Bowling	270
Swimming (¼ mph)	300
Walking (3¾ mph)	300
Vigorous activity	over 350
Chopping or sawing wood	400
Tennis	420
Squash and handball	600
Cycling (13 mph)	660
Running (10 mph)	900

Adapted from *Exercise and Weight Control*, Committee on Exercise and Physical Fitness of the American Medical Association and the President's Council on Physical Fitness in cooperation with the Lifetime Sports Foundation. Prepared by Robert E. Johnson, M.D., Ph.D., and colleagues, Department of Physiology and Biophysics, University of Illinois, August, 1967.

Additional needs are possibly 2 to 5 per cent. The bulky, heavy clothing required for outdoor wear impedes movement and this increases the amount of energy used in moving. The muscular action of shivering also increases a person's energy needs. Shivering can usually be prevented by adequate clothing and exercise. If the body is chilled, additional energy is needed to rewarm it. Hence, the ravenous need for hot nourishing food when you come in out of the cold. (The energy you have probably expended in walking briskly or skating or skiing has something to do with it, too.)

People who work at physical labor in environments where the temperature is above 30° C (86° F) have additional energy requirements and require more energy-giving foods to offset the effects of increased metabolism and lessened mechanical efficiency. The body's metabolism is speeded up with higher temperatures, and more energy is required. There is also a lessening of mechanical efficiency and there may be a loss of fluids and electrolytes from sweating (see Chapter 17). People who live in hot climates (tropical or subtropical climates) usually find that it is a lot of work just to move about in very hot weather. They curtail their physical activities, which effectively cuts down on their energy requirements. The languor associated with South Sea Islands, then, has a physiological basis.

Recommended Daily Food Guides

Recommended daily requirements of specific nutrients have been established both in the United States and in Canada (and in many other countries). International standards have been issued by the United Nations Food and Agriculture Organization and the World Health Organization (FAO/WHO). Food guides have also been developed to help people to select foods that will ensure that they have an adequate supply of essential nutrients in their daily diets.

The Guide To Good Eating, developed by the United States Department of Agriculture, and Canada's Food Guide, issued by the Department of National Health and Welfare, are shown on pages 264–265. Both guides recommend specified amounts to be included in a daily diet from each of four basic food groups: (1) milk (and milk products), (2) meat (and alternates), (3) vegetables and fruits, and (4) breads and cereals. The two guides list essentially the same foods, and the recommended amounts are similar with minor variations. Both provide the foundation for a good diet. A practical guide to food selection, based on the U.S. and Canadian guides, is shown on page 266. You will note that it shows the average percentage contribution of the different food groups to nutrient requirements in North American diets, as well as some practical suggestions in applying the food guides.

NUTRITIONAL NEEDS THROUGHOUT THE LIFE CYCLE

Major factors affecting nutritional needs throughout the life cycle were included in the discussion of needs requiring particular attention at each stage of the life cycle in Chapter 13. At this point, we are going to enlarge on these to discuss how changes in growth and development affect specific requirements in each age group.

The Pregnant Woman and the Fetus

The developing fetus receives its nourishment from the mother, in whose body the fertilized ovum is implanted. The fetus is supplied on a priority basis before the mother; in cases of severe malnutrition, both will suffer. Malnutrition, especially from the second trimester on, may cause fetal abnormalities and impair brain development. Some of the more common nutritional problems that affect the growing fetus are insufficient intake of calcium on the mother's part, insufficient intake of protein, and insuffi-

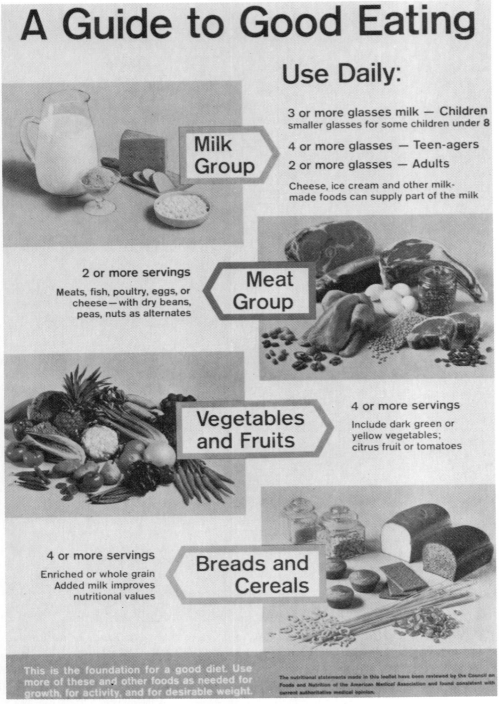

A Guide to Good Eating

Use Daily:

Milk Group

3 or more glasses milk — Children
smaller glasses for some children under 8

4 or more glasses — Teen-agers

2 or more glasses — Adults

Cheese, ice cream and other milk-made foods can supply part of the milk

Meat Group

2 or more servings

Meats, fish, poultry, eggs, or cheese — with dry beans, peas, nuts as alternates

Vegetables and Fruits

4 or more servings

Include dark green or yellow vegetables; citrus fruit or tomatoes

Breads and Cereals

4 or more servings

Enriched or whole grain Added milk improves nutritional values

This is the foundation for a good diet. Use more of these and other foods as needed for growth, for activity, and for desirable weight.

The nutritional statements made in this leaflet have been reviewed by the Council on Foods and Nutrition of the American Medical Association and found consistent with current authoritative medical opinion.

(Courtesy of National Dairy Council, Chicago.)

cient intake of calories. An insufficient intake of calcium will impair ossification (formation of bones and teeth), and will decalcify the mother's teeth as the needed mineral is drawn from the mother's existing supplies. If the expectant mother does not have a sufficient quantity of protein in her diet, the rate of physiological growth of the fetus is impaired. It is generally believed that if the pregnant woman's intake of calories is insufficient, the fetus (and newborn infant) are less resistant to disease.

Numerous studies have shown that the quality

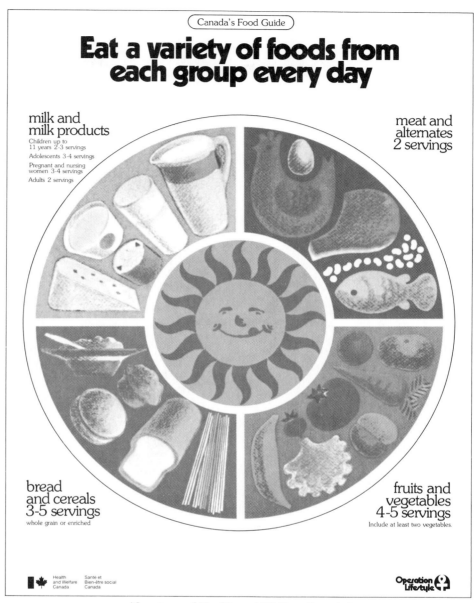

(Courtesy of Health and Welfare Canada.)

of the expectant mother's diet is a very important factor in the healthy mother and baby both before and after delivery. Women in these studies who had a good diet had fewer complications at delivery and fewer miscarriages, stillbirths, or premature deliveries than mothers with poor diets.

During the first few months of pregnancy nausea and early morning vomiting, which are believed to be due to hormonal changes, may interfere with an adequate intake of food. If these persist into the second trimester, they can be serious problems. During pregnancy it is felt that nutrient requirements for calcium are increased by 50 per cent and for most other nutrients by 20 per cent. The expectant mother should have approximately 32 fluid ounces of milk (or the equivalent in alternate foods) daily, and should also have three servings of meat or its alternates daily. The pregnant woman should include a good supply of fruits and vegetables in her diet. Her caloric needs are increased, although the additional allowances suggested by various experts are not large, ranging from 200 to 700 calories per day.

Common nutritional problems of pregnancy include deficiencies of specific nutrients, particularly calcium, protein, and vitamins A, B_6, B_{12},

PRACTICAL GUIDE TO FOOD SELECTION

Food Group	Recommendations United States	Canada	Practical Hints	Average percentage contribution of food groups to nutrient requirements on North American Diets*
Milk and Milk Products				
Children up to about 11 years	3 glasses	2–3 glasses (20 fl. oz.)	For variety substitute the following for ½ cup of milk: ¾ cup ice cream; ½ cup milk pudding; ½ cup cottage cheese 4 oz. yogurt; ¾ oz. cheddar cheese (1 in. cu. = ¾ oz); 1 oz. processed cheese; 1 serving of cream soup made with milk	76% of calcium 41% of riboflavin 24% of protein 12% of vitamin A
Adolescents	4 or more glasses	4 glasses (32 fl. oz.)		
Adults	2 or more glasses	2 glasses (12 fl. oz.)		
Expectant and nursing mothers	4 glasses	3–4 glasses (32 fl. oz.)		
Fruits and Vegetables				
Fruit to include source of vitamin C, such as oranges, tomatoes, vitaminized apple juice	4 or more servings	4–5 servings	1 serving of fruit could be: 1 orange, apple, or banana; ½ grapefruit; ½ cup canned fruit; ½ cup fruit juices; 4 stewed prunes	94% of vitamin C 54% of vitamin A 19% of iron 20% of thiamin 17% of niacin (applies to both fruits and vegetables)
Vegetables to include dark green or yellow vegetables, often raw			1 serving of vegetables could be 1 potato; ½ cup tomato juice: ½ cup of canned or frozen vegetables, peas, green beans, etc.; 1 serving of vegetable soup	
Meat and Alternates				
Meat, fish, poultry, eggs, or cheese—with dried beans, peas, nuts, and seeds as alternates	2 or more	2 servings	3 oz. of boneless cooked meat, fish, or poultry constitute 1 serving. The following can be substituted for 1 oz. of meat: 2 tbsp. peanut butter; ½ cup baked beans; 1 egg	40% of niacin 41% of protein 30% of iron 24% of thiamin 22% of riboflavin 18% of vitamin A
	(extra serving for expectant mothers)			
Breads and Cereals				
Enriched whole grain (added milk improves the nutritional value)	4 or more	3–5 servings	The following are substitutes for 1 slice of bread (whole wheat, white enriched, rye, etc): ¾ cup of oatmeal, cooked; 1 cup ready-to-eat enriched cereal; ¾ cup macaroni, spaghetti, noodles, cooked (enriched); ½ cup rice, cooked	40% of thiamin 32% of iron 25% of niacin 21% of protein 20% of riboflavin
Vitamin D				
	400 international units (I.U.) for all growing persons up to 22 years, including breast-fed babies, expectant and nursing mothers		400 I.U. in 30 fl. oz. of enriched milk or 4 tbsp. of fortified margarine. If enriched milk not available use vitamin D supplements	

*Based on Statistics Canada data.
Adapted from *Selected Nutrition Teaching Aids*. Ottawa, Department of National Health and Welfare, 1976.

C, D, and E. Many experts feel there is a link between protein deficiency and toxemia of pregnancy. Other problems affecting an adequate nutritional intake include nausea and vomiting (as noted above) and dyspepsia. We will be discussing these problems in more detail later in the chapter. Most pregnant women find it is easier to tolerate small, frequent meals rather than three large ones. Regarding the food cravings reported by many women during pregnancy, there is still no definite answer to whether these indicate a real physiological need or are prompted by cultural or psychological influences.

The Nursing Mother and the Infant

The woman who is breast feeding her infant has higher requirements for most nutrients than the expectant mother, including those for energy, proteins, minerals, and vitamins. These are needed to cover the demands made on the mother's body for the production of the milk as well as the nutrients secreted in the milk that provides nourishment to the infant. Energy requirements are estimated to be between 600 and 900 calories a day higher than for those of pregnant women, with the addition of 1000 calories over that for nonpregnant women recommended for the lactating mother. The need for additional nutrients increases as the infant grows and demands more nourishment.

The diet recommended for lactating mothers is essentially the same as for pregnant women and should include plentiful supplies of milk and alternate calcium and protein sources. The nursing mother needs a lot of fluids to provide for the water content of breast milk (2 to 3 quarts are suggested).

A common problem in nursing mothers is a deficiency of calcium and phosphorus, due to the high content of these minerals in the milk secreted. Because of the higher requirements, existing nutritional problems the mother may have had are likely to become more severe. This is not the time for the mother to go on a reducing diet. Her weight will normally stabilize without extra dieting. As most nursing mothers soon become aware, what they eat and drink affects the infant they are nourishing. It is recommended that they avoid highly spiced foods, alcohol, and artificial sweeteners. Drugs should be taken only on the recommendation of the physician, including those commonly sold over the counter in drug stores, such as laxatives, aspirin, and sedatives.

The normal newborn infant usually loses approximately 5 per cent of its birth weight during the first 2 to 3 days of life, owing to adjustments in total body water. With adequate nutrition (120 calories per kg. per day), the normal healthy infant should gain 20 to 25 grams per day during the first 4 months of life. Adequate nutrition during infancy is important to prevent permanent damage to the central nervous system, as well as to promote the optimal growth and development of other body tissues. The gastrointestinal tract of infants is relatively immature. Breast milk, which is the baby's natural food, provides the most easily digested source of nourishment. Breast milk is also the most complete food, needing only to be supplemented by vitamin D for the first few months. However, many babies have been raised to healthy adulthood on cow's milk, goat's milk, and formulas made from these or other substances (soybeans, for example). Many good formula preparations are available on the market. The formula used must be tailored to the needs of each individual infant.

Most nutrition experts now recommend that solid foods not be added to the infant's diet until he is 4 to 6 months of age. Until that time, the tongue projects, which makes swallowing food difficult. It is also believed that exposure to certain foods (especially those high in protein) in early infancy may lead to later allergies. Solids should be introduced gradually, with one new food at a time, in soft, or pureed form.

During the first year of life, the infant's rate of growth and development is quite remarkable. It slows down during the second year, however, and the mother may notice that the 1-year-old's appetite is not as great as it was. She should be reassured that the loss of appetite of the typical 1-year-old is normal. It is during the second year of life, too, that the child moves from breast or bottle feeding and soft food supplements, to drinking from a cup and eating table foods.

The Child

In the toddler and preschool years the child's physical and social skills related to eating develop rapidly. A summary of their skills from approximately 3 months to 6 years is shown on page 268. The child needs the same types of foods as the adult, with quantities adjusted to meet his smaller size. Because their independence is rapidly developing also, small children much prefer foods that they can manage themselves, usually foods that can be eaten with the fingers. Good eating habits can be established at this time, with a pattern of regular meals and a sufficient but not excessive intake of nutritious food.

Malnutrition in childhood results in growth failures and, as we have noted earlier, renders the child more susceptible to infections. In addition, iron-deficiency anemia can occur.

Excess intake of vitamins, particularly vitamins A and D, has become a common problem, presumably because many mothers mistakenly believe that their children can only benefit from consuming large amounts of vitamins. A good diet can provide the minerals and vitamins the child requires, although physicians and baby clinics often recommend supplements when the child is going through a growth spurt, when his appetite is poor during illness, or if certain foodstuffs are not eaten because the child does

DEVELOPMENT OF A CHILD'S PHYSICAL AND SOCIAL SKILLS

Age	Physical Skills	Social Skills
3–6 months	Tongue projects so swallowing food is difficult. Fingers foods.	
6–12 months	Uses hands. Uses tongue and lips when eating. Chewing movements start. Takes juice and water from cup but spills when cup is removed.	Perceives size, shape, weight, and texture. Reads facial expressions and gestures. Very demanding of person who feeds him.
12–18 months	Grasps and releases finger foods. Grasps spoon, inserts in dish but filling poor. Spoon often upside down when reaches mouth. Release of cup and spoon poor and drops frequently.	Demands everything in sight at table. Refuses milk from bottle. Loves an audience.
18 months–2 years	Drop in appetite. Uses both hands when feeding. Drinks well from cup but release still poor Tongue can lick off chin. Turns spoon in mouth.	Ritualistic. Refusals and preferences. Easily distracted.
2–3 years	Drinks with small glass held with one hand. Spoon is grasped between thumb and index finger and goes into mouth without turning. Considerable spilling.	Finicky and fussy eaters. Spotless eaters may demand to be fed. Messy eaters won't accept help. Food jags. Ritualistic. Dawdles. Demanding: — of *whole* foods; — of between-meal-snacks; — of candy if in home. Dislikes: — food mixtures; — vegetables. Food is the most important part of second birthday.
3–4 years	Holds cup by handle. Tilts head back to empty cup. Pours from pitchers. Uses fork. Little spilling. Little assistance needed. Chews more foods.	Conforming and assentive. Fair appetite: — milk intake increase; — vegetables are slowly accepted. Asks for favourite foods. Able to choose between two alternatives. Birthday cake is important part of third birthday party.
4–5 years	Use knife and fork. Tilts cup to empty it.	Assertive. Lively mind. Very social. Fair to very good appetite. Food jags or strikes. Reacts to incentives, e.g., "eating to be big." Sets table and cooks.
5–6 years	Able to feed himself.	Influenced by group and social pressures outside home. Still prefers plain foods.

From *Selected Nutrition Teaching Aids*. Ottawa, Department of National Health and Welfare, 1976.

not like them (or cannot tolerate them) or because some foods are not available or too expensive, as for example, fresh fruits and vegetables at certain times of the year.

The school-age child's rate of growth is slower than it was in infancy or will be again in adolescence. However, it is critically important that his nutritional needs be met to promote his optimal growth and development. A nutritious breakfast that includes a good source of protein is particularly important for the school-age child to ensure good work performance and good concentration in the late morning hours. Teachers of special education classes for children with emotional problems have found that the most troublesome youngsters were those who had come to school without eating breakfast.

School-age children are also developing their social skills and enjoy inviting another child home to share meals with them. At this age children also begin to enjoy experimenting with different food tastes and add to the variety of foods they will eat, although they still prefer plain foods and those they can eat with their fingers.

Among the common problems of childhood, iron deficiency is the most prevalent deficiency, and deficiencies in calcium and vitamins C and D are also problems in many children's diets. Socioeconomic factors play a large part in the dietary sufficiency of children, with those from higher income families generally having a more adequate intake of essential nutrients, and those with the least income and education having the most problems. Obesity is fairly common in all racial groups, and among rich and poor, during the pre-adolescent stage. It is often caused by poor eating habits such as eating too many non-nutritious snacks and overeating, particularly high carbohydrate foods. There is, however, some feeling now that one cannot rule out heredity as a factor in obesity.

The Adolescent

During adolescence, both boys and girls undergo growth spurts, and their nutritional needs are greatly increased. Again, they require the same essential nutrients as other people, with increased quantities of those particularly required for growth. They especially need larger quantities of the milk food group. Parents may be amazed at the amount of food teen-agers, especially boys, can consume and, if they are active, remain slim. Adolescents, as they begin to assert their independence from parental control, often begin to make decisions about the foods they will eat. Peer pressure is a very strong influence, and diet fads may be taken up by a group (or sometimes just by one adolescent) who may become vegetarian, or adopt a diet that contains only organically grown foodstuffs.

Obesity is a major health problem in this age group. Diabetes, the onset of which often coincides with puberty, becomes a major cause of death and disability in the United States from the age of 15 years onward. The relationship between obesity and diabetes is currently undergoing considerable study. Obese adolescents, as a general rule, tend to be less active physically than those of normal weight, and this seems to be especially true of girls.

Some adolescents, particularly girls, develop an obsession with being thin, and a condition known as anorexia nervosa (a loss of appetite due to emotional problems) has become a serious problem in this age group. It may be caused by other problems, such as anxiety or depression

(which may, or may not, be related to obesity). If unchecked, anorexia nervosa can lead to abnormal water and temperature regulation and deranged hormonal changes. (Whether the hormonal changes are cause or effect is currently under study.) If severe, the anorexia can lead to death, as the teen-ager literally starves herself to death.

Teen-age girls are particularly vulnerable to iron-deficiency anemia, as the monthly loss of blood begins to occur with puberty. Adolescents, both boys and girls, experience a rise in gastric acidity, which is felt to be caused by hormonal changes. They are also prone to abdominal pains of vague origin. It is not wise, however, to ascribe them always to "growing pains." Persistent or severe abdominal pain should always be investigated.

The Adult

Growth continues into the early years of young adulthood, although not at such a rapid rate as during adolescence. The young adult needs a good supply of proteins, minerals, and vitamins, although not in such large quantities as teen-agers. This is the age when good eating habits need to be strengthened to maintain health and to prevent illness in the future. Young adulthood is often a turning point, when the individual is setting up housekeeping away from parental influences. He is on his own, then, to make decisions regarding the foods he will eat or not eat, and to establish his own eating habits. Many young adults, because of pressures of work or other commitments, or just not bothering to make sure they eat properly, slip into poor dietary habits that will affect their future health. Good nutritional counseling is an important measure in helping young adults protect themselves against problems such as obesity, heart attacks, hypertension, and the like in their middle and later years.

Caloric needs usually decline, as does the need for extra supplies of protein when a person reaches full adulthood, but his vitamin and mineral requirements do not. A common nutritional problem in adults is obesity, which is considered to be the most prevalent health problem in North America. Anemia, due to inadequate intake of iron, is a common problem in women. Diabetes, which surfaces as a major killer in the adolescent years, is one of the leading causes of death in the United States in the 25- to 44-year-old group. The development of gallstones, believed to be due to excessive intake of cholesterol, is another common problem that affects both men and women. Anorexia nervosa continues to be a problem in young adulthood, particularly in women, although it is not as common a problem as in the teenage years.

During the middle years there is usually a gradual slowing down of activity, and the individual requires fewer calories than he did in his young adult days. Often, people tend to eat the same amounts, however, with the result that they put on weight, and obesity is a major problem. As a person gets older, there is a decrease in digestive enzymes, and heartburn (dyspepsia) is a common problem among middle-aged and older adults. If good oral hygiene has not been practiced, problems with teeth and gums may develop and lead to poor nutrition. Gallstones continue to be another major problem in older adults, as does diabetes. With the aging process, there is a loss of skeletal calcium (a condition known as osteoporosis), and a good intake of calcium and vitamins is required. Women are particularly prone to this problem after the menopause because of changes in hormonal secretions.

Older Adults

The nutritional needs of the elderly are the same as those of other adults, although they do require fewer calories, again, because of lessened activity. Their nutritional problems usually stem from a lack of adequate intake. Older adults often have deficiencies of proteins, vitamins, and minerals in their diet. Calcium (for the reason noted above) is particularly important. A lack of Vitamin D leads to a condition called osteomalacia (softening of the bones). Vitamin D–fortified milk and margarines help to combat this problem

● The failure of many older adults to eat an adequate diet may be due to a number of factors including a lack of money for food, out-of-date nutrition information, physical handicaps that make shopping or cooking difficult, feelings of loneliness, rejection, or apathy, and physical changes such as a loss of appetite, poorly fitting dentures, and troubles with constipation. Good nutrition counseling is very important. Older adults can be helped to get the most out of their dwindling food dollar, and to prepare nutritious meals simply. They should be encouraged to share meals with friends and to engage in activities that will stimulate the appetite, such as walking in the fresh air or mild exercise. The development of "Meals on Wheels" programs has been a boon for the housebound elderly and those who find preparing a substantial meal difficult. Volunteers who have participated in these programs often remark that the friendly visit of the person delivering the meal seems to mean as much to the individual as the food. It is sometimes difficult to get away and deliver the rest of the meals on time.

FACTORS AFFECTING NUTRITIONAL STATUS

A person's nutritional status reflects the balance that is maintained between the body's requirements for nutrients and energy and the actual intake of food. It depends, then, on three major factors: the requirements of the individual for nutrients and energy, his intake of food, and the efficiency of his bodily processes for absorbing, storing, utilizing, and excreting nutrients. We have already discussed nutrient and energy requirements in health throughout the life cycle, and we will be talking about nutritional needs of the sick later in the chapter, so let us now look at the other factors.

Intake

If a person eats more food than the body requires, or, conversely, he does not eat enough to meet his energy and nutritional requirements, problems develop. A number of factors—economic, physical, and psychosocial—affect food intake.

In Chapter Four, in discussing major health problems, we mentioned affluence as being a contributing factor in the widespread prevalence of overweight or obesity in North America. We also mentioned the serious poverty that exists in many countries, and in parts of our own, that prevents people from having sufficient food to meet their nutritional needs.

Among the physical factors affecting food intake, the condition of a person's teeth, gums, and the mucous membranes of the oral cavity are important factors for nurses to consider in assessing a patient's nutritional status. A person with no teeth or with poorly fitting dentures, or one whose mouth is in poor condition, has difficulty in biting or chewing food and will limit his intake to those foods he can handle easily. Other physical factors to be considered are the person's general state of health and specific health problems he may have. (These are discussed in more detail in subsequent sections.) There are also biological variations in the ability to tolerate certain foods. Many people have allergies to specific foods. Milk, chocolate, shellfish, and berries are some of the foods to which many people are allergic.

The need for milk and milk products to provide sources of protein and calcium is not the same for people in all racial groups. Adults in many racial and ethnic groups cannot tolerate milk. Research has indicated that the reason for this is the absence of the enzyme lactase (which digests the milk sugar, lactose). Without this enzyme, lactose in milk ferments in the gastro-intestinal tract, and the individual may complain of diarrhea, a bloated feeling and discomforts due to the formation of gas. It is felt that one reason for the deficiency may be the dropping of milk from the diet after childhood in many cultures. It has been estimated that between 50 and 75 per cent of blacks, Orientals, Hindus, Eskimos, and American Indians show lactose intolerance, as do approximately 10 to 25 per cent of adults of European descent. To improve nutrition for these people, sharp cheese (aged over 60 days), yogurt, and tofu (soy bean curd) may be used, since the lactose in these foods has been converted to lactic acid, which can be digested.[2]

One has to be careful in recommending beans as an alternate source of protein, too. One type of bean, the fava bean (broad or horse bean) can cause hemolytic anemia in persons who have a deficiency in glucose-6-phosphate dehydrogen-ase (G-6-PD), which is an important enzyme in the breakdown of glycogen in red blood cells. An absence of this constituent in the blood evolved in people who lived in malaria-infested areas as a protection against that disease. It is estimated that over 100 million people have this deficiency in their blood—among them a large number of blacks.

A person's emotional status will also affect his intake of food. We have already mentioned this point in connection with anxiety, such as the "knots" and "butterflies" in the stomach, and the pre-examination nausea or vomiting. In one psychiatric hospital setting, the dietetic staff observed interesting correlations between food intake and the general anxiety level of both patients and staff. When they were upset by changes in their environment, such as staff changes, hospital policy changes, and holidays, the consumption of such "security foods" as bread and milk went up, as did the amount of food left on plates. When things settled down, eating patterns returned to normal.[3]

Some people use food as a source of comfort and security; they may eat excessively because of their anxieties or because of a lack of fulfill-ment of the basic needs of love and belonging.

Other emotions besides anxiety will also affect a person's appetite and, hence, his intake of food. The depressed patient does not want to eat; the happy individual usually does, unless he is too excited by happiness to eat.

The attractiveness of a meal and the environ-ment in which it·is served also contribute to a person's enjoyment of food, and encourage peo-ple to eat, as all restaurant managers realize.

As we noted at the beginning of this chapter, cultural, moral, and religious values play a con-siderable role in the food people eat. Food habits are learned, and eating habits vary considerably in different cultures and among different reli-gious groups. They also vary from one family to the next, and from individual to individual.

Among cultural groups, food habits usually have their origins in types of food that are available in the part of the world in which the group lived. Potatoes are plentiful in many parts of North America; hence, they form a staple of the diet in many homes. In many countries, rice is the staple food and forms a part of the culture. When people from one culture move to another part of the world, they usually carry their food habits with them. In North America, where peo-ple from all over the world have settled, it is important for the nurse to be aware of the cul-tural food heritage of patients and of their reli-gious backgrounds as well, since many religions have specific food rules.

Many people are vegetarian in their diet choice, because of religious beliefs or personal preference. (It is not unusual in an East Indian household, for example, to find both vegetarian and non-vegetarian family members.) Orthodox Hindus subscribe to the doctrine of "ahimsa," which means not killing. Many other religious groups also espouse vegetarianism. The largest group in North America are members of the Seventh Day Adventist Church. Other people are also becoming vegetarians for moral reasons (not wanting to kill animals for food), for health reasons (to reduce cholesterol, or because of a declining tolerance of meat with advancing age), or simply from personal preference. It is possible to have a vegetarian diet that fulfills, or even exceeds, recommended nutrient requirements. A four food group guide for a balanced vegetar-ian diet suggests:[4]

1. Grains, legumes, nuts and seeds—6 or more servings daily (including yeast-raised, whole grain bread, beans and a few nuts and seeds)

2. Vegetables—3 servings or more daily (one or more of dark, leafy greens)

3. Fruit—1–4 servings daily (including a raw source of Vitamin C)

4. Milk and eggs—2 or more glasses daily for adults, 3 or more for children (other dairy prod-ucts and an egg may make up part of the require-ment, with eggs optional—up to 4 per week)

There are different forms of vegetarianism. Some people do not eat red meat, but will eat poultry and fish. Some will not eat any animal products, including poultry, fish, milk, and eggs. Because the cow is sacred in India to both Hindus and Sikhs, cow's milk and products made from it are not consumed. (Milk from the water buffalo is used instead in India.) It is important in caring for people to find out the particular foods they do eat, as well as those they do not. The most common nutritional problems among vegetarians include deficiencies of iron and vitamin D. Acceptable sources of protein include milk and dairy products (if eaten), and the meat alternates. Soybeans and peanuts (and foods made from these) are a very important source of dietary protein in many parts of the world. To ensure an adequate intake of iron, it is good to encourage the use of eggs (if permitted), of fruits and vegetables containing iron, and whole grain and enriched cereals. To increase the Vitamin D content of vegetarian diets, eggs and vitamin D–fortified milk and margarine, or a regular intake of vitamin tablets, may be suggested. Children and expectant and lactating mothers are particularly vulnerable to nutritional disorders because of their additional nutrient needs. In addition to the problems mentioned above, they may have a deficiency of calcium if milk and milk products are not included in their diet. It is often necessary to use calcium tablets as a supplement.

Other dietary restrictions are found in different cultural groups. Many religious groups do not eat pork, as, for example, people of the Islamic, Jewish, Seventh Day Adventist religions. Non-vegetarian Hindus and Sikhs will usually not eat beef or veal because of the sacredness of the animal from which these meats come.

Then, too, there is the matter of food preparation. For people of some religious faiths, the preparation of food is a ritual. Orthodox members of the Jewish sect will only eat foods that are *kosher*, that is, *prepared according to prescribed ritual*. Many Islamic people will eat meat only if the animal has been ritually slaughtered. Kosher meat may, however, be acceptable.

Besides following formal restrictions, many people limit their diets to food prepared in styles customary to their own culture. In most Asian countries, meat, poultry and fish are usually cut up into small pieces and cooked (as you will probably have noted in meals prepared in Chinese restaurants). A large steak, or piece of chicken, or fish, then, may not be acceptable to the Oriental patient. Many people from other cultures are used to foods that have been highly spiced, as, for example, the Indian curries, the hot Mexican chilis, and the kimchee* of Korea. People from these cultures often find the typical North American diet very bland and unappetiz-

*Kimchee is known as the Korean salad, and contains a mixture of vegetables and large amounts of garlic and spices.

ing. They usually like to add a very hot sauce to most foods to improve the flavor.

Then, too, food habits vary from one family to another, even if all other factors are constant. In some households, breakfast is a sketchy or non-existent affair, whereas in others it is considered one of the main meals of the day. The patterns of eating that were learned in the home have a considerable influence on the food habits children maintain later in life, and are handed down from one generation to the next.

There is, however, also the matter of individual differences in taste and preference for food, as anyone from a large family knows. From the moment of birth, various factors, such as good or poor digestion, allergies, and differences in taste, imagination, education, and the food habits in the home, will influence the individual's set of eating habits.

Health problems also affect a person's intake of adequate nourishment. In addition to allergies and poor digestion, most physical and emotional problems affect food intake in some way, often by bringing on anorexia or nausea and vomiting. We will be discussing these problems later in this chapter, but perhaps we should mention here three common health problems that can interfere with a person's taking sufficient nourishment to meet his requirements. These are *alcoholism*, drug *addiction*, and *smoking*.

The alcoholic often drinks instead of eating, and his nutritional status suffers as a result. Serious nutritional problems are found in many alcoholics, and these require prompt intervention.

Drug addicts too can have serious nutritional problems. The addict may opt to buy drugs instead of food with his limited funds, or he may not feel the need for food when he is "high" on whatever drug that he is taking.

Smokers often substitute coffee and a cigarette for food at mealtime. Smoking diminishes the sense of taste and leaves a person with a bad taste in his mouth. People who have stopped smoking often remark on how good food tastes again.

Efficiency of the Body in Processing Food

Any factor that interferes with the body's ability to retain, absorb, store, utilize, or excrete nutrients will adversely affect a person's nutritional status. Disease processes, congenital problems, or injury to any part of the gastrointestinal system may therefore result in nutritional problems. Probably the most common type of illness affecting the gastrointestinal tract is infection, especially gastroenteritis, which is a major cause of death in many underdeveloped countries, and a very common cause of illness in both the United States and Canada. A number of other disorders, which the nurse will learn about in her courses in medical-surgical nursing, are also specific to the gastrointestinal system. Congenital problems are usually discussed thoroughly in pediatric nursing courses, so we will not go into these further at this point, except to note that there are both congenital malformations, that is, defects or abnormalities in the anatomical structures of the system, and congenital disorders affecting the physiological processes involved in the digestion and absorption of food.

Illnesses involving parts of the body other than the gastrointestinal tract may also cause disturbances in the processing of food, as well as altering the body's needs for energy and for specific nutrients. This aspect of nutrition will be discussed in the next few paragraphs.

FOOD AND THE SICK PERSON

Food as a source of nourishment is particularly important for those who are ill. Nearly all sick persons have some disturbances in gastrointestinal functioning. They may lose their appetites or be unable to tolerate food and fluids; there may be a problem in the digestion of food or in the absorption of nutrients from the gastrointestinal tract. Whatever the problem, the sick person's nutritional needs are usually different from those of the well. Lack of exercise because of illness may decrease the body's need for energy-giving foods but, at the same time, there is a greater need for tissue-building nutrients.

The nutrients that are taken into the body, normally via the gastrointestinal tract, are digested and then absorbed into the blood stream and taken to the cells of the body. In the cells, metabolic activity takes place. Metabolism has two phases: catabolism and anabolism. In *catabolism* the glucose derived from carbohydrates and the ketones and glycerol derived from fat, are broken down into carbon dioxide, water, and energy. Proteins are broken down into carbon dioxide, water, urea, and energy. In *anabolism* this energy is used in the synthesis of enzymes and proteins needed by the body cells. The restructuring of amino acids to form protein elements of the body is a particularly important part of anabolism.

In the well person, the processes of anabolism and catabolism are normally equal. In the sick, particularly those who are incapacitated, the catabolic activities are increased, which leads to a breakdown of cellular materials and a subsequent deficiency of protein. Thus, there may be a decreased need for food to meet energy requirements but an increased need for specific nutrients in the person who is ill. Additional protein foods are important for almost all sick people. There are, of course, some conditions in which a high-protein diet is contraindicated, but the foregoing statement is a good general rule.

There are certain conditions, too, in which metabolic activity, both anabolic and catabolic, is increased, as in patients with a fever, and in these cases there is a need for additional energy-giving foods as well as proteins.

In a good many disease conditions, the patient may be unable to tolerate food or fluids, or may lose these through vomiting, diarrhea, or other means. In these cases, the replacement of lost fluids and nutrients is an important part of the patient's therapeutic care. In some disease conditions, there is interference with the absorption of food. These cases require special adaptation of the diet.

Types of Diet for the Ill

As a part of the patient's therapeutic regimen, food is usually prescribed in the form of a diet. There are many kinds of diet. For example, the average patient is on a regular or full (normal) diet. This means that he eats any or all of the foods that he normally eats in health. Generally, fried and highly seasoned foods are not served to patients because of the difficulty many people normally have in digesting them. A modification of the full, or regular, diet is the light diet. The foods on this diet are cooked simply, with an avoidance of fried foods, rich desserts, and other fat-laden foods. Coarse gas-forming foods, such as corn, turnips, radishes, onions, cabbage, cauliflower, and cucumbers, are also usually avoided.

A third type of diet is the soft diet. This diet consist of food that requires little chewing and contains no harsh fiber or highly seasoned foods. Because soft-diet foods are easily digested, they are often indicated for people who have gastrointestinal disorders or difficulty in masticating food.

A fourth kind of diet is the liquid diet. There are usually three types of liquid diet: full liquid, clear liquid, and bland liquid. A clear liquid diet permits water, tea with lemon, coffee, juices, clear bouillon, carbonated beverages, and clear gelatin desserts. A full liquid diet is free of irritating condiments and cellulose. Often included in a full liquid diet are all the foods on a clear liquid diet plus such others as strained

FORM A-72A
66725 - 15M - REV. 10-73

DIET CHANGES

VANCOUVER GENERAL HOSPITAL
FOOD SERVICES DEPARTMENT

DATE	Meal B.L. or D.	STANDARD DIET SPECIFY CONSISTENCY					THERAPEUTIC DIET (Doctor Must Prescribe) SPECIFY CONSISTENCY					HOLD TRAY	NO TRAY TO O.R.	NO TRAY	Resume Tray. Specify Consistency	FORCE FLUID	NUR. INIT.	DIET. INIT.
		REG-ULAR	ADV. SOFT	REST. SOFT	FULL FLUID	CLEAR FLUID	REG-ULAR	ADV. SOFT	REST. SOFT	FULL FLUID	CLEAR FLUID							
10/11	B	✓											✓					R.S.

BED NO. R 42 A   PATIENT'S NAME   MRS. ANN YOUNG

A sample change of diet form. (Courtesy of the Vancouver General Hospital.)

FORM A-72
66720
24M - REV. 10-73

DIET LIST

VANCOUVER GENERAL HOSPITAL
FOOD SERVICES DEPARTMENT

DATE	NUR. INIT.	DIET. INIT.	PATIENT LIKES	PATIENT DISLIKES
9/11	KS		BACON FOR BREAKFAST MILK, TEA ORANGE JUICE	EGGS COFFEE GRAPEFRUIT JUICE

DIET SIGNALS

(PURPLE) - STANDARD DIETS
YELLOW - THERAPEUTIC
RED - CALCULATED
ORANGE - CHANGE (ATTN. DIETITIAN)
BLACK - FORCE FLUIDS

NOURISHMENT (FOOD SERVICES DEPT. USE ONLY)

1000 HRS. JUICE

1400 HRS. TEA

2000 HRS. COCOA

DOCTOR R. L. S
COMMENTS:
AGE: 29 YRS.
UNIT NO.: R 4295

THIS SPACE FOR FURTHER
RESTRICTION - E.G.
ISOLATION, FEED, ETC.

BED   NAME (SURNAME ONLY)
42A   YOUNG

REG-ULAR	ADV. SOFT	RESTR. SOFT	FLUID	CLEAR FLUID	THERAPEUTIC

A sample diet form. (Courtesy of the Vancouver General Hospital.)

soups, simple puddings or custards, refined cooked cereals, and milk. A bland diet is the same as full liquid but without coffee, tea, colas, and soups made with meat or those that are highly seasoned.

Therapeutic diets are special diets designed for the needs of the individual patient and vary greatly in their composition and purpose. Many special diets are designed to eliminate substances that are irritating to the gastrointestinal tract. The amount and kind of nutrients may be varied or certain nonnutritive compounds eliminated. For example, restrictions may be placed on the flavoring or seasoning used or on the amount of cellulose to be consumed. There are also diets that restrict the amount of sodium, sugar, or protein. There are high calorie diets and low calorie diets, high protein diets and low protein diets. There are also diets which control the quantity and type of fats. Each therapeutic diet is ordered by the physician to meet the patient's specific needs. The quantity of each kind of food is calculated by the dietitian or nutritionist, and each meal is served carefully in the prescribed amounts of specific foods.

Regardless of the kind of diet, it is important that the patient understand why he is served certain foods. The nurse and the nutritionist can help gain the patient's cooperation and thereby his acceptance of the specified food as part of his prescribed therapy.

COMMON PROBLEMS

We mentioned many of the common nutritional problems to which people in various age groups are vulnerable when we were discussing nutritional needs throughout the life cycle. Because the problems of dyspepsia, anorexia, nausea, and vomiting are commonly seen in patients, and because they are particularly open to nursing interventions, we will discuss these in considerable detail.

On a global basis, the most common problems associated with nutrition throughout the world are malnutrition, starvation, and obesity. Although malnutrition is often regarded as an affliction of only underdeveloped and poor countries, it is also of great concern to health workers in North America.

At least 30 per cent of the United States population have diets that fail to measure up to standards for one or more nutrients, especially iron, calcium, vitamin A, vitamin C, riboflavin, and calories. Malnutrition can show up as anemia or obesity, or in close association with diseases related to poor nutrition, such as heart

disease, hypertension, stroke, diabetes, severe dental and periodontal disease, and digestive diseases. Especially vulnerable to malnutrition are young children, adolescents, young pregnant women, families of the poor, handicapped persons, and people over 65 years of age. A national study[5] in Canada revealed many nutritional problems in that country also. Iron deficiencies were so widespread that remedial food enrichment practices and a national nutrition education program were recommended. Protein deficits were found in a substantially large proportion of pregnant women, and protein and/or calorie deficits among a small but noteworthy group of children under the age of 5 years. Shortages of calcium and vitamin D were found to be a problem in the daily diets of many infants, children, and adolescents, and a moderate thiamine deficiency was revealed among adults. A deficiency of vitamin C was found in the Inuit (Eskimo) group, and, to a lesser extent, among the native Indian population. The survey also revealed that a large proportion of adults in the country have a problem of overweight.

There are many causes of malnutrition. In poor and underdeveloped nations, the climate and terrain may be such that those crops that do grow well are neither sufficient in quantity nor nutritionally adequate for the resident population. Overpopulation is often a concomitant factor in such cases. Most foods have to be imported and are, therefore, costly, so that only the very rich can afford to eat well. Indeed, the situation in some countries is so extreme that many people starve to death. The United States and Canada, with other countries and international organizations (such as UNESCO, UNICEF, and WHO, for example), are participating in food distribution programs to countries in need and providing agricultural specialists to advise on food cultivation and processing.

Nutritional problems are a major concern in industrialized nations as well. In countries where food is abundant, many people suffer from inadequate nutrition, often in the form of obesity. Obesity may be caused by simple overeating, but more often than not it is a symptom of malnutrition. Contrary to popular belief, people do not necessarily choose naturally the foods their bodies need. In fact, most people choose their foods according to cost and preparation time. The so-called convenience foods, which are relatively expensive, are highly processed and take little or no preparation. They are also usually high in carbohydrates and low in protein. Foods rich in carbohydrates occur abundantly in nature and therefore are usually inexpensive in comparison with protein-rich foods, such as meat and dairy products. With the escalating cost of living, therefore, the average person is likely to eat more rice and potatoes and less meat, and more canned and fewer fresh fruits and vegetables.

Many common diagnostic tests and treatments for the ill interrupt a person's normal dietary pattern, and as a result he may not have a sufficient intake of essential nutrients and energy-giving foods. Meals may be withheld for tests that are ordered, the person may be allowed nothing by mouth for long periods of time and maintained on low-calorie infusions, or a nutritionally inadequate diet may be required in his treatment. The term *hospital malnutrition* has been applied to this increasingly prevalent nutritional problem. The nurse working in an acute care facility needs to be aware of the need for a careful assessment of her patients so that remedial measures can be instituted promptly.

Dyspepsia, Anorexia, Nausea, and Vomiting

Among the most common problems nurses will encounter in patients in their day-to-day practice are dyspepsia, anorexia, nausea, and vomiting. *Dyspepsia* is the technical term for indigestion. It is often the first indication that something is wrong with gastrointestinal functioning.

A loss of the desire for food often leads to nausea and vomiting, unless the source of stress is removed and the body's normal equilibrium is restored. The inability to take in food and fluids, or the body's rejection of them, poses a serious threat to homeostasis and involves all areas of functioning of the human body.

Indigestion is common among people of all ages, but most prevalent in older adults. It seems to be one of the annoying and, often, distressing accompaniments of the aging process.

Gastroenteritis, which is a common cause of anorexia, nausea, and vomiting, still remains one of the most common types of short-term illness in North America. It is a very common problem in infants and small children. It is still one of the major causes of death in infants under one year in North America, and in children under 5 years in Middle and South America and in most developing countries throughout the world. It is also a distressing problem for many international travelers, whose gastrointestinal tracts are exposed to foods and fluids that are not a part of their normal diet. In addition, anorexia, nausea, and vomiting frequently accompany so many health problems that the nurse should be acquainted with the physiolog-ical mechanisms involved in these disturbances, and be able to take appropriate interventions to assist patients with these problems.

Physiological Considerations. Indigestion is characterized by pain and distress in the epigastric region. It may be accompanied by other symptoms, such as eructation (burping) or flatulence (the excessive formation of gases in the stomach or intestine; flatus is the term used for gas expelled through the anus). Many pregnant women and older adults complain of heartburn, which is characterized by a burning pain located behind the sternum. It is caused by a regurgitation of acid contents of the stomach into the esophagus, the burning sensation being due to irritation of the mucous membrane lining the esophagus.

Anorexia, nausea, and vomiting are varying degrees of distress of the upper gastrointestinal tract. Anorexia means loss of appetite, or lack of desire for food, and it involves the subjective perception of a distaste for food. The individual often expresses this by saying, "I don't feel like eating." Anorexia may precede nausea. In nausea, not only is there a distaste for food but the mere thought of food becomes repelling. In addition, the individual usually complains of an uncomfortable sensation in the region of the stomach. Vomiting, the forceful ejection of the stomach's contents, is usually preceded by nausea.

Although anorexia, nausea, and vomiting are considered by many to be sequential stages of the same physical phenomenon, any one of the three may occur by itself in the absence of the other two.

Anorexia has been defined as a loss of appetite. Appetite is the pleasant sensation of a desire for food. Although appetite and hunger frequently occur together, they are not the same. Hunger is an uncomfortable sensation that indicates a physiological need for nourishment, whereas appetite is a learned response. As such, appetite is closely related to cultural and social values. To a large extent, one's appetite is conditioned by previous pleasant experiences with food. A number of different stimuli will arouse the appetite. These include olfactory stimuli, such as the pleasant odor of something cooking; visual stimuli, such as an attractively served meal; auditory stimuli, including the clatter of pots and pans in the kitchen as dinner is being prepared; or gustatory stimuli, as when one tastes a sample of food and finds it agreeable, and the appetite is whetted for more.

When a person loses his appetite, specific visceral changes occur. There is usually a hypofunctioning of the stomach; gastric tone is lessened, and the secretion of hydrochloric acid is decreased. It has also been observed that the stomach of the anorectic patient is pale in comparison with those of people with normal appetites.

These same physiological findings have been observed in individuals suffering from nausea, except that in the case of the nauseated person, they are more pronounced. In nausea, there is a relaxation of the walls of the stomach, and gastric secretions and muscular contractions cease. Because of this relaxation, the stomach is usually situated lower in the abdominal cavity than it normally is. At the same time as the muscles of the stomach are in a relaxed state, the muscular wall of the intestine shows increased contractility, and contents from the duodenum may be regurgitated back into the stomach. *Retching*—that is, an unproductive attempt at vomiting—may occur several times before vomiting actually takes place.

The act of vomiting involves a sequence of events that culminates in the forceful ejection of the stomach's contents. Initially there is a relaxation of the upper portion of the stomach, including the cardiac sphincter. This is followed by strong contractile waves in the lower portion of the stomach, which effectively close off the pyloric sphincter and prevent the stomach contents from passing into the duodenum. Subsequently, the diaphragm and the abdominal muscles contract. The strong contractions of these muscles during the act of vomiting account for the feeling of "soreness" that many people experience as an aftereffect of vomiting. With the simultaneous contraction of the diaphragm and the abdominal muscles, intra-abdominal pressure is greatly increased and the stomach is literally squeezed between the two sets of muscles. The contents in the relaxed upper portion of the stomach are then forced upward through the esophagus and out through the mouth. Normally, the glottis is closed and respirations cease during the act of vomiting in order to prevent the vomitus from being aspirated (entering the lungs).

Indigestion is caused by the body's inability to process the foods that are taken into it. It may result from diminishing ability to chew food properly. Or, it may result from putting too much of a load on the system by overeating, by eating too quickly, or by eating highly spiced foods or foods that are foreign to the gastrointestinal tract. It is often associated with eating certain foods. Foods that contain a lot of fat or are cooked in fats or oils are particularly troublesome to many people, as are gas-forming foods (lettuce, cabbage, and beans, for example) and milk in those unable to tolerate it. Smoking may be a factor because it stimulates the secretion of acid gastric juices in the stomach.

Factors Causing Anorexia, Nausea, and Vomiting. The primary center controlling vomiting is located in the medulla oblongata. It is thought that stimulation of this center may give rise to anorexia, nausea, or vomiting, depending on the degree or intensity of the stimulus. Thus, a person who does not feel like eating may become nauseated at the sight of food and may vomit if he tries to eat it. However, vomiting is not always preceded by nausea, and it is believed, therefore, that only certain areas in the vomiting center are directly involved with nausea. The vomiting center may be stimulated by a number of factors. These include chemical stimuli (drugs and other toxic substances), impulses from the cerebral cortex (strong emotions), and impulses arising from receptors in the viscera (internal factors).

Drugs and Other Toxic Substances. Two of the most common causes the nurse may see in community practice and in the emergency unit of acute care facilities are food and drug poisonings. Toddlers and small children are particularly vulnerable to both because they will often eat or drink food that is left on a counter or table, or ingest household products (such as bleach or insecticides) or their parents' pills, if these are within reach.

A number of different chemical agents may give rise to anorexia, nausea, and vomiting. Many common drugs also cause anorexia, nausea, and vomiting, including digitalis (frequently used in the treatment of people with heart conditions); a number of the narcotics, such as morphine; and many drugs used as anesthetics. When giving a patient any medication, in fact, it is important to note whether nausea and vomiting are listed as possible side effects of the drug, and, if so, to watch for these symptoms in the patient. The drugs apomorphine and syrup of ipecac, because of their specific action on the vomiting center, are often administered when it is considered desirable to rid the stomach of its contents—if, for example, the individual has ingested a poisonous substance. Other toxic substances that are circulating in the blood stream, such as bacterial toxins in infections or in food poisoning, may also stimulate the vomiting center.

Food Poisoning. Every year, a number of deaths from food poisoning receive a great deal of publicity, but countless more cases occur, many of them unreported. Food poisoning is always a potential problem in large gatherings, such as picnics, where food may be held for long periods of time at temperatures conducive to the growth of bacteria.

If food poisoning is suspected, it is important to find out what the person has eaten and also whether any other person who ate the same food is affected as well. The symptoms of food poisoning usually occur within 1 to 5 hours after the contaminated food is eaten. They usually develop abruptly and may include nausea, vomiting, abdominal cramps, and diarrhea. Most cases of food poisoning last no more than 5 to 6 hours, or 24 hours at the most. They will usually subside on their own as the body rids itself of the offending substance. The individual should be watched for signs of shock and for the development of neurological symptoms, which occur with certain types of food poisoning, including botulism, shellfish poisoning, and mushroom poisoning. Shock may be caused by excessive food loss (from vomiting and diarrhea), by bacterial toxins, or by an allergic reaction to the food ingested. Shock is discussed in Chapter 17.

Botulism (caused by the *Clostridium botulinum* organism) is the most serious food poisoning because it is fatal in about 60 per cent of cases. Although cases receive a great deal of publicity, fortunately its occurrence is relatively rare. The most frequent cause is improperly home-preserved vegetables, although preserved fruits, fish, and meat products may also be sources of botulism.

The organism releases gas as it grows and is sometimes evidenced by a bulging can or lid of a jar. The symptoms of botulism usually develop 12 to 36 hours after the food has been eaten, but may be delayed up to 4 days. The early symptoms are similar to those of other food poisonings, with the addition of weakness, dizziness, visual disturbances, and dryness of the mouth and throat. Often the person will complain of headache. Other neurological symptoms, such as paralysis, limitation of eye movements, dilated pupils, decreased tendon reflexes, and impaired speech, often follow. The cause of death is usually respiratory paralysis. If botulism is suspected, the person should be referred for emergency medical treatment immediately.

Shellfish poisoning can also cause neurological symptoms, through the transmission of toxins from the plankton on which they feed. Particularly dangerous are shellfish harvested during the so-called "red tide." Fortunately, the mortality rate is not so high as in botulism, although rates ranging from 5 to18 per cent have been reported in some outbreaks. The symptoms may develop as soon as 20 minutes after eating, with *paresthesia* (abnormal sensations such as prickling or tingling) of the hands and mouth, weakness of the arms and legs, and a feeling of floating. The person may also notice *ataxia* (a failure of muscle coordination), headache and vomiting. Respiratory or *bulbar paralysis* (due to effects of the toxin on motor centers in the medulla oblongata) may ensue. Prompt medical attention is important. No specific treatment is known as yet; the measures used are those for respiratory paralysis. If the person survives the first 12 hours, he is likely to recover.

Another common type of food poisoning, particularly in the spring, late summer, and early fall, is that caused by certain "wild" varieties of mushrooms. In mushroom poisoning, the individual usually has an acute attack of nausea, vomiting, and diarrhea starting about 2 to 3 hours after eating. Hallucinations and intoxication reactions may follow. Some varieties of mushrooms are more poisonous than others and may lead to kidney and renal failure. It is important, then, to find out what kind of mushrooms were eaten, how many, and where. If possible, the nurse should get a sample of the mushrooms or save any emesis for analysis. The individual should be hospitalized so that he can be watched for delayed reactions. Often, the stomach is washed out, and a strong laxative is given to speed the mushrooms through the gastrointestinal tract.

Psychosocial Stressors. Indigestion may be caused, or aggravated, by psychosocial factors. A meal that is taken when a person is under stress, for example, is not easily digested. If a person is angry, or worried about something, he may feel that his stomach is "tied up in knots," excessive acid secretion may ensue, and he may also suffer from excessive gas formation and resultant distention in the stomach and intestines.

Stressful situations may give rise to anorexia, nausea, or vomiting. The event or situation need not necessarily be unpleasant. An individual may be "too excited to eat." Infants and toddlers will often vomit if overstimulated, particularly after a meal. Older children, too, may become nauseated or vomit, if excited or fearful. However, it is in connection with unpleasantly stressful situations that the symptoms of anorexia, nausea, and vomiting are most often noted. Worry over a pending examination, pain, anxiety, and fear may all give rise to these symptoms. Similarly, other psychic factors such as the sight of something particularly abhorrent, unpleasant odors, or even extremely loud noise can also take away one's appetite, make one feel nauseated, or cause vomiting.

Anorexia Nervosa. Earlier in this chapter, we mentioned anorexia nervosa as a common problem affecting nutrition in the adolescent and early adulthood years. Although it does affect some boys and a few older adults, it is particularly prevalent among girls 14 to 17 years old. This disorder is felt to be due to psychosocial stressors. One of the characteristic accompaniments of the loss of appetite, however, is amenorrhea due to decreased levels of the female hormones. There has, therefore, been a great deal of controversy about whether the poor nutritional state resulting from the anorexia causes the drop in female hormones or the drop in female hormones causes the loss-of-appetite syndrome. At the present time, most experts feel there is not sufficient evidence to support the physiological theory of hormonal disturbance as the root cause of anorexia nervosa. They tend to feel that it is a mental disorder, characterized by a distorted perception of body size. The individual thinks she is much bigger and fatter than she really is and becomes obsessed with the need to lose weight. Appetite lessens and self-induced vomiting may occur.

Internal Factors. The parts of the body containing receptors that initiate vomiting are the stomach, duodenum, uterus, kidneys, heart, pharynx, and semicircular canals of the ear. The stimuli that give rise to anorexia, nausea, and vomiting include irritation of the receptors, as, for example, the tickling of the back of the throat to induce vomiting; the eating of irritating foods; stretching of the organ, as occurs when a child stretches his stomach by overeating and promptly vomits; or pressure on the receptors. Irritation of the gastrointestinal tract by infectious, chemical, or mechanical agents, and distention of, or trauma to, other viscera also affect the vomiting center.

A disturbance in motion, such as one experiences with the rolling motion of a ship at sea, or with any rapid change in direction of the body, stimulates receptors in the labyrinth of the ear. These receptors send out impulses that are carried by the vestibular nerve to the cerebellum, and thence to the vomiting center in the medulla.

Indigestion is often caused by problems in the gastrointestinal tract, where a disturbance in structure or functioning, inflammations, or new growths (such as tumors), either in the tract itself or in its accessory organs, may interfere with the body's ability to process and utilize foodstuffs. In older persons particularly, chewing may be difficult if the person gradually loses teeth or if ill-fitting dentures prevent proper mastication. The motility of the gastrointestinal tract also lessens with age—food is not processed as quickly.

The heartburn frequently experienced in the second and third trimesters of pregnancy is usually caused by a lessened stomach capacity and a slowing of the digestive processes as the growing fetus exerts pressure on organs in the abdominal cavity. In older adults, it is due in many cases to a slowing down of the digestive processes and a diminished ability to handle food.

ASSESSMENT

Subjective Data

● In order to assess the nutritional status of an individual, the nurse needs information about all the factors that affect an individual's state of nutrition. These include age and stage of development, sex, height, usual weight, present weight, usual habits with regard to daily activities and current activity level, usual dietary pattern and any recent deviations from it, and present status with regard to food and fluid intake. She should know whether he is on a special diet and, if so, if he is adhering to it. She should also know the person's religious affiliation, his ethnic origin, whether he subscribes to any special beliefs about food, and his attitude toward food.

She should determine the patient's socioeconomic status and that of the family and learn something about their lifestyles. She should be aware of the person's general physical condition and his emotional status. She should also know about any health problems he may have that could cause alterations in his nutritional needs or interfere with his digestive processes. If the patient is female, the nurse should obtain information about the menstrual history and determine if she is pregnant or a nursing mother.

Much of this information is available to the nurse in the data gathered during the nursing history and in the initial nursing clinical appraisal. Information about the patient's current health status and health problems, special diet orders, and status relative to pregnancy or lactation should be available from the patient's record.

The nurse supplements the information she has gathered about the patient from other sources by talking with him and through her observations.

CHARACTERISTICS OF GOOD NUTRITION AND POOR NUTRITION*

Good Nutrition	Poor Nutrition
About average *height* for age	Body undersized or poorly developed
About average *weight* for height	Thin (more than 10 percent underweight) or fat and flabby (more than 10 percent overweight)
Good layer of *subcutaneous fat*	Subcutaneous fat lacking or in excess
Muscles well developed and firm	Muscles small; pot belly
Skin turgid and of healthy color	Skin pale, sallow, or rough (hyperkeratosis): edema; seborrhea; dermatitis
Guns firm and *mucous membranes* of mouth reddish pink	Mucous membranes pale; tongue abnormally red or smooth; lesions at corners of mouth; gums swollen or bleeding
Hair smooth and glossy	Hair rough and without luster; thin; easily plucked
Eyes clear, good night vision	Angular lesions of eyelids; reddened or thickened, opaque conjunctivae; night blindness
Legs straight	Bowed legs; knock-knees; beaded ribs
Appetite good	Appetite poor; diminished taste acuity
General health excellent	Susceptible to infections; lack of endurance and vigor
Good-natured and full of life	Irritable, overactive; or phlegmatic, listless, unable to concentrate

*A number of these signs are nonspecific; that is, they may relate to more than one nutrient and to other conditions of health besides nutritional state. Taken in conjunction with a good history, however, they provide a reasonable index of nutritional state.

From Briggs, G. M., and Calloway, D. H.: *Bogert's Nutrition and Physical Fitness.* Philadelphia, Saunders College Publishing, 1979, p. 447.

DESIRABLE WEIGHTS FOR MEN AND WOMEN — IN POUNDS ACCORDING TO FRAME (IN INDOOR CLOTHING)

Men of Ages 25 and Over

Height (With Shoes On), 1-Inch Heels Feet	Inches	Small Frame	Medium Frame	Large Frame
5	2	112–120	118–129	126–141
5	3	115–123	124–133	129–144
5	4	118–126	124–136	132–148
5	5	121–129	127–139	135–152
5	6	124–133	130–143	138–156
5	7	128–137	134–147	142–161
5	8	132–141	138–152	147–166
5	9	136–145	142–156	151–170
5	10	140–150	146–160	155–174
5	11	144–154	150–165	159–179
6	0	148–158	154–170	164–184
6	1	152–162	158–175	168–189
6	2	156–167	162–180	173–194
6	3	160–171	167–185	178–199
6	4	164–175	172–190	182–204

Women of Ages 25 and Over*

Height (With Shoes On), 2-Inch Heels Feet	Inches	Small Frame	Medium Frame	Large Frame
4	10	92–98	96–107	104–119
4	11	94–101	98–110	106–122
5	0	96–104	101–113	109–125
5	1	99–107	104–116	112–128
5	2	102–110	107–119	115–131
5	3	105–113	110–122	118–134
5	4	108–116	113–126	121–138
5	5	111–119	116–130	125–142
5	6	114–123	120–135	129–146
5	7	118–127	124–139	133–150
5	8	122–131	128–143	137–154
5	9	126–135	132–147	141–158
5	10	130–140	136–151	145–163
5	11	134–144	140–155	149–168
6	0	138–148	144–159	153–173

*For girls between ages of 18 and 25, subtract 1 pound for each year under 25.

Courtesy of Metropolitan Life Insurance Company.

ADULT WEIGHT IN KILOGRAMS FOR WOMEN, ACCORDING TO FRAME, IN INDOOR CLOTHING*

Height in cm (With 5-cm Heel Shoes)	Small Frame	Medium Frame	Large Frame
147 (4'10")	41.3–44.5	43.5–48.0	47.0–54.0
148	41.7–44.8	43.9–48.6	47.4–54.4
149	42.1–45.3	44.3–49.2	47.8–54.8
150	42.6–45.8	44.7–49.8	48.2–55.3
151	43.1–46.3	45.2–50.3	48.7–55.8
152	43.6–46.8	45.7–50.9	49.3–56.4
153	44.0–47.4	46.2–51.5	49.8–56.9
154	44.5–47.9	46.7–52.0	50.3–57.5
155	45.0–48.4	47.2–52.6	50.8–58.0
156	45.5–48.9	47.7–53.2	51.4–58.6
157	46.0–49.4	48.2–53.7	51.9–59.1
158	46.4–50.0	48.7–54.3	52.4–59.7
159	46.9–50.5	49.2–54.8	53.0–60.2
160	47.4–51.0	49.7–55.4	53.5–60.8
161	48.0–51.6	50.3–56.1	54.1–61.5
162	48.6–52.3	50.9–56.8	54.8–62.2
163	49.2–53.0	51.5–57.6	55.5–62.9
164	49.9–53.7	52.2–58.3	56.2–63.7
165	50.5–54.4	52.8–59.0	56.8–64.4
166	51.1–55.0	53.4–59.8	57.5–65.1
167	51.7–55.7	54.0–60.5	58.2–65.8
168	52.4–56.4	54.6–61.2	58.9–66.5
169	53.0–57.0	55.3–62.0	59.5–67.2
170	53.6–57.7	56.0–62.7	60.2–68.0
171	54.3–58.5	56.7–63.4	60.9–68.8
172	55.0–59.2	57.4–64.2	61.6–69.6
173	55.7–60.0	58.1–65.0	62.3–70.4
174	56.5–60.7	58.9–65.7	63.1–71.2
175	57.2–61.5	59.6–66.5	63.8–72.1
176	57.9–62.3	60.3–67.3	64.5–72.9
177	58.6–63.0	61.0–68.0	65.3–73.7
178	59.3–63.8	61.7–68.8	66.0–74.6
179	60.0–64.5	62.5–69.5	66.7–75.4
180	60.8–65.3	63.3–70.3	67.5–76.2
181	61.6–66.1	64.0–71.0	68.2–77.0
182	62.4–66.9	64.8–71.8	69.0–77.9
183	63.2–67.7	65.6–72.6	69.7–78.7

From Koh, E. L.: Height-Weight Correlation in the Metric System. *Canadian Medical Association Journal,* 110:1044, 1974.

Objective Data

There are many outward signs of both good nutrition and malnutrition that are readily observable to the trained eye. Characteristics that the nurse can observe in people with good nutrition and those with poor nutrition (a comparison) are shown in the table on page 280. Particularly important aspects to note, then, are the person's height and weight and the condition of the hair, the eyes, the mouth, (especially the teeth and mucous membranes), the skin and its underlying fat and muscle tissues, and the limbs. The person's general appearance, the pace and vigor with which he carries out activities, and his general emotional tone should be noted. Is he fat or thin? Does he look emaciated? Does he appear listless and apathetic, or does he tackle things with enthusiasm? Is he good-natured, irritable, or depressed?

In severe cases of malnutrition, the heartbeat may be accelerated and its rhythm altered. The person's blood pressure may be elevated and he may lose his sense of position—it may be difficult to sit up or stand erect. The lips and tongue may be red and swollen; the gums may be spongy and may bleed easily; and the nails may become spoon-shaped, brittle, and ridged. The face may look drawn, with hollow cheeks and dark circles under the eyes and on the cheeks. The parotid glands and the thyroid glands often become swollen. The person may become confused, and he may have a burning or tingling sensation in the hands and feet. His muscles may appear wasted and the joints swollen.[6]

The patient's current weight is compared with his usual weight. Weight tables provide a good general guide to desirable body weight, but they must be considered in terms of the individual's body frame and the amount of fatty tissue the person has in subcutaneous layers of skin.

Body frame is usually divided into three categories—small, medium, and large. One can generally assess the type of body frame by looking at the person. A more accurate assessment is made by measuring the wrist size. The wrist is measured at its smallest circumference, and compared with the individual's height (without shoes). A person with a medium frame would be expected to have the following:[6]

Height	Wrist Measurement
4'8" to 5'2"	5½ to 5¾ inches
5'2" to 5'5"	6 to 6¼ inches
5'5" to 6'	6¼ to 6½ inches

Measurements below the average range (for the person with a medium frame) would be considered to have a small frame; those above, a large frame.

ADULT WEIGHT IN KILOGRAMS FOR MEN, ACCORDING TO FRAME, IN INDOOR CLOTHING*

Height in cm (With 2.5-cm Heel Shoes)	Small Frame	Medium Frame	Large Frame
157 (5'2")	50.5–54.1	53.2–58.6	56.9–63.5
158	51.0–54.6	53.7–59.1	57.4–64.2
159	51.6–55.2	54.3–59.7	58.0–64.9
160	52.2–55.8	54.9–60.3	58.6–65.6
161	52.8–56.4	55.5–60.9	59.2–66.3
162	53.3–56.9	56.0–61.5	59.7–67.0
163	53.9–57.5	56.6–62.1	60.3–67.7
164	54.5–58.1	57.1–62.7	60.9–68.4
165	55.1–58.7	57.7–63.3	61.5–69.2
166	55.7–59.4	58.3–64.0	62.1–70.0
167	56.3–60.1	58.9–64.7	62.8–70.7
168	57.0–60.8	59.5–65.4	63.5–71.4
169	57.6–61.5	60.2–66.1	64.2–72.2
170	58.2–62.2	60.8–66.8	64.9–73.0
171	58.9–62.9	61.4–67.5	65.6–73.7
172	59.6–63.6	62.0–68.2	66.3–74.5
173	60.2–64.4	62.7–69.0	67.0–75.3
174	60.9–65.2	63.4–69.8	67.7–76.1
175	61.6–66.0	64.1–70.7	68.4–77.0
176	62.3–66.8	64.9–71.5	69.2–77.8
177	63.0–67.6	65.6–72.4	70.0–78.7
178	63.8–68.4	66.4–73.2	70.7–79.5
179	64.5–69.2	67.2–74.1	71.5–80.4
180	65.3–70.0	68.0–75.0	72.2–81.2
181	66.0–70.7	68.8–75.9	73.0–82.0
182	66.7–71.5	69.6–76.8	73.8–82.9
183	67.5–72.3	70.4–77.6	74.7–83.8
184	68.2–73.1	71.2–78.5	75.5–84.7
185	69.0–73.9	72.0–79.4	76.4–85.6
186	69.7–74.7	72.8–80.3	77.2–86.5
187	70.5–75.5	73.6–81.2	78.1–87.5
188	71.2–76.4	74.4–82.1	79.0–88.4
189	72.0–77.3	75.3–83.0	79.8–89.3
190	72.7–78.2	76.1–83.9	80.6–90.3
191	73.5–79.2	77.0–84.8	81.5–91.2
192	74.2–80.2	77.9–85.8	82.4–92.2
193	75.0–81.2	78.7–86.8	83.3–93.2

*From Koh, E. L.: Height-Weight Correlation in the Metric System. *Canadian Medical Association Journal,* 110:1044, 1974.

Another measurement that is frequently used is the mid–upper arm circumference, which is indicative of the mass of skeletal muscle. The assessment of body fatness can be done in a number of different ways. One that is commonly used is the measurement of the thickness of folds of skin and fat. The measurement is usually taken on the inside of the upper arm (called the triceps skinfold measurement).

Special instruments have been developed for measuring subcutaneous fatty tissue, but whether these are available for nurses to use, and whether the nurse or some other health professional takes these measurements are matters of agency policy.

A complete physical examination may be undertaken on an initial assessment by a nurse practitioner or a physician, with particular attention being paid to palpation of the various organs of the digestive tract and its accessory organs.

Laboratory Tests. Blood and urine tests are considered the most reliable means of assessing nutritional status.

Blood tests that are commonly ordered include those for hemoglobin and hematocrit (for iron deficiencies), total serum protein (for protein deficiency), and cholesterol (for excessive amounts). If it is suspected that there is a dysfunctioning of the thyroid gland, a test for protein-bound iodine (PBI) is usually ordered.

Urine is usually tested for protein, glucose, and acetone. Normally, the findings are negative for all three. The presence of protein is usually indicative of a dysfunctioning of the kidneys in processing metabolic wastes from protein consumed. The presence of glucose and acetone may be indicative of diabetes mellitus. Other tests that may be ordered if diabetes is suspected include fasting blood sugar and glucose tolerance tests. Both of these are blood tests that assess the ability of the body to process carbohydrates and to utilize glucose. Other tests on a 24-hour sample of urine may be ordered if further investigation is indicated to assess nutritional status. A urinary urea nitrogen test is used as an indication of the person's catabolism and nitrogen balance. A creatinine test may be ordered to assess the degree of muscle protein depletion.

Indigestion, Anorexia, Nausea, and Vomiting

Because it is often difficult to differentiate indigestion from other, more serious health problems, particularly in older persons, complaints of indigestion should never be dismissed lightly. If the symptoms are persistent or particularly severe, or if you are just not sure, the individual should be referred to his physician for further investigation of the problem.

In assessing the individual suffering from indigestion, anorexia, nausea, or vomiting, the nurse may gather information from both the patient and his family. Pertinent information includes the nature of the patient's discomfort, the length of time the person has had these symptoms, the severity of the symptoms, and their relationship to eating habits, personal lifestyle, and emotional stress. Specific causal factors should be identified, if possible. For example, has the patient eaten something that disagreed with him? Is he taking any medication that may have gastrointestinal side effects? Is he under emotional stress? Does the patient have

cultural, moral, or religious beliefs that are affecting his appetite? For example, the Orthodox Jewish patient may not want to eat dairy products and meat at the same meal. The Chinese person may prefer rice and tea with his meals, and may leave the standard hospital food untouched. The nutritional status of the patient should be assessed.

Subjective Observations. Dyspepsia, anorexia, and nausea are subjective feelings; hence, their identification is highly dependent on the individual's ability to express his discomfort. The person who has indigestion may complain of pain in the epigastric region. The nurse should identify the location of the pain, its nature, its intensity, when it occurs, and its frequency. Is it related to eating certain foods? Is it relieved by any particular measures? Often the patient says he has "a little indigestion" or "heartburn." He may complain of a "burning" feeling or a bloated feeling in his abdomen, "gas on the stomach," or flatulence.

In assessing the person who reports indigestion, it is important to remember that many heart attacks start with what the victim thinks is indigestion. Also it is often difficult to differentiate the pain of indigestion from that of a stomach or intestinal ulcer. Particularly anxiety-provoking to the patient is the pain of heartburn, which, as the name suggests, is located usually behind the sternum in the region around the heart. It is frequently confused with the pain of angina pectoris (an acute pain in the chest resulting from decreased blood supply to the heart.) The symptoms of indigestion, however, are usually directly related to the intake of food. They are not relieved by the ingestion of more food (as is the case of peptic ulcers, which are often soothed by milk or bland foods) or by nitroglycerine (a drug often ordered for patients with angina pectoris). Heartburn is often relieved by taking an antacid. Uncomplicated indigestion is often relieved by drinking a carbonated beverage, which aids in the eructation of gas. Indigestion is usually more acute when the trunk is bent, as in sitting, or when the person is lying down. Mild exercise, such as walking, often relieves the distress by helping to hasten the passage of food through the digestive tract, to prevent or relieve indigestion. In angina pectoris, on the other hand, the pain is often brought on or aggravated by exercise, as with many older persons who shovel snow or indulge in a strenuous physical exercise. The epigastric pain of indigestion may radiate up towards the neck, but seldom down the arm as it does in angina.

Patients with anorexia may say that they are not hungry or that they "just don't feel like eating.'' The nauseous person may complain simply of "feeling sick" or may specifically locate the sensation of nausea as being in the epigastric region. An uncomfortable feeling in this area is usually accompanied by other symptoms of a distressing nature. Frequently there is increased perspiration and greatly increased salivation. The person may state that his mouth is full of "spit." Some people feel faint, and some complain of vertigo (dizziness) or tingling sensations in the fingers or toes. After vomiting, a person often complains of a soreness in the stomach area.

Objective Observations. The nurse can supplement the patient's observations by noting his reactions to foods. Do reports of heartburn, indigestion, or flatulence occur after the patient eats certain foods? Does he simply toy with food, and actually eat very little? Does he push the food away at mealtime without touching it? Such behavior can indicate that a person is anorectic and perhaps nauseated. The nurse may note that the patient expresses no interest in his food and appears apathetic and listless.

The person who has indigestion is usually obviously uncomfortable, as is the one who is nauseated. The nauseated person, and the one about to vomit, usually show pallor and increased perspiration. Beads of perspiration may be evident on the person's forehead, or upper lip. If you take the person's pulse, you may note that it is markedly increased and that he is breathing rapidly. The pulse rate may increase at first, but it usually then drops to below normal. If you take the blood pressure, you will usually find that it has dropped.

In projectile vomiting, the impulse to vomit is very sudden, occurring with little or no warning (that is, with no symptoms of nausea beforehand). Moreover, the ejection of the stomach's contents is more forceful than in ordinary vomiting. This type of vomiting is often seen in infants with disorders of the gastrointestinal tract and in patients with head injuries.

Vomiting should be assessed in terms of both the nature of the vomiting and characteristics of the vomitus (material vomited). In relation to vomiting, the nurse should determine its type—that is, whether it is projectile or regurgitated (ordinary vomiting); whether it is preceded by feelings of nausea; its frequency; and its occurrence in relation to intake of food, the administration of drugs, and the individual's emotional state. Characteristics of the vomitus that should be noted are amount; color; consistency (that is, watery, liquid, or solid); the presence of undigested food, blood or other foreign substances; and odor (see Chapter 9).

Gastrointestinal disturbances quickly result in deterioration of the patient's nutritional status. Food and fluids, especially the chloride ions, are lost as a result of vomiting of gastric juices. Prolonged deficiency in nourishment and in fluid intake results in malnutrition and dehydration; dehydration, in turn, can cause constipation. The patient can be expected to be constipated because of the fluid withdrawn from the feces in an effort by the body to compensate for the lowered fluid intake or excessive fluid loss. There will probably also be a decrease in the amount of urine excreted, and the urine is more concentrated.

A person who suffers from anorexia or nausea over a period of time loses weight and, in addition to showing signs of dehydration and malnutrition, will become weak and listless owing to inadequate intake of nutrients. The individual who has experienced prolonged vomiting will show more pronounced effects due not only to the lack of intake but also to the loss of food and fluids through vomiting. This individual may show a marked weight loss and rapidly progressive signs of weakness and prostration, as well as signs of fluid and electrolyte imbalance (see Chapter 17). Prolonged vomiting in children is more serious than in adults because of the relatively greater loss of fluids and electrolytes in proportion to body weight.

In people with anorexia nervosa, the weight loss can be very rapid, with a girl who started out weighing 121 lb. (55 kg.), for example, dropping to 77 lb. (35 kg.) in 2 to 3 months.[7] As we mentioned earlier, menstruation ceases. The person has an obsessive fear of becoming fat and may induce vomiting in herself after eating. The individual usually becomes irritable, impatient, and depressed. In severe cases, she will look emaciated, will be apathetic and weak, and will suffer from severe depression.

Diagnostic Tests and Examinations. Specific diagnostic tests and examinations may be ordered by the physician. The most commonly ordered x-ray studies to assess the internal structure and functioning and to detect the presence of tumors or stones in the digestive tract and its accessory organs are the gastrointestinal (GI) series and the gallbladder series. The upper GI series is a visualization of the esophagus, stomach, and duodenum. It is also called a barium meal because the patient is asked to drink a glass of barium sulfate (a radiopaque substance), and its passage is followed through the upper gastrointestinal tract in a series of x-ray films, or projected onto a fluoroscope screen. It is used to assess the motility and integrity of the tract; any structures, dilatations, or outpouchings impeding passage of the barium through the tract; the presence of abnormal growths or tumors; or evidence of other organs pressing on the tract.

X-rays are frequently ordered to detect obstructions such as gallstones (calculi) or tumors in the gallbladder, the cystic bile duct, and the common bile duct and its accessory ducts. The examinations may include a cholecystogram, which is an x-ray of the gallbladder, and a cholangiogram, which is an x-ray of the cystic, hepatic, and common bile ducts. Both the GI and gallbladder series may be done on an outpatient basis.

Often a specimen of the vomitus is sent to the laboratory for examination to ascertain its contents. Frequently it is examined for blood. Microscopic examination may reveal occult blood, that is, blood that is present in the specimen but hidden to the naked eye. The nurse's responsibility includes seeing that a correctly labeled specimen is sent to the laboratory in the designated container. In some cases, contents of the stomach are removed by suction for analysis.

Blood chemistry tests can also be significant. The patient who is vomiting is losing hydrochloric acid (HCl) and therefore H^+ ions. He is in danger then of developing alkalosis. An examination of the blood gases may be ordered to determine the acid-base balance (see Chapter 17). A decrease in blood chlorides (hypochloremia) is also likely to occur as Cl^- ions are lost along with the H^+ ions. Prolonged vomiting may cause severe sodium depletion as well.

PRIORITIES FOR NURSING ACTION

Priority situations with regard to nutritional problems are those in which the individual's nutritional status is jeopardizing his general health or causing other health problems. The grossly overweight individual, as we have mentioned, should be referred for medical assistance, whether or not he or she is showing signs of other health problems. Malnourished individuals are also referred for medical assistance because of the possibility that malnourishment may be caused by another health problem. Severely malnourished individuals require prompt intervention by health professionals. In some situations the nurse may be responsible for initiating treatment—for example, if she is working in a community where no doctor is available. However, in this situation the nurse needs additional preparation for coping with such circumstances, and this type of training is usually included in more advanced courses in nursing. The nurse should nevertheless be alert to the signs of severe malnourishment in individuals, whether they are ill and in an inpatient facility, or in an ambulatory setting in the community.

People who are severely malnourished, or whose nutritional status is threatened because they are unable to take sufficient food and fluid on their own, usually require that nourishment be provided either in lieu of, or supplementary to, their oral intake by means such as intravenous feedings (see Chapter 17) or gastric gavage, which is discussed later in this chapter.

The patient who is vomiting needs prompt attention, directed first of all at making sure that he does not aspirate the vomitus. A person who is lying down and starts to vomit should be helped to a sitting position if this is possible and not contraindicated. Otherwise, the head should be turned to the side and the person positioned so that the vomitus will drain from the mouth. It is particularly important to watch helpless patients, such as those who are unconscious, semiconscious, or paralyzed, to make sure that the airway is not blocked. Other priorities in nursing care of the vomiting patient are to relieve the symptom and to provide comfort and support to the patient.

With most patients who are anorectic or nauseated, the immediate problem is usually to prevent aggravation of the symptoms. The nauseated individual usually feels better lying down in a cool and quiet room with adequate ventilation. If this is not possible, the person should be encouraged to sit quietly and take a few deep breaths. This helps to relax the diaphragm. Measures to take the person's mind off his gastrointestinal problems may also help.

With the person who is suffering from acute indigestion, the first priority is to rule out the more serious problem of a heart attack. If there is doubt, a physician should be consulted.

If food poisoning is suspected, it is advisable to notify a physician right away. Often, the stomach may have to be washed out, or the person may need monitoring for signs of delayed reactions. Laboratory testing may be needed. People who may have botulism, shellfish poisoning, or mushroom poisoning should be taken to an acute care facility as quickly as possible.

GOALS FOR NURSING ACTION

The long-range goals for people who have actual or potential problems of nutrition are basically one or more of the following:

1. To maintain adequate nutrition and hydration of the individual
2. To promote his optimal nutrition
3. To restore the individual to a satisfactory

PRINCIPLES RELEVANT TO NUTRITION ✓

1. An adequate intake of essential nutrients and energy-giving foods is required for optimal health.
2. An individual's nutritional status is determined by the adequacy of the specific nutrients and energy-giving foods taken into the body, absorbed, and utilized.
3. Nutritional needs depend on an individual's age, sex, body frame, amount and kind of daily activity, the secretions of endocrine glands, and health status.
4. Nutritional needs are usually altered in illness.
5. Food has psychological meaning for people.
6. Food habits are learned.
7. Food habits are related to cultural, religious, and moral beliefs.

---

nutritional status if his nutritional balance has been disturbed

4. To prevent indigestion, anorexia, nausea, and vomiting whenever possible

5. To maintain the safety, comfort, and hygiene of patients with anorexia, nausea, and vomiting

SPECIFIC NURSING INTERVENTIONS

Teaching

The nurse in the community does much nutritional counseling in the course of her work, sharing this responsibility with the nutritionist, the physician, and others. Many of the nutritional problems the nurse encounters require the specialized assistance of another health professional. The overweight person, for example, needs advice about reducing diets and exercise programs, and usually requires much support to adhere to them. Some people have found "Weight Watchers" clubs a help in this regard. Grossly overweight people need medical supervision if they wish to undertake a reducing program; it can be dangerous to lose too much weight too quickly. Fatty tissue helps to support

some of the body's internal structures and, if the fat is removed too quickly, there may be serious problems.

The overweight but malnourished individual needs assistance in changing his eating habits to ensure a properly balanced diet containing all the essential nutrients. Malnourished individuals should have a thorough physical examination to rule out health problems other than nutrition, and to ascertain the specific causes and extent of the malnourishment.

Many people, however, simply want help in planning meals to ensure that they and their families have an adequate, nutritious diet. The nurse works closely with the nutritionist and the health educator in teaching people about basic nutrition needs.

Some of the important points to stress in basic health teaching about nutrition are:

1. The need for a nutritionally balanced diet to promote optimal health (the national food guides are very helpful in this regard)

2. The special needs of children, adolescents, and expectant and nursing mothers to promote their optimal growth and development

3. The need for regular mealtimes to foster the development of good eating habits

---

PRINCIPLES RELEVANT TO ANOREXIA, NAUSEA, AND VOMITING ✓

1. The loss of food and fluids through vomiting can seriously disturb the body's nutritional status and fluid and electrolyte balance.
2. Food is a very common carrier of organisms that cause illness in man.
3. Drugs and other toxic substances, disturbances of motion, psychosocial stressors, and internal stressors can all stimulate the vomiting center.
4. Bacteria will grow rapidly in food, given a suitable temperature and medium.
5. Openings to the esophagus and to the trachea are in close proximity in the throat.
6. Dyspepsia, anorexia, nausea, and vomiting can often be prevented.

4. The need for a good breakfast to start the day

5. The need for good oral hygiene to promote an adequate intake of essential nutrients

6. The need for good standards of cleanliness in the preparation, storage, and serving of food to prevent infections

Changing Food Habits

It is sometimes necessary for a person to change his food habits because of illness. He may be told by the physician that he can no longer use salt to flavor his food, or he may have to give up eating a favorite dish. The patient may be put on a low-fat diet, or any one of a number of special diets. In these situations, people react differently. Some accept the restrictions of a special diet fairly easily; others are less amenable to change.

One of the most common reasons for failure of a patient to adhere to a diet is lack of understanding of why it is necessary. Another underlying cause may be fear resulting from the loss of a familiar food. The person who has been used to eating pasta all his life, and for whom this represents a basic security food, will find it difficult to adjust to a diet on which this is banned. An individual may rebel against being told what to eat or may resent the loss of personal choice in the matter.

There are other factors that must be taken into consideration also. These include socioeconomic factors; the cultural, religious, and moral values of the patient; and the matter of control over the purchase and preparation of food in the home.

The most influential member of a household in regard to purchasing and preparing the food that is eaten in the home is, in most instances, the mother. Younger, better-educated homemakers usually have the best nutritional knowledge and are more adaptable, but it is often necessary to work with others who may be more resistant to change.

Many older people find it hard to alter the eating patterns they have been used to all their lives, yet often they are the ones on whom dietary restrictions are imposed. Then, too, in most "new American" and "new Canadian" families, it has been recognized that food habits from the homeland are retained long after language, clothing, and other aspects of daily living are altered.[8] Often, strong resistance may be encountered to suggested changes involving the removal or alteration of familiar foods.

It is usually better to work within the framework of the individual's existing food habits, and to suggest modifications wherever possible rather than complete change. The elderly person's protein intake may be increased, for example, by the addition of cheese to his lunch of tea and toast. Supplementing a familiar diet of beans and rice by the addition of meat and milk may be accepted more readily by the Puerto Rican family than the suggestion of a completely different way of eating.

Another important item to consider is the effect of the patient's diet on other members of the family. Can the family afford to buy the special foods that are required for the patient? What problems may develop as a result of the need for preparing a different meal for one individual?

Providing Nourishment for the Ill

Food for the sick person is both therapeutic and a source of pleasure and nourishment. Most patients, if they are not too ill, look forward to mealtimes; meals provide diversions in a sometimes otherwise monotonous day and a pleasant change from the necessary treatments that many people must undergo when they are ill.

Usually other personnel are employed in a health agency to prepare and, often, serve food to the patient. The nurse, however, has important responsibilities with regard to the patient's nourishment.

Illness, as we have mentioned, has a very great bearing upon a person's acceptance of food. Those who are nauseated, dyspeptic, or in pain or who have a fever are less desirous of food than are healthy people. The nurse has a responsibility to modify these factors as much as possible so that the patient will accept nourishment. Small, frequent meals are often more acceptable to the sick person than larger servings at regular mealtime hours.

The sedentary patient is less likely to have a big appetite than the patient who exercises regularly. If a patient is able to perform some activity he should be encouraged to do so, for it will stimulate his appetite. It is important, however, that this activity be carried out well before meals, not directly afterward, and that the amount of exercise is not exhausting.

It is also necessary to cater to the particular tastes of the individual, to find out what he does and does not like in the way of food, in order to encourage him to take a sufficient amount of nourishment.

Then, too, anxiety may affect a patient's desire for food, as well as his ability to digest it. Sometimes anxiety is manifested in complaints about the food. The coffee is cold, the meat may be too well done. Often these complaints are a vocalization of a deeper anxiety. Understanding

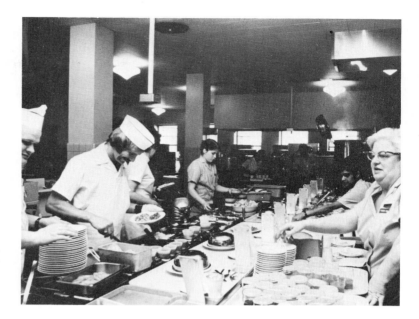

In addition to the special diets which are designed for particular illnesses, the kitchen staff must cater to a wide variety of individual preferences in preparing meals.

and acceptance on the part of the nurse can do much to help the patient to accept his illness and his diet.

The amount of food that patients eat and the amount of fluids they drink are sometimes very important therapeutically. It is the nurse who observes how much he eats and drinks and who has the responsibility for communicating this knowledge to other members of the health team. Many health agencies have a standard form (in addition to the Intake and Output chart in the patient's record) that is kept at the patient's bedside so that fluid consumption can be recorded. Often the patient can help to keep the bedside record himself. Once the record is completed, the information is transferred to the "I and O" form in the patient's record.

The nurse is also responsible for helping the patient to get ready for his meals. The patient is offered a bedpan or urinal and is provided with facilities for washing his hands prior to eating. Often a patient who has an unpleasant taste in his mouth will find his appetite improved if he brushes his teeth before eating.

Another factor which affects a person's appetite is the environment in which he eats. If a patient is served in his room, the air should be fresh and free from unpleasant odors. In addition, the patient's unit should be free of unpleasant sights. Bedside treatment trays are neatly covered and any unnecessary equipment is removed.

The nurse can also see that the patient is free from pain at mealtimes and that he is not subjected to unpleasant treatments immediately before or after meals. Enemas and dressing changes should be carried out at a time when they will have little effect on the patient's appetite.

Some patients like to get out of bed to eat their meals. If this is allowed, the nurse can help the patient to get up a few minutes before his tray arrives. Patients find it very difficult to eat and to swallow when they are flat in bed. If a patient cannot be raised to a sitting position, he will be more comfortable lying on his side while he eats. A comfortable position with adequate support helps make meals more enjoyable experiences.

Some patients prefer company at mealtime. Pleasant conversation with visitors or members of the nursing staff often relaxes the patient, so that the meal is more pleasurable and his appetite and digestion are improved. If the nurse stops to talk with a patient, she is guided by the patient's wishes in regard to mealtime conversations.

Tray Service

Although dining-room service for patients is becoming popular, most patients in hospitals still receive their food on trays in their rooms. Patients are not always physically able to go to a dining room, and not all hospitals have such facilities for their patients.

The nurse may need to work with the dietary department or aides to help promote good standards for tray service. The following standards should be adhered to:

1. The tray should be large enough to hold the dishes and utensils needed for the patient's meal and, at the same time, small enough to fit on the patient's overbed or bedside table.

2. Food must be served at the proper temper-

SPEEDISET   MOORE BUSINESS FORMS   3

FOR APPROXIMATE MEASUREMENTS ONLY

CREAMER, "TETRA PAK" _____ 20CC	★ CUP, PAPER DRINK (7 OZ) _____ 190CC
TRAYPACK CEREAL MILK OR CREAM (3 OZ) ___ 90CC	POT BEVERAGE-INSULATED PLASTIC 200CC
TRAYPACK MILK (8 OZ) _____ 240CC	SOUP BOWL (4 OZ LADLE) INSULATED 120CC
★ TRAYPACK FRUIT JUICE 4 OZ _____ 120CC	★ JUG, STAINLESS STEEL (S-100) _____ 960CC
GLASS JUICE 4 OZ _____ 100CC	★ JUG, BLUE PLASTIC _____ 850CC
ONE SIP _____ 10CC	★ JUG WATER DISPOSABLE _____ 850CC
★ CUP, CROCKERY TEA _____ 150CC	CUSTARD (120 GRAMS) _____ __ 90CC
★ CUP, PAPER DRINK-(3 OZ) _____ 70CC	JELLO (90 GRAMS) _____ 85CC
-(5 OZ) _____ 130CC	JUNKET (100 GRAMS) _____ 80CC
★ MEASURES TAKEN ½" FROM RIM OF CONTAINER.	30CC = 1 OUNCE = 2 TBSP = 6 TSP

FORM M - 186
REV. 4 - 76
61860

December 4/77   B4
DATE   NURSING UNIT

Bed No.
206A

MRS
MR. MISS MRS.   UNIT NUMBER

DUVAL   MARIE
SURNAME   GIVEN NAME

Intake Required
2500cc

DR. A.S. SMITH
DOCTOR   BLOCK CAPITALS

ALL MEASUREMENTS IN CCs.

DAY			AFTERNOON			NIGHT		
HOUR	INTAKE	OUTPUT	HOUR	INTAKE	OUTPUT	HOUR	INTAKE	OUTPUT
0700		250	1500			2300		
0800	430		1600			2400		
0900			1700			0100		
1000	120	300	1800			0200		
1100			1900			0300		
1200	370		2000			0400		
1300		200	2100			0500		
1400	190		2200			0600		
Total	1000	750						

VANCOUVER GENERAL HOSPITAL
FLUID INTAKE AND OUTPUT   **DAY**

A simple bedside fluid intake and output record. (Courtesy of the Vancouver General Hospital.)

ature; that is, hot food should not be allowed to cool and cold food should not be allowed to warm.

3. Food should always be covered when it is being carried to the patient's bedside. Covering food helps not only to maintain the proper temperature but also to prevent drying out, which affects the flavor, texture, and appearance of food.

4. Food should be served as attractively as possible, in arranged portions, with garnishes to give color appeal. Small portions are more stimulating to the appetite than large portions.

5. The napkins, dishes, utensils, and the tray itself should be spotlessly clean.

6. The arrangement on the tray should be neat and organized. Any spilled food should be replaced.

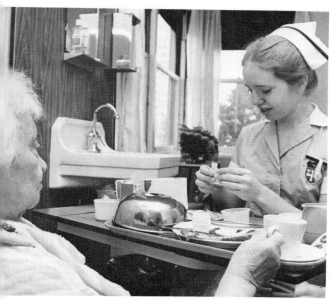

A relaxed, unhurried atmosphere and an attractively arranged tray contribute to the patient's enjoyment of a meal.

7. China and utensils should be attractive and in good condition.

8. The patient should always get the right tray with the right diet. Each tray has a card with the patient's name, bed number, and type of diet. If the nurse has any doubts as to the correctness of a patient's tray, she can check the diet orders before the patient is served.

Feeding the Patient

If it is necessary for the nurse to feed the patient, a few simple rules will make him more comfortable:

1. Whenever possible, use the utensils that are normally used for the food being served.
2. Never hurry the patient. Sit down to feed him whenever possible.
3. Offer the patient small rather than large amounts of food.
4. Offer the food in the order that the patient prefers.
5. Note whether any food or liquid is hot and

There are several types of drinking cups available commercially which can be useful to people who are ill.

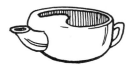

if it is, warn the patient to take only small portions or sips.

6. A straw or drinking cup will often help a patient to take liquids.
7. If the patient can hold bread or toast, let him manage it himself.
8. Be careful not to spill food. Wipe the patient's mouth and chin whenever necessary. Always protect the patient with a napkin.

After the patient has finished his meal, the tray is removed promptly. A patient is never hurried with his meal. If his fluid intake is to be recorded, the amounts are noted on his fluid sheet. The nurse should be familiar with the amount of fluid contained in the commonly used containers. Estimated volumes of consumed fluids suffice in most situations.

Patients should be provided with facilities for washing their hands and brushing their teeth after meals. This offers a good opportunity for the nurse to teach oral hygiene and the correct method for brushing teeth.

Preventive Measures

Dyspepsia. Preventive measures for the person with an actual or potential problem of indigestion are really common-sense measures related to eating habits. These include:

1. Eating small meals rather than large ones. Dividing the total daily food intake into five small meals—breakfast, lunch, a mid-afternoon snack (the British afternoon tea), a light supper, and a snack before bedtime—is often helpful for older people. Children, with their smaller stomach capacities, often do better with smaller meals and snacks at mid-morning and mid-afternoon and before bedtime than with three large meals. Pregnant women also benefit from having smaller, more frequent meals, as the growing fetus presses on the abdominal organs to effectively lessen stomach capacity.
2. Avoidance of coffee, tea, cola drinks, and other drinks containing caffeine.
3. Avoidance of fried foods and those high in fat content.
4. Avoidance of highly spiced foods.
5. Avoidance of any foods that the person has found to give him indigestion.
6. Having some mild exercise, such as walking, after meals.

Anorexia, Nausea, and Vomiting. The prevention of anorexia, nausea, and vomiting always involves a consideration of both the patient and his environment. Nursing measures that are effective in preventing these problems are often specific to the causes that have been discussed.

The nurse can often help the patient to identify situations and stimuli that are causing the problem. She can then help to modify or eliminate these. Frequently the patient is aware of events or subjective experiences, such as pain, which cause nausea and vomiting.

An environment that is clean and pleasant is helpful in stimulating the appetite and preventing nausea and vomiting. If the patient eats while he is in bed, the nurse can provide him with a clean table that is free of equipment. The emesis basin should be kept out of sight. If the patient feels more secure with it nearby, it can be kept within easy reach.

Unpleasant odors, sights, and sounds are noxious stimuli that may contribute to anorexia, nausea, or vomiting. To dissipate unpleasant odors, a well-ventilated room is important, and the use of deodorants may be necessary at times. Vomitus is always removed immediately and treatment trays are covered and placed as inconspicuously as possible.

Personal cleanliness is particularly important in the case of the person who has anorexia or a tendency to become nauseated. Other preventive measures include those described in the section earlier in this chapter on provision of nourishment for the sick.

In discussing measures that prevent anorexia, nausea, and vomiting, the use of tonics to improve the appetite and of antiemetic drugs to control nausea and vomiting must be included. Most physicians have their own preferences about tonics to improve the appetite. These are usually ordered 20 to 30 minutes before meals or may be given once or twice daily. Antiemetic drugs have a specific action on the vomiting center, and they may be given 20 to 30 minutes before mealtimes or otherwise as ordered. Many people who are susceptible to motion sickness travel much more comfortably if they take an antiemetic medicine shortly before embarking on a plane trip or other journey. It is well to remember that these drugs usually produce some drowsiness as a side effect.

Food Poisoning.   The prevention of food poisoning involves teaching people measures in regard to selecting, preparing, and storing foodstuffs and cooked foods to prevent unsafe quantities of disease-carrying bacteria (or their toxins) from being consumed. Such measures include:[9]

1. Buy from reputable dealers. Patronize only clean stores.
2. Keep hot foods hot (140° F, 60° C, or higher) and cold foods cold (40° F, 4° C, or lower).
3. After marketing, place frozen foods in the freezer compartment of your refrigerator or in a deep-freeze until ready for use.

4. Do not buy foods supposed to be frozen but which are thawed. Frozen foods that have been completely thawed or have been held at the refrigerator temperature more than one or two days should not be refrozen.
5. Heat pre-cooked frozen foods, like TV dinners and meat pies, for the time and temperature recommended on the labels. Read the labels.
6. Refrigerate "left-overs" from prepared dishes within an hour and keep refrigerated until re-serving or re-heating. Store left-over poultry and stuffing separately.
7. After preparing foods containing eggs, meat, milk, gravy, salads with dressing, such as sandwiches, picnic or buffet dishes: serve them within two hours or else refrigerate.
8. If canning foods at home: (a) always follow professional directions carefully; (b) never can non-acid foods such as meat, fish, meat-vegetable mixtures, soups, or non-acid vegetables like beans, peas, asparagus and corn, unless a pressure-cooker, properly attended, is used.
9. Do not taste foods from bulging and leaking cans, or cans whose contents spurt out or are bubbly, off-colour or off-odour.
10. Do not eat foods that have an "off" flavour.
11. Keep everything in your kitchen clean.

Safety, Comfort, and Hygiene Measures

In caring for seriously ill patients, who may not be fully conscious, the nurse should make sure that they are able to swallow before attempting to give them fluids or food. In assessing the swallowing reflex, the presence of the gagging reflex should be established first. A standard method of testing for the gagging reflex is to touch the back of the throat with an applicator or tongue depressor. If the gagging reflex is present, the person may be given small sips of water first, while the nurse watches for the swallowing movements in the neck. It is helpful to support the person's shoulders and head to make swallowing easier.

The nurse can assist the vomiting patient by holding a curved basin (emesis basin) under his chin to catch the vomitus, and supporting his head and shoulders. Most people find it easier to vomit when they are in a sitting position with the head bent over the basin. If the patient is lying down, his head should be turned to one side and his body placed in a side-lying position if possible. Again, the head should be supported. The patient who is lying on his back can choke and aspirate vomitus unless his head is raised and supported so that the vomitus can drain out of the mouth. In postoperative vomiting, the patient will find it less painful if the nurse supports his incision with her hands while he vomits.

The nurse should stay with the patient while he is vomiting. Vomiting is an unpleasant experience. Not only is it physically distressing but there is a loss of control and dignity which most people find embarrassing. The nurse can do much to reassure the patient by a calm acceptance of the situation and sympathetic yet efficient ministrations. For the patient's own feelings of dignity, and because most people find it distressing to watch someone vomiting, the patient should be screened from the view of others. Curtains can be quickly drawn around the patient's bed, or the door of his room closed to ensure privacy.

While the patient is vomiting, the nurse should provide him with tissues and help him to wipe his mouth. After he has stopped vomiting, mouth care and a hand and face wash will help him to feel more comfortable. Any linen that has been soiled should be changed promptly. The room should be aired and the patient allowed to rest.

If the patient is unable to tolerate food or fluids, frequent mouth care is essential to prevent complications (see Chapter 25).

Maintenance of Hydration and Nutritional Status

Helping the patient to maintain a satisfactory hydration and nutritional status is an important nursing function. Encouraging the individual to take fluids regularly helps him to attain adequate fluid intake. If he has difficulty in retaining fluids, giving him small amounts of fluid at frequent intervals is preferable to giving a large volume all at once. Patients who have been vomiting are usually permitted only clear fluids until vomiting subsides. Ginger ale and clear tea are frequently tolerated much better than other fluids when the stomach is upset. When other fluids are introduced into the patient's diet, those that are high in carbohydrate and protein are preferable because of the body's need for energy and tissue-building nutrients. For infants and small children, clear apple juice is often tolerated when milk is not. High carbohydrate fluids are also available on the market specifically for infants and small children.

People who are anorectic or nauseated may become more so when confronted with large servings of food. Small portions, attractively served, are usually more appealing. It is often necessary to cater to the individual's particular food preferences to encourage him to eat. Patients should also be assisted with their meals if they are unable to manage alone.

For patients who are unable to tolerate food

and fluids by mouth or are taking an insufficient quantity, fluids may be given intravenously. In some cases the patient is fed through a tube which is inserted into the stomach. This latter method of feeding is called a *gastric gavage*.

Many patients with gastrointestinal problems require gastric suction. This is a method of removing the gastric contents by means of suction apparatus. Patients on gastric suction are usually maintained with intravenous feedings to provide them with fluids and nourishment.

In some instances, it may be necessary to cleanse the stomach before further food and fluids can be taken, particularly if the individual has ingested some noxious substance. The procedure for washing out the stomach is called *gastric lavage*. This procedure is also frequently carried out prior to gastric surgery.

The description of a technique for carrying out each of these measures is detailed below.

In maintaining fluid and electrolyte balance, the accurate recording and reporting of fluid intake and output is essential. Both parenteral and oral intake must be accurately assessed. The patient can often help in recording the amount of fluid he drinks. If the patient is receiving gastric tube feedings, the amount given must be recorded accurately. On the output side, the amount of emesis should be measured or estimated when measurement is not feasible. In addition, drainage and suction returns should be included in the total output.

When the patient is receiving supplementary fluids, such as intravenous or interstitial therapy, the nurse is also responsible for the care specific to this therapy (see Chapter 17).

Gastric Intubation. The primary reasons for the insertion of a tube into the stomach or the intestine are:

1. To establish a means of draining the stomach by suction. This is often done when a patient has an obstruction of the gastrointestinal tract or has undergone surgery of the tract
2. For diagnostic purposes—for example, to identify the constituents or the volume of stomach contents or to identify malignant cells or microorganisms such as the tubercle bacillus in the gastric washings
3. To aspirate or wash out the stomach contents, as when a person has taken poisonous materials
4. To establish a route for feeding the patient who is unable to take nourishment by mouth

Four types of tubes that are commonly used for gastric intubation are (1) Levin tube, (2) Ewald tube, (3) Jutte tube, and (4) Rehfuss tube. The *Levin tube* is the one most commonly

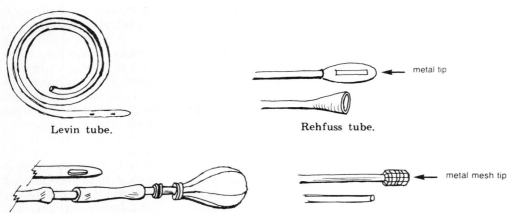

Types of gastric tubes. (From Rambo, B. J., and Wood, L. A.: *Nursing Skills for Clinical Practice.* 3rd ed. Philadelphia, W. B. Saunders Company, 1982, Vol. 2.)

used for gastric intubation. Both plastic and rubber tubes are available. The tip of the tube is solid, but there are several holes on the side. It is normally passed through the nose of the patient into his stomach. The insertion of a Levin tube may be either a physician's or a nurse's responsibility, depending on the policy of the health agency.

The *Ewald tube* is a rubber tube with a large opening (lumen) which is used to withdraw contents from the stomach. The *Jutte tube* has a small metal mesh tip. The *Rehfuss tube* also has a metal tip (not mesh). The metal, of course, is used to augment the force of gravity in facilitating passage of the tube down through the gastrointestinal tract. Usually, there are three markers on the tubes (in the form of black rings) to indicate how far the tube has been inserted: one band into the stomach, two bands into the pylorus, and three bands into the duodenum.

The Insertion of a Gastric Tube. Before the insertion of a gastric tube, the procedure is explained to the patient. Not only do most patients want to know how they can help, but explanations frequently allay fear. The passage of a tube is painless, but it sometimes stimulates the gag reflex as it passes over the nasopharyngeal area. If the patient breathes deeply at the first sign of gagging, he is less likely to become nauseated and vomit.

In the preparation of the equipment, if a rubber tube is used, it is placed in a bowl of chipped ice. This makes the tube more rigid (because cold causes contraction) and thus more easily directed on insertion. It also lubricates the tube. Usually a plastic Levin tube is sufficiently rigid for insertion, but it must also be lubricated with water.

In addition to the ice and the Levin tube, a protective covering, a kidney basin, tissues, a syringe, a cup, and a straw are required. A stethoscope is optional. The syringe is used to withdraw the stomach's contents after the Levin tube has been inserted. This also determines that the tube is positioned in the stomach. The cup and straw are to give the patient a drink of water to facilitate swallowing the tube.

If it is possible, the patient should be in Fowler's position. In this position the passage of the tube is facilitated by the pull of gravity; it is also easier for the patient in this position to spit out vomitus if this becomes necessary during the insertion of the tube.

The kidney basin and tissues are required because the patient may vomit. As noted previously, stimulation of the glossopharyngeal nerve endings in the posterior pharynx transmits impulses to the vomiting center in the medulla of the brain.

As a guide to the distance to which the tube is to be inserted, the nurse measures the distance from the patient's nose to an earlobe and then to the umbilicus. This distance is roughly equal to the distance from the lips to the stomach. The nurse then marks this distance on the tube with a piece of adhesive tape.

As a lubricant for the Levin tube, water has two advantages: (1) it moistens the tube and thus permits smoother passage of the tube over the mucous membranes, and (2) if the tube enters the lungs, the water is not likely to become a focus of irritation. Some agencies suggest that a water-soluble lubricant be used; such lubricants are less dangerous to the lungs than oil-base lubricants. The tube is inserted along the floor of the nose, as shown on page 293.

The Levin tube is never forced upon encoun-

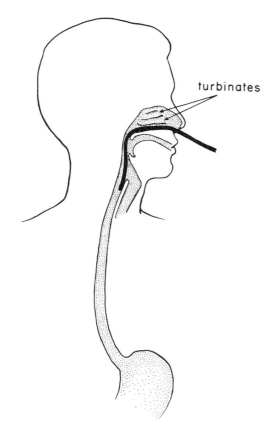

Insertion path for nasal tubes is along the floor of the nose. (From Wood, L. A., and Rambo, B. J.: *Nursing Skills for Allied Health Services*. 2nd ed. Philadelphia, W. B. Saunders Company, 1980, Vol. 3.)

tering an obstruction. Not only is force unpleasant to the patient, but damage to the mucous membrane that lines the gastrointestinal tract can easily occur and can provide a likely site for infection.

To facilitate the passage of the tube, the patient is given a mouthful of water to swallow as the tube in inserted into the esophagus. Swallowing helps to pass the tube down the esophagus into the patient's stomach by setting up peristaltic waves.

The stomach is never empty; it always contains at least a little gastric juice, which is secreted by the glands in the walls of the stomach. Therefore the position of the tube can be ascertained by aspirating with the syringe. The obtaining of gastric contents verifies that the tube is positioned in the patient's stomach. If gastric juice cannot be obtained, the following tests may be performed:

1. Place the free end of the tube in a container of water. An absence of bubbles indicates that the tube is in the stomach. Rhythmic bubbling usually indicates that the tube is in the patient's lungs.

2. Hold the end of the tube to the ear. A crackling sound usually indicates that the tube is in the patient's lungs.

3. Ask the patient to hum. If the tube is in the patient's lungs he will not be able to do this.

4. Inject a small amount of air with the syringe and then listen to the epigastrium with a stethoscope. A popping noise can be heard as the air enters the stomach.

If the patient coughs during the insertion of a tube, it should be removed immediately. Cyanosis and dyspnea usually indicate that the tube has entered the trachea. Once it has been ascertained that the Levin tube is in the patient's stomach, the tube is secured to the patient's face with a small piece of adhesive tape.

The Irrigation of a Levin Tube. The purpose of irrigating a Levin tube is to wash the lumen of the tube in order to maintain a clear passage. Usually this is not a sterile procedure unless the patient has just had stomach surgery. (If the patient has had surgery, it is important to maintain aseptic technique in all procedures involving the operative area.) The order to irrigate the Levin tube is issued by the physician. Irrigations are ordered for regular intervals, or they are done only when the tube becomes blocked. In either case it is important to watch the patient closely and note whether the tube becomes blocked. If the patient is on gastric suction, the most obvious sign of blockage is a lack of gastric returns from the tube. In addition, the patient is likely to feel uncomfortable and his abdomen will be distended.

After the nurse has provided the explanation that the patient requires and has reassured him that this is a painless measure, she assembles the necessary equipment. She requires a syringe, usually a 20 or 30 ml. syringe, or an Asepto syringe; the irrigating solution specifically ordered (often water or normal saline); and a receptacle for the returned irrigation fluid.

Between 15 and 30 ml. of fluid is injected into the tube before the plunger is gently drawn back to withdraw the fluid. Because the mucous membrane lining of the stomach is easily damaged, the fluid is injected and withdrawn very gently. This measure is repeated until the tube is cleared. If fresh blood appears as a result of the irrigation, the measure is terminated and the information is reported to the physician. During the irrigation the nurse observes the color and consistency of the returning fluid. This is recorded on the patient's chart.

Gastric Suction. The purpose of gastric suction is to remove the contents of the patient's stom-

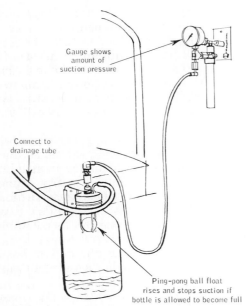

Wall-mounted suction apparatus. (From Sutton, A. L.: *Bedside Nursing Techniques in Medicine and Surgery*. 2nd ed. Philadelphia, W. B. Saunders Company, 1969.)

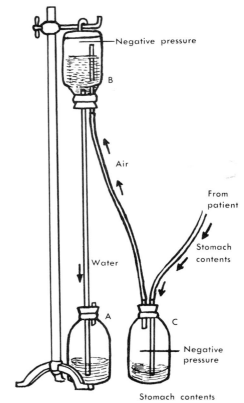

The water displacement method of producing suction.

ach. It is indicated as a measure to prevent or relieve distention and vomiting, to remove blood postoperatively, and to remove the stomach contents of patients who have gastrointestinal obstructions. It may also be used as a measure to cleanse the stomach prior to gastric surgery.

Generally speaking, there are two types of gastric suction: continuous and intermittent. Continuous suction is applied continuously (as the name indicates); intermittent suction is turned on and off as the patient requires or, usually, on the physician's order.

There are four basic ways of supplying suction. The first is by using the electric suction machine, which is portable and can be brought to the patient. It is run by electricity and the amount of suction can usually be regulated. The second method of supplying suction in acute care hospitals today is by means of suction apparatus built into the wall. There are usually suction outlets at the head of the patient's bed. The pressure of wall suction systems can be regulated by the nursing personnel.

The third method of supplying suction is by the use of the principle of displacement of water. Systems based on this method do not require electricity and are simple to construct. There are both two- and three-bottle systems. Simply explained, the water falls by gravity from bottle B to bottle A (see the accompanying illustration). This creates a vacuum in bottle B. If bottle B is connected directly to the patient's gastric tube, the vacuum is transmitted to his stomach, with

the result that the stomach's contents flow to bottle B, that is, from a high pressure area to a low pressure area. If, on the other hand, bottle B is connected to bottle C, and bottle C is connected to the patient's gastric tube, the stomach contents will be received in bottle C.

A Gomco Thermotic pump. (From Sutton, A. L.: *Bedside Nursing Techniques in Medicine and Surgery*. 2nd ed. Philadelphia, W. B. Saunders Company, 1969.)

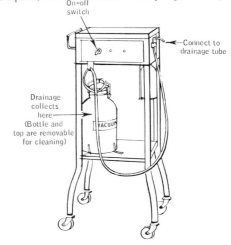

A fourth means of supplying suction is by the Gomco Thermotic pump, which is electrically operated but is motorless. This pump provides intermittent suction through the alternate contraction and expansion of air.

When a patient requires gastric suction, he will probably find the constant presence of the gastric tube irritating to his throat, and it is likely that he will not be able to take fluids by mouth. Therefore, he requires special care for his mouth and nose so that they do not become dry, cracked, and subsequently infected. To ease the irritation by the tube on the patient's throat, the patient is often allowed to have throat lozenges or to chew gum.

Since gastric suction returns are an important part of the patient's fluid output, the nurse measures the amount of drainage accurately, and she notes the clarity, color, and consistency of the drainage. These observations are reported on the patient's record. Any untoward changes in the patient's suction returns, such as bright red returns, or in the patient's condition, such as an accelerated pulse, are reported promptly so that the physician can be notified.

Gastric Lavage. Gastric lavage is the washing out of the stomach. It is done prior to some types of gastric surgery or to remove noxious substances from the stomach. It is often an emergency procedure, carried out in the emergency unit of a hospital or in a doctor's office.

For a gastric lavage an Ewald tube frequently is used. It has a larger lumen than the Levin tube, and it may have a funnel at one end to facilitate the administration of the fluid for washing the patient's stomach. Because the lavage tube has a larger lumen than the Levin tube, it is usually inserted through the patient's mouth into his stomach. When a Levin tube is used, it can be inserted through the patient's nose or through his mouth.

The equipment required for a gastric lavage consists of the lavage tube and funnel, the solution ordered by the physician, a pail to receive stomach contents, ice in which to place the tube if a rubber one is used, a kidney basin for vomitus, and a protective covering for the patient.

Usually 500 ml. of solution is administered into the patient's stomach, and the funnel is then inverted to allow the stomach's contents to empty into the pail. To create a siphon, the tube is pinched while some of the fluid is still in it. Then it is lowered and inverted below the level of the patient's body and held inside the pail. Gravity drains the fluid from the tubing, and the vacuum thus established in the tubing draws the liquid from the patient's stomach. The washing is repeated until it is considered that the stomach is satisfactorily cleansed.

During the lavage the nurse notes the reaction of the patient, the amount and kind of solution used, and the amount, color, and consistency of the returns. These observations are reported in the patient's record. Following gastric lavage, the patient usually needs a mouthwash.

Gastric Gavage. A gastric gavage is a feeding given to a patient through a tube which is inserted either through his nose or through his mouth into his stomach. It is done when the patient is unable to take food orally. The feeding can be given in two ways: at intervals as ordered (for example, every 4 hours), or as a continuous drip over the 24-hour period. The latter method is usually indicated when the patient has diarrhea, gastric irritability, or a reflex bowel disturbance.

The food used for a gavage feeding is usually given as a thick liquid. A typical tube feeding might include powdered milk, cream, cereal, strained meats and vegetables, orange juice, corn oil, sugar, iodized salt, vitamin compounds, and water, blended into liquid form. The feeding may be made up using different amounts of various nutrients in order to meet the patient's dietary needs.

It is the physician's responsibility to order the type of nourishment that the patient requires. In some health agencies a regular house diet is mixed in a blending machine so that it can be fed by gavage tube.

A gastric gavage or tube feeding is frequently given when the patient is unable to take food orally.

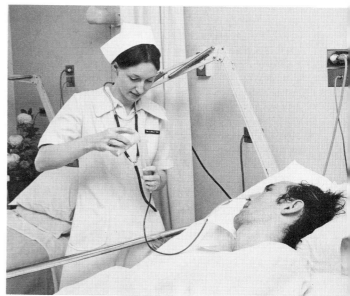

Often the patient who is to receive a gavage feeding has a Levin tube already inserted. If this is not the case, the tube may be inserted by the physician or the nurse, depending on agency policy. The nurse explains to the patient that feeding through the tube is painless and will provide him with adequate water and nourishment.

The nurse heats the feeding to room temperature. Sometimes it is ordered that the stomach be aspirated prior to a new feeding to determine if the food is being passed into the intestinal tract. Before commencing the feeding the nurse should raise the head of the bed, unless this is contraindicated. She then injects a small amount of water into the tube to make sure that the lumen is clear. A disposable feeding bag may be used or the feeding may be injected by syringe. If a disposable bag is used it may be hung on an intravenous standard, and the rate of flow adjusted as desired. If the syringe method is used, care is taken to allow as little air as possible to be injected into the patient's stomach. The feeding should always be given slowly. Usually the gavage feeding flows through the tubing by gravitational force. However, if it does not do this readily, slight pressure can be applied on the plunger of the syringe. After the completion of the feeding, a small amount of water is again inserted into the tubing in order to clear the lumen of the tube of the gavage feeding. This prevents souring of any formula in the tube. Some patients learn to administer their own gavage feedings.

The nurse records the amount of the gavage feeding that the patient has taken, as well as the amount of water that was administered. Should the patient start to gag or vomit during the gavage feeding, the feeding is terminated, and the situation is reported to the physician and recorded in the patient's record.

If the patient is to have a continuous gavage, a Baron food pump or a burette (glass or plastic container) and tubing may be used. The burette is hung to the side of the patient at a level just above him. The nurse adjusts the rate of flow of the gavage feeding as ordered. She also maintains a level of gavage fluid in the burette. The patient is observed at frequent intervals for any untoward signs resulting from the feeding.

Total Parenteral Nutrition (Hyperalimentation). When the body is seriously depleted of nutrients, it is often necessary to replace these by giving greater than normal amounts. If the person is unable to take these orally, they are frequently given by intravenous infusion. The terms *total parenteral nutrition* (or simply the

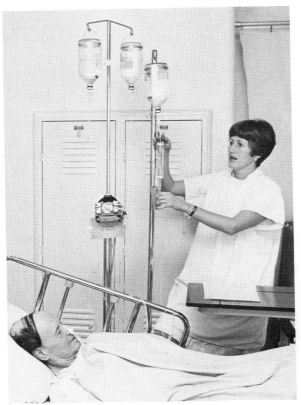

Hyperalimentation is a method of giving large amounts of nutrients via the intravenous route to patients whose nutritional reserves have been seriously depleted.

initials TPN) and *parenteral hyperalimentation* are used to refer to the intravenous administration of hypertonic nutrient solutions. The solution is administered slowly through a central venous catheter directly into the superior vena cava, where it is rapidly diluted by the large blood flow there. Because the danger of infection is very great, it is important that the sterility of the entire system be maintained. The number of people mixing the solutions, changing the bottles, and changing the dressing at the site of the infusion is restricted as much as possible.

Planning and Evaluating Specific Nursing Interventions

The long-range goals for nursing action, as we have mentioned before, provide general directions for nursing care. The patient who is reluctant to eat, for example, might be expected to achieve an outcome such as "eats all of his meals each day," or the objectives might be less than that to start with and gradually increased. For people taking in a less than adequate amount of fluids, the target intake should be specific and, again, a gradual increase in daily targets may be helpful. It is essential that the patient be involved in the planning unless he is too ill to be, and, if possible, encouraged to assist in keeping track of his food and fluid intake.

Evaluation of the expected outcomes depends on targets set by the nurse and the patient cooperatively. It is helpful if these have been specifically stated. Some of the questions for the nurse to keep in mind, however, are:

1. Is the individual eating his meals?
2. Does he enjoy them?
3. Is his intake of food and fluids adequate to meet his daily requirements?
4. How do you know that it is?
5. If the patient is on a special diet, is he adhering to it?
6. If he is in hospital, does he select foods that are compatible with his prescribed diet from the diet menu?

The nurse also observes the patient to assess his nutritional status and the progress made toward achieving the long-range goals. Comparison of her observations of the patient with the characteristics of good nutrition and poor nutrition are again helpful in this regard.

Dyspepsia, anorexia, nausea, and vomiting may be actual or potential problems. They may be accompanied by, or lead to, other problems. The problems of malnutrition, dehydration, and fluid and electrolyte imbalance must always be considered if any of these problems persist. In infants and small children, all three can develop very quickly, particularly in the child who is vomiting. Other problems that often occur are pain and discomfort and problems associated with dehydration, such as dryness of the mucous membranes lining the oral cavity and parched, dry, or cracking lips (see Chapter 17).

When specific problems have been identified, expected outcomes for nursing intervention need to be developed. For example, for the person who is vomiting, one expected outcome might be stated as "takes small amounts of clear fluids every hour and retains them." The outcome may be subsequently changed to "tolerates a full liquid diet," if the vomiting does not persist. (In this case, the vomiting might become a potential problem, rather than an actual one.) In many instances, the expected outcome of nursing intervention is the absence of the problem, which may be stated in terms of prevention, as in "prevent further weight loss," or more positively, as in "maintains present weight" or "shows consistent weight gain daily." The identification of the problem is followed by the selection of appropriate nursing measures to resolve it. Many nursing interventions are directed toward teaching the individual measures to ameliorate the problem or to prevent its recurrence. There are usually many teaching tasks when diagnostic or therapeutic measures, such as those described later in the chapter, are necessary.

Evaluation is dependent on the outcomes expected from nursing intervention. A guide to evaluating the effectiveness of nursing intervention is included at the end of the chapter. You may want to add other questions that relate to specific problems you have identified in patients and their expected outcomes.

GUIDE TO ASSESSING NUTRITIONAL STATUS

1. What are this person's age, sex, height, type of body frame, usual weight, and present weight?

2. How does his weight compare with national standards for height and weight?

3. What are his usual habits with regard to eating?

4. What are his usual daily activities? His current activity level? What is his present status with regard to food and fluid intake?

5. Is his intake of food and fluids adequate to meet his daily requirements for nutrients and energy-giving foods?

6. What is his general physical condition? Does he appear obese? thin? emaciated?

7. Does he show characteristics of good nutrition? of poor nutrition? of severe malnutrition?

8. What do the results of his latest physical examination show relative to his nutritional status? What diagnostic tests or examinations were done (blood, urine, x-ray studies)? What were the results?

9. Does he have a health problem which may be affecting his intake of food, or his digestive abilities?

10. What is his emotional status? His attitude toward food?

11. Does the patient have cultural, religious, or moral beliefs or values concerning food which conflict with his dietary needs?

12. Is the individual on a special diet?

13. Does he understand the purpose of it? Is he adhering to it?

14. Does the patient need extra fluids?

15. Does he need help with his meals?

16. Are there foods the patient needs to avoid or to eat?

17. Does the patient or his family need help with planning meals to provide optimal nutrition? Will altering existing patterns of dietary intake because of a special condition cause any problems? Do they need help with basic nutrition matters?

GUIDE TO ASSESSING THE PATIENT WITH DYSPEPSIA, ANOREXIA, NAUSEA, OR VOMITING

1. What is the nature of the patient's problem? Is he anorectic, is he nauseated, or has he been vomiting? Is he suffering from indigestion?

2. If the patient is vomiting, is the airway clear? Can vomitus drain from the mouth? What is the nature of the vomitus? its amount? How often does he vomit?

3. How long has he had this problem? Is it related to a specific cause, such as particular foods, medications, or stressful situations?

4. Does the patient have other distressing symptoms, such as headache or pain?

5. How much food and fluid is the patient taking?

6. Does he show signs of poor nutritional status? of dehydration?

7. Have specific laboratory tests or examinations been ordered? If so, what are the nurse's responsibilities relative to these? What learning needs does the patient have with regard to them?

8. Have specific diagnostic or therapeutic measures been prescribed? If so, what is the nurse's responsibility relative to these? What are the patient's learning needs with regard to these?

9. Are there factors in the environment that contribute to the patient's discomfort? Can these be modified?

10. What nursing measures can contribute to the patient's safety, comfort, and hygiene?

GUIDE TO EVALUATING THE EFFECTIVENESS OF NURSING INTERVENTIONS

1. Has the patient adopted better eating habits, including an adequate, nutritious diet?

2. Have the symptoms of digestive disorders been alleviated? That is, has vomiting stopped? Is nausea less troublesome? Is the patient beginning to regain his appetite? Is he free from indigestion?

3. If he is still vomiting, is the patient safeguarded from aspirating any vomitus?

4. Is the patient comfortable?

5. Is he able to retain fluids for gradually extended periods of time?

6. Is he able to take and retain adequate food and fluids for his nutritional needs?

7. Do results of laboratory tests reflect adequate nutrition?

STUDY SITUATION (1)

Susan James, aged 20, works at a day-care center and lives on a communal farm at the edge of town with five other people. All the members of the commune are vegetarians, their staple diet consisiting of rice, whole-grain cereals, and organic fruits and vegetables which they grow on the farm. Susan has not been feeling well for the past few days. She was admitted to hospital this morning suffering from severe abdominal pains and diarrhea, with a tentative diagnosis of regional enteritis. She is 5 feet 2 inches (157 cm.) tall. Her wrist measurement is 6 inches (15.24 cm.), and she weighs 95 lbs. (43.1 kg). She looks thin and pale. Laboratory test results show that her blood levels of hemoglobin, hematocrit, and serum protein are below normal. The physician has ordered bed rest and a high calorie, high protein diet with a vitamin B_{12} supplement for Susan. He has also ordered an iron preparation to be given parenterally.

1. What are some of the factors contributing to Susan's nutritional problem?

2. What information would you need to be able to help Susan?

3. Where would you obtain this information?

4. What are some of the objective signs you might observe in Susan?

5. How much is she below the average weight for her height and body frame?

6. What subjective observations might you note?

7. What factors would you take into consideration in developing a plan of care for Susan?

8. What specific nursing interventions would you consider in Susan's care?

9. How would you evaluate the effectiveness of these interventions?

STUDY SITUATION (2)

Mrs. W. Stanley had her appendix removed 3 days ago. Since she returned from the operating room, she has been nauseated continually and vomits after every meal. Mrs. Stanley says she has severe pain in her operative area, and she is reluctant to eat and to get out of bed. The doctor has ordered that she get up and walk to the bathroom at least three times a day and that she have food and fluids as tolerated.

1. What are the possible reasons for this patient's nausea and vomiting?

2. What nursing interventions might help her?

3. What specific observations should the nurse make about the patient?

4. When the patient says she does not want to get out of bed, what should the nurse do?

5. How could the nurse possibly increase Mrs. Stanley's appetite?

6. What dangers and complications might result from the vomiting?

7. By what criteria can the nurse evaluate the effectiveness of her nursing care?

SELECTED READINGS

Asian Diet Fact Sheet: Cultural and Religious Backgrounds. *Nursing Times, 73*:108–110, November 10, 1977.

Baldwin, W.: Anorexia Nervosa. *Nursing Times, 71*:134–135, January 23, 1974.

Chung, H. J.: Understanding the Oriental Maternity Patient. *Nursing Clinics of North America, 12*:67–75, March, 1977.

Ciseaux, A.: Anorexia Nervosa: A View from the Mirror. *American Journal of Nursing, 80*(8):1468–1470, August, 1980.

Claggett, M. S.: Anorexia Nervosa: A Behavioral Approach. *American Journal of Nursing, 80*(8):1471–1472, August, 1980.

Colley, R., and Wilson, J.: Meeting a Patient's Needs with Hyperalimentation. *Nursing '79:* Part 1, 9(5):76–83, May, 1979; Part 2, 9(6):57–61, June, 1979; Part 3, 9(7):50–53, July, 1979; Part 4, 9(8):56–63, August, 1979; Part 5, 9(9):62–69, September, 1979.

Diekelmann, N. L.: The Young Adult: The Choice Is Health or Illness. *American Journal of Nursing, 76*(8):1272–1277, August, 1976.

Gillis, D.: Adapting Foodstyle: Counseling Tips. *Canadian Nurse, 77*(3):19, March, 1981.

Hoppe, M.: The New Tube Feeding Sets: A Nursing '80 Product Survey. *Nursing '80, 10*(3):25–33, March, 1980.

Iveson-Iveson, J.: Prevention: How to Stay Healthy: The General Picture and Diet (Part I). *Nursing Mirror, 149*:27, September 13, 1979.

Johnson, M.: Folk Beliefs and Ethnocultural Behavior in Pediatrics. *Nursing Clinics of North America, 12*:77–84, March, 1977.

Keithley, J. K.: Proper Nutritional Assessment Can Prevent Hospital Malnutrition. *Nursing '79, 9*(2):68–72, February, 1979.

Kornguth, M. L.: When Your Client Has a Weight Problem: Nursing Management. *American Journal of Nursing, 81*(3):553–554, March, 1981.

Langford, R. W.: When Your Client Has a Weight Problem: Teenagers and Obesity. *American Journal of Nursing, 81*(3):556–559, March, 1981.

McCreary, C. S., et al.: When Your Client Has a Weight Problem: Pickwickian Syndrome. *American Journal of Nursing, 81*(3):555, March, 1981.

Melton, J. H.: A Boy with Anorexia Nervosa. *American Journal of Nursing, 74*:1649–1651, September, 1974.

Miller, B. R.: When Your Client Has a Weight Problem: Jejunoileal Bypass: A Drastic Weight Control Measure. *American Journal of Nursing, 81*(3):564–568, March, 1981.

Misik, I.: Dr. Evans, Obsessed with Food, Was Starving Himself. *Nursing '80, 10*(3):54–56, March, 1980.

Mojzisik, C. M., et al.: When Your Client Has a Weight Problem: Gastric Partitioning. The Latest Surgical Means to Control Morbid Obesity. *American Journal of Nursing, 81*(3):569–572, March, 1981.

Naish, J.: Discomfort after Food. *Nursing Times, 71*:2060–2062, December 25, 1975.

Parker, C.: Food Allergies. *American Journal of Nursing, 80*(2):262–265, February, 1980.

Richardson, T. F.: Anorexia Nervosa: An Overview. *American Journal of Nursing, 80*(8):1470–1471, August, 1980.

Salmond, S. W.: How to Assess the Nutritional Status of Acutely Ill Patients. *American Journal of Nursing, 80*(5):922–924, May, 1980.

Schmidt, M. P. W., et al.: Modifying Eating Behavior in Anorexia Nervosa. *American Journal of Nursing, 74*:1646–1648, September, 1974.

Scogna, D. M., and Smalley, R.: Chemotherapy-induced Nausea and Vomting. *American Journal of Nursing, 79*(9):1562–1565, September, 1979.

Shubin, S.: Nursing Patients from Other Cultures. *Nursing '80, 10*(6):78–81, June, 1980.

Speck, P.: East Comes West. *Nursing Times, 72*:662–664, April 25, 1976.

When Your Client Has a Weight Problem: Overeaters Anonymous. *American Journal of Nursing, 81*(3):560–563, March, 1981.

White, J. H., et al.: When Your Client Has a Weight Problem: Nursing Assessment. *American Journal of Nursing, 81*(3):549–553, March, 1981.

Williams, E. J.: Food for Thought: Meeting the Nutritional Needs of the Elderly. *Nursing '80, 10*(9):60–63, September, 1980.

Yen, P. K.: Fast Food . . . Is It Junk? *Geriatric Nursing, 2*:184, May-June, 1982.

REFERENCES

1. Briggs, G. M., and Calloway, D. H.: *Bogert's Nutrition and Physical Fitness.* Philadelphia, Saunders College Publishing, 1979.

2. Overfield, T.: Biological Variation Concepts from Physical Anthropology. *Nursing Clinics of North America, 12*:19–26, March, 1977.

3. Chappelle, M. L.: The Language of Food. *American Journal of Nursing,* 72:1294–1295, July, 1972.
4. Robertson, L., et al.: *Laurel's Kitchen: A Handbook for Vegetarian Cookery and Nutrition.* Petaluma, California, Nilgiri Press, 1976.
5. Report of Nutrition Canada National Survey, 1970–1972. Ottawa, Department of National Health and Welfare, 1975.
6. Keithley, J.: Proper Nutritional Assessment Can Prevent Hospital Malnutrition. *Nursing '79,* 9(2):68–72, February, 1979.
7. Russell, G. F. M.: Anorexia Nervosa. In Wyngaarden, J. B., and Smith, L. H.: *Cecil Textbook of Medicine.* 16th ed. Philadelphia, W. B. Saunders Company, 1982, pp. 1379–1382.
8. Lowenberg, M. E., et al.: *Food and Man.* New York, John Wiley & Sons, 1968.
9. *Selected Nutrition Teaching Aids.* Ottawa, Department of National Health and Welfare, 1976.

15

The Nurse Should Be Able to:

- Discuss the importance of adequate urinary elimination to the health and well-being of the individual
- Describe normal functioning with regard to urinary elimination in infants, children, and adults
- Discuss factors that may cause disturbances of urinary functioning
- Assess a person's urinary elimination status
- Identify common problems people have with urinary elimination
- Identify situations requiring immediate nursing intervention in the care of patients with problems of urinary functions
- Apply relevant principles in planning and implementing nursing interventions in patients
   a. to promote optimal urinary functioning
   b. to prevent potential urinary problems
   c. to restore normal voiding patterns in patients with alterations in urinary elimination
- Evaluate the effectiveness of nursing interventions

URINARY ELIMINATION NEEDS

CHAPTER 15

INTRODUCTION

In order to maintain effective functioning, the human body must rid itself of wastes. The body has four principal mechanisms for the removal of wastes products: from the urinary tract as urine, from the gastrointestinal tract as feces, through the skin as perspiration, and through the lungs in expired air. Each mechanism has its specific function in clearing the body of wastes resulting from the processing of nutrients and their subsequent utilization in the cells.

In this chapter, we will discuss urinary elimination, the common problems associated with it, and measures that nurses can use to help people with these problems. We will discuss bowel elimination in Chapter 16, the mechanism of perspiration as a means of waste removal in Chapter 17, and the removal of wastes through the lungs in Chapter 18.

Most of the nitrogenous wastes of cellular metabolism are excreted in the urine. In addition, the urinary system plays an important role in maintaining the fluid and electrolyte balance of the body. Both of these functions are essential in the maintenance of physiological homeostasis.

The act of voiding is also an important area of independent functioning for an individual. Control over voiding is learned early in childhood, and actual or potential loss of independence in regard to this vital function constitutes a serious threat to the individual's social and emotional well-being. If such a loss occurs, he fears it will mean a return to the dependent state of infancy, and his feelings of self-esteem are markedly jeopardized.

Most people have difficulty in discussing urinary functioning and problems they may have in connection with it. In our culture, there are social taboos about the subject of elimination and, once a child has been toilet-trained, he is taught that this topic is not talked about in polite company. The act of voiding is also done privately in our society. Then, too, the intimate anatomical relationship between the urinary and the reproductive tracts contributes to making urinary functioning a sensitive topic. Necessary intervention is a potential source of embarrassment for both the nurse and the patient, particularly if one is male and the other female. If the nurse can discuss urinary elimination and carry out necessary nursing measures matter-of-factly, without showing signs of embarrassment herself, this can go a long way towards putting the patient at ease.

ANATOMY AND PHYSIOLOGY OF THE URINARY TRACT

The urinary tract consists of the kidneys, the ureters, the bladder, and the urethra. Normally, a person has two kidneys. These are situated in the back part of the abdominal cavity, behind the peritoneum and just below the diaphragm, one on either side of the spinal column.

The kidneys are complex organs whose chief functions are the elimination of waste products of body metabolism and the control of the concentration of the various constituents of body fluid, including the blood. These functions are accomplished through an efficient filtering system that removes the excess water, acid, and other wastes from the blood as it passes through the kidney. The blood retains the essential elements needed by the body through selective reabsorption. Blood comes to the kidney through the renal artery and is filtered in the glomeruli of the nephrons. The filtrate contains water, the waste products of metabolism, electrolytes, and glucose. These products pass along the nephron's tubules, where some solutes and water are reabsorbed. The tubules also secrete substances such as drugs into the urine.

The body can continue to function effectively even though a considerable amount of kidney tissue has been damaged—indeed, even if one kidney is absent or does not function at all.

The ureters are long, narrow muscular tubes

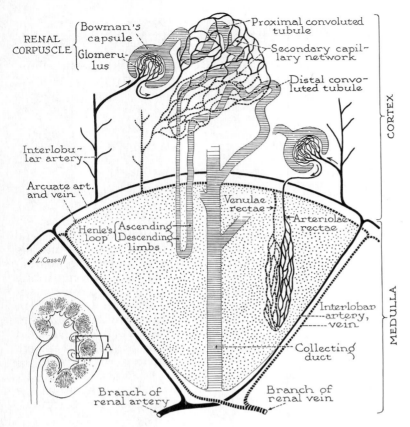

RENAL CORPUSCLE { Bowman's capsule / Glomerulus }

Proximal convoluted tubule

Secondary capillary network

Distal convoluted tubule

Interlobular artery

Arcuate art. and vein

Henle's loop { Ascending / Descending limbs }

Venulae rectae

Arteriolae rectae

CORTEX

MEDULLA

Interlobar artery, vein

Collecting duct

Branch of renal artery

Branch of renal vein

L.Cassell

A

A nephron. (From King, B. G., and Showers, M. J.: *Human Anatomy and Physiology*. 6th edition. Philadelphia, W. B. Saunders Company, 1969.)

The urinary system.

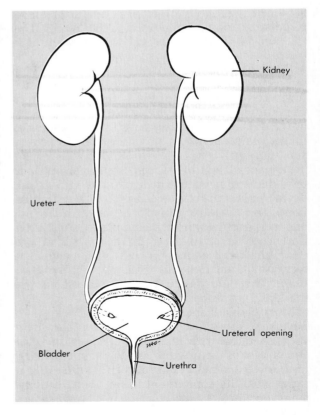

Kidney

Ureter

Ureteral opening

Bladder

Urethra

which serve to transport urine from the kidneys to its storehouse, the bladder.

The chief function of the bladder is to retain urine until it can be excreted. The average adult bladder holds 300 to 500 ml. of urine; however, the bladder has been known to hold 3000 to 4000 ml. of urine. The bladder is a hollow muscular organ whose efficient functioning depends upon the maintenance of muscle tone in the bladder wall and upon the integrity of the nervous system innervating the bladder.

The bladder, when empty, lies in folds in the pelvic cavity. As urine enters it in rhythmic spurts from the ureters, the walls of the bladder expand and it expands into the pelvic cavity, thrusting upwards in the abdominal cavity. When a sufficient amount of urine has accumulated in the bladder, normally 300 to 500 ml. in the adult, sensory impulses are sent to the spinal cord and thence to higher centers in the brain. The individual becomes aware of the urge to void. If there are no inhibiting factors, the muscle of the bladder wall contracts and the internal sphincter at the base of the bladder relaxes, allowing urine to flow into the urethra. The stimulus allowing this act is a stretch reflex that is evoked by increase in pressure as the bladder fills with urine. The action is essentially a cord reflex, although it may be facilitated or inhibited by higher centers.

Micturition—the act of voiding—is normally under voluntary control after about the age of 3 to 4 years. This control is exerted via a second external sphincter muscle. The external sphincter is located about the middle of the urethra—in men, just as the urethra enters the glans penis.

The urethra itself is a short, muscular tube whose function is to carry urine from the bladder to its exit point from the body. In women, the urethra is approximately 3 to 5 cm. (1¼ to 2 inches) long; it opens just above the vagina. In men, the urethra is about 20 cm. (8 inches) long from its origin in the bladder to its external opening in the glans penis. It crosses the length of the penis and carries the products of both the urinary tract and the reproductive tract in the male. Meatus is the term used for the external opening of the urethra in both men and women.

The entire urinary tract is lined with a continuous layer of mucous membrane that stretches from the meatus to the pelvis of the kidney.

NORMAL URINARY FUNCTIONING

The average adult usually excretes between 1000 and 1500 ml. of urine in a 24-hour period. The total volume varies with the amount of fluid intake and also with the amount of fluids lost through other routes, such as sweating, vomiting, or diarrhea.

The pattern of voiding—that is, the number of times a person voids during the day and the amount eliminated each time— is highly individualized. In depends on a number of factors, such as early childhood training, habitual response to the urge to urinate (nurses are noted for delaying their response to this impulse in themselves), the amount of fluids consumed, and the capacity of the individual's bladder, among other things. Most people void first thing in the morning, possibly four to six times during the day, and again before retiring. A person does not usually have to get up at night to void unless he has consumed a large amount of fluids prior to bedtime.

In appearance, normal urine is clear and straw-colored or light amber. The darker the color, the more concentrated it is. The specific gravity of urine has a normal range of 1.003 to 1.030. Usually, the first urine voided in the morning is more concentrated than that excreted at other times of the day.

Normal urine has a pH of 4.8 to 8.0; it is usually slightly acidic (with a pH around 6) in people on normal diets. When left to stand, urine gradually becomes alkaline, owing to the disintegration of its constituents, and a cloudy sediment develops.

Freshly voided urine has a faintly aromatic odor, which becomes stronger on standing. Normally urine contains creatinine, uric acid, urea, and a few white blood cells. It does not normally contain bacteria, red blood cells, sugar, albumin, acetone, casts, pus, or calculi (stones that form in the urinary tract).

VARIATIONS IN URINARY FUNCTIONING THROUGHOUT THE LIFE CYCLE

The normal newborn infant voids within the first 24 hours of life. If the infant has not voided by the end of 24 hours, this usually indicates a serious problem. It is important then to note whether the infant is wet or dry each time it is changed during the first 24 hours. The voiding may have been missed if it occurred during delivery, but if there has been no voiding, attention should be drawn to the fact. The newborn infant has a limited capacity to concentrate or dilute urine and the small infant may void up to 18 times a day or more. The urine of infants is usually dilute and odorless. The frequency of voiding usually decreases gradually during infancy, although this is highly dependent on the amount of fluids consumed and on the surrounding temperature. The body temperature of the infant is much more affected by environmental temperatures than that of adults, and more fluids are needed for internal body processes when body temperature is high (see Chapter 19).

The infant's renal reserve capacity is much smaller than that of adults. By the end of the first year, however, the kidneys have reached their full functional capacity.

By the time a child has reached early childhood, the specific gravity and other urine findings are similar to those in adults. Children usually have to void more frequently than adults do, because of their smaller bladders. The urge to void is usually more urgently felt in children too, although if they are busy they may not heed it at first and then have to race to the bathroom.

The neurophysiological pathways necessary for voluntary control of the bladder mature later than those for bowel control. Most children become physiologically ready to stay dry in their third year.

By the time the child goes to school, he has pretty well mastered the art of controlling his bladder, although accidents may still happen if the child is under stress or gets too busy, particularly with outdoor activities, to get to a bathroom in time.

In children, a proportionately larger amount of body weight is in a fluid state than in adults. Children, therefore, excrete a greater volume of urine in proportion to body weight. The school-age child (from 6 to 12 years) voids as much as some adults—up to 1000 ml. in a day, which is the low range of normal for adults. Because of their smaller bladders, however, they still need to void more frequently than do adults.

As the child grows, his bladder also grows and its capacity increases. The proportionate amount of his weight that is in fluids decreases. His urinary elimination usually settles into an adult pattern well before adolescence. Unless problems develop, the pattern continues through adulthood, with variations as noted below.

The pregnant woman usually finds that she has to void more often and with great urgency, particularly during the early and late stages of her pregnancy. These problems are due to pressure by the enlarging womb on the bladder and, also, it is felt, to hormonal changes that are taking place within her body. There is a dilation of the urinary system, which is partly due to pressure, but there is also a relaxation of smooth muscle due to hormonal changes. This dilation may lead to stasis (or slowing down) of urine flow, with a resultant increased vulnerability to urinary tract infections.

During the middle years of adulthood, many women who have had children begin to have difficulty in retaining urine within the bladder as the muscles of the pelvic floor, weakened by childbirth, begin to lose their tone. A small amount of urine may leak out of the bladder if the person laughs heartily, coughs, or sneezes.

A generalized loss of muscle tone and lessened efficiency of the kidneys contribute to the need many older people (both men and women) have to void more frequently than younger adults, usually with increased feelings of urgency.

Toilet Training of Children

Many times, you, as a nurse, will be asked by mothers of toddlers about toilet training. One of the most important considerations is to help the mother to have a relaxed attitude toward toilet training. In our North American culture, a great deal of emphasis has been placed on the ritual of toilet training. In many other parts of the world, little children run around bare-bottomed until the age of 4 or so, and no one seems to worry about it. Toilet training is not a big deal. While having a child run around without diapers or pants is not recommended for public health reasons, there is something to be said for the relaxed manner in which mothers in other cultures approach the task of toilet training. We have used the word mother throughout this discussion, but the father often takes part in the

training too, and sometimes a grandmother or baby-sitter is responsible for it.

The nurse who is advising should remember the principles of learning (see Chapter 11). Toilet training is a learning experience for the child, and the same principles apply as in any learning experience. Mother is the teacher of the child.

Toilet training should not begin until the child has reached the stage when voluntary control over elimination is possible. The neuromuscular structures are not developed sufficiently for bowel control until the age of 15 to 18 months. "Exceptional" children may use the potty before this age but, in most instances, it is mother who has been trained to put the child on the potty at certain intervals, or at a time of day when he usually has a bowel movement. (When the child is ready for toilet training, the mother can take advantage of this regularity if a pattern has evolved, as it does in most children.) Children who are trained too early are often the ones who rebel during the "terrible twos" stage and refuse to use the potty. Some 2-year-old children have been known to go up to 5 days without a bowel movement (when they normally had one a day) in stubborn defiance. This is one area where the child, not the mother, has the control.

The ability to control voiding is usually not present until a little later. When the child stays dry for 2 hours or more is usually a good indication, as is the child's ability to associate the puddle on the floor with something he did. The child by this time is usually able to tell mother that he needs to void.

Parents should invest in a small potty chair or a specially designed child's training seat that fits over the big regular one. The low potty chair has the advantage of allowing the child's feet to rest on the floor and aids in defecation. Many children have a fear of flush toilets. By this age, they have probably tried putting something in the toilet and watching it go down the drain when the toilet is flushed. If they sit on the toilet seat, they may think they will fall in and go down that hole too. Some children seem to enjoy sitting on the big toilet, however; it is a new experience and the child is usually rewarded by mother with praise and a big smile.

It is advisable to get a good supply of training pants and put the child in these during the day. Diapers are associated with wetting and having a bowel movement whenever the urge is felt; you want to extinguish this association and have the child associate wearing pants with going to the potty when the rectal or voiding reflex occurs and the urge is felt.

The child should not be left on the potty for long periods of time. His attention span is short, and he gets restless and bored quickly. You do not want him to associate the potty with the frustration of being confined too long.

The child should be praised when the desired results are obtained (the principle of reward for desired behavior). Parents should not show annoyance or displeasure if the child does not void or have a bowel movement but should remove the child from the potty and let him go about his play.

Results should not be expected right away. At first the child has no idea of why he is being asked to sit on the potty, but will do so since it seems to please mother. Gradually, sitting on the potty will become associated with having a bowel movement and voiding, and the learning is reinforced by mother's obvious pleasure in what he did.

Parents should not scold the child or frown if he continues to wet his pants or have his bowel movements in them. In the beginning, most children will come and tell mother after the fact, rather than before. The child should be changed promptly and matter-of-factly so that he associates the comfort of being clean and dry with wearing pants. The unwanted behavior will be more easily extinguished if it is not reinforced with a lot of attention (the principle of extinction of learning by non-reinforcement). This approach also substitutes a desirable behavior—one that achieves reward—which is a more effective reinforcement to learning than punishment. Some parents have been known to apply behavior modification theory by using tangible rewards, such as a cookie or other small treat.

Each child is different. A parent may be concerned because a mother down the street, or a friend, has a child who is completely toilet trained, while her own is nowhere near it at the same age. Each child has his own pattern of physical and psychosocial growth and development. The nurse can reassure the mother that her child will get there—faster if the mother does not become anxious about it. The mother's anxiety is usually conveyed to the child. Girls usually seem to find the learning easier than boys do, and this point should be kept in mind by the mother of a boy whose next-door neighbor has a girl.

The child's diet should include enough fluids so that bowel movements are soft and the child does not associate discomfort (from hardened stools or the slight burning that comes with concentrated urine) with having a bowel movement or voiding while sitting on the potty.

When the child is able to go to the bathroom on his own, a small stool will make it easier for him. The little boy needs to be high enough that his penis is over the toilet bowl, so that he can direct the stream of urine into the bowl instead of onto the floor. Sitting on the toilet seat with his feet on something solid makes defecation easier. Both boys and girls find the stool a help in getting onto most toilet seats, which are designed for adults, not children.

Fathers, of course, have an important role in helping to provide a model for little boys in bladder training and other matters too. Most mothers in single parent families feel the need to enlist the aid of a father substitute in helping little boys to identify with a male role model.

Children learn faster if they have a slightly older sibling whose activities they like to imitate.

Most children have achieved control over bowel and bladder elimination during the day by the time they are between 3 and 4, but it may be achieved later. Night-time control is usually gained by the age 4 or 5, but later in some cases.

If the child continues to have "accidents" just when you think he has finally achieved control, he should not be shamed by being put back in diapers. This will only cause resentment and hostility. He may have been just too busy playing to go to the bathroom, or he may have a bit of diarrhea that makes the urge to defecate more urgent than usual. A goal of the training is to encourage the development of self-esteem in the child. When a new sibling arrives on the scene, the child of 3 or 4 may be resentful and may want to be put in diapers again, because the baby gets all mother's attention when his diapers need changing.

FACTORS AFFECTING URINARY FUNCTIONING

Under conditions of good health, a number of factors may affect the volume of urinary output and the pattern of voiding, as well as the characteristics of urine excreted. These factors should be taken into consideration in the nurse's assessment of an individual's urinary elimination status.

Urine carries away most of the body's excess water. Hence, as mentioned earlier, both fluid intake and the amount of fluids lost through other routes will affect the volume and usually also the frequency of urinary output.

In addition to the changes in urinary function that we have noted throughout the life cycle, there are also inborn differences in anatomical structure and physiological functioning. Some people have a larger bladder capacity than others or a seemingly more efficient urinary system. They may not, then, need to void as often as others. Early childhood training also plays its part in an individual's response to the urge to urinate. Because voiding is under voluntary control, however, people may alter their voiding patterns because of situational factors such as the availability of toilet facilities, the pressures of work, mealtimes, and the like. In social situations, women are often more reluctant to excuse themselves to answer nature's call, thus contributing to higher rates of urinary infection in females than in males.

A person's diet may affect the constituents of urine. A vegetarian diet, for example, will cause the urine to be alkaline. Drugs will sometimes change the appearance of urine. For example, Mandelamine, a urinary antiseptic, when given in conjunction with a sulfonamide (an anti-infective), will cause the urine to be turbid.

Emotional factors may also cause urinary disturbances. Anxiety, for example, often stimulates the urge to void more frequently (as in a nervous person waiting in an airport for his plane to depart, or a student waiting for an examination to begin). Strong fear may cause a person to void involuntarily. Pain, on the other hand, may inhibit voiding.

In addition to the normal factors that may affect urinary elimination, a number of abnormal conditions may cause dysfunctioning of the urinary system.

Infection is one of the most common causes of urinary disturbances. Because the entire urinary system is lined with a continuous mucous membrane, an infection that begins in one part of the system can travel rapidly to all parts of the tract. Bacteria commonly found in the large intestine (Escherichia coli, for example) are common causes of urinary tract infection. The proximity of the outlets of the gastrointestinal and the urinary tracts contributes to this transfer.

During infancy and childhood, urinary tract infections are common. These are usually caused by fecal organisms although other types of infections (such as streptococcal infections) may occur and give rise to serious kidney problems. Urinary tract infection continues to be a problem in adolescence and young adulthood, particularly in women. Its frequency of occurrence increases with sexual activity (a bladder infection sometimes called "honeymoon cystitis" or "bride cystitis" often occurs after initial sexual activity in girls). Women are particularly prone to bladder infections because of the shortness of the female urethra. Stasis of urine in the bladder as a result of retention is another factor predisposing to infections and also the formation of bladder stones. We mentioned that pregnant women are particularly vulnerable to urinary tract infections because of the predisposition to stasis of urine in the bladder.

Disturbances in the circulatory system also can have an effect upon kidney function. Heart disease and diseases of the venous and arterial systems often interfere with the circulation of blood to the kidneys. Normally, 170 liters of blood are filtered through the adult kidneys in one day. From this filtration process approximately 1 to 1.5 liters of urine are formed and excreted. Any disease that interferes with the circulation of blood through the kidney can result in the impairment of kidney functioning.

Obstructions may occur in almost any part of the urinary tract. Most commonly they are seen in the pelvis of the kidney, in the ureter, and, in the male, in the prostatic section of the urethra. Blockage of the urinary tract, whether by a malignancy or stones, hinders the excretion of urine.

Congenital problems such as structural anomalies may cause blockage of the urinary tract or give rise to other functional problems. Many congenital problems are discovered in infancy and early childhood and surgical or other therapeutic measures taken to correct them. These problems are dealt with in pediatric nursing courses. Some anomalies, however, may not give rise to early signs and symptoms and may not cause problems until later in life (or not at all). A person with only one kidney, for example, may not discover this fact until an x-ray of the abdomen is taken for some other purpose.

Hormone disturbances, such as those resulting from dysfunctioning of the adrenal or pituitary glands, can also have an adverse effect upon the kidneys. The antidiuretic hormone, aldosterone, and possibly norepinephrine affect the reabsorption of fluid within the kidney tubules.

A generalized trauma to the body, such as hemorrhage, burns, or shock, or a systemic infection can also affect the kidneys. For example, in severe dehydration there is a depletion in the amount of fluid within the body, which can severely disturb kidney function, even to the point of failure.

Any generalized muscular disturbance can also affect urinary tract function. Specific dysfunctions of the muscles of the bladder, the ureters, or the urethra can cause urinary problems, such as retention of urine or poor urinary control.

Neurological factors can interfere with normal kidney and bladder function. Drugs that depress the central nervous system, for example, can cause a loss of voluntary control over micturition. Hence, patients under heavy sedation and those undergoing general anesthesia may void by reflex action when the bladder is full. Damage to the spinal cord or to the pathways that trans-

dysuria - difficulty (w/ pain)
nocturia - during sleep you have to get up

mit impulses from the spinal cord to the brain may also result in the loss of voluntary control over voiding, as may damage to the brain itself.

COMMON PROBLEMS

Disturbances in urinary functioning may cause localized alterations in voiding patterns or generalized problems resulting from impairment of elimination of waste products from the body.

Localized Problems

Of the localized problems, the following are among those most commonly seen: urinary incontinence, difficulty in voiding (dysuria), pain or a burning sensation upon voiding, frequency, urgency, the need to void at night (nocturia), excessive output of urine (polyuria), distention from urinary retention, scanty urine output, diminished urinary output (oliguria), and foreign substances in the urine.

Urinary incontinence, or involuntary voiding, is a common urinary problem among the ill. Sometimes there is a complete inability to control the flow of urine and, as a result, a constant dribbling occurs. Not only is this demoralizing and embarrassing to the individual, but the urine can also be a source of irritation to the skin in the anogenital area. Urinary incontinence sometimes occurs temporarily after an operation. It can also result from diseases of the nerves and muscles of the bladder. We mentioned that many middle-aged women with weakened muscles of the pelvic floor have difficulty retaining urine within the bladder, and this often leads to *Stress incontinence*, the excretion of small amounts of urine involuntarily with exertions such as coughing or laughing.

The term *dysuria* refers to difficulty in voiding or pain on voiding and may be caused by a number of factors. It can result from a blockage in any part of the urinary tract, from trauma, from muscular abnormalities of the bladder, ureters, or urethra, from infection of the urinary tract, or from psychogenic factors. In older men, hypertrophy (increase in size) of the prostate gland, which surrounds the urethra, is a common cause of difficulty in voiding.

A burning (or scalding) sensation on voiding may be caused by the excretion of a more highly concentrated urine than normal; it is also a frequent problem in people with infections of the urinary tract.

Frequency—that is, voiding more often than usual—may be caused by very benign factors such as drinking an excessive amount of fluids.

As mentioned earlier, it is a common problem during pregnancy and, while inconvenient, is usually not indicative of serious urinary dysfunction. Anxiety, as also noted above, can stimulate voiding and cause distressing frequency, at times with loss of control. On the other hand, frequency, particularly combined with urgency, is also commonly seen in people with infections of the urinary tract.

Urgency, the urge to void in a hurry, is an embarrassing problem. Its most common cause is infection of the urinary tract, although it may also be due to the same causes that produce frequency.

Having to get up from sleep in order to void (*nocturia*) may be due simply to drinking a large amount of fluids prior to bedtime, but it may also be caused by disturbed kidney functioning, particularly with regard to the kidney's inability to concentrate urine. Nocturia is not to be confused with *enuresis*, or bedwetting, which is a fairly common childhood and sleep disorder (see Chapter 20).

The passage of an increased amount of urine, called *polyuria* or *diuresis*, can be caused by failure of the tubules to reabsorb water or by disturbances in the hormonal balance of the body. Certain drugs, called *diuretics*, are often given to increase urinary elimination in people who suffer from fluid retention; these drugs cause a temporary polyuria.

Distention caused by *urinary retention* is another common problem. In retention, the urine is formed in the kidneys, but the person is unable to excrete it from the bladder. As a consequence, his bladder becomes distended and he feels increasingly uncomfortable. Some patients have retention with overflow; they void small amounts of urine frequently but continue to have distended bladders. Urinary retention predisposes a person to bladder infection (*cystitis*).

The passage of a lessened amount of urine (*oliguria*) can be caused by dehydration or by an impairment of the circulation of blood to the kidney. A lowered efficiency of the kidney or a blockage within the urinary tract can also result in oliguria.

A complete absence of urine output may indicate *renal anuria* (suppression of urine) a condition in which there is an absence of urinary excretion from the kidneys. It usually indicates serious kidney impairment. If this condition is prolonged, toxic substances build up within the body and the patient eventually dies. In both renal anuria and urinary retention, the patient is unable to void. However, in urinary retention the urine is retained in the bladder, and the distended bladder can be felt on palpation of the

enuresis - bedwet

abdomen. In renal anuria, the urine never reaches the bladder.

● Foreign substances in the urine may be found upon examination in the laboratory. Blood in the urine *(hematuria)* may be due to kidney damage or to infections of the urinary tract. Infections frequently cause the urine to contain pus *(pyuria)* or albumin *(albuminuria)*. The presence of protein in the urine *(proteinuria)* is usually due either to tissue disintegration or to an increase in glomerular permeability. *Casts,* on the other hand, are coagulated protein from the lumen of the kidney tubules. Sugar in the urine *(glycosuria)* is seen when the body is unable to utilize all the sugar which is ingested.

Generalized Problems

In addition to the localized problems related to urinary dysfunctioning, generalized problems occur that affect many body systems. When there is severe reduction in the ability of the kidneys to function, the patient usually develops *uremia.* This condition may result from trauma or infection, for example, or because of a chronic kidney disorder. The impairment in renal functioning has several effects on the body, in addition to a lessened amount of urine excretion (oliguria), which progresses (if not checked) to complete urine suppression (anuria). Water is retained, and there is a resultant edema of body tissues. The acid-base balance is disturbed, and the patient may develop acidosis owing to failure of the kidneys to remove the acidic products of metabolism. Potassium excretion is impaired, with a resulting high concentration of potassium in body fluids. This may give rise to neuromuscular irritability, as evidenced by an irregular pulse, for example. There is usually retention of the nonprotein nitrogenous waste products of metabolism as well, particularly of urea, whence the condition derived its name.

Thus, there are significant changes in blood chemistry. The concentration of urea in the blood (blood urea nitrogen, or BUN) may be increased from a normal value of 15 to 25 mg. per 100 ml. to as much as 200 mg. per 100 ml. in severe cases of uremia. Similarly, the blood creatinine level may rise from a normal value of 1.2 mg. per 100 ml. to 13 mg. per 100 ml. The extent of the increase in blood levels of these substances provides an indication of the severity of the kidney impairment.

Other problems may also accompany impaired kidney functioning as a result of the body's attempts to rid itself of wastes normally excreted in the urine by utilizing other channels. Perspiration is increased and deposits of salts may accumulate on the skin *(urea frost)*; the skin becomes pale and powdery, and the patient may have problems such as itching *(pruritus)* and an offensive odor on the skin due to the urea deposits.

When the kidneys are inhibited in the elimination of excess acid from the body, the lungs attempt to compensate for this; there are respiratory changes involving the character and depth of respirations. The respirations become deeper, the rate of respirations increases, and sometimes the patient's breath has the odor of urine.

ASSESSMENT

In assessing the patient's urinary elimination, the nurse needs information about the patient's usual voiding pattern (bladder habits) and any deviations from the normal that he is having at the time of admission to the health agency. She considers these in terms of the patient's age, his usual food and fluid intake, and disturbances that he has now with regard to taking sufficient food and fluids to maintain optimal urinary functioning.

She takes into consideration the patient's mental status: Is he confused? What is his level of consciousness? She also considers the possibility of potential or actual sources of anxiety he may have, which might cause or contribute to disturbances in urinary functioning.

Most of this information will be available from the nursing history and the clinical appraisal. In addition, the nurse needs to be aware of the nature if the patient's health problem(s) (if identified), and the physician's diagnostic and therapeutic plans of care for the patient. If diagnostic tests or examinations have been carried out, the nurse will find these reports very helpful in her assessment of the patient. Information from these sources is supplemented by the subjective and objective data she gathers in her observations.

Subjective Observations

People who have urinary problems are usually considerably distressed; their symptoms are often uncomfortable, sometimes inconvenient, and occasionally embarrassing. Often people are reluctant to talk about their urinary problems, and they may need encouragement in order to verbalize them. It is important to minimize the individual's feelings of embarrassment by ensuring privacy and a quiet place for discussion.

The patient may describe sensations of pain related to voiding, for example, or he may have noted disturbances in the normal pattern of voiding. The patient may be distressed by frequency or urgency in the need to void, or conversely, he may find micturition difficult. Patients are usually aware, too, of changes in the amount of urine. When there is either suppression of urine formation in the kidneys or retention of urine in the bladder, the amount of urine voided may be small. On the other hand, in some types of disease conditions, there may be copious amounts of urine formed and excreted. Some patients find that their sleep is disturbed because of the need to urinate. The patient may also be the first to notice abnormalities such as the presence of blood or pus in the urine.

Objective Observations

The nurse also makes specific observations from which she gathers objective data. The characteristics of the patient's urine (color, odor, consistency, amount, and the presence of abnormal constituents) are observed; these should be checked against the normal ones. If the urine is lighter than normal in color, this may be due to either an abnormally high intake of fluids or a diminution of the concentrating power of the kidneys. A dark, brownish color usually indicates a more concentrated urine. Urine may also be almost orange in color in some conditions owing to the presence of bile salts. Drugs may also change the color of the urine. Urine sometimes has a sweetish odor, often described as "fruity," which is characteristic of the presence of acetone. Blood in the urine may be observed as bright red, or the urine may be smoky in color. Another abnormal constituent which may be noted by visual observation is pus, which often gives a cloudy appearance to the urine.

The nurse should also note carefully the patient's intake and output and relate these to her other observations about the patient's voiding pattern and the characteristics of the urine. Urinary retention, for example, can be identified by checking the amount and frequency of voiding. If the patient voids 30 to 50 ml. of urine every 1 to 2 hours, he is probably retaining urine. In addition, a distended bladder can often be palpated. With the patient in the dorsal recumbent position, palpation just above the symphysis pubis reveals a firm distention, and percussion with the fingers causes the dull sound indicative of a full bladder.

In addition, the nurse should be alert to manifestations of generalized problems in relation to urinary dysfunctioning as they have been described in the preceding section.

One of the primary responsibilities of the nurse in caring for patients with urinary problems is assessment and recording of pertinent observations. The early detection of edema, of changes in the pigmentation of the skin, or of signs of central nervous system or neuromuscular dysfunction can contribute significantly to the total plan of care for the patient.

An important part of the assessment includes taking exact measurements of the patient's fluid intake and output. These fluids are usually measured in milliliters and recorded on a fluid balance sheet on the patient's chart. Occasionally it is also necessary to record the amount of fluid ingested as a part of the patient's food and the amount lost in perspiration and feces, but these are rare situations. Normally fluid output includes all liquid drainage (for example, gastric suction, vomitus, bleeding, or diarrhea) and urine excretion.

Diagnostic Examinations

Tests are performed on urine to evaluate kidney function. Some tests indicate the rate of glomerular filtration, tubular reabsorption, and excretion by the kidneys.

A routine urinalysis is probably the most common urine examination. It includes microscopic examination and tests of pH, specific gravity, albumin, and sugar.

Urine Test	Normal Results
pH	4.8 to 8.0
Specific gravity	1.003 to 1.030
Albumin	Negative
Sugar	Negative
Microscopic examination	(Female) few red blood cells; few casts
	Straw to light amber in color

Blood in urine may be obvious or hidden. Laboratory tests can detect red blood cells and dissolved hemoglobin (hemoglobinuria).

Nurses are frequently called upon in the clinical areas to perform some of the more routine laboratory tests on urine. Thus, a nurse may be requested to carry out a test for specific gravity or to test the patient's urine for the presence of sugar or acetone.

Tests of renal function include the concentration and dilution tests, and the tests for specific chemicals such as creatinine, urea, and nonprotein nitrogen. Generally speaking, most of these tests have special requirements for the food and fluid intake of the patient, the hours when urine specimens are to be collected, and, perhaps, definite times when blood specimens are to be collected. For some tests, a 24-hour urinary output must be collected. It is important

MEDICAL PLAN NO. (FOR O.P.D. USE ONLY)	▶				
ABNORMAL APPEARANCE			pH FRESH SPECIMEN	6	
SPECIFIC GRAVITY	*1.010*				
PROTEIN	*nil*				
REDUCING SUBSTANCES	*nil*				
GLUCOSE	*nil*				
KETONES					
DEPOSIT	MI. URINE	CENTRIFUGED			
W.B.C.					
PUS.	*3-5*		} H.P.F.		
R.B.C.					
CASTS/HYALINE					
CASTS/GRANULAR			} L.P.F.		
CASTS/CELLULAR					
CASTS/WAXY					
EPITH. CELLS	*1-3*		H.P.F.		
CRYSTALS					

January 31, 1982   JC5
Mrs.   82-1320
Doe   Jane
RONALD J. SMITH
                                 2.5

DIAGNOSIS   *Frequency ? UTI*

URINE VOIDED: DATE *Feb 1/82* TIME *0700*

**ORDER ALL OTHER TESTS ON
URINE CHEMISTRY FORM M110A**

ORIGINAL AND DUPLICATE TO BE SENT TO LABORATORY
RETAIN TRIPLICATE COPY ON NURSING UNIT

FORM M-110 REV 2-75   61100

50M

VANCOUVER GENERAL HOSPITAL
URINALYSIS ROUTINE   *82-8321   R.T. Jones Feb 1* 19 *82*
LAB. NO.   TECHNICIAN   DATE
RETURN TO NURSING UNIT

A sample laboratory urinalysis report form. (Courtesy of Vancouver General Hospital.)

that the patient understand what he should do to prepare for these tests and how he can help with them.

Urine cultures are done to determine the presence of pathogenic microorganisms. A catheter specimen may be required for culture, but usually a midstream specimen will suffice. Urine is normally sterile.

This nurse is checking the sugar content in her patient's urine by comparing its color to the color chart provided in a Clinitest set. (See Appendix II for detailed instructions.)

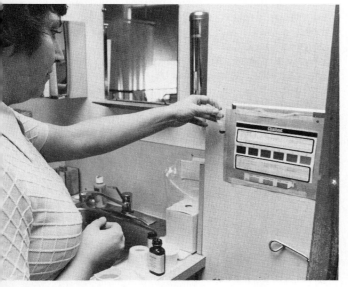

When a midstream specimen from the male patient is needed, the patient cleanses the urinary meatus with an antiseptic solution. He voids some urine, which is discarded, and then collects the midstream urine in a sterile container. The remainder of the stream is also discarded.

Obtaining a midstream specimen from a female patient is more difficult. The labia and vestibule should be thoroughly cleansed with soap and water or antiseptic solution. If soap is used, it must be rinsed off. The patient then voids. The first part of the stream is discarded, the midstream specimen is caught in a sterile container, and the remainder of the urine is also discarded. Most female patients find it easier to obtain this specimen when the toilet is used for discarded urine. For some tests a 24-hour sample of urine is used. The first urine voided in the morning is usually discarded and collection begins with the next urine voided. All urine voided during the subsequent 24 hours is collected (including the first urine of the following morning) in one large container. Disposable cardboard containers are frequently used these days, although a large gallon glass container serves the purpose as well. Urine must be stored properly during the 24 hours.

Some blood tests are also indicative of kidney function. The non-protein nitrogen (NPN) test measures the ability of the kidney to remove urea, creatine, and so forth, from the blood. The blood urea nitrogen (BUN) test is a more sensitive test of kidney function. For each of these tests, 5 ml. of venous blood is collected.

There are many examinations of the urinary tract. A cystoscopy is the examination of a patient's bladder with a lighted instrument which is inserted up the urethra. The intravenous pyelogram and retrograde pyelogram outline the pelvis, calices, urethers, and urinary bladder by means of a contrast medium which is visible on x-ray.

PRIORITIES FOR NURSING ACTION

If the patient has a problem that causes interference with the excretion of urine from the bladder, it is important that he be watched for signs of urine retention. Although some adult bladders have been known to hold up to 3000 to 4000 ml. of fluid, not all bladders will contain this quantity, and there is a danger of rupture when the bladder content is considerably below this point. The early detection of urinary retention is therefore vitally important. It should be reported promptly so that appropriate medical or nursing intervention can be started. Frequently, it is left up to the nurse to initiate action; that is, the physician may leave an order for catheterization as necessary. When needed, it should be done promptly. A patient should never be left with a distended bladder.

When a patient has an impairment in kidney functioning, the body's ability to eliminate the nitrogenous waste products of protein metabolism is decreased. The accumulation of these waste products within the body constitutes a serious threat to the patient's life. One of the most important aspects of nursing care for patients with urinary problems is the constant monitoring of fluid intake and output. If there is a decrease in fluid loss below the levels considered safe, this fact should be reported promptly so that appropriate therapy can be instituted. In assessing the safety levels for the patient, the nurse is guided by the physician's estimate for this particular patient, but it is helpful for her to remember that the normal urine output in an adult is approximately 1000 to 1500 ml. per day. An output of less than 25 ml. per hour (600 ml. in a 24-hour period) is considered inadequate for a normal adult.

GOALS FOR NURSING ACTION

The basic goals for nursing action in helping patients with their needs for urinary elimination are:

1. Maintenance of normal urinary elimination
2. Re-establishment of a normal voiding pattern
3. Facilitation of elimination of urine from the bladder
4. Assisting with measures to reduce the workload of the kidneys in patients with impaired urinary functioning
5. Assisting with measures to minimize the effects of impaired urinary functioning on the body

One of the most important nursing responsibilities in the care of people who are ill is helping them to meet their very basic elimination needs, both to void and to have bowel movements. In caring for people who are having problems in urinary elimination, the urgent need to void is often a very distressing accompaniment to other problems. The nurse's prompt attention to their needs and sympathetic understanding of their distress can go a long way towards relieving both their physical and mental discomfort.

SPECIFIC NURSING INTERVENTIONS

Measures to Maintain Normal Urinary Elimination

People who are ambulatory can take care of their elimination needs by using bathroom facilities. Often sick patients need the nurse's help to get to the bathroom and to use the facilities. Many hospitals and other inpatient facilities are equipped with specially constructed toilets, washbasins, and supportive bars to help patients who find the use of ordinary bathroom equipment difficult. Measures the nurses uses to assist the patient in getting out of bed, in walking, and in sitting on the toilet seat are described in Chapter 23.

The ill person, however, is often confined to bed and must use the bedpan or the urinal for elimination purposes. Women patients use the bedpan for both urination and defecation. Male patients need the bedpan for defecation and the urinal for voiding. Having to use these articles for such a basic need is embarrassing for most people, and the nurse does everything possible to assure the patient's privacy, to avoid unnecessary exposure of bodily parts that are considered by most people to be very private, and to make the procedure as safe and as comfortable as possible for the patient, both physically and psychologically.

To ensure privacy, the curtains are drawn around the patient's bed, or the door of a private

PRINCIPLES RELEVANT TO URINARY ELIMINATION

1. Most of the nitrogenous wastes of cellular metabolism are eliminated by the kidneys.

2. The kidneys play an important role in maintaining the fluid and electrolyte balance of the body.

3. The suppression of urine formation in the kidneys threatens the life of an individual.

4. The kidneys normally mature to full functioning ability by the end of the first year of life.

5. The necessary neuromuscular structures for voluntary control of voiding are not usually sufficiently developed until the age of 2 to 3 years.

6. Loss of voluntary control over voiding is a serious threat to an individual's self-esteem.

7. The average adult voids 1000 to 1500 ml. of urine in a 24-hour period; the average school age child voids up to 1000 ml. in 24 hours.

8. A larger proportion of body weight in children is composed of fluids.

9. Awareness of the need to void normally occurs in the adult when the bladder contains 300 to 500 ml. of urine.

10. The lining of the urinary tract consists of a continuous layer of mucous membrane.

11. The intimate anatomical relationship between the urinary and reproductive tracts makes urinary functioning a sensitive topic for most people.

12. The location of the urinary meatus in close proximity to the anus and to the external sex organs makes the urinary tract vulnerable to infection from these sources.

13. Urinary output of less than 25 ml. per hour (600 ml. in a 24-hour period is considered inadequate for adults.

---

room is closed. If the patient can use the bedpan or urinal himself, the nurse may wait outside the curtain or door if she feels the patients might need assistance. Otherwise, she places the patient's call signal within easy reach for him.

Unnecessary exposure can be avoided by folding back one corner of the bedcovers for easy insertion of the pan or urinal. Methods of assisting the helpless or semi-helpless patient onto a bedpan are described in Chapter 23. Other measures for aiding the patient in using a bedpan are discussed in Chapter 16.

The procedure can be made as comfortable as possible for the patient by using the proper equipment and handling it competently. Assistance is given to the patient as needed, e.g., cleansing the perineal area. Male patients, however, do not usually need cleansing after using the urinal, since the urine does not normally dribble onto the skin. The nurse provides the patient with the means for washing his hands after he has finished. The entire procedure should be handled in a matter-of-fact manner. Since the bedpan is extremely uncomfortable to use, the patient should never be left on it any longer than necessary. Thus, the call signal must be answered promptly.

In the sick person, urine may contain harmful microorganisms. To prevent cross-infection, a separate bedpan and urinal are kept for each patient's use in almost all agencies today. They are stored in the patient's bedside locker, in an adjoining bathroom, or, in some agencies, in a separate room on the nursing unit.

Metal bedpans and urinals usually become cold when they are stored, so they need to be warmed before being used. Rinsing them with warm water helps to eliminate this problem and lessens the patient's discomfort. The nurse's hands should also be warmed if they are coming in contact with the patient's skin. Recently, more agencies are using disposable equipment that is used for one patient only, and then discarded. If this is not the case, or if there is multiple usage, the equipment must be sterilized after every use.

The nurse helps to prevent infection in the patient, herself, and other patients and workers by washing her hands before and after assisting patients. The patient should always be provided with the opportunity to wash his hands after using these articles (as he would at home after voiding).

The male urinal was designed to fit over the

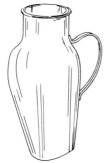

A male urinal. (From Rambo, B. J., and Wood, L. A.: *Nursing Skills for Clinical Practice.* 3rd ed. Philadelphia, W. B. Saunders Company, 1982, Vol. 2.)

patient's penis so that urine could be excreted without spillage. It has a handle for convenience (specially designed urinals are available for patients who have the use of only one hand) and it is usually flat on either one side or the bottom so that it can be set down on a flat surface after use without the contents spilling.

The patient can use the urinal when in the supine position, the lateral position (either side), or Fowler's position, or when standing at the side of the bed. If at all possible, patients prefer to use the urinal without help, particularly if the nurse or other attendant is female. He sometimes needs the nurse's help, however, and this should be given without embarrassment and treated as any other procedure with which the patient needs help.

The patient should be exposed only as much as necessary. The patient's legs are separated sufficiently to allow the urinal to be placed between them. Holding the urinal with one hand, the nurse gently inserts the penis into the urinal sufficiently far to prevent urine from leaking out onto the bedclothes or the patient's skin. The nurse holds the urinal in place if the patient cannot do so.

A female urinal may be used for some patients. It is similar in design to the male urinal, but has a long, wide top, shaped like a spout. The patient may stand at the side of the bed to use this article, sit on the edge of the bed, or sit in bed. If necessary, it may be used when the patient is in a side-lying position. Because of its shape, the spout must be in contact with the patient's skin or urine will leak out. The spout end should point towards the rectum and the handle should be on top so that it can be easily grasped.

If the patient is on measured intake and output, the contents of the bedpan or urinal are examined and urine measured before they are disposed of in the toilet (in rooms with adjoining bathrooms) or in the hopper, if this system is used in the agency.

Measures to Assist in the Re-establishment of a Normal Voiding Pattern

Some patients with urinary problems have difficulty in voiding; others may suffer from urinary incontinence. For those patients whose ability to control voiding has been lessened, the nurse can often assist them to train their bladders to function at regular and predictable times. For the nurse to be able to assist the patient in this, she should know his normal pattern of voiding. What are the times when he voids and when is he usually dry?

The patient is encouraged to assume as natural a position as possible for voiding and to void at regular times, preferably at his normal voiding periods. There is considerable debate whether the effort involved in getting on and off the bedpan exceeds that involved in getting out of bed and using a commode. Many women patients find it easier to void when they use a bedside commode, and male patients find it easier if they stand at the side of the bed to use a urinal. If permissible, these measures often help the patient in regaining a normal pattern of voiding.

The patient can be assisted to void by the various means just described. In addition to those already mentioned, digital pressure at the side of the urinary meatus or a circular movement over the bladder can often stimulate urination. If the patient has had a catheter in place over a period of time, he will need to have it clamped for intervals of 2 to 3 hours in order to increase the muscle tone before bladder training is initiated. The patient can expect accidents during a bladder training regimen; nevertheless, many people do develop a regular voiding pattern.

It has already been mentioned that the patient

A female urinal. (From Wood, L. A., and Rambo, B. J.: *Nursing Skills for Allied Health Services.* 2nd ed. Philadelphia, W. B. Saunders Company, 1977.)

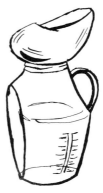

should be encouraged to void as soon as he feels the urge to do so. The importance of having nursing personnel answer the patient's call signal promptly cannot be overemphasized. The patient should not be kept waiting or allowed to become incontinent because his request for a bedpan or a urinal went unheeded.

If an accident does occur, the patient's bedding should be changed at once. If it is not allowed to stay wet this has the psychological advantage of encouraging the patient to keep his bed dry. Changing wet linen also helps to prevent skin irritation and the development of unpleasant odors.

In a bladder retraining program, it is essential that the patient have an adequate intake of fluids to stimulate the secretion of sufficient urine to distend the bladder enough so that the micturition reflex is initiated at regular times. The provision of fluids at regular intervals helps to ensure an adequate intake; under normal circumstances, a minimum of 2000 ml. per day has been suggested, although 3000 ml. or more is preferred if the patient can tolerate a larger amount.

Patients on a bladder retraining regimen have much need for both physical and emotional support. They usually require physical assistance from nursing personnel when they need to use a bedpan, commode, or toilet. The dependence on others and the lack of control over such a basic function as voiding can be very distressing to the patient. Since both the patient and his family will probably need help, the nurse must understand the meaning that urinary problems have for them. Sympathy, tolerance, and patience are all required of the nurse in helping patients with urinary problems.

Retraining for Bowel and Bladder Control

Incontinence of both urine and feces is a common problem for people who have had spinal injuries. It is an altogether too common problem among the elderly who are in nursing homes and other extended care facilities. In the older person, incontinence may be the result of a stroke or other health problem that damages integrity of the neuromuscular structures involved in voluntary control of voiding and defecation. Or, the incontinence may be due to diminishing strength of the muscles of bladder and bowels and the respective sphincters controlling elimination. Nursing personnel in long-term care facilities spend countless hours and expend considerable energy changing bed linen and the clothes of incontinent patients. Yet numerous programs have demonstrated that a good

bladder and bowel retraining program can effectively resolve the problem for many people, and minimize it for others.

The key to effective retraining is consistency over different times of the day or night and over the days of the week. A program that is carried out on the day shift Monday to Friday but not followed through at night or on the weekends and holidays is not likely to succeed. There may be less staff on at these times, but it is important to get the priorities in order. The program must have the wholehearted support of all staff involved in caring for the patient—and the patient's cooperation—to be effective.

Retraining, like the toilet training of children, is a learning process. It takes a long time for people in whom the voluntary control has been lost for a long period of time. It usually takes weeks, and may take months, but it is well worth the effort. Success is very rewarding for both the patient and the nursing staff.

It is important that the nurse and other personnel who are working with the patient in establishing the program know the patient well and have a good working relationship with him. This helps to lessen anxiety for the patient and the embarrassment of the lapses into incontinence that do occur. Because it is the patient who is learning to regain control, his cooperation is most important to the success of the program. Nursing personnel are there to help in the learning process.

Only positive reinforcement should be given—the individual is very sensitive to any sign of displeasure on the part of staff. Punishment by look, gesture, or words will only result in more frequent incontinence, and should never be used.[1]

A program that may be used for people in whom the incontinence has a physiological basis and one for an individual whose urinary incontinence has a psychological cause are shown in the table on page 317.

Measures to Facilitate the Elimination of Urine From the Bladder

Maintenance of adequate urinary elimination is important to physiological functioning. For the patient who has difficulty in voiding, there are certain nursing measures that can be provided to assist him. In addition to urinary catheterization, which is carried out as ordered by the physician, there are also measures to stimulate the act of voiding. Some ways in which this is done are:

1. Helping the patient to assume a natural position for voiding

RETRAINING FOR BLADDER CONTROL

Example programme for an individual whose urinary incontinence has a physiological cause:

1. Observe and record every incidence and time of incontinence, over a 24 hour period each day for 4–5 days (minimum). Graph this baseline data. Check for pattern in graph. (This may save a great deal of time and frustration when setting up interval scheduling for the retraining programme.)
2. The programme is set up on a 24 hour basis, regardless of how many times the patient must be aroused at night. *Consistency is imperative.*
3. Establish the interval schedule—q 1 h is a common one with which to start.
4. An accurate 24 hour record of fluid intake and output is kept, with the time as well as amount recorded.
5. On every hour help the patient into an upright sitting or standing position (if possible) making sure that strict privacy is afforded. Manual expression of the bladder is used if necessary. The patient should be taught this technique since he will be responsible for doing it and it allows him some measure of independence. Use a commode or toilet when possible since most people have difficulty using a bedpan.
6. Allow the patient to assist with this procedure as much as possible within his capability, i.e., record keeping, cleaning himself, etc.
7. Use positive verbal reinforcement after each successful attempt and encouragement when the attempt is not successful.

Example programme for an individual whose urinary incontinence has a psychological cause:

1. Set up an interval schedule using your baseline, as derived in step 1 above. For children this is done, at first, only for the waking hours.
2. Record fluid intake and output (with time indicated) accurately.
3. Carefully select a consumable reinforcement for the individual. This is always paired with verbal praise. Juice is excellent since it increases the incidence for relearning to take place.
4. *Each* time the person is successful immediately reinforce.
5. When incontinence occurs the individual should clean himself if possible, otherwise the nurse can do this with as little attention as possible.
6. When the frequency of incontinence decreases the consumable reinforcement is decreased gradually but the verbal praise is continued until incontinence is extinguished.
Note: It is imperative that no attention, or as little attention as possible, is given for incontinence since it will raise the frequency of the behaviour.

Modified from McEachern, J.: Retraining Bowel and/or Bladder. Surrey, British Columbia, paper prepared for Douglas College Nursing Programme, 1975.

2. Providing a commode or, preferably, assisting the patient to the bathroom if this is possible (male patients frequently find it easier to void when they are standing rather than sitting or lying down)
3. Running water within the patient's hearing
4. Providing water in which he can dangle his fingers
5. Providing privacy and setting aside a time for voiding
6. Providing a warm bedpan or urinal
7. Applying a warm hot water bottle to the patient's lower abdomen (this may require a doctor's order)
8. Pouring warm water over the perineum (the water must be measured)
9. Relieving pain

It has long been accepted that warmth applied to the bladder and perineal areas will help to relax the muscles used in voiding and therefore facilitate this process.

There is always the possibility of introducing an infection into the urinary tract when catherization is done. Hence the procedure is being carried out less often than it was formerly. Unless the physician has expressly ordered the insertion of a urinary catheter, alternative measures are tried before catheterization is considered.

Patients who cannot void or those who void without control are usually embarrassed as well as anxious. The nurse can offer support by providing explanations of the reason for the problem. The patient should be encouraged to respond to the urge for voiding promptly, rather than waiting. It is important, in this regard, for the nurse to answer the patient's call signal promptly so that the patient is not kept waiting for a urinal or a bedpan. At no time should the nurse show impatience or a lack of understanding of the patient's distress.

Urinary Catheterization of the Female Patient. A urinary catheterization is the introduction of a narrow tube, called a urinary catheter, through the urethra into the bladder in order to remove urine. It is ordered by the physician, although it is usually carried out by a female nurse for the female patient and by a male nurse, an orderly, or the physician for the male patient. This does not mean, however, that a female nurse might not find it necessary to catheterize a male patient on occasion.

The purpose of urinary catheterization may be to obtain a sterile urine specimen for laboratory examination or to empty a patient's bladder preoperatively so that the danger of incising the bladder is lessened. A urinary catheterization is also ordered postoperatively for a patient who is unable to void. Normally the act of voiding is a spinal cord reflex subject to voluntary control by the cerebrum. After surgery, however, some patients have difficulty in voiding. This is particularly true when anxiety is mediated through the hypothalamus and the sympathetic nervous system to the nerves that supply the bladder muscles.

Another reason for a urinary catheterization

is to insert a retention or indwelling catheter in order to prevent uncontrollable voiding or voiding upon an operative area. A patient who has surgery on her perineum will probably have an indwelling catheter inserted postoperatively in order to prevent the urine from irritating the operative area.

Equipment. A catheter is a hollow tube made of rubber, plastic, glass, metal, or silk. Plastic catheters are becoming increasingly popular. Catheters are graded in size according to the French scale; No. 14 and No. 16 catheters are commonly used for the catheterization of the adult female patient. The larger the number, the larger is the lumen of the catheter. It is, of course, safest to use the correct size of catheter for each patient, but should the nurse be unsure about which size to use, she should use a smaller size in order not to harm the mucous membrane of the urethra or to cause the patient discomfort. The larger the lumen of the catheter, the more quickly will urine flow from the bladder, but usually this is not of great importance unless the patient's bladder is greatly distended. In any case, a clamp can be used to regulate the flow of urine according to the physician's order.

There are many kinds of catheters available. Retention or indwelling catheters are inserted into the patient's bladder and are kept in place by an inflated balloon or a rubber ring that is larger than the bladder orifice. These catheters may have a single lumen, as in the mushroom catheter, a double lumen, or even a triple lumen, as in the Foley-Alcock catheter. The latter type of catheter is used for continuous irrigations, in which the fluid flows continuously up one lumen to the bladder and down a second lumen into a receptacle. The third lumen is connected to the inflated balloon that keeps the catheter in place. A straight catheter is usually used when the purpose of the catheterization is to remove urine rather than to have the patient retain the catheter.

The equipment for a urinary catheterization should be sterile. Because the mucous membrane lining the urinary tract is continuous and because the warm mucous membrane is a likely place for the propagation of bacteria, an aseptic technique is carried out throughout the entire catheterization procedure. Disposable, prepackaged catheterization sets are available, but if these are not used, the set that is to be used is checked to make sure that it is sterile.

A catheterization set contains, at a minimum, the catheter, a receptacle for the urine, and materials for cleansing the labia and urinary meatus of the patient. Some agencies suggest that the nurse use sterile rubber gloves during the catheterization procedure, whereas others suggest that sterile forceps may be used for the insertion of the catheter. In either case it is important that the catheter remain sterile during its insertion up the urethra into the patient's bladder.

The nurse needs to have a good light in order to visualize the urinary meatus and prevent contamination. Either an extension lamp or an extendable lamp can be used to illuminate the perineal area.

Since urinary catheterization can be an embarrassing measure, it is important that the nurse protect the patient from unneccessary exposure. The positions that are most often used for the catheterization are the dorsal recumbent and lithotomy positions, although some authorities advocate a side-lying position with the patient's knees flexed and the upper leg higher than the lower. Once the patient assumes the position that is to be used, she is covered with drapes in such a way that her legs and body are adequately covered. Then only the perineal area is exposed. In her explanation to the patient, the nurse assures her that the catheterization is usually painless but that the patient may experience a feeling of pressure and of wanting to urinate because the catheter irritates the urethra. Discomfort is minimized if the patient is relaxed.

Preparation of the Patient. In explaining a urinary catheterization, the nurse must be guided by the needs of the patient. Some patients want a detailed explanation; others simply want assurance that it is a painless measure. From inexperience many patients want to know whether it will hurt, how long it will take, and where the tube goes. The nurse should rarely assume a knowledge of anatomy on the patient's part; indeed, she may be surprised at some of the beliefs people have. That sterile technique is maintained is important to the patient's safety, but the patient probably has little awareness of this.

If the patient needs a retention catheter, she probably requires reassurance that she will be able to move about freely in bed and, very often, will still be able to get out of bed. The length of time a retention catheter remains in place depends upon the reason for its insertion; the physician determines when it is to be removed. Points that can prove helpful to the patient with a retention catheter are:

1. Usually the patient should drink a large amount of fluid, approximately 3000 ml. per day
2. The patient may move freely in bed
3. The patient should not lie on the catheter tubing
4. It is normal to have a feeling of wanting to void for a while while the catheter is in place

After the patient has been properly draped, a sterile towel is placed between the patient's legs to make it easier to maintain sterile technique. The receptacle for the urine is then placed on the towel near the urinary meatus. This receptacle should be lower than the patient's bladder so that the urine will flow easily from the bladder to the receptacle by the force of gravity. All the equipment is placed conveniently.

Cleansing the Perineal Area.

Trauma to the mucous membrane of the urinary tract and the admission of bacteria to the urinary tract can result in a local or a generalized infection. Therefore, the patient's perineal area is cleansed thoroughly. There are many different ways suggested to do this; soap and water and a variety of antiseptics are used. Regardless of the method used, the patient's labia must be as clean as possible, and the urinary meatus as free from bacteria as possible.

The following are guides to cleansing the perineal area:

1. If the area is obviously soiled wash with soap and water and then dry; all soap is carefully removed, because it can inactivate some disinfectants

2. Use a mild, nonirritating disinfectant

3. Use each swab just once, cleansing from the cleanest area (near the symphysis pubis) toward the most contaminated area (near the rectum)

4. Cleanse the outer labia, the inner labia, and then the vestibule of the perineum; a minimum of five sponges is needed.

5. Once the vestibule has been cleansed, the labia must not touch it until the catheter has been inserted. It is necessary to keep the labia separated with the fingers for adequate visualization and to prevent unwanted contamination of the catheter.

Insertion of the Catheter.

The catheter used in a urinary catheterization should be smooth so that it will not damage the mucous membrane of the urethra. In order to facilitate the passage of the catheter up the urethra, a water soluble lubricant is used. The lubricant is applied to the catheter prior to its insertion into the urethra.

With sterile forceps, sterile gloves, or sterile gauze, the urinary catheter is picked up approximately 10 cm. (4 inches) from the tip and inserted gently into the urethra. The catheter should be inserted 3 to 5 cm. (1¼ to 2 inches) into the urethra—that is, the distance from the urinary meatus to the bladder. If any resistance is met during the passage of the catheter, it is withdrawn and the situation is reported to the physician.

The other end of the catheter lies in the sterile receptacle between the patient's legs and is held in place until the patient's bladder is empty or until the urine specimen has been obtained. If the patient has a large amount of retained urine, the distended bladder should be emptied gradually. Not all fluid should be drained off at once or there is danger of decompressing the bladder too quickly. The sudden release from pressure may result in injury to the organ itself or may cause a generalized reaction within the body, characterized by chills, an elevated temperature, and, occasionally, shock. These complications can be avoided by clamping off the catheter at intervals to allow time for the bladder to adjust to the changes in pressure caused by withdrawing the urine from it. Once the urine has been obtained, the catheter is pinched and withdrawn slowly. The patient is assisted with drying the perineal area and assuming a comfortable position before the equipment is removed.

A description of the urine is recorded. This includes the amount, the color, the clarity, and any unusual characteristics. If the urine has an unusual odor, if the nurse encountered any difficulty during the urinary catheterization, or if the patient experienced any unusual discomfort, these observations are also recorded.

Urinary Catheterization of the Male Patient.

Usually this measure is carried out by a male nurse or nursing orderly, however, on occasion a female nurse may have to catheterize a male patient (and vice versa). This can be particularly embarrassing to the patient, but he will be helped by an understanding, competent manner on the part of the nurse. The equipment that is necessary is similar to that used for a female urinary catheterization. The use of sterile rubber gloves is advised to facilitate the maintenance of sterile technique.

The downward curvature of the prepubic urethra of the male can be straightened by lifting

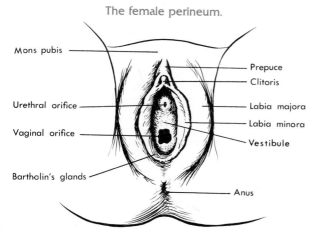

The female perineum.

Mons pubis

Prepuce

Clitoris

Urethral orifice

Labia majora

Labia minora

Vaginal orifice

Vestibule

Bartholin's glands

Anus

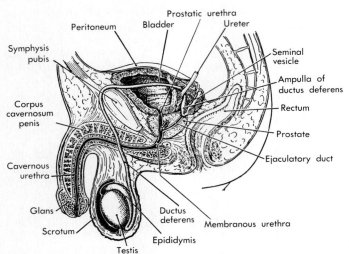

Symphysis pubis

Peritoneum

Prostatic urethra

Bladder

Ureter

Seminal vesicle

Ampulla of ductus deferens

Rectum

Prostate

Ejaculatory duct

Corpus cavernosum penis

Cavernous urethra

Glans

Scrotum

Testis

Epididymis

Ductus deferens

Membranous urethra

The male urogenital system.

the penis and, with slight traction, holding it perpendicular to the patient's body. The patient lies in the dorsal recumbent position, his knees flexed and his legs slightly rotated externally to expose the penis. The draping and placing of the equipment are similar to that used for a female catheterization.

After the catheter and the urethral orifice are lubricated, the penis is extended as described and the catheter is then inserted to a distance of approximately 20 cm. (8 inches)—that is, into the patient's bladder. When, in the course of the insertion, the catheter meets the resistance of Guérin's fold or the pouch of the fossa navicularis, the resistance can be bypassed by twisting the catheter. If the catheter encounters resistance at the vesical sphincters, it should not be forced, but held firmly until the sphincters relax. Once the catheter is in place the procedure is similar to that for catheterization of a female patient.

Insertion of a Retention Catheter.   If a patient requires an indwelling catheter, a syringe, sterile water for the inflation of the balloon of the catheter, connecting tubing, and a receptacle for the draining urine are needed, in addition to the equipment used in a simple catheterization. After the indwelling catheter is inserted into the patient's bladder, the balloon is filled with the amount of sterile water that it is designed to hold. After the water has been injected, slight tension is placed upon the catheter to make sure that it is in place and that is will not come out of the patient's bladder easily. If the balloon is in the patient's urethra, the nurse will encounter considerable difficulty in filling the balloon and the patient will complain of discomfort. In such cases, the catheter is inserted a little farther into the bladder and the fluid is again injected into the balloon.

Once the indwelling catheter is safely in the

patient's bladder, it is attached to the connecting tubing, the other end of which is in a receptacle, which is often attached to the patient's bed. Sterile technique is maintained in connecting the tubing.

The receptacle for the urine is situated at a level lower than the patient so that the urine flows readily by force of gravity. The tubing should not loop below the receptacle, because a kink may be formed that occludes the lumen. In addition, the urine then would have to flow against gravity. The tubing is pinned to the bed in such a manner that the lumen of the tubing is patent. This can be accomplished by pinching a piece of sheet on either side of the tubing and pinning the sides over the tubing. The tubing that lies on the top of the bed should be kept flat to facilitate drainage. Sometimes the catheter tubing is taped to the patient's thigh to avoid pulling on the catheter as the patient moves about in bed. The nurse should make sure that the patient's leg is never resting on the tubing, since this will occlude the lumen. Also, the lowest point of the tubing should always be above the level of urine in the drainage bottle, or, as already stated, the urine is forced to run uphill, against the force of gravity.

For the patient with an indwelling catheter, the physician may order continuous or intermittent drainage. If he orders continuous drainage, the catheter is attached to the tubing, and the urine is allowed to drain freely into the receptacle that is provided. If intermittent drainage is ordered, the tubing is clamped at designated intervals.

Urine receptacles are available commercially which attach to the upper leg and can be used to receive urine from a catheter while the patient is walking around. These leg bags are usually disposed of when they accumulate urine and are replaced by clean, sterile bags.

When the patient requires continuous or intermittent drainage, many agencies use disposable closed drainage sets. When these are used, the urine bag is simply emptied when full, or at regular intervals, and the tubing is left untouched until the entire set is either removed or changed. Urine meters are often used when the measurement of hourly urine outputs is required. The meters are usually rigid plastic containers that attach (in most instances) to a drainage bag. The meters are calibrated to measure small amounts (200 ml. or less) of urine.[2] If closed drainage sets are not used, it is necessary to change the tubing and urine receptacle regularly to prevent the accumulation of salt deposits and the development of unpleasant odors. Often the urine receptacle is changed daily and the tubing every few days.

When tubing is changed or the catheter is disconnected from the tubing for a period of time—for example, when the patient is to be up and walking around—or when a bladder irrigation is to be done, it is vitally important that the sterility of both the catheter and the tubing be maintained. Small disposable urinary adaptor protectors are now available. These provide a sterile cover for both tubing and catheter when these are disconnected.

Urinary catheters are usually changed at the physician's order. They are never changed without good reason because of the danger of infection to the patient. If there is any obstruction to urine flow which is not cleared by an irrigation, the catheter should be replaced. Other signs that a catheter may need to be changed are:

1. Insufficient urine in the drainage bottle in comparison with the fluid intake of the patient

2. Abdominal distention just above the symphysis pubis, which on palpation indicates a full bladder (see discussion of urinary retention, p. 321).

Male External Drainage. An external urinary appliance is often used for men instead of a retention catheter for patients who are unable to control voiding. (Protective pants may be used for women; these have a nonabsorbent plastic or rubberized lining. They can be worn over an absorbent pad.) The external appliance for men is a rubber condom with a short tube that can be connected to a drainage bottle or bag. Known by various names, such as urosheath or "Texas condom," it provides a convenient and relatively safe method of collecting urine from patients who are incontinent. It is considered much safer than risking the chance of infection through the use of a retention catheter. It also makes bladder retraining easier, since the condom can be left off for gradually increasing periods of time so that the patient feels more "normal." This psychological effect in itself is important for the patient.

The condom is disposable, relatively inexpensive, and easily applied so that it can be changed frequently. It is rolled over the penis so that the narrow tube opening at the end is over the urinary meatus at the tip of the penis. The tube is then connected to a drainage tube and attached to a bottle or other container for the urine.

Urinary Bladder Irrigation ("Internal"). The procedure of bladder irrigation is not used as commonly today as in times past. It is now felt by many authorities that the danger of introducing infection into the bladder during the course of the irrigation is sufficiently great to offset many of the benefits. When a bladder irrigation is ordered, the importance of maintaining sterile

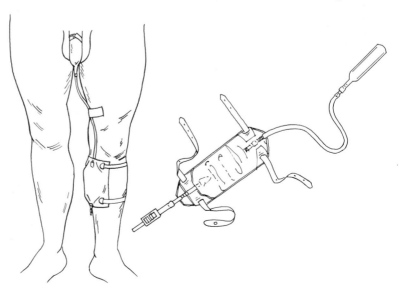

An external urinary appliance. The urine is collected in a bag that can be attached to the calf or the thigh.

technique during the procedure cannot be over-stressed.

A physician might order urinary bladder irrigations for a patient who has an indwelling catheter. The purpose of the irrigations is to cleanse the bladder or to apply an antiseptic solution to the lining of the bladder.

This nursing measure is a sterile procedure similar to urinary catheterization. The equipment required includes a container for the irrigation solution, a receptacle for the returned irrigation solution, and a syringe with a tip that fits into the urinary catheter. The solutions that are used for irrigations vary considerably; sterile water, sterile normal saline, and many antiseptic solutions are used. The irrigating fluid is usually administered at room temperature unless the physician orders otherwise.

Sterile equipment is used for the bladder irrigation, and sterile technique is maintained throughout this nursing measure. The end of the catheter and the end of the tubing are kept sterile while the bladder is irrigated. Frequently they are put in a sterile container placed close to the patient's leg.

After the tubing has been disconnected from the catheter, a small amount of sterile solution is introduced into the bladder. This is done by using either a funnel or an Asepto syringe. The amount of solution that is recommended for insertion varies in different agencies, with many suggesting that no more than 50 ml. be introduced at any one time for an "internal" bladder irrigation, 30 ml. for an irrigation done through a retention catheter. The solution is always administered gently in order not to damage the mucous membrane lining. The fluid should be allowed to run in slowly and the syringe or funnel should be kept low to prevent exerting undue pressure on the walls of the bladder. The catheter is pinched off before the syringe (or funnel) is completely empty to prevent the introduction of air into the bladder. The fluid is then withdrawn by permitting it to drain from the catheter into a basin. This procedure—the administration of fluid and its return—is repeated until all the solution ordered has been used or until the return flow is clear.

In recording this nursing measure the nurse notes and records the strength and kind of solution used in the bladder irrigation and the character of the return flow. Was the return flow cloudy or colored? These observation are reported in the patient's record.

Assisting With Measures to Reduce the Workload on the Kidneys

The principal functions of the kidneys are to control the concentration of the various constituents of body fluid and to eliminate the waste products of metabolism, chiefly the nitrogenous wastes of cellular metabolism. When kidney function is impaired, various measures may be instituted to relieve them of some of their workload. Often the patient is put to bed to minimize activity and, hence, lessen cellular metabolism. Unless the patient is losing large amounts of protein in the urine (which occurs in some conditions), he is usually given a low-protein diet, again to minimize the amount of nitrogenous wastes from protein metabolism that need to be eliminated. There may also be restrictions placed on the sodium and potassium in his diet, since sodium contributes to fluid retention, and the accumulation of potassium, which a damaged kidney cannot excrete (or has a lessened ability to excrete), may cause serious neuromuscular disturbances. The patient's fluid intake may be limited to prevent or lessen edema. It is important for the nurse to see that instructions regarding both food and fluid intake for the patient are followed exactly. Patients with renal disorders often suffer from anorexia and may need encouragement to eat their meals. The patient should be made aware of the importance of adhering to the diet and fluid intake that has been ordered for him, since this is part of his therapy. Many patients can help to keep track of their fluid intake; by encouraging them to participate in their care in this way, the nurse can often gain their cooperation.

Sometimes, in order to put the kidneys at rest and give them a chance to recover when there has been extensive tissue damage, or to maintain patients whose kidneys are no longer functioning, an artificial kidney is used. In the artificial kidney, blood is continually removed from an artery and allowed to circulate through a channel with a thin membrane through which a *dialyzing fluid* removes the impurities from it before it is returned to the patient through a vein. This process is called *renal dialysis*. There are several different types of machine for renal dialysis now available on the market, including units for home use. Some patients require renal dialysis for a short period of time, to tide them over an acute episode, but many people without functioning kidneys have been maintained over a period of years with an artificial kidney. Frequently, these patients come into an outpatient department or a clinic for dialysis every few days. In addition to renal dialysis, other methods of removing impurities from body fluids are occasionally used, such as peritoneal or gastrointestinal dialysis. In these techniques, large amounts of dialyzing fluid are injected into the peritoneal cavity or inserted into the gastrointestinal tract and later removed. Dialysis occurs in these cases through the mucous membrane.

For detail on the use of the renal dialysis machine, the nurse is referred to a medical-surgical nursing text.

When there is impairment of kidney function, the individual's fluid and electrolyte balance is disturbed. There is usually a retention of fluid in the tissues, and the patient's fluid intake is frequently restricted to minimize this tendency. When edema is present, the nurse should remember that edematous tissue is more prone to break down than normal tissue is, and therefore nursing measures to maintain the integrity of the skin are especially important. Patients who are confined to bed require particular attention to prevent the development of pressure areas. Fluids tend to collect in dependent parts of the body, such as the sacral area in bed patients, and also the lower limbs. These areas should be carefully watched for signs of impending tissue breakdown, and measures should be taken to prevent this. (See Chapter 25 for a discussion of measures to prevent the formation of decubitus ulcers.)

Meticulous skin care is important in the care of patients with renal impairment, not only as a factor in maintaining skin integrity, but also to cleanse the skin of perspiration and to get rid of the unpleasant odor from the increased elimination of nitrogenous wastes by this route. Bathing is particularly important for the patient's cleanliness and comfort.

To compensate for the lessened ability of the kidneys to excrete excess acid, an increased amount of carbonic acid is eliminated through the respiratory tract. Measures to facilitate breathing are therefore important. When the patient is in bed, his position should be such that maximum expansion of the chest is possible. The room should be well-ventilated, and an adequate supply of oxygen ensured (See Chapter 18).

The accumulation of nitrogenous wastes due to the kidneys' lessened ability to excrete these may cause disturbances in neuromuscular functioning. Headache and lethargy are not uncommon, and in severe cases of renal impairment, the patient may become disoriented and subsequently comatose. In these cases, the safety needs of the patient must be especially kept in mind. Although the sensorium usually remains clear even in patients with considerable kidney damage, it is always wise to watch for signs of mental confusion, particularly in older patients. Measures such as side rails to protect the confused patient from injuring himself and the application of mitts to prevent him from pulling at catheters or other tubing are frequently needed (see Chapter 24).

Weakness of the muscles may result from the retention of potassium ions, and the patient usually fatigues easily.

Because the heart is a muscular organ, it is usually affected by potassium retention. Readings of the apical heart beat are frequently ordered to assist in monitoring cardiac function in patients with renal disorders.

The experience of undergoing renal dialysis can be very frightening for the patient at first. Often the individual is very ill, and the machinery that is used can provoke much anxiety. Many large acute care hospitals now have a renal dialysis unit, often with a nurse in charge of the unit. A number of people may be involved in operating the machine, in taking samples for laboratory analysis, and in supervising technical details, and this too can be alarming to the patient. An explanation of the procedure beforehand helps the patient to understand what is happening to him, but the nurse should be aware that the patient needs continuing encouragement and supportive care. The presence of someone who is interested in him as an individual as well as in the technical aspects of his care can be very reassuring.

GUIDE TO ASSESSING URINARY ELIMINATION STATUS

1. What is the age of the patient?
2. If a child, has he achieved voluntary control over voiding during day time? night time?
3. What is the patient's usual voiding pattern? present pattern?
4. Is he having problems with voiding? If so, what are they?
5. What is the patient's usual food and fluid intake? Has this changed recently?
6. Is he on any medications that might affect urinary functioning, e.g., diuretics?
7. Are there any factors that might be affecting his voiding pattern?
8. Does he have a diagnosed health problem that is causing urinary dysfunctioning?

9. Is he voiding an amount of urine that is normal in relation to his intake and sufficient to promote health?

10. Does he show signs of localized urinary problems? generalized problems?

11. Is the urine normal in color, amount, odor, consistency? Does it contain observable abnormal constituents, such as blood or pus?

12. Has a urinalysis been done? If so, are the findings within normal ranges?

13. Have other urine tests or blood tests been ordered to assess renal functioning? If they have been performed, what were the results?

14. Have specific interventions been ordered, such as catheterization?

15. Does the patient have difficulty in discussing his urinary problems?

16. Does the patient need help in re-establishing a normal voiding pattern?

17. Does he need help with this diet and fluid intake?

18. Does he need an explanation of laboratory tests and nursing care measures?

19. Does the patient or his family need skills or knowledge in order to prevent a recurrence of his problem or improve his health?

GUIDE TO EVALUATING THE EFFECTIVENESS OF NURSING INTERVENTION

1. Is the patient taking the required amount of fluids to maintain adequate fluid balance? Is he voiding an adequate amount?

2. Are the laboratory test results showing improvement?

3. Is the patient's skin in good condition?

4. Is he getting sufficient rest?

5. Is he taking an adequate diet?

6. Is he comfortable—free from pain, restlessness, and anxiety?

STUDY SITUATION

Mrs. Smith needs an indwelling catheter prior to her surgery tomorrow. Mrs. Smith is an intelligent person; she understands the purpose of her surgery, but she has never had a urinary catheterization. The catheter is to be inserted the next morning.

That afternoon Mrs. Smith's husband comes to the nursing unit desk greatly disturbed. His wife has told him that she has to have a tube inserted and he does not understand why. In talking with Mr. Smith, the nurse learns that his mother had had a tube inserted and she died 2 days later.

1. What factors should the nurse consider in her explanation?

2. What should the nurse include in her explanation to Mr. Smith? Why?

3. What principles guide the nurse in carrying out a urinary catheterization?

4. Why is a urinary catheterization a distressing measure?

5. What nursing care interventions would be essential for Mrs. Smith as a result of the indwelling catheter?

6. How can the nurse evaluate the effectiveness of her nursing care after the catheterization?

SUGGESTED READINGS

Brink, C.: Promoting Urine Control in Older Adults: Assessing the Problem. *Geriatric Nursing*, 1:241–245, November-December, 1980.

Butts, P. A.: Assessing Urinary Incontinence in Women. *Nursing '79*, 9(3):72–74, March, 1979.

Demmerle, B., and Bartol, M. A.: Promoting Urine Control in Older Adults: Nursing Care of the Incontinent Patient. *Geriatric Nursing*, 1:246–250, November-December, 1980.

Finkbeiner, A. E., et al.: Promoting Urine Control in Older Adults: Helpful Drugs: Nursing Implications of Drug Therapy. *Geriatric Nursing*, 1:270–274, November-December, 1980.

Grant, R.: Washable Pads or Disposable Diapers. *Geriatric Nursing*, 3:248, July-August, 1982.

Gurevich, I.: The New Urine Meters: A Nursing '80 Product Survey. *Nursing '80*, 10(12):47–53, December, 1980.

Hartman, M.: Intermittent Self-Catheterization: Freeing Your Patient of the Foley. *Nursing '78*, 8(11):72–75, November, 1978.

Kinney, A. B., et al.: Promoting Urine Control in Older Adults: Urethral Catheterization . . . Pros and Cons. *Geriatric Nursing*, 1:258–263, November-December, 1980.

Reed, S. B.: Giving More Than Dialysis. *Nursing '82*, 12(4):58, April, 1982.

Ruble, J. A.: Childhood Nocturnal Enuresis. *American Journal of Maternal Child Nursing*, 6:26–31, January-February, 1981.

Wells, T.: Promoting Urine Control in Older Adults: Scope of the Problem. *Geriatric Nursing*, 1:236–240, November-December, 1980.

Wells, T., and Brink, C.: Promoting Urine Control in Older Adults: Helpful Equipment. *Geriatric Nursing*, 1:264–269, November-December, 1980.

REFERENCES

1. McEachern, J.: Retraining Bowel and/or Bladder. Surrey, British Columbia, paper prepared for Douglas College Nursing Programme, 1975.

2. Gurevich, I.: The New Urine Meters: A Nursing '80 Product Survey. *Nursing '80*, 10(12):47–53, December, 1980.

16

The Nurse Should Be Able to:

- Discuss the importance of adequate bowel elimination to the health and well-being of the individual
- Describe normal functioning in regard to bowel elimination in infants, children, and adults
- Discuss factors that may cause disturbances in bowel functioning
- Identify common problems people have in bowel functioning
- Assess a patient's status in regard to bowel functioning
- Identify situations requiring immediate nursing intervention in the care of patients with problems of bowel functioning
- Apply relevant principles in planning and implementing nursing interventions in patients
    a. to promote optimal bowel functioning
    b. to prevent potential problems in bowel elimination
    c. to restore normal elimination patterns in patients who have problems in meeting their bowel elimination needs
- Evaluate the effectiveness of nursing interventions

BOWEL ELIMINATION NEEDS

INTRODUCTION

During the process of digestion, food and fluids taken into the body are mixed and processed, nutrients are selected and absorbed for utilization of body tissues, and the waste products of digestion are excreted. The principal portions of the digestive tract concerned with the excretory function are the colon and the rectum. The colon receives digestive products in the liquid form of chyme, further processes this, and transports the resultant waste products to the rectum for removal from the body through the anal opening. In the colon, much of the water from the chyme is absorbed, so that, as the waste products pass through, they take on a semisolid and finally solid form. Sodium and chloride ions are absorbed during the process, and potassium and bicarbonate ions are excreted.

Interference with the normal functioning of gastrointestinal elimination has serious repercussions on the body's total functioning. The individual is usually uncomfortable and often distressed. If normal functioning is not restored, all body systems will eventually be affected. Complete stoppage of bowel functioning is a medical emergency, and surgical intervention is usually necessary to overcome the problem.

In dealing with disturbances of bowel elimination, as with urinary problems, nursing intervention is a potential source of embarrassment for both the nurse and the patient. The nurse can help put the patient at ease by discussing elimination without showing embarrassment herself and by carrying out necessary nursing measures in a relaxing manner.

ANATOMICAL AND PHYSIOLOGICAL CONSIDERATIONS

The rectum is a narrow muscular tube that is a continuation of the lower (sigmoid) colon. In the adult it is approximately 15 to 20 cm. (6 to 8 inches) in length and 2.5 to 4 cm. (1 1/2 inches) in width at the anal opening. The walls of the rectum consists of three transverse folds and folds that are vertical. The transverse folds are believed to assist in keeping the feces in the rectum until defecation is initiated. The vertical folds each contain an artery and a vein. The anal canal forms approximately the last 2.5 cm. (1 inch) of the rectum. Two muscular sphincters control the discharge of feces from the anus. The inner sphincter is composed of smooth muscle and is involuntary, responding to distention of the rectum; the external sphincter is composed of striated muscle and is under voluntary control.

Food passes through the gastrointestinal tract in wavelike propulsions called peristalsis. As the distal portion of one part of the tract becomes distended, a reflex is triggered to propel the food along to the next portion. There are three principal reflexes involved in this process: the gastrocolic reflex (propelling food from the stomach to the small intestine), the duodenocolic reflex (from small to large intestine), and the rectal reflex, which is initiated when the rectum is full and gives rise to the urge to empty it. Peristalsis occurs in the large intestine at infrequent intervals. Peristalsis is stimulated by the intake of food and fluids into the gastrointestinal tract. When food enters the duodenum from the stomach, approximately half an hour after ingestion, there is a mass peristaltic action as the gastrocolic reflex sets up a chain reaction throughout the system. The products of digestion move through the small intestine and the duodenocolic reflex is initiated. This pushes what was there into the large intestine. There is a mass peristaltic action in the large intestine and the waste products are propelled forward. In this movement, the part of the colon that is distal to the bolus (waste products) relaxes while the portion of the colon that is proximal to the bolus

327

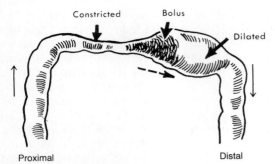

Constricted   Bolus

Dilated

Proximal   Distal

Waste products pass through the large bowel as shown here.

contracts. Thus, the waste products are propelled forward. Feces are pushed forward to distend the lower bowel and pass into the rectum. Distention of the rectum and lower colon stimulates parasympathetic nerve endings that transmit impulses to initiate the rectal reflex. At the same time, parasympathetic nerve impulses travel up the spinothalamic tract to a center in the medulla. The internal sphincter of the anus relaxes and the colon contracts. The urge to have a bowel movement is felt.

Although the rectal reflex is stimulated by the presence of waste products in the rectum and lower colon, the act of defecation itself is controlled voluntarily. Therefore, a person may or may not respond to the stimulus. During the act of defecation, a number of accessory muscles are brought into play. These are primarily the muscles of the abdominal wall, the diaphragm, and muscles of the pelvic floor. Contraction of the muscles of the abdominal wall, and fixing of the diaphragm, increase pressure within the abdominal cavity to force contents of the lower colon and rectum downward. Closing of the glottis (by holding the breath) also increases intra-abdominal pressure. If a forced expiration against the closed glottis is done, the pressure is greatly increased. Contraction of the muscles of the pelvic floor, and simultaneous relaxation of the anal sphincter, help in pushing the fecal mass through the anal canal. If a person does not respond to the stimulus to defecate, the urge will disappear.

NORMAL BOWEL ELIMINATION

The feces that are discharged through the anal orifice are the accumulated wastes from the intestines. The bulk of the feces consists of digestive residues and water, with water making up 60 to 80 per cent of the total. The digestive residues include those from undigested and unabsorbed foods and from digestive secretions. In addition, the feces also contain the debris of cells and mucus sloughed off the lining of the gastrointestinal tract and small amounts of material that have been secreted into the intestines, as well as bacteria and their products.

The intestines are the principal route for the excretion of some minerals, notably calcium and iron, as well as a large portion of the body's excess potassium. The usual brown color of stools is due to the presence of bile salts, chiefly urobilinogen, which is excreted via this route.

Between one tenth and one third of fecal matter consists of living and dead bacteria and their products. Bacteria are normally resident in the intestinal cavity. The usual resident bacteria are often referred to as the normal intestinal flora. It is felt that some of these aid in the digestive process through the synthesis of certain vitamins. To the bacteria normally present, then, are added those that have been taken into the gastrointestinal tract (through food and fluids, from fingers, or in swallowed air, for example) and the end products of bacteria from other parts of the body. All in all, it is estimated that between 50 billion and 500 billion living and dead bacteria are excreted in a person's feces in the course of a 24-hour period.

As the feces pass through the rectum, they assume the shape of that tubelike structure. Normal stools are soft and solid in consistency and cylindrical in shape. The amount of fecal matter excreted is highly dependent on the coarseness of the foodstuffs consumed. It may vary from 100 to 200 gm. per day in a person whose diet contains a large proportion of refined food to 300 to 400 gm. per day in the person who eats a diet that is high in fiber content. The number of bowel movements a person has also varies considerably from one individual to another, with the normal range considered to be between one bowel movement every 2 to 3 days and three bowel movements per day.

If the waste products are propelled too rapidly through the intestines, the resultant stools will be loose and watery. This is due to the shorter than normal amount of time available for the absorption of water from the intestines. If, on the other hand, there is undue delay in evacuation of the waste products, an excessive amount of water may be absorbed from them, with resultant stools that are dry and hard.

VARIATIONS IN BOWEL FUNCTIONING THROUGHOUT THE LIFE CYCLE

The first bowel movement the newborn infant has is the passage of meconium, a black, tarry substance that is present in the gastrointestinal tract of the full-term fetus. The stools gradually change from black to yellowish brown during the first week of life. There is a considerable variation in the pattern of bowel movements in infants. One may have a bowel movement several times a day, another once every 2 to 3 days. Young babies may have four to seven bowel movements in a day. In breast-fed babies the stools are usually looser and lighter yellow in color and do not have as strong a fecal odor as those of bottle-fed babies. Breast-fed babies also rarely develop constipation, although they may do so when they are weaned if their fluid intake is not sufficient. With the addition of solids to the diet, the stools become fewer in number, darker in color, and firmer in consistency.

Infants and small toddlers normally have a bowel movement whenever the rectum is full, in response to the rectal reflex. The necessary neuromuscular control for voluntary control is usually not present until the age of about 15 to 18 months. (Most child care specialists do not advocate starting to train the child until he is 1½ to 2 years old.) By the time they are 3 to 4 years old, most children have fairly good control over defecation, although accidents may still happen if the child is in a stressful situation, is too busy to go to the bathroom, or has diarrhea.

During the preschool years a pattern of bowel habits is established that the individual will usually carry with him throughout his lifetime, unless a conscious effort is made to change them. These patterns vary widely from one person to another, as we have already noted.

In school-age children, adolescents, and young adults, the elimination pattern of the individual tends to remain fairly constant. However, there are some variations in pregnant women, in middle-aged women who have borne children and in older people that should be noted.

During pregnancy, the entire gastrointestinal tract becomes more sluggish as pregnancy has a relaxing effect on smooth muscle. Constipation is common and may be caused by the flaccidity of muscles due to hormonal changes or, in the latter stages of pregnancy, to pressure on the abdominal organs. Changes in body structure, too, make it difficult for the pregnant woman to bend over to increase intra-abdominal pressure and facilitate defecation. Hemorrhoids, which are enlarged veins in the rectal area, are not infrequently seen in pregnant women and add to the discomfort of bowel evacuation.

During the middle years of adulthood (and later if the problem is not corrected), women in whom the muscles of the pelvic floor have been stretched from childbirth may have difficult in evacuating the rectum, or they may have a problem in controlling the anal sphincter, with a resultant small bit of incontinence if they cannot get to a bathroom in time to respond to the urge to defecate.

In old age, a loss of muscle tone and decreased exercise may lead to constipation. Older people may require a high fiber diet and a good intake of fluids to increase peristalsis and to keep the consistency of the feces soft.

FACTORS AFFECTING BOWEL FUNCTIONING

A great many factors will affect a person's bowel functioning in addition to the variations that occur at different stages in the life cycle.

The food a person eats and the amount of fluids he consumes have a great deal to do with both the nature of the bowel movements he has and the frequency with which these occur. An adequate amount of fiber in the diet, such as that found in whole grain cereals and raw fruits and vegetables, is important in providing sufficient bulk to stimulate the peristaltic action of the intestines. People whose diet consists mostly of highly refined foods usually have fewer bowel movements and the stools are likely to be firmer and darker in color than those who ensure that they include whole grain cereals and breads and some raw fruits and vegetables in their daily diet. Then, too, some foods are notoriously gas-

A diet containing adequate fluids and fiber will promote normal bowel functioning in most persons.

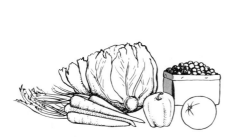

Vegetables and fruit

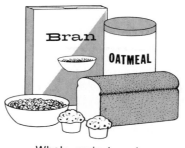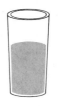

Whole grain breads and cereals

Adequate fluids

forming, such as cabbage, turnips, lettuce, and beans. Some fried foods, as well as meats with a high fat content, are particularly hard to digest. Food-borne infection may also cause gastrointestinal upsets (see Chapter 14).

● The water content of the body needs continual replenishment to keep up with the body's internal needs and to cover the amount of water excreted in body wastes. If there is an inadequate intake of fluids, the body's internal needs will be taken care of first, on a priority basis, with lessened amounts of water being excreted in urine and feces. The urine becomes more concentrated as a result, and the feces become drier and harder than usual.

The principal source of water replenishment for the body is the fluid that one drinks. It is important, then, to ensure an adequate intake of water and other fluids to maintain the soft consistency of the feces. Many a sturborn case of constipation has been cured by making sure that the person had six to eight glasses of water a day. It is one of the simplest and, often, most effective means both to maintain the soft consistency of the feces and to promote peristaltic action in the intestines.

A person's habits regarding bowel evacuation are a factor that must be considered too. The act of defecation is voluntary after the age of about 3 to 4 years in normal, healthy people, and a conditioned response is established to a certain time of the day, or after meals for example (when the gastrocolic reflex occurs and the rectal reflex is subsequently stimulated). Many people use aids such as taking a glass of hot water with lemon juice or a cup of hot tea or coffee before breakfast to stimulate having a bowel movement. Many maintain their faith in eating prunes or drinking prune juice at breakfast or eating a bowl of bran flakes before going to bed at night to promote regularity. (Both are good, natural aids to elimination.) Some people habitually take laxatives, or will use suppositories on a regular basis, while some have been known to give themselves a daily enema to clear the rectum.

A person's lifestyle also affects his bowel functioning. Regular mealtimes and a regular time for defecation help in establishing maintaining a regular pattern. Making sure that a person has some exercise every day helps to improve muscle tone. In Chapter 14 we mentioned that light exercise after meals, such as walking, helps to stimulate peristaltic action and promote digestion. Prolonged inactivity contributes to constipation, and prolonged sitting is conducive to hemorrhoids. People who are bedridden lose tone in their muscles very rapidly, and constipation is a very common problem among the sick. Constipation may also be a problem in people like nurses and others who do shift work, since the individual's biological time clock is constantly being readjusted to fit changing schedules.

Medications that a person is taking may also affect his bowel functioning. Drugs that depress the nervous system may lessen the motility of the intestines. Some drugs are irritating to the gastrointestinal system and may cause hypermotility, with resultant diarrhea.

Nor should we forget the effects of emotions on a person's bowel functioning. Stress and anxiety may lead to either increased or decreased motility of the gastrointestinal tract. Anger, too, particularly if it is not expressed openly, may cause disturbances of functioning, often with excessive gas formation and resultant distention.

There are also many congenital abnormalities, injuries, and disease processes that affect bowel functioning. Some infants are born with an imperforate anus, for example, which must be corrected by surgery before normal bowel movements can occur. Some may have other abnormalities of the structure of functioning of the gastrointestinal tract that interfere with normal bowel elimination. (These conditions are usually covered extensively in pediatric nursing courses.) In patients who have had spinal cord injuries, the rectal reflex, which is normally transmitted from the rectum to the sacral area by the parasympathetic nerves, may be destroyed. They may also lose control of the voluntary muscles concerned with defecation. This may happen, too, with a patient whose brain has been damaged by the effects of a stroke. With special training, however, these people can usually achieve a regularity of bowel habits that enables them to be free of the constant fear of incontinence.

COMMON PROBLEMS

The nurse is likely to encounter problems of bowel dysfunction in both young and old people and in both community and institutional practice. Among the common problems are: constipation, diarrhea, abdominal distention, flatulence, pain or discomfort associated with elimination, impacted feces, bowel incontinence, and parasitic infestations. In addition, the nurse is likely to care for people who, because of a health problem, have an artificial opening made into the intestine for the removal of the waste products of digestion. Because the first six of the problems we have named tend to occur in combination, we will discuss them under the two headings of constipation and diarrhea.

Constipation

Constipation is a very common problem among otherwise healthy people of all ages, as well as in the ill. Constipation is difficulty or infrequency in passing stools. Stools that are harder and drier than usual are more difficult to pass. As we mentioned earlier in this chapter, stools may become hard and dry if there is an undue delay in the evacuation of feces. It stands to reason, then, that anything that causes undue delay in the passage of feces is likely to result in contipation.

A breakdown in the conditioned reflex for defecation is by far the most common cause of delay of evacuation. In many people, the act of defecation is under voluntary control and is conditioned to time and activity. When the urge to defecate is overcome by voluntary muscle contraction, the rectum adjusts itself to the increased tension or may even return stools to the sigmoid. If this is habitually done, the normal conditioned reflex is lost. This may be due to habits developed in early childhood or to failure on the part of adults to respond to the normal defecation urge because of the pressures of time and daily activities. Pain on defecation, such as that associated with hemorrhoids or rectal surgery, will also interfere with the normal conditioned reflex.

Another common cause of constipation is excessive tone of the circular muscle of the intestines, which is thought to be due to an imbalance of the autonomic nervous system. Strong emotions are believed to cause constipation through the increased production of epinephrine, with resulting inhibition of peristalsis. Some drugs, among them morphine and to a lesser extent codeine, decrease motility in the small intestine and the colon because of their depressant action on the central nervous system.

Disturbances in reflex peristalsis may be due simply to the lack of sufficient fluids or bulky foods in the diet. An inadequate intake of foods such as cereals and vegetables may result in insufficient bulk in the residue of waste products to stimulate the reflex for defecation. The excessive use of laxatives may cause constipation owing to overstimulation of the bowel and a "wearing-out" (accommodation) effect on the nerves initiating the reflex action. People who habitually use laxatives frequently have to change the type taken to overcome this effect. Disease processes, including inflammation of the pelvic or abdominal viscera and tumors, may also cause a disturbance in reflex peristalsis.

Mechanical disturbances that can also cause constipation include weakness of the intestinal muscles as a result of a lack of essential vitamins (notably the B group) or electrolytes (particularly potassium), disease processes, or old age; weakness of the voluntary muscles controlling defecation; and weakness in any of the abdominal, pelvic, or diaphragmatic muscles. Obstruction in any part of the gastrointestinal tract will also delay or prevent the passage of feces. Obstruction may be caused by disease processes, tumors, or congenital abnormalities.

The person who is constipated may have other problems as well as the hardened feces. He may complain of a "bloated feeling." This is caused by abdominal distention, which results when the waste products remain too long in the gastrointestinal tract. The distention is caused by air that remains in the large intestine and the fluid that moves back into it when waste products have been there for a long time.

Flatus results from swallowed air, the consumption of gas-forming foods, or bacterial action within the large intestine. If not expelled, the air accumulates in the intestine and often causes generalized discomfort and crampy pain. The patient who is constipated may also complain of a headache, anorexia, and nausea. These usually disappear upon evacuation of the rectal contents.

Another frequent complaint of the constipated person is that of *tenesmus*, which is frequent painful straining in unproductive attempts at defecation. Pain on defecation may be associated with hemorrhoids, which are common among pregnant women and among older people. Anal fissures (linear ulcers at the mrgin of the anus) will also make defecation painful.

If stool remains in the rectum for a long period of time, it may develop into a large, hardened mass that is difficult to expel. The term impacted feces is used to describe this condition. Sometimes there is seepage around the mass, with a resultant discharge of small amounts of liquid stool. This is important to remember, particularly in bedridden patients, because there is the possibility that constipation may be overlooked when it has been noted that the patient has had a bowel movement.

Diarrhea

Diarrhea is the discharge of loose, watery stools due to inordinate speed in the passage of waste products through the gastrointestinal tract. It has many causes. Some diarrheas are due to direct stimulation or irritation of the central or autonomic nervous system. Diarrhea resulting from tension is an example. Diarrhea may be the most obvious manifestation of anxiety in a stable individual. Pre-examination diarrhea is a fairly common occurrence among students, as is pre-battle diarrhea among soldiers.

Certain drugs, such as reserpine, which is used for the treatment of hypertension, may also cause hypermotility of the intestine by acting on the autonomic nervous system, with resultant diarrhea.

Probably the most common set of causes of diarrhea, however, result from irritation of the gastrointestinal tract. These lead to a reflex type of diarrhea, the reverse of the mechanism that occurs in constipation. The irritation may be mechanical, as that caused by dietary indiscretions such as eating coarse foods or an excessive amount of seasonings; it may be chemical, as in some food and drug poisonings; or it may be, in some individuals, an allergic reaction to certain foods. For example, many people have allergic reactions after eating shellfish. Inflammation of the intestinal mucosa due to pathogenic infection is a very common cause of diarrhea. It is believed that the diarrhea experienced by many international travelers is caused by changes in the normal bacterial flora of the colon. Certain drugs, termed cathartics, cause formation of loose stools through irritation of the intestinal mucosa.

There are a few conditions producing diarrhea that may be considered to be defects in the anatomical processes necessary for defecation. Some disease conditions may cause an increase in the neuromuscular excitability of the intestine. Certain "malabsorption syndromes" also exist, in which the problem is one of failure on the part of the intestines to absorb water or nutrients as the digestive products pass through it.

The person who has diarrhea often complains of generalized abdominal pain. This is usually caused by flatus, which distends the large and small intestines. He may also have pains of a piercing, gripping nature. These are usually spasmodic, and are caused by the strong peristaltic contractions of the intestinal musculature as the waste products are propelled precipitously through the gastrointestinal tract. These pains are frequently accompanied by a feeling of urgency in the need to defecate. Although an increase in the number of stools is not always an indication of diarrhea, it often occurs with diarrhea. Again, as in constipation, there may be frequent, painful straining, which, in the case of the person with diarrhea, may produce a small watery discharge rather than formed stool. Redness and *pruritus* around the anal area, due to constant irritation, may add further to the person's discomfort.

If the diarrhea is prolonged, the individual will show signs and symptoms of fluid and electrolyte loss, such as poor tissue turgor, weight loss, thirst, and malnutrition (see Chapter 17). He complains of fatigue, weakness, and general malaise. Nausea and vomiting frequently accompany diarrhea and further aggravate the loss of fluids and electrolytes.

Incontinence

Incontinence of feces frequently occurs in combination with incontinence of urine. It is a common problem in people who have been paralyzed as a result of spinal cord injuries, as we have mentioned. It is also common in people who have had a stroke or other problem in which centers in the brain controlling voluntary movement or the neural pathways transmitting impulses from the sacral area to the brain have been impaired. If the person has lost consciousness, incontinence will occur as a result of loss of voluntary motor control in any case. However, if measures are taken to restore normal bowel and bladder functioning as soon as the person regains consciousness, the incontinence need not be a continuing problem. Unfortunately, many post-stroke patients are plagued with the problem of incontinence for months or years because the proper measures are not taken during the acute stage of the illness. Incontinence is a very prevalent problem among elderly residents in nursing homes and other extended care facilities. In the older person, it may be the result of health problems, such as a stroke, or it may be due to loss of strength in the muscles controlling defecation. Sometimes, the incontinence is psychological in origin. This is more common in children than in adults.

Whatever the cause, incontinence is a very distressing problem for an individual. It reduces him to the dependent state of an infant, and his self-esteem is shattered. It is very embarrassing for the patient, his family, and his visitors. For the person who has always been fastidious in his habits, it can be very demoralizing. He may become extremely anxious about his bowels, wanting reassurance from nursing personnel that he is "clean."

Incontinence seriously restricts an individual's social activities. He is fearful of leaving the confines of the nursing home (sometimes even his room) in case he has an accident. Inconspicuous devices to collect urine for men and protective undergarments for women help to make socialization easier but, especially in the case of fecal incontinence, there is always the problem of unpleasant odors. In a large percentage of patients, continence can be restored with a good program of bladder and bowel retraining, as has been demonstrated in rehabilitation programs for people with paralysis from spinal cord injuries and in numerous studies undertaken in long-term care facilities for the elderly.

Artificial Openings into the Intestine

Some people are unable to have a normal bowel movement because of a disease process or obstruction that makes it impossible for feces to pass normally through the colon, into the rectum, and out through the anal canal. For these people, an artificial opening from the colon to the surface of the abdomen may be created surgically. The procedure may also be done for people who are paralyzed from a spinal cord injury when it is considered advisable to divert the fecal matter before it reaches the rectum. In an ileostomy, the opening is from the ileum to the surface of the abdomen. This may be performed because of surgical excision of part of the bowel, chronic inflammatory conditions, or tumors of the bowel. The consistency and contents of the fecal matter that flows from the openings made in the two procedures are different. In the ileostomy, the fecal matter, being higher in the bowel, is more liquid in consistency and, since it also still contains digestive enzymes, is more irritating to the skin of the abdomen. A great deal of sensitivity is needed by nurses who are caring for the patient on whom such a procedure has been done. The patient needs much emotional reassurance and support to accept the idea of the operation and also to accept it as part of himself once it has been done.

Parasitic Infections

Parasitic infestations are prevalent throughout the world. There are no longer geographical limitations to their boundaries, because of the rapidity with which people move about in the world these days, as well as the migration of large groups of people from one part of the globe to another. Some types of intestinal parasites, however, are more common in some geographical areas than in others. In North America, among the most common are the helminths, or parasitic worms, which cause infections in the gastrointestinal tract. Pinworms, roundworms, hookworms, and tapeworms are four that are not uncommonly seen. Children are particularly vulnerable to worm infestations because they will often pick up dirt on their fingers, which gets transferred to the mouth. They also often go barefooted and can pick up infections through the soles of the feet, especially if there is a cut or scratch on the foot. Pinworms are prevalent throughout the world, although they are most commonly found in large families, in poor areas, and in schools and dormitories where one person may infect another. Roundworms and hookworms are prevalent in tropical regions and in temperate zones up to 40° latitude (including the southern United States). Tapeworms are common in the United States, Canada, and many other parts of the world. Parasitic infections are

SUMMARY OF BASIC FEATURES OF FOUR HELMINTHIC INFECTIONS

Features	Roundworm	Pinworm	Tapeworm	Hookworm
Causative agent	Ascaris lumbricoides	Enterobius vermicularis	Taenia saginata or solium	Necator americanus
Mode of transmission	Ingestion of ova in dirt contaminated by human feces. Hand contamination from infested household dust.	Inhaled from infested air; ingested from hands that had contact with infested anal skin or fomites.	Ingested from handling or eating infested beef or pork.	Penetration of bare feet.
Clinical manifestations	May be asymptomatic. Fever and malaise; restless, disturbed sleep. Abdominal distention and discomfort; vomiting. Anemia. Infested stools; steatorrhea; intestinal obstruction. Peritonitis.	Perianal itch. Nose picking. Restless and irritable.	Varied symptoms: Abdominal cramping or pain, nervousness, insomnia, anorexia, weight loss. Sometimes asymptomatic.	Severe anemia. Occult blood in feces. Abdominal colic, malnutrition, intestinal or bile duct obstruction. Intestinal mucosa and liver damage.
Diagnostic findings	Positive stool culture for ova and parasites.	Microscopic viewing of parasite on scotch tape strip removed from perianal area.	Positive stool culture for ova and parasites.	Positive stool culture for ova and parasites.
Medical treatment	Piperazine derivative (Antepar).	Piperazine derivative (Antepar) or Povan.	Stabrine or Yomesan.	Tetrachloroethylene or Hexylresorcinol.

From Tackett, J. J. M., and Hunsberger, M.: *Family Centered Care of Children and Adolescents.* Philadelphia, W. B. Saunders Company, 1981.

usually discussed thoroughly in pediatric nursing texts.

The worm infestations cause irritation of the intestinal tract, often with resultant diarrhea, pruritus around the anal area, and the presence of worms in the stools. They may also lead to more serious problems, including intestinal obstruction, anemia, and damage to the liver, brain, and heart.

ASSESSMENT

In assessing a person's bowel functioning it is important to know the age of the person and his general state of health. As a baseline for her assessment, the nurse needs to know about the usual bowel habits and the normal patterns of defecation of the individual. People vary in both frequency of defecation and nature of stools; what is normal for one person may not be normal for another.

A knowledge of the patient's pattern of bowel elimination includes the frequency of defecation and a description of the color, odor, and consistency of stools (hard, soft, or liquid). Feces may contain foreign matter that the patient may be able to describe, such as blood, worms, pus, or mucus. Most people become anxious if they think there is blood in the stools. Black stools may indicate the presence of old blood, and red stools, fresh blood. However, certain foods and medications can also discolor feces. For example, beets can color feces red, and iron (in a medication) can color feces black.

It is important to find out if the patient is having any current problems, and if so, the nature of these problems as he sees them. Has he had them long? Does he get them often? Does he have a colostomy or ileostomy?

The nurse should also determine whether the patient uses laxatives or other aids to elimination, such as suppositories or enemas, and, if so, what kind is used. Some people use laxatives or other aids regularly. Some feel that a "good purge" or "cleaning out" every once in a while is beneficial to the system, and they will use a strong cathartic for this purpose, even if they are not constipated.

Food habits are also pertinent in assessing the person's bowel functioning. Failure to ensure that the diet has sufficient bulk or fluids may lead to constipation. The ingestion of irritating foods may cause diarrhea. It is important to know then what the individual's dietary intake has been in the immediate past and also what his normal food habits are.

Since emotions play such an important role in the causation of many cases of bowel dysfunction, it is helpful to determine if the patient has been under any particular stress.

The nurse should also find out something about the person's lifestyle. Does he eat regular meals? Does he take time to go to the bathroom when he feels the need to have a bowel movement? Does he exercise regularly? Does he do shift work?

Much of this information will have been gathered in taking the nursing history. The nurse also needs to be aware of the nature of any health problems the patient has that may affect bowel functioning, and of the physician's plans of care for the patient. These data can usually be found in the patient's record. The nurse supplements these data with her own observations.

Subjective Observations

Control over defecation and urination is taught in early childhood and may be associated with values of good and bad. In some cultures, control over bladder and bowel functioning is expected early, and there may have been much tension and anxiety associated with early teaching.

Many people are embarrassed to talk about their elimination problems. In discussing these problems, then, the nurse should ensure privacy, since it is often difficult for patients to talk about their bowel habits in the presence of other people. The nurse, too, may find it hard to ask the personal questions that are necessary. Questions should be phrased in simple, nontechnical language that assists the patient to give pertinent information in his answers and yet maintains his own feelings of personal dignity in doing so.

If the person has indicated that he is having a problem, the nurse should ask him to describe the nature of the problem. He may say he is "all bound up" or hasn't had a bowel movement for 3 days. She should also ask if he has any of the other problems discussed earlier in this chapter that are frequently associated with constipation. Most people use the term diarrhea, although some may say frequent, loose stools. It is important to find out if the problem is associated with any foods the person has eaten recently. Is he having pain or any of the other problems associated with diarrhea that were discussed earlier in this chapter? Are other people in the family affected too?

In caring for a small child it is important to know the stage he has reached in regard to toilet training and the words the child uses to express his elimination needs. It is important to continue the toilet-training schedule maintained at home. With more and more hospitals permitting and encouraging parents to stay with children, the mother or father at the bedside can be very helpful in this regard.

✔ CHARACTERISTICS OF NORMAL FECES

Consistency	Soft, formed
Shape	Cylindrical
Color	Brown
Amount	100–400 gm./day depending on coarseness of diet
Frequency	1–3 times a day to once every 2–3 days

Objective Observations

The patient with bowel problems may not be able to communicate his discomfort verbally to the nurse. She should, therefore, be alert to the signs and symptoms that indicate this discomfort. The patient may have had no bowel movement for several days, he may have abdominal distention, and he may be passing large amounts of flatus by rectum or by mouth. The hospitalized patient is particularly prone to constipation because of lack of exercise and the alterations in daily activity and, often, in diet that are imposed by being confined to hospital. These interfere with the normal conditioned reflex for defecation.

In observing the feces of the patient, it is important to note the consistency, color, size, shape, and odor of the fecal matter and compare them with the normal. The presence of foreign matter, as described earlier, should also be noted.

The person who is constipated may show signs other than the passage of hardened feces, as we discussed earlier, and the nurse should be alert to these. In abdominal distention, for example, the patient usually has a swollen abdomen, which on palpation feels hard and unyielding. Pain on defecation may be noted by the difficulty the individual appears to be having when he tries to have a bowel movement.

Pertinent observations in the case of the patient with diarrhea include the frequency and consistency of the stools, as well as their odor and the presence of foreign matter. Undigested food is sometimes present in the feces because of the speed with which it is propelled through the gastrointestinal tract. Signs of localized irritation around the anus may be present. These include redness and pruritus. If the diarrhea is prolonged, the patient will show signs and symptoms of fluid and electrolyte imbalance as well as poor nutrition.

It is essential that an accurate record of the patient's intake and output be maintained. This will include the number of bowel movements and the approximate amount of fluid lost through the feces. The nurse should also note the patient's ability to tolerate foods and fluids. It is very important to determine the patient's nutritional status and to observe for signs of weakness and fatigue.

Diagnostic Tests

Among the diagnostic tests for persons with bowel dysfunction is the laboratory examination of a specimen of feces. It is often the responsibility of nursing personnel to collect the specimen and send it to the laboratory, where it may be examined for such substances as blood, microorganisms, parasites, and other abnormal constituents, as well as for fat, nitrogen, urobilinogen, which feces normally contain.

Blood from the lower gastrointestinal tract is usually bright red, whereas old blood from the upper tract may appear black. On the other hand, blood may be present but occult, that is, hidden to the naked eye.

The specimen can usually be kept at room temperature. Sometimes, however, it is frozen for transport to the laboratory and sometimes it is placed in a preservative solution.

Excess fat in the stools can be indicative of gastrointestinal disease, as can the presence of undigested food and urobilinogen. Normally there is a considerable amount of the latter in feces, but in cases of an obstruction in bile flow the feces may be clay-colored and negative for urobilinogen.

X-ray and fluoroscopic examinations of the gastrointestinal tract may also be done. A lower

NORMAL VALUES FOR FECES

Bulk	100–200 gm./24 hours (may be up to 300–400 depending on coarseness of diet)
Dry matter	32–64 gm./24 hours
Total fat	Less than 6.0 gm./24 hours
Total nitrogen	Less than 2.0 gm./24 hours
Urobilinogen	40–280 mg./24 hours
Water	Approximately 60–80%

Modified from Beeson, P. B., et al. (eds.): *Cecil Textbook of Medicine.* 15th ed. Philadelphia, W. B. Saunders Company, 1979.

GI series is often done to visualize the colon and rectum. In this case, the barium sulfate is introduced in the form of an enema. Scans and ultrasound techniques may also be used, as well as radioactive isotope tracings for diagnostic purposes.

It is often necessary to examine the inner cavity of the anal canal, the rectum, and the lower colon to look for disease processes, tumors, fissures, or hemorrhoids. In order to visualize the cavity, a tubular instrument with a light at the end of it is commonly used. An *anoscopy* is an inspection of the anal canal by this means: a *proctoscopy* is this type of examination of the rectum, and a *sigmoidoscopy* (or *proctosigmoidoscopy*) is such an examination of the rectum and sigmoid colon. For some examinations, a speculum is used, either alone or in combination with the lighted tube. These instruments may be called anoscopes, proctoscopes, or sigmoidoscopes, depending on the examination for which they are designed. An enema or a suppository is usually given before the examination to clear the tract of fecal material. The patient is asked to get into a knee-chest position. If he is unable to do this, Sims's position may be used. The patient should be draped carefully so that he is suitably covered, and the center fold of the drape can be raised to expose the anus. These examinations are both embarrassing and uncomfortable for the patient. The nurse can help the person by making sure that he does not have to wait too long in the required position, by ensuring that the drapes cover him well so that he is not unnecessarily exposed, and by reassuring him that the discomfort is of short duration.

PRIORITIES FOR NURSING ACTION

People are uncomfortable when they need to empty their bowels. Elimination is a very basic physiological need. When people are well, they can usually take care of their own needs for bowel elimination by going to a bathroom and using the toilet facilities. When they are ill, however, they are often dependent on the help of nursing personnel to meet this very basic need. They may need help to get to the bathroom, or if confined to bed, may have to use a bedpan. Often, with sick people, the need is urgent and takes precedence over other matters. It is important that the nurse promptly answer the patient's request for a bedpan or for help to get to the bathroom.

If the person is having problems with bowel elimination, the nurse also has to assess the acuteness of the problem in determining priorities for nursing action.

In determining priorities for nursing action in the care of patients with problems of bowel functioning, the nurse must take into account

◢ PRINCIPLES RELEVANT TO BOWEL FUNCTIONING ▇▇▇▇▇

1. **The function of the bowels is to eliminate the waste products of digestion.**
2. **Normal bowel elimination is essential to efficient body functioning.**
3. **The body's fluid and electrolyte balance can be seriously affected by disturbances in bowel functioning.**
4. **Obstruction of the bowel poses a serious threat to life.**
5. **The oral intake of food or fluids stimulates a mass peristaltic action in the gastrointestinal tract.**
6. **The urge to defecate results from stimulation of the rectal reflex by distention of the lower colon and rectum.**
7. **The act of defecation is normally under voluntary control after the age of 3 to 4 years.**
8. **The necessary neuromuscular structures are not sufficiently developed for voluntary control over bowel elimination until the age of 15 to 18 months.**
9. **Once achieved, control over defecation is an important area of independent functioning for the individual.**
10. **The number of stools an infant has per day varies considerably, with four to seven per day being average for young babies.**
11. **The normal pattern of bowel elimination in individuals after infancy varies from one bowel movement every 2 to 3 days, to three bowel movements per day.**
12. **Patterns of bowel elimination and consistency of feces are highly dependent on an individual's food and fluid intake.**
13. **Stress, anxiety, and other strong emotions may interfere with bowel functioning.**

the acuteness of the condition. In the severely constipated patient, there may be an immediate need to end the patient's discomfort through bringing about a bowel movement. Complete stoppage of the bowel is a medical emergency requiring surgical intervention. With the patient who is acutely distressed with diarrhea, nursing intervention will be directed first to carrying out measures to control the discharge of stools. There may also be an urgent need to replace lost fluids and electrolytes.

SPECIFIC NURSING INTERVENTIONS

Measures to Re-establish Normal Bowel Functioning

In People Who Are Constipated. Constipation is a problem for many people, both sick and well. It is almost always a problem for patients confined to bed, and care should be taken to direct nursing action toward its prevention in patients who are ill. Because bowel habits are learned early in childhood and each individual's pattern of elimination is different, the nurse must develop a plan of care in conjunction with the patient, taking into consideration the individual's previously established pattern.

Important factors to consider in preventing constipation or in overcoming a long-standing problem of constipation include regularity of time for defecation; prompt attention to the urge to defecate; a diet that contains sufficient laxative food, sufficient bulk, and a sufficient intake of fluids; and an adequate amount of exercise.

Because the gastrocolic reflex is usually strongest after breakfast, immediately after the morning meal is a good time to encourage the patient to move his bowels. Affording privacy is important. Sufficient time should be allowed for the process, and the patient should not be hurried. If his condition permits, the individual should be allowed to go to the bathroom or to use a bedside commode. Most patients find it awkward to use a bedpan to have a bowel movement. If a bedpan has to be used, the patient should be in a sitting position unless this position is contraindicated.

The patient may need to be helped to increase his sensitivity to the stimulus for defecation. Drinking hot fluids helps to activate mass peristalsis and, particularly if they are taken before breakfast, helps to stimulate the gastrocolic reflex and subsequently the rectal reflex. The patient should be given an explanation of the process of elimination with stress placed on the importance of responding to the urge to defecate. The individual can sometimes be helped to defecate by massaging the abdomen in a circu-

lation motion, moving downward over the descending colon on the left side of the abdomen. Slight pressure on the side of, or posterior to, the anus sometimes helps expel feces. Nursing personnel use cotton gauze or digital pads for this measure.

Through repetition of these measures at the same time each day or as frequently as the patient is in the habit of having a bowel movement, regular habits can often be re-established. Glycerin suppositories or enemas are also used in some situations to facilitate defecation, particularly when regularity is being established. Their use is then gradually withdrawn as a regular pattern is set. Laxative drugs and stool softeners, such as mineral oil, may also be used sometimes to help in developing regularity; again, their use is gradually terminated as the patient gains improved colonic functioning.

The individual may require help also in establishing dietary patterns that give him a sufficient amount of laxative foods, foods containing fiber, and adequate fluids for normal bowel functioning. Fluid intake, it is usually suggested, should be 2000 to 3000 ml. per 24 hours, depending on the person's tolerance. The diet should contain sufficient bulk to stimulate reflex activity, as well as other foods which the individual finds have a laxative effect on him. Prunes, figs, prune juice, and, to a lesser extent, acid fruit juices from citrus fruits and previously cooked dried fruits are particularly good to stimulate intestinal motility. It should be noted that older people are not always able to tolerate the roughage contained in many fresh fruits and vegetables. For them, increasing bulk through whole grain breads and cereals and encouraging them to increase their fluid intake are often helpful.

Constipation is aggravated by inactivity and poor muscle tone. A regular program of activity designed for the individual can be planned and the patient assisted to carry it out. Strengthening of the abdominal muscles is particularly important.

In People with Diarrhea. In attempting to re-establish normal bowel functioning in the patient with diarrhea, it is important to know the cause of the diarrhea. The most common cause is irritation of the gastrointestinal tract; removal of the irritant will therefore stop the symptoms in most cases. Specific drugs may be ordered to decrease intestinal motility or to coat the irritated membranes of the intestines. If the diarrhea is psychological in origin (for example, if it is caused by anxiety or tension), it will often disappear when the stressful situation is over. If, however, it is a chronic problem, medical intervention is usually necessary to help the patient to resolve his problems. Some diarrheas are the result of defects in the anatomical processes necessary for defecation. These conditions require medical or surgical therapy.

In People with Artificial Openings into the Intestine. For people who have had a colostomy, elimination may be allowed to follow the person's normal pattern with the fecal matter being collected in a pouch or bag that is fitted over the stoma and changed as necessary. Or, control over elimination may be attempted by using irrigations at regular intervals.

There is, however, no way to control the flow of fecal matter from an ileostomy, so that a pouch or bag over the stoma is the traditional way of coping with the problem.

Diet is, of course, very important in regulating the content of the fecal matter and the production of gas in the intestines. In the matter of food, each person has to determine what is best for him. Generally speaking, foods that are irritating or gas-forming are best avoided, and those that have a laxative effect should be taken with caution. Foods that the person knows from past experience give him trouble are best avoided. It is usually through a process of trial and error that a person determines what foods he can enjoy without distressing aftereffects.

Common measures that may be carried out by first-year nursing students are changing a colostomy dressing and irrigating a colostomy. These measures are described later in the chapter in the specific nursing interventions.

In People with Parasitic Infections. The principal measures used in re-establishing normal bowel functioning in people with parasitic infections are directed toward ridding the gastrointestinal tract of the parasite and preventing further infestations. Specific antihelminthic drugs are used in the treatment of worm infections. Sometimes enemas are used to assist in ridding the colon of the parasite. If hospitalized, the person is put on enteric isolation precautions (see Chapter 26), which must be strictly carried out. In the case of persons with pinworms, it is usually necessary to treat the whole family. The disinfection of clothing and bed linens is also recommended. In the case of tapeworms, which may be transmitted through meats, such as pork and beef, careful washing of the hands after handling meat, cleaning of the chopping board before reuse, and thorough cooking of the meat are important preventive measures. Roundworms may lurk in dirt contaminated by infected feces, and the careful washing of fruits and vegetables, particularly in areas where these worms are prevalent, is a good preventive measure. Hookworm infestation is usually accomplished through penetration of the soles of the

feet; hence, in areas where these worms are prevalent, it is not a good idea to go around barefooted. Measures to prevent further recurrence for all types of worm infection include good hygiene and sanitary measures.

Well-enforced government regulations help to ensure that our food supplies are safe, but it is important that the consumer take adequate precautions as well. The measures suggested in Chapter 14 to prevent food poisoning are important in preventing helminthic infections, as well. One cannot stress too much, however, the importance of good personal hygiene and good hygienic practices in the kitchen, nor of cooking meats (in particular pork) thoroughly. Great caution should be used in eating meats that are not government inspected, such as that from wild animals and, even with government inspection, of pork and pork products where worms can lurk undetected.

The Use of Bedpans

As we discussed in Chapter 15, patients who are not ambulatory must use bedpans and urinals in elimination. Many of the principles discussed in Chapter 15 also apply to bowel elimination. The nurse should do all that is possible to insure the privacy, safety, and comfort of the patient who is using a bedpan for defecation. The procedure can be made as comfortable as possible for the patient by using the proper equipment and handling it competently. Assistance is given to the patient as needed, such as cleansing the rectal area. Since the bedpan is extremely uncomfortable to use, the patient should never be left on it any longer than necessary. Thus, the call signal must be answered promptly.

Excretory products from the gastrointestinal tract contain a very large number of microorganisms. To prevent cross-infection, almost all agencies keep a separate bedpan and urinal for each patient's use. They are stored in the patient's bedside locker, in an adjoining bathroom, or, in some agencies, in a separate room on the nursing unit.

Metal bedpans usually become cold when they are stored. Rinsing them with warm water helps to eliminate this problem and lessens the patient's discomfort. The nurse's hands should also be warmed if they are coming in contact with the patient's skin. Many agencies use disposable bedpans that can be discarded after use by one patient. Equipment that is used for more than one patient must be sterilized after every use.

The nurse helps to prevent infection in the patient, herself, and other patients and workers by washing her hands before and after assisting patients. The patient should always be provided with the opportunity to wash his hands after defecating. After use of the bedpan, the perineal and rectal area is cleansed with toilet paper or washed with soap and water.

The nurse protects the patient's safety at all times when helping the patient with a bedpan. In addition to being uncomfortable, bedpans are also awkward to use. The patient should be helped to a secure position on the pan and supported to ensure that his balance is not going to be upset. The toilet paper should be within easy reach if the patient can use it himself. The patient may need something to hold onto to support himself if he is going to get off the pan himself; the siderails may be helpful in this regard.

It is more comfortable for the patient to be in a sitting position for using the bedpan. The head of the bed is elevated unless this is contraindicated. The bedpan can be used in the supine position if necessary; measures to assist the helpless or semi-helpless patient onto the bedpan are discussed in Chapter 23 in connection with helping the patient to raise his buttocks.

An alternative measure, which may be used with some patients, is to have the bed flat, with the side rail up on the far side of the bed from the nurse. The patient is instructed or assisted to roll onto his side and grasp the side rail. The bedpan is placed in position under the patient's buttocks, and the patient is then returned to the back-lying position. The head of the bed should then be elevated, if permissible, to bring the patient into a sitting position. The position of the bedpan may need some slight adjusting for the patient's comfort and to prevent spillage.

A fracture (or slipper) pan, which is smaller, both in diameter and in height, than the standard bedpan, may be used when patients are unable to use the regular sized one. It is slipped under the patient's buttocks from the front of the body. It is easier to use if the patient is in a squatting position with the legs wide enough apart to permit the pan to be placed between them and then slipped under the buttocks. Care must be taken not to injure the patient's skin in using this fracture pan; this is important with all bedpans, but particularly important to keep in

mind when the fracture pan is used, because it is very narrow at the base that is slipped under the patient and could easily tear tissues.

Measures to Relieve Distressing Symptoms

Patients who have bowel dysfunction often have associated problems such as abdominal distention, excess flatus, and pain. With the person who is severely constipated, there is always the danger of impacted feces.

The constipated patient is usually relieved of his discomfort and concomitant distressing problems when a satisfactory bowel movement is effected. This may be brought about by the administration of a laxative or by the use of a rectal suppository, an enema, or a colonic irrigation. At times, manual extraction of feces is necessary. If laxatives are ordered, these are usually given at bedtime so that they will act after breakfast the following morning.

Medications to coat and soothe the lining of the intestines (emulsive drugs) or to reduce muscular spasm (antispasmodic drugs) are often prescribed for patients with diarrhea. Some of these drugs are taken at regular intervals during the day; other are taken after each bowel movement. If the diarrhea is caused by an infectious agent, appropriate therapy to combat the infection is prescribed by the physician.

Relief of abdominal distention and excess flatus can often be accomplished through the insertion of a rectal tube. Sometimes an enema may be ordered for this purpose also. Pain on defecation is often relieved by measures that soften the feces to permit their easier passage through the anal canal. Ensuring an adequate intake of fluids and sufficient bulk in the diet is helpful. For the specific pain of hemorrhoids, analgesic suppositories are often used (such as dibucaine suppositories). If other measures are not effective, surgery is sometimes indicated both for hemorrhoids and for anal and rectal fissures, if palliative therapy (treatment affording relief of symptoms) is not effective.

The Enema.   An enema is the injection of fluid into the rectum. Generally its purpose is to aid in the elimination of feces or flatus from the colon. This may be done to relieve constipation or remove fecal impaction, to cleanse the rectum and colon prior to examination, or as a safety measure to prevent possible infection in patients who are undergoing surgery or who are about to deliver. It may, however, be used for other purposes, such as to reduce fever or cerebral edema.

Enemas may act by stimulating evacuation by distention, by stimulating peristalsis by irritation, or by lubrication to make evacuation easier.

A fracture (slipper) pan. (From Rambo, B. J., and Wood, L. A.: *Nursing Skills for Clinical Practice.* 2nd ed. Philadelphia, W. B. Saunders Company, 1982, Vol. 2.)

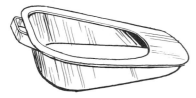

Cleansing Enemas. Cleansing enemas are given chiefly to remove feces from the colon. There are many kinds of cleansing enema: The soapsuds enema usually contains 1000 to 1500 ml. of soap solution. The saline enema contains 1000 ml. of normal saline. A third kind of cleansing enema that is often used is the tap water enema, which contains 100 to 1500 ml. of tap water. No more than 300 ml. is given to a child, and less to an infant.

These enemas, because of the volume of fluid used, serve to distend the rectum and lower colon, thereby stimulating the evacuation reflex. The soapsuds enema also has an irritating effect, due to the chemicals contained in the soap, and this enhances the action of the enema.

Disposable enemas are commonly used in many home and hospital situations. These contain hypertonic solutions, usually of sodium phosphate and biphosphate compounds. Their action is predominantly irritating, although the distention produced by the injection of the fluid also helps to stimulate peristalsis.

Oil Enemas. An oil enema may be given in cases in which there is severe constipation or the patient has a painful anal condition. The oil acts principally as a lubricant to make evacuation easier. Various oils, such as mineral, olive, or cottonseed oil, may be used. The amount given is small, usually 150 to 200 ml., and it is usually intended that the patient retain the enema for approximately an hour. Often a cleansing enema is ordered following an oil retention enema.

Other Types of Enemas. Other enemas may be given for a multiplicity of purposes. An antihelminthic enema may be used to assist in removing parasitic worms from the colon. An astringent enema may be ordered to contract tissue and to stop hemorrhage. An emollient enema may be given to coat the mucous membrane of the colon and to soothe irritated tissue. Sedative and stimulant enemas are sometimes given. Paraldehyde is not uncommonly used for sedative enemas, whereas 90 to 180 ml. of black coffee is sometimes used as a stimulant enema. Magnesium sulfate, 120 ml. of a 50 per cent solution, reduces cerebral edema. Ice water is sometime used as an enema to reduce fever.

Equipment and Supplies. Enema equipment and solutions are obtainable in disposable sets. If these sets are not available, the patient requires certain clean equipment. Rectal tubes are usually made of rubber; however, plastic rectal tubes are also available today. Rectal tubes vary in diameter; they are measured on the French scale. A No. 22 or No. 24 French is the size commonly needed by an adult. Also needed are

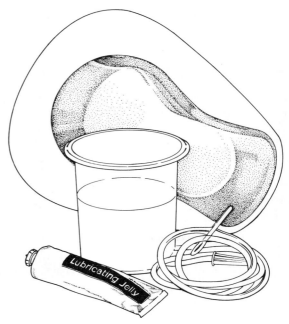

Equipment used in administering an enema includes a rectal tube, a container for the enema solution, tubing to connect the rectal tube to the container, a clamp, a lubricant, and a bedpan.

a container for the enema solution, tubing to connect the rectal tube to the container, a clamp, a small receptacle for extra fluid, and a lubricant for the rectal tube. The patient will also need a bedpan if he cannot use a toilet.

Administration. Before the enema equipment is taken to the patient, he will probably require some explanation about this measure. The patient's active help is important to the effectiveness of the enema. For maximum results he should try to hold the solution for 10 minutes. If the patient is in bed the head of the bed is lowered to make the bed level so that the fluid will flow in by force of gravity. It may not always be possible to have the bed completely flat; for example, if the patient is short of breath, the head of the bed should be no lower than is safe for him.

The top bedding is fan-folded to the foot of the bed and the patient is provided with a drape for warmth and comfort. For the administration of the enema, the patient is usually placed on his left side with both knees flexed, the top leg slightly higher than the lower one. It is felt that in this position, the descending colon being on the left side, the injection of fluid is facilitated by the force of gravity. However, this position may be varied according to the patient's condition and his wishes.

The usual temperature of a solution for an enema is 105°F (40°C). This temperature is not

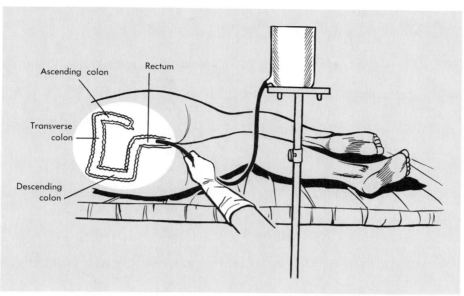

To have an enema administered, the patient lies on the left side.

harmful to the mucous membrane lining the colon and rectum. The rectal tube is well lubricated (usually with a water-soluble lubricant) in order to facilitate its insertion into the rectum and to lessen the irritation of the mucous membrane. Prior to the insertion of the tube the equipment is connected and a small amount of fluid is run through the tubing to expel the air. Then the tubing is clamped, and the rectal tube is inserted approximately 5 to 7.5 cm. (2 to 3 inches) into the rectum. If the patient is a child, the tube should be inserted only 2.5 to 3.75 cm. (1 to 1½ inches). The rectum of the average adult patient is 15 to 20 cm. (6 to 8 inches) in length. If the patient takes a deep breath while the tube is being inserted, the anal sphincter relaxes and the rectal tube can be inserted more easily. The tube must be inserted beyond the internal sphincter. If any obstruction to the insertion is encountered, the tube is withdrawn and the physician is notified. A rectal tube should never be forced because it might damage the mucous membrane or aggravate a disease process.

The solution for an enema is released slowly for the patient's comfort and to avoid damage to the mucous membrane. The higher the solution container is held, the greater is the pressure exerted. Hence, the solution container should not be more than 60 cm. (2 feet) above the level of the bed. For gynecological patients, the container is suspended at the patient's hip level in order to lessen the pressure on the adjacent reproductive organs. If the patient complains of discomfort while the solution is flowing, the flow is stopped for a few minutes and then recommenced cautiously. Any further discomfort demands the termination of the measure.

Following the administration of the solution, the rectal tube is pinched and removed. The patient retains the enema for 10 minutes if possible. In the case of an oil retention enema, the length of time for retention of the fluid is usually one hour.

When the enema is expelled, the nurse makes certain observations. She observes the color and consistency of the feces, the approximate amount of fluid returned, the general amount of flatus that is expelled (large, small), and the general reaction of the patient. All these observations are recorded in the patient's chart. The nurse also takes particular note of any unusual findings in the enema return, for example, blood, mucus, pus, or worms. Following the expulsion of the enema, the patient is made clean and comfortable. The equipment is then rinsed in cold water and washed in hot soapy water. In hospitals, equipment is sterilized after each use to avoid the transfer of organisms. Disposable equipment is placed in a paper bag or other suitable container for removal.

Siphoning an Enema. If the patient cannot expel the enema within a half hour after its administration, it is usually necessary to siphon off the enema. This is generally a nursing decision. To siphon off an enema is to withdraw the enema solution from the patient by using positive-negative pressures and the force of gravity. The equipment and supplies required include a rectal tube and water soluble lubricant, a small amount of warm tap water (105°F or 40.6°C) a receptacle for the enema solution, and a funnel.

The patient lies on his right side with his hips drawn to the edge of the bed. In this position the descending colon is uppermost, a situation that facilitates the removal of the enema solution by force of gravity. The receptacle for the enema solution is placed at a level lower than the patient's hips, often on a chair at the side of the bed.

The rectal tube is first connected to the funnel and then well lubricated with the water soluble lubricant. The funnel is then half filled with water while the tubing is pinched to prevent leakage. The rectal tube is inserted into the patient in the same manner as for an enema. The pressure on the tubing is released and a small amount of fluid is allowed to run into the rectum. Then the funnel is quickly inverted and lowered over the bedpan. The negative pressure of the fluid in the tube and funnel produces a siphon, which draws the enema fluid from the patient's colon.

After the removal of the enema fluid, the patient may require assistance regarding his comfort and hygiene. The enema fluid is observed for its color and consistency, and these observations are charted on the patient's record.

The Rectal Tube. The purpose of the insertion of a rectal tube is to facilitate the expulsion of flatus. The equipment required for this measure includes the rectal tube, a receptacle for the end of the tube, a lubricant, and adhesive tape. The adhesive tape is used to hold the rectal tube in position.

After the patient's need for information about this measure has been met, he is asked to lie in the same position as for an enema. The rectal tube is lubricated and inserted 5 to 7.5 cm. (2 to 3 inches) into the rectum. It is then taped in place, and the free end of the tube is put in a container placed near the patient's buttocks. A rectal tube is usually left in place for half an hour.

After the tube has been removed and the patient has received any needed assistance, the approximate amount (large, small) of flatus that was expelled is noted. Usually the patient can describe this. In addition, since the patient who has flatus usually has a hard distended abdomen, the nurse can palpate his abdomen to note any change. These observations are then recorded on the patient chart.

The Manual Extraction of Feces. The manual extraction of feces is the removal by hand of impacted feces from the rectum. A fecal impaction is a large hardened mass of feces that has accumulated in the rectum, usually owing to prolonged constipation. The equipment required for manual extraction includes a rectal glove, a container for the glove, a lubricant, and a bedpan. After the measure has been explained to the patient, he lies on his left side.

The nurse puts on the rectal glove and thoroughly lubricates her second or third finger. She inserts this finger carefully into the rectum and manually breaks the impacted feces. The lubricant is used to facilitate the insertion of the nurse's gloved finger and to protect the rectal mucosa from abrasion. When the feces have been broken, they are removed by hand to the bedpan. The manual extraction of feces is often followed by a cleansing enema. This is ordered by the physician or the nurse in charge. After this nursing measure, the nurse charts the amount, color, and consistency of the feces. She also notes the presence of any flatus and the patient's general reaction (pallor, fatigue, and the like).

The Rectal Suppository. A rectal suppository is a small conical sphere that is designed to slip easily through the anal canal into the rectum. It melts at body temperature. A glycerin or medicated rectal suppository may be administered as a local irritant to facilitate elimination, as a vehicle for the administration of a sedative, or as an antispasmodic. The equipment needed for the insertion of a rectal suppository consists of a rectal glove, lubricant, the suppository, and a container for the suppository. The patient may need information about the function of the suppository and its insertion as well as the nursing techniques that are involved. The patient lies in the same position as for an enema.

With a gloved hand, the suppository is inserted one fingerlength, approximately 7.5 to 10 cm. (3 to 4 inches) into the rectum in adults, and half that distance in children. It is usually possible to tell when the suppository is in place because the rectal sphincter "grabs" or "sucks" it in and closes. If the purpose of the suppository is to aid in the explusion of the rectal contents, the patient should try to retain the suppository for about 20 minutes. If the suppository is administered for other purposes, it is retained indefinitely. When inserting the suppository, the nurse must exercise care to be certain that the mucosa of the rectum is not torn and that the suppository is not forced when any resistance in the rectum is met. The suppository must contact the bowel wall; it should not be inserted into a bolus of stool.

After the suppository has been administered, this fact is recorded, as are the effects of the suppository. These can often be observed 15 to 30 minutes after administration, depending upon the medication.

Colostomy Care

Irrigation of a Colostomy. The purpose of a colostomy is usually to divert feces from the

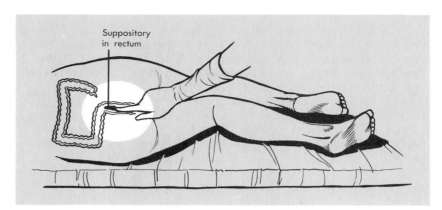

The insertion of a rectal suppository.

intestinal tract through an artificial opening to the abdomen. It may be done as a temporary measure to give the bowel below the incision a chance to heal, or it may be permanent.

In a permanent colostomy there is usually only one opening (stoma); in a temporary colostomy there may be two. The one closer to the stomach is called the proximal stoma; it is from this opening that the feces are discharged. If there is a second stoma it is farther from the stomach (closer to the anus) and hence is referred to as the distal stoma. There should be some direction in the nursing care plan as to how the nurse may distinguish between the proximal and distal stomas. An irrigation is generally prescribed for the functioning proximal stoma; only occasionally is a solution (an antiseptic solution, for example) instilled into a distal stoma.

The purpose of a colostomy irrigation is to cleanse the colon of fecal matter by injecting fluid into the colon through the colostomy open-ing. The equipment required for this nursing measure is similar to that needed for an enema, with the addition of a small rectal tube, a large glass Y connector, and unsterile waste gauze. The person who has a colostomy often needs careful instruction with regard to both the colostomy dressing and the colostomy irrigation. Most people can, with guidance assume the responsibility for carrying out these measures themselves. There are several methods of irrigating a colostomy. One method is detailed here.

The nurse's approach to these nursing measures is extremely important. The patient is often anxious about this adjustment to the change in his life pattern as a result of this surgery, and any revulsion on the part of the nurse could be particularly disturbing to the patient and his family. Patients often feel embarrassed and find the colostomy hard to accept. They may not want to watch the nurse irrigate it at first, or they may be angry that this has happened to them. The nurse may also have strong feelings

The administration of an irrigating solution to a colostomy by means of a Y tube.

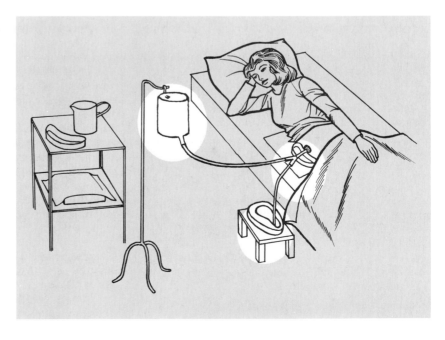

of dislike at doing this procedure which may show in her facial expression. Her calm acceptance of the situation and her care to protect the patient's feelings of dignity can do much to reassure the patient.

At the commencement of a colostomy irrigation, the patient lies on the side toward which the colostomy opening has been made, or sits upright so that the expulsion of feces is more easily accomplished. If he is in bed, the lower bedding is protected by a waterproof towel and the top bedding is fan-folded down to expose the colostomy opening. A bedpan is placed conveniently at a level lower than the colostomy opening. The container for the irrigating solution is placed not more than 30 cm. (1 foot) above the patient's pelvis in order to keep the pressure of the fluid low enough not to damage the mucous membrane of the intestine. A narrow rectal tube is connected to the irrigating container and a small amount of the irrigating solution is permitted to run through the rectal tube in order to expel the air in it.

The rectal tube is lubricated, and then inserted gently into the colostomy stoma. The irrigating fluid is allowed to run slowly into the colon. After a small amount is administered, the intake tubing is clamped and the output tubing is released so that the return flow drains into the bedpan. This process is repeated until the returns from the colostomy are clear.

The returns of the irrigation are observed for color and consistency of the fecal matter. The condition of the operative area is also noted. Throughout this nursing measure the patient should be encouraged to participate actively. Most patients learn to carry out a colostomy irrigation while they are in the hospital so that they can eventually do this independently.

Stoma cones can be used to guide the insertion of the catheter. A stoma cone is a plastic cup that fits over the colostomy stoma. The cup has a hole for the catheter and a detachable plastic

In irrigation of a colostomy, the catheter is often inserted through a stoma cone.

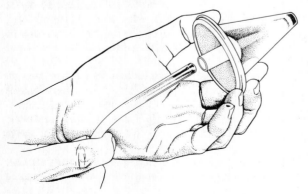

sheath that guides the fluid and feces into a receptacle. One of the advantages of these is the complete enclosure of the fluid and feces during the irrigation. Using the cone also reduces the risk that the bowel will be perforated during the procedure.

The Colostomy Dressing. The colostomy dressing is a clean procedure rather than a sterile one. The dressing on the colostomy stoma is changed as often as necessary in order to keep the patient clean and his skin free from fecal matter. It is important that the skin surrounding the stoma be protected from irritation. Usually a protective lubricant, such as zinc oxide, is used for this purpose.

The equipment that is needed for a colostomy dressing includes unsterile gauze, unsterile dressings, lubricant, a tongue depressor, and a container for the disposal of the soiled dressings. Nursing personnel may use rubber gloves if they desire. As with the colostomy irrigation, the nurse's approach to this task is important. Most people require considerable reassurance and a calm acceptance of the task. The patient can be helpful; in fact most people learn to change their own dressings. Therefore, each time the nurse dresses a colostomy she should be conscious of the learning needs of the patient.

The patient sits in a comfortable position for changing his dressing. If he is in bed, the bottom bedding is protected with waterproof material and the bedclothes are fan-folded to expose the colostomy stoma. The patient is draped for warmth and comfort. The soiled dressings are removed and the skin around the colostomy stoma is cleansed with soap and water. A protective substance is then applied generously to the skin around the stoma, and a clean dressing is applied. The first layer of dressing usually consists of gauze, then unsterile surgical dressings are applied. Adhesive ties are used to hold the dressing in place. The color, the consistency, and the amount of fecal matter on the old dressing are recorded. The nurse also records the appearance of the colostomy stoma and the presence of any excoriated areas. (*Excoriation* is the loss of superfical tissue, such as epidermis.)

Plastic colostomy bags are also available commercially. They have attachable, specially designed belts that are worn around the waist or bags that stick directly to the skin. These bags are disposable are changed whenever they become soiled.

Colonic Irrigation. A colonic irrigation (*enteroclysis*) is a measure designed to wash out the lower colon. Its purpose may be merely to cleanse the large intestine, or it may be to stimulate peristalsis and relieve distention. Other uses of the colonic irrigation are to relieve inflammation and to reduce body temperature. In the latter two instances the temperature of the solution is usually cooler. The equipment required for a colonic irrigation consists of the solution, a solution container, a colonic irrigation tube (No. 30 French is suggested), a lubricant, a catheter (No. 20 French is suggested), and a bedpan.

Initially the colonic tube is marked 5 to 7.5 cm (2 to 3 inches) from the tip; adhesive tape can be used for this purpose. The catheter is marked 12.5 cm. (5 inches) from the tip in the same manner. These marks serve as a guide to the distance to which the tubes should be inserted. The type and temperature of the solution are prescribed by the physician.

This is not a painful measure, but patients usually require information about it. The patient turns on his right side with his hips toward the edge of the bed. This position facilitates the drainage of fluid from the colon. He is provided with drapes. The tubing and the catheter are connected to the solution container and the solution is allowed to run through the tubing before it is clamped. Both the colonic tube and the catheter are lubricated; the tip of the catheter is then placed in the opening or eye on the side of the colonic tube. The other end of the colonic tube is placed in a receptacle at the patient's bedside. Holding the two tubes together, the nurse gently inserts them into the rectum up to the 7.5 cm. (3 inch) mark on the colonic tube. Next the catheter is drawn back sufficiently to free its tip from the colonic tube and it is then inserted to the 12.5 cm. (5 inch) mark. The solution is allowed to flow gradually and continuously so that the inflow and outflow are equal. If the patient has pain, the flow is stopped for a few minutes. If the pain persists, the irrigation is discontinued and the discomfort is reported.

When the irrigation returns are clear, the irrigation is discontinued, but the colonic tube is kept in place until drainage ceases. If at any time the colonic tube becomes blocked, it must be removed and cleansed, then reinserted.

The character of the return flow is observed. Particular note is made of the presence of mucus, blood, pus, or feces. The observations are recorded on the patient's chart.

Maintenance of Fluid and Electrolyte Balance

Patients who have diarrhea need extra fluid intake to compensate for the fluid lost through the gastrointestinal tract. In diarrhea, fluids and electrolytes are lost because of hypersecretion of mucus from the membrane (due to irritation) and because of lack of reabsorption by the bowel of fluids ingested and of fluids secreted into the bowel. Normally, 8 liters of fluid are secreted into the bowel in a 24-hour period. Most of this fluid is reabsorbed. Severe diarrhea depletes the body's potassium levels and lowers the amount of sodium chloride. The initial effect of this electrolyte loss is acidosis as a result of the loss of base; however, with prolonged potassium loss, alkalosis is eventually accompanied by a chloride loss.

In constipation there is a need for additional fluid intake both as an aid in activating peristalsis and to keep the feces soft. Often merely ensuring that the patient is taking enough fluids is sufficient to relieve constipation.

Maintenance of Adequate Nutritional Status

Maintaining adequate nutrition can be a particular problem for the patient who has diarrhea. Because the food moves quickly through the gastrointestinal tract, many food constituents are not absorbed. The ingestion of small amounts of nonirritating food at frequent intervals is often helpful in preventing diarrhea and facilitating absorption. Usually a bland diet is ordered to prevent further irritation of the gastrointestinal mucosa.

The constipated patient, on the other hand, may be anorectic and need help to stimulate his appetite. The diet for the constipated patient should be planned to meet his needs for fluids, extra bulk, and for foods that have a laxative effect.

Maintenance of Comfort and Hygiene

Meeting the comfort and hygiene needs of the patient with elimination problems is a valuable contribution to his sense of well-being. Cleanliness is essential. The sight and odor of fecal material is repugnant, and the high bacteria count in feces makes it a possible source of contamination. The patient should be given the opportunity to wash his hands after he has had a bowel movement (as he would normally do at home). The rectal area should be cleaned and the patient assisted with this if he is unable to do it himself. Soiled linen should be removed immediately.

Some patients with diarrhea feel more secure if the bedpan is close at hand. In these cases, the pan can be kept covered and placed inconspicuously within reach. Care should be taken that the pan is emptied and cleaned after each use.

After the patient has had a bowel movement, his room may require ventilating and freshening to eliminate unpleasant odors. Since such matters can be embarrassing to the patient, the nurse should take the initiative in these measures.

Many patients with bowel problems develop irritation of the skin and mucous membranes in the anal area. Cleanliness is important to prevent infection, and emollient creams help to keep the skin intact and to soothe the irritated area.

An important factor to consider in the care of patients with constipation or diarrhea is the nurse's reaction to these patients and their problems. It is helpful if the nurse can accept her own feelings and not communicate these to the patient.

GUIDE TO ASSESSING BOWEL FUNCTIONING

1. How old is the patient?

2. What is the patient's normal pattern of bowel movements? their frequency? consistency? color? odor? Is he in the habit of using laxatives, suppositories, or enemas? What does he use? How often?

3. Does he have a colostomy or ileostomy?

4. If the individual is a child, has he reached the stage where he can control his bowel movements? If so, is he toilet-trained?

5. What is the patient's normal diet? What is his usual amount of exercise or activity? How much water does he usually drink per day? Does he have a regular time to go to the bathroom? Is he on shift work?

6. Is the patient now having constipation, diarrhea, or associated problems such as abdominal distention, flatulence, abdominal pain, pain on defecation, rectal bleeding, or incontinence of feces? Are there abnormal constituents in the stools such as blood, pus, or worms? Absence of color?

7. On examination, does the abdomen look swollen? Does it feel hard and unyielding on palpation? Is there evidence of irritation around the anal area, e.g., redness or breaks in the skin? Does the patient complain of itching in that area? Are there signs of fecal impaction, as, for example, the passage of small amounts of seepage instead of formed stool?

8. How long has the patient had these problems? Has he been eating any irritating foods lately? Is he under any stress? What is his nutritional status? State of hydration? Does he have a health problem that could be affecting his bowel functioning? Is he on any medications? If so, what are they?

9. Does he require immediate medical or nursing intervention to relieve any of his problems?

10. Has a stool specimen been ordered for laboratory examination? Have the results come back yet? Are they normal?

11. Have other diagnostic tests or examinations been ordered? Have reports from these been completed? What do they show?

12. What are the patient's learning needs in relation to re-establishing a normal pattern of bowel movement? prevention of recurrence of problems? diagnostic tests or examinations?

GUIDE TO EVALUATING THE EFFECTIVENESS OF NURSING INTERVENTION

1. Is the patient comfortable? Is he free from distressing symptoms?

2. If the patient has been constipated, has a successful bowel movement been accomplished? If he has had diarrhea, have the stools returned to normal in consistency and frequency? If he has had distention, does the abdomen feel soft?

Have flatulence, abdominal pain, and pain on defecation been relieved? Are stools clear of worms?

3. Has a normal pattern of elimination been established?

4. Is the patient's nutritional status satisfactory? Is his fluid and electrolyte balance normal? Is he taking sufficient exercise?

5. Does the patient's diet contain a sufficient amount of bulky foods to ensure stimulation of the defecation reflex? Is he taking enough fluids?

6. Is the patient aware of his dietary and fluid needs to ensure adequate fecal elimination? Does his selection of foods and his fluid intake indicate this?

7. Does the patient practice good hygiene? For example, does he wash his hands after a bowel movement?

STUDY SITUATION

Mr. S. Norris is a 70-year-old man living at home who has abdominal pain. He has been retired for 5 years after an active life as a house painter, and he now spending most of his time watching television. Mr. Norris lives alone in a small house just outside the city. He has three grandchildren who live a few miles away and he visits them on Sundays.

Mr. Norris has been increasingly uncomfortable because of constipation during the past few years. He says he never took medicines when he worked but now has to take a laxative every day. Because he does not like to cook, he generally eats frozen TV dinners, sandwiches, and cookies, and occasionally eggs. His doctor has asked you to assist Mr. Norris in regulating his bowel habits.

1. What factors should you take into consideration before assisting Mr. Norris?

2. What questions would you ask Mr. Norris about his bowel habits?

3. For what reasons might Mr. Norris be constipated? What associated problems might he have?

4. What interventions would you think best to try? Outline the expected outcomes of nursing interventions for Mr. Norris.

5. What would you include in your teaching program for this patient? How would you evaluate the effectiveness of your teaching?

6. Mr. Norris's physician has ordered an enema for the patient. How would you explain this measure to him?

7. Describe the position most desirable for the administration of an enema and why it is desirable.

8. What observations should you record regarding the enema?

SUGGESTED READINGS

Aman, R. A.: Treating the Patient, Not the Constipation. *American Journal of Nursing,* 80(9):1634–1635, September, 1980.

Beber, C. R.: Freedom for the Incontinent. *American Journal of Nursing,* 80(3):482–484, March, 1980.

Mahoney, J. M.: What You Should Know about Ostomies: Guidelines for Giving Better Postop Care. *Nursing '78,* 8(5):74–79, May, 1978.

Schramm-Nortridge, J. A.: Helpful Hints for Assessing the Ostomate. *Nursing '82,* 12(4):72, April, 1982.

Vigliarolo, D.: Managing Bowel Incontinence in Children with Meningomyelocele. *American Journal of Nursing,* 80(1):105–107, January, 1980.

Wilpizeski, M. D.: Helping the Ostomate Return to Normal Life. *Nursing '81,* 11(3):62–64, March, 1981.

Yen, P. K.: Nutrition: Why Eat a Fiber Rich Diet? *Geriatric Nursing,* 2:436, November-December, 1981.

17

The Nurse Should be Able to:

- Discuss the importance of fluid and electrolyte balance to an individual's health and well-being
- Describe the distribution of fluid and the major electrolytes in the body
- Discuss the normal methods of fluid and electrolyte intake and output to and from the body
- Explain the principal mechanisms that maintain the body's fluid and electrolyte balance
- Identify factors that may affect an individual's fluid and electrolyte balance
- Discuss fluid and electrolyte needs throughout the life cycle
- Assess a patient's fluid and electrolyte status
- Apply relevant principles in planning and implementing appropriate nursing interventions in patients
    a. to maintain fluid and electrolyte balance
    b. to assist in restoring balance if a disturbance has occurred
- Evaluate the effectiveness of nursing interventions

FLUID AND ELECTROLYTE NEEDS

INTRODUCTION

Water has been called the indispensable nutrient. Approximately 50 to 70 per cent of the total body weight of an adult is made up of water and its dissolved constituents; 70 to 80 per cent of the total body weight of the infant is similarly in a fluid state. The fluid system plays an essential role in the body. Its principal functions are (1) the transportation of oxygen and nutrients to the cells and the removal of waste products from them, and (2) the maintenance of a stable physical and chemical environment within the body. Important in the latter function are the *electrolytes*. You will recall from your chemistry courses that electrolytes are compounds that in water solution separate into particles, each capable of carrying an electrical charge. Sodium (Na^+), for example, carries a positive charge; it is therefore a cation. Chlorine (Cl^-), with which it combines to form salt (NaCl), carries a negative charge; it is an anion. The electrolytes in body fluids are important in the chemical reactions that occur within the cells. They also help to regulate the permeability of cell membranes, thus controlling the transfer of various materials across the membrane. They are vital to the maintenance of the body's acid-base balance and are also essential in the transmission of electrical energy within the body. Without the calcium ion, for example, muscle contraction could not occur.

Under normal circumstances, the body maintains a very precise fluid and electrolyte balance. Both the volume and the constituents of body fluids vary but little from day to day, and usually return to a state of equilibrium within a very few days following any minor disturbance.

Serious fluid and electrolyte imbalance may occur as a result of a number of health problems. The nature of the imbalance may be either an excess or an insufficiency. An individual may retain an excess amount of fluid in the tissues and become *edematous*. On the other hand, he may lose an inordinate amount of fluids (through persistent vomiting, for example) and become *dehydrated*. Whenever fluids are lost or retained in excessive amounts, there is an accompanying loss or retention of electrolytes, so that both fluid and electrolyte balances are disturbed. Disturbances in fluid and electrolyte balance can cause serious repercussions within the body. Both the transportation and regulatory functions of the fluid system are likely to be affected. The cells may not get sufficient nourishment, for instance, or there may be an accumulation of waste products owing to inefficiency of the mechanism for their removal. The body's acid-base balance may be upset and temperature regulation impaired (see Chapter 18). There may also be interference with the transfer of materials

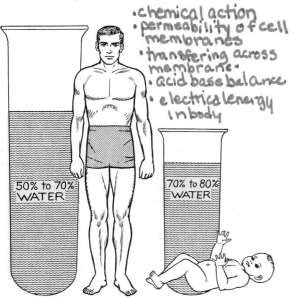

- chemical action
- permeability of cell membranes
- transfering across membrane
- acid base balance
- electrical energy in body

50% to 70% WATER

70% to 80% WATER

across the cell membrane, so that a shift occurs in the distribution of fluids and electrolytes. Activities within the body that depend on the transmission of electrical energy, such as muscle contraction and the relay of nerve impulses, may also be impaired.

Whenever there is a disturbance in fluid and electrolyte balance, the body attempts to compensate for the lack or the excess, whichever the case may be, by bringing into play various adaptive mechanisms. A very common example of this occurs in the person who perspires heavily on a hot day and then finds that he is thirsty for extra fluids to replace those he has lost through sweating. The body has a number of adaptive mechanisms in addition to thirst; we will discuss these later in this chapter.

If the imbalance is too great, however, or persists over a prolonged period of time, the body's adaptive mechanisms may not be able to cope. In this event, the body's defenses collapse and prostration ensues. This may happen, for example, when there is a continuous loss of fluids with no replacement, or a very sudden large loss, as in massive hemorrhage.

THE PHYSIOLOGY OF FLUID AND ELECTROLYTE BALANCE

In order to understand the physiological processes involved, it is perhaps easier to consider different aspects of fluid and electrolyte balance under separate headings:

1. The distribution of fluid and electrolytes within the body
2. The modes of transport of fluids and electrolytes
3. The balancing of fluid intake and output
4. Mechanisms regulating fluids and electrolyte balance
5. Maintenance of the body's acid-base balance

The Distribution of Fluid and Electrolytes

Fluid within the body is generally considered to be distributed in what may be termed two basic compartments. First, body fluids are found within the cells of the body. This type, termed *intracellular fluid*, accounts for approximately 40 to 50 per cent of the total body weight. Second, fluid occurs outside the cells of the body; this is *extracellular fluid*. There are two kinds of extracellular fluid. One is the fluid in the spaces between the cells; called *interstitial*

	EXTRACELLULAR FLUID	INTRACELLULAR FLUID
Na^+	142 mEq/l.	10 mEq/l.
K^+	5 mEq/l.	141 mEq/l.
Ca^{++}	5 mEq/l.	<1 mEq/l.
Mg^{++}	3 mEq/l.	58 mEq/l.
Cl^-	103 mEq/l.	4 mEq/l.
HCO_3^-	28 mEq/l.	10 mEq/l.
Phosphates	4 mEq/l.	75 mEq/l.
SO_4^{--}	1 mEq/l.	2 mEq/l.
Glucose	90 mgm.%	0 to 20 mgm.%
Amino acids	30 mgm.%	200 mgm.% ?
Cholesterol Phospholipids Neutral fat	0.5 gm.%	2 to 95 gm.%
Po_2	35 mm.Hg	20 mm.Hg ?
Pco_2	46 mm.Hg	50 mm.Hg ?
pH	7.4	7.0

The electrolyte content of body fluids. (From Guyton, A. C.: Function of the Human Body. 4th Ed. Philadelphia, W. B. Saunders Co., 1974.)

fluid, this component accounts for approximately 15 per cent of the total body weight of an adult. The other component, *intravascular fluid*, is the fluid in the blood and lymph vessels: it makes up approximately 5 per cent of total body weight in an adult.

There is a constant shift of fluid from one compartment to another as it performs its function of transporting nutrients and oxygen to the cells and removing wastes and manufactured products from the cells. In health, the amount of fluid in the circulating blood and the total amount of fluid within the cells must be maintained at a fairly constant volume. In cases of dehydration the body fluid is drawn from within the cells and routed into the blood vessels. This explains why a patient who is unable to retain fluids owing to prolonged vomiting soon loses the elasticity of his subcutaneous tissue, his skin becoming loose and flabby.

The principal electrolytes and their concentrations in extracellular and intracellular fluid are given in the accompanying illustration. It can readily be seen that the electrolyte composition of the two types of fluid is quite different. The fluid contained within the cells is essentially a potassium solution, whereas extracellular fluid is high in sodium ions. Both types of fluid also contain specified quantities of other electrolytes, as shown in the illustration.

The electrolyte composition of the two types of extracellular fluid (that is, interstitial and intravascular) is essentially the same insofar as principal electrolytes are concerned. The fluid within the blood vessels does, however, contain a much greater concentration of protein than is found in the interstitial fluid.

Modes of Transport

In the process of body functioning, fluid and electrolytes are constantly moving from within the cells to the extracellular compartments and vice versa. This transfer is accomplished by several different means, the three most common being osmosis, active transport, and diffusion.

Osmosis is the movement of a solvent, such as water, through a partition separating solutions of different concentrations. The solvent tends to pass from a solution with a lesser concentration to one with a higher concentration to equalize the concentrations of both solutions. This movement is possible when a semipermeable membrane separates the two solutions. Cell membranes and the walls of capillaries are examples of semipermeable membranes. However, some of the dissolved substances in body fluid do not move between the membranes as readily as water. Electrolytes are examples of this.

Therefore, when it is necessary for the body to transfer electrolytes from the cells to the extracellular fluid—to achieve a balance, for example—an *active transport mechanism* is brought into play. Although this mechanism is not yet completely understood, it is believed that a substance known as *adenosine triphosphate (ATP)* is released from the cell. This substance appears to give the electrolytes the energy required to pass through the semipermeable membrane. The transfer of sodium, potassium, and a number of other ions, including amino acids, is believed to take place via this mechanism.

Diffusion is a process whereby molecules and ions tend to distribute themselves equally within a given space. When used in connection with gases, it refers to the process by which the molecules of the gases interpenetrate and become mixed; this occurs because of the incessant motion of the molecules. The exchange of oxygen and carbon dioxide that occurs in the alveoli and capillaries of the lungs takes place through a process of diffusion.

Balancing of Fluid Intake and Output

A person derives fluid and electrolytes from three main sources: the fluid that is ingested in liquid form, the fluid content of the various foods that are eaten, and the water that is formed as a byproduct of the body's oxidation of foods and body substances. The total daily intake of water under normal circumstances is approximately 2100 to 2900 ml. The average amount of fluid gained by an adult in a 24-hour period from each of the sources listed above is:

Ingested fluids	1000 to 1500 ml.
Ingested food	900 to 1000 ml.
Metabolic oxidation	200 to 400 ml.
Total	2100 to 2900 ml.

Normally the body maintains a precise balance between fluid intake and fluid output. The average daily intake of fluids from various sources and output via various routes are shown here. (From Sheridan, E., Patterson, H. R., and Gustafson, E. A.: *Falconer's The Drug, the Nurse, the Patient.* 7th Ed. Philadelphia, W. B. Saunders Co., 1982.)

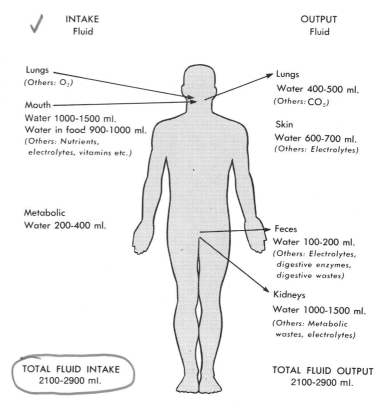

INTAKE
Fluid

OUTPUT
Fluid

Lungs
(Others: O_2)

Mouth
Water 1000-1500 ml.
Water in food 900-1000 ml.
(Others: Nutrients,
electrolytes, vitamins etc.)

Metabolic
Water 200-400 ml.

Lungs
Water 400-500 ml.
(Others: CO_2)

Skin
Water 600-700 ml.
(Others: Electrolytes)

Feces
Water 100-200 ml.
(Others: Electrolytes,
digestive enzymes,
digestive wastes)

Kidneys
Water 1000-1500 ml.
(Others: Metabolic
wastes, electrolytes)

TOTAL FLUID INTAKE
2100-2900 ml.

TOTAL FLUID OUTPUT
2100-2900 ml.

Water is lost from the body through the skin by perspiration, through the lungs in expirations, and from the kidneys in the urine. In addition, a small amount of fluid is excreted in the feces. The total daily loss of water from the body in normal circumstances is approximately 2100 to 2900 ml., depending largely upon the amount of fluid intake. It is lost as follows:

In urine	1000 to 1500 ml. daily
In feces	100 to 200 ml. daily
From the skin	600 to 700 ml. daily
From the lungs	400 to 500 ml. daily
Total	2100 to 2900 ml.

The balance between the fluid taken in and the fluid excreted is maintained within a very narrow range. The intake usually equals the output over a 3-day period even though it may not always be equal over a single 24-hour period.

Mechanisms Regulating Fluid and Electrolyte Balance

The main forces at work in holding water within the various compartments of the fluid system of the body are generated by proteins and electrolytes. In the intravascular compartment (blood vessels) the force is generated largely by the serum albumin, in the intercellular fluid by the sodium ion, and within the cells by protoplasm. Water passes freely through the capillary walls and membranes, but the protein molecules and the sodium ions do not move as freely. These substances exert an osmotic pressure that tends to hold water in the respective compartments. Osmotic pressure is that pressure exerted by particles which tends to draw a solvent toward it. A patient who has lost a great deal of serum albumin through malnutrition tends to become edematous, since fluid is drawn from the blood plasma into the intercellular spaces. This happens because the main force holding the water in the blood vessels has been lost.

By far the most important regulatory mechanism operating to maintain the body's fluid balance is the kidneys. When the intake of fluid is insufficient or when there is an excessive loss of fluid from the body, the amount of urine that is excreted is decreased. Conversely, when an excess amount of fluid is ingested, urine output increases. This is accomplished through the selective reabsorption of water in the tubules of the kidney.

The kidney also exerts the main control over the sodium and potassium balance of the body through the selective reabsorption of these ions in the tubules. When sodium and potassium need to be retained, increasing amounts are reabsorbed. Excess sodium and potassium are excreted in the urine. If there is an acute shortage of sodium in the body, the excretion of this ion through the urine may be cut to almost zero. In the case of potassium, however, there appears to be an obligatory excretion of a certain amount in the urine.[2] Thus, there is always some potassium in the daily urine output, even though the body reserves may be dangerously low. This factor is taken into account by the physician when he is planning replacement therapy.

The control of fluid and electrolyte balance by the kidneys is influenced by two sets of hormones. The antidiuretic hormone (ADH), which is produced primarily in the anterior hypothalamus and stored in the pituitary gland, is a major factor in controlling water reabsorption. When the body takes in an insufficient quantity, or there is water deprivation from other sources, the secretion of ADH is stimulated. This in turn causes increased reabsorption of water in the kidney tubules and a lessened volume of urinary output. Aldosterone, one of several steroid hormones produced in the adrenal cortex, exerts a major influence in promoting the retention of sodium and the excretion of potassium. Aldosterone secretion appears to be stimulated by such factors as a lessened sodium intake, an excess of potassium, muscular activity, trauma, and emotional tension.[2]

The gastrointestinal tract also helps to regulate fluid and electrolyte balance. The manner in which this is done is similar to the action of the kidneys—that is, through the selective reabsorption of water and solutes, the reabsorption taking place principally in the small intestine. Although the volume of digestive juices secreted into the gastrointestinal tract each day is considerable (approximately 8200 ml.), all but about 100 to 200 ml. of fluid is reabsorbed. Under normal circumstances, only a small amount of the body's daily fluid loss is from the gastrointestinal tract in the feces, and the loss of electrolytes by this route is normally negligible. Both fluid and electrolytes may be lost in considerably quantity, however, in such conditions as vomiting and diarrhea.

Thirst is another of the regulatory mechanisms operating to maintain fluid balance. Thirst is the desire for more fluids. It usually indicates a basic physiological need for water, although it may sometimes occur as a result of dryness of the mucous membranes of the mouth and throat from other causes, such as mouth-breathing. In cases in which thirst is due to a simple dryness of the oropharynx rather than a basic lack of water in the body, it may be relieved by measures to keep the mucous membranes moist. Good oral hygiene can usually relieve this dryness.

"True thirst," due to a basic lack of water, usually occurs when body cells are dehydrated, extracellular volume is lessened (as in a hemorrhage), or certain centers in the hypothalamus are stimulated.[2] It is thought that the thirst mechanism is closely related to the control of water balance by the antidiuretic hormone (ADH). When the body is suffering from a lack of water, the thirst mechanism operates to increase the intake of water, while ADH restricts the loss of water through urinary output.

The *lungs* are also important in the regulation of fluid and electrolyte balance. Ordinarily, the amount of water lost from respiration is quite small. Whenever respirations are increased in rate and depth, however, the amount of water lost via this route is also increased and may become a significant factor to consider. This may occur, for example, with strenuous muscular exercise, in fevers or any condition in which respirations are considerably increased, or when the air that is breathed is very dry. This last point is important to remember in the administration of inhalation therapy. Oxygen or other substances given by inhalation should always be humidified in order to counterbalance the loss of water through expiration. The loss of electrolytes through respiration is normally minimal, although the lungs can play an important role in maintaining the acid-base balance of the body, as discussed later.

Maintenance of Acid-Base Balance

Intimately connected with the fluid and electrolyte balance of the body is the maintenance of acid-base (or H^+) balance. You will recall from your chemistry courses that acids carry hydrogen ions, which can be released to combine with other substances. Alkalis (base substances) do not carry hydrogen ions, but can combine with the hydrogen ions released by an acid. The relative acidity or alkalinity of body fluids is expressed in terms of pH, which refers to the concentration of hydrogen ions in the fluid. The pH is measured on a scale of 1 to 14. Water, which is considered a neutral substance (being neither acid nor alkaline), has a pH of 7.0. The pH scale is based on a negative logarithm, and acidic solutions have a pH lower than 7 and alkaline solutions a pH higher than 7.

Normally, the acid-base balance (or H^+ concentration) of body fluids is maintained by means of four mechanisms. A local small buildup of extra acid or base may be corrected

by a simple process of *dilution*—that is, the circulating fluid picks up the extra ions and takes them away from the trouble spot; they become diluted in the total volume of fluid circulating. The excess acid accumulated in a muscle after exercise, for example, may be removed in this way. The body also has a system of *buffers*, which operate within the fluid system to correct a tendency toward either acidity or alkalinity. Buffers are pairs of substances consisting of a weak acid and its salt, which act as sponges to absorb extra hydrogen or base ions, as required. The principal buffering agents in body fluids are the carbonic acid–bicarbonate system, which operates mainly in the extracellular fluid; the phosphate buffer system, which operates predominantly in the intracellular fluid; and the protein buffer system, which operates in both (proteins can act as either acids or bases as needed). If the first two mechanisms fail to effect a balance, the body has two other regulatory mechanisms that may be brought into play—namely, the *kidneys* and the *lungs*. The kidneys can vary the acidity of the urine in response to the body's need to throw off excess acid or base. They act principally by controlling base bicarbonates. The lungs aid in maintaining acid-base balance through their control of carbonic acid. They can eliminate either more or less carbonic acid (in the form of carbon dioxide and water), thus either ridding the body of excess acid or conserving it. When you have engaged in strenuous exercise, for example, you may find that you are breathing more quickly and more deeply than usual, as the body attempts to rid itself of the extra acid from the waste products of muscle cell metabolism.

When large amounts of fluids are lost or retained in the body, there can be disturbances of acid-base balance. The balance can swing in the direction of a higher concentration of either acid or base. The term *acidosis* refers to a swing toward the acid side, through either a retention of excess acid (H^+ concentration) in the body or a depletion of the body's alkaline reserves. The normally basic state of body fluids becomes more acidic; a pH below 7.35, the lowest point on the normal range for blood, is generally considered to indicate acidosis. *Alkalosis* is the opposite of acidosis; there is either a lessening of the acid (H^+ concentration) of body fluids or an excess of alkaline reserves. When the pH of the blood exceeds 7.45, the highest point in the normal range, the condition is called alkalosis. When acidosis or alkalosis results from disturbances in metabolism, the term metabolic acidosis or metabolic alkalosis is used; when it results from disturbed respiratory functioning, it is called respiratory acidosis or respiratory alkalosis.

FACTORS AFFECTING FLUID AND ELECTROLYTE BALANCE

There are many factors that will disturb the body's fluid and electrolyte balance. It is perhaps helpful here to discuss these factors under the following general headings:

✓ Insufficient Intake

The sources of water and electrolytes for the body are the food and fluids ingested. Any disturbance in the source of nourishment is reflected in the body. People who do not take in a sufficient amount of food and fluids, either because these are not available or because of illness, will usually show a disturbed fluid and electrolyte balance, particularly if the insufficient intake is prolonged.

✓ Disturbances of the Gastrointestinal Tract

A very large volume of fluid in the form of digestive juices is secreted into the gastrointestinal tract each day. Almost all of this fluid is reabsorbed during the process of digestion. Interference with the normal processes of secretion and reabsorption can result in serious fluid and electrolyte imbalance. The nature of the imbalance depends to a large extent on the portion of the gastrointestinal tract affected. In order to appreciate the significance of this point, it is helpful to keep in mind the volume, the pH, and the electrolyte composition of the various digestive juices. The approximate volumes and pH of the principal digestive juices per day are as follows:

	Daily Volume	Usual pH
Saliva	1500 ml.	6.7
Gastric secretion	2500 ml.	1.0–2.0
Intestinal secretion	3000 ml.	7.8–8.0
Pancreatic secretion	700 ml.	8.0–8.3
Bile	500 ml.	7.8
Total	8200 ml.[3]	

The major components that are involved in electrolyte and acid-base balance are found in the gastric and intestinal secretions. Gastric juice contains large quantities of hydrochloric acid and a significant amount of sodium. Gastric mucus contains a high proportion of sodium and chloride, small but significant amounts of potassium, and a relatively small amount of carbonate. Thus, when fluids are lost from the stomach through vomiting, there may be a significant loss of acid as well. Prolonged vomiting may cause severe sodium depletion and loss of the chloride ion also. The body's reserves of potassium may be lessened also. Gastric suctioning removes hydrochloric acid and fluids; gastric washings can severely deplete the store of chloride ions, particularly if these washings are done with water rather than normal saline. All gastric tube irrigations as well as gastric washings should therefore be done with isotonic saline to prevent the depletion of these electrolytes.

Pancreatic juice, bile, and the intestinal secretions are predominantly basic and contain relatively large amounts of carbonate, as well as sodium and chloride. In addition, a large proportion of the total volume of potassium excreted from the body daily is via the gastrointestinal tract in the feces. Thus, diarrhea generally results in the loss of fluids, and of sodium and chloride ions, as well as of the base secreted in the intestine. Severe diarrhea depletes the body's potassium also.

✓ Disturbances of Kidney Function

Because the kidney is so intimately concerned with the regulation of fluid and electrolyte balance, any impairment in renal function may disturb this balance. Damage to the kidney itself may interfere with its ability to reabsorb water and electrolytes in the tubules. An imbalance in the antidiuretic hormone (caused by pituitary gland dysfunction, for example) affects kidney functioning, particularly the reabsorption of water. Similarly, an imbalance in aldosterone (which may result from steroid therapy) affects sodium retention and potassium excretion by the kidneys. The kidneys are also affected by disturbances in cardiovascular functioning. An insufficient flow of blood through the kidneys due to a poorly functioning heart, for example, hampers the efficiency of the kidneys in that there may not be enough blood circulating through the kidneys to produce an adequate amount of glomerular filtrate. Retention of fluid in body tissues may then occur. This is evidenced by edema, which is a frequent accompaniment of many cardiac conditions.

Excessive Perspiration or Evaporation

One of the largest variables in the amount of water lost from the body daily is the volume of perspiration. This may range from zero to several liters per day, depending on such factors as the amount of physical activity of the individual, the temperature of the environment, and the presence of fever. When there is excessive perspiration, two protective mechanisms are brought into play: thirst, which increases the amount of fluid intake, and adjustment of the water output by the kidneys.[2]

When fluids are lost through sweating, there is a loss of sodium chloride as well. Hence, people who live in hot climates, and those who must work in temperatures above normal often find they need more salt in their food to replace that lost through perspiration. As a person becomes acclimatized to higher environmental temperatures, however, the body usually adjusts by lessening the salt content of sweat so that the loss of sodium and chloride ions by this route is minimized.

Hemorrhage, Burns, and Body Trauma

In hemorrhage, not only fluid but also a percentage of all the blood elements is lost. The total circulatory volume is decreased and, in a large hemorrhage, the body's adaptive mechanisms may collapse and shock may ensue.

In burns, as well as in some trauma to the body (including surgical trauma), fluids and electrolytes are lost from the general circulation, as these tend to accumulate in the interstitial spaces. Fluids are removed from the plasma, sodium is depleted throughout the body generally, and potassium is released in excessive amounts from the damaged cells. Proteins are also depleted. Therefore, there is a need to replace not only fluids but also sodium, potassium, and proteins in order to restore a balance.

FLUID AND ELECTROLYTE NEEDS THROUGHOUT THE LIFE CYCLE

The pregnant woman's circulatory system must take care of the unborn infant's oxygen needs, and its fluid and electrolyte needs, as well as her own. To cope with these demands, her total blood volume is increased by approximately 50 per cent, the production of red blood cells in her body is stepped up by almost one third, and total cardiac volume is increased by approximately 10 per cent. The pregnant woman's heart must also beat faster (her resting pulse rate increases) with the extra demands on her circulatory system. There is also a marked increase in the body's water content. An average of 6.5 to 7 liters is gained, including 3.5 liters for the needs of the fetus and the balance for the mother's bodily needs.

Many pregnant women complain of fluid retention, which may be caused by such factors as changes in hydrostatic and osmotic pressure, an increase in capillary permeability, and a tend-

ency to retain sodium. Some edema is common, particularly in the late stages of pregnancy. Some women develop a pregnancy-induced hypertension (toxemia of pregnancy), a complication that can cause problems for both fetus and mother. The hypertension is related to sodium and water retention.

As mentioned at the beginning of the chapter, 70 to 80 per cent of a newborn's body weight is water. Until the age of around 2 years, fluids continue to make up a greater proportion of total body weight than they do in older children and adults. Much of the additional fluid is extracellular, and is rapidly lost in the event of illness, a factor that makes the infant very vulnerable to fluid and electrolyte and acid-base imbalances. The infant also has a high metabolic rate, because of its greater proportional body surface area, its growth needs, and its relatively large body organs. The high metabolic rate means that there is more rapid turnover of water in the body of children than in adults, and children need a larger amount of fluids proportional to body weight. Another factor contributing to the infant's vulnerability to fluid and electrolyte imbalances is the immaturity of its homeostatic mechanisms. The kidneys in infants, for example, have a limited ability to concentrate and dilute urine, a mechanism that is important in maintaining fluid balance.

By the time the child is around 2 years of age, fluid volume as a percentage of total body weight, as well as its distribution in the body, is similar to that in an adult. The basal metabolic rate gradually decreases through childhood until maturity, and the water turnover gradually slows down to adult levels. Throughout childhood, however, the individual continues to need a

RANGE OF AVERAGE WATER REQUIREMENT OF CHILDREN AT DIFFERENT AGES UNDER ORDINARY CONDITIONS

Age	Average Body Weight in kg.	Total Water in 24 Hours, ml.	Water per kg Body Wt. in 24 Hours, ml.
3 days	3.0	250– 300	80–100
10 days	3.2	400– 500	125–150
3 months	5.4	750– 850	140–160
6 months	7.3	950–1100	130–155
9 months	8.6	1100–1250	125–145
1 year	9.5	1150–1300	120–135
2 years	11.8	1350–1500	115–125
4 years	16.2	1600–1800	100–110
6 years	20.0	1800–2000	90–100
10 years	28.7	2000–2500	70– 85
14 years	45.0	2200–2700	50– 60
18 years	54.0	2200–2700	40– 50

From Vaughan, V. C., III, McKay, R. J., and Behrman, R. E.: *Nelson Textbook of Pediatrics*. 11th ed. Philadelphia, W. B. Saunders Company, 1979, p. 175.

NORMAL BLADDER CAPACITY AND VOIDING

Age	Approximate Capacity	Number of Voidings in 24 Hours	Average Quantity at Each Voiding in cc.'s
Birth	60 cc.	14	30
Birth to 3 months	60–115 cc.	13–14	30
3–6 months	115–150 cc.	20	30
6–12 months	150–280 cc.	16	45
1 year	280 cc.	12	60
6 years	500–700 cc.	7–8	120–150
12 years	850 cc.	7–8	180–240

From Tackett, J. J. M., and Hunsberger, M.: *Family Centered Care of Children and Adolescents.* Philadelphia, W. B. Saunders Company, 1981, p. 1382.

greater volume of fluids proportionate to his body weight than an adult does, and he also loses a proportionately greater volume in urine.

In children there is also a greater exchange of fluids in the gastrointestinal tract than there is in adults. This factor is important because it is through this exchange that water and sodium are reabsorbed and potassium is excreted. Thus, problems interfering with the reabsorption of fluids in the gastrointestinal tract can cause major fluid losses in children. They can become dehydrated quickly with even minor gastrointestinal upsets. Edema is often seen in refugee children who are starving. In this case the fluid flows from the blood vessels into the tissues because lowered levels of plasma protein are insufficient to hold the fluid.

With adolescence, there is a maturing of all body systems and the homeostatic mechanisms for regulating fluid and electrolyte balance begin to function as they do in adults. In fluid and electrolyte balance, as in so many other aspects of physiological functioning, there is a difference between males and females, with women having a tendency to retain fluids during the 2 or 3 days immediately prior to the menstrual period. Just before the menstrual period, there is an increase in the level of the hormone progesterone. This hormone is related in chemical composition to aldosterone and has a similar effect in promoting the retention of sodium, which, in turn, leads to the retention of water in the body.

Throughout adulthood, there is a gradual decrease in the functional capacity of the cardiovascular system as blood pressure increases and the individual becomes more vulnerable to cardiovascular diseases. A gradual lessening in efficiency of the fluid and electrolyte regulating mechanisms contributes to making the older adult slower to recover from imbalances than he was in his younger days.

During the menopause many women have a problem with fluid retention. Although a number of theories have been postulated, no single definitive cause has been isolated. Generally it is usually considered to be "idiopathic," that is, due to no known cause.

In the elderly, the prevalence of hypertension and the incidence of cardiovascular disease increase. The arteries thicken and become less elastic. Many older people have a problem with varicose veins, which, if deep, will cause swelling of the ankles. It is usually difficult to get older people to drink a sufficient amount of fluids to meet their bodily needs, particularly when they are ill. It is important to make a point of offering extra fluids between meal times and encouraging them to drink more water, milk, and juices.

COMMON PROBLEMS

A great many problems may result from disturbances in fluid and electrolyte balance. All other systems in the body are dependent on the effective functioning of the fluid system. It serves not only as the transport mechanism for moving nutrients and removing wastes, but also provides an optimal environment for the efficient functioning of body cells.

As a result of fluid and electrolyte imbalance, then, problems may arise in any of the body's functional areas. These problems often require medical or nursing intervention. The type of problem and the intervention required depend to a large extent on the specific nature of the imbalance and the extent of the disturbance. The most common problems that the nurse will encounter are those associated with dehydration, edema, and accompanying disturbances in acid-base balance.

Dehydration is a general term used to designate a condition in which the body or tissues are deprived of water. It may result from a number of causes, such as an insufficient intake of fluids, an excessive loss of fluids, or other disease conditions, as discussed earlier in the section on factors affecting fluid and electrolyte balance.

Edema is a condition in which there is excessive fluid retained in the tissues; it may be either generalized or localized. It may result from disturbances in kidney function, disturbances in circulatory function (as, for example, in people with cardiac conditions), inflammation, increased permeability of the cell membranes, or a number of other health problems.

ASSESSMENT

In order to assess the patient's fluid and electrolyte status, the nurse should be aware of factors in the patient's history which could cause an imbalance. She should be alert to signs and symptoms in the patient that could be indicative of fluid and electrolyte imbalance, and she should be able to identify significant laboratory findings. In addition, the nurse should know the physician's plan of therapy for the patient and understand the rationale on which this plan is based.

The patient's medical history provides the nurse with much valuable information about existing or potential fluid and electrolyte problems. The person who has had a history of nausea and vomiting over several days, for example, is likely to show disturbances resulting from the loss of fluids generally, the loss of acid from gastric secretions, and possibly a depletion of the sodium ions as well. The patient who is admitted for surgery may develop fluid and electrolyte imbalance postoperatively and will need careful observation on the part of the nurse to detect signs and symptoms of impending imbalance. The baseline data entered by the physician, other nurses, and other members of the health team on the patient's record can alert the nurse to the presence of any of the health problems discussed in the section on factors affecting fluid and electrolyte balance.

Subjective Observations

Significant factors in the patient's history that may alert the nurse to the possibility of fluid and electrolyte imbalance include recent changes in the individual's usual patterns of intake and output or the presence of any one of the health problems already mentioned. When taking the nursing history, the nurse should obtain information about the patient's normal habits of food and fluid intake and output. How many glasses of water does he usually drink per day, for example? How many cups of tea or coffee? What types of fluids does he like? What foods does he usually eat? This type of information not only provides baseline data with

which to compare but also helps the nurse to plan the patient's care to prevent fluid and electrolyte imbalances from developing or to assist in correcting those that have occurred.

In addition to obtaining information about usual habits, the nurse should ascertain if there have been any recent alterations in the individual's pattern of intake and output. For example, has the patient been suffering from anorexia, and not taking the usual amount of food and fluid? Has he noticed that he is not voiding as much as usual or, conversely, has been voiding more than usual? Is he taking any medications that could affect fluid and electrolyte balance, as, for example, steroids? Has he experienced any changes in his food intake or fluid output as a result of illness recently? Has he noticed that he is particularly thirsty lately? Is he aware of any recent rapid gain or loss in weight, or gradually increasing obesity? Has he noticed any weakness in his muscle strength, or signs of muscular irritability, such as tremors or twitching of the muscles?

Objective Observations

Although fluid and electrolyte disturbances are usually the result of other disorders in the body, they may in themselves give rise to specific problems.

Of particular importance to the nurse is an awareness of the early signs of dehydration in a patient. His tongue is often dry and furry. He may complain of thirst, his skin tissues usually appear to be loose and flabby (loss of tissue turgor), and the mucous membranes appear dry. The patient frequently also complains of fatigue. The nurse will note that the patient's urine is scanty in amount and darker in color than normal urine. If the dehydration progresses, evidence of a greater degree of imbalance may be noted. Fluid is first drawn from the interstitial spaces and then from within the cells in order to maintain an adequate blood volume. However, as dehydration advances, the blood volume may also be lessened, and the patient's pulse may then become weak and his blood pressure low. He may experience a feeling of faintness, and sometimes signs of mental confusion are evident. With moderately advanced dehydration, the individual's temperature is usually elevated and there is a marked weight loss as well. In the most extreme cases of dehydration, the patient may go into shock, which progresses to a comatose state.

Also important to the nurse is the early recognition of retention of fluid in the body tissues. Edema may be localized or generalized. Gener-

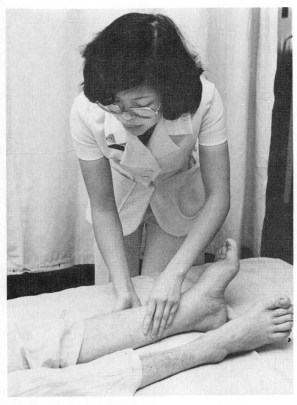

The nurse checks for signs of edema in this patient.

alized edema can usually be observed first in the soft tissues around the eyes and in dependent areas of the body. If the individual is up and walking around, the edema may be noted first in the feet and ankles. With bed patients, the nurse may notice edema particularly around the sacral area. The patient's skin appears puffy and soft to the touch. The edematous patient usually shows a gain in weight, which is due to the extra fluid he is retaining. When there is marked edema, the blood volume becomes increased, with a resultant rise in blood pressure. The lungs may be affected, since the lungs are a low pressure area in the circulatory system and extra fluids tend to accumulate there. Thus, the patient may show symptoms of dyspnea, with moist and noisy breathing. When there is a retention of fluids, there is usually a lessened volume of urine output.

Diagnostic Tests

Diagnostic tests for patients who have potential or actual fluid and electrolyte problems usually involve the laboratory examination of specimens of blood and urine. Electrolyte levels in the blood serum can be determined after the collection of approximately 5 ml. of venous blood. Potassium, sodium, calcium, and magnesium concentrations are frequently measured. Normal blood values for these elements in adults are:

Potassium	3.5 to 5.0 mEq./L
Sodium	136 to 145 mEq./L
Calcium	8.8 to 10.5 mg./100 ml.
Magnesium	1.5 to 2.5 mEq./L

A blood gas analysis is often carried out to assess the acid-base balance. For this, 5 ml. of arterial blood is withdrawn. Measurement of the pH, Pco_2, and standard Pco_3 is usually ordered. The pH indicates the overall acid-base balance of the body (normal, 7.35–7.45). Pco_2 is the pressure of carbon dioxide dissolved in the plasma and indicates carbonic acid retention (normal, 35–40 mm. Hg). Standard Pco_3 measures the amount of bicarbonate buffer (normal, 25–29 mEq./liter). Often a Po_2 reading is requested; it measures the oxygen tension, normally 95 to 100 mm. Hg.

Diagnostic tests of the urine are done to measure the fluid and electrolyte balance. Tests for acetone and diacetic acid may indicate a disturbance in the metabolism that results in a type of acidosis. Urine is examined to test for the excretion of chlorides and sometimes potassium. The specific gravity of urine indicates the concentration of dissolved materials, such as waste products, and can reflect the degree of hydration of the patient. Other urine and kidney tests are more likely to assess kidney functioning, which may or may not be a contributing factor to fluid and electrolyte imbalance.

PRIORITIES FOR NURSING ACTION

Disturbances in fluid and electrolyte balance can have serious effects on body functioning. The nurse must be particularly alert in noting early indications of *imbalance*. These should be drawn to the attention of the attending physician promptly so that appropriate therapy can be instituted to correct the situation before it becomes too advanced. The consequences of marked imbalances of fluids and the major electrolytes in the body have been documented throughout this chapter. It should be stressed, therefore, that all measures to maintain or restore fluid and electrolyte balance should receive priority from the nurse.

The individual with an elevated temperature is especially vulnerable to disturbances in his fluid and electrolyte balance. His fluid requirements are higher than normal (at least 3000 ml. of fluid is believed to be required by the person with pyrexia), and his fluid losses are usually also in excess of the normal (see Chapter 19).

Children, in particular, show signs of dehydration with accompanying electrolyte imbalance very rapidly in acute illnesses. A child who has been running a temperature, or who has had diarrhea for even a few days, may be brought into the hospital in a state of acute dehydration. He will need immediate medical and nursing intervention.

The nurse should also always be alert to the possibility of _circulatory collapse, or shock_, which occurs when the body's fluid system is not able to cope with major disturbances. Shock is always considered a medical emergency and requires prompt intervention. It may be caused by a sudden, extensive loss of fluids from the body, such as occurs in hemorrhage or in severe burns, or by prolonged dehydration. It may also result from severe trauma of any kind, surgery, heart conditions, infections, allergic reactions, or toxicity from drugs. Shock may occur immediately after an injury, or its appearance may be delayed.

It should be noted that in the case of a sudden hemorrhage, there is no time for the development of early symptoms and the patient may show signs of circulatory collapse very suddenly. Again, prompt intervention is essential to save the person's life. It is important to remember that any injury produces shock, which may range from mild to severe—so severe, in fact, that the patient may die from the effects of shock itself rather than from the disturbance that caused it.

Shock is frequently present in persons admitted to the emergency unit of a health agency. It is also a possible complication in many conditions for which people are hospitalized as, for example, surgery or cardiac conditions. It may, however, just as easily occur in people on the street, at home, or in a physician's or dentist's office. The subject of shock will be treated in much more detail in courses you will take later

✔ SHOCK

Subjective Observations	Objective Observations
Patient may complain of:	Nurse may observe:
Feeling of faintness	Pallor
Dizziness	Cold, clammy skin
Blurring of vision	Profuse sweat
Thirst	Rapid, weak, thready pulse
Apprehension	Low blood pressure
	Rapid, shallow breathing (may progress to air hunger)
	Nausea, possibly vomiting
	Patient may be drowsy, lapse into unconsciousness

in your nursing program. However, as a first-year student you should:

1. Be able to recognize the existence of shock in a patient, and indications of impending or worsening shock
2. Be aware when prompt intervention is needed and summon assistance
3. Be able to take steps to facilitate the institution of emergency measures

The signs of shock evident in a patient may vary somewhat, depending on its cause, its severity, and the length of time the patient has been in shock. However, there are some classic signs and symptoms with which the student should be familiar. These may be divided into those which the patient may be aware of (subjective data) and those which the nurse may observe (objective data) as listed in the table above. Any or all of these signs and symptoms may be present.

If you suspect that a patient is going into shock, you should alert the nurse in charge so that prompt action can be taken to obtain emergency intervention. Most health agencies have a standard routine for such emergencies and a well-stocked cart available for treatment needs.

PRINCIPLES RELEVANT TO FLUID AND ELECTROLYTE BALANCE

1. **The average adult requires 2100 to 2900 ml. of fluid in a 24-hour period.**
2. **Children require a greater volume of fluids, proportional to body weight than adults.**
3. **Normally, fluid intake is balanced against fluid loss.**
4. **When fluids are lost or retained in excessive amounts, there is an accompanying loss or gain of electrolytes.**
5. **The signs and symptoms accompanying electrolyte imbalance vary according to the excess or deficiency of the specific electrolyte.**
6. **The specific electrolytes lost from the body in any fluid loss depend on the route of the loss.**

The recommended treatment for patients in shock has undergone considerable revision in recent years, and opinions vary with regard to the use of different drugs to aid in the restoration of blood pressure. There has also been controversy over the positioning of the patient. It is, therefore, a good idea to acquaint yourself with the specific routine of the agency in which you are having experience and also with the contents of the emergency cart. It is generally recommended at present that the patient be placed flat in bed (dorsal recumbent position) with the feet and legs slightly elevated, unless there are contraindications to this position, as in the case of the cardiac patients, for example. You are usually safe in assuming that intravenous therapy will be started (to raise the volume of circulating fluids) and the necessary equipment should be gathered. Oxygen equipment and intubation equipment may also be required, so these should be available.

Medical anti-shock trousers (MAST) are now quite extensively used in the pre-hospital emergency care of injured persons, particularly those in shock or hemorrhaging. Sometimes called "trauma trousers" or "MAST suit," these are inflatable pants that are used to apply an even pressure to the body below the waist, thus helping to control hemorrhage or to prevent circulatory collapse or both. The trousers can be assembled around the patient, then zipped together in sections and inflated. Care must be taken that the trousers are not deflated too quickly, or circulatory collapse may ensue. Usually the physician will direct the deflating process. If the trousers are used in your community, all nurses should be given instruction on them by the local emergency services agency.

The patient is usually very apprehensive and frightened. Therefore, he needs to be reassured. A calm, unhurried, manner and competent actions on the part of the nurse can help to prevent the patient from becoming anxious and also help to reassure worried family members who may be present. The key to appearing calm and competent lies in knowing what to do in an emergency. It is important then to learn the procedures and policies of the agency in which the nurse is working.

GOALS FOR NURSING ACTION

The basic goals of care for the patient with actual or potential fluid and electrolyte problems are to assist the patient to maintain a homeostatic balance insofar as this is possible or to restore a balance that has been disturbed.

SPECIFIC NURSING INTERVENTIONS

Measures to Maintain Fluid and Electrolyte Balance

Ensuring Adequate Food and Fluid Intake. Of primary importance in the nursing care of the patient with fluid and electrolyte problems is the maintenance of a therapeutic fluid intake. In many instances the physician orders the exact amount of oral fluid for a patient. Sometimes, however, it is a nursing function to judge the oral fluid needs of the patient. For example, the nurse determines that the patient with a fever or an infection requires large amounts of fluid (at least 3000 ml. per day).

Generally speaking, if the patient is dehydrated or has lost an excessive amount of fluids, he should be encouraged to take extra fluids. Additional fluid intake may be contraindicated in some cases, however. If the patient is nauseated or vomiting, for example, it is not reasonable to expect that he can tolerate oral fluids. Patients with kidney or heart conditions may require restriction of their fluid intake. The nurse should be aware of the physician's objectives in medical therapy and never push or force fluids beyond the limit prescribed.

People normally get electrolytes from the food and fluids they ingest. Therefore, to maintain good electrolyte balance, adequate nutrition is essential. When the patient is deficient in certain electrolytes or extra are needed in the body, these may be administered by medication. For example, calcium tablets are frequently ordered for pregnant women because of the heavy demands for additional calcium to promote growth of the fetus.

In addition, it is not unusual for restricted electrolyte intake to be prescribed; for example, the physician might order a salt-free or low-salt diet for a patient. The usual purpose here is to restrict the oral intake of sodium (Na^+). It is frequently the nurse's responsibility to help the patient to understand the necessity for the restriction and to help him plan meals with this in mind. Most people are able to assume the responsibility for restricting their diets. Nevertheless, in hospitals it is not unknown for a "helpful" roommate to lend his salt shaker to a person on a restricted salt diet.

Monitoring Fluid Intake and Output. With patients who have existing or potential fluid and electrolyte problems, it is essential to monitor fluid intake and output accurately. When the physician wishes to know the fluid intake of a particular patient, accurate measurements are made of all the fluids he is given. This includes fluid given orally, intravenously, interstitially, and rectally. Most hospitals provide chart forms for recording fluid balance.

Body fluids are normally excreted through the kidneys, the intestine, the lungs, and the skin. In recording the amount of fluid output, the nurse measures the amount of the patient's urine accurately. In addition, she measures any drainage, such as bile drainage and suction returns.

In some instances, significant amounts of fluid lost in the feces, from wounds, or by perspiration are also recorded.

It is difficult to obtain an exact record of fluid intake and output in all cases. Most hospitals have charts or written material that show the estimated fluid content of the drinking glasses, cups, soup bowels, and other utensils usually used in the agency. However, it requires the

---

2-8738   RIVERSIDE HOSPITAL OF OTTAWA

NORTH   JANE   SP 1249
223 TREE RD   OTT   234-7566-600
NORTH   RICHARD   HUS
SAME
1.9.77 1PM F 30 M SURG   RC
        420   1

TOTAL 24 hr Intake _4090cc_ Date _Sept 1/77_

2330–0730			0715–1545			1545–2345		
Time	Type	Amount	Time	Type	Amount	Time	Type	Amount
2400	I/v 5%D/w	200cc	0800	Juice	100	1700	I/v 5% D/W	200cc
	I/v 5%D/s 1000cc put up.	—		Coffee	130		absorbed & discontinued	
				H2O	150			
0015	H2O	100 cc	0830	I/v D/s 5%	150cc	1730	Soup	170
				I/v D/w 1000cc put up.			Tea	130
							Milk	200
0700	i/v D/s	850 cc	1000	Milk	100cc	2030	Tea	130
0715	Tea	130 cc	1200	Soup	170		Gingerale	200
				Tea	130			
			1530	H2O	50			
				I/v D/w 5%	800			
Total		1280cc	Total		1780 cc	Total		1030 cc
Oral		230	Oral		830	Oral		830
I.V.		1050	I.V.		950	I.V.		200
T.B.A.		150cc	T.B.A.		200cc	T.B.A.		—

Total 24 Hr Output

Time	Type	Amount	Time	Type	Amount	Time	Type	Amount
2400	Urine	300	0900	Urine	200	1800	Urine	300
0700	Urine	700	1200	Urine	600	2200	Urine	600
			1500	Urine	500			
Total		1000cc	Total		1300cc	Total		900 cc
Urine		1000	Urine		1300	Urine		900
Other		—	Other		—	Other		—

Large Glass = 200 cc
Small Glass = 100 cc

Soup Bowl = 170 cc
Cup = 130 cc

A sample fluid balance work sheet. (Courtesy of the Riverside Hospital of Ottawa.)

cooperation of all personnel to maintain an accurate record of the patient's total fluid intake. The patient can often help to keep his own record, particularly if he understands the need for doing this.

An accurate recording of output is usually more difficult. For example, the amount of fluid loss from perspiration may be considerable in the patient with a fever, yet measuring this is almost impossible. The nurse should, however, record the fact that the patient is perspiring profusely and draw this to the attention of the physician. Often the amount of fluid lost from wounds can only be estimated. Sometimes the number of dressing pads that are soaked through is helpful in assessing the extent of wound drainage.

When drainage tubing is irrigated, or such procedures as gastric washings or bladder irrigation are done, the amount of fluid inserted must always be included in the calculations of fluid intake and output.

Keeping an accurate record of urine output can also present some problems. When patients have bathroom privileges, it is necessary to place a measured container in the bathroom and to enlist the patient's cooperation in collecting urine and, if feasible, measuring the amount voided. Patients who are incontinent of urine and feces present additional problems in the assessment of fluid losses. The nurse must watch these patients carefully for fluid retention or excessive fluid loss.

The urine output of the average adult is 1100 to 1700 ml. in a 24-hour period. When urine output is less than 25 ml. or more than 500 ml. per hour, it generally is abnormal. Abnormalities of either excess or inadequate urine output should be drawn to the attention of the patient's physician so that appropriate therapy can be instituted.

Observing for Signs and Symptoms of Imbalance. In assisting in the maintenance of fluid and electrolyte balance, the nurse must be alert to early indications of imbalance. Observations of the degree of hydration of the patient are noted and recorded. The nurse should watch particularly for early signs of dehydration or fluid retention, as these were outlined in the section on assessment of the patient.

When observing for indications of electrolyte imbalance, the nurse should have an understanding of the patient's medical condition and the potential problems that may occur. If she is aware, for example, that the patient has a condition involving dysfunction of the adrenal cortex or impairment of renal function, she should observe him carefully for signs of sodium and potassium imbalance. Most of the body potassium is normally in the fluid within the cells, yet the potassium in the blood plasma is maintained at a fairly constant volume even when there is a significant loss of the ion from the cells. Thus the body may be seriously depleted of potassium before significant changes can be noted in the blood plasma level, which is the only tabulated measurement. Therefore, the nurse should be alert to the early signs and symptoms of potassium deficiency such as muscular weakness, irregularities of the pulse, or nervous irritability.

When the nurse is aware of potential problems, her observations are more directed and purposeful. She knows what to look for, and her observations can be of inestimable assistance to the physician in diagnosing the patient's condition and planning therapy.

Assisting in the Restoration of Fluid and Electrolyte Balance

General Considerations. Whenever a disturbance in fluid or electrolyte balance occurs, steps must be taken to restore homeostasis. Since the principal sources of fluid and electrolytes are the foods and fluids a person takes in, adjustments in diet or fluid intake or both may be sufficient to rectify a mild imbalance. In the case of deficiencies of specific electrolytes, supplements may be given in the form of medications. Often, however, fluid loss is too extensive and the accompanying loss of electrolytes too great to be corrected by oral intake alone, or this method of replacement may be contraindicated. Fluids and electrolytes may then be administered by other routes, by intravenous infusion, by blood transfusion, or by interstitial or rectal infusion. The decisions of route to be used and the type of solution to be administered are made by the physician. His decisions are based on his knowledge of the patient's condition and the particular factors causing the imbalance.

The care of the patient with fluid and electrolyte problems includes good supportive nursing measures as well as assistance with curative measures. Hygiene is of particular importance for patients with these problems. The patient's physical comfort is largely dependent upon his feeling of cleanliness and freshness. Profuse diaphoresis may necessitate frequent changes and baths; dry, scaly skin and mucous membranes are lubricated with emollient creams. One of the dangers of cracked lips and dry mouth is the increased risk of secondary infections.

The overhydrated patient, in particular, should turn in bed regularly to promote circulation and adequate nourishment to all tissues. The presence of edema or even the weight of·

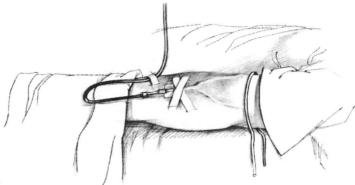

The site of an intravenous infusion.

Intravenous Infusion. The infusion of fluids directly into the peripheral veins is often indicated when a patient is unable to take fluids orally. Infusion permits the patient to obtain many fluids, electrolytes, and nutrients that are necessary to life. In addition, it has the advantage of rapid absorption, which is particularly important in the administration of some medications.

Many kinds of intravenous fluid are available for infusion. The physician decides which kind of fluid the patient needs. For example, a patient may require 5 per cent dextrose in water, normal saline, or 10 per cent dextrose in normal saline. Usually intravenous fluid is provided in 250, 500, or 1000 ml containers.

In some agencies, only the physician is permitted to start an intravenous infusion; in others it is a responsibility of the graduate nurse. Often hospitals have policies regarding the kinds of infusions that nurses can initiate. Sometimes the physician orders the addition of drugs such as norepinephrine, vitamin C, potassium chloride, Neo-Synephrine, or nitrogen mustard to an intravenous solution. It is the responsibility of the nurse to know which she is permitted to add and which drugs the physician must administer.

The choice of site for an intravenous infusion is dependent upon a number of factors. The condition of the patient's veins as well as his comfort must be considered. The *cephalic* and *basilic* veins in the inner aspect of the elbow are used most frequently. These sites may require extension of the patient's arm, which can be uncomfortable after a prolonged period. If, however, these veins are entered along the shaft of radius and ulna (bones of the forearm), the bones provide a natural splint and make extension of the elbow unnecessary.

Prior to starting an intravenous infusion, the tubing is attached to the intravenous flask. Ster-ile precautions are taken throughout this procedure in order to protect the patient from infection. In addition to the flask and the intravenous tubing, the nurse requires a tourniquet, an antiseptic swab, a sterile syringe, a standard to hold the flask, and a receptacle for the discarded fluid.

After the tubing has been attached to the intravenous flask, the flask is hung upon the standard and the fluid is then run through the tubing before the tubing is clamped. By running the fluid through the tubing, air is removed so that it will not be introduced into the patient's vein. Air injected into a vein can result in an air embolus. An embolus is a clot or plug that has been transported by the blood from a larger blood vessel to a smaller one, which can result in the blocking of blood flow.

A tourniquet is applied to the patient's arm above the intravenous site. At the same time, the patient clenches and unclenches his fist. These measures distend the veins in his arm to make them more accessible for venipuncture. The injection site is cleansed with antiseptic, and a sterile needle (No. 18, 19, 20, or 21) is then attached to the syringe and inserted at a 45-degree angle, bevel up, into the vein. Some resistance to the needle is encountered at the skin, but the subcutaneous tissues and veins offer very little resistance. The patient perceives pain when the needle goes through the skin but little discomfort thereafter. The plunger of the syringe is drawn back to ascertain that the needle is in the vein (indicated by obtaining blood). The syringe is disconnected, and the tubing is attached to the needle. The rate of flow is then established. Depending upon the patient's condition, the rate of flow may range from 40 to 100 drops per minute. The usual rate is 80 drops per minute. The rate of flow for an intravenous infusion is often ordered by the physician.

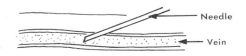

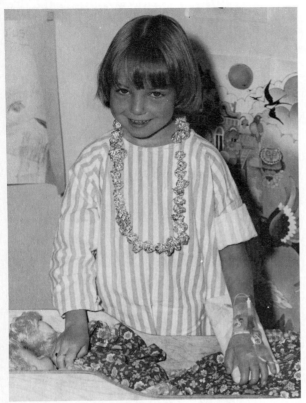

The intravenous needle and tubing are held in place with tape, and an armboard is used to immobilize the joint.

The tubing and the needle are then attached to the arm by adhesive tape. The patient can be provided with an armboard to immobilize his arm if this is necessary. Whenever the site of the needle insertion is near a joint, as, for example, the elbow or the wrist, it is wise to use an armboard to prevent the needle from being dislodged with the patient's movement. It is very difficult to maintain immobility of a part without support such as a board provides. To be effective, the armboard usually should reach from above the elbow joint to the end of the fingertips, although sometimes the fingertips are curved over the end of the armboard. The board should always be padded for the patient's comfort and safety.

If intravenous fluids are to be administered over a prolonged period of time, polyethylene tubing (Intra-cath) may be used instead of a needle for an infusion; the tubing fits through the needle, which is removed after the tubing has been inserted into the vein. Tubing is more flexible than a needle, but it must be checked to make certain that it does not become dislodged and move down the patient's vein, particularly when it is being removed. In some agencies, Intra-caths are inserted only by physicians.

Often with children, and sometimes with adults whose surface veins are inaccessible or unsuitable for infusion, it is necessary to make a small incision in order to locate an appropriate site for the needle insertion. In these cases, a "cut-down" will be used by the physician. This technique is not carried out by nursing personnel, although the nurse should have the equipment ready and assist the physician as needed.

It may be necessary to vary the height of the intravenous flask according to the pressure with which one wishes the fluid to enter the vein. The higher the flask, the stronger is the gravitational pull on the fluid, and the greater the pressure it exerts. Usually 1 meter (3 feet) above bed level is an adequate height for most intravenous infusions.

Frequently it is the nurse's responsibility to adjust the rate of flow of the intravenous solution. Various methods of deriving the number of milliliters per minute are used, the objective being to divide the total amount of solution equally over the time period prescribed for the infusion. For example, if 250 ml. of fluid is to be given over a 2-hour period, the rate of flow should be approximately 2 ml. per minute to allow all of the fluid to run through in 2 hours.

During an intravenous infusion, the patient is observed for any untoward effects. Specifically, the nurse should note the entry site of the intravenous needle or catheter for swelling, redness, blanching, or pain. These reactions can indicate that the needle has slipped out of the patient's vein, with the result that the fluid is flowing into the surrounding tissues. The I.V. should be stopped immediately. Patients are also observed for signs of overhydration or cardiac overload. A faster pulse rate, an increase in blood pressure, or dyspnea can indicate cardiac overload and consequently are reported to the physician immediately. If the fluid appears to be running too quickly or the patient shows signs of overhydration or cardiac overload, the flow should be slowed down.

The nurse records on the patient's chart the amount and the kind of intravenous fluid being administered, as well as the name of the person who initiated the procedure. The site of the intravenous puncture and the rate of flow are also recorded. In this way another site can be chosen for the next infusion. Generally the sites are chosen by starting from the lower part of the arm and working upward so that previous infusion sites will not impede the flow of solution in the veins.

Several problems may be encountered in the administration of intravenous fluids. If the fluid stops running or flows spasmodically, the needle may have become dislodged, or the bevel of the needle (or the end of the plastic tubing) may be resting against the wall of the patient's vein. Slight alteration of the position of the needle or tubing can often correct this. If the intravenous solution flows into the interstitial spaces, the infusion must be restarted with another sterile needle. The nurse can tell if the infusion has gone into the interstitial spaces by the edema that forms around the injection site when fluid infiltrates the subcutaneous tissues. Another problem is the appearance of air bubbles in the tubing. When this happens the tubing can be disconnected at the needle and the fluid allowed to run through the tubing until the bubbles are expelled. Another method of removing an air bubble is to "flick" the tubing with the finger, while holding the tubing taut, until the bubble rises in the container.

Adding Medications to Intravenous Infusions. Medications are frequently added to intravenous infusions. This method of administration is particularly useful when a slow, continuous infusion of a medication is desired.

An antibiotic, for example, might be administered by this route to a patient who has a massive infection. The route is also useful in fluid and electrolyte maintenance or replacement. Potassium chloride is often administered this way. Medications administered by this route are called intravenous *admixtures*. They may be added to the solution before an intravenous is started, or while it is running.

Sometimes, the drug to be added cannot be mixed with the intravenous solution or may need to be given slowly or intermittently. In these cases, a second intravenous set may be used. A *"piggy-back" set* is used for the intermittent administration of a drug into an intravenous infusion. A small bottle containing the drug is suspended (on an extension hook) from the same pole used for the primary intravenous bottle and is connected to the upper opening (upper Y-port) of the primary set by means of a short tube. The bottle containing the drug must be suspended at a higher level than the primary bottle, so that the pressure of the flow from the

"Piggy-back" and secondary sets can be used for intravenous infusion of drugs that are not mixed directly with the primary intravenous solution.

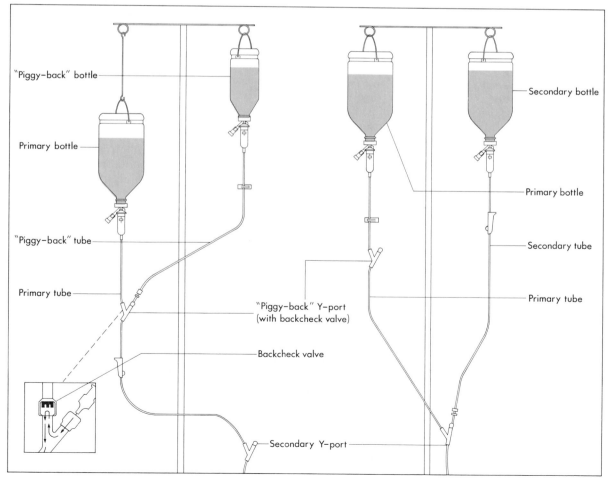

bottle containing the drug is greater than that from the primary bottle. When the flow clamp on the "piggy-back" tube is opened, the difference in pressure causes the backcheck valve in the upper Y-port to cut off the flow of the primary solution until the level of the drug in the "piggy-back" tube falls to a point lower than the drip chamber of the primary bottle.

A *secondary set* can be used for either intermittent or simultaneous administration of a drug solution. Any size intravenous fluid container may be used to hold the drug. The bottle is suspended at the same level as the primary bottle. The attachment is made at the lower Y-port of the primary tube.

Discontinuing an Intravenous Infusion.

To discontinue an intravenous infusion, an antiseptic swab for cleansing the open area is needed. The intravenous tubing is clamped, and then the adhesive tape on the patient's arm is loosened. The needle is removed quickly from the patient's vein, the antiseptic swab is placed over the puncture wound, and digital pressure is applied until the bleeding stops. If plastic tubing has been used instead of a needle, it is withdrawn carefully and checked to make sure that none of the tube remains in the patient's vein. Since the length of the tube that was inserted is often recorded in the patient's chart, the length of the removed tube can be checked against this record.

Whenever bleeding persists from the intravenous site, pressure is prolonged by means of a small dressing in order to prevent bleeding into the tissues and resultant bruise. Subsequently, the kind and amount of fluid that was infused is recorded, as is the time the intravenous infusion was terminated.

Blood Transfusion.

Prior to a blood transfusion, the patients blood is typed. There are many blood groups besides the basic A, AB, B, and O types. The Rh factor is determined along with the blood group. Usually 5 ml. of blood is taken for typing.

Blood transfusions are usually started by a physician or a specially qualified nurse. Initiating a transfusion is similar to starting an intravenous infusion. A careful check is always made to be certain that the patient is getting the right blood. Usually this means that two nurses check the number on the blood bottle against the number on the duplicate request form on the patient's record, and the name on the requisition against the name on the patient's record and identification band. In some hospitals it is also necessary to check the patient's hospital identity number on the blood bottle, the blood requisition, the chart, and the identification band.

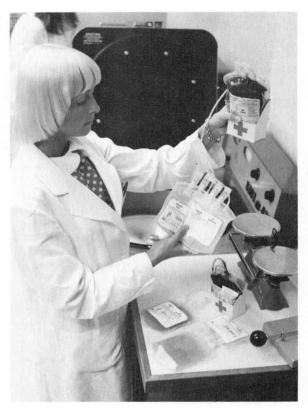

Proper identification of blood for transfusion is essential.

A No. 18 needle is usually used for a blood transfusion, and the rate of flow of the blood is normally 40 drops per minute. Special note is made of the patient's reaction and condition; at any sign of urticaria, chills, backache, or respiratory or circulatory distress, the transfusion is terminated and the physician notified. The patient's temperature and blood pressure are taken, and a sample of urine is obtained for laboratory analysis. The urinalysis is done to look for evidence of the lysis of red blood cells, which occurs when there is incompatibility of donor and recipient blood. Because most reactions to a blood transfusion occur within a short time after it has been started, the nurse should stay with the patient for the first 15 minutes.

Recording the initiation of a blood transfusion should include the time it was started, the amount of blood, the number on the bottle of blood, and the name of the person who initiated the transfusion. Termination of the blood transfusion is similar to the termination of the intravenous infusion.

On occasion a patient requires a phlebotomy, that is, an opening into a vein in order to remove blood. This measure is carried out by the physician, usually to decrease blood volume (in order to relieve dyspnea caused by congestion of blood in the lungs, for example). For this procedure, empty bottles to receive the blood are required, in addition to the equipment that is needed to enter a vein.

Interstitial Infusion. Interstitial infusion, hypodermoclysis, and subcutaneous infusion are synonymous terms referring to the administration of large amounts of fluid into subcutaneous tissue. This measure is not used often; it is utilized when a patient is unable to take fluids orally, rectally, or intravenously. Its purpose is to supply the patient with fluids, electrolytes, and occasionally nourishment. Hyaluronidase (Wydase) is often added to the fluid to hasten its absorption. This enzyme breaks down the hyaluronic acid of the connective tissue.

Whether the initiation of an interstitial infusion is the responsibility of the nurse or the physician depends on the policy of the specific agency. The usual sites for the administration of an interstitial infusion are just below the scapula, the abdominal wall above the crest of the ilium, the lower aspect of the breast, and the anterior aspect of the thigh.

The equipment that is used is similar to that used in intravenous infusions. A No. 19, 20, 21, or 22 needle is used. Usually, two sites are used simultaneously. After the equipment has been set up (see Intravenous Infusion), the needle is inserted into the skin at a 20-degree angle. It is then taped in place and the flow of the fluid is adjusted in accordance with the physician's order. The usual rate of flow for an interstitial infusion is 60 to 120 drops per minute. The rate is dependent upon the ability of the individual to absorb the fluid. Thin people usually absorb fluid more easily than obese people, because they have fewer fat cells.

The nurse assists the patient in assuming a comfortable position, since this treatment is often lengthy. Observations are indicated to detect untoward symptoms, particularly those related to circulatory collapse (for example, an accelerated, weak pulse). The patient should also be watched for signs of respiratory difficulty

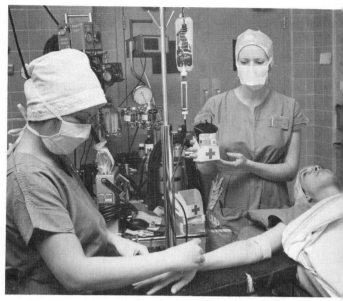

Ready reserves of blood must be available during surgical procedures.

that could indicate overhydration, such as dyspnea or moist and noisy breathing. Sometimes the infusion is poorly absorbed and the nurse may notice that tissues at the site of injection are becoming edematous. If untoward symptoms develop, the infusion should be stopped and the physician notified promptly. Because of the site of interstitial infusions, adequate draping is necessary for the patient's comfort.

At the termination of an infusion the needle is removed and a small antiseptic dressing is taped over the wound with slight pressure to prevent leakage of the fluid. The nurse records the time of initiation and termination of the infusion, as well as the type of fluid, the amount of fluid absorbed, the addition of any medications, the rate of low, and the patient's reaction to the treatment. Again it is wise to record the site of the infusion so that the injection sites can be changed for subsequent infusions.

GUIDE TO ASSESSING FLUID AND ELECTROLYTE STATUS

1. How old is the patient?

2. What is the patient's usual pattern of fluid intake and output?

3. Have there been any recent changes in this pattern? Has the patient been anorectic, for example, and not taking the usual amount of food and fluid? Has the patient had a lessened amount of urine output? an increased amount?

4. Has the patient had any loss or gain in weight recently? Can he tolerate food and/or fluids by mouth?

5. Does he have a health problem which could cause fluid and electrolyte imbalance? For example, has he been nauseated or vomiting, has he had diarrhea? Does he

have a kidney problem? a cardiac condition? Has he lost large amounts of fluid from any cause?

6. Is he taking any medication that could affect fluid and electrolyte balance?

7. Does he show signs or symptoms of dehydration? of fluid retention?

8. Do laboratory tests show findings indicative of fluid or electrolyte imbalance?

9. Has measurement of intake and output been ordered for this patient? If so, are the totals of intake and output normal for a 24-hour period?

10. Are there restrictions on the patient's fluid or electrolyte intake? Does he need help to plan a diet to meet these restrictions?

11. Is the patient receiving medications to supplement or replace electrolytes?

12. Have parenteral fluids been prescribed? If so, why have they been ordered? What are the nurse's responsibilities in their administration? Are there special precautions to be observed with any of these?

13. Have intravenous admixtures been ordered? How are they to be added?

14. What does this patient or his family need to know about maintaining or restoring his fluid and electrolyte balance?

GUIDE TO EVALUATING THE EFFECTIVENESS OF NURSING INTERVENTION

1. Is the patient taking adequate food and fluids to meet his fluid and electrolyte needs?

2. Is his urine output compatible with his fluid intake?

3. If there are restrictions on the patient's fluid or electrolyte intake, are these being observed?

4. If parenteral fluids have been prescribed, have they been given at the correct time? Have sterile precautions been observed in their administration? Is the infusion flowing at the proper rate?

5. Is his skin in good condition? his mouth?

6. Do the patient and his family have all the information they need to assist in maintaining or restoring his fluid and electrolyte balance?

STUDY SITUATION

Mr. R. Miller is admitted to a medical nursing unit of a large city hospital late one evening. His diagnosis was tentatively given as dehydration and emaciation. The physician has directed that the patient be given food and fluids as tolerated. He has ordered various laboratory tests. He has also ordered an intravenous infusion of 1000 ml. of 5 per cent dextrose in normal saline to be started at midnight and to be run at 80 drops per minute. Mr. Miller is 70 years old and is on Social Security. He has no family and lives alone in a rooming house, where he cooks on a small hot plate. A friend accompanied him to the hospital. Mr. Miller is very thin and says he has not eaten well in many months. He appears frightened; this is his first admission to a hospital.

1. What is dehydration?

2. What subjective and objective observations might you anticipate? Why?

3. How long can you expect this patient's intravenous infusion to run?

4. What factors should be taken into consideration in explaining the intravenous infusion to this patient?

5. What observations should you make regarding his intravenous infusion?

6. Outline a nursing care plan for this patient.

7. How can you evaluate the results of your planned nursing interventions for this patient?

SUGGESTED READINGS

Aspinall, M. J.: A Simplified Guide to Managing Patients with Hyponatremia. *Nursing '78*, 8(12):32–35, December, 1978.

Felver, L.: Understanding the Electrolyte Maze. *American Journal of Nursing*, 80(9):1591–1595, September, 1980.

Freshwater, M. F.: "Dutch Boy" Technique Helps During I.V. Insertion. *RN*, 39:7, March, 1976.

Grant, M. M., et al.: Assessing a Patient's Hydration Status. *American Journal of Nursing*, 75:1306–1311, August, 1975.

Managing I.V. Therapy. Nursing Photobook Series. Horsham, Pennsylvania, Intermed Communications Inc., 1979.

Monitoring Fluid and Electrolytes Precisely. Nursing Skillbook Series. Horsham, Pennsylvania, Intermed Communications, Inc., 1978.

Reed, G. M., and Sheppard, V. F.: *Regulation of Fluid and Electrolyte Balance.* 2nd edition. Philadelphia, W. B. Saunders Company, 1977.

REFERENCES

1. Falconer, M. W., et al.: *The Drug, the Nurse, the Patient.* 6th ed. Philadelphia, W. B. Saunders Company, 1978.
2. MacBryde, C. M., and Backlow, R. S. (eds.): *Signs and Symptoms: Applied Pathologic Physiology and Clinical Interpretation.* 5th ed. Philadelphia, J. B. Lippincott Company, 1970.
3. Metheny, N. M., and Snively, W. D., Jr.: *Nurses' Handbook of Fluid Balance.* 2nd ed. Philadelphia, J. B. Lippincott Company, 1974.

18

The Nurse Should Be Able to:

- Elaborate on the statement, "Oxygen is essential to life"
- Describe the physiology of respiration including the five basic processes involved
- Discuss factors that may interfere with the normal functioning of these processes
- Discuss variations in oxygen needs throughout the life cycle
- Assess a patient's respiratory functioning status
- Identify common problems
- Identify signs of impending respiratory failure in a person and take appropriate action
- Apply relevant principles in the planning and implementation of nursing interventions to:
   1. Maintain patency of the patient's airway
   2. Increase ventilatory efficiency
   3. Ensure adequate oxygen intake
   4. Decrease bodily needs for oxygen
   5. Minimize the patient's anxiety
- Evaluate the effectiveness of nursing intervention

OXYGEN NEEDS

CHAPTER 18

INTRODUCTION

Oxygen is essential to life. All cells in the body require it, some being more sensitive to a lack of oxygen than others. Nerve cells are particularly vulnerable; a few minutes of severe oxygen deprivation may cause irreversible damage to brain cells. Longer periods of even less severe deprivation can lead to death, or to permanent damage of brain tissues.

Normally, oxygen is taken into the body through the air we breathe. It is carried to the cells by the blood, which also returns the waste material, carbon dioxide, to the lungs for disposal in the expired air. The term *respiration* is used to describe the exchange of oxygen and carbon dioxide between the atmosphere and the cells of the body. Two major systems are involved in the process—the pulmonary system and the cardiovascular system. Problems in either system or insufficient oxygen in the atmosphere can interfere with satisfaction of the very basic need for oxygen.

A person whose oxygen needs are being met adequately is not normally aware of the process of respiration. Respiration can, however, be altered voluntarily. Eating and drinking, for example, may involve voluntary changes in the breathing pattern. Similarly, speaking and singing require a certain amount of control over respiration. Some people develop considerable skill in adjusting their breathing patterns to produce specific effects with the voice. Singers and actors are usually particularly adept at this. Under normal circumstances, however, most people are not aware of the regular pattern of breathing in and breathing out, which occurs rhythmically 12 to 18 times per minute in the normal adult.

When a person has difficulty in meeting his oxygen needs, he usually becomes acutely aware of his respirations and attempts to control their rate and depth. He also becomes very anxious. The inability to obtain oxygen and to control a function that is essential to life can be terrifying.

Prompt attention to the patient's needs is imperative, not only because of the vital role of oxygen in sustaining life, but also because the anxiety induced by difficulty in breathing can in itself affect a person's respirations and further aggravate the situation. The competence of the nurse in knowing what to do in the situation and in helping the patient to feel that he has some control over the situation are important supportive measures in caring for the patient who is having difficulty meeting his oxygen needs.

THE PHYSIOLOGY OF RESPIRATION

The physiology of respiration can be divided into five logical sections:

1. The provision of oxygen from the atmosphere
2. The mechanisms that regulate the respiratory process
3. The passage of air from the atmosphere to the alveoli of the lungs and from the alveoli to the atmosphere
4. The diffusion of oxygen and carbon dioxide between the alveoli and the blood and between the blood and the tissue cells
5. The transportation of oxygen to the cells and carbon dioxide away from the cells by the blood stream

1. Basic to the respiratory process is the availability of oxygen. Normally, the atmosphere supplies all the oxygen an individual requires. The air at sea level contains approximately 20 per cent oxygen and 0.04 per cent carbon dioxide. These concentrations appear to be the most conducive for normal breathing.

2. A number of factors regulate the respiratory process. The principal mechanism of control is the *respiratory center* located in the medulla. The respiratory center contains both inspiratory and expiratory centers. Generally speaking, these operate as an "alternating circuit" type of

mechanism; when one is active, the other is inactive.

Impulses from a number of specialized receptors in the body are transmitted to the respiratory center to effect changes in respiration. The well-known Hering-Breuer reflex is initiated by impulses from *stretch receptors* located principally in the visceral pleura around the lungs. At a specific point in inspiration, these receptors transmit impulses to the respiratory center, which promptly inhibits inspiration and triggers the expiratory phase of respiration. The reverse takes place during expiration. Chemical receptors in the respiratory center, aorta, and carotid sinuses are called *chemoreceptors*. These receptors are sensitive to changes in the chemical composition of blood and tissue fluid. A lowered concentration of oxygen, a higher concentration of carbon dioxide, a lowered blood pH (increased acidity), and an elevation in blood temperature will all stimulate increased respirations. An alteration in the arterial blood pressure affects *pressoreceptors* in the aorta and carotid sinuses, and these receptors then transmit impulses to the respiratory center. A sudden rise in arterial blood pressure inhibits respirations. Respiration may also be affected by impulses arising from *proprioceptors* located in the muscles and tendons of movable joints. These receptors are stimulated by movements of the body. Active exercise is a powerful stimulant to respiration, as you will know if you have recently joined a physical fitness class, started jogging or running, or for that matter, if you engage in any type of active exercise.

Emotions also have an effect on the character of respirations. Anxiety, for example, can cause a prolonged state of respiratory stimulation. Pain, fear, and anger usually cause an increase in the rate and depth of respirations. Exercise and emotional upsets both increase cardiac output, thereby causing an increased production of carbon dioxide. With the CO_2 level in the blood raised, the respiratory center is stimulated.

With exercise, cellular metabolism is also speeded up, with a resultant buildup of metabolic waste products, including lactic acid and carbonic acid. The latter disintegrates into carbon dioxide and water and becomes another factor contributing to the increased respiratory rate of a person who is engaged in active exercise.

3. The passage of air from the atmosphere to the alveoli of the lungs, the exchange of gases there, and the subsequent return of air to the atmosphere are collectively referred to as *ventilation*. During ventilation, the air passes through the nasal passages, pharynx, larynx, trachea, bronchi, and bronchioles to the alveoli and then back. In its passage to the lungs the air is humidified, cleansed of foreign materials, and warmed. The respiratory tract is lined with mucous membrane, part of which contains cilia and excretes mucus to trap organisms and other foreign material.

4. Once oxygen enters the alveoli of the lungs, it passes into the blood as a result of the difference in the pressures of the gases on either side of the alveolar membrane. Since the partial pressure of oxygen in the inspired air is higher than the pressure of the oxygen in the venous blood, the oxygen passes from the area of higher pressure to the area of lower pressure. The same principle holds for the passage of carbon dioxide from the blood to the alveoli.

5. Once the oxygen enters the blood, it combines with hemoglobin to form oxyhemoglobin and is carried by the arteries to the capillaries throughout the body. From there it is transported via the interstitial fluid to the tissue cells, again because of the difference in the pressures. It is apparent that the delivery of oxygen to the cells depends on the hemoglobin level in the blood plasma and the adequacy of the blood circulation.

FACTORS AFFECTING RESPIRATORY FUNCTIONING

It would seem logical to discuss the factors that affect respiratory functioning in relation to the same five headings we used in the previous section, that is, those factors that affect each of the five components of the physiological process of respiration.

Availability of Oxygen

A decrease in the availability of oxygen from the atmosphere can cause serious respiratory problems. The term "ambient anoxia" is used to describe this condition. At high altitudes, where the pressure of oxygen in the air is low, a person will experience considerable difficulty in breathing until he becomes acclimatized to the rarefied atmosphere. Once he is acclimatized, his breathing rate may be seven times as fast as at sea level in order to provide him with sufficient oxygen.

The presence of noxious gases in the air will displace the oxygen normally present and lessen the amount available for respiration. In most fires, for instance, suffocation from smoke is usually as great a hazard as bodily injury from

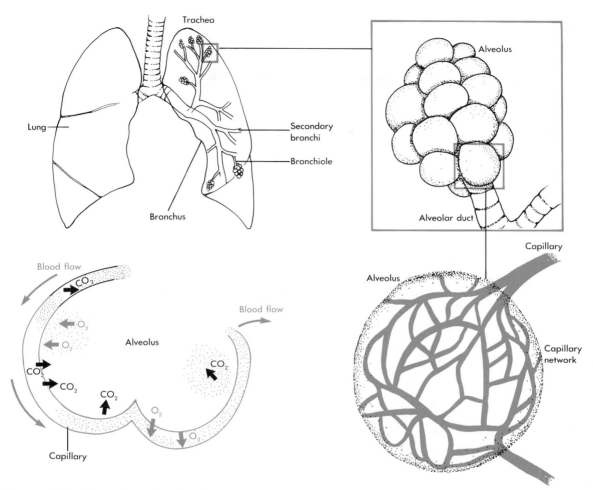

Oxygen (O_2) diffuses from the alveolus into the capillary, while carbon dioxide (CO_2) diffuses from the capillary into the alveolus.

the flames. In heavily industrialized areas, a combination of gaseous wastes from industrial plants and the exhaust fumes from automobiles may pollute the atmosphere to a level that it is dangerous to health. Many cities now have a pollution monitoring system. When the pollution level reaches a point that is considered dangerous, industries in the area may be restricted in their operations until the pollution level is relatively safe again.

Control Mechanisms for Breathing

Respiratory problems may also be caused by anything that interferes with the control mechanisms for breathing. A number of different factors may depress or totally inactivate the respiratory center in the medulla. Depressed respirations almost invariably accompany a

head injury and are believed to be due to cerebral edema. The edema causes increased pressure within the cranial cavity, which depresses the activity of the respiratory center. Drugs and anesthetics that act as depressants on the central nervous system will also depress respirations and may, when administered in large dosages, cause respiratory arrest. Morphine is usually cited as an example of a drug that depresses respirations, although any central nervous system depressant will decrease respirations as well as depress other parts of the central nervous system.

As discussed earlier in the section on the physiology of respiration, the respiratory center is sensitive to chemical stimuli resulting from changes in the composition of blood or tissue fluids. If a person faints, or voluntarily holds his breath until he faints, the accumulation of carbon dioxide in the blood quickly triggers the mechanism for inspiration and the patient automatically begins to breathe again. A lessened quantity of oxygen in the blood acts more slowly than an increased amount of carbon dioxide as a respiratory stimulant. This is because the blood normally carries an amount of oxygen greater than that which is needed for immediate use. It takes a longer period of time for the body to feel the need for more oxygen and to respond to the oxygen lack. Increased acidity of the blood (a lowered pH) will increase both the rate and depth of respirations as the body attempts to "blow off" acid through the expired carbon dioxide. In patients with a fever, the accelerated rate of metabolism caused by the higher than normal body temperature leads to an increase in the amount of end products of metabolism, which are acid in character. The respiratory response is an increase in the rate and depth of respirations.

Ventilation

The passage of oxygen from the atmosphere to the alveoli and the passage of carbon dioxide from the alveoli to the air require an unobstructed airway. Anything that interferes with the patency of any part of the respiratory tract can interfere with the efficiency of respirations. Normally the cough is a mechanism by which the respiratory tract is cleared of foreign materials. Obstructions in the pharynx, larynx, trachea, and bronchi can stimulate the cough reflex.

Some patients have difficulty in clearing mucus from the bronchial tree, perhaps because it is painful to cough, because of lack of strength, or because of unconsciousness. At any rate, fluids can accumulate and require nursing intervention for their removal. Continual bed rest and maintaining a prone or supine position can contribute to this difficulty by limiting chest expansion and alveolar ventilation. Also, certain drugs and diseases of the nervous system interfere with muscle control and the normal methods of clearing the respiratory system. The principle muscles concerned with respiration are the muscles of the chest wall and the diaphragm. These include the internal and external intercostals, the sternocleidomastoid, the scalenes, the thoracohumeral, and the thorascapular muscles. In addition, in forced breathing, the abdominal muscles may be brought into use. Trauma to any of these muscles, as may result from accidental injury or from surgery, will impair respiration. Similarly, any disease process that weakens or paralyzes these muscles (such as poliomyelitis) will affect the individual's ability to breathe normally.

Diffusion of Oxygen and Carbon Dioxide

Under certain circumstances, oxygen and carbon dioxide are impeded from crossing through membranes of the alveoli, the capillaries, or red blood cells. This impediment is referred to as "alveolocapillary block." For example, the distance the gases have to travel may be increased owing to pulmonary edema or inflammation. The successful exchange of gases depends on the efficient functioning of the two major pump systems in the body, the lungs and the heart.

Any malfunctioning of the lungs or the muscles of respiration because of injury or disease will interfere with the transfer of oxygen and carbon dioxide. For example, conditions that disturb the balance of the partial pressures of these gases can result from disturbed passage through the airway, such as occurs in asthma, in which expired air is obstructed in the bronchioles. In addition, any decrease in the elasticity of the lung tissue can impair respiration. For example, in emphysema (a condition common among heavy smokers in which the alveoli are chronically distended) extra effort must be made to deflate the lungs because of the inelastic tissue.

Transport of Oxygen and Carbon Dioxide to and from Cells

A great many factors may affect the efficient functioning of the heart. In some conditions there may be inadequate force to pump the blood through the lungs, or there may be an impediment in the return flow of blood from the lungs to the heart, causing a slowing up (stasis) of blood in the small vessels that surround the alveoli. Such conditions will interfere with respiration by disturbing the balance of partial pressures of oxygen and carbon dioxide within the blood circulating through the lungs.

Similarly, any condition affecting the circulation of blood to the tissues can interfere with the transportation of oxygen from the lungs to the cells. This would include all types of heart disease and arterial or venous disorders, as well as blood dyscrasias. Since hemoglobin carries the oxygen in the blood stream, a reduction in the amount of hemoglobin, such as in anemia, lessens the amount of oxygen carried to the cells.

Among the major diseases affecting the cardiovascular system are those which cause the blood vessels to narrow and deteriorate. This results in inadequate oxygenation, and subsequent damage of tissues in vital organs, such as the heart, the brain, the kidneys, or other parts of the body. Most of the damage is caused by four major types of heart disease—atherosclerosis (hardening of the arteries), hypertension (high blood pressure), rheumatic heart disease, and congenital defects. These diseases may lead to congestive heart failure, myocardial infarction, and stroke.

OXYGEN NEEDS THROUGHOUT THE LIFE CYCLE

During pregnancy, the diaphragm is pushed upward as the fetus grows and the uterus expands in the abdominal cavity. The lungs of the mother are gradually squeezed as space in the chest cavity decreases. Pregnant women usually find that they are breathing more rapidly than usual and may experience dyspnea after mild exertion.

The infant in utero receives its needed oxygen from the mother, the supply being transferred from the mother's circulation to the placenta and, thence, via the umbilical cord to the fetus. In the fetus, blood flows through four channels that normally close after birth: (1) the umbilical arteries and veins, (2) the ductus venosus in the liver, (3) the foramen ovale, which lies in the atrial cardiac septum and (4) the ductus arteriosus, which connects the pulmonary artery with the descending aorta (pp. 376–377).

Although intermittent, shallow, and rapid respiratory movements have been observed in infants in utero, it is felt that these movements are due to electrical activity in the cortex—the fetus does not breathe through its lungs. Indeed, well-developed terminal air saccules are not present until about 38 weeks gestation, and the lungs, in any case, are partially (approximately 40 per cent) filled with fluid until birth. This fluid is a mixture of swallowed wastes and amniotic fluid. If, for any reason, the supply of oxygen from mother to fetus is cut off, there may be resultant brain damage to the child. This problem is most likely to develop during the late stages of labor. Two conditions that may result from fetal asphyxia (suffocation) are mental retardation and cerebral palsy. The latter is a persisting motor disorder that shows up before the age of 3 years and is characterized by uncoordinated motor functioning.

With the first breath of life, air replaces fluid in the infant's lungs. The newborn infant breathes only through his nose; hence, congestion in the nasal passages can create a major problem. The infant breathes much more rapidly than an adult, with 35 to 50 breaths per minute being the normal range. The rate remains high through the first months of life, slowing down

gradually to about 20 to 40 breaths per minute at 12 months. The higher rate is, of course, due to the smaller lung capacity. A normal full term infant has a total lung capacity of only 300 ml. and a tidal volume of 25 ml.

Some newborns develop acute respiratory distress (ARD). The distress may be caused by a hyaline membrane, which has been found on autopsy to line the alveoli, the alveolar ducts, and the bronchioles of some newborns who have died with ARD. The membrane prevents the exchange of oxygen and carbon dioxide across the alveolar wall. Sometimes, however, there is no known cause. Infants with hyaline membrane disease usually die within a few days after birth. Infants who develop the idiopathic type of respiratory distress may, however, survive. Premature infants, children of diabetic mothers, and infants delivered by cesarean section are more vulnerable to the respiratory distress syndrome than others.

Respiratory infections are a major cause of infant and childhood deaths. Newborns are usually immune, because of antibodies received from the mother, until they are about 3 months old. By the age of 6 months, however, virtually all infants have had at least one attack of acute respiratory disease. During the first 2 to 3 years of his life, a child usually has 8 to 9 respiratory infections per year, as he gradually builds up his active immunity to the organisms normally prevalent in his environment. Immunization (which confers passive immunity) to whooping cough is routinely started in infancy to protect the child from this disease, which used to cause many deaths in infancy and early childhood.

Infants continue to be obligatory nose breathers through the first year of life. Hence, nasal congestion presents problems, especially when the child is being fed.

During childhood the diameter of the upper respiratory tract is small, and obstruction caused by the accumulation of secretions from an infection, an allergy, or the inhalation of a foreign body can be disastrous. Peanuts are a particular hazard for preschool children.

With adolescence, there is a rapid increase in lung capacity as the chest expands. Boys show a greater increase than girls, the shoulders of the male becoming broader, and the chest cavity larger than those of his female counterpart. Although fewer teenagers are smoking cigarettes than formerly, a great many begin to smoke in their teens, thus endangering their future health.

The functional capacity of an individual's respiratory system gradually declines as he gets older. Adults who remain physically active, however, maintain higher aerobic capacities than do sedentary individuals. In most physical

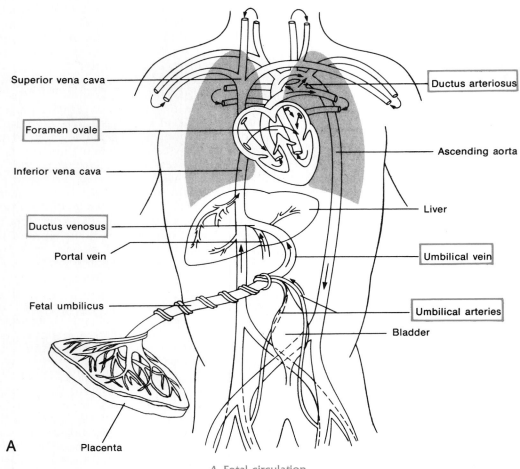

Superior vena cava

Ductus arteriosus

Foramen ovale

Ascending aorta

Inferior vena cava

Ductus venosus

Liver

Portal vein

Umbilical vein

Fetal umbilicus

Umbilical arteries

Bladder

A

Placenta

A, Fetal circulation.

Illustration continued on opposite page

fitness classes, emphasis is placed on aerobic exercises (such as running, jogging, and strenuous calisthenics), which are designed to improve cardiovascular and respiratory fitness (see Chapter 23).

Respiratory infections, in the form of colds, bronchitis, and pneumonia, continue to be a major cause of short-term illness throughout adulthood. Most people appear to be most resistant to these infections in the late middle years. It is at this time, however, that the chronic respiratory ailments become more prevalent. The term *chronic obstructive lung disease* (COLD) is used to refer to disorders of the respiratory tract such as emphysema, chronic bronchitis, and asthma.

In old age, a person's chest shrinks in size, and respiratory efficiency is reduced. Older people often notice that they have a little more difficulty breathing, particularly after exertion, than they did before. They are also, once again, more susceptible to respiratory infections. Mucous secretions tend to accumulate more readily in the older person. You will probably notice that older people seem to clear their throat a lot; they may need to cough and bring up sputum more often than younger adults.

ASSESSMENT

Subjective Data

One of the prominent indications of respiratory distress is the feeling of difficulty in breathing experienced by the patient. This is termed *dyspnea*.

Difficulty in breathing is a subjective symptom. It is, therefore, difficult to assess totally by objective observation, although it is sometimes necessary to do so. A person who is choking or unconscious is obviously not able to tell you about his respiratory problems. Nor are infants and small children able to communicate their distress in words. In these cases, the nurse has to rely on her powers of observation to detect difficulty the patient is experiencing.

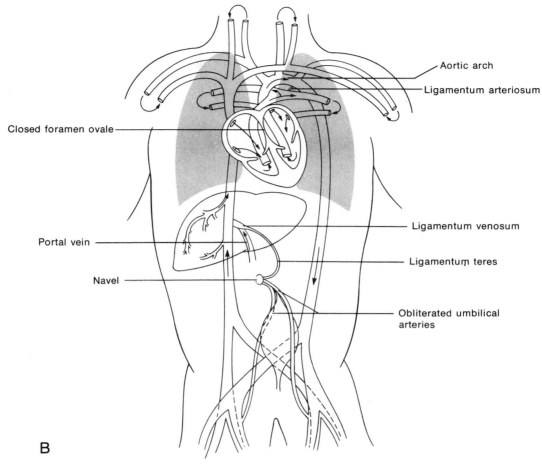

B, Neonatal circulation. Note the closure of the foramen ovale, the ductus venosus, the ductus arteriosus, and the umbilical vein and arteries after birth. (From Tackett, J. J. M., and Hunsberger, M.: *Family-Centered Care of Children and Adolescents.* Philadelphia, W. B. Saunders Company, 1981, pp. 530–531.)

As part of the nursing history, the nurse gathers information about any health problems the patient has and, in her initial clinical assessment, she observes the patient's respirations (see Chapter 9).

If the patient has indicated that he is having respiratory problems, or if the nurse has noted deviations from the normal breathing pattern when she was taking the vital signs, the matter should be pursued further. A good place to start is to find out how long the patient has had the problem, the nature and extent of the respiratory distress, and whether it is brought on or relieved by specific factors. It is also important to find out if the patient is currently taking any medications. If so, the name of the drugs and the dosage should be carefully noted on the patient's record, as part of the nurse's observations. It is also important to find out if the patient has been using any breathing aids at home, (or in another agency, if the patient has been transferred).

Many people with chronic respiratory problems use oxygen at home (portable units are available), and they often use humidifiers, nebulizers, and other aids as well. These, too, should be noted on the patient's record.

Specific problems the patient has identified should be investigated by further questioning. Common complaints include: dyspnea, fatigue, coughing, sneezing, wheezing, hiccuping, sighing, fainting, dizziness, and chest pain. Factors that precipitate the distress, and those that relieve it, should be noted.

People whose oxygen needs are not being met often complain of dyspnea on exertion. They may find it difficult to climb a flight of stairs or walk a block to the corner store without finding it hard to breathe. Often, the person finds it more difficult to breathe when he is lying flat (orthopnea). Asthmatic patients, those with chronic obstructive lung disorders, and those with heart conditions frequently use numerous pillows to raise themselves to a sitting position for more comfortable sleeping. The sitting position promotes maximum expansion of the chest and, also, prevents the pooling of blood in the large abdominal vessels. Excessive fatigue is commonly experienced, as even normal daily activities tire the patient out when he does not have enough oxygen to supply his body needs.

Coughing is the body's mechanism for ridding the respiratory tract of irritations and obstructions, which it does by means of an explosive expiration. Sneezing is a similar mechanism, but is confined to the nose. *Wheezing* (commonly noted in patients with COLD) indicates that air in the respiratory passages is passing through a narrowed lumen. *Hiccupping* (hiccoughing) is a spasmodic contraction of the diaphragm, which may be caused by irritation of the respiratory or digestive systems. *Sighing* involves a prolonged inspiration followed by a long expiration. In *yawning* there is a deep, long inspiration usually caused by mental or physical tiredness, although it may be due to a deficiency of oxygen in the atmosphere. Both sighing and yawning are mechanisms by which the body attempts to increase the amount of oxygen taken into the lungs.

Many patients with respiratory problems complain of pain in the chest. The pain may or may not be associated with the act of breathing. Pain may be caused by a number of different factors, such as inflammation, the presence of space-occupying lesions, or increased muscular activity as the patient works harder to breathe. The presence or absence of chest pain should be noted. A description of the pain (for example, sharp, dull, intermittent, or steady) should be reported, as should its location and its relationship to breathing.

Other pertinent information to gather from the patient includes his smoking history and his employment history. Smoking, as we have mentioned numerous times, is a frequent offender in the development of respiratory problems. If the patient is, or was, a smoker, pertinent information includes how long he has smoked, and how many cigarettes per day. With regard to employment history, many chronic respiratory problems have been traced to pollutants in the atmosphere of the work environment. Particularly at risk are miners (the process of drilling causes fine particles of metal and rock to pervade the atmosphere) and people who work with asbestos or chemicals.

Also to be considered are the patient's other health problems. You will remember that there are two major systems involved in respiration— the respiratory and the cardiovascular. Therefore, any heart or circulatory problems the patient has can interfere with his ability to meet his oxygen needs.

The patient's family history is also pertinent. Researchers are finding more and more evidence that the same health problems appear in successive family generations. The assumption is that there is a certain amount of genetic predisposition to problems in a specific body system. Therefore it is important to know of family members who have had allergies, asthma, chronic bronchitis, frequent bouts of pneumonia, or the like.

Objective Data

Observations should be directed and purposeful. They are based on the nurse's knowledge of the physiological mechanisms involved in respiration, her ability to identify deviations from the normal, and her understanding of the disease process affecting the patient.

Pertinent observations include an assessment of the character of the patient's respirations, his color, his behavior, and the presence of pain, cough, or sputum, as well as observations related to his general physical status.

In observing the character of the patient's respirations, the nurse should note the rate and rhythm of breathing. The normal rate for adults is 12 to 18 per minute, and normal breathing is silent and effortless. Labored breathing may be observed in the use of accessory muscles for inspiration or expiration and in the flaring of the nostrils on inspiration. Distention of the neck veins may also may be present. Difficult breathing is often accompanied by abnormal sounds. Wheezing, which we have already mentioned, is caused by a narrowed lumen. *Rhonchi*, a rattling in the throat or a dry coarse rale in the bronchial tubes, may be caused by a partial obstruction. A squeaky or grating sound may indicate a *friction rub*—caused by the rubbing together of irritated surfaces of the pleura—as in "dry" pleurisy (inflammation of the pleura). *Rales*, short bubbling sounds, are indicative of fluid in the respiratory tract. An obstruction of the upper airway may result in *laryngeal stridor*, a coarse, high-pitched sound that accompanies inspiration.

The nurse should also note the movements of the patient's chest on breathing. Normal respiration results in deep and even movements. Labored respirations may be persistently shallow, or there may be alterations in rhythm and depth. For example, in *Cheyne-Stokes breathing* there is a regular pattern of gradually decreasing depth to the respirations followed by a cycle of increasing depth. The pattern of inspiration and expiration may be varied also. Normally, the inspiratory phase is shorter than the time for expiration (1.0 to 1.5 seconds for inspiration, 2 to 3 seconds for the expiratory phase). Both are shorter, of course, in children. Often the expiratory phase is prolonged in people with chronic obstructive lung problems.

Air hunger is one of the symptoms associated with *hypoxia*, a condition in which there is a reduced oxygen content of the tissues. In air hunger the respiratory rate and the depth of respirations are markedly increased as the body attempts to obtain more oxygen to augment the depleted reserves in the tissues.

The patient's color is frequently an important indication of respiratory distress. *Cyanosis*, a bluish tinge in the skin and mucous membranes, is frequently associated with respiratory distress. Cyanosis may appear as a general duskiness of the skin surface, but more frequently it is observed as a bluish tinge in the lips, or around them (circumoral cyanosis), in the earlobes, under the tongue, and in the beds of the nails. It is not, however, considered a very reliable sign of respiratory distress, since its presence depends on a number of factors, including the tissue blood flow and volume, tissue oxygen uptake, the hemoglobin content of the blood, and skin color.

Cyanosis is not always present in respiratory insufficiency. There are some conditions in which an oxygen deficiency may cause the patient's skin to show an increased reddish tint. This may occur as a result of prolonged anoxia in which there has been damage to the kidneys. The damage may result in an excessive output of the substances that stimulate the production of red blood cells, with a resultant ruddy skin coloring.

When an obstruction occurs in the respiratory tract, coughing is usually stimulated. The cough is a protective mechanism of the body. To *expectorate* is to bring up mucus from the lungs. *Hemoptysis* is the expectoration of blood-streaked sputum. *Sputum* consists mostly of mucus that is brought up from the lungs. It usually also contains leukocytes, epithelial cells, secretions from the nasopharynx, bacteria, and dirt. Patients with respiratory diseases frequently expectorate sputum. Sputum should be observed for amount, color, consistency, odor, and the presence of foreign material such as blood or pus. The character of the sputum is often specific to the type of disease the patient has. People with emphysema, bronchitis, and other chronic obstructive disorders usually have a thick, tenacious sputum. The sputum from people with pulmonary edema is usually pink in color with an aerated, frothy appearance.

If the patient has a cough, the nurse's observations should include its frequency and time of occurrence, its relationship to activity (that is, if it is present on exertion or under some other condition), whether it is productive of sputum, and whether there are specific factors that induce cough or effectively relieve it. People suffering from oxygen lack are usually restless and they look anxious.

Because nervous tissue is very sensitive to oxygen deficiency, the patient with respiratory problems may show signs of impaired brain functioning. An early sign is faulty judgment, which may progress to confusion and disorientation. Safety precautions such as using side rails on the bed should be taken to protect the patient. Other signs that the brain is suffering from oxygen lack include headache, *vertigo* (dizziness), *syncope* (fainting), and drowsiness. The nurse should be alert for signs of mental confusion, drowsiness, or abnormal behavior in the patient. It is important to remember that these symptoms are reversible.

Additional observations the nurse may note are tachycardia and increased blood pressure, as the cardiovascular system attempts to keep up with the body's demands for oxygen. Because of the vital role of respiration in total body functioning, other systems may also be affected, and signs and symptoms indicative of their impaired functioning may be present. Because muscular activity, for example, demands increased oxygen consumption, the patient tires easily, particularly with any extra exertion.

Diagnostic Tests and Examinations

A complete assessment of the patient's respiratory functioning usually includes a total physical examination with particular focus on the lungs, various x-ray procedures, and laboratory tests. Sometimes, scans are done after radioactive isotopes are inhaled or injected. Another diagnostic tool is *thoracentesis*, or aspiration of fluid from the pleural cavity.

Nursing responsibilities with regard to diagnostic tests ordered for the patient include explaining the purpose of the test to the patient, giving him a description of the procedure, and telling him what is expected of him. Many anxieties and fears can be allayed by a simple explanation in nontechnical terms that the patient can understand. The nurse may also be asked to assist in carrying out these tests. She should know the purpose of the test and the significance of the results. The laboratory findings are important not only for assessing the patient's nursing problems, but also as an aid in evaluating the effectiveness of therapy.

Physical Examination of the Lungs. In the physical examination of the lungs, all of the basic methods of observation we discussed in Chapter 9 are used. A visual inspection of the chest is done to look for scars, abnormalities in the dimensions of the chest or the sternum, and abnormal chest movements. Scars may indicate that the person has had chest surgery or an injury, either of which could affect his respiratory functioning. Normally, the chest is smaller from front to back than it measures from one side of the body to the other. People with COLD often develop a *round* or a *barrel chest*; that is, the anterior-posterior dimension and the lateral dimension are approximately the same. Sometimes the sternum protrudes anteriorly, the so-called *pigeon chest*. This condition comes from a softening of the ribs, from rickets, or, sometimes, from emphysema. Sometimes, the softening of the ribs causes the lower part of the sternum to sink into the chest, however, giving the chest a funnel-like appearance *(funnel chest)*.

Palpation of the chest, using the palms of the hand and the fingertips, may be done to assess the inspiratory and expiratory movements of the lungs and, also, to check for *fremitus,* or vibrations that can be felt. Percussion is done to listen for abnormal sounds in the lungs. Normally, the lungs are resonant, emitting a hollow sound that is moderate to loud in intensity and low in pitch. A stethoscope is used to amplify the breath sounds in the airways and lungs and to listen for sounds in the pleural cavity. The examiner is listening for *adventitious sounds* (those not normally present), such as those we described earlier in the chapter, as well as for subtle variations in the normal sounds emanating from the respiratory tract.

X-ray and Other Procedures. The standard x-ray, the CAT scan, fluoroscopy, bronchography, and bronchoscopy are all means by which the lungs may be visualized. In fluoroscopy the chest movements can also be observed.

In *bronchography* an iodized oil is instilled into the bronchial tree as a contrast medium so that, when a chest x-ray is made, the structures of the lung are visualized.

Bronchoscopy is the examination of the bronchial tree with a lighted instrument. A local anesthetic is sprayed on the patient's pharynx and he is usually sedated before the examination. In preparation for bronchoscopy, the patient does not take food or fluids for at least 6 hours beforehand. If he wears dentures, they are removed before the examination.

Isotopic procedures may be done to assess lung functioning, or to detect abnormalities such as pulmonary embolus, tuberculosis, lung cancer, or COLD. Radioactive xenon (the compound ^{133}Xe) may be given as an inhalation in a test to measure the adequacy of ventilation of regions of the lungs, or it may be injected for a test to measure regional blood flow in the lungs. Radioactive iodine (^{131}I) may be given intravenously and a lung scan done to detect abnormalities in the lungs.

The *examination of sputum* is a common diagnostic test. Normally a sterile wide-mouth vial or Petri dish is used to collect the sputum. Sputum is best collected early in the morning, when there is more of it and it is most easily expectorated. The sputum should be coughed up from the lungs, not from the back of the throat. Sometimes a 24-hour specimen of sputum is ordered. If this is the case, the quantity is usually to be measured. The sputum should be collected in a graduated container. If an ungraded one is used, the nurse can put into the container a measured amount of saline solution. The specimen when collected can then be poured into a graduated container and the quantity of saline subtracted from the total to give an accurate estimate of the amount of sputum in the 24 hour period.

For *nose and throat cultures,* a sterile, cotton-tipped applicator is touched to the inside of the nose or throat and then returned to a sterile test tube. Separate swabs and containers are used for the nose and throat.

A hemoglobin test is important in assessing oxygenation of the blood. Another important laboratory test that is performed frequently is the measurement of *partial pressures of blood gases.* For this test, a sample of arterial blood is drawn and sent to the laboratory for analysis. The analyses of blood gases reflect the efficiency of ventilation and of the transport system for oxygen and carbon dioxide, and the rate of metabolism in the cells, as well as the state of the buffer systems. Normal values for Po_2 are 95 to 100 mm. Hg and for Pco_2 are 35 to 45 mm. Hg. The P stands for partial pressure—that is, the pressure of the gas dissolved in the blood. (The particular gas is only a part of the total volume of gases in the blood, hence the term "partial pressures.") It is important that the sample be taken to the laboratory immediately. The container is usually surrounded by ice to ensure that the gases remain in solution.

There are a number of *tests of pulmonary function* which may also be ordered for the patient. Among those that are commonly done are *maximum voluntary ventilation* (MVV) and *forced vital capacity* (FVC).

The measurement of maximum voluntary ventilation is a good indication of a person's ability to take air into his lungs. It measures the maximal amount of air a person can breathe in one minute. The normal for adult males is 125 to 150 liters per minute; for females, 100 liters per minute.

Forced vital capacity (often referred to simply as vital capacity) measures the volume of expired air which the patient exhales following deep inspiration. This test requires the expenditure of less effort on the patient's part and yields essentially the same information as the MVV. Sometimes the results are given as a ratio of vital capacity (VC) to maximum voluntary ventilation (MVV). A ratio below 75 per cent indicates obstruction in the airway.

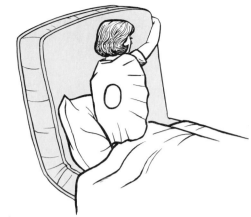

For thoracentesis, the patient assumes a sitting position with her arm across her chest in order to enlarge the intercostal spaces.

Thoracentesis. A thoracentesis is the aspiration of fluid from the pleural cavity. Normally there is just enough fluid present to lubricate the pleura so that the lungs can move freely. Pleural fluid is serous. The pleural cavity is a potential space which under normal conditions does not contain any fluid or air except the few milliliters of pleural fluid. The pressure in the pleural cavity is normally negative (-4 mm. of mercury), and because of this the lungs are kept from collapsing.

A thoracentesis may be indicated for either diagnostic or therapeutic purposes. In a diagnostic thoracentesis, a specimen of pleural fluid is obtained in order to identify an infecting microorganism or the presence of abnormal cells. Therapeutically, a thoracentesis is performed to remove fluid that is causing pressure upon the chest organs or to remove air that is inhibiting respirations.

If the patient has not had a thoracentesis previously, he will need an explanation of the procedure beforehand. The patient usually assumes a sitting position so that the fluid collects at the bottom of the pleural cavity. He places his arm over his head or in front of his chest in order to extend the intercostal spaces. The patient is warned not to cough or to move suddenly during the procedure because of the danger of the needle's becoming dislodged and piercing his lungs.

The equipment that is required for a thoracentesis consists of an aspirating set, an airtight drainage bottle, tubing, suction machine or pump in order to obtain a negative pressure within the drainage bottle, local anesthetic, syringe, sterile gloves, mask, and discard basin. Before the doctor begins the thoracentesis, the nurse establishes negative pressure in the drainage bottle in order to draw the fluid from the pleural cavity. Because there is some negative pressure within the pleural cavity, it is necessary to have greater negative pressure in the drainage bottle before fluid can be drained. It is also essential to prevent air from getting into the pleural cavity because it produces pneumothorax (the accumulation of gas or air in the pleural cavity), which causes collapse of the lungs. The thoracentesis needle has an attachable stopcock which can be opened and shut in order to prevent air from getting into the pleural cavity. A syringe can be attached to the stopcock to obtain fluid for laboratory examination.

After the patient assumes a sitting position and is draped comfortably, the physician wipes the area of insertion with disinfectant. The thoracentesis is done below the surface level of the fluid, often in the frontal plane in line with the crest of the ilium. The doctor determines the level of the fluid by percussion. The area is anesthetized locally and then the long thoracentesis needle is inserted through the intercostal space into the pleural cavity. The tubing is connected to the stopcock and to the source of negative pressure, and upon a signal from the doctor the valves are opened to let the fluid flow into the drainage bottle.

During the procedure the nurse watches the patient carefully for any signs of respiratory distress—for example, cyanosis or dyspnea. If the fluid is removed quickly the patient may faint. Puncturing a blood vessel with the needle is a complication that can result in a lung hemorrhage.

After the needle is withdrawn, pressure is applied over the site, collodion is often used to seal the skin over the puncture wound, and a sterile dressing is applied. The patient is observed frequently for several hours after the thoracentesis for any signs of respiratory embarrassment or shock. Damage to the lungs may be indicated by the presence of frothy, blood-tinged sputum (hemoptysis), by excessive coughing, or by difficulty in breathing.

The nurse records on the patient's chart the time; treatment; name of the doctor; amount, color, and consistency of the fluid obtained; and the condition of the patient. If the thoracentesis is successful therapeutically, the patient will probably find breathing easier because the fluid is no longer present to exert pressure upon his lungs.

COMMON PROBLEMS

In discussing pertinent subjective and objective data to be gathered, we have already noted many of the common problems with which the nurse can help people who are having trouble meeting their oxygen needs. In summary, these problems include:

1. Dypsnea, which may be due to a number of causes, the principal ones being an obstructed airway; inadequate ventilation of the lungs; an inadequate supply of oxygen in the atmosphere; impaired circulatory efficiency; increased demands of the body for oxygen; pressure on, or trauma to, the respiratory center in the medulla; and anxiety (or strong emotion of any kind).

2. Coughing, which may be due to irritation of the respiratory tract, increased secretions, or foreign bodies in the tract.

3. Sputum, which may be due to increased amount of secretions (often the result of an inflammatory process) or a slowing down or stasis of blood in lungs.

4. Fatigue and muscle weakness due to inadequate oxygenation of muscle tissue.

5. Vertigo, fainting, or disturbances in thought processes due to inadequate oxygenation of the brain.

6. Chest pain, which may or may not be related to breathing and may be caused by such factors as inflammation, pressure from tumors, increased muscular activity in breathing, or trauma.

PRIORITIES FOR NURSING ACTION

Difficulty in breathing is a distressing symptom. It always requires immediate attention by nursing and medical personnel. Early and prompt intervention can often minimize attacks and prevent the need for radical measures. The nurse should therefore observe the patient closely for any changes in his condition that

PRINCIPLES RELEVANT TO OXYGEN NEEDS

1. Oxygen is essential to life.
2. A person can survive only a few minutes without oxygen.
3. An insufficient supply of oxygen impairs functioning of all body systems.
4. Irreparable brain damage may result from prolonged periods of inadequate oxygen.
5. Cells of the cerebral cortex begin to die as soon as they are deprived of oxygen.
6. Air at sea level containing approximately 20 per cent oxygen and 0.04 per cent carbon dioxide is normally adequate to meet man's oxygen needs.
7. Carbon dioxide concentrations between 3 and 10 per cent increase the rate and depth of respirations.
8. The body's ability to meet its oxygen needs depends on the adequacy of functioning of the cardiovascular and the respiratory systems.
9. A patent airway is essential to normal respiratory functioning.
10. The respiratory tract is lined with mucus-secreting epithelium.
11. Coughing, swallowing, and sneezing are mechanisms by which the body attempts to rid itself of foreign materials in the respiratory tract.
12. Difficulty in breathing provokes anxiety.

indicate increasing difficulty with respiration. These should be reported immediately, and appropriate measures instituted. Severe distress in breathing is a medical emergency. Signs of impending respiratory failure include rapid, shallow breathing; rapid, thready pulse; fear and apprehension; restlessness; and confusion. Restlessness often occurs early and is an important sign to watch for in patients. Cyanosis may or may not be present.

If respiratory failure seems imminent, the nurse should make certain that the patient's airway is clear; institute ventilation by mechanical means; and obtain assistance. Measures for the resuscitation of patients with respiratory failure are detailed in a later section.

GOALS FOR NURSING ACTION

Principal goals of nursing action in the care of patients who are having difficulty in breathing include the following:

1. Maintaining the patency of the airway
2. Increasing ventilatory efficiency
3. Ensuring that the patient has an adequate supply of oxygen
4. Decreasing the demands of the body for oxygen
5. Minimizing the patient's anxiety

SPECIFIC NURSING INTERVENTIONS

Measures to Maintain a Patent Airway

A patent airway is essential to adequate respiration. Suctioning, positioning, and coughing are measures used to maintain the patency of the air passages. Suctioning is done to clear mucus and other secretions from the upper airway. One of the surest indications of partial blockage of air passages by mucus (or other secretions) is the sound of "wet breathing." As the air passes through the secretions it creates a typical gurgling sound. The frequency with which a patient needs suctioning is variable, but if the patient tends to accumulate fluids, a suction catheter should always be nearby for immediate use. The procedure for throat suctioning is described later in this chapter.

For the conscious patient, medications in the form of nose drops or aerosol sprays may be used to help liquefy secretions and facilitate their removal from the air passages.

Body position also effects patency of the airway. The unconscious patient should be placed in a semiprone position (Sim's position) without a pillow for his head and with the mandible extended forward and up. This position prevents the tongue from falling back and permits the drainage of fluids from the mouth. For the conscious patient, Fowler's position allows maximum chest expansion and helps to make the expectoration of sputum easier. Helping the patient to change his position frequently while he is in bed permits expansion of all areas of the lungs and helps to promote the drainage of secretions. When a patient is lying on his left side, he is not able to expand his left lung to its maximum capacity.

Coughing is an important means by which a person clears his respiratory tract of secretions and foreign material. For the patient who finds it painful to cough, the pain will be eased if the nurse supports the painful area, such as an operative incision, firmly while he coughs. The patient can accomplish the same purpose by holding a small pillow firmly over the painful area, unless he is unable to do so. A folded bath towel inside a pillow case makes an effective "splint pillow" for this purpose.

Artificial Airways. An artificial airway is inserted into a patient's throat in order to keep his tongue forward and the airway patent. Artificial airways are usually made of plastic or rubber. There are long and short airways for deep and shallow intubation. In deep intubation the airway extends through the pharynx into the trachea. This type of airway is usually inserted by a doctor. In shallow intubation the airway extends behind the tongue and terminates in the pharynx. This type of airway is often inserted by the nurse.

In shallow intubation the patient's tongue is brought forward and the airway is placed in his mouth with the base of the curve against his tongue. The airway is then turned so that the base of the curve is against the soft palate. It is then in position in the pharynx.

The insertion of a shallow airway.

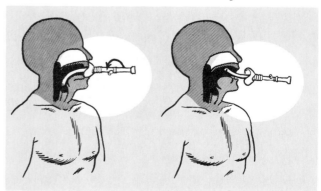

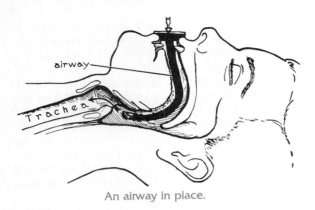

An airway in place.

If there is serious obstruction in the upper airway (nose, mouth, or throat), an artificial opening may be made into the patient's trachea (a tracheotomy) and a tube inserted to facilitate breathing. This procedure may be done when there has been injury that impedes the passage of air in the upper airway, for example, or a tumor blocking the passage.

Throat Suctioning. Oxygen reaches the alveoli of the lungs by passing through the mouth, the nose, the pharynx, the larynx, and the bronchi and bronchioles. A patent airway is essential to the passage of air through this route. The purpose of throat suctioning is to help a patient clear his airway by removing secretions and foreign materials from his nose, mouth, and pharynx. In most instances, the patient needs an explanation of the procedure. He can be reassured that this is a painless measure that will relieve his breathing so that he will be more comfortable. If the patient can cough while the suction is applied, it will facilitate the removal of mucus.

The equipment required includes a throat suction, a container for cold water, and a clean catheter. In hospitals, catheters are sterilized after each use. The catheter has a narrow lumen with a fine tip and several openings along the sides. The openings prevent irritation of the mucous membrane in any one area by distributing the negative pressure of the suction over several areas. Whenever there is any indication that a person might require emergency suctioning, this equipment is kept nearby.

The respiratory tract is lined with mucous membrane, which can easily be injured by mechanical means; therefore the catheter is never forced against an obstruction. Normally the catheter is inserted by the nurse as far as the pharynx for suctioning; deeper suctioning is generally a physician's procedure.

The catheter is attached to the suction machine and then lubricated with water. Water is drawn through the catheter in order to ensure the patency of the lumen. The patient assumes a position with his head turned to one side, facing the nurse. In this position his tongue falls forward and does not obstruct the entry of the catheter. The catheter is then gently inserted through the nose or mouth into the pharynx, rotated gently and withdrawn. Suctioning is begun when the catheter is in place. This procedure is repeated until the airway is clear. If the patient coughs while the catheter is in place, it helps to remove the mucous accumulations and foreign materials.

A Y tube is sometimes used with suction equipment. One stem of the Y is closed off with a finger to apply suction through the catheter. When this stem is left open, the suction is stopped in the catheter. This method does away with the repeated insertion and removal of the catheter, and thus minimizes trauma to the mucous membranes of the air passages.

Measures to Increase Ventilatory Efficiency

The principal factors that impede ventilation are obstruction of the airway and inadequate expansion of the chest. Measures to ensure patency of the airway, as just discussed, are therefore essential to increasing ventilatory efficiency.

Measures that assist in optimal expansion of the chest include positioning of the patient (as already noted) and the alleviation of pain or discomfort associated with breathing. The chest is sometimes splinted to relieve painful respirations, or the physician may leave orders for analgesics to be given. Usually these are given at the nurse's discretion. Coughing may also interfere with respirations. The administration

Suctioning a patient's throat to remove mucus that is obstructing the airway.

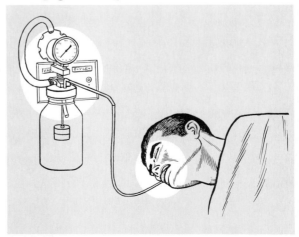

of cough mixtures will usually provide relief from this discomfort. Frequently cough mixtures are left at the patient's bedside to be taken as needed.

Deep breathing at frequent intervals should be encouraged. Exercise helps to improve ventilatory functioning, and active or passive exercise within the patient's level of tolerance should be promoted. Abdominal distention should be prevented by giving the patient small, frequent meals of easily digestible food. Foods that are gas-forming (see Chapter 14) should be avoided. The patient's garments should be loose-fitting, and bed coverings should not be tucked in tightly.

Postural Drainage. Postural drainage is done to facilitate the drainage of secretions from the respiratory tract to assist in maximum ventilation. The position of the patient for postural drainage depends on the areas of the lung to be drained. For drainage from the lower lobes, the patient assumes a position in which his chest is lower than his hips, so that gravity will assist the movement of the mucus. Several special postural drainage beds are now available. If a special bed is not available, one way of assuming this position is for the patient to lie in a prone position across the bed with the waist at the edge of the bed. The upper part of the body is supported by the arms, which rest on a chair at the side of the bed. A receptacle for sputum is put on the chair in front of the patient.

Another position assumed by hospital patients who require postural drainage is a prone position over the knee break of the bed. The patient lies facing the bottom of the bed so that his waist is at the knee break and his head and chest incline downward.

Postural drainage is carried out to drain sputum from the lungs and to obtain a specimen of sputum. For therapeutic purposes it is ordered by the physician, usually for 10 to 15 minutes, three to four times daily.

Percussion of the chest helps to dislodge mucus and is frequently done prior to the treatment. For more detailed instructions on techniques used in postural drainage, the student is referred to a medical-surgical nursing textbook.

Mechanical Ventilation of the Lungs. When an individual's own respiratory apparatus is not functioning normally, it is sometimes necessary to use mechanical aids to ventilate the lungs. Depending on the extent of respiratory dysfunction, either "assisted" or "controlled" ventilation may be used. "Assisted" ventilation is the term used to describe a mechanically generated airflow that is initiated by the patient's own efforts at inspiration and serves to increase his

inadequate breathing. In "controlled" ventilation, the airflow is delivered according to a preset cycling pattern that is not influenced by the patient's own breathing.

Basically, ventilators can be divided into two groups, those operating on the principle of negative pressure and those employing positive pressure. The negative-pressure machines generate a suction (negative pressure) on the outside of the chest. This creates within the thorax a pressure gradient with the atmosphere, so that air flows into the lungs. The positive-pressure ventilators, on the other hand, force air into the lungs by means of a power-driven source, thereby creating intrathoracic pressure (positive) that causes the lungs and chest to expand. A variety of ventilators are now available on the market. The Bird and Bennett respirators are examples of positive-pressure machines; the Emerson cuirass, which is a shieldlike appliance that fits over the body, is now more commonly used for negative pressure than the Drinker respirator (iron lung) used formerly.

Measures to Ensure Adequate Oxygen Intake

General measures to ensure an adequate supply of oxygen include the provision of fresh air. The patient's room should be kept well ventilated. Many patients with respiratory problems like to have the bed placed beside a window so that they can get fresh air. These patients are often particularly sensitive to alterations in the temperature and humidity of the environment. Atmospheric oxygen may need to be supplemented by inhalation aids, such as oxygen tents, oxygen masks, nasal cannulae, and nasal catheters. The use of these aids is discussed later in this chapter.

Inhalation Therapy
Humidity Therapy. The provision of air that has a high water content is a form of therapy that has been used for people with respiratory problems for many generations. Traditionally this has taken the form of steam inhalations, but there are now many techniques available to provide a high humidity environment for those who require this form of therapy. The purpose of humidity therapy is to provide extra moisture to the mucous membranes lining the respiratory tract. The moisture helps to soothe irritated mucous membranes, and also helps to dilute thick secretions and to loosen the crusts that frequently form on the mucous membranes as a result of respiratory infection. The secretions and crusts can then be coughed up or aspirated more easily. The moisture may also be used as a vehicle for administering a medication directly

to the respiratory tract. In this case, the water vapor is passed over the medication from which it picks up molecules that are then inhaled with the vapor.

A high humidity environment may be established in oxygen tents, in specially constructed plastic hoods, and in entire rooms; however, the most common method of increasing the humidity in the atmosphere immediately surrounding the patient is by means of a humidifier (steam kettle). Many types of humidifiers are manufactured commercially, and both hot and cold humidifiers are available. In the home, a small commercially bought humidifier or an electric kettle may be used to supply steam. Whatever type of equipment is used in the home or in the hospital, most patients require some help with it.

The physician may order continuous *humidity therapy* (or steam inhalations), or he may order it for one-half hour every 4 hours (humidity therapy, ½ hour q4h).

Nursing care measures relevant to *humidity therapy* include:

1. Explaining the equipment to the patient and advising him to breathe in the water vapor (steam) deeply
2. Taking safety precautions to protect the patient from burns if heated humidity (hot steam inhalations) is used; the patient should be warned not to touch any of the equipment that may become hot, and the humidifier (kettle) should be kept well out of reach if the patient shows any signs of mental confusion
3. Arranging the humidifier so that the water vapor surrounds the patient's head
4. Preventing drafts, which could be chilling
5. Changing linen when it becomes damp
6. Encouraging the patient to expectorate mucus during the inhalations and providing him with a container for the sputum

Oxygen Inhalation Therapy.

It is necessary under some circumstances to provide the patient with a concentration of oxygen that is higher than that found in the air. The physician orders the method of administration of the oxygen, the concentration, and the length of time that the patient is to receive the oxygen. The latter factor is sometimes left to the nurse's judgment, the order simply stating "oxygen as necessary."

Oxygen is generally supplied in two ways, from tanks or from wall outlets (piped-in oxygen). Oxygen from the latter source is stored in a central storage area. Most newer hospitals employ the piped-in method of supply. In the home, oxygen is supplied in portable tanks.

Oxygen tanks are steel cylinders in which the oxygen is stored under a pressure of 2200 pounds per square inch at 70° F (21° C). There are different sizes of oxygen tanks: the larger ones store 244 cubic feet of oxygen; the smaller tanks store less oxygen but are readily portable. Each tank has a pressure reduction valve that enables the oxygen to be released at a pressure lower than that within the tank. An oxygen tank normally has two gauges: one indicates the amount of oxygen in the tank (the pressure) and the other indicates the amount of oxygen being released (in liters per minute).

The oxygen gauges are generally attached to the tank before it is brought to the patient. In most hospitals respiratory (inhalation) technologists usually supply and service the oxygen equipment. The following steps are followed in order to attach the gauges to the tank:

1. Open the cylinder valve slightly and then close it quickly to remove any dust in the outlet ("cracking the tank"; this produces a loud hissing sound, which can be frightening when not explained beforehand)
2. Connect the regulator valve to the cylinder outlet and tighten the nut with a wrench
3. Make sure that the liter flow valve is in the "off" position
4. Open the cylinder valve slowly until the pressure gauge registers the pressure in the cylinder
5. Adjust the liter flow valve to the desired rate of flow

There are a variety of liter flow indicators. The gauge type and the ball float type are two that are commonly seen.

Piped-in oxygen is usually under low pressure, between 50 and 60 pounds per square inch. Usually only a liter flow valve is needed. To attach the equipment for piped-in oxygen:

1. Make sure that the liter flow valve is in the "off" position
2. Attach the valve to the outlet—some valves are attached by a screw nut; others are inserted directly into the wall outlet

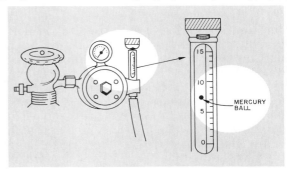

An attachment for an oxygen tank showing the pressure gauge and the liter flow gauge (mercury-ball type).

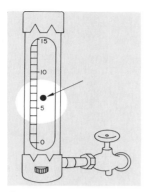

An attachment for an oxygen wall outlet with a mercury-ball liter flow gauge.

3. Slowly turn the liter flow valve to the desired liter flow

Fears and Precautions in the Use of Oxygen Equipment. When nursing a patient who is receiving oxygen inhalations, there are certain precautions, practices, and facts with which the nurse needs to be familiar. The administration of oxygen is often a frightening experience for the patient and his family. To many patients, it denotes a serious illness; a surprising number of patients remember a relative or a friend who died while receiving oxygen. Oxygen is essential to life and to have to depend upon equipment in order to live is in itself anxiety-producing. This is a situation over which the patient often has little control, and, because he is so completely dependent upon others even for the air he breathes, he feels helpless.

Such fears can often be allayed. Explanations about the oxygen equipment are geared to the patient's needs. Some people want to understand in great detail; others are satisfied with a simple explanation. If the patient is well enough to help with his therapy, the nurse can teach him to administer the oxygen himself and thus help him to feel that he has some control over the situation.

Some patients fear suffocation when using inhalation equipment; many dislike the feeling of having something cover their nose and mouth when a mask is used. Children in croupettes and patients in oxygen tents often feel isolated from their fellow patients. In addition, the necessity of depriving the patient of everyday pleasures such as the use of cigarettes, facial creams, and perfumes adds to his or her feelings of helplessness. Cigarettes are never permitted because a spark could readily start a fire in the presence of concentrated oxygen. Creams and perfumes with an alcohol base are not used because they can contribute to a fire.

When handling oxygen equipment the operator's hands should be free of oils and alcohol, which are highly flammable. Normally the use of electrical equipment around oxygen is restricted to appliances that have been checked and found safe—that is, appliances that will not spark or start a fire.

Lotions and liquids for the patient's use should have a water rather than oil or alcohol base. Special mouth care solutions and back rub lotions that are not flammable must be used in the presence of oxygen equipment.

Principles Relevant to the Administration of Oxygen. *Oxygen is a colorless, odorless, and tasteless gas that is essential to life.* Because oxygen can be neither seen, tasted, nor smelled, the equipment gauges are relied upon to indicate that oxygen is being supplied. The concentration of oxygen in a tent can be tested by an analyzer. The patient who is receiving oxygen is interrupted as little as possible in order to decrease oxygen loss and promote rest.

Oxygen dries and irritates mucous membranes. Most patients who are receiving oxygen require special mouth care in order to maintain good oral hygiene. The provision of fluids for the patient is also important; often the patient is dependent upon the nurse for the administration of fluids. Oxygen is always humidified before it is supplied to the patient.

Oxygen supports combustion. It is essential to the patient's safety that there be no smoking within 4 meters (13 feet) of oxygen equipment. This applies to patients and visitors and usually requires continual explanation and enforcement. Oxygen is not explosive, but a spark created in the presence of a high concentration of oxygen can ignite a fire quickly.

Methods of Administering Oxygen. There are four basic methods of administering oxygen: tent, nasal catheter, face mask, and nasal cannulae (nasal prongs).

The oxygen tent. Tents were at one time the most common method of administering oxygen. Today they are seldom used for adults except in instances in which the patient requires a high humidity environment in addition to supplemental oxygen. The tents are still used frequently with children; in this case they are referred to as *croupettes.*

Oxygen tents are usually made of a clear plastic material that does not permit the diffusion of oxygen or air through it. The motor unit of the tent is usually electrically driven; it circulates the air in the tent and cools it to the desired temperature.

The oxygen concentration in a tent can generally be kept between 50 and 60 per cent, although each time the tent is opened oxygen is lost. Oxygen analyzers are instruments which measure the concentration of oxygen inside the tent. These measurements should be done regularly—for example, every four hours.

A temperature between 68 and 70° F (20 to 21° C) in the tent is comfortable for most people. The ventilation fan can be set at a moderate speed in order to provide sufficient circulation of air. The minimum liter flow of oxygen for the tent is generally 8 liters per minute. However, some patients require a more rapid flow to meet their oxygen needs, whereas the flow should be limited to a maximum of 4 liters per minute for patients with emphysema.

To set up an oxygen tent, the following steps are performed:

1. Turn on the motor and set the liter flow to the desired level
2. Arrange the canopy over the patient's head so that most of the space in the tent is in front of the patient's face
3. Tuck the canopy under the mattress and secure the canopy over the patient's thighs with a drawsheet folded lengthwise and tucked in on each side of the bed
4. Flush the tent for 20 minutes to bring the concentration of oxygen up quickly to 50 per cent; warn the patient that this makes a hissing noise
5. Provide the patient with a mechanical bell for calling nursing personnel

Because oxygen supports combustion, precautions are taken to prevent fires. Patients do not smoke in an oxygen tent, nor are any electrical devices used inside the tent, such as electrically controlled signal lights, hearing aids, transistor radios, and electric shavers. "No smoking" signs should be placed on the door of the patient's room and visitors should be counseled not to smoke. The patient in the tent may feel cold because of the circulating air. The temperature can often be raised and extra covers provided.

Patients should be discouraged from plugging the oxygen outlet of the tent with towels in order to close off drafts.

Nursing measures for the patient in an oxygen tent are planned so that the tent is opened as infrequently as possible. Each time the tent is opened oxygen is lost, and the patient consequently receives less than the desired concentration of oxygen.

Patients in oxygen tents often feel isolated from fellow patients; however, they have the same needs to communicate and feel a part of a group. Tent motors today are usually so quiet that patients can hear reasonably well inside them. People can normally be heard by the patient if they speak distinctly.

The nasal catheter. Oxygen catheters are made of plastic and are disposable. They have a series of six or eight holes on the sides and are about 45.7 cm. (18 inches) long. A No. 14 French catheter is usually used for an adult patient. Because oxygen dries and irritates mucous membranes, the oxygen is passed through water (humidified) before it is administered by catheter.

The advantage of the administration of oxygen by catheter is the freedom of movement that it affords the patient. Patients receiving oxygen by this method can obtain about a 50 per cent concentration of oxygen. The minimum liter flow of oxygen by catheter is generally 6 to 7 liters per minute, except for the maximum limit of 4 liters per minute used in treating patients with emphysema.

The catheter is lubricated before insertion, preferably with water. An oil base lubricant is dangerous because it can be aspirated and subsequently irritate the lungs. The catheter is inserted to a distance about equal to the distance from the patient's nose to his earlobe. It is inserted until the tip is opposite the uvula in the oropharynx (seen through the mouth) and is

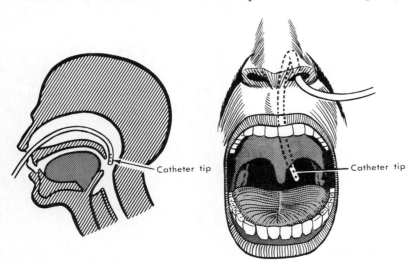

The position of the nasal catheter for oxygen administration. Note that the tip of catheter is opposite the uvula.

Catheter tip

Catheter tip

then taped in place as illustrated. It is never forced against an obstruction. In another technique of shallow insertion, a nasal catheter is inserted approximately 3 inches—that is, into the nasopharynx.

Oxygen catheters are removed every 8 hours, and a clean catheter is inserted into the other nostril. Patients receiving oxygen by catheter require special mouth and nose care. The catheters tend to irritate the mucous membranes, thereby stimulating secretions, which must be removed. Water base lubricants will soothe irritated nares.

The face mask. A variety of inhalation masks are available for use. The lightweight plastic mask that covers the patient's nose and mouth is used extensively today. It provides a concentration of oxygen of about 50 per cent with a minimum liter flow of 8 liters per minute. There are also several non-rebreathing masks in use that can provide an oxygen concentration as high as 95 per cent.

After the liter flow valve is turned on, the mask is applied to the patient's face. Oxygen masks come in different sizes; the mask selected should rest comfortably on the patient's face. Patients who are receiving oxygen by mask are assisted in taking fluids and performing hygienic measures to protect the skin and mucous membrane of the face and mouth from irritation.

Positive-pressure masks are used when oxygen is administered under pressure. These masks apply pressure on exhalation only. A variety of positive-pressure masks are available. With the meter mask, the concentration of oxygen is regulated by a dial on the flow meter. The rebreathing mask has a bag below the mask that permits the partial rebreathing of exhaled air along with the oxygen.

Nasal cannulae (nasal prongs). Nasal cannulae provide a convenient and comfortable method of administering oxygen. Usually made of a soft plastic material, they consist of two tubes approximately one-half inch in length that are fitted into the patient's nostrils and are held in place with a light elastic halter. A concentration of approximately 37 per cent oxygen in the alveolar air may be achieved with a flow rate of 5 liters per minute; a concentration of about 40 per cent is achieved with a flow rate of 8 liters per minute. Oxygen applied in this way is always humidified; the cannulae are changed frequently and nasal care is provided as needed.

Carbon Dioxide Inhalation. The administration of carbon dioxide is sometimes used to increase the rate and depth of respirations. It is also administered as a treatment for singultus (hiccups).

Carbon dioxide is usually supplied in cylin-

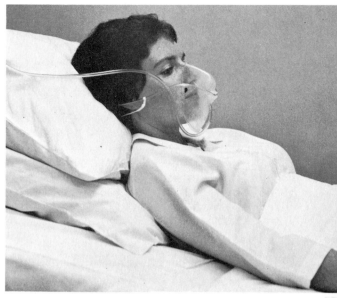
A plastic oxygen mask.

ders in combination with oxygen; this mixture is called carbogen. It is usually administered by mask as a 5 per cent concentration in 95 per cent oxygen. Today in many hospitals CO_2 is given by means of an Adler Rebreather, which eliminates the use of the heavy cylinders. The treatment is generally ordered by the physician for 10- to 15-minute periods several times a day, repeated no oftener than q1h.

In carrying out this treatment, the nurse alternates the application of the mask with periods of normal atmospheric breathing during the 10- to 15-minute intervals. That is, the nurse applies the mask for a few minutes, then removes it and lets the patient breathe without it for several respirations, then reapplies the mask. This procedure is repeated during the interval designated for the treatment.

In administering carbon dioxide, the nurse must watch for the signs and symptoms of CO_2

Oxygen nasal cannulae (nasal prongs).

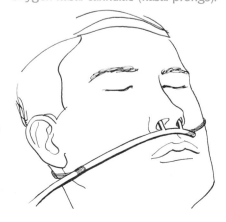

toxicity. At the first indication of vertigo, dyspnea, nausea, or disorientation, the treatment is stopped and the condition reported to the physician.

Aerosol Therapy.   Aerosol inhalation (nebulization) is a method by which a nonvolatile drug is inhaled into the respiratory tract. A stream of oxygen or compressed air is passed over a solution of the drug and picks up small particles to form a spray. The patient breathes in the spray deeply to force the tiny particles to travel deep into the respiratory tract. Different kinds of aerosols are marketed for use, some of which attach to a face mask that the patient wears during the treatment.

Most aerosol treatments are given by IPPB (intermittent positive-pressure breathing), but a similar spray can be formed by means of a hand atomizer for use in the home. When the bulb of the atomizer is squeezed, air passes over the medicine and picks up small particles to form the spray which the patient inhales. The particles formed by the hand atomizer are usually larger than the particles formed in a nebulizer.

When the physician orders aerosol inhalation, he also orders the type of drug to be administered, the quantity of the drug, and the frequency of the treatment. The liter flow of oxygen that is necessary for aerosol therapy is usually 6 to 8 liters per minute. The exact flow is determined by the density of the spray. A treatment usually lasts 15 to 20 minutes; more exactly, it lasts until all the medicine has been inhaled.

When intermittent aerosol therapy is ordered, the treatment is usually carried out by a respiratory technologist, but in some instances it may be a nursing responsibility. The nurse should then be familiar with the equipment and its use. The most commonly used machines for this type of therapy are the Bird and the Bennett respirators.

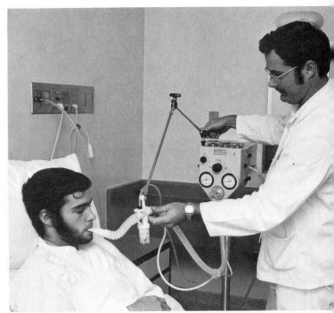

A patient receiving a treatment with a Bennett respirator. The respiratory technologist is assisting the patient.

Measures to Decrease Bodily Needs for Oxygen

The need for oxygen by the body is related to the rate of metabolism of the tissue cells. Factors affecting metabolic rate include physical activity, disease processes, and emotional reactions. Although a certain amount of activity is essential to promote optimum ventilation of the lungs, excessive activity should be avoided. The patient's level of tolerance must be carefully assessed and care taken that the patient does not overexert himself.

An elevated body temperature increases the basal metabolic rate and contributes to respiratory distress. Care should be taken then to prevent the patient from developing an infection, and measures taken to keep body temperatures within normal limits.

Emotional tension is also a factor to be considered in patients with respiratory problems. Anxiety, for example, may be mediated through the parasympathetic nervous system and result in constriction of the smooth muscles of the bronchioles. The expression of other emotions, such as fear, anger and grief, is also closely related to respiration. Strong emotions such as anger and fear initiate responses to prepare the body for action, and respirations become faster and deeper.

Measures to Minimize Anxiety

Anxiety almost invariably accompanies dyspnea. To be unable to breathe easily and normally is a frightening experience. The person with chronic respiratory problems may live in constant fear that his next breath may be his last one.

The patient's anxiety contributes to his respiratory problems, and a vicious circle may develop. The patient becomes dyspneic; his dyspnea produces anxiety; the anxiety results in more dyspnea. It is essential that this circle be broken.

Helping to establish the patient's confidence in the care he is receiving is an important factor in alleviating anxiety. Prompt attention to the patient's needs, such as answering his call-light immediately and attending to his wants without delay, can often prevent or minimize an attack of dyspnea. It is important in this regard to remember that anxiety is not always expressed openly. The patient may not necessarily say "I am frightened," but his actions convey this meaning to the astute and observant nurse. The patient may make a seemingly excessive number of requests, or attempt to keep the nurse engaged in conversation. The physical presence of someone competent who can help him if need be is reassuring to the patient.

Efficient handling of equipment and skillful execution of procedures contributes to the patient's feeling that he is in good hands. The

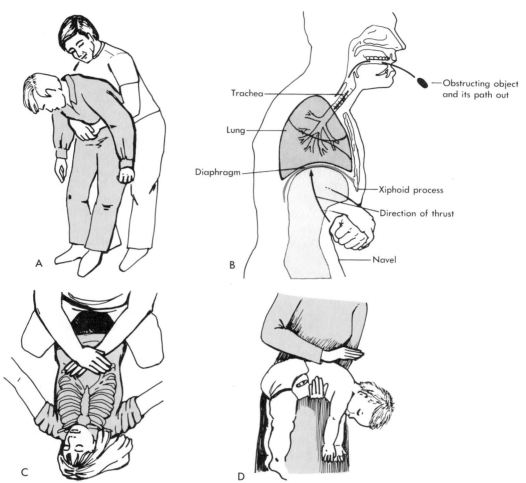

The Heimlich maneuver.

A, If the victim is upright, stand behind the victim and place both arms around his waist. Make a fist with one hand and place it against the victim's abdomen just above the navel, below the rib cage. Place your other hand over your fist and give a sharp quick upward thrust to the abdomen. The action is done by sharp flexion of the elbows, by a "bear hug," which compresses the rib cage.

B, The action has the effect of elevating the diaphragm. The sudden elevation of the diaphragm compresses the lungs and the air pressure ejects the food or other foreign object from the victim's windpipe.

C, If the victim has collapsed and you are unable to lift him, a variation of the maneuver can be done. With the victim lying on his back, you kneel astride his hips, facing him. With one of your hands on top of the other, place the heel of your bottom hand on the abdomen slightly above the navel and below the rib cage. Press into the victim's abdomen with a quick upward thrust. Repeat several times if necessary. If the victim vomits, quickly turn him to his side and wipe out his mouth to prevent aspiration.

D, When the victim is an infant or small child, have the child bend over or place him face down over your forearm, supporting his chest. With the heel of the other hand, give him four rapid slaps between the shoulder blades. For a child, if the obstruction remains, grasp him from behind and follow the instructions in part *A*.

nurse should be familiar with the equipment used in the care of patients with respiratory problems and should have confidence in her own ability to perform the necessary procedures.

Caring for the patient who has difficulty in breathing can be anxiety-provoking for the nurse. Knowing what measures to take and how to use equipment contributes to her feelings of confidence in giving care.

Measures to ensure the patient's comfort and improve his sense of well-being are also valuable adjuncts in the care of patients with respiratory problems. Good personal hygiene is important, and the patient who experiences dyspnea on exertion may need assistance from the nurse in this regard. Many patients with respiratory disorders are "mouth-breathers" and good oral hygiene is needed. Because of the drying effects of oxygen, patients who are on oxygen therapy require special mouth care to maintain hydration of the tissues in the oral cavity and prevent the development of infection or other complications.

Difficulty in breathing is often related to emotional problems. Distressing situations may provoke attacks of difficulty in breathing. The nurse should be alert to conditions that appear to precipitate such attacks and should report these to the physician.

Emergency Situations

Choking. Choking on food can be easily recognized. Victims are unable to speak or breathe. Their faces become pale, followed by a blue or purple discoloration, and the victim finally collapses. Death may occur in 4 to 5 minutes. A person who is choking will grasp at his throat, and this action will help to distinguish choking from other conditions with somewhat similar symptoms, such as heart attacks.

A first aid procedure called the *Heimlich maneuver* can save people who are choking. It can be done by any informed person and needs no special equipment. The procedure is shown on page 391.

In most cases, choking on food occurs during inspiration, which means that the piece of food is sucked in against the opening into the larynx; the lungs are partially expanded. If you suddenly push the diaphragm up, the lungs compress and push air up through the trachea, causing the object to "pop" out. If the object that is causing the choking is only partially dislodged but not expelled, you can shove a finger inside the victim's mouth to the base of his tongue and use a hooking action to move the object to the front of the mouth.

To Avoid Choking:

1. Cut food into small pieces; chew slowly and thoroughly
2. Avoid laughing and talking while chewing and swallowing
3. Avoid excessive intake of alcoholic beverages before and during meals
4. Do not allow children to walk, run, or play with food or foreign objects in their mouths
5. Keep foreign objects (such as marbles, beads, and thumbtacks) away from infants and small children

Artificial Respiration. Among the several methods of resuscitation for respiratory failure, the most widely used are: (1) the oral method (mouth-to-mouth or mouth-to-nose), (2) the revised Sylvester method, and (3) the self-inflating bag-mask method. The oral method is the simplest to use and is generally considered the most effective in first aid situations. It can be used by and with almost all age groups and in most situations. As an alternative method when physical, religious, or esthetic reasons preclude use of the oral method, the revised Sylvester method (Brosch modification) is internationally advocated for first aid situations when mechanical aids are not available. When the equipment is available (as, for example, in hospitals or first aid stations) the self-inflating bag-mask method is generally preferred.

Oral Method

1. Place the patient flat on his back if possible
2. Ensure an open airway—lift the patient's neck and press his forehead so that head is tilted backward; life the chin upward

AIRWAY CLOSED   AIRWAY OPEN
(HEAD HYPEREXTENDED)

3. Remove any foreign materal from mouth and throat

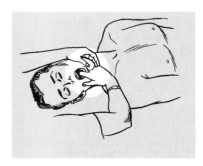

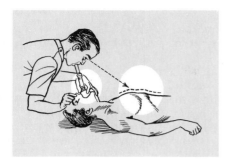

Mouth-to-mouth resuscitation using an airway.

4. If an airway such as the Brook airway is available, insert it in the patient's mouth over his tongue (see the section on artificial airways earlier in this chapter)

5. Occlude the patient's nostrils (by pinching them together) and blow into his mouth by placing your mouth directly over the patient's; observe the rise of the patient's chest

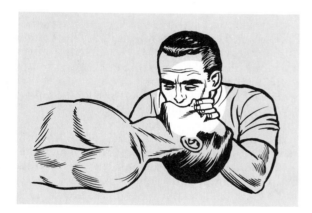

6. After each inflation, raise your mouth from the patient's and allow the patient to exhale

7. Repeat this procedure approximately 12 to 15 times each minute; continue until normal breathing is restored

If it not possible to achieve an airtight seal between your mouth and that of the patient, the mouth-to-nose method may be used. Bring your hand that is holding the patient's chin up over his mouth to seal it off. Blow directly into the patient's nostrils. When using the oral method with infants and small children, bring your mouth over the nose *and* mouth of the child. Repeat the procedure 20 to 30 times per minute, using gentle puffs of air to avoid undue pressure which could damage the lungs.[1]

Revised Sylvester Method. The procedure recommended by the St. John Ambulance Association is as follows:

Quickly place the casualty on his back, elevating the shoulders with a folded coat or other suitable padding. Extend the neck and tilt the head straight back as far as possible in order to raise the tongue off the back of the throat, thus *opening the airway*. Make sure his airway is not obstructed.

Compression Phase: Kneel at the casualty's head, grasp his wrists, and cross them over the lower half of the sternum (breastbone). Rock forward, pressing firmly downward upon the casualty's chest, thus forcing the air out of his lungs. This phase should take about two seconds. . . . Count *one and two and. . . .*

Expansion Phase: Release the downward pressure and draw the casualty's arms upward, outward, and backward. This pulls the chest wall into the expanded position and sucks air into the lungs. Count *three and four and. . . .*

Now return the wrists to their original position across the sternum. . . . Count *five.*

Timing: In order to simulate normal breathing, movements should be repeated in a rhythmic manner—about 12 times each minute for an adult, somewhat faster for a child. The First Aider should watch for signs of obstruction in the airway or change in the color of the face of the casualty and adjust his movements when the casualty shows signs of voluntary breathing. Care should be taken to use a reasonable amount of pressure in relation to the age and physical build of the casualty.

If an assistant is available, have him maintain the

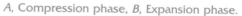

A, Compression phase, *B,* Expansion phase.

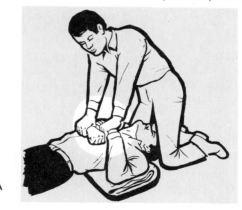

A

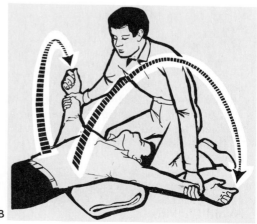

B

position of the casualty's head—tilted well back—and watch for the presence of any obstruction, such as stomach contents, in the mouth. He may relieve the First Aider since this method of Artificial Respiration is physically demanding.[1]

Self-Inflating Bag-Mask Method.

The self-inflating bag-mask unit consists of a mask, system of valves, self-inflating bag, and oxygen tube-connector. The mask is designed to form an airtight seal around the patient's mouth and nose. When squeezed and released, the bag reinflates itself rapidly. The valves permit air to enter the mask when the bag is squeezed; an exhaust valve carries the exhaled air away so that it does not enter the bag. The unit can be used with or without supplemental oxygen.

To use this unit effectively, an airtight seal must be maintained between the patient's face and the mask. In addition, the patient's head must be tilted, keeping the jaw in a forward position.

1. Place the patient in a supine position with shoulders elevated and neck extended

2. Stand at the head of the patient and apply mask over his nose and mouth; hold the mask with the thumb and index finger on the top of the mask and the third, fourth, and fifth fingers on the patient's jaw (the pointed end of the mask goes over the nose)

3. With the other hand, squeeze the bag firmly and continue squeezing until you see the patient's chest rise, then release your grip on the bag and allow it to expand on its own; do not remove the mask from the patient's face; repeat the procedure 12 to 15 times per minute

With this method, you must be particularly alert to signs of vomiting or regurgitation. If the patient vomits or regurgitates food, quickly re-

The basic position of the hands in holding a bag mask in place is demonstrated. A tight seal should be maintained between the mask and the patient's face with one hand while the bag is squeezed with the other hand. The patient's airway must be kept open by keeping the neck extended as shown.[2]

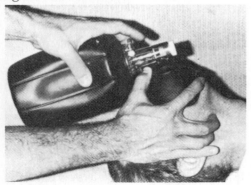

move the mask, turn the patient's head to the side, and use your finger or a suction unit to clean out the mouth. Then resume the ventilation.[2]

Cardiopulmonary Resuscitation.

The methods of artificial respiration described above are used when a person has stopped (or almost stopped) breathing. When, in addition, a person's heart stops beating, a technique called *cardiopulmonary resuscitation* (CPR) is used. CPR simply means restoring heart and lung action when it has stopped or severely decreased. The techniques of CPR can present some danger to the victim, so they must be learned and practiced on a mannikin in a supervised class. Many hospitals require every staff member to take a refresher course at least once a year.

To help you remember the steps in CPR, the American Heart Association recommends using the ABC's. The letter *A* stands for airway, the letter *B* for breathing, and the letter *C* for circulation.

Airway.

If you find a person who appears to have collapsed, first find out whether he is conscious. Look at the person closely, shake him gently by the shoulders and shout, "Are you all right?" If the person does not respond, yell for help. Then open the victim's airway. If the person is not lying on his back, roll him over, so that he is on a flat firm surface. Follow the instructions for establishing an airway given above; that is, lift up the neck or chin gently with one hand while you push down on the forehead with the other hand to tilt the head back. When the airway is open, check whether the person is breathing. Put your ear close to his mouth and *listen* for breathing, while you *look* at his chest to detect motion. Do you *feel* any breath on your cheek? If you cannot hear, see, or feel his breath, the victim is not breathing and you must start to provide artificial respiration.

Breathing.

The fastest and most direct way to provide breath is by the mouth-to-mouth technique. Place your hand on the victim's forehead and use the thumb and index finger to close off his nostrils. (Keep the heel of your hand on his forehead so that his head remains tilted.) Take a deep breath, open your mouth wide, and place it tightly over the victim's mouth. No air should be able to escape. Immediately give four quick full breaths to the victim.

Circulation.

Quickly check the victim's pulse. It is fastest to check the carotid pulse, because your hands are at his head, and because the carotid pulse can be checked without removing the person's clothing. While you keep one hand on the victim's forehead (to keep the head tilted and airway open), feel the carotid artery with the other hand. If you do not find a pulse, you must provide artificial circulation in addition to breathing. Artificial circulation must be provided because simply supplying oxygen to the lungs will not save the patient unless the oxygen can get from the lungs to the heart and into the bloodstream to be carried to the rest of the body, especially the brain. Artificial circulation is provided by means of *external cardiac compression*. Look at the illustration below. In effect, when you apply rhythmic pressure to the lower half of the victim's sternum you are forcing his heart to pump blood. To perform external cardiac compression, kneel at the victim's side near his chest. Locate the notch at the lowest portion of the sternum. Place the heel of one hand on the sternum 1 1/2 to 2 inches above the notch. Place your other hand on top of the hand in position. Be sure to keep your fingers off the victim's ribs. Align your shoulders over your

hands, keeping your elbows straight. Depress the sternum about 1 1/2 to 2 inches for an adult victim. Then relax pressure on the sternum *completely*. Do not remove your hands (keep them in position), but allow the victim's chest to return to its normal position between compressions. If you are the only rescuer, you must provide both breathing and cardiac compressions. If another person is with you, one person can breath for the victim, while the other person performs compressions. If there is one rescuer, you must provide 15 compressions for every two quick breaths. That means you must provide compressions at a rate of 80 per minute: When there are two rescuers, one person gives a breath to the victim after every fifth compression. The compressions are given at the rate of 60 per minute.

If your are by yourself, keep giving CPR for one minute, then yell for help again, and check the victim's pulse. Telephone quickly for help if necessary, but resume CPR immediately. If there are two rescuers, you can switch tasks when the person giving compressions gets tired.

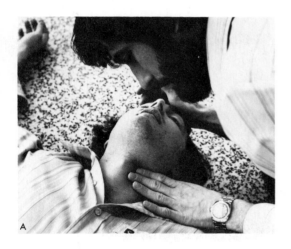

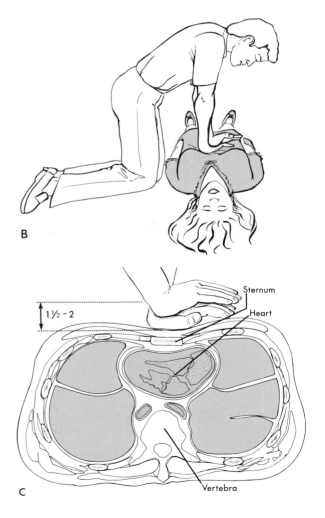

Cardiopulmonary resuscitation (CPR). *A,* The victim's carotid pulse must be checked to determine whether artificial circulation is needed. (Photo by Victor Wong. Copyright Studio Impact, Ottawa, Ontario.) *B,* The person performing CPR should kneel beside the victim and lean forward so that his arms are straight while the hands push down on the sternum. *C,* Pressure from the heel of the hand compresses the chest cavity, providing artificial circulation. The rescuer's fingers should be kept off the victim's chest.

The technique for cardiac compression is different in children and infants. For infants only the tips of your fingers are used. The sternum is depressed 1/2 to 3/4 inch at a fast rate of 80 to 100 times a minute. For children, the heel of your hand is used, and the sternum is depressed 3/4 to 1 1/2 inches, depending on the size of the child.

CPR is continued until other life support help arrives, the victim begins to breathe spontaneously, the rescuers cannot continue, or the victim is pronounced dead by a physician.

GUIDE TO ASSESSING OXYGEN NEEDS

1. Does the patient complain of difficulty in breathing? How long has he had this condition?

2. Is he anxious about his ability to breathe? What can the nurse do to alleviate his anxiety?

3. What are his respirations like in rate, depth, regularity, and sound? Is he using accessory muscles of respiration in breathing?

4. What is his position in bed or on a stretcher?

5. Does he show signs of cyanosis?

6. Does his condition require immediate medical or nursing intervention? What measures should the nurse institute first?

7. Has the specific causal factor for the dyspnea been identified? Which of the five processes involved in respiration have been impaired in function?

8. Is the patient's airway clear? Does he need suctioning or other measures to clear the airway?

9. Is the patient receiving an adequate supply of oxygen? Has oxygen therapy been ordered? If so, by what method of administration?

10. What position is best for this patient to promote maximal ventilatory efficiency?

11. Is the patient distressed by coughing?

12. Is he bringing up sputum?

13. Is the patient showing signs of restlessness? of mental confusion?

14. Have diagnostic tests and examinations been ordered for this patient? What are the patient's learning needs relative to these? What are the nurse's responsibilities?

15. Has the patient or his family other learning needs (for example, needs relating to the patient's activities, measures to prevent dyspnea, or the use of equipment for his treatment)?

GUIDE TO EVALUATING THE EFFECTIVENESS OF NURSING INTERVENTION

1. Is the patient breathing more easily?

2. Has his anxiety been relieved?

3. Is his airway patent?

4. Has his ventilatory efficiency been improved?

5. Have distressing symptoms such as coughing been relieved?

6. Has cyanosis been lessened?

7. Is the patient able to bring up sputum sufficiently to clear the bronchial tree?

8. Are his activities commensurate with his level of tolerance?

9. Has he (or his family) gained the knowledge and skills necessary to prevent further attacks or to continue his treatment at home?

STUDY SITUATION

Mr. R. S. Rowlands is a 38-year-old patient who has been in the hospital for 3 weeks. His medical diagnosis is acute bronchial asthma. When he was admitted his breathing was dyspneic, he appeared cyanotic, and his respiratory rate varied from 28 to 34 respirations per minute.

Mr. Rowlands did not want his bed to be flat; he demanded five pillows from the nurse and spent most of his time bent forward in bed. He was thin and appeared anxious. The physician ordered an oxygen mask for Mr. Rowlands, who liked to use the oxygen and to turn it on and off himself.

1. What factors should be taken into consideration in explaining to this patient how to use the oxygen equipment?

2. By what means can the patient's need for oxygen be assessed?

3. For what reason might the patient demand five pillows, and why would he like to handle the oxygen himself?

4. What nursing interventions might ease this patient's breathing?

5. How can the effectiveness of these measures be evaluated?

6. What objectives could help to guide the nursing care of this patient?

7. What observations should you make about this patient?

8. What are his nursing problems? How would you resolve these problems?

SUGGESTED READINGS

Cohen, S.: Pulmonary Function Tests in Patient Care. *American Journal of Nursing*, 80(6):1135–1161, June, 1980.

Fuchs, P. L.: Understanding continuous mechanical ventilation. *Nursing '79*, 9(12):26–33, December, 1979.

Fuchs, P. L.: Getting the Best out of Oxygen Delivery Systems. *Nursing '80*, 10(12):34–43, December 1980.

Hart, R.: A Review of CPR for Adults. *Nursing '79*, 9(2):54–59, February, 1979.

Kirilloff, L. H., and Maszkiewicz, R. X.: Guide to Respiratory Care in Ill Adults. *American Journal of Nursing*, 79(11):2005–2012, November, 1979.

Matheny, L.: Emergency! First Aid for Cardiopulmonary Arrest. *Nursing '82*, 12(6):35, June, 1982.

Nielsen, L.: Mechanical Ventilation: Patient Assessment and Nursing Care. *American Journal of Nursing*, 80:2197–2217, December, 1980.

Rifas, E. M.: How You . . . and Your Patient . . . Can Manage Dyspnea. *Nursing '80*, 10(6):34–41, June, 1980.

Sears, D. A.: Adult Respiratory Distress Syndrome: A True Test of Nursing Skills. *Nursing '80*, 10(5):51–56, May, 1980.

Standards and Guidelines for Cardio-Pulmonary Resuscitation (CPR) and Emergency Cardiac Care (ECC). *Journal of the American Medical Association*, 244(5):453–509, August 1, 1980.

Tecklin, J. D.: Positioning, Percussing, and Vibrating Patients for Effective Bronchial Drainage. *Nursing '79*, 9(3):64–71, March, 1979.

Voyles, J. B., et al.: Pulmonary Problems in Infants and Children. *American Journal of Nursing*, 81:509–532, March, 1981.

Weaver, T. E.: New Life for Lungs through Incentive Spirometers. *Nursing '81*, 11(2):54–58, February, 1981.

REFERENCES

1. *First Aid*. Third Canadian edition. Ottawa, St. John Priory of Canada Properties, 1974, with amendments to May, 1979.

2. *Emergency Care and Transportation of the Sick and Injured*. Chicago, American Academy of Orthopaedic Surgeons.

19

The Nurse Should Be Able to:

- Explain in simple terms the heat-regulating mechanisms of the body
- Discuss factors affecting body temperature
- Discuss variations in temperature regulation throughout the life cycle
- Identify common problems of disturbed temperature regulation
- Identify and intervene appropriately in emergency situations involving people with marked disturbances of body temperature
- Apply relevant principles in planning and implementing appropriate nursing interventions in the care of patients with disturbances of body temperature
- Apply relevant principles in planning and implementing therapeutic interventions involving heat and cold applications
- Evaluate the effectiveness of nursing interventions

TEMPERATURE REGULATION NEEDS

CHAPTER 19

INTRODUCTION

The surface temperature of the body varies with environmental changes, and man has had to learn to dress appropriately to protect himself from both the hot tropical sun and the cold northern winds. Over the centuries, he has also developed the ability to modify his immediate surroundings to provide an environmental temperature most comfortable for him.

With regard to the internal, or core, temperature of the body, however, man is homeothermic, or warm-blooded, with inborn mechanisms for maintaining a stable temperature within the body. These mechanisms include those concerned with both the production of heat within the body and its dissipation.

Usually the heat-regulating mechanisms of the body maintain a precise balance between heat production and heat loss. In this way the internal body temperature is kept within a very narrow range, usually varying not more than a degree or so in a day. The heat-regulating system, as we mentioned in Chapter 9, is one of the body's most important homeostatic mechanisms.

Every once in a while, however, the balance is upset and deviations outside the normal range of body temperature occur. Many people who are ill have an elevated temperature. It is, indeed, one of the cardinal signs of illness, often being one of the first observable indications that there is a disturbance of body function. The maintenance of a higher than normal temperature puts considerable stress on the body's adaptive mechanisms, and is very debilitating.

The balance may also be upset in the opposite direction from fever. Mild degrees of lowered body temperature apparently do not do as much harm to the body as fever does. Everything simply slows down and when the body warms up, it will commence to function at normal levels again. However, the problem of accidental *hypothermia* (excessively low body temperatures) due, in most cases, to prolonged exposure to cold environmental temperatures has been receiving increasing attention. It appears to be more common than was once thought. *Frostbite*, which involves freezing of the skin tissues in one area of the body, such as exposed earlobes, the tip of the nose, fingers, or toes, has always been a problem in cold climates. This and *chilblains*, which are a mild form of frostbite, are a common source of discomfort, particularly to older people who live in cold, damp climates and whose homes are not equipped with central heating.

Applications of both heat and cold have been used for centuries to treat various disorders of the human body. Both have systemic and localized effects on body tissues and are still frequently utilized in therapy.

THE BODY'S MECHANISMS FOR TEMPERATURE REGULATION

Body heat results from the energy released by foods in the process of cellular metabolism. Heat is lost from the body through a variety of means: direct contact with cooler objects in the immediate environment (principally air) by the process of *conduction*, which is enhanced by the *convection* (movement) of air currents circulating around the body; the *evaporation* of moisture from the surface of the body; and the transfer of heat, in the form of electromagnetic waves, from the body to cooler objects in the environment by *radiation*.

The regulatory mechanisms controlling body temperature are located in the preoptic area of the hypothalamus. Neurons in this area respond to changes in the temperature of the blood circulating through the area by sending impulses either to the anterior heat-losing center (in the hypothalamus) or to the posterior heat-promoting center. These centers have a reciprocal effect on each other; when one is activated, the other is depressed.

The body has various adaptive mechanisms to promote heat if body temperature falls too low, or to lose excess heat if the temperature goes too high.

Stimulation of the heat-producing center increases wakefulness and stimulates muscular activity. If the individual does not engage in some form of exercise in response to this, the body will initiate its own muscular activity involuntarily in the form of shivering, which can produce a considerable amount of heat within the body. At the same time, stimulation of the sympathetic nervous system facilitates the release of both epinephrine and norepinephrine into the blood stream. As a result, cellular metabolism is speeded up, which increases heat production.

Stimulation of the sympathetic nervous system also results in the phenomenon of *piloerection*, which means that the hairs literally stand on end. In human beings, this can actually occur but most often a milder reaction takes place, evident in the "gooseflesh" appearance of the skin. In animals with long hair, this mechanism serves to entrap a layer of warm air next to the skin. In human beings, the mechanism is not so effective in providing insulation, but it occurs nonetheless. Cessation of sweating usually occurs as well, to reduce the amount of heat lost through evaporation of water from the body surface.

Concomitantly, vasoconstriction occurs and blood is drawn from surface vessels to minimize the amount of heat lost through conduction, convection, and radiation. The individual becomes pale and his skin is cold to the touch; he also feels cold.

With prolonged exposure to colder temperatures than normal (as in cold climates in the wintertime) the thyroid gland is stimulated to increase production. This increases the metabolic rate, thereby increasing heat production. However, this is a slower process, which occurs over a period of weeks.

Stimulation of the heat-losing center, on the other hand, has an inhibitory effect on the mechanisms for heat production, and the reverse effect is seen. Muscular activity is decreased; metabolism is slowed down; circulation to the skin is increased; and the rate of production of thyroxin by the thyroid gland gradually decreases.

The body also has two other mechanisms to facilitate heat loss; these are sweating and panting. In lower animals, rapid shallow breathing (panting) increases the amount of heat lost by evaporation of moisture from the respiratory tract or tongue. Rapid shallow breathing in dyspneic patients has the same effect. In human beings, however, the principal mechanism for cooling the body is by increasing perspiration. This greatly facilitates the loss of heat from the body through the process of evaporation of moisture from the skin. If the environmental temperature is above body temperature, perspiration is the only mechanism available to the person for heat loss.

FACTORS AFFECTING BODY TEMPERATURE

Under conditions of good health, a number of normal activities and physiological processes affect body temperature. Any factor that increases the metabolic rate will raise the temperature of the body; conversely, a decreased metabolic rate will lower body temperature. In exercise, muscular activity increases body temperature as a result of heat production by body muscles. Heavy muscular exercise may increase the body temperature by as much as 2.2° C (4° to 5° F). When the temperature begins to rise, the body's heat regulating mechanisms start to function. Blood is drawn to the surface for cooling and the person starts to perspire. Usually an elevated temperature due to exercise quickly returns to normal with the cessation of exercise.

Strong emotions, such as anger, will also raise body temperature because of stimulation of the sympathetic nervous system. The "heat of anger" and "feverish with excitement" are common expressions and they can, indeed, be physically true. One notices this particularly with children, whose body temperatures are more labile (that is, they fluctuate more easily) than those of adults.

Disturbances in the production of thyroxin by the thyroid gland also affect body temperature. An excess production of thyroxin (due to an overactive thyroid gland) increases the basal metabolic rate, thereby stimulating heat production. People with a thyroid deficiency, on the other hand, have a lower metabolic rate, and consequently a body temperature that is usually at the low end of the normal range.

An increase in body temperature itself will stimulate the cells to increase the rate of cellular metabolism and heat production. For each 1° C rise in temperature, the rate of heat production increases 13 per cent, and the metabolic rate may be forty times as much as normal. As a result, an increased temperature by itself tends to heighten a fever. A lowered body temperature has the reverse effect of decreasing metabolism, which will in turn lessen body temperature still further.

The specific dynamic action of foods also affects body temperature. The body's metabolic rate is stimulated by the intake of food and remains elevated for several hours after a meal. Foods differ in their specific dynamic qualities. Proteins increase the metabolic rate much more than fats and carbohydrates do, and the increase remains high over a longer period of time. This is the reason that a breakfast with high protein content will sustain you longer than one containing carbohydrates only (such as orange juice and toast).

Besides the factors that increase the metabolic rate, a number of other factors, some of which were discussed in Chapter 9, will also influence body temperature.

The environment has a pronounced effect upon body temperature. Not only permanent changes, such as those encountered when moving to a hot or cold climate, but also temporary changes, such as a brief hot spell, affect the body by raising or lowering its temperature. The body's ability to withstand high environmental temperatures is dependent on the humidity of the atmosphere. When the air is dry and there are sufficient air currents to carry away heat from the body by convection, an individual can stand very high temperatures with little or no increase in body temperature. If, on the other hand, the humidity is high, the amount of heat lost through evaporation from the surface of the body is decreased and body temperature begins to rise quickly. This explains why one feels so uncomfortable on hot, "muggy" days.

Similarly, a cold environment decreases body temperature. Cold, damp weather is much more chilling than cold dry weather, and when there is considerable amount of air movement, increasing amounts of heat are carried away from the body. The "wind chill" factor can then produce the effect of a temperature much lower than that which is registered on the outdoor thermometer.

Clothing, of course, decreases the effects of environmental temperatures on body heat. The insulation of the body by adequate, warm clothing lessens the impact of cold temperatures. In warm climates, cottons are more comfortable to wear because they absorb moisture. Synthetic fibers and wool do not absorb as well; hence, they inhibit the removal of perspiration from the body.

Although normal processes can cause mild fluctuations in body temperature, many illnesses also cause deviations from the normal. Most frequently, these are in the direction of an elevated temperature. The most common of these illnesses are infections, diseases of the central nervous system, neoplasms, and metabolic disorders. The prolonged use of some drugs, among them morphine and LSD, may also give rise to fever.

TEMPERATURE REGULATION THROUGHOUT THE LIFE CYCLE

Early in pregnancy, there is a slight rise in the body temperature of most women, which continues until about the fourth month. There is then a gradual fall in body temperature, which usually remains slightly below normal levels throughout the remainder of pregnancy. The lowered body temperature corresponds to a lower metabolic rate in the pregnant woman.

During the early months of pregnancy, it is important that the mother be safeguarded as much as possible from developing a fever. High fever in the mother during the first 4 months of pregnancy can be teratogenic, that is, it can cause the development of physical defects in the infant in utero, particularly in the brain in its early stages of development.

Normally the infant is maintained for 9 months in the warm, protected environment of the mother's uterus. Immediately after birth, the newborn's temperature usually falls 1 to 2° C because of the evaporation of amniotic fluid from the skin as the infant's total body surface is exposed to the cooler environment outside the mother's body. Further heat loss is prevented in the delivery room by drying the infant and placing him under radiant heat immediately. The newborn's temperature is unstable because the heat regulating system is not yet fully developed. Hence, it is important to maintain a stable environmental temperature. A "neutral thermal environment" (32° C or 89.6° F) is considered best because it requires minimum oxygen consumption at rest. This point is particularly important in the care of premature infants, whose heat-regulating mechanisms are even less mature than those of a full-term infant.

During the first year of life, the infant continues to be highly dependent on environmental temperature to maintain its own internal temperature because of immaturity of the heat-regulating system. The shivering mechanism does not usually begin to function until after the first year and heat must be produced through increasing the basal metabolic rate. It is important, then, that infants be protected from becoming too cold, or too warm, with changes in the environmental temperature. Appropriate clothing for the climate is essential (warm "woolies" for winter weather, and cool cottons for summer or in the tropics).

Infants can develop a high fever very rapidly, and this frequently occurs with the acute respiratory infections that are so common in early childhood. The high fever may produce convulsions—a very frightening experience for the new mother. Rubbing the infant with wet hands is one method advocated for reducing temperature without causing shock. The friction of rubbing brings blood to the surface for cooling and the evaporation of water from the surface of the body aids in the process.

During childhood, the body temperature averages approximately 37° C (98.6° F). The child's temperature is more labile than that of adults. A child can run a fever with excitement, for example; however, fever in children is usually secondary to infection, and is often the first indication that they are ill. It is not until adolescence that sweating in the axilla occurs; children do not have this mechanism to assist in cooling the body.

With onset of the menses, girls experience a cyclical rise and fall of body temperature, which continues through the childbearing years. There is a fall in the early morning temperature of most women just after the onset of menstruation. The temperature remains at this lower level until ovulation takes place. There is then an abrupt rise of 0.3 to 0.4° C (0.5 to 0.75° F), which continues until the start of the next menstrual period.

Women also experience variations of body temperature during the menopause. Once ovulation has ceased, secretion of the female hormones, the estrogens, declines rapidly. One of the distressing side effects is a disturbance in temperature regulation that gives rise to the characteristic "hot flushes" (or "hot flashes") experienced by middle-aged women. During one of these episodes, the individual suddenly feels very warm, her skin becomes extremely flushed, and she often finds herself being drenched with perspiration. The attacks usually last for only a few minutes, but they may continue, occurring at irregular intervals for a number of years. Countless women have been relieved of this distressing symptom by taking a low dosage of estrogen on a cyclical basis, that is, 3 weeks out of 4, on prescription from their physician. Recently, however, there has been some concern that the estrogens may cause a proliferation of endometrial tissue in the menopausal woman, thus predisposing her to cancer of the uterus. Many physicians are advising women not to take estrogens for too long a period.

The basal metabolic rate gradually decreases with age, so that older people of both sexes usually have a lower body temperature than young adults. The decreasing efficiency of most body systems that accompanies the aging process also renders the older person more vulnerable to the effects of changing environmental temperatures. The sweating and circulatory systems become sluggish, and older people do not cope very well with heat. There is decreased peripheral circulation, for example, owing to changes in the aging skin. The shivering reflex is also not as effective, and hypothermia can be a problem.

COMMON PROBLEMS IN TEMPERATURE REGULATION

Fever

The physiological mechanisms responsible for fever are not known for all disease processes. It is generally felt that fever may be caused by abnormalities in the brain itself or by toxic substances that affect the heat-regulating mechanisms.

A number of stimuli may activate the hypothalamic centers. Important among these are the substances called pyrogens, which are secreted by toxic bacteria or released by degenerating tissue. It is believed that these substances stimulate the release of a second substance, endogenous pyrogen, from the leukocytes that have been drawn to the diseased area. The endogenous pyrogens then act on the thermoregulatory centers.[1]

There is evidence to support the belief that fever caused by pyrogens has some beneficial effects in helping the body to combat infection. It is felt that the fever acts in two ways: (1) It creates an undesirable temperature for the survival of bacteria; and (2) the increased rate of metabolism in the cells increases their production of immune bodies and also their ability to phagocytize foreign bodies, thus impeding bacterial invasion.

Dehydration can also affect the hypothalamic centers directly so that the temperature rises to febrile levels. Part of the elevation is due to lack of fluids for sweating, which deprives the body of one of its principal mechanisms for losing excess heat.

Fever may occur postoperatively owing to any one of a number of causes. It may be due to excessive heat production, as in the case of pathogenic infection, but is usually thought to be due to inadequate heat elimination.

Fever frequently accompanies a head injury and is often seen in patients with spinal cord

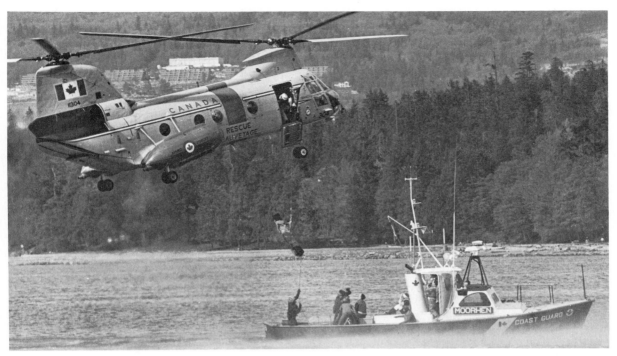

Hypothermia is often a prime factor to be treated in rescue operations. (*Vancouver Sun* photo. Used with permission.)

injuries. In these cases, it is felt to be caused by pressure on, or injury to, the hypothalamus or the tracts leading to and from the heat-regulating centers.[2]

Hypothermia

The most common cause of hypothermia is prolonged exposure to cold environmental temperatures, although a lowered body temperature may be induced artificially sometimes for the purpose of cardiac or vascular surgery, or in the treatment of some poisons.

People vary considerably in ability to withstand cold temperatures. Persons with darkly pigmented skin, aged people, and those in poor physical condition are more affected by the cold than others. The amount and type of clothing worn for insulating the body are also important. Multiple layers of lightweight clothing serve to entrap warm air close to the skin and have been found to be more effective than fewer layers of bulky, heavy clothing for keeping the body warm. Water acts as a heat conductor, and damp clothing therefore conducts heat away from the body. The "wind chill" factor, as we mentioned, considerably increases the effect of cold environmental temperatures on the body. Rarefied atmospheres, as experienced by mountain climbers, also magnify the effect of cold on the body.

ASSESSMENT

Usually the first thing that is done to a person on admission to a health agency is to take his temperature. Indeed, fever is such a universal sign of illness that it is important to observe all patients for the signs and symptoms of disturbed body temperature. In order to have baseline data on which to judge whether a person's temperature is above, or below, his normal, it is helpful to take the temperature over a period of several successive days at different times of the day and to plot the readings on a temperature graph (flowsheet).

Many inpatient agencies have specific policies for the taking of temperatures. Some require that all patients have their temperature taken once, or sometimes twice, a day to screen for fever. If once a day, it is usually considered that early evening is the best time, since in many patients with a fever, this is time when the temperature is most elevated. If temperatures are taken in the morning, this should be done an hour or so after the patient wakens, when the body temperature is stabilized. When a patient has a fever, the temperature should be taken at more frequent intervals. If it is abnormally elevated, as often as every 15 minutes is sometimes indicated. All newly admitted patients should have a temperature taken, as well as all preoperative and postoperative patients. Postoperatively, the temperature is usually taken every 4 hours for the first 48 hours. In addition to these general guidelines, the nurse should be alert to signs and symptoms indicating the presence of fever and should take the patient's temperature if she thinks it may have changed. The temperature should be evaluated in relation to such factors as the patient's usual normal temperature, the time of day, the environmental temperature, and the normal physiological processes that may affect body temperature. Details on the methods of taking body temperature are given in Chapter 9.

If the patient is admitted to the health agency running a fever, it is important to find out how long he has had it, how high the temperature has been, and whether the person has had any other signs and symptoms of illness. In the case of children, it is particularly important to ask if they have been exposed to a communicable disease, so that they may be isolated to protect other children on the unit. Some agencies have a policy of putting all children with an elevated temperature on admission on isolation precautions for 24 hours to observe them for development of a rash or other indication of one of the childhood diseases.

When a person is admitted with a cold-weather injury, the nurse should find out the circumstances of the accident. How long was the exposure? Under what conditions? What parts of the body are affected? What first aid measures were used to treat the person before he was admitted? It is also helpful to know how old the person is, his general physical condition, and any existing health problems that he has. The patient's history, taken on admission, and observations noted in the clinical appraisal of the patient and recorded on the patient's chart can furnish data to aid the nurse in her assessment.

In order to know what to look for in making her observations and the relevant questions to ask the patient (or family or significant other), the nurse needs to understand a little more about the mechanism of fever—the types of fever commonly encountered, and the stages a person goes through when he has a fever. She should also understand what is happening to body tissues affected by cold and be able to make pertinent observations.

Fever

A term that is frequently used synonymously with fever is *pyrexia*. *Hyperpyrexia* and *hyperthermia* are used interchangeably to designate an abnormally high fever—that is, 40.6° C (105° F) or over. *Habitual hyperthermia* refers to a condition in which the average daily temperature is slightly above normal limits.

Although prolonged fevers are not seen as commonly today as in the years before the use of antibiotics, it is well for the nurse to know the technical terms used for different types of fevers. The terms are descriptive and explain the nature of the fever.

An *intermittent* or *quotidian* fever is one in which the temperature rises each day but falls to normal sometime during the 24-hour period, most usually during the early morning hours. A *remittent* fever is one which shows marked variations in the temperature readings during a 24-hour period, the lowest reading, however, always being above the patient's normal level. In a *relapsing* fever, the patient's temperature may be normal for 1 or 2 days, then elevated for varying periods. These periods of normalcy are interspersed irregularly throughout the course of a relapsing fever. The term *hectic* or *septic* may be used to describe an intermittent fever in which there are wide fluctuations in daily temperature readings. It is not unusual for the temperature to vary as much as 2.2° C (4° F) within a 24-hour period in this type of fever. Another type of fever is called a *constant* fever. In this type, the patient's temperature remains at essentially the same level over a period of days or weeks.

The Stages of a Fever. The typical stages of fever occur in response to the physiological processes that are taking place within the body. There are three distinct stages to a fever: (1) the *chill* phase, or period of rising temperature; (2) the *course* of the fever, when the temperature is maintained at an elevated level; and (3) the *termination*, or period when the temperature falls to normal. During the three stages, different sets of mechanisms are operating, giving rise to the signs and symptoms characteristic of each stage.

The Chill Phase. During the onset of a fever, it is thought that there is a resetting of the body's internal "thermostat" at a higher level.[1] This may be a response to the presence of pyrogenic substances, or to any one of the other causes listed in the section on the etiology of fever. The resetting of the internal thermostat brings the body's heat-producing mechanisms into play as an attempt is made to bring the temperature up to the "desired" level. The person experiences what is known as a *chill*. Muscular activity is increased, in the form of shivering, which may vary in severity from merely a feeling of being cold, with slight shivering, to violent muscular contractions (shaking chills).

At the same time as the shivering mechanism is induced, the rate of cellular metabolism increases, and the waste products of metabolism, carbon dioxide and water, are formed in greater quantities. The increased carbon dioxide level in the blood stimulates the respiratory center and the person breathes faster and more deeply. This leads to extra fluid loss, and the patient feels thirsty. Also, as metabolism is accelerated, there is an increased demand by the cells for more oxygen and glucose. The heart beats more rapidly (in response to this demand), and the nurse will note that the patient's pulse rate is higher than normal.

Concomitantly, heat-conserving mechanisms are instituted. Vasoconstriction occurs and the patient becomes pale, and his skin is cold to the touch. He also feels cold and may ask for extra blankets. Often, there is a "gooseflesh" appearance to the skin as "piloerection" takes place. Sweating usually also ceases.

During the chill phase, the rectal temperature rises steadily, although the elevation is usually not evident by oral thermometer until the end of a chill. Body temperature may be increased by as much as 1.1 to 4° C (2 to 7° F).[2] A chill may last for a few minutes or as long as an hour. In mild cases of fever, such as one sees with the common cold or in light cases of influenza, the chill phase is usually brief.

The Course of a Fever. During the second stage of a fever, or when the fever is "running its course," the temperature has reached the preset level and there is a balance between heat production and heat loss. Because of the increased body temperature, the skin feels warm to the touch and there is usually a generalized flushing of the skin. The increased metabolic rate required to maintain the elevated temperature puts heightened demands on the body for more oxygen and glucose. The heart and respiratory rates remain high, and water loss through respiration increases the patient's feeling of thirst. The elevated temperature also increases nervous irritability. Headache, photophobia (sensitivity to light), and restlessness or drowsiness (or both) are not uncommon symptoms. An abnormally high fever is often accompanied by a state of mental confusion, which may progress to delirium. The patient becomes disoriented as to time and place. He may not know where he is or, often, what day it is. Sometimes the patient may have hallucinations. He may become quite irrational and combative. Finally, prostration (collapse) may ensue. In young children, a convulsion not infrequently accompanies fever, usually at the outset.

The maintenance of an elevated temperature is very debilitating to the patient. During the first week or so of a fever, there is always some destruction of body protein and *albuminuria* (protein in the urine) is usually noted in the laboratory findings of the febrile patient.[1] The patient often complains of a generalized weakness and is not inclined to much activity. Aching of the muscles and joints is also frequently present. In addition to the destruction of tissue protein, it is believed that the parenchyma of many cells begins to be damaged when the body temperature rises above 40° C (105° F).[1] In sustained high fevers there may be permanent damage to nervous tissue, since this tissue does not regenerate. The upper limit for survival has been estimated by various experts to be a body temperature of 46° C (114.8° F).[2]

Febrile patients usually lose weight. Although the increased metabolic rate maintained during the course of a fever increases the body's need for nourishment, most patients have little interest in food. This loss of appetite (*anorexia*) may give way to nausea and vomiting as the fever progresses. The combination of increased need for food and lack of interest in it leads to a loss of weight.

Usually during the course of a fever, the temperature does not remain at a constant level but tends to fluctuate. Thus, periods when body temperature is rising are usually interspersed with periods when it is falling, even though the lowest temperature reached may always be above normal. When the temperature is falling, mechanisms for additional heat loss are dominant. Vasodilatation occurs and the skin becomes flushed and warm. Sweating (*diaphoresis*) is usually present to maximize heat loss through evaporation. The body thus loses more fluids, and the possibility of dehydration presents a problem.

When fever is prolonged, the problem of dehydration is more likely to occur. This is due to a number of factors, including the greater loss of water through increased respirations and the further loss of fluids from sweating during periods when the body temperature is falling. There is often a lessening in the output of urine as more than the usual amount of fluid is lost through the skin and lungs. Other evidences of dehydration may be noted. The skin and mucous membranes may appear parched and dry. The patient's lips may become cracked and sore, and lesions may occur at the corners of the mouth. These lesions are termed *herpes simplex,* but are often referred to as "fever blisters" because they are so frequently seen in patients with fever. The nurse may note other signs and symptoms of dehydration, as discussed in Chapter 17. It is well to remember that young children, in particular, become dehydrated very quickly if there is a sustained fever.

The Termination of a Fever. When the cause of the elevated temperature has been removed, as for example when antibiotics have "taken hold" and removed the cause of infection, the body's thermostat is reset at its original level. The mechanisms for increased heat production cease to operate, and mechanisms for increased heat loss are instituted. These are the same mechanisms that have already been described as operating during the course of a fever when the temperature is fluctuating and there is a temporary drop. The patient's temperature may drop to normal quickly, over a period of hours (by crisis), or gradually over a period of days or weeks (by lysis).

Hypothermia

The basic physiological mechanism operating in hypothermia is a constriction of the blood vessels in the peripheral tissues of the body. With the vasoconstriction, there is a decreased flow of blood to the area and consequently a decreased supply of oxygen to the tissues. The decreased blood flow results in diminished local sensation (a numbness is perceived) and a weakness of the muscles. The skin feels cold and becomes pale. The walls of blood vessels in the area may be directly damaged by the cold, with the result that plasma fluid leaks into interstitial spaces. The area becomes swollen. The blood in the vessel then becomes more concentrated and small clots begin to appear, giving a typical mottled look to the tissues. Eventually, the clots will close off the vessel completely and the area becomes avascular (without blood supply). A pulse can no longer be felt. If there is a quick freezing of the tissues, as sometimes happens in very cold climates to exposed noses, cheeks, or ears, the affected part becomes white and shiny, sometimes with a blue tinge.

The skin is the first tissue to be cooled and the most likely to be damaged. Blood vessels, nerves, and muscles are also very vulnerable and easily damaged. Bones, connective tissue, and tendons are more resistant to damage from cold exposure. The areas of the body that are most vulnerable to damage from the cold are those that are most exposed, such as the hands, the face—especially the cheeks and the nose—the ears, and the feet.

In addition to the localized reactions to cold, the person who has suffered from exposure under conditions of extreme cold may develop cold exhaustion. In response to the cold, his physical and mental responses slow down. He begins to lose the ability to move his limbs as well as normally and he finds that he is stumbling often. His speech becomes slurred and his vision impaired. Often he becomes irritable, and he may become irrational. Muscular cramps and shivering are common and, as long as the shivering mechanism is still operating, he will have an increased pulse and respirations.

If body temperature drops below 25° C (77° F), the person's breathing will become slow and shallow and his pulse rate very slow. He becomes drowsy and will usually fall asleep. If he is not rescued, death will ensue. It is felt that the lowest limit for body temperature is about 20° C (68° F).

PRIORITIES FOR NURSING ACTION

In determining priorities for nursing action, the nurse must assess the severity of the patient's condition. If the patient's temperature is abnormally high, there is an immediate need to lower it. The patient should be put to bed, if he has been up and around, and the physician notified promptly. There are a number of measures that may be used to bring about a rapid reduction in body temperature. These include the use of antipyretic drugs, which have a systemic action and various techniques for "surface cooling" of the body.

Other disturbances in the body's homeostatic heat balance that require prompt intervention include heat cramps, heat exhaustion, heat stroke, and accidental hypothermia.

Heat cramps may occur in hot climates or hot weather as a result of prolonged, excessive sweating. This depletes the sodium chloride in body fluids and results in pallor, extreme thirst, nausea, and dizziness. The body temperature may be normal or slightly elevated, and, if the salt depletion is excessive, severe muscular cramps result. Putting the person in a cool room and giving fluids with salt added (as, for example, lemonade with salt in it), salt in the form of tablets, or a hypotonic solution of table salt and baking soda (1 level teaspoon of salt and ½ teaspoon of baking soda in 1 liter of water) will relieve mild cases.

Heat exhaustion may result from lengthy exposure to heat, especially if combined with high humidity. The person usually becomes very pale, with a cold, clammy skin and lowered blood pressure. The person shows signs of shock (pale, cold and clammy skin, lowered blood pressure, rapid, weak pulse, generalized weakness, and often nausea and vomiting). Generally moving the person to cooler and less humid surroundings and giving fluids will relieve this

SUBJECTIVE AND OBJECTIVE DATA IN PATIENTS WITH DISTURBANCES OF BODY TEMPERATURE

Subjective Data	Objective Data
Fever	
Chill Phase	
Feeling of being cold	Skin cool to touch
Intermittent chills	Pale gooseflesh appearance
Apprehension	Observable shivering or shaking
	Increased pulse rate
	Increased respiratory rate
	Increased rectal temperature
Course of the Fever	
Feeling of being warm	Skin flushed
Thirst	Hot to touch
Lips sore	Perspiration (may be profuse)
Feeling of generalized weakness	Elevated temperature (may fluctuate)
Restlessness, drowsiness	Dry mouth and lips
Headache	Fever blisters
Sensitivity to light	Tongue coated, "furry"
Aching muscles and joints	Scanty urine
Anorexia, nausea, vomiting	Lethargy
	With high fever, may show disorientation
	Delirium, with hallucinations
	Irrational combative behavior
	Convulsions (in children)
	Loss of weight
	Dehydration
Termination of fever	
Feels improved	Bodily functions return to normal
	Skin flushed
	Sweating (diaphoresis) often profuse
	Increased respiration
	Increased pulse
	Dropping temperature
	Clearing sensorium
	Return to normal functioning.
Hypothermia	
Exposed area feels cold	Skin cold to touch
Diminished local sensation (feeling of numbness)	Pale—becoming white or blue-tinged
Weakness of muscles	Sometimes mottled appearance of skin
Inability in flex joints	Absence of pulse
Tiredness	Swelling
Drowsiness	Slow, often stumbling movements
	Sometimes irrational behavior
	Vision impaired
	Breathing slow and shallow
	Pulse rate slow

condition. Stimulants, such as strong black coffee, may also help.

Heat stroke, a condition of severe prostration, may be caused by prolonged exposure to high environmental heat temperatures. It is most frequently seen in the elderly and is believed to be due to failure of the heat regulatory centers in the brain. The condition is characterized by very high fever, coma, and the absence of sweating. It requires immediate action to lower the body temperature as quickly as possible. Prompt medical intervention is needed and the individual should be hospitalized.[3]

On the other side of the temperature spectrum, the common priority problem is accidental hypothermia.

Hypothermia is a chilling of the whole body from exposure to cold. If the core temperature of the body is below 34°C (94°F), treatment of the hypothermia takes precedence over other problems because of the threat to a person's life.

In cases of *accidental hypothermia,* the body temperature has been known to go down as low as 69.8°F. and the person survived.[4] The individual in this case was a 24-year-old woman in Tennessee, so it is not always the elderly who are the victims (although they are more vulnerable), nor does accidental hypothermia only occur in cold, northern climates or in people who have been caught in a snowstorm in the mountains. If the person is in the early stages of hypothermia, that is, if he is suffering from cold

PRINCIPLES RELEVANT TO TEMPERATURE REGULATION

1. The surface temperature of the body varies with environmental changes.

2. The internal, or core, temperature is maintained within a very narrow range, normally fluctuating no more than a degree or so in a given individual.

3. Upper and lower limits of body temperature for survival are considered to be 46°C (114.8°F) and 20°C (68°F).

4. Heat is generated in the body through the process of cellular metabolism.

5. Heat is lost from the body through the mechanisms of radiation, conduction, convection, and evaporation.

6. The generation and loss of heat is controlled thermostatically in the hypothalamus.

7. An elevated temperature is often one of the first signs of illness.

8. The maintenance of a temperature above the normal level requires the expenditure of an increased amount of energy by the body.

9. A high body temperature may in itself stimulate further heat production.

10. Body cells are damaged by excessively high surface or internal temperatures.

11. Body tissues freeze when exposed to excessively low environmental temperatures.

12. Irreparable tissue damage can result if prompt intervention is not taken.

13. Cell destruction can be avoided if prompt intervention is taken.

14. Both infants and older people are more susceptible to changes in environmental temperatures than other people.

---

exhaustion, he should be protected from the elements and, also from the cold and possibly wet ground. If possible, the individual should be wrapped in dry clothing and put into a sleeping bag to protect him from further exposure and to promote gradual warming of the body. Sudden warming, as, for example, with hot water bottles or an electric blanket, is to be avoided because it can cause dilatation of superficial blood vessels and a resultant withdrawal of blood from vital internal organs. If the person is conscious and you have him in a warm place, he may be given hot liquids and a warm bath. Sweet liquids are advocated, because prolonged exposure to cold reduces the body's supplies of sugar.

If the person has become stuporous or unconscious and it is necessary to transport him to medical facilities, he should be placed between blankets and care taken to protect him from further cold en route. The condition requires prompt medical intervention and hospitalization. For this condition, there have been many new developments in treatment; warming of the body by internal means—that is, by warming the blood rather than applying external heat— is now being advocated by many authorities.

GOALS FOR NURSING ACTION

The principal goals of nursing action in the care of the patient with a fever are:

1. To reduce the amount of heat produced within the body

2. To facilitate heat elimination from the body

3. To minimize the effects of fever on the body

The goals of nursing action for the patient with excessive lowering of surface or core body

Sometimes a cool, moist cloth on the forehead helps the patient with a fever to feel more comfortable.

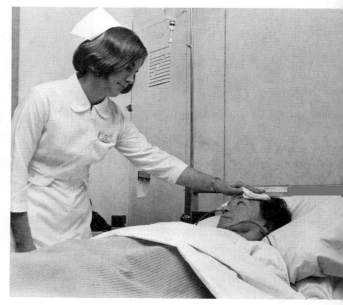

temperature, depending on the severity of the problem, are:

1. To thaw tissues
2. To prevent tissue damage
3. If necessary, to obtain medical intervention as soon as possible

SPECIFIC NURSING INTERVENTIONS

General Measures

The patient who has an elevated temperature needs rest. Rest and inactivity decrease the rate of the metabolic process and also muscular activity and thereby decrease the amount of heat produced in the body. Usually, the patient is restricted to bed in order to curtail his activities. Rest, however, involves more than restrictions of physical activity; it also means mental rest. Sometimes the simple act of taking a patient's temperature may itself give rise to anxiety on the part of the patient. An elevated temperature may mean that surgery is postponed, or that a much anticipated return to home and family is delayed. The patient needs to be assured that all is being done for his welfare and that he is in competent hands. Anticipating the needs of the patient helps him to relax. Very often, a simple explanation of procedures and treatments can alleviate many anxieties.

The patient with a fever needs a cool, quiet environment. He is often irritable and may be hypersensitive to stimuli. An effort should be made to minimize noise and provide the patient with the opportunity for rest. A cool, comfortable room increases heat elimination and helps the patient to rest more easily. Sometimes a fan is used to increase the circulation of air in the room and facilitate the removal of heat from the body through conduction and convection. Care should be taken, however, that the patient does not become chilled. The bedclothes of the patient with a fever should be light and comfortable, since heavy coverings inhibit heat elimination.

Measures to Minimize the Effects of Fever on the Body

The presence of a temperature above the normal level puts stresses on the body's adaptive mechanisms. The patient is usually uncomfortable; he is losing more than the normal amount of fluids and using more energy than usual to maintain the elevated body temperature. Nursing action should then be directed toward relieving discomfort, maintaining hydration, and maintaining the patient's nutritional status.

Comfort Measures. Good hygiene is important to the patient's health and comfort. Diaphoresis (profuse sweating), a common accompaniment of fever, is uncomfortable. Bathing the patient and assisting him to change his gown and bedding so that he is clean and dry are important contributions to his physical well-being. Because sweat glands are more numerous in the axilla and around the genitalia, these areas need particular care when the patient is bathed. Flannelette sheets, because of their greater absorbency, are often used in place of ordinary cotton (muslin) ones on the beds of patients who are perspiring profusely.

Maintaining Hydration. The hydration of the patient is of primary importance. Diaphoresis and the loss of additional fluids through increased respirations increase the amount of fluid eliminated from the body, and this fluid needs to be replaced. In addition, during a fever, there is increased production of metabolic waste products, which must be eliminated. The necessity for removing these products from the body, together with any toxic substances that may be present, emphasizes the importance of fluids. Generally 300 ml. per day is considered a desirable fluid intake. If the patient is unable to take fluids orally or in sufficient amounts, parenteral fluids may be ordered.

An accurate record of the patient's fluid intake and output must be maintained. Intake records should include all fluids taken orally and those given parenterally. In computing output, urine should be measured accurately and a note made of the extent of sweating and the loss of any fluids through vomiting or diarrhea. Suction returns should also be included in the output calculations.

The patient should be observed carefully for signs of dehydration. When a patient becomes dehydrated during the course of a fever, his skin often becomes dry and scaly. The application of creams helps to keep the skin in good condition. Dehydration frequently results also in cracks in the patient's lips, tongue, or mucous membrane lining of the mouth. Good oral hygiene is imperative to prevent infection from developing and also to contribute to the patient's comfort. There is a need to cleanse, hydrate, and lubricate the mouth and lips. If the patient is unable to clean his own teeth with a toothbrush, he may be helped by the nurse, who uses a toothbrush or a tongue depressor with gauze and mouthwash. If ordinary mouthwash is ineffectual, the nurse may need to use a stronger solution, such as half-strength hydrogen peroxide or milk of magnesia.

Frequent intake of fluids helps to maintain hydration of the oral cavity. Rinsing the mouth with water (or mouthwash) and chewing gum also help to preserve hydration. If the patient is unable to take fluids orally, to rinse his mouth, or to chew gum, the nurse may meet this need for the patient by cleaning the mouth with swabs. Glycerin and lemon swabs, or swabs dipped in milk of magnesia, are used in many places for this purpose.

Lubrication may be accomplished by the application of creams or petrolatum to the lips. If the patient is unable to apply lubricating cream himself, the nurse can meet this need by applying sterile petrolatum to the lips. The petrolatum should be sterile because there are frequently splits or cracks in the lips due to the fever, which provide a portal of entry for infection.

Maintaining Nutritional Status.

The old adage of "feed a cold and starve a fever" has been proved wrong. Indeed, because of the body's increased metabolic rate and the increased destruction of tissues that are so often a concomitant of fever, there is a need for both proteins and carbohydrates. Proteins aid in the formation of body tissue; carbohydrates supply the body with much-needed energy. Frequently these products are supplied in the liquids taken orally or given parenterally. The patient's weight should be checked at frequent intervals, and the physician should be kept informed of the patient's nutritional status so that appropriate therapy may be instituted.

Rest is essential to minimize the patient's energy requirements. Physical activity should be kept to a minimum. During the convalescent stage, activity should be increased gradually to prevent tiring the patient unduly.

An important function of the nurse is the communication of her observations to other members of the health team. The nutritional status of the patient with a fever must be carefully monitored by the nurse and accurately reported and recorded. See Chapter 14 for the signs of good and poor nutritional status to watch for in patients.

Measures to Reduce Heat Production and Facilitate Heat Loss

Antipyretic Drugs. Antipyretic drugs, such as aspirin, are often ordered to reduce a patient's fever. These drugs have a specific action on the heat-regulating centers but do not eliminate the cause of the fever. Their administration may be designated at specific times or the order may leave the time of their administration to the nurse's judgment. It is not unusual for antipyretic drugs to be given when a patient's temperature reaches 38.9° C (102° F). When a patient who has a fever is receiving antibiotics, these are usually administered at regular intervals in order to maintain a therapeutic drug level in the patient's body. The use of antibiotics for patients with infections reduces the fever by eliminating the cause of it—that is, the infection within the body.

Tepid Sponge Bath. When it is considered desirable to lower the patient's temperature rapidly, a tepid sponge bath may be given. This is a simple and reliable nursing measure that can be employed either in a home situation or in the hospital. It is carried out on the order of a physician. The technique is based on the principle that the body loses heat through the mechanisms of conduction to a cooler substance, in this case the tepid water, evaporation of water from the surface of the body, and convection of the heat away from exposed body surfaces during the bathing process.

Prior to the bath, the temperature, pulse, and respirations are taken. These observations are important for the subsequent evaluation of the effectiveness of the bath. There are many ways of giving a tepid sponge bath. One way is described here.

The equipment required for the tepid sponge bath consists of a basin of water 30 to 38°C (85 to 100°F), towels, wash cloth, bath blanket, and isopropanol rubbing compound. To initiate this nursing care intervention the top bedclothes are fan-folded to the foot of the bed, and the patient is draped with his bath blanket. Then his gown is removed and his body is sponged. Heat is lost from the body as water is sponged onto the body surface and some of the water is permitted to evaporate. Large areas are sponged at a time, for example, one side of the leg, one side of the arm, the chest and the abdomen. Long strokes are used on the legs and on the back. Because the blood vessels are close to the body surface in the axillae, the wrists, and the groins, the cooling effect of the bath is enhanced by applying the wet cloths there for an extended period of time, that is, by slowing down the bathing process in these areas. A gentle patting motion is used to dry each area; brisk rubbing increases the activity of the cells and therefore the rate of heat production. The back of the patient is then gently rubbed with the isopropanol rubbing compound before the gown and covers are replaced.

The temperature, pulse, and respirations are taken 20 minutes after the sponge bath. The bath is usually repeated until the patient's temperature has reached the level designated by the physician. If the physician's order does not in-

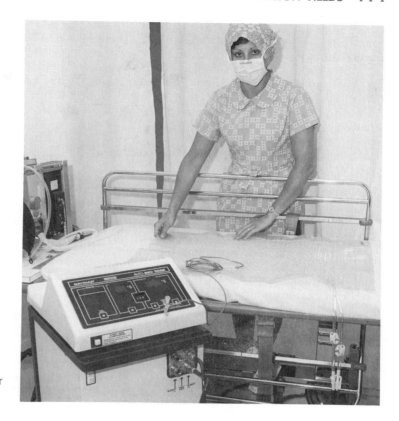

Hypothermia machines are used to lower body temperatures quickly.

clude the temperature at which treatment is to be discontinued, the bath should be stopped before the normal temperature is reached. A further drop in temperature may be expected to occur after it is discontinued.

Sometimes an alcohol bath is ordered, because alcohol evaporates at a lower temperature than water and thus hastens the cooling process. In this case, isopropanol is substituted for the water or, in some instances, may be added to the water. If alcohol is used, the procedure is always terminated before the temperature reaches normal.

A nursing intervention which is somewhat similar to the tepid sponge bath is the use of a wet sheet and a fan to increase heat elimination from the body. The patient is covered only by a sheet that has been dampened with water. A fan is so directed that there is constant movement of air over the sheet. This measure promotes evaporation and convection and thereby increases heat loss from the body. This is a rather drastic measure and is used only in exceptional circumstances.

Hypothermia Machines. Many hospitals have a hypothermia machine, which is used for rapid surface cooling of the body. This machine may be used for patients who have temperatures of 39.4°C (103°F) and over when it is felt that it is essential to bring the body temperature down

quickly or when there has been brain damage to the heat-regulating centers and it is necessary to maintain artificial cooling of the body over a prolonged period of time.

This technique uses the mechanisms of radiation and conduction. The patient is placed on or between cooling blankets, which are attached to a refrigerating machine. The blankets contain coils in which a refrigerant circulates. A considerable amount of heat is lost from the body through direct conduction to the cooling substance and through the radiation of heat waves from the body to the cooler blankets.

Because some people shiver in response to the application of the hypothermia blanket, drugs are sometimes given to minimize shivering. Patients receiving hypothermia treatment frequently need a great deal of reassurance and explanation about the treatment. It is a most uncomfortable procedure, according to people who have experienced it.

Applications of Heat and Cold

Applications of heat and cold as therapeutic measures are probably well known to the student before she commences her nursing education. Applying a hot water bottle or a heating pad to cold feet is a comfort familiar to many, particularly to those who live in cold climates.

The application of ice as a means of stopping nosebleed (epistaxis) is a common therapeutic measure carried out in the home. In addition, rubbing the chest with a decongestant ointment or a liniment is a traditional remedy for the treatment of colds in many families. The student herself has probably already had firsthand experience with many of these therapeutic measures.

Generally speaking, applications of heat and cold are used in health agencies and in the home as therapeutic measures. In the hospital, these measures are carried out at the direction of the physician. Occasionally heat and cold also serve as comfort measures. If this is the sole reason for their use, it is often left to the judgment of the nurse and patient whether and how to apply them. The nurse therefore needs a knowledge of the physiological reactions resulting from these measures and of the untoward reactions which may occur. If the nurse is ever in doubt about the use of heat or cold, she should consult the physician before she applies these measures.

Applications of heat and cold are also used in the course of physical medicine as part of rehabilitation programs. In these instances physical therapists use such measures as paraffin baths and whirlpool baths on the advice of the physician.

Types of Applications. Heat and cold are relative degrees of temperature dependent to some extent upon the perception of the individual. The temperature at the surface of the skin of the torso is generally 33.9°C (93°F).

Applications at this temperature are usually undifferentiated as either cold or hot, but applications that are 11.1°C (20°F) below or 8.3°C (15°F) above this level excite cutaneous nerve fibers. Local tolerance is thought to range between 4.4°C (40°F) and 43.3°C (110°F). Generally any application that is above or below these levels can be the cause of tissue damage.

Temperature is perceived in gradations: cold to cool, tepid, indifferent, and warm to very, very hot. Different areas of the body have varying sensitivity to changes in heat and cold. For example, the back of the hand is not particularly sensitive to changes in temperature. Also, people perceive the temperature more acutely when the temperature of the skin is changing. That is why a hot bath feels hotter at first than it does after the skin becomes adjusted to it. Extremes in temperatures, both hot and cold, are perceived as painful (see Chapter 21).

Many different types of hot and cold applications can be used as therapeutic measures. Both heat and cold can be applied as dry treatments or as moist treatments, and the source can be varied according to the purpose. Moreover, irritants and counterirritants are quite similar in action to applications of heat. An *irritant* is a substance that, when applied to a patient's skin, produces a local inflammatory reaction through its chemical action. An irritant becomes a *counterirritant* when the purpose of its application is a reflex action in underlying tissues, that is, when the purpose of the treatment is to initiate a physiological reaction in tissues underlying the skin. Mustard is a common example of a counterirritant that has had a long history of use as a local application (mustard plaster) to relieve congestion in the chest.

The choice of the kind of application that is to be used is dependent upon a number of factors:

1. The purpose of the application
2. The age of the patient and the condition of his skin
3. The general physical health of the patient
4. The area of the body that is affected
5. The duration of the treatment
6. The availability of equipment

Reasons for the Application of Heat. Heat is applied to the body for any of several reasons. It can be applied to produce a local or a systemic effect or both. A local effect is one that is specific to a defined area of the body, for example, to relieve local muscle spasm. A systemic effect is one that is reflected in the body as a whole—for example, general warmth felt throughout the body.

Heat is known to relieve pain. Thus, pain that is caused by the contraction of muscle fibers is relieved when the muscle spasm is reduced by heat. Heat also increases circulation to an area and can thereby relieve the pain of ischemia (lack of blood). Sometimes the collection of fluid in an area can cause pain because of the increased pressure. The swelling can be reduced by the application of heat. As blood circulation improves, fluid is more easily absorbed from the tissues and consequently swelling or edema is reduced. Frequently hot applications to a swollen area, such as the ankle, are alternated with cold applications, because heat and cold are most effective while the temperature of the area is changing. The cold in this instance reduces the flow of fluid to the swollen area.

Toxins and waste products are also thought to be causes of discomfort which can be relieved by an increase in blood circulation to the irritated tissues.

The fact that heat helps to alleviate many types of pain does not mean that it is indicated for all instances of pain. Heat can hasten the suppurative (pus-forming) process, and in the case of an inflamed appendix it could cause the appendix to rupture. Although the physician supplies the directions regarding the application of heat, the nurse must always be aware of the purpose of the treatment and alert to possible untoward actions. There is, for instance, always a danger that a burn may result from the local application of heat, or that deeper-lying tissues may be affected and an inflammatory process aggravated. Inflammation is the reaction of tissues to injury; it is characterized by pain, swelling, redness, and local heat.

Heat increases circulation to the area of the body to which it is applied. It therefore can be applied to improve the oxygenation and nourishment of tissues, thus aiding tissue metabolism and subsequent healing. For example, heat applied to an infected surgical incision not only hastens suppuration but also increases the nourishment of the tissue cells and the healing process. Improved circulation in this case also enhances the elimination of toxic and waste substances via the blood stream.

Another purpose of applying heat locally is to soften exudates. An exudate is a discharge produced by the body tissues. Sometimes the discharge from an open wound forms hardened crusts over the area. Hot moist compresses are often used to soften these crusts so they can be easily removed. It has already been mentioned that heat is also used as a comfort measure. It can be used to promote the relaxation of skeletal muscles and thereby to promote general comfort and rest.

Reasons for the Application of Cold. Cold is applied to the body for both systemic and local effects. For systemic purposes, cold is applied to slow the basal metabolic rate. This is indicated in certain kinds of heart surgery, because a low basal metabolic rate results in a lessened demand of the body tissues for oxygen and nourishment and thus decreases the work of the heart. For a similar reason a patient's limb may be packed in ice prior to amputation. The cold slows the speed of the circulation of the blood and thus enables the surgeon to control bleeding more easily during the operation.

Cold can also be applied to stop hemorrhage, since it constricts the peripheral arterioles and increases the viscosity of the blood, in addition to contracting the muscles and depressing cardiac action. The nurse often sees ice bags applied routinely to patients after a tonsillectomy as a prophylactic measure against hemorrhage.

Cold applications slow the suppurative process and the absorption of tissue fluids. They also reduce swelling, such as that in a sprained ankle, and slow other inflammatory processes, such as inflammation of the eye.

Because cold contracts the peripheral blood vessels, it raises the blood pressure. This is more usually a side effect than the sole reason for cold applications.

Pain can also be relieved through the use of cold applications. Cold restricts the movement of the blood and tissue fluids; therefore it relieves pain caused by an increased amount of fluid moving into the tissues, as in the case of a sprain. In addition, intense cold numbs pain receptors. As a result cold is used as a local anesthetic. There is, however, a danger in the prolonged use of intense cold: it interferes with the supply of oxygen and nourishment to the tissues and may result in tissue death.

PRINCIPLES RELEVANT TO THE THERAPEUTIC USE OF HEAT AND COLD

1. Heat is distributed throughout the body by the circulating blood and by direct conduction throughout the tissues.
2. Heat is lost from the body chiefly through conduction, convection, and evaporation at the surface of the skin.
3. The amount of heat that is lost from the body is directly proportional to the amount of blood that is circulating close to the surface of the skin.
4. The amount of blood that circulates close to the surface of the skin is influenced by the dilatation and constriction of peripheral arterioles.
5. Applications of heat and cold influence the dilatation and constriction of peripheral blood vessels.
6. Moisture conducts heat better than air.
7. People vary in their ability to tolerate heat and cold. People at both extremes of the age spectrum—that is, the very old and the very young—are particularly sensitive to heat and cold.
8. People become less sensitive to repeated applications of heat and cold.
9. The length of time of exposure to extremes in temperature affects the body's tolerance of the temperature.

Local Applications of Heat. Heat can be applied to a patient as radiant heat, conductive heat, or conversive heat. *Radiant heat* is heat whose wavelength is in the infrared portion of the electromagnetic spectrum.[5] A commonly used example is the infrared lamp. *Conductive heat* is heat transferred by direct application—for example, by a hot water bottle or hot compresses. *Conversive heat* is heat converted from primary sources of energy—for example, from short wave or ultrasound wave energy. The application of this latter type of heat is classified as medical diathermy; it is utilized to provide heat to deep tissues. Radiant and conductive heat provide heat to the superficial tissues only.

Both moist and dry forms of heat can be applied to the skin or mucous membranes. Usually it is necessary to apply superficial heat for 20 to 30 minutes in order to obtain the desired effect.

Since patients become accustomed to heat after prolonged applications, they should be cautioned against turning up a heating pad or refilling a hot water bottle without checking the temperature. All patients are observed closely for any untoward reactions to heat applications, such as a prolonged erythema (redness), blister formation, or discomfort.

The Hot Water Bottle. The hot water bottle has long been a vehicle for applying dry heat to the body. It is used as both a therapeutic and a comfort measure, although therapeutically its use is being surpassed by the electrical heating pad. Some hospitals and other inpatient health agencies have prohibited the use of hot water bottles because of the ever-present danger of burns to patients.

The water for a hot water bottle is tested for its exact temperature. Fifty-eight degrees C (135° F) is generally considered to be a desirable temperature for an adult whose sensations and circulation are intact. A temperature of 50° C (120° F) is considered safe for children and for adults who are unconscious or debilitated or who have impaired circulation. The water for a hot water bottle can usually be obtained from the hot water tap; its temperature is checked by the thermometers that most hospitals provide for measuring the temperature of unsterile solutions.

The hot water bottle is filled one-half to two-thirds full, and the air is expelled from the remainder of the bottle by pressing the sides together before the top is applied. In this way the hot water bottle remains fairly light and is easily molded to the patient's body.

After the outside of the hot water bottle has been dried, it is tested for leakage and then placed in a cloth cover before it is taken to the patient. The cover slows the transmission of heat, absorbs perspiration, and thereby lessens the danger of burning. The stopper of the hot water bottle is well covered, because it can become sufficiently hot that on direct contact it will burn a person's skin.

The hot water bottle is placed on the desired area and molded to the patient's body. If the hot water bottle is given to a person who burns easily, it is wise to place a sheet or blanket between the person and the bottle. When continuous heat is to be applied, it is usually necessary to change the hot water bottle every 1½ to 2 hours in order to maintain the desired temperature.

When hot water bottles are not in use they are hung upside down with the top unscrewed. This allows the bottle to dry inside and prevents the sides of the bottles from sticking together.

The Electric Pad. Electric pads and electric blankets are frequently used as a means of providing dry heat. They have the advantages of being light, of being easily molded to the patient's body, and of providing constant heat. Their disadvantages are related to cleaning and to the danger of short circuits, particularly when they are used with oxygen equipment. The heating pads that are used in hospitals are frequently covered with a plastic material that can be easily and effectively cleaned. It is often possible to lock the mechanism for setting the temperature of the heating pad so that it cannot be changed without the nurse being aware of it.

The Infrared Lamp. The infrared lamp, which supplies radiant heat, is used to provide heat to a localized area of the body. Infrared radiation penetrates 3 mm. of tissue at the most; thus it provides surface heat only.

The action of infrared heat is to increase blood circulation (hyperemia), thereby increasing the supply of oxygen and nourishment to the tissues. An infrared lamp is frequently used in the treatment of decubitus ulcers (bedsores). It is also often used in obstetrical and gynecological cases to promote the healing of a suture area on the perineum.

Before applying heat from an infrared lamp, the nurse makes sure that the patient's skin is dry and clean. This lessens the danger of burning the skin. A small infrared lamp is placed 45 to 60 cm. (18 to 24 inches) from the area of skin that is to be treated; a larger lamp is placed 60 to 75 cm. (24 to 30 inches) away. The heat is provided for from 15 to 20 minutes, but the patient is checked after the first 5 minutes to make sure that he is not being burned. At the end of the treatment the patient's skin is generally moist, warm, and pink.

The danger in the use of the infrared lamp is

that the patient will be burned. The nurse should frequently observe the patient's reaction to the application of infrared heat and terminate the treatment at the first sign of reddening or pain. In addition the patient should be warned that the lamp will become hot after it has been on for a few minutes. Placing an infrared lamp under the bedclothes is inadvisable because of the danger of fire.

The "Baker" (Heat Cradle).

The "baker" is another means of providing radiant heat. In this case the heat is less localized; it is often applied to large areas, such as the abdomen, chest, or legs. The baker is a metal cradle into which are installed several electrical sockets for luminous bulbs. The metal acts to reflect the heat from the bulbs toward the patient. Often the baker is covered by the top bedding in order to hold in the heat and to prevent cooling by the circulating air. The temperature of the baker should not exceed 52° C (125° F).

Steam Inhalations.

In the care of patients with respiratory conditions, steam inhalations are frequently used to loosen congestion and to help liquefy secretions. Both hot and cold steam are used. The topic of inhalations was discussed in Chapter 18.

The Hot Compress.

Hot compresses, which utilize the principle of heat conduction, can be either sterile or unsterile moist applications. Generally gauze is soaked in the solution ordered, the excess fluid is wrung out of the gauze,

Heat in the form of steam inhalations is often used to relieve the congestion of a cold. A young child must be protected against contact with the hot water and steam.

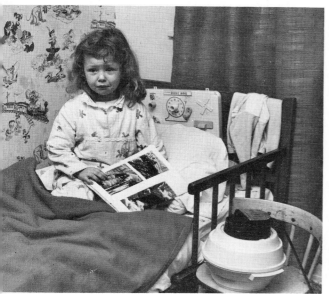

and the gauze is then applied to the specified body surface. The compress should be moist but not so wet that the solution drips from it. Sterile precautions are indicated when the compress is to be applied to an open wound or to an organ such as the eye. In such cases, sterile gauze is soaked in a sterile or antiseptic solution, and sterile forceps or sterile gloved hands are used to wring out the compress. The compress is applied at the hottest temperature that the patient can tolerate. Frequently an insulating waterproof cloth is placed over the compress in order to hold in the heat. In some situations heating pads or hot water bottles are placed over the compress to provide additional heat.

Hot compresses are often indicated to hasten the suppurative process and to improve the circulation of blood to the tissues. Normal saline and antiseptic solutions are frequently ordered by the physician.

Compresses generally retain heat poorly, the length of time that they remain hot being somewhat dependent upon the thickness of the material, the temperature of the solution, and the use of insulating materials. Ordinarily compresses are ordered every hour or every 2 hours; however, if constant applications of hot moist compresses are ordered, the nurse or the patient should change them every 10 to 15 minutes.

The Hot Pack.

A hot pack, which is sometimes referred to as a hot fomentation or foment, is a piece of heated moist flannel or similar material that is applied to a patient's skin in order to provide superficial moist heat. It is used for a larger area than the hot compress. Because intense heat can be applied in this manner, there is a danger that the patient may be burned. This danger is minimized if the hot pack is sufficiently dry that water does not drip from it.

A hot pack can be prepared by boiling or steaming pieces of flannel or by heating commercially prepared packs. If the flannel is boiled it is necessary to wring it out before applying it. There are hot pack machines available which steam the flannel to prepare it for application. Once the foment has been heated, it is applied directly to the patient as hot as he can tolerate it. If the hot pack is shaken slightly before it is applied, there is little danger of burning the patient and it is more comfortable for him. Sometimes petrolatum is applied to the skin beforehand to serve as a protective coating and to slow the transfer of heat. The hot foment is covered with an insulating waterproof material and then secured to the patient with a towel or binder. Often a hot water bottle or heating pad is applied over this to provide additional heat.

A hot pack usually keeps hot for 10 to 15 minutes. Once it has cooled it is removed and, if continuous heat is required, it is replaced with another pack. If the patient does not need another application for some time, his skin is dried.

Hot packs are frequently indicated to relieve muscle spasm, as when a patient has poliomyelitis. They are also applied to hasten the suppurative process and to decrease muscle soreness.

Upon the application of a hot pack, an erythema of the skin is to be expected as a result of the dilatation of the local blood capillaries. Blistering of the skin should be avoided.

Body Soaks.   Body soaks and arm and foot soaks are therapeutic measures ordered by the physician to provide warmth or to apply a solution to cleanse an area of the body. Generally they are indicated to hasten suppuration, to cleanse an open wound, or to apply a medicated solution to a designated area.

Special portable containers, including both arm and foot baths, are available commercially for this purpose. These containers can be sterilized in order to provide a sterile environment when one is indicated, as when burned areas need to be soaked.

The solution for a body soak is ordered by the physician. Often sterile normal saline or sterile water is used. The temperature of the solution should be 47.2° C (115° F) unless otherwise ordered by the physician for a specific reason.

The patient's dressings are removed and his limb is immersed gradually into the solution. The dressings may need to be soaked before removal to avoid trauma to the tissues. The limb is immersed slowly in order to acclimatize the patient to the temperature of the solution. The patient assumes a comfortable position during the treatment to avoid fatigue and muscle strain. The length of the treatment is usually 20 minutes. The temperature of the solution is checked every 5 minutes, and additional solution is supplied when necessary. After the soaking is completed, the patient's limb is dried and dressings are replaced as necessary.

If the patient has an open wound, aseptic technique is carried out. The container, the solution, and the towels are sterile. In some agencies, the nurse wears a mask when carrying out this procedure. Sterile dressings are applied after the soak (see Chapter 27).

During and after soaking of an area of the body, the nurse observes the condition of the patient's wound and the amount and character of any discharge. It is expected that the heat of the solution will cause some vasodilatation and erythema and that the solution itself will cleanse and soften exudates. These observations are then recorded.

The Therapeutic Bath.   Therapeutic baths are provided to supply warmth, to cleanse, and to apply a medication. They are indicated chiefly for people who have skin diseases or who have had certain kinds of perineal or rectal surgery.

The solutions that are used are ordered by the physician; the most common are saline, tap water, sodium bicarbonate, starch, and oatmeal. The last three, often called colloid baths, can now be purchased commercially in special preparations.

The temperature for the therapeutic bath can vary from 4.4 to 47.2° C (40 to 115° F). The temperature ranges of the baths are generally classified as follows:

Hot bath 40.6–47.2° C (105–115° F)
Warm bath 38.9–40.6°C (100–105° F)
Tepid bath 36.7° C (98° F)
Cold bath 4.4–21.1° C (40–70°F)

Unless otherwise ordered, the bath is generally given at a temperature of 36.7° C (98° F)—a tepid bath.

A bathtub contains approximately 30 gallons of fluid when it is two-thirds full. The nurse may need this information in order to calculate the correct amount of medication to be added to a bath. For example, a normal saline solution requires 40 g. of sodium chloride to 4 liters of water (1½ ounces to 1 gallon). The following quantities of medication are for a bathtub two-thirds full.

Medication	Amount or Strength
Sodium bicarbonate	250 g.
	(8 ounces)
Potassium permanganate	1:20,000
Sodium chloride	1200 g.
	(45 ounces)
Tar	60 ml.

Once the patient's bath is drawn, the ordered medication is added and the temperature is checked. Then the patient is assisted into the tub. Generally a male patient prefers an orderly or male nurse to help him. Usually the patient remains in the bath for 15 minutes, and he is checked regularly for any untoward reactions. If the patient complains of vertigo (dizziness) or syncope (fainting), the bath should be terminated at once. The water should be drained off and the patient assisted from the tub as soon as he is over the attack. The nurse should not attempt to move the patient when he is feeling dizzy or faint. She should always obtain assistance as needed to ensure the patient's safety.

The patient's skin is patted dry with a soft towel after a medicated cutaneous bath. If dressings are necessary, new ones are applied.

The sitz bath is a special bath the purposes of

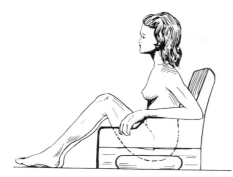

Adequate support aids the patient in being as comfortable as possible in a sitz bath. (From Lucile A. Wood and Beverly Rambo, eds.: *Nursing Skills in Allied Health Services.* Vol. 1. Philadelphia, W. B. Saunders Co., 1977.)

which are chiefly to provide warmth, to cleanse, and to provide comfort to the patient's perineal area. It is often indicated after rectal or perineal surgery.

There are several commercially manufactured sitz baths available. Some models fit over toilets, on chairs, or on beds. There are also comfort seats that can be placed in bathtubs, as well as separate sitz bath units.

The sitz bath is generally ordered with saline solution or tap water. The temperature is 38.9° to 40.6° C (100° to 105° F), and the patient stays in it for 10 to 20 minutes. The nurse makes sure that the perineal region of the patient is immersed if he is seated in a bathtub or that his perineal area is being irrigated if he is seated in a commercial sitz bath.

Usually patients who require sitz baths have recently had rectal or perineal surgery and therefore comfort is an important concern. Adequate support during the bath is also essential. The patient may require help during the bath, particularly if there is any doubt about his ability to tolerate the bath. The patient's pulse is taken 5 minutes after the start of the bath; if it is unduly accelerated or irregular, he should return to bed, and the nurse then reports this to the physician.

In recording a sitz bath on the patient's chart, the nurse records the appearance of the patient's wound, the amount and character of the discharge, and any untoward reactions experienced by the patient, as well as the time of the treatment and the nature of treatment itself.

The Ultraviolet Lamp.
Ultraviolet radiation is also used clinically to treat wounds and skin diseases. The sun is a natural source of ultraviolet light, but artificial sources are used therapeutically. The hot quartz mercury lamp, the carbon arc lamp, and, of course, the sun lamp are all used.

Generally, ultraviolet radiation is carried out

in a special department, such as the physical therapy department. The normal skin reaction produces an erythema, tanning, and a proliferation of the cells of the epidermis.

If the patient needs ultraviolet treatments, the physician generally orders them every other day for maximum effect. Fair-skinned people are more sensitive to ultraviolet radiation than dark-skinned people. Sulfanilamide medications increase this sensitivity.

Diathermy.
Medical diathermy is the provision of heat to the deep tissues of the body by transforming certain kinds of physical energy into heat in the deep tissues. It is usually done in a physical therapy department under the direction of a physician.

Various types of high frequency currents are used: short wave, microwave, and ultrasound. The treatment is painless, the patient's chief perception being one of warmth. It is used for much the same reasons as superficial heat.

Local Applications of Cold

The Ice Bag.
The ice bag or ice cap and the ice collar are commonly used means of applying dry cold to the body. An ice collar is a long narrow rubber or plastic bag that fits around the neck.

Ice bags are usually made with an opening through which small pieces of ice are inserted. Once the ice bag is filled, the air is expelled before the top of the ice bag is secured. The air is removed in order that the ice bag can be molded to the patient's body.

Before the flannel cover is put on, the bag is dried. The cover retains cold for more gradual application and it absorbs the water formed by atmospheric condensation. The bag is placed on the area of the body to be cooled.

Generally, ice bags need to be refilled when all the ice has melted or as ordered. If continuous ice applications are ordered, the ice bag is checked once an hour to see that the cold is maintained.

When an ice bag is in place, the pressure of the bag should not cut off circulation. At the first sign of tissue numbness and a mottled bluish appearance, the bag should be removed and the physician notified. These signs could be the result of either the cold or pressure upon the tissues.

Cold applications are often alternated with hot applications, or the cold applications are spaced in such a way that the tissue warms between applications. The alternate contraction and dilatation of the blood vessels is a highly effective method of inducing hyperemia and increasing tissue fluid absorption.

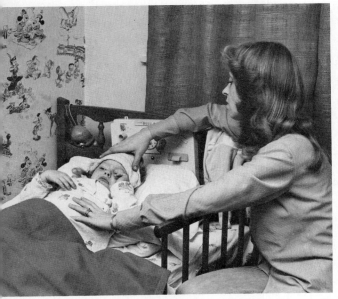

A moist cold compress is used by this mother to soothe her feverish child.

When ice bags are not in use they are stored with the tops removed so that the air will dry the inside and prevent the sides from sticking together.

The Ice Compress.   Moist cold can be applied by means of ice compresses. These are frequently used to terminate a nosebleed (epistaxis) or to supply moist cold to the eye.

An ice compress is usually made of gauze or other cloth material. The gauze is cooled over ice chips, wrung out, and then applied. It is replaced as it becomes warm. Another method of applying a moist cold compress is to place some chipped ice in a cloth bag, which is then placed directly over the area to be cooled. The disadvantage of this is that as the ice melts the water drips on the patient.

Just as in the application of the ice bag, the patient's skin is observed for any signs of untoward effects of the cold. Prolonged vasoconstriction can result in venous congestion and subsequent tissue anoxia. If the patient's skin maintains a bluish, mottled appearance for several hours, there is danger of permanent damage to the cells.

Most hospitals have ice-making machines and ice crushers to break the ice into small pieces. The chips of ice are used in ice applications because they mold easily to the body and are more comfortable.

The Ice Pack.   Ice packs are used occasionally to lower the body temperature or to lower the temperature of a patient's limb prior to surgery.

It is done in some types of open heart surgery, and it is usually carried out in the operating room.

On a hospital nursing unit the nurse occasionally sees a patient's limb packed in ice in preparation for amputation. A special container is available commercially for this purpose. The patient's leg (or arm) is wrapped in cloth and placed in the container. Chips of ice are then packed around the limb. It is important that the patient be given the explanation of the procedure that he requires and that the ice be kept around the limb for the prescribed length of time.

Applications of Irritants and Counterirritants.   Many kinds of preparations are available for administration as irritants. The purpose of some irritants is merely to cause hyperemia through surface vasodilatation (rubefacients), whereas others have been used to produce blisters (vesicants) or abscesses (pustulants). The latter two kinds of irritants are rarely used today.

An irritant is applied gently to the designated surface area. Following its application the area is observed every 5 minutes, the irritant being left on for 20 minutes unless otherwise specified. Irritants are washed off gently with warm water and soap and the skin is patted dry.

An irritant becomes a counterirritant when its primary purpose is to relieve underlying congestion or pain.

Of the many counterirritants that were used in the past, such as the linseed poultice, flaxseed poultice, and mustard plaster, the mustard plaster is the one still used occasionally today. The mustard plaster (mustard sinapism) is a mixture of mustard, flour, and warm water. Hot water is not used because it inactivates enzymes in the mustard. The proportions vary according to the age of the individual:

Infant: 1 part mustard, 12 parts flour
Child: 1 part mustard, 8 parts flour
Adult: 1 part mustard, 3 parts flour

The skin is observed after the application has been on for 5 minutes; if it is reddened, the plaster is removed. At the end of the treatment (20 minutes) the skin should appear reddened but not blistered. People with fair skin tend to burn easily and should be checked frequently to make sure that the skin does not show signs of burning. After the mustard plaster has been removed and the patient's skin has been washed and dried, petrolatum or olive oil is applied to the skin to soothe it.

Mustard plasters can be purchased commercially. The precautions just mentioned should also be followed when using these preparations.

GUIDE TO ASSESSING DISTURBANCES OF BODY TEMPERATURE

1. What is the patient's temperature? His pulse and respiratory rate?
2. Are these abnormal in view of the time of day, the patient's activities, and other physiological factors that might cause a slight or temporary deviation from the normal TPR?
3. Has the patient had prolonged exposure to excessively hot or cold environmental temperatures?
4. Is immediate nursing or medical intervention indicated?
5. Does the patient show signs that he is having a chill?
6. What is the color of the patient's skin? Does it feel warm? cool to the touch? or cold?
7. Is the patient perspiring?
8. Does he complain of any physical symptoms such as headache or fatigue? pain? absence of sensation in any part of the body?
9. Is the patient able to tolerate food and fluids?
10. Is the patient losing excessive amounts of fluid through perspiration or increased respirations? Is his urine normal in color and amount?
11. Does he appear dehydrated?
12. What does his tongue look like?
13. Is the patient restless, irritable? Are there signs of mental confusion?
14. What medications have been prescribed for this patient?

GUIDE TO EVALUATING THE EFFECTIVENESS OF NURSING INTERVENTION

1. Has the patient's temperature come down? gone up? Is it within safe limits?
2. Is his fluid intake adequate for his needs?
3. Is his nourishment adequate?
4. Is the patient comfortable?
5. Is he getting sufficient rest?
6. Is his skin in good condition? His mouth?

GUIDE TO ASSESSING THERAPEUTIC APPLICATIONS OF HEAT OR COLD

1. Does the patient understand the purpose of the treatment?
2. What precautions need to be taken to protect the patient from harm?
3. Is he aware of the dangers?
4. Does the patient require added safety precautions because of his age, his general physical condition, the condition of his skin or his mental state?
5. Is the patient able to participate in his treatment? Is this desirable?

6. Are there specific skills that the patient (or his family) needs to learn or knowledge that he needs to gain in order to carry out the treatment at home?

7. Is the patient safe during the application?

8. Is he comfortable?

9. Is the hot or cold application producing the desired physiological effect, for example, increased circulation to the part, or relief of pain?

STUDY SITUATION (1)

Mrs. S. James is a 34-year-old woman who works as an aide in one of the city hospitals. She is married and has a 5-year-old son. Mrs. James is admitted to the hospital with an elevated temperature of unknown etiology. Her temperature at admission was 39.1° C (102.4° F), her pulse 100, and her respirations 24. The patient had a chill during her first evening in the hospital, when her fever rose to 40° C (104° F). The following morning she felt improved, but she still perspired profusely and in the evening appeared restless and flushed.

The doctor left orders that Mrs. James was to have a tepid sponge bath and aspirin gr. x̄ if her temperature rose above 39.4° C (103° F). He also asked the patient to drink at least one glass of fluid every hour of the day.

1. What factors are relevant to your explanation of a tepid sponge bath to this patient?

2. How can the patient's production of body heat be minimized?

3. How can the loss of body heat be facilitated?

4. What is the action of aspirin gr. x̄?

5. How should you evaluate the effectiveness of the nursing care?

6. Why did the doctor want Mrs. James to drink at least one glass of fluid every hour?

7. What observations would indicate to the nurse that the patient is taking insufficient fluid?

8. Describe an environment which would be therapeutic for this patient.

STUDY SITUATION (2)

Mrs. J. Watson has an infected cut on her right hand. She is at home and the physician has ordered hot soaks for her hand. As the public health nurse you have been asked to assist Mrs. Watson. This patient is 75 years old and she has poor blood circulation.

1. What are the specific problems of this patient in relation to her infected cut?

2. What factors should you take into consideration in helping to plan this patient care?

3. What physiological reactions are to be expected as a result of the hot soaks?

4. How could the effectiveness of the soaks be evaluated?

5. What specific precautions should be taken? Why?

6. Outline the objectives and a plan of care for this patient.

SUGGESTED READINGS

Burn Care. Nursing Photobook. Dealing with Emergencies. Intermed. Communications.

Capobianco, J. A.: How to Safeguard the Infant against Life-threatening Heat Loss. *Nursing 80,* *10*(5):64–67, October, 1980.

Castle, M., and Watkins, J.: Fever: Understanding a Sinister Sign. *Nursing 79, 9*(2):26–33, September, 1980.

DeLapp, T. D.: Taking the Bite out of Frostbite and Other Cold Weather Injuries. *American Journal of Nursing, 80*(1):56–60, January, 1980.

Eoff, M. J., and Joyce, B.: Temperature Measurements in Children. *American Journal of Nursing, 81*:(3):1010–1011, March, 1981.

Gedrose, J.: Prevention and Treatment of Hypothermia and Frostbite. *Nursing 80, 10*(2):34–36, October, 1980.

Schumann, L.: Commonsense Guide to Topical Burn Therapy. *Nursing 79, 9*(3):34–39, March, 1979.

REFERENCES

1. Guyton, A. C.: *Textbook of Medical Physiology.* 6th ed. Philadelphia, W. B. Saunders Company, 1981.

2. MacBryde, C. M., and Blacklow, R. S. (eds.): *Signs and Symptoms: Applied Pathologic Physiology and Clinical Interpretation.* 5th ed. Philadelphia, J. B. Lippincott Company, 1970.

3. Cain, H. D.: *Flint's Emergency Treatment and Management.* 6th ed. Philadelphia, W. B. Saunders Company, 1980.

4. Carswell, H.: Accidental Hypothermia: A Matter of Turning the Scoreboard Around. *The Medical Post,* November 12, 1974, p. 15.

5. Rusk, H. A.: Rehabilitation Medicine. 2nd ed. St. Louis, C. V. Mosby Company, 1964.

20

The Nurse Should Be Able to:

- Discuss the importance of comfort, rest, and sleep to the health and well-being of the individual
- Describe the characteristics of the five stages of sleep
- Discuss normal patterns of rest and sleep throughout the life cycle
- Explain the relationship between illness and sleep disturbances
- Identify factors interfering with a patient's comfort, rest, and sleep
- Identify common sleep problems
- Determine priorities for nursing actions related to the patient's comfort, rest, and sleep
- Apply relevant principles in planning and implementing nursing interventions in patients
    a. to promote their comfort, rest, and sleep
    b. to prevent problems from developing
    c. to restore normal patterns of rest and sleep in people with problems in this regard
- Evaluate the effectiveness of nursing interventions

COMFORT, REST, AND SLEEP NEEDS

CHAPTER 20

INTRODUCTION

Comfort has been defined as "a state of ease or well-being."[1] When a person is comfortable, he is at ease with himself and with his environment. Rest is synonymous with repose or relaxation and implies freedom from emotional tension as well as physical discomfort. Sleep is a period of decreased mental alertness and lessened physical activity which is a part of the rhythmical daily pattern of all living creatures.

Discomfort can result from stimuli of both psychosocial and physical origin. A person who is afraid or worried is uncomfortable, as is one who is cold or in pain.

There are innumerable causes of emotional discomfort; many have been mentioned earlier in this text. For example, the newly admitted hospital patient is subjected to the stresses that accompany going into any strange environment. The ill person often fears pain, death, and disability, and he worries about his ability to cope with forthcoming stresses. Neglect by the nursing staff or care by an unyielding, unconcerned nurse also contributes to a patient's discomfort. The patient looks to the nurse for understanding and support in order to attain some degree of psychological comfort.

Physical discomforts can cause mental distress and interfere with a person's psychosocial equilibrium. Pain, nausea, heat, and even an untidy environment are stimuli that the patient finds uncomfortable and sometimes unbearable. By the selection of appropriate interventions, the nurse can prevent the development of many situations that could be a source of discomfort. Many discomforts can be alleviated if they do occur. The nurse should, therefore, be alert to the earliest signs of discomfort in a patient and aware of interventions that can be used to relieve discomfort or prevent it from increasing.

The nurse has many resources at her disposal to relieve a patient's discomfort, but it is only through a systematic approach to the problem that the effective measure or measures can be selected. It is important that the nurse record her observations of the results of her nursing interventions in order that other members of the health team may be made aware of her findings and can avail themselves of this knowledge for the patient's benefit. For example, some people like the head of the bed elevated to a certain degree; others like it flat. If there are no therapeutic reasons to the contrary, the bed should be maintained at the elevation the patient finds most comfortable.

Interventions vary in their effect from one person to another. Consequently the nurse should find the measure or combination of measures that is most effective for a specific patient.

Rest does not necessarily mean inactivity. People often find a change of activity as relaxing as sitting or lying down to rest. The person who has a sedentary job, for example, may find that physical activity in the form of a leisurely walk, skating, or swimming is relaxing and restful for him. The person who has been physically active all day may obtain his rest in watching television, reading, playing cards, or just sitting down and talking with his family or friends. People who are ill also find these same activities sometimes more restful than lying in bed with nothing to do.

Freedom from anxiety is important in rest, as it is in comfort. This subject is discussed in Chapter 30, so we will not go into it further here.

Sleep is an essential part of our lives and takes up approximately one third of our time. All body cells need a period of inactivity to refresh and renew themselves. It has been found, too, that sleep is essential for growth and the repair of body tissue. The secretion of the human growth hormone is increased during sleep, as is that of some other hormones (for example, testosterone in early puberty).[2]

Whether everyone needs the full recommended 8 hours of sleep a night is currently under debate. A survey by Hartmann and others at the Sleep and Dream Laboratory in the United States would seem to cast some doubt on this. These investigators found that people who usually sleep less than 6 hours a night appeared better able to cope with their daily activities than those who slept for long periods. The "short-sleepers" were generally efficient, energetic people who worked hard, felt good in the morning, and were socially adept, decisive people who were happy with their lives and their work. "Long sleepers," that is, those who slept 9 hours or more, tended to be worriers. They also had many aches and pains, discomforts, and concerns, and were not very sure of themselves, their careers, or their lifestyles.[3]

NORMAL FUNCTIONING IN REGARD TO SLEEP AND REST

Human bodily functions follow a pattern over the course of a 24-hour period that has been called a "circadian rhythm," a term derived from two Latin words: *circa,* meaning "about," and *dies,* meaning "day." It is as if the human body had been constructed with a biological time clock that regulates its activities. Body temperature, pulse rate, and blood pressure all fluctuate during the course of a day, usually being lowest during the early morning hours. The circadian rhythm varies in different individuals. Some people awaken bright and alert in the morning; others do not begin to function at their best until 9 or 10 o'clock. It is believed that this is due to temporal differences in the low point of an individual's temperature. People whose lowest body temperature occurs late in their sleep period find it difficult to get up in the morning and take longer to "get going." These are the ones who are irritable and cross, or uncommunicative, until after their legendary first cup of coffee. In general, however, reaction time for most people is slower in the early morning than later in the day. Efficiency peaks about 11 a.m. when body temperature is usually approaching its highest. At this time, a person's metabolism is up and his energy reaches its greatest level.

Our sleep and wakefulness periods occur in a regular cyclical fashion. The human "biological clock" is made up of cycles of approximately 90 minutes in length. Infants are believed to have a biological cycle of 60 minutes. Elephants, if you are interested, are said to have a biological cycle of 120 minutes.

Stages of Sleep

Sleep occurs in 90-minute cycles in the adult human being. There are usually four to six 90-minute cycles in a person's normal sleep time. In addition, there are believed to be five stages in each 90-minute sleep cycle. These stages have been identified from readings on an electroencephalogram (EEG), which provides a graphic representation of the electrical waves emanating from the brain.

As an individual is dropping off to sleep, he begins to feel relaxed and drowsy. His vital signs, such as heart and pulse rate, become slower, and his body temperature becomes lower. Alpha waves begin to form on the EEG. As he enters the first stage of sleep, the individual may experience a sudden jerk.

In *Stage 1 sleep,* the vital signs become even slower and the muscles more relaxed. The EEG reading becomes very flat. At this point, however, the individual is easily aroused.

He becomes a little harder to waken as he enters *Stage 2 sleep.* Some activity appears on the EEG and the individual can still be aroused fairly easily, although he is in a more completely relaxed state.

A person in *Stage 3 sleep* is difficult to rouse. His blood pressure and body temperature have dropped and the EEG waves appear larger and slower.

As the individual enters *Stage 4 sleep,* delta waves begin to appear on the EEG. The person is completely relaxed and may not move. It is extremely difficult to awaken a person in this stage of sleep. It is believed that it is during this stage that the increase in release of the hormone regulating growth and promoting tissue healing occurs. Bedwetting and sleepwalking are most likely to occur during this stage.

After the individual has completed Stage 4, it is thought that he retraces the cycle back to Stage 2 and then enters REM sleep, that is, *Stage 5.* REM sleep is a light sleep; this is the time when dreaming occurs. Vital signs fluctuate and the eyes move rapidly back and forth, which is the reason for the name given to this stage (rapid eye movement or REM for short). There is, however, increased muscular relaxation, particularly in the face and neck. The EEG reading is similar to that of a person in a waking state in deep

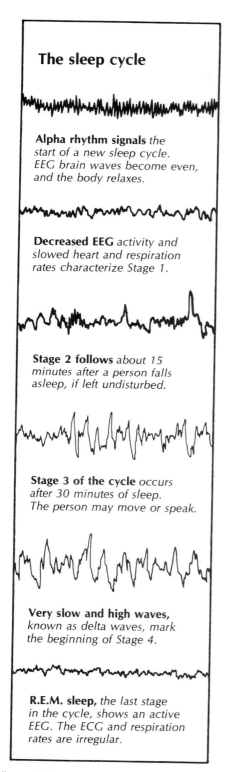

The sleep cycle

Alpha rhythm signals *the start of a new sleep cycle. EEG brain waves become even, and the body relaxes.*

Decreased EEG *activity and slowed heart and respiration rates characterize Stage 1.*

Stage 2 follows *about 15 minutes after a person falls asleep, if left undisturbed.*

Stage 3 of the cycle *occurs after 30 minutes of sleep. The person may move or speak.*

Very slow and high waves, *known as delta waves, mark the beginning of Stage 4.*

R.E.M. sleep, *the last stage in the cycle, shows an active EEG. The ECG and respiration rates are irregular.*

From Albert, I. B., and Albert, S. E.: Penetrating the Mysteries of Sleep and Sleep Disorders. RN, 37:36–39, August, 1974, p. 37.

concentration. During this stage adrenal hormones are released into the blood stream in spurts; these affect vitality, fatigue, metabolism, and the ability to resist infection. They also influence the transmission of nerve impulses. Dreams, which occur during this stage, are believed to promote the psychological integration of daily activities.

With the completion of the REM stage, approximately 90 minutes after falling asleep, the individual recommences the cycle at Stage 2, follows the sequence to Stage 4, returns to Stage 2, and experiences the REM stage. In the final cycle, the individual continues beyond REM to Stage 1, and the individual wakens.

During the first few hours of sleep, the individual will spend more time in Stage 4 than in later cycles, and the length of the REM stage increases toward morning. Hormonal activity also increases toward morning.

Sleep Deprivation

Sleep deprivation has profound effects on an individual's functioning abilities, whether he is in good or ill health. A person deprived of sleep is likely to appear irritable, nervous, or anxious, or he may be apathetic. His thought processes may be impaired; he may have difficulty remembering things, and often he will not respond appropriately to stimuli. Minor troubles may become major problems. His sensory perception may be distorted and he may experience delusions or even hallucinations. It is believed that after 48 hours of sleep loss, the body produces a stress chemical that may account for the behavioral changes.

Deprivation of REM sleep can be especially disturbing for the individual. The adrenal hormones enter the blood stream but not at the proper biological time, causing the person to feel depressed and fatigued, and to have poor powers of concentration. It has been shown that when a person experiences gross deprivation of REM sleep, his body will try to catch up and he may enter the REM stage almost immediately after falling asleep instead of following the stages as they normally occur.

Deprivation of Stage 4 sleep results in a decrease of the growth hormone in the blood stream and will cause the individual to feel tired, depressed, and generally unwell. As this hormone promotes tissue healing, deprivation of Stage 4 sleep can be particularly harmful to persons recovering from illness or injury.

In some instances, it is thought beneficial to depress REM sleep, as in the case of persons suffering from certain heart conditions or peptic ulcers, since most nocturnal attacks occur during the REM stage of sleep.

FACTORS AFFECTING COMFORT, REST, AND SLEEP

Most people have a bedtime ritual that forms part of their sleep habits. It has been reported that a substantial proportion of adult Canadians like to watch the 10 p.m. (10:30 in Newfoundland) national news on television and this is one of their nightly rituals. Many people enjoy a light snack before going to bed. Some like a cup of coffee or tea and find that, for them, it does not interfere with getting to sleep. For many people, a warm bath or shower is part of their nightly ritual. Each person has his own habits in regard to going to bed and getting ready for sleep. Most people also have a particular position they find most comfortable for sleeping. Some like to curl up in a ball; some are "tummy" sleepers; still others prefer a back-lying position.

Interference with these bedtime habits is likely to cause a disturbance in sleep patterns. People who are in a strange environment often find it hard to get to sleep the first night or so. A major change in habit patterns can disturb all body functions, as we mentioned in Chapter 2 in connection with the stress of change. Nurses in the course of their work frequently have to work evening or night shifts, and this disturbs their normal circadian rhythm. It usually takes a few days to accustom oneself to sleeping in the daytime and having one's first meal late in the day. Other people who work shifts also have the same problems.

Excessive stimulation, that is, more excitement than one is usually accustomed to, will make it harder to get to sleep for most people, unless they are exhausted by the stimulation. A lack of sufficient exercise may be another reason some people find it difficult to sleep; the muscles are not tired enough. A person who is hungry often cannot rest. On the other hand, an excessive intake of food, particularly highly seasoned food that may cause problems in digestion, may also interfere with sleep. A larger than usual amount of fluid intake before retiring usually means that an individual has to get up during the night to relieve a distended bladder.

Noise and other disturbances when a person is asleep may arouse him and disturb the cyclical pattern of his sleep. If he is suddenly awakened from deep sleep, he is likely to be confused and disoriented, a condition that has been de-

scribed in the literature as "sleep drunkenness." It appears to be most pronounced in children and in people with sleep disorders.

Many sources of excessive sensory stimulation disturb the comfort, rest, and sleep of hospital patients (see Chapter 22). Often, environmental factors are a problem, such as the warm temperatures of most hospital rooms, the hardness of most hospital pillows, the lights that are turned on, or forgotten to be turned off, the noise of nurses at the nursing station, and the sudden stillness after patients have been awakened by some noise.[4]

Other things that often disturb rest are medications that must be taken at night, and the early morning awakening that is still part of the routine in many hospitals, often followed by a long delay before breakfast is served.

Discomfort of any kind interferes with a person's ability to rest and to sleep. A number of causes of discomfort were discussed in the introduction to this chapter. Pain is, of course, always a deterrent to rest and sleep. Often, however, it is the minor irritations and discomforts that are most troublesome to patients. Discomfort may be physical or psychological. *Anxiety,* about big or little things, is probably the most common cause of inability to rest. A person lies awake and worries, and the worries magnify as sleep eludes him.

Illness and sleep problems go hand in hand. Illness disturbs the normal rhythm of sleep and wakefulness. People who are ill require more sleep because of their need for increased growth hormone to promote tissue repair, but as just stated, their normal sleep pattern is usually disturbed. Sleep deprivation, as we mentioned, can itself be a cause of illness. It is interesting to note that people who have been deprived of sufficient REM sleep usually spend more time in this stage when they are catching up on lost sleep. Apparently dreaming is a very necessary part of our lives.

Drugs will also distort sleep patterns. The reticular formation in the brain is believed to control sleep. Cerebral depressant drugs that induce sleep work in one or more of several ways:

1. They may depress the reticular formation so it no longer responds to stimuli
2. They may depress the response of the cerebral cortex to stimuli from the reticular formation
3. They may cause a specific reduction in the response to stimuli producing wakefulness (for example, anxiety, depression, or pain). Alcohol, for instance, has this effect, as do many of the tranquilizing drugs.

Barbiturates have been widely used for people with sleep problems although they are now being used less frequently. They have a tendency to depress REM sleep, so that the person has an abnormal sleep cycle. A person who is taken off these drugs after having taken them for several days, or fails to take them, usually has a considerable increase in dream activity, and he may be convinced that he never slept at all. Barbiturates also depress parts of the brain that are responsible for inhibitory activity. Hence, they not infrequently have an excitatory effect, somewhat like alcohol. Older people are particularly susceptible to this reaction and may become confused and excited instead of going to sleep when they are given barbiturate sedatives.

SLEEP AND REST THROUGHOUT THE LIFE CYCLE

Often, one of the first changes in bodily function noticed by a pregnant woman is that she is sleepy most of the time. Women seem to require extra sleep during pregnancy, particularly during the first and third trimesters. Their sleep is frequently interrupted, however, because of the need to void, which is caused by a decreased bladder capacity (see Chapter 15). Additional rest is important throughout pregnancy, and a short nap sometime during the day, or a rest lying down, is usually advocated. Keeping the feet elevated when resting helps to combat the mild edema many women experience, particularly during the later stages of pregnancy. Often, however, the woman has difficulty finding a comfortable position for resting when she is "heavy with child" and having difficulty moving her bulky body. Lying on the left side is said to be helpful because it takes pressure off the vena cava and is felt to help in reducing ankle swelling and, also, to increase circulation to the fetus.

The developing infant is said to sleep in utero or, at least, to have rest periods. Newborns fall into a deep sleep almost immediately after birth. Most newborns sleep for an average of 16 hours a day, with the longest uninterrupted sleep being a little over 4 hours. Approximately half of the newborn's sleep is active, characterized by rapid eye movements, a total relaxation of postural muscles, irregular breathing, frequent small movements, sucking, and smiling. The other half of the newborn's sleep is quiet and characterized by a slow and regular pulse, a lack of conjugated (working in unison) eye movements, regular breathing, and a partial relaxation of postural muscles.

The infant continues to spend a large part of his time sleeping throughout the first year of life. It is during this time, however, that diurnal patterns are established and the sleep cycle gradually takes on adult characteristics. By about 6 weeks of age, most infants are sleeping for longer periods during the night than during the day, and by 4 months most are sleeping through the night, with the longest sleep period averaging around 8½ hours. The pattern of the sleep cycle in the 3-month-old infant is beginning to resemble that of the adult. Approximately two thirds of the infant's total sleep is quiet sleep by this time. Most infants are comfortable lying on the stomach, and this position is often advocated because of the disadvantages of sleeping on the back. The back-lying position tends to flatten the infant's head (the bones being still soft and malleable). There is also the danger that the infant can aspirate vomitus and choke when in this position.

Toddlers generally sleep 10 to 14 hours a day in total, and many require two naps a day until they are around 2 years old. During the toddler stage, bedtime rituals become very important. Most children seem to have an extra burst of energy and become overly active when they get tired and, as all mothers know, they become irritable. In establishing good sleeping habits, it is helpful to have a quiet period for the toddler before bedtime, such as reading a story to the child, or engaging in some other quiet activity. A quiet period and consistent bedtime routines are important for all children. Preschool-age children are often apprehensive about being left in the dark, and may need a night light. Nightmares and bedwetting, or enuresis, as mentioned above, are common problems that usually disappear as the child matures (see Chapter 15). By the time a child has reached school age, he is usually sleeping about 11 to 12 hours a night. the amount of sleep required gradually diminishes to around 9 to 10 hours at age 12. Teenagers seem to require longer periods of sleep once again, which is possibly related to their growth needs.

The average healthy adult sleeps about 7 hours a night. As a person gets older, the amount of sleep required seems to lessen. Although the need for rest periods during the day increases, people over the age of 65 years generally sleep less than younger adults, and usually have frequent periods of wakefulness during the night.

COMMON PROBLEMS OF SLEEP

The most common sleep problems are insomnia (inability to get to sleep, or excessive wakefulness), hypersomnia (excessive sleeping), narcolepsy (sudden, irresistible sleep attacks), somnambulism (sleepwalking), enuresis (bed-wetting), and night terrors.

Most people have problems in getting to sleep at some time or another, usually during periods of stress and anxiety; for many people this is a serious problem. *Insomnia* may be symptomatic of illness, or may be caused by anxiety, nervous tension, habitual lifestyle patterns, or any one of a number of causes. People for whom bedtime was not a pleasant experience when they were children—going to bed may have been used as a form of punishment—may become insomniacs later in life. Insomnia is by far the most common of all sleep disturbances.

It is felt that people who have a tendency to *sleep excessively* may be using this as a defense mechanism to escape from anxieties or frustrations in the fulfillment of their basic needs. This, of course, is not always the case; a person who seems to require more than the average amount of sleep should always be referred to a physician for a complete medical examination to see if there are other reasons for the excessive sleeping.

Narcolepsy is a problem that affects a small but significant number of people. The irresistible sleep attack may last from 10 to 20 minutes. The person often has vivid dreams and may often be unable to move on awakening. Accidents are more common among narcoleptics than among the general population, as one might expect. People with this problem are usually prohibited from working with machinery or at occupations where their problem could be a safety hazard. They should also be under medical supervision.[5]

Sleepwalking is more common among men than women. It is also fairly common among children. There is usually a familial tendency to sleepwalking. It tends to occur during Stages 3 and 4 of the sleep cycle; hence people who are sleepwalking are usually confused and disoriented. It is not wise to waken them, but the person should be protected from harming himself.

Nightmares and *night terrors* are common sleep problems in children, reaching their peak in the preschool years. *Nightmares* are felt to be caused by psychological factors, and are, basically, a manifestation of anxiety. They occur during active sleep. When having a nightmare, the child moves restlessly in bed, he may whimper or cry, he grimaces, or his face has an anxious expression. He may or may not wake up. If he does, he is usually easily reassured and goes back to sleep quickly. *Night terrors* are felt to be due to physiological reasons; immaturity of the central nervous system is given as the

probable cause. They occur during deep sleep. The child either sits bolt upright in bed or assumes a bizarre crouching posture, and screams. The child is terrified. His pulse and respirations are rapid, and the pupils of his eyes dilated (manifestations of the flight-fight reaction to danger). Often he is disoriented. Although he may not seem to recognize the person who answers his cries, he can usually be soothed by cuddling and a low, gentle voice reassuring him.[7]

Enuresis, or bedwetting, is a common problem in children and may occur in some adults. It is generally found more frequently in males and in emotionally disturbed children. Some reports indicate that enuresis is more prevalent among children in low socioeconomic groups than in higher ones. It is believed to be caused in many cases by immaturity of the bladder, and many children just "grow out of it." Enuresis should, however, always receive medical attention because it may not be just a developmental problem, but could be a sign of other health problems.[6]

ASSESSING COMFORT, REST, AND SLEEP STATUS

Making sure that patients are comfortable, that they receive sufficient rest, and that they are able to sleep are among the nurse's most important responsibilities. In order to assess the individual's status with regard to comfort, rest, and sleep, the nurse needs information about his usual sleep and rest patterns, specific sleep problems he may have, and the nature of any health problems that may be causing alterations in his sleep patterns.

She also needs to be aware of any restrictions that have been placed on his mobility. Is he confined to bed, for example? Or is he restricted to a certain position in bed for therapeutic reasons or because of the nature of his illness? People with heart conditions and those with respiratory problems are usually most comfortable when sitting up in bed or in a semi-sitting position. This then would be best for them therapeutically. The person with a fracture may have to be flat on his back, as Mr. Jordan (Chapters 8–9) was, or he may have to have the injured appendage maintained in a specific position. The nature of the surgical intervention a patient has had often determines the position he must take in bed. Even an intravenous infusion limits the patient's position in bed.

The nurse also needs to know the physician's plan of care for the patient. She must be aware of the medications the patient is receiving, and the nature of the diagnostic and therapeutic measures planned for the patient. Anxiety is such a common cause of sleep and rest problems that the nurse needs to know if there are any particular worries he has in connection with his health, real or imagined health problems, and whether he has reasons for worry about these. It is helpful also to know of any other stresses which may be causing the patient anxiety (see Chapter 30).

Information about usual sleep patterns, chronic disorders, and the present comfort, rest, and sleep status of the patient are available to the nurse from the nursing history and the initial nursing clinical appraisal. The patient's record provides information about the nature of his current health problems, and the physician's plan of care. Reports of diagnostic tests will also be found there, as well as requests for consultation by specialists and their reports. Medication the patient is receiving will be listed on the doctor's order sheet; the nurse needs to be aware also of medications the patient may have been taking at home, since drugs may distort sleep patterns, as we discussed above.

The nurse supplements this information through her objective observations. Many people are aware of the sources of their discomfort, and, when given the opportunity, will make them known. The nurse who communicates her understanding of the patient's problems and who takes the time to listen to him can frequently identify specific sources of worry and discomfort. Then she can take steps to relieve them.

There are other avenues of expression besides the verbal ones, of course. The patient who is uncomfortable may appear restless, pale, or tense; he may perspire profusely or lie rigidly in bed. All in all, there are a multitude of ways of expressing discomfort, and the nurse needs to be aware of them and alert to their possible meanings.

The person who is unable to sleep may communicate this verbally to the nurse, but she must also watch for the signs of sleep deprivation in the patient, as previously described. Nurses make frequent rounds of patients when they are on the night tours of duty and they note patients who are having difficulty getting to sleep or are wakeful during the night. Nurses on the day staff always check the night nurse's report to see if their patients had disturbed sleep during the night. The nurse also observes patients during the day and evening shift to see if they are getting sufficient rest and the extra sleep needed in illness.

PRIORITIES FOR NURSING ACTION

All aspects of promoting comfort, rest, and sleep are priority items insofar as nursing action is concerned. Particularly with ill patients, in whom rest and sleep are essential components of their therapy, the nurse must do everything possible to ensure that factors causing the patient discomfort or interfering with his rest and sleep are eliminated, or minimized if they cannot be eliminated entirely. Factors that will increase comfort, and promote rest and sleep, should be well known to the nurse so that she can assess the relative merits of specific actions to help each particular patient. This aspect of nursing care is considered so important that, in some agencies, the nurses have developed "sleep care plans" for patients.[4] This would seem to be a good way of ensuring that a definite series of nursing activities are planned to help each patient obtain adequate sleep. Interventions that nurses have found helpful for a particular patient are communicated to others so that there is consistency in the approach used by all nursing personnel.

GOALS FOR NURSING ACTION

The principal goals of nursing action with regard to the patient's comfort, rest, and sleep status are:

1. To promote comfort
2. To prevent discomfort
3. To alleviate discomfort
4. To ensure that the patient has rest
5. To assist the patient to obtain an adequate amount of sleep to meet his requirements.

NURSING INTERVENTIONS TO PROMOTE COMFORT, REST, AND SLEEP

There are innumerable nursing interventions that nurses have found helpful in making patients comfortable and promoting their rest and sleep. Every experienced nurse has a repertoire of interventions that she has tried with patients and can tell you those that she has found to be successful. The beginning nurse must learn these, and she will find older, more experienced nurses very good sources of information about comfort measures and aids to promoting rest and sleep for patients.

Some general considerations might prove helpful to the student; these will be given first, and then we will discuss specific nursing interventions.

PRINCIPLES RELEVANT TO COMFORT, REST, AND SLEEP

1. **Definite periods of sleep are an essential component of the circadian rhythm in human beings.**
2. **Adequate amounts of sleep are needed for optimal physical and psychosocial functioning of the individual.**
3. **Growing persons require more sleep than others.**
4. **Individual needs for sleep vary with age, growth patterns, health status, and individual differences.**
5. **Lack of sufficient sleep impairs a person's physical functioning, his mental alertness, and his social relationships.**
6. **Individual habits vary with regard to bedtime rituals.**
7. **Sleep patterns may be disturbed by changes in a person's normal daily living patterns, by social and emotional problems, by physical problems, and by minor irritations or discomforts, as well as by pain.**
8. **Sleep patterns are almost invariably disturbed by illness.**

General Considerations

People usually get to sleep more quickly and sleep better when their lifestyle permits regular habits for mealtimes, work or school hours, periods of relaxation, and bedtime hours. Adequate nutrition and adequate exercise are important in promoting restful sleep. People should be encouraged to pursue restful and relaxing activities prior to preparing themselves for sleep. Many people have found specific relaxing techniques helpful (see Chapter 30). Tea and coffee are both stimulants, and most people find it best to avoid these prior to bedtime. Almost everyone has an occasional sleepless night. If the sleeplessness continues, however, for more than one or two nights, one should consult a physician for a thorough investigation of the problem and assistance in resolving it.

The sick person finds his normal patterns of daily living disrupted. It is helpful to provide diversional activities during the day, if these are not ruled out by his health problem, so that he does not sleep too much in the daytime and find himself unable to sleep at night. Morning naps are considered to be more beneficial than afternoon ones, because they are a continuation of the light REM sleep, whereas if a person sleeps in the afternoon, it is often a heavy sleep from which he wakens feeling groggy.

If some of the usual bedtime rituals can be maintained for the patient, he will feel more secure and better able to rest. The dietary department should be alerted to his usual bedtime snack and, if he is used to having a bath or shower before retiring, he should be given opportunity to continue this practice if his condition permits.

Patients should be offered a bedpan or a urinal if they are unable to go to the bathroom themselves, or should be assisted to the bathroom, so that they can wash their hands and face and clean their teeth, which are part of most people's bedtime rituals at home.

Some people are very fond of their own pillow, and may find hospital pillows hard. There would seem to be no reason why the patient could not have his own pillow if he so desired. A familiar object or routine helps to promote security. A person may like the pillows arranged in a certain way; the head of the bed elevated to a certain angle; his position just so; his clock turned so he can see it during the night. It is small things like these that contribute so much to a person's comfort.

The nurse will find that it is worthwhile to spend a few extra minutes "settling" patients and attending to all the small details that are important to them. They will rest better and they are not so apt to need additional help later on in the evening or during the night.

Most people find a back massage soothing and an aid to sleep. For some, relaxing techniques are helpful. Besides the relaxing exercises, a number of techniques for learning to control tension in the muscles and bring relaxation have been developed. The nurse will find reference to some of these in articles listed in the suggested readings at the end of the chapter.

If hypnotic (sleep-inducing) drugs have been ordered, they should be given a few minutes before the lights are turned out. Analgesics to relieve pain should be administered sufficiently early for them to take effect before the hypnotic is given. This enhances the effects of the hypnotic.[4]

When the patient is "settled," and all details attended to, the lights should be dimmed. Noise should be kept to a minimum, and the patient not disturbed unless absolutely necessary.

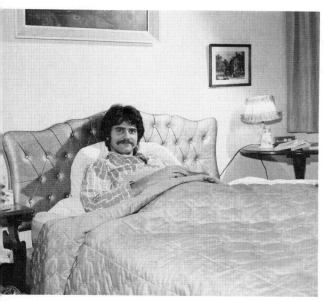

For the person who is ill at home or in the hospital, much of his comfort depends on the condition of his bed.

The Bed of the Ill Person

The bed is especially important to most people who are ill. To the patient in the hospital, the bed may be the one thing that he feels is entirely his. Moreover, much of a patient's comfort is dependent upon the condition of his bed, particularly if he is in it for long periods of time. When a patient appears to be unduly particular about his bed, the nurse should remember that he may spend 24 hours of his day in it. To him a neat, clean, and wrinkle-free bed is necessary for comfort. Other patients who are exacting in regard to their beds and bed units may be clinging to a position from which they can control some aspect of their environment at a time when they believe that many decisions and activities are beyond their control. The ill patient's horizons often narrow, and matters about which he normally would have no concern become important.

Traditionally, the hospital bed is made in the morning after the patient's bath. When the bed is made, soiled linen is changed and the entire bed is aired and remade. It is equally important that linen be changed whenever it becomes damp or soiled. Soiled or wet linen predisposes a patient to skin breakdown and to infections.

Types of Beds According to Purpose. There are several ways of making a bed and each has its purpose. The *closed bed,* which is defined as an empty bed, is made after its occupant is discharged from the hospital. In a closed bed the spread extends over the bedclothes to the top of the mattress and the pillows are placed on top of the spread. In some hospitals the spread covers the pillows as well as the entire mattress.

The *open bed* refers to a bed that has been assigned to a patient. It may be prepared for a new patient, or may be made for any patient who is out of bed. The spread is folded back with the blankets, and the top sheet is turned back on the spread. One side of the top bedclothes is sometimes turned back so that the patient can get into the bed easily.

The *occupied bed,* as its name implies, refers to a bed that is occupied by a patient. Generally in this situation the person must remain in bed continuously, even while the nurse is making the bed. It is important for the nurse to learn to change linen and make a bed smoothly and quickly while the patient remains in it. Often the patient in an occupied bed is seriously ill and a great deal of activity is contraindicated.

The *anesthetic bed* or *recovery bed,* a variation of the basic hospital bed, is used for the patient immediately after surgery. Its purpose is to provide a clean area into which a patient can be easily moved. It is also important that the bed linen can be easily changed, with a minimum of disturbance to the patient. Frequently this type of bed is made in such a way that a part of it can be changed without remaking the entire bed; for example, a separate short sheet might be placed under the patient's head in such a manner that it can be removed when it is soiled without disturbing the rest of the bedclothes.

The *diagonal toe bed* is designed to expose the leg or foot of the patient and at the same time to provide warmth and adequate covering. A variation of the open bed, it is often used to air wet casts and for the patient whose leg is in traction. In the latter situation, ropes and pulleys extend from the patient's leg over the end of the bed, thus making it impossible to completely tuck the covers under the mattress at the foot of the bed.

Linen for the Hospital Bed. The linen required for the basic hospital bed comprises two sheets, two pillowcases, one plastic or rubber drawsheet (optional), one cotton drawsheet (optional), one or two blankets, and one spread. (Blankets are also optional.)

Cotton and rubber drawsheets have been traditionally used on the sick person's bed for two reasons: They are easier to change than the bottom sheet, and they protect the mattress. With the availability of plastic-covered mattresses, however, an increasing use of cotton mattress pads (similar to the ones that are commonly used in the home), the routine use of drawsheets, both rubber (or plastic) and cotton, is disappearing. In many agencies the use of drawsheets is now reserved for the beds of patients who need them; they are no longer put on every bed.

When a plastic or rubber drawsheet is used, it is placed under a cotton drawsheet since the rubber (or plastic) retains heat and is uncomfortable. The drawsheet usually extends from above the patient's waist to his midthigh. Thus it can serve to absorb secretions in cases of urinary or fecal incontinence.

The cotton that is used for sheets, pillowcases, and drawsheets must be of a heavy weight that wears well in spite of strong pulling and frequent washing. Moreover, because linen is often washed in disinfectant solutions in order to kill microorganisms, a heavy weight is necessary to withstand the laundering.

The blankets that are used in hospitals and most other health agencies are frequently made of a loose cotton weave or a mixture of flannel and cotton. The blankets should be able to withstand frequent washings without damage or shrinkage. In many hospitals, the temperature of patients' rooms is such that no blankets are needed. However, blankets are sometimes necessary for warmth. Usually one or two blankets suffice. An extra blanket is sometimes used as a throw blanket over the spread. Blankets should never be used by more than one patient because of the danger of transferring microorganisms from one patient to another. The extra blanket can be rolled and stored at the foot of the bed, fanfolded down to the bottom of the bed, or put in the patient's closet until he wishes to use it. Elderly patients are often more sensitive to the cold than younger patients and require more covers for warmth.

Changing the Hospital Bed. There are two basic procedures in changing a hospital bed: stripping the bed and making the bed. When the nurse is changing a bed, she should remember that microorganisms are present in the environment and be aware of the methods by which they are spread. The following principles should be kept in mind.

1. Microorganisms are present on the skin and in the general environment.
2. Some microorganisms are opportunists; that is, they can cause infections when conditions are favorable. For example, a break in the skin or mucous membrane of the patient may become a site of infection.
3. Patients are often less resistant to infections than healthy people because of the stress resulting from an existent disease process.
4. Microorganisms can be transferred from one person to another or from one place to another by air, by inanimate objects, or by direct contact among people. The nurse should therefore avoid holding soiled linen against her uniform, should never shake linen, and should wash her hands before going to another patient.

The use of good body mechanics is also important in making a bed. The principles that underlie body movements in helping the patient to move are equally applicable in bedmaking (see Chapter 23). Some guides based on these principles are useful here:

1. *Maintain good body alignment.* For example, the nurse stands facing the direction in which she is working and works in such a way that she does not twist her body.
2. *Use the large muscles of the body rather than the small muscles.* For example, flexing the knees in order to bring the body to a comfortable working level is preferable to bending at the waist. The former uses the large abdominal and gluteus muscles, whereas the latter puts strain upon the back muscles and shifts the center of gravity outside the base of support.
3. *Work smoothly and rhythmically.* This is less fatiguing because the muscles are alternately contracted and relaxed.
4. *Push or pull rather than lift* because it requires less effort.
5. *Using your own weight to counteract the weight of an object decreases the effort and strain.* If the nurse shifts her weight when she is pulling a mattress, it requires less effort than if she pulls the mattress with her arms. In addition, she places little strain upon her back and arm muscles.

The method used for stripping and making a bed differs from place to place. Basically, however, every health agency wants the end product to be neat, clean, comfortable, and durable, and the bed-changing process to be economical in use of time, equipment, and the patient's and nurse's energies. The following methods are suggested as guides to the student.

Stripping the Bed. Stripping a bed necessitates removing the linen and detachable equipment from the bed.

1. *Obtain the necessary equipment.* Usually the nurse brings the linen and equipment needed to make the bed at the same time as that required to strip it. Clean linen for the bed and equipment for patient hygiene can often be collected at the same time. The fresh linen is placed on the bedside chair in the order in which it is to be used. Generally all that is needed to strip a bed is a receptacle for soiled linen. Some

hospitals provide a small hamper cart, which the nurse takes to the door of the patient's room and into which she places the soiled linen. Care must be taken that microorganisms are not transferred by means of the hamper cart from one patient to another. Ideally, a linen hamper is provided for each patient.

If hampers are not provided, the nurse can tie the bedspread by its corners to the post at the foot of the bed to serve as a receptacle for soiled linen. Placing soiled linen on the floor increases the possibility of spreading microorganisms.

The nurse can avoid extra trips by taking several bundles of linen out to the linen hamper at one time. The nurse would also be wise to bring all her clean linen and clean equipment at one time in order to save time and effort. (See the procedures for making the open bed.)

2. *Remove the equipment from the bed.* First the nurse places the patient's bedside chair beside his bed. The back of the chair is in line with the foot of the bed and the front faces the head of the bed. Sufficient room is left between the chair and the bed for the nurse to pass in order to save her steps when she goes around the foot of the bed. If a chair is not available, a movable table may be used. The patient's call light, refuse bag, and so on are detached from the bed and placed on the bedside table. The patient's pillows are placed on the seat of the bedside chair; soiled pillowcases are put in the linen hamper.

3. *Remove the linen from the bed.* Starting at the head of the bed, the nurse loosens the top and bottom bedding from the mattress as she walks around the bed. When she returns to the first side of the bed, she grasps the spread at the center and near side and folds it to the bottom of the bed. She then picks up the spread at the center and lays it folded in quarters across the back of the bedside chair. This step is repeated for the blankets and the sheets, if they are to be reused. None of the linen should touch the floor.

If drawsheets are used they are folded with as little contact as possible and then picked up in the center and placed over the back of the chair. The reason for folding linen in such a manner is that it is ready to be placed back on the bed with a minimum of movement. Conservation of energy and movement is important to a nurse's efficiency and to the quality of her care. The remaining linen that is not to be reused is rolled into itself and discarded into the laundry hamper or linen bag.

4. *Turn the mattress.* After the linen has been removed from the bed, the mattress may be turned from side to side, if the nurse feels this is needed, and pulled to the head of the bed. By grasping the lugs at the side of the mattress and

by using good body mechanics, the nurse can turn a mattress with little effort.

5. The nurse washes her hands when she has finished stripping the bed and before putting on the clean linen. The used linen and the mattress harbor microorganisms that should not be transferred to clean linen.

Making the Open Bed. Frequently patients who are in bed much of the day are able to get up while the nurse makes the bed. However, the decision regarding the patient's activity is usually the physician's, and the nurse should not help a patient out of bed unless there is a written order. Because a patient states that he feels well enough to get up is not sufficient reason for him to do so. On the other hand, even though the patient has permission to get up, his condition may change and the nurse may suggest that he stay in bed.

1. *Make the bed.* The bottom sheet is placed on the bottom half of the mattress in such a way that the open edge is away from the center and the sheet just hangs over the bottom edge of the mattress. The sheet is then opened to the head of the bed and centered over the mattress. The sheet is tucked under the mattress at the head of the bed and the corner is mitered or squared on one side. The sheet is then tucked in smoothly along the sides. To miter the corner of a sheet the following steps are performed.

a. Tuck the sheet in securely under the mattress at the head of the bed.
b. Lift the sheet at A (see illustration above), and bring it along the side of the mattress.
c. Grasp the sheet at B and bring this point directly up, releasing the sheet at A.
d. Tuck in the part of the sheet that hangs below the mattress.
e. Bring B down firmly and tuck under the mattress. The underfold of the corner (C) should be even with the edge of the mattress.

To square a corner means to tuck in the end of the sheet and then to fold the side under so that the fold runs parallel to the corner and gives a boxed appearance to the corner.

After the bottom sheet has been tucked in on one side of the bed, the drawsheets are placed on the bed if they are indicated. They are tucked in on the near side.

The top sheet is then placed across the foundation near the foot and opened so that the bottom half of the bed is covered. It is then carried to the head of the bed until the edge of the sheet is even with the edge of the mattress. The blankets and bedspread are applied in the

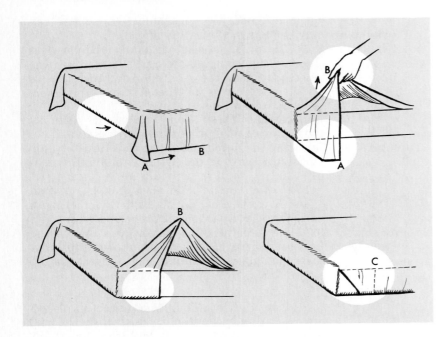

Mitering a corner.

same manner but are brought to within approximately 23 cm. (9 inches) of the edge of the mattress.

When the bed has been made completely on one side, the other side is made up in the same manner. The foundation is pulled tight so that it is free of wrinkles. Wrinkles are uncomfortable and can be irritating to the skin. Many agencies now use contour (fitted) sheets, which make it easier to provide a firm wrinkle-free foundation for the bed.

The head of the bed is completed by folding back the top covers. The pillows are replaced on the bed.

2. *Replace the equipment.* Before the nurse leaves the bedside she replaces any equipment that the patient requires. This includes attaching the signal light to the bed, placing the bedside chair beside the bed, and arranging the bedside table within the patient's reach. All unnecessary equipment is removed, and small articles that the patient is not using are placed safely in his bedside table. The nurse should ask the patient's permission before discarding any of his belongings, including flowers.

Making the Closed Bed. The procedure is usually carried out by staff of the housekeeping department. In some situations, however, it may be a nursing responsibility. To make a closed bed the nurse follows the same method as for an open bed except that the spread is brought to the head of the bed so that it is even with the top sheet, and the top sheet and blanket are not folded back. There are many variations of this pattern in hospitals.

Making the Occupied Bed. Making an occupied bed is similar to making an open bed except that the nurse is concerned with maintaining the patient's body alignment, safety, and comfort. It is preferable to make the bed while the bed is level; however, some patients are unable to assume the supine position because of their condition—for example, because of difficulty in breathing. In such cases, the nurse is challenged to make a comfortable, neat bed while the head of the bed is elevated. Although the physician usually orders the position in which the patient is to be maintained, it is often the nurse's decision whether the patient's position can be changed while the bed is made.

When a bed is stripped while the patient remains in it, a pillow is left for the patient's comfort. After the spread and blankets have been removed, a bath blanket is placed over the top sheet, which is then removed by drawing it down from under the bath blanket. If the patient is to be washed, it is done at this time, before the foundation of the bed is changed, to prevent the clean sheet from becoming damp or soiled during the bath.

It is easier to change the foundation of the bed if the patient is moved to the far side of the bed. The foundation on the near side is loosened. If the linen is to be removed, it is folded to the center of the bed. Clean linen is placed on the near side of the bed and tucked in. The patient then rolls over the folded linen to the near side of the bed. The soiled linen is removed, and the clean linen is pulled tightly across the bed and tucked in.

The patient is assisted to the center of the bed

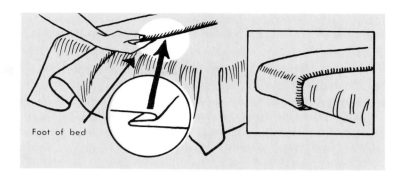

Foot of bed

A vertical toe pleat is made while the nurse is standing at the foot of the bed.

and the second pillow is replaced. The top covers are replaced as for an open bed. The nurse must remember to withdraw the bath blanket after she has put on the top sheet. For some patients, as for example, orthopedic patients in traction, the bed may be made from top to bottom rather than from side to side.

When the nurse replaces the top covers, she should allow sufficient room for the patient to move his feet. Toe pleats in the top covers will provide this extra space for the patient. To make a vertical toe pleat, the upper sheet and the blankets are raised and a 5 cm. (2 inch) fold is made in the sheet and blankets parallel to the foot of the bed. The linen is then tucked in. As an alternative, the nurse can loosen the top covers at the foot of the bed, or the patient can cross his feet before the corners are mitered in order to ensure sufficient foot room.

After the nurse completes the bed she tidies the unit. This involves putting away personal utensils that the patient is not using and placing articles such as his water glass and radio within easy reach. The hospital patient's signal cord is attached to the bed so that it is always within easy reach. It gives the patient a feeling of security to know that the nurse may be easily and quickly summoned.

Today, hospitals often employ a housekeeping staff which is responsible for cleaning the patient's unit. It is the staff's responsibility to clean the bed-unit tables, change the patient's drinking water, and look after his flowers. Floor washers are assigned to clean the hospital floors regularly. In a hospital where a specialized staff is not employed for these purposes, these duties may very likely become the nurse's responsibility. In any case, the nurse is often responsible for checking that the patient's environment is clean and comfortable. It is a good idea for the nurse to stand back and check that everything is neat and tidy and that the patient is comfortable.

Making the Anesthetic Bed (Recovery Bed).

The anesthetic bed is an adaptation of the basic hospital bed. It is customarily made directly after the patient goes to surgery. If the patient is to go to the recovery room (postanesthetic room or P.A.R.) after surgery, the bed is usually taken there so that the patient is transferred to his own bed immediately after the operation is over.

The purpose of the anesthetic bed is to provide a safe, comfortable, and convenient bed for the postsurgical patient. Usually the foundation for an open bed is completed, and then one or two rubber (plastic) and cotton drawsheets are placed over it to protect the bottom sheet. This is done because a short drawsheet is more easily changed than an entire bottom sheet; therefore the patient will be disturbed less if it is necessary to change any part of the foundation of the bed.

The top covers on the anesthetic bed are generally folded back in order to make it easier for the patient to be transferred into the bed. One method of arranging the top covers is to fold the bedclothes up on both sides and both ends. Then all the covers can be quickly folded to one side or the other when the patient is transferred to the bed.

The anesthetic bed is always made with clean linen, as free from microorganisms as possible. A clean bed lessens the danger of infection and is generally more comfortable. If a pillow is needed for the postoperative patient, it should have a plastic covering to protect it from any vomitus and drainage. In many agencies today, all pillows have plastic covers for easy cleaning.

The bed unit for the postoperative patient is arranged for efficiency of care. The patient's personal belongings are put safely away, and the bedside table is left clear. Tissues should be immediately available and a kidney basin should be nearby so that it can be obtained quickly if it is needed. Side rails should be attached to the bed. An intravenous standard should be either attached to the bed or available in the patient's room. Blood pressure equipment is needed also. Since oxygen or suction equipment is often required at the bedside, the nurse must check that a space is set aside for this equipment and that the equipment is ready for the patient when he returns from the operating room.

The Mattress. There are many different kinds of mattresses available for both therapeutic and comfort purposes. The regular mattress for the hospital bed is firm and often covered with a plasticized material. Patients who are allergic to these mattresses require mattresses made of foam rubber. This type offers the patient support but molds somewhat to his body. The foam rubber mattress also has an advantage in that it places less pressure upon the patient's bony prominences. Because of this it is often used in the prevention and treatment of decubitus ulcers in patients who must remain in bed for long periods of time.

Also available are split foam rubber mattresses. These mattresses are divided horizontally into three sections. The sections at the head and foot of the bed are approximately ¾ meter (2½ feet) in length and the middle section ½ meter (1½ feet) in length. The middle section is in turn divided lengthwise into two parts, one of which can be pulled out in order to insert a bedpan without moving the patient. The split foam rubber mattress is generally used for debilitated patients and for those who are unable to move.

A third type of mattress is the alternating pressure mattress, which is run by a small motor. This mattress can be filled with either air or water. Areas of the mattress are alternately deflated and inflated, with the result that there is a continual change in the pressure upon the various parts of the patient's body. These alterations of pressure stimulate circulation to the skin, thus facilitating the nourishment of tissues and the removal of waste products. Before a patient is placed on an alternating pressure mattress he requires an explanation of the use of the mattress and reassurance about his safety. Some patients feel nauseated initially because of the motion, but this usually disappears within several hours. The nurse must also warn the patient and staff to be careful not to prick the mattress with safety pins or sharp instruments. This bed is more effective with only a single layer of linen between the mattress and the patient. Care must be taken not to pinch or shut off the tubing to the motor when the bed is being made.

Another type of bed, the air-fluidized bed, uses the flotation principle to provide uniform support to all parts of the body. The mattress portion of the bed is made of very fine medical-grade optical glass spheres. Air is blown through these spheres to keep them constantly moving,

and the patient experiences a comfortable sensation of floating without feeling unstable.[8]

Sawdust mattresses are also used by some agencies for patients whose movement is limited, to provide more equal distribution of pressure. Gel flotation and Silastic flotation pads are frequently used when the patient is transferred to a normal bed. These pads are often used in home care.

It should be noted that the use of any of these special mattresses or pads is *not* a substitute for nursing care. Patients still need frequent turning, good skin care, and proper positioning, topics we will discuss shortly.

The Overbed Cradle

The overbed cradle is a device that attaches to the mattress of the bed and extends over the top of the bed. It is used to keep the top bed covers off the patient. Some overbed cradles are hoop arrangements which extend from one side of the bed to the other; others extend only to the midline of the bed. Overbed cradles are usually made of metal or plastic.

The primary purpose of the overbed cradle is to keep the weight of the top bedclothes off the patient. Patients who have burns, uncovered wounds, or wet casts often need to keep the top bedclothes away from the injured area. When the nurse is applying a cradle to the patient's bed, she should ensure that it is securely fastened to, or under, the mattress. The cradle is carefully positioned so that the area of the patient's body that is to be free from the weight of the top bed covers is directly under the cradle. The top bedclothes must be pulled up higher than normally so that they cover the shoulders of the patient.

The Footboard

The footboard is a device that is placed toward the foot of the patient's bed to serve as a support for his feet. Some footboards fit onto the bed frame across the foot of the bed; others attach to the sides of the bed frame and thus may rest on the mattress at any point along the bed. Footboards are usually made of wood, plastic, or heavy canvas.

Footboards are also used to keep the weight of the top bedding off the patient's feet as well as to support the patient in maintaining his feet in a neutral position. Normally the feet of the patient who is lying in the dorsal position will be bent into plantar flexion (see Chapter 23). In time, if his feet are not exercised or supported, they may become fixed in plantar flexion. This condition, known as footdrop, is the result of contractures of the gastrocnemius or soleus muscles. With this complication, the patient is unable to stand with his heels on the floor. Footdrop is usually treated by physiotherapy, but sometimes it can be modified only by surgery.

When the nurse applies a footboard to the bed, it is placed so that the patient can rest the soles of his feet against it while the rest of his body is in good alignment. The top bedclothes need to be brought higher up on the bed so that they cover the patient's shoulders. The footboard is securely fastened to the frame of the bed; it usually has to be removed when the foundation of the bed is stripped.

A *footblock* is a block of wood or a box that is placed at the foot of the bed. Its purpose is the same as that of the footboard. The footblock has a disadvantage: it is not adjustable to the height of a patient. On the other hand, it is easily obtainable for the patient who is confined in bed at home.

The Fracture Board

The fracture board (bed board) is a support that is placed under the patient's mattress to give added rigidity to the mattress. It is usually made of wood or of wood and canvas and is constructed to fit the standard hospital bed. One type of fracture board has hinges so that the head and knee gatches of the bed can be used with the board in position. Another type is made of slats, which provide for flexibility so that the head and knee gatches of the bed can be raised or lowered if desired.

The fracture board is used in situations in which the patient needs additional support for his back. Patients who have spinal injuries often have fracture boards ordered by the physician.

The fracture board is easily applied to an unoccupied bed. Usually an orderly can slide the fracture board from a stretcher to the bed, making sure that the hinged joints of the board correspond to the gatches of the bed. The nurse should explain to the patient that the purpose of the board is to provide firmness and thus should not be modified by the extensive use of pillows.

The Balkan Frame

The Balkan frame is a frame made of wood or metal that extends lengthwise above the bed and is supported at either end by a pole. A trapeze may be attached to the frame just above the

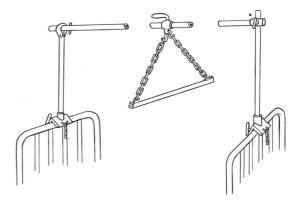

A Balkan frame with trapeze.

patient's head as an aid to the patient in lifting himself up in bed. Often the Balkan frame serves as an attachment for the pulleys and weights of traction equipment, which is used for patients who have fractures of the lower limbs, particularly the femur.

Often the sole purpose of the Balkan frame is to provide a trapeze. Some frames use only one pole when it is necessary to support only a trapeze. The nurse can show the patient how to use this as an exercise device or as an aid in moving.

The Bradford Frame

The Bradford frame is a canvas, stretcher-like device that is supported by blocks on the foundation of the bed. It is often used to immobilize patients who have injured spines. The canvas is divided into three parts so that the small center portion can be removed to insert a bedpan. In many fracture beds the canvas covering of the frame is in strips to facilitate care of the patient.

One of the nurse's responsibilities is to reassure the patient that he is not likely to fall off the frame and that he should lie quietly. Brad-

The Bradford frame. Note the removable canvas strip in the center to allow insertion of a bedpan.

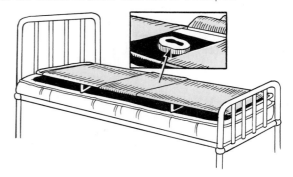

ford frames have been replaced in many instances by Stryker frames and Foster beds.

A number of other beds have been devised for patients who will be helpless for long periods of time and for those with specific health problems, as, for example, the CircOlectric bed, the HighLow Tilt bed, the Rocking bed, and the Chair bed. These are usually discussed in medical-surgical nursing courses and the student is directed to texts in this field for additional information.

Positioning the Patient

Generally patients assume the positions that are most comfortable for them. For the patient who can move easily and freely in bed without therapeutic considerations, the nurse's chief responsibility in regard to his position is his comfort. The astute use of pillows and the provision of a firm foundation will help him remain comfortable.

Patients assume positions for therapeutic reasons as well as for comfort. There are many possible reasons for positioning a patient therapeutically; to maintain good body alignment, to prevent contractures, to promote drainage, to facilitate breathing, and to prevent the development of skin breakdown over bony prominences are but a few.

The physician often prescribes the appropriate therapeutic position for a patient. There are many situations, however, in which the nurse used her judgment as to which position is best. Intelligent assessment of a patient's problems and a knowledge of anatomy and physiology are important bases for such judgments. Also, the nurse needs to be aware of the variety of positions that it is possible for the patient to assume and the supportive measures that promote his comfort in these positions.

The following are guides with which the nurse should be familiar in assisting patients to assume different positions:

1. Positions as close as possible to the basic anatomical position provide good body alignment, which is, of course, desirable.

2. Joints should be maintained in a slightly flexed position. Prolonged extension creates undue muscle tension and strain.

3. Positions should be changed frequently, at least every 2 hours. Prolonged pressure on one area of the skin may cause the skin to break down, with resultant pressure sores (decubitus ulcers). The tolerance of the skin of individual patients is not generally known.

4. All patients require daily exercise unless it is medically contraindicated.

5. When a patient changes his position, his joints should go through the full range of motion unless this too is medically contraindicated.

Anatomical Position. The anatomical position will be discussed in Chapter 23. In positioning patients in bed, the principles of the anatomical position are maintained—that is:

1. Good alignment of all body parts
2. Equal weight distribution of body parts
3. Maximal space in body cavities for internal organs
4. Joints in functional position (for walking, grasping objects, etc.)

Certain positions that do not follow the therapeutically anatomical position fully may be best for some patients. The basic principles should be kept in mind and applied insofar as is possible, however.

Supine (Dorsal Recumbent) Position. In the supine (dorsal recumbent) position the patient lies on his back with his head and shoulders slightly elevated. Usually one pillow suffices for this purpose. The lumbar curvature of the back is best supported by a small pillow or a folded towel if necessary.

If the patient does not have support for his thighs, they will tend to rotate outward. Two rolled towels or a rolled bath blanket tucked in at the lateral aspects of the thighs under the trochanter of the femur will maintain the patient's legs in alignment. His legs should be slightly flexed for maximal comfort. This is attained by placing a small pad under his thighs just above the popliteal space. Direct pressure should be avoided upon the popliteal area because of possible interference with circulation to the extremities and injury to the popliteal nerve. The *trochanter roll* (or hip roll) is often used for this purpose; it is made from a bath

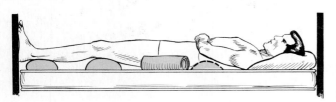

Supine (dorsal recumbent) position with padding for support and to prevent pressure on bony prominences.

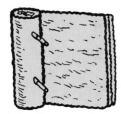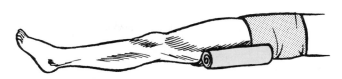

A trochanter roll can be used to prevent external rotation of the hip. The safety pins used to secure the roll initally are placed so that they face away from the patient.

towel. The towel is folded lengthwise once and then rolled to within 6 inches of one end. The roll is secured by two safety pins that are fastened between the body of the roll and the tail of the roll. To support the thigh of the patient so as to prevent external rotation, the tail of the roll is placed under the patient's thigh, with the safety pins away from the patient. The roll is then firmly secured along the patient's leg. Trochanter rolls may also be used to raise a patient's heels off the foundation of the bed.

In the supine position, the patient's feet will normally assume a plantar flexion position. Prolonged positioning in plantar flexion, however, can result in footdrop, a condition in which the gastrocnemius and the soleus muscles remain involuntarily contracted. Preventive measures for this complication include the use of the footboard, which helps the patient to maintain his feet in dorsal flexion and removes the weight of the bedclothes from his toes, and the heel protector, which supports the foot's position as well as providing protection for the heel. Flexion, extension, and circumduction of the patient's ankles help maintain muscle tone and ankle joint mobility.

When the patient is lying in the supine position (and in all positions described subsequently), care should be taken to maintain the fingers in a functioning position, that is, fingers flexed and thumb in opposition. A small hand

The heel protector supports the foot in dorsal flexion and protects the heel simultaneously. (From Lucile A. Wood and Beverly J. Rambo: *Nursing Skills for Allied Health Services*. Vol. 1, 2nd Ed. Philadelphia, W. B. Saunders Co., 1977.)

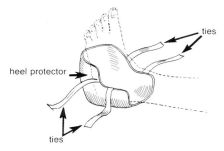

roll may be placed in the palm of the hand and the fingers curved around it. This is particularly important for unconscious patients and for those who have difficulty of movement in one or both hands. Wristdrop must also be prevented. The hand should never be left in a dependent position. It should be supported so that it is in a straight line with the lower arm.

Sponge rubber pads, sheepskin pads, and *small pillows* also serve as supportive devices. Placed under bony prominences, they relieve pressure; placed in the lumbar curve or under a limb, they support or elevate an injured part. A small sponge rubber pad placed in the patient's hand can be used as an exercise implement. It can also be used to prevent severe flexion of the hand and to separate skin surfaces in conditions of spastic contraction. The size of the pad allows slight flexion of the hand and fingers, with the thumb comfortably placed in its normal anatomical position.

Sandbags also serve as a means of providing support to the patient. They are firmer than trochanter rolls and, because of their weight, are less easily moved. For this reason, sandbags are desirable when body alignment must be maintained—for example, in fractures. Sandbags should be pliable so that they can be shaped to the contours of the body.

In some cases, the patient's head and shoulders are not elevated by pillows and rolls. The patient lies on his back with his head and shoulders on the flat surface. Supports similar to those just described are used when indicated.

This position is frequently prescribed for patients who have had spinal anesthetics.

Prone Position. The prone position is a position in which the patient lies on the abdomen with the head turned to one side. Many people are relaxed and sleep well in this position; some find it most comfortable to flex their arms over their heads.

Supportive measures for the patient in this position include a small pillow or pad, as needed, under the abdomen at the level of the diaphragm in order to give support to the lumbar curvature and, in the case of the female patient,

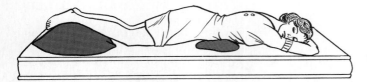

Prone position with padding for support and to prevent pressure on bony prominences. Note that the head is turned to the side and no pillow is provided.

to take weight off the breasts. A small pillow or towel roll under each shoulder helps to maintain the anatomical position. In addition, a pillow under the lower legs elevates the patient's toes off the bed and permits slight flexion of the knees. Alternatively, the patient can extend the toes over the end of the mattress to take the weight off the toes. Plantar flexion is minimized if the patient's lower legs are also supported. When the patient is in a prone position, there is pressure on the knees. A small pad under the thighs can be used to relieve this pressure. Sheepskin or sponge rubber pads may also be used under the knees.

The patient may prefer a pillow for his head. Unless the physician wishes the patient's head on a flat surface, in order to promote drainage of mucus, for example, a small pillow is often more comfortable; however, it should not be so thick as to hyperextend the patient's head.

Lateral (Side-Lying) Position. In the lateral position, the patient lies on his side with both arms forward and his knees and hips flexed. The upper leg is flexed more than the lower leg. Weight is borne by the lateral aspects of the patient's ilium and by his scapula.

The upper knee and hip should be at the same level; the upper elbow and wrist should be at the same level as the upper shoulder to prevent the limbs from being in a dependent position. The patient's heels and ankles may be protected by using small pads (for example, of sheepskin or sponge rubber) to keep them from rubbing on the bedclothes.

If the patient's upper arm falls across his chest, his lung capacity may be restricted; a pillow to support the patient's arm permits greater chest expansion and enables the nurse to readily observe the character and rate of his respirations.

Lateral position. Notice the pillow supporting the patient's upper arm in order to allow for chest expansion.

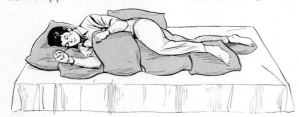

The person who lies laterally will probably prefer a pillow for his head. A pillow of proper depth should prevent lateral flexion of the head. Frequently the patient will also require the support of a pillow placed lengthwise behind his back.

The lateral position is prescribed in order to take weight off the sacrum of the patient; in addition, the patient can eat more easily in this position than in the supine position. It also facilitates some kinds of drainage. Finally, many people find it a relaxing position.

Fowler's Position.* Fowler's position is probably one of the most frequently assumed positions. It is a sitting position in which the head gatch of the patient's bed is raised to at least a 45-degree angle.

In Fowler's position the patient is usually comfortable with at least two pillows for the back and head. The first pillow is best placed far enough down the patient's back to provide support for the lumbar curvature. A second pillow supports the head and shoulders. An emaciated patient will probably need three pillows. For patients who are very weak, pillows placed laterally will support the arms and help to maintain good body alignment.

Small pillows or a pad under the patient's thighs permits slight flexion of the knees, and a footboard permits dorsal flexion and prevents the patient from sliding toward the foot of the bed. Occasionally the knee gatch of the bed is

_____
*In some agencies, Fowler's position refers to the elevation of the upper part of the body without flexion at the hips; any elevation with hip flexion is referred to as the semi-Fowler position.

Fowler's position. Pillows can be provided for the patient's arms if such support is required.

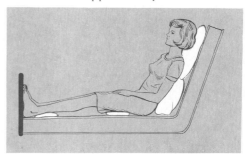

used to support flexion of the knee. If the knee gatch is used, it should not be flexed too much because of the danger of putting pressure on the popliteal nerve and major blood vessels that are close to the skin surface in the popliteal area. Prolonged pressure can cause serious interference with both nerve supply and circulation to the lower limbs. Hence, the knee gatch is seldom used for patients now.

In Fowler's position the main weight-bearing areas of the patient are the heels, sacrum, and posterior aspects of the ilium. The nurse should pay particular attention to these areas when she gives skin care.

Fowler's position is indicated for patients who suffer either cardiac or respiratory distress, since it permits maximal chest expansion.

Two variations of Fowler's position are the *semi-Fowler* and *high Fowler* positions. The semi-Fowler position refers to an elevation of the head of approximately 30 degrees. This is a comfortable position for the patient who must remain with his head and chest slightly elevated. The high Fowler position refers to the full sitting position, that is, with the head of the bed elevated to a 90-degree angle. The head gatches of most hospital beds can be elevated to this height. A position somewhat similar to the high Fowler is the sitting position in which the patient leans over an overbed table upon which several pillows have been placed for comfort. Some patients with respiratory problems find this position makes breathing easier for them. Patients who have difficulty exhaling tend to lean forward to compress the chest for additional force on expiration. The pillows on the overbed table provide support for the arms and help to maintain the individual in as erect a position as possible to increase his total lung capacity.

Sim's Position (Semiprone or ¾ Prone Position). Sims's position is similar to the lateral position except that the patient's weight is on the anterior aspects of the patient's shoulder girdle and hip. The patient's lower arm is behind him, and his upper arm is flexed at the shoulder and elbow. The upper leg is acutely flexed at

the hip and knee, and the lower leg is slightly flexed at the hip and knee.

A rolled pillow placed laterally and in front of the patient's abdomen will support the patient in this position. Pillows for the patient's upper arm and upper leg will prevent adduction of these limbs, and a small pillow for the patient's head will prevent lateral flexion. If, however, the patient is unconscious and the nurse wants to promote mucus drainage from the mouth, a pillow under his head is contraindicated.

In Sims's position the patient's feet naturally assume the plantar flexion position. If the patient is to maintain Sims's position for some time, supports should be provided in order that his feet assume the dorsal flexion position. A footboard or sandbag can be used for this purpose.

Sims's position can be established on both the left side and the right side. The patient's position should be changed frequently; if he is unable to move himself, the nurse can help him turn every 2 hours, or oftener as needed. When turning the patient who is unconscious, the nurse should be sure that the patient's eyelids are closed to prevent the possibility of the cornea's being scratched by the bedclothes. Good skin care, particularly to the anterior aspects of the patient's ilium and shoulder girdle, is also indicated.

This position is prescribed for patients who are either unconscious or unable to swallow. It permits the free drainage of mucus. Sims's position also allows maximal relaxation and is therefore a comfortable sleeping position for many people.

Trendelenburg Position. This position is used for some kinds of surgery and occasionally in situations involving shock and hemorrhage. In the modified Trendelenburg position shown on page 442, the patient lies on her back. The foot of the bed is elevated at a 45-degree angle so that the patient's hips and legs are higher than her shoulders.

This adaptation of the Trendelenburg position is sometimes used for a patient who requires vaginal irrigation. In this procedure it is important that the patient's hips be higher than her chest in order that the irrigating fluid will reach the posterior fornix of the vagina. Draping for this position is similar to that used in the lithotomy position (see Chapter 9).

In a regular Trendelenburg position the foot of the bed is elevated but the patient is not flexed at the waist. This position is also used in some situations when the patient is in shock.

There are other positions for patients, and the nurse will see them used in the nursing unit

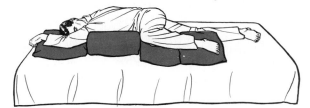

Sims's position (semiprone position). A small pillow may or may not be placed under the patient's head.

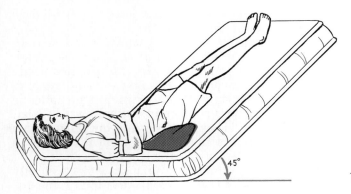

45°

The modified Trendelenburg position.

and in the operating room. But, regardless of the position of the patient, certain principles apply: In positioning the patient in bed, it is most important that the nurse drape the patient adequately. In many situations it is equally important that she change the patient's position frequently. Adequate exercise, good skin care, and supportive measures for maintaining good body alignment should also be carried out.

The Back Massage (Back Rub)

In helping the patient relax in preparation for sleeping, after his bath and at other times as indicated, the patient's back is rubbed with an emollient lotion or cream. Although alcohol was for many years the traditional solution for rubbing the backs of patients in hospital, and is still used in some agencies, it is no longer recommended as a back rub. Alcohol dries and hard-

A soothing back rub helps to relax the patient and promotes comfort and rest.

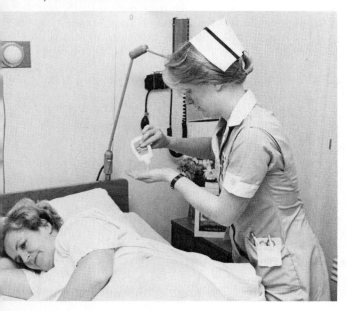

ens the skin, leaving it more susceptible to cracking. This is a particular hazard in the elderly, whose skin tends to be dry and thin, and in patients whose nutritional status or hydration is poor. Emollient creams and lotions are considered preferable. Most agencies have their own preference as to the type of cream or lotion used for back care.

When the nurse gives the patient a back rub, the best position for the patient is the prone position. The side-lying position is the next most preferable. These positions permit the nurse to use long, firm strokes, which are both soothing to the patient and stimulating to the blood circulation. A circular motion over the body prominences of the shoulder blades and at the base of the spine helps to keep the skin in good condition.

When giving a back rub, the nurse should warn the patient that the solution may feel cold. It is more comfortable for the patient if the nurse warms the solution in her hands before she applies it to the patient's back. The nurse starts at the shoulder area and, using the palms of her hands and her fingertips, rubs the patient's neck with circular motions extending to the hairline. This helps to relax the shoulder and neck muscles, which so often are tensed in anxious people. She then moves her hands to the sacral area and repeats the circular motions with the palms of her hand and her fingertips. Then, starting at the sacrum, she rubs up the center of the back to the hairline, using long smooth strokes, then over to the shoulders, where she proceeds down the sides of the back, using broad circular motions. The circular motions are made to increase circulation to these bony prominences. The pressure of the nurse's motions should be sufficiently firm to stimulate the muscle tissue. However, if the patient is very thin or the skin is in poor condition, the nurse should be careful not to use undue pressure in rubbing or massaging. After the circular motions over the shoulders, the nurse brings her hands down to the lower edge of the patient's buttocks and to the patient's

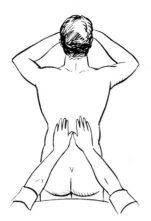

Long, smooth, circular motions increase the blood circulation to the skin.

PLANNING AND EVALUATING NURSING ACTION

Interventions to promote comfort, rest, and sleep are an integral part of nursing care for all patients. A specific "sleep plan," or a sleep and rest plan, is helpful in focusing attention on these important aspects of patient care and in facilitating communication about each individual's needs, preferences, and problems with regard to comfort, rest, and sleep. Expected outcomes for specific interventions are related to each of these three needs. The expected outcomes of comfort measures might be that the patient is comfortable at all times, as evidenced by facial expression, by absence of restlessness and of other outward signs indicative of discomfort, and by verbal expressions that communicate to the nurse that he is comfortable. A decrease in frequency of requests for analgesics (or requests for other things) also helps to indicate to the nurse that the patient is comfortable.

Expected outcomes of interventions to promote rest and sleep relate to the amount of rest and undisturbed sleep the patient has, and to the ease with which he is able to get to sleep. The outcomes then might be expressed in terms of the amount of additional rest considered desirable for the patient, the time taken to get to sleep, the number of hours slept, and the number of times his sleep is interrupted by wakeful periods. A decrease in the last-named might be a criterion for measuring the effectiveness of the nursing interventions taken.

As with nursing interventions used with other problems, the setting down in writing of the expected outcomes in sufficient detail that they can be used as criteria for evaluation by all nursing personnel helps to direct observations used in both assessing and evaluating the patient's comfort, rest, and sleep status.

sacrum, continuing with the broad circular motions. This process is continued until the circulation to the skin has been stimulated and all lotion is rubbed in well. The nurse also rubs the patient's knees, elbows, heels, and any other reddened areas on bony prominences. Care should be taken, however, not to massage reddened areas on the patient's thighs or lower legs. Sometimes, when circulation is poor, a person may develop a clot in one of the blood vessels supplying the limbs. Surface areas in the vicinity of the clot often become reddened, warm to the touch, and tender. Massage may loosen the clot and cause it to circulate in the blood stream. This can be dangerous because the clot may subsequently block another vessel (for example, in the heart), where it can cause much damage. The nurse should always report the presence of reddened areas on the patient's skin and particularly those that may be indicative of clot formation in the blood vessels below the surface.

GUIDE TO ASSESSING COMFORT, REST, AND SLEEP STATUS

1. What are the patient's usual habits in regard to sleep and rest (e.g., usual hours for sleeping, taking naps, snacks at bedtime, hygiene practices before retiring, placement and number of pillows, sleeping position, other aids for sleeping)?

2. Does he have any long-standing problems with resting and sleeping? Has he any problems now?

3. Does he have a health problem(s)? If so, what is the nature of the problem or problems? What are the diagnostic and therapeutic plans of care for him? If diagnostic reports have been received, what do they indicate about this patient's problem(s)?

4. Have hypnotic drugs been ordered for the patient? Analgesics? Was the patient using any medications before admission to this agency? If so, what drugs were they?

5. Are there any restrictions on the patient's mobility? Has a therapeutic position been prescribed?

6. What potential or existing sources of anxiety does this patient have? (See Chapter 30 for further questions in this regard.)

7. What position is best for this patient? Does the patient need assistance to maintain a position of good body alignment?

8. Does he need help with meeting his needs for elimination? If so, what kind of help does he need?

9. Does he say that he is uncomfortable, unable to rest or to sleep? If so, what things are causing his discomfort? Is he in pain? Is his bed comfortable? Does his dressing need changing? Can he reach everything he needs?

10. Do you observe any signs of discomfort in the patient (e.g., is he restless? pale? tense? perspiring profusely? lying rigidly in bed? Are his bed and his unit neat and tidy? Is the foundation of the bed firm and free of soiled or damp linen? Does he look uncomfortable?)?

11. Does he have difficult getting to sleep at night? Is he wakeful during the night?

12. Is he getting sufficient rest and sleep?

13. Is the environment conducive to sleeping and resting?

STUDY SITUATION

Mrs. R. Rogers is a 56-year-old woman who was admitted to the hospital with acute rheumatoid arthritis involving her back, her knees, and her feet. Mrs. Rogers is an obese woman and she finds it difficult to breathe when the head of her bed is flat. She complains of pain in her joints continually. Mrs. Rogers has a limited income and lives by herself in a small apartment. Her husband died 4 years ago, and her one daughter lives out of town and finds it difficult to visit her mother frequently.

The physician has ordered that Mrs. Rogers be maintained in good body alignment at all times. Her position is to be changed every four hours. She is on a low calorie diet. Her medications include acetylsalicylic acid (0.6 gm. four times a day) and Seconal (50 mg. at bedtime).

1. What factors might cause Mrs. Rogers to have problems with regard to comfort, rest, and sleep?

2. How would you assess Mrs. Rogers' present comfort, rest, and sleep status?

3. What objective signs would indicate to you that Mrs. Rogers is uncomfortable, is not resting, or is not sleeping well?

4. What subjective observations by Mrs. Rogers might you note?

5. What other members of the health team are, or might be, involved in helping Mrs. Rogers? For what purpose?

6. What positions do you think might be most comfortable for Mrs. Rogers?

7. What supportive devices might make Mrs. Rogers more comfortable? How should you use them?

8. Outline a nursing care plan for Mrs. Rogers.

SUGGESTED READINGS

Feinberg, I.: Changes in Sleep Cycle Patterns with Age. *Journal of Psychological Research*, 10:283–306, October, 1974.

Felton, G.: Body Rhythm Effects on Rotating Work Shifts. *Nursing Digest*, 4:29–32, January-February, 1976.

Hayter, J.: The Rhythm of Sleep. *American Journal of Nursing*, 80(3):457–461, March, 1980.

Landry, R. F.: Offbeat Rhythms and Biological Variables. *Occupational Health and Safety*, April, 1981.

Tom, C., and D. Lanuza (Guest Editors): Symposium on Biological Rhythms. *Nursing Clinics of North America*, 11:4, December, 1976.

Zelechowski, G. P.: "Helping Your Patient Sleep: Planning instead of Pills. *Nursing '77*, 7(5):64–65, May, 1977.

REFERENCES

1. The American Heritage Dictionary of the English Language. New College Edition. Boston, Houghton Mifflin Company, 1976.
2. Editorial: Sleep. *Lancet*, 1:963, April, 1975.
3. Quig, J.: Morning Becomes Who? *The Canadian*, December 20, 1975.
4. Grant, D. A., and Klell, C.: For Goodness' Sake, Let Your Patients Sleep. *Nursing '74*, 4:54–57, November, 1974.
5. Albert, I. B., and Albert, S. E.: Penetrating the Mysteries of Sleep and Sleep Disorders. *RN*, 37:36–39, August, 1974.
6. Lowy, F H.: Recent Sleep and Dream Research: Clinical Implications. *Canadian Medical Association journal*, 102:1069–1077, May, 1970.
7. Tackett, J. J. M., and Hunsberger, M.: *Family-Centered Care of Children and Adolescents*. Philadelphia, W. B. Saunders Company, 1981.
8. Harvin, J. S., and Hargest, T. S.: The Air-Fluidized Bed: A New Concept in the Treatment of Decubitus Ulcers. *Nursing Clinics of North America*, 5:181–186, March, 1970.

21

The Nurse Should Be Able to:

- Discuss the importance of pain as a protective mechanism for the body
- Describe the physiological mechanisms for receiving, transmitting, and interpreting pain sensations
- Explain present thinking regarding the cause of pain by various types of stimuli
- Discuss factors affecting an individual's perception of pain and his reaction to it
- Discuss variations in pain perception and pain reaction throughout the life cycle
- Assess the patient's pain status
- Identify situations requiring immediate action to relieve a patient's pain and intervene appropriately
- Apply relevant principles in planning and implementing nursing interventions
    a. to prevent potential problems of pain
    b. to relieve a patient's pain
    c. to help him to cope with it
- Evaluate the effectiveness of nursing interventions

PAIN AVOIDANCE

CHAPTER 21

INTRODUCTION

Pain is a sensation that is caused by the action of stimuli of a harmful nature. It is one of the most common causes of discomfort in an individual, and both Maslow and Kalish have included pain avoidance among the first priority physiological needs. Pain avoidance would seem to be almost an instinctive reaction to harmful factors in the environment. Certainly, newborns are capable of avoiding pain and will withdraw from it if possible. If one leg of a newborn is stroked, for example, the other leg will cross over and push the offending hand away.[1] People who have pain experience varying degrees of distress, from a mild feeling of discomfort to an acute feeling of agony that obliterates all other sensations.

Although distressing, pain is in most instances a protective mechanism that warns the individual that body tissues are being damaged or are about to be damaged. The point at which pain is first felt is called the *pain perception threshold*. In controlled laboratory experiments, it has been found that this threshold is remarkably similar in most individuals under normal circumstances; that is, people subjected to an increasing amount of a painful stimulus, such as an increasing degree of heat applied to an area of the body, report feeling pain at almost exactly the same point of intensity of the stimulus. However, this threshold may be altered by a person's physical condition or by his emotional state at the time the pain is experienced.

Then, too, each person's *reaction to pain* is highly individualistic. Pain is also one of the most common and, probably, the most important of all the signs and symptoms of illness. Some people accept pain with stoical indifference; others react to similar pain with weeping or other outward displays of suffering. Also, the same individual may react to pain differently under different circumstances. The way in which an individual reacts to pain at any given time appears to be influenced by a number of factors: physical, emotional, and cultural.

The reasons for the anomalies in both the perception of pain and the reaction of people to it has intrigued physiologists, psychologists, and sociologists for many years. Although pain is such a common symptom of illness, there are still large gaps in our knowledge concerning the mechanisms for receiving, transmitting, interpreting, and reacting to pain sensations. Recent research in the fields of neurophysiology, experimental psychology, sociology, and nursing has increased our understanding of the phenomenon of pain and contributed to our ability to help people in pain. However, there are still many unanswered questions for which different theories have been proposed.

THE PHYSIOLOGY OF PAIN

It is generally agreed that pain begins with stimulation of sensory nerve endings located on the body's surface or in the deeper structures. Although it has been traditionally assumed that there were specific receptors for pain, as for touch and temperature, there seems to be evidence that pain is not a pure sensation. Rather, it may be caused by intense stimulation of all types of sensory receptors. Thus, a hot water bottle may feel comfortably warm in one instance but in another—if the temperature of the water it contains is too high—the heat may be painful. Similarly, stroking or patting of the skin with a light pressure may be soothing, whereas rough massage can hurt.

The sensory nerve endings appear to be differentially sensitive to painful stimuli; that is, some are more sensitive to pain than others. Also, some areas of the body are richly supplied with free sensory nerve endings that are sensitive to painful stimuli, while other areas are not.

447

The skin has an abundant supply, as have some of the internal organs, such as the arterial walls, the joints, and the periosteum. Other organs have fewer receptors that are sensitive to pain; the brain and the alveoli of the lungs have none.

Once a pain impulse is initiated by the stimulation of a sensory receptor, the impulse is transmitted rapidly via first-level neurons to the lateral portion of filaments in the spinothalamic tracts of the spinal cord and thence to the thalamus. In the thalamus, there is a crude sorting-out and evaluation of the pain impulses, which are then transmitted via third-level neurons to higher centers in the brain. Between the thalamus and the sensory areas of the cerebral cortex where pain is perceived, it is believed that there is a further sorting-out and evaluation of the sensory impressions. Not all impressions reach the cortex; a person can only focus his attention on a limited number of stimuli at any one time. It is believed that the reticular system of the brain performs the function of evaluating the sensory impressions received in the thalamus and forwarding on to the cortex those of sufficient importance to merit attention.[2] Once the impression reaches the cortex, the person becomes aware of the pain. Action is then set in motion to counteract the noxious stimulus that has caused the pain.

In some instances, the stimulus is of sufficient intensity for a response to be initiated at the cord level. For example, the slightest touch of a hot stove causes a reflex reaction, and the individual withdraws his hand immediately.

Sometimes pain is perceived in one area of the body although the stimulus was in another area. Pain that is initiated in a deep visceral organ, for example, may be perceived by the individual on a surface area, or sometimes pain appears to be transferred from one surface area to another. This is called referred pain. The pain of myocardial infarction (a blockage in one of the blood vessels supplying the heart muscle) typically gives rise to feelings of pain in the left shoulder and down the left arm of the afflicted individual, in addition to the pain felt in the region of the heart.

The physiological mechanism of referred pain is more complicated than the mechanism just described for the perception of pain. In referred pain, the fibers carrying pain impulses from the viscera are believed to synapse (join together) with other neurons in the spinal cord. If the pain stimulus from the visceral organs is sufficiently intense, the sensation tends to spread over into some areas that normally receive stimuli only from the skin. Thus the individual has the sensation of pain coming from the skin rather than, or as well as, from the viscera.

THE SPINAL-GATING HYPOTHESIS

An interesting theory about pain which has received a considerable amount of attention in recent years is the spinal-gating hypothesis. The proponents of this theory, Ronald Melzack and Patrick Wall, contend that the mechanism of pain is not so simple as the explanation given above would indicate. In Melzack and Wall's "gate control theory,"[2] they propose that a neural mechanism, located in the substantia gelatinosa of the dorsal horns of the spinal cord, acts as a gate that can increase or decrease the flow of nerve impulses from peripheral fibers to higher centers in the brain.

Pain impulses are carried by two types of fibers in the spinal cord—one large in diameter, the other small. The large fibers conduct rapidly and adapt quickly; they become inactive in the absence of stimulus change. Input from these fibers has an excitatory effect on the spinal gating mechanism, causing it to close. Sharp, immediate pain is thought to travel via the large fibers and, since it travels quickly, some input will pass through the gate before the mechanism is activated to close. The small fibers conduct more slowly than the large fibers, and are slower to adapt; they are tonically active. Prolonged pain, it is thought, travels through the smaller fibers (because the larger ones adapt quickly when there is no change in stimulus); input from these fibers has an inhibiting effect on the gating mechanism, causing the gate to open (or remain open).

Additional factors in the operation of the gate controlling mechanism are the motivational and cognitive influences from the higher centers of the brain. These influences, which include such factors as attention, anxiety, expectations, suggestion, and memory of previous experiences (including cultural and social background), descend from the brain and modulate the pain impulses traveling upward from peripheral sites. Through a process of comparison of the input from the sensory systems and from the central control (the brain), the spinal-gating mechanism will be excited and close, or be inhibited and open.

Beyond the gating mechanism are transmission cells. When the amount of information passing through the gate to the transmission cells reaches a critical level, these cells fire, thus activating the neural areas responsible for pain perception and response.

The gate-control theory provides a plausible explanation for some of the puzzling features of pain. For example, rubbing or otherwise stimulating a painful area, according to this theory, reduces the perception of pain because the

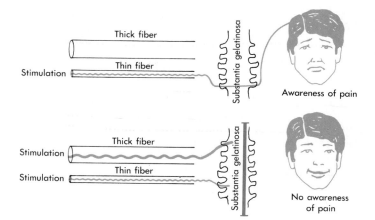

Stimulation of thick nerve fibers, which may be done by nursing measures such as massage, may stimulate the release of endorphins so that pain impulses from thin nerve fibers are blocked in the substantia gelatinosa.

change in stimulus activates the large fibers (which had adapted), causing the gate to close. In pathological pain syndromes, where, in some cases, the larger fibers have been destroyed, more input is carried through the smaller fibers, which have an inhibitory effect on the spinal-gating mechanism. With regard to spontaneous pain or delayed pain, this theory suggests that a summation of input from the smaller fibers (which conduct more slowly) occurs in the transmission cells, causing a latent response.

Endorphins

Although many neurophysiologists disagree with parts of Wall and Melzack's theory, subsequent research tends to substantiate the basic contention that pain impulses are sorted out in the spinal cord before being sent on to the brain.[3] Substances found in the substantia gelatinosa of the cord, such as opiate receptors and endorphins, would seem to bear out this contention.

Endorphins are substances that have been found in the synapses between nerve fibers. It is believed that they have the ability to inhibit the transmission of pain impulses by blocking their passage across the synaptic space. The mechanism works like this: If a pain signal being carried by a neuron arrives at a synapse, it is normally transmitted across the space and carried upward toward the brain. However, a descending impulse from the brain can trigger the release of endorphins onto opiate receptors in the afferent neuron carrying the pain impulse. The net effect is to block transmission of the signal across the synapse, so that it does not reach the brain.

It is believed that many traditional nursing interventions, such as those designed to relieve anxiety, stimulate the release of endorphins, thus helping to prevent pain.

COMMON CAUSES OF PAIN

Generally speaking, any stimulus that causes tissue damage, or is perceived by the individual as potentially causing injury to body tissues, causes pain. Thus, pain may result from a number of different kinds of damaging stimuli, including irritating chemical substances, mechanical trauma, thermal extremes, or ischemia (lack of blood flow to a part), as well as from psychogenic factors.

Chemical Irritants

Direct stimulation of free sensory nerve endings by irritating chemical substances will cause pain. A common example of this is the pain that occurs when one spills a drop of acid on the skin. Also, it is now believed that whenever tissues are damaged, certain chemical substances are liberated by the injured cells. Some of these substances trigger the inflammatory response (see Chapter 26). Others, it is thought, excite pain receptors in the damaged area. These substances are believed to include histamine and peptides of the bradykinin group. They are sometimes referred to simply as kinins.[4] Thus, in the case of the acid burn, there is usually an initial sharp, stinging pain, caused by the chemical irritation of the nerve endings by the acid, followed by a longer-lasting pain that is due to the action of substances released by cells that have been damaged by the acid.

Ischemia

Other chemical irritants that are believed to cause pain are the acidic waste products of cellular metabolism. When these substances accumulate, as, for example, in areas of the body where blood supply to a part is not sufficient to carry them away, pain is believed to result from the irritating effect of these substances on free nerve endings. This helps to explain the pain in ischemic areas where blood supply has been cut off or impaired and metabolic waste products accumulate. Another factor in the pain of ischemia is the death of tissue cells in the area, resulting from the loss of blood supply. The decaying cells also liberate irritating chemical substances, as already discussed, and this would contribute to the pain.

Mechanical Trauma

Pain may be incurred by physical force or other mechanical means. When an individual is driving a nail into the wall, for example, the hammer may accidentally hit the thumb instead of the nailhead. The resulting bruise and painful thumb are familiar to most of us. The pain is felt to be caused in this instance by pressure on the nerve endings initially, with chemical irritation from the kinins released by damaged cells as a factor in the continued pain of the bruised tissues.

Pain may also result from *stretching or contraction* of body tissues, or from prolonged pressure on the tissues. Distention of a hollow organ such as the stomach is a common example of stretching of the tissues. If a person eats a very big meal (as at Thanksgiving or Christmas), he may develop considerable discomfort in the region of his stomach. It is believed that stretching of the tissues causes pain because of two possible factors: stretching of the nerve endings in the sensory receptors and the occlusion of small blood vessels in the stretched tissue, which results in localized ischemia.

When *tissues are contracted* (as, for example, in a muscle spasm), there is constriction of small blood vessels in the area with, again, localized ischemia resulting. There may also be stretching of the nerve endings. In addition, in prolonged muscular contraction, cellular metabolism is greatly increased, with a resultant buildup in metabolic waste products, which the constricted blood vessels cannot carry away. As already stated, these metabolic waste products are believed to be chemically irritating to sensory nerve endings and therefore to cause pain.

Continued pressure on any body structure causes tissue damage and concomitant pain. The pain is thought to be due to pressure on the nerve endings and also to localized ischemia resulting from the occlusion of small blood vessels in the tissues being pressed. Even the prolonged pressure of sitting too long in the class-

room may cause pain unless one changes position or stretches occasionally. Normally a person alters his position every few minutes. This is a conditioned response to the perception of pain sensations, which are felt whenever pressure is exerted on any one area for too long. People who have impaired pain perception—for example, unconscious or paralyzed patients—may not feel these pain sensations. The individual does not therefore of his own accord alter his position, and pressure areas can easily develop. For this reason, it is particularly important that the patient be turned frequently and that other measures be taken to prevent prolonged pressure on any part of the body (see Chapter 24).

Heat and Cold

Extremes of heat and cold cause pain. They also damage body tissues. Everyone is familiar with the burn that is caused by excessive heat, and with the pain that results from even a small burn on the tip of the finger. Here, the initial burning pain probably results from the intensity of the thermal stimulus. The lingering after-pain is believed to be due to the destruction of tissue and the release of irritating chemical substances from the injured cells. Because burns are one of the most frequent causes of accidental injury to patients, the nurse must be ever alert to protect patients from the danger of solutions that are too hot, heating pads that are set at too high a temperature, and the like (see Chapter 24). Again, these precautions are especially important when the patient's pain perception is impaired.

Extreme cold, particularly if there is freezing of body tissues, as in frostbite, also causes tissue damage and accompanying pain. Cold constricts the blood vessels in the affected tissue and may completely cut off the blood supply. The pain in a frostbitten nose or finger is most severe when the blood flow is returning and the constricted vessels are being dilated.

Psychogenic Pain

Pain may be experienced by an individual in the absence of any physiological basis for it. This occurs in a *conversion reaction*, for example, in which emotional disorders are experienced by the patient as bodily symptoms rather than as mental ones. Pain may also arise from the physiological accompaniments of psychogenic disorders, as in the tension headache caused by contraction of the muscles in the back of the neck and dilatation of blood vessels in the head.

TYPES OF PAIN

Pain can be classified as superficial, deep, or visceral. *Superficial pain* is usually described as having either a burning or a pricking quality. It arises from stimulation of receptors in the skin or the mucous membranes of the body. As a rule, an individual is able to localize surface pain fairly accurately because of the large number of free sensory nerve endings on the surface of the body.

Deep pain arises from the deeper structures of the body, such as the muscles, tendons, joints, and fasciae. It is usually described as dull, aching, cramping, gnawing, or boring. Muscles and tendons are particularly sensitive to pain and may give rise to pain of considerable intensity.

Visceral pain may be perceived as originating in the organ itself, or pain may be felt at a site far removed from the affected viscera through the mechanism of referred pain. It is usually more difficult to localize visceral pain because there are fewer sensory nerve endings in the viscera than on the skin or mucous membranes. The nature of the pain experienced is sometimes highly specific to the particular organ involved and the pathological process that is taking place. In myocardial infarction, for example, the pain is often described as constricting, viselike, or compressing. Pain in hollow muscular organs frequently gives rise to sensations of gripping, cramping, or twisting. In the case of a peptic ulcer, the patient often describes pain as having a gnawing, burning, or sometimes knifelike quality.

An accurate description of the nature of the pain as reported by the patient often helps the physician to diagnose the cause of the patient's condition. The nurse should be careful, however, not to put her own interpretation on the patient's description nor to suggest words for the patient to use. It is far better to record and report the patient's pain as he describes it in his own words.

The nurse may also hear the term "*central pain*" used. This type of pain arises from injury to sensory nerves, the neural pathways, or the areas in the brain that are concerned with pain perception. It is often very difficult for the patient to describe this type of pain since it is usually unlike anything he has experienced before. Some people have, however, described it as gnawing, burning, or crushing.[4]

There are also causes of *phantom pain* such as the pain that a patient feels in his toes after the limb has been amputated. This is thought to be due to the persistence of the pain sensation or a "pain memory" after the cause for it is removed.

PAIN RECEPTION AND PAIN REACTION

There are always two aspects to pain: pain perception and pain reaction. The pain perception threshold, although remarkably the same in most individuals under normal circumstances, may be altered by certain physical and emotional factors. Pain reaction, or the way in which a person reacts to pain, varies considerably from one individual to another and within the same individual under different circumstances. The two aspects of pain can be dissociated. For example, in certain conditions a physician may not be able to do anything about a person's perception of pain, but he may be able to treat the reaction to pain.

Pain Perception

The ability to perceive pain is dependent upon the integrity of the nerve fibers that receive, transmit, and interpret pain impulses. Thus, injury to sensory nerves, the sensory tracts in the spinal cord, the thalamus, or sensory areas in the cerebral cortex will interfere with pain perception. A patient who has had a spinal cord injury, for example, and is paralyzed from the waist down does not feel pain in the lower half of his body. This patient must then be protected from harmful stimuli to which a person with normal pain perception would respond by taking suitable action to prevent injury to body tissues. For example, paraplegic patients must be taught to alter their position frequently when they are sitting in a wheelchair, or they soon develop decubitus ulcers. The nurse must also take special precautions to protect paralyzed or unconscious patients from the pressure of tight bed coverings, which may cause foot drop, among other distressing effects.

Sometimes pain perception seems to be facilitated. In some disease conditions affecting the central nervous system (for example, in a neuritis in which the nervous tissue is inflamed), the individual often becomes hypersensitive to painful stimuli. Also, with the prolonged application of painful stimuli, the neural pathways appear to become worn and the pain perception centers hypersensitive. Thus, a person who suffers from continuous pain becomes more, rather than less, sensitive to it.

Areas of the body adjacent to injured areas are usually more sensitive to pain than normal tissue is. The skin adjacent to a wound area, for example, is usually very tender. It is thought that in these cases there is a spillover of pain impulses into neighboring pathways, much the same as in the case of referred pain. There is also the factor of engorgement of the tissues in the wounded area owing to the inflammatory process, and this may cause pressure on sensory nerve endings in the surrounding tissue.

Tissues that are already damaged react to additional painful stimuli, even of minimal intensity, much more readily than does normal intact tissue. The sensitivity of the sunburned skin is usually cited as an example of this phenomenon, which might be considered as a case of stimulus overload.

On the other hand, intense pain in one part of the body may raise the pain threshold in other areas. A person who is suffering considerable pain from a broken leg, for example, may not be aware of pain from an abrasion on his elbow. This is probably due to selective perception, the stimulus of greater priority (or intensity) taking precedence in attention over the less intense, or less significant, stimulus.

The pain perception threshold is also altered by an individual's level of consciousness. The unconscious person—for example, the patient under a general anesthetic—does not feel pain. The ability to perceive pain, as tested by a person's reaction to a pinprick or to supraorbital pressure, is frequently used to determine a patient's level of consciousness. Both pain perception and pain reaction may be altered by the emotional state of the individual and by the amount of attention that is focused on the pain. These points are discussed later.

Pain Reaction

There are both physiological and behavioral manifestations in the reaction to pain. The *physiological manifestations* are those of the "alarm reaction" of the body to the threat of danger from any harmful stimulus (see Chapter 2). Among the signs and symptoms that the nurse can observe are pallor, elevated blood pressure, and increased tension of the skeletal muscles. Gastrointestinal functioning may also be impaired. The person in pain usually does not want to eat, and nausea and vomiting are not uncommon accompaniments of pain. Restlessness and irritability are frequently seen. The patient who is in pain cannot rest and he cannot sleep.

With severe pain of any sort, the body's defenses may collapse. In such an event, the nurse may observe signs of weakness and prostration in the patient. His blood pressure may drop and his pulse become weak and slow. There may be increased pallor, and the patient is often described as being "white as a ghost." Collapse and loss of consciousness may ensue.

The *behavioral responses to pain* differ much more widely from one individual to another than do the physiological manifestations. Everyone has observed the individual who "never flinches" even though the pain he experiences is intense. Such behavior is usually much admired in our Western society. On the other hand, some people react to pain with loud groans, weeping, screaming, thrashing about, or violent attempts to remove themselves from the source of pain.

A person's reaction to pain is influenced by a number of factors. The individual's physical condition, his emotional state, and the way in which he has been conditioned to respond to pain will all affect his reaction to pain in a particular situation.

If a person is tired, or weakened physically, his resistance and control over his reactions are lessened. He may then react to a minimal stimulus with an exaggerated response that is all out of proportion to the intensity of the stimulus. When one is tired, even a small cut on the finger may seem too much to endure, and tears or profanity may be evoked. Thus, the harassed mother who is attempting to cook dinner and, at the same time, look after small children may suffer a slight burn at the stove and promptly burst into tears.

Conversely, in extreme exhaustion, the individual's attention span is markedly reduced and he may not be able to concentrate his attention on any one stimulus for a sufficient length of time to react to it. Thus, the severely sunburned sailor who has been adrift in an open boat may not complain of pain at all, or if he does, his mind soon wanders from it to other things.

The emotional state of the individual also modifies his reaction to pain. Anxiety and fear aggravate it. This is understandable, since anxiety, fear, and pain all provoke the same physiological "alarm reaction" in the body in response to stimuli that threaten the individual's safety. Certainly, if anxiety is relieved, the patient's reaction to pain is considerably lessened. As we mentioned earlier, it is believed that anxiety-relieving measures are associated with the release of endorphins that block the transmission of pain impulses. If there is a strong emotional response to stimuli other than the pain-producing one, however, this emotional state may block out the awareness of pain. A

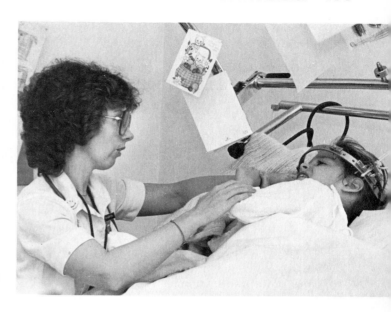

The nurse comforts a young patient who is in pain.

football player injured during a game may not notice that he has been hurt until the game is over. In this case, excitement and the desire to win may be so intense as to demand the individual's full attention, so that the sensory impressions of pain from the injury become of lesser priority and he does not perceive them. A similar explanation could account for the numerous reports of soldiers wounded in battle who state that they did not feel pain even though they had injuries of considerable extent. The overriding fear during the battle and the necessity for self-preservation at all costs may take precedence over impressions from any other sensory stimulation, so that pain is not perceived. It is felt that the distracting circumstances stimulate endorphin release through the action of descending impulses from the brain. Pleasurable emotions tend to nullify pain perception, so that the person who is in a happy or contented mood does not usually seem to feel pain to the same extent as the worried patient.

Then, too, an individual's emotional makeup, his cultural and social background, and his early home and school training have a great deal to do with his behavior in response to painful stimuli. There has been much study by sociologists, for example, of the differing reactions of various cultural groups to pain.[5] The North American Indian is often cited as an example of a member of a cultural group in which stoical indifference to pain is a highly valued characteristic. Among people of Latin origin, on the other hand, an open display of suffering is usually permitted as the socially approved response to pain.

In our Western society, very strong values are placed on bravery, endurance, and the ability to bear pain with silent fortitude. Children in our culture are taught very early that they are expected not to cry when they are hurt. "Be brave," "Don't be a sissy," and "Only babies cry," are the frequent admonishments of mothers to young children. Even children from ethnic groups in which the open display of suffering is permitted soon learn from their teachers and from their peer groups in school and on the playground that they must react to pain in the accepted North American manner or be scorned by their fellows.

The nurse who has been raised in this framework of "only babies cry" may find herself reacting negatively to the patient who does not handle his pain in the "approved" manner. If she realizes that her reaction is normal and a reflection of her social values, which are different from those of the patient, she is in a better position to analyze and accept her own feelings. These feelings then need not interfere with her acceptance and support of the patient.

PAIN AVOIDANCE THROUGHOUT THE LIFE CYCLE

Newborn infants, as we mentioned at the beginning of the chapter, will try to get away from pain if it is at all possible. The action appears to be a reflex response to a harmful or potentially harmful stimulus. Other than withdrawing or trying to push the painful stimulus away, however, the infant has few means at his disposal to protect himself from pain. By crying, he can alert the people who are looking after him that all is not well, but he is highly dependent on his caretaker to diagnose his problem, locate its source, and assess its severity, as well as take the necessary steps to relieve his pain. As the mother becomes accustomed to her infant, she usually becomes very astute in differentiating a hunger cry from one indicating other discomfort or one indicating a desire to be picked up and cuddled. Mothers very quickly learn, too, to interpret the behavioral manifestations of pain in their offspring. An infant who draws his legs up is usually having abdominal pain, for example. An older infant who puts his hand up to an ear frequently probably has an earache.

Even as newborns, boys appear to be less sensitive to pain than girls. They are also, as a general rule, more active and stronger.[1] As toddlers, boys tend to be rougher and more venturesome in their play, and consequently they have more cuts, scrapes, and bruises than girls do. It is perhaps just as well that they are a little less sensitive to pain.

Adolescence is a period when the young person is struggling for control of his emotions and his behavior, and adolescents, as a general rule, do not tolerate pain very well. The prompt administration of medications to relieve pain is, therefore, important in their care. There have been some remarkable exceptions to the general rule of teenagers' inability to tolerate pain, however. One is often impressed by the fortitude displayed by teenagers in the face of a lengthy painful illness.

By the time a person has reached adulthood, he has usually learned to control his reactions to pain so that they fit the norms of his culture. As he gets older his sensory perception gradually decreases and, with this decline in functioning ability of the sense organs, his sensitivity to pain is reduced.

ASSESSMENT

Pain is probably the most personal and the most distressing of all the symptoms of disease. Only the individual who is experiencing the pain really knows what it is like. The primary source of information about the pain he is having, then, is always the patient. Other sources the nurse can use include her own observations of the patient and those of other members of the health team.

Objective Data

In gathering information about the patient's pain, the nurse should ascertain, whenever possible, the following aspects of the pain experience:

1. The quality of the pain
2. The location of the pain
3. The intensity of the pain
4. The time the pain occurs and its duration
5. Any factors that appear to precipitate the pain
6. Any measures which relieve it or measures with which the patient has tried to relieve it

Quality. Patients use many descriptive terms when talking about pain. A number of the terms commonly used have been mentioned earlier in the chapter in the section on classification of pain. Frequently patients describe pain in terms of something that is familiar to them. Thus, pain may be likened to the cutting action of a knife, if it is a sharp, piercing pain; or to "hammers pounding inside the head" in certain types of headache. In recording and reporting pain, the nurse should use the exact words the patient has used in order to convey an accurate description of the pain as the patient perceives it.

Location. The patient is usually able to localize superficial pain fairly accurately and also pain arising from bones, muscles, joints, and blood vessels. Visceral pain is more difficult to localize. Often, the patient complains of pain generally in the epigastric region, or in the lower part of the abdomen, in the chest, or in the lower back when a visceral organ is affected. Often, too, the pain from viscera is referred to a surface area. An exact description of the location of the pain is of considerable assistance to the physician in diagnosing the patient's condition, and to the nurse in planning her care.

Intensity. The degree of pain felt by the patient is also important in assessing his nursing needs and the need for medical or nursing intervention. Certain tissues are more sensitive to pain than others; for example, muscle tissue appears to be highly responsive to painful stimuli, and the pain from bruised or ischemic muscles may be excruciating. Hence, it is necessary to use great care in moving patients who have disorders involving the musculoskeletal system.

When the intensity of the patient's pain changes abruptly, it is usually an indication that the nature of his condition has altered. For example, when an inflamed appendix ruptures, or a peptic ulcer perforates, the patient usually experiences very sharp and severe pain, which persists and is quite different both in quality and intensity from the pain felt previously.

Time and Duration. An accurate description of the patient's pain should include when it occurs, how long it lasts, and whether it is an intermittent pain that recurs or a steady pain that continues. Pain is often most severe at night, when a person is alone. A possible explanation for this is that, in the absence of other people or activities to distract him, the individual's full attention is then focused on his discomfort. The duration of the pain is very important. An example of this may be found in obstetrics, in which the length of the interval between pains and the time each pain lasts are significant in assessing the patient's progress in labor, the muscular contractions of the uterus becoming stronger and closer together as delivery becomes imminent.

Precipitating Factors. Pain is often related to the patient's activities. In some cardiac conditions, pain may be brought on by exertion, and in planning the patient's care, it is important to know how much activity the patient can tolerate. Sometimes it is necessary to space nursing measures to allow the patient to rest between activities. For example, it may be wise in some cases to leave the patient's bath until an hour or so after breakfast in order to give him time to rest after the exertion of eating a meal. With patients who have musculoskeletal problems, pain is frequently associated with movement of the affected structure. Again, it is important to know exactly what movement precipitates pain, both for medical assessment of the patient's condition and for planning care to minimize the patient's discomfort. Pain in the gastrointestinal tract may be precipitated by eating certain foods. Again, pain may be related to an intolerance of factors in the environment. Noise may bring on a headache, for example. Very often the patient is able to identify the specific factor or factors that cause pain, and these should be recorded and reported,

again using the patient's own words in preference to an interpretation of what he says. Often, it is helpful to ask the patient what he was doing when he first noticed the pain. The answer may give you a clue to the precipitating cause. Arguing with a teenage son, for example, could have raised the patient's blood pressure and precipitated a violent headache, or waiting for a job interview might have activated his stomach ulcers.

Measures That Relieve Pain. Frequently, the patient has tried a number of measures to relieve his pain before he seeks medical help. The nurse should ascertain the measures he has tried and the effectiveness of these in relieving his pain. For example, does rest relieve the pain that is brought on by exertion? Does holding the limb in a certain way prevent pain on movement? This type of information is of value both to the physician in assessing the patient's condition and developing a plan of therapy, and to the nurse in her determination of nursing measures which will help to alleviate pain.

Subjective Data

The nurse can supplement the information she obtains from the patient with her observations of his reaction to the pain. She should be alert to the physiological manifestations of pain as these have just been described. Very often the patient's facial expression and posture will indicate that he is having pain. The patient in pain often has a typical facial grimace: his brows are knotted, his facial muscles are tense and drawn, and his mouth is often drawn downward. In addition, he may assume a characteristic position to minimize the pain. With abdominal pain, the patient may draw up his knees and curl into a ball; for a sore arm he may hold the

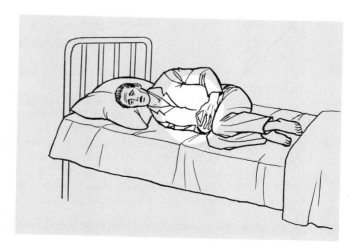

A person who is experiencing pain may assume a position indicative of the site of the pain.

affected part. In severe pain patients sometimes lie rigidly because any movement intensifies the discomfort. Some patients, because of their training to bear pain in stoical silence, do not like to complain of pain. As a result, the nurse may find it difficult to identify even the existence of pain. Pallor, muscular tension (as in the drawn facial muscles or a clenching of the fists), posture, inactivity, and profuse perspiration may be the only outward evidences of pain in these people.

The nurse may, however, often note other behavior in patients who are having pain. Restlessness and increased sensitivity to stimuli in the environment, such as noise and bright lights, are frequently indicative of pain. The patient in pain often shows evidence of increased emotional tension as well; he may react with irritability and bad humor to people or things that disturb him. Pain usually prevents people from sleeping or resting comfortably, and, because pain is usually worse at night, insomnia may be a problem. Nursing measures to ensure that the patient is relieved of pain are important in order to enable him to rest.

Information from Other Sources

Frequently pain is the principal symptom that prompts people to seek medical help. The physician then has usually investigated the nature of the patient's pain, and the nurse can often obtain much information from the patient's physician or from the notes made on the patient's record. Of particular importance are notations made regarding factors that precipitate pain, since the nurse may be able to institute measures to eliminate or minimize these factors.

The observations made by all members of the nursing team who are caring for the patient contribute to the total picture of the patient's pain. These observations should be accurately reported and recorded so that all staff members are aware of measures that prevent, minimize, or alleviate the patient's pain, as well as factors that aggravate it.

In addition, other members of the health team, such as the physical therapist, can often contribute information about the patient's pain. The physical therapist usually assists in assessing the patient's mobility and functional ability and can provide guidance to nursing personnel on activities that the patient can tolerate without pain. The patient's family too can be helpful in regard to the nature of the patient's pain, factors that precipitate it, and measures that help to alleviate it. Some people are reluctant to admit that they have pain, or may try to minimize its severity when talking to medical personnel, usually again because of their cultural background; yet they have often confided the extent of their suffering to their wife or husband. Or, the wife may be aware of such evidences of her husband's discomfort as his inability to sleep or his restlessness and increased irritability.

PRIORITIES FOR NURSING ACTION

The relief of pain is always a matter of priority for nursing action. However, there are some circumstances in which it is more urgent than in others, when the prompt treatment of pain is essential to save a person's life or to prevent damage to body structures. Severe pain can cause a collapse of the body's adaptive mechanisms. Hence, the presence of severe pain in a patient requires immediate intervention. The nurse's judgment of the patient's condition is extremely important. If she observes signs of weakness and prostration, such as markedly increased pallor, a lowered blood pressure, and weakened pulse in a patient who is having pain, the physician should be notified immediately so that his (or her) guidance can be obtained on the measures to be taken. He may wish the administration of analgesics discontinued and

PRINCIPLES RELEVANT TO PAIN

1. **Pain has a protective function in warning a person of present or potential damage to body tissues.**
2. **Pain may be caused by a number of different kinds of stimuli.**
3. **Tissues of the body differ in their sensitivity to painful stimuli.**
4. **Severe pain can cause collapse of the body's adaptive mechanisms.**
5. **The ability to perceive pain is dependent upon integrity of the neural structures which receive, transmit, and interpret pain impulses.**
6. **Pain perception may be altered by certain physical and emotional factors.**
7. **A person's reaction to pain is highly individualized and depends on a number of factors—physical, emotional, and cultural.**

other measures such as intravenous infusion with supportive drug therapy instituted. Or he may feel that the patient's condition warrants immediate surgical intervention.

The action of pain-relieving drugs is more effective if these are administered before the pain reaches a peak. Early intervention at the beginning of pain, then, can often prevent a serious attack. This is important in such conditions as myocardial infarction, or biliary or renal colic (stones in the bile duct or the ureter of the kidney), in which the pain can mount to agonizing proportions. The patient's request for pain relief should be answered without delay.

Another situation in which the prompt relief of pain is imperative is the care of the surgical patient. The restlessness that accompanies increasing pain can cause damage to newly sutured tissues. The patient should therefore be kept comfortable at all times during the immediate postoperative period. Analgesics for the relief of pain are usually prescribed every 3 to 4 hours as needed (p.r.n.) for the first 48 hours following surgery. The nurse's judicious administration of these medications can make the patient's recovery from surgery much easier.

The relief of pain is not always, of course, a matter of administering a medication. Many times nursing measures such as changing the patient's position, straightening his bed, or helping him to overcome his anxiety are equally effective in alleviating pain. In exercising judgment as to the appropriate measures to be taken, the nurse utilizes her knowledge about the pa-

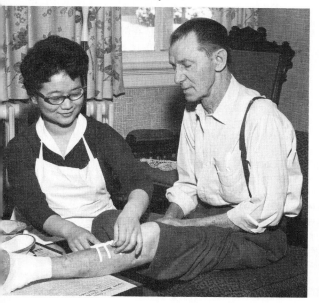

Changing a patient's dressing helps to eliminate irritating stimuli that can cause pain.

tient's medical condition and also her knowledge of each individual patient and his reaction to pain.

GOALS FOR NURSING ACTION

Nursing action for the patient who is having pain is directed primarily toward three goals:

1. Eliminating or minimizing the stimuli that are causing pain.
2. Alleviating pain
3. Assisting the patient in coping with pain

SPECIFIC NURSING INTERVENTIONS

Measures to Eliminate or Minimize Painful Stimuli

Whenever possible, it is always better to prevent pain than to treat it. One cannot always do this, of course. Many times pain is the chief reason a person has sought medical help. Investigation of the cause of pain and elimination of its source frequently constitute a major part of the patient's total care. The nurse can often help to control the extent of suffering, however, through eliminating or minimizing known causes of pain and discomfort.

Pain is usually a warning signal that body tissues are being damaged or are about to be damaged. When exertion brings on pain, the patient's activities may need to be curtailed to prevent further injury to body cells. The patient with a heart condition, for example, must learn to moderate his activities to prevent further damage to the heart and concomitant pain. The activities of the surgical patient, to use another example, are usually restricted until the wounded tissues have healed sufficiently that normal movement will not disturb the healing process.

It is not possible to curtail all movement that is painful, though, nor is it always wise. The dangers of immobility in people who are sick have been well documented. The postoperative patient, for example, must move about and must breathe deeply and cough to prevent respiratory complications, even though these activities cause him some pain. The nurse's actions are then directed toward minimizing the patient's discomfort. Supporting the patient's incision can lessen pain when he coughs or breathes deeply. The nurse may use her hands to support the incision, or sometimes a pillow held firmly against the operative area will accomplish the same purpose. A binder may be needed to provide support to the operative area when the patient is up and walking around.

Whenever it is necessary to lift or turn a patient for whom movement is painful, the utmost gentleness should be used. The nurse should always make certain that she has sufficient help in moving the patient so that he is not subjected to unnecessary pain or discomfort. Supporting a painful limb while turning the patient can help to minimize his discomfort. In addition, devices such as a "turning sheet," which is placed under the patient, can sometimes be used to advantage to prevent excessive handling of painful limbs.

All the comfort measures discussed in Chapter 20 are important in eliminating sources of pain for the patient. For example, helping a patient to change his position relieves muscle strain and also prevents pressure on any particular part of the body for too long a period of time. Positioning to maintain good body alignment aids in preventing painful muscular contractures. A soothing back rub will often help to relax a patient and ease muscular tension. Also, helping the patient to stay dry and comfortable and relieving any sources of irritation can aid in eliminating stimuli that can cause pain.

The nurse should remember too that helping the patient to meet his basic physiological needs can eliminate many existing or potential sources of pain. For example, food can prevent or relieve the uncomfortable muscular contractions of an empty stomach. Seeing that the patient is taking sufficient fluids helps to prevent the distressing effects of dehydration (see Chapter 17). The pain caused by a distended bladder and the discomfort of constipation are both preventable by nursing action and may be relieved by specific nursing techniques (see Chapter 15). Ensuring that the patient gets sufficient rest and sleep is an important consideration also, since fatigue lowers a person's resistance and control, thereby increasing his reaction to painful stimuli.

Measures to Alleviate Pain

Since time immemorial, man has sought measures to relieve pain. Innumerable drugs have been concocted and elaborate rituals developed to help people bear suffering. It is only in recent years, however, that research in the field of neuroanatomy has given scientific credence to many of the traditional methods, developed through a process of trial and error, that people use to alleviate pain.

Acupuncture, for example, which has been used for centuries in Asian cultures for pain relief, has become a standard part of medical therapy in the Western world, and we are beginning to understand why it works. Similarly, we have found that there is a scientific basis for many of the traditional comfort measures nurses have used over the years, such as the soothing back rub. Essentially, there are three types of nursing interventions that have been found particularly useful in helping people in pain. These are: distraction, relaxation techniques, and cutaneous stimulation. You may hear them referred to as *noninvasive techniques*. They are often effective alone, or they may be used to enhance the effectiveness of other measures, such as the use of analgesic drugs.

Distraction. Distraction is a useful tool for helping to alleviate acute pain as well as pain that persists over a long period of time. It works by lessening an individual's awareness of painful stimuli. The individual whose attention is diverted to something else has a number of sensory impressions competing for his attention, and his awareness of pain sensations is lessened. McCaffery, a consultant in a nursing care of people with pain, calls it a kind of "sensory shielding".[6]

Specific techniques that have been found helpful for acute pain include:

1. Getting the patient to talk about an exciting experience he has recently had. It might be a football game he has seen, or a race, the plot of a movie he has watched, or a story he has heard. If the patient is a child, you might ask him to count, or recite a rhyme, or participate in a game with you. The key points are that the activity is something that keenly interests the person and something in which he takes an active part.

2. Teaching the person active listening techniques. Tapping in rhythm to loud, fast music is one method. Closing the eyes and concentrating on the music is helpful in this one.

3. Getting the person to participate in rhythmic singing exercises. Chants or simple songs with a strong beat (such as ones you learned around the fire at summer camp) are good to use with both adults and children. Adults are usually more self-conscious than children, however, and often prefer to mouth the words silently. Tapping the foot, or a finger, for emphasis, is an additional distraction that can be added to this technique.

4. Teaching the person slow, rhythmic breathing exercises. One technique, which can be taught easily to people who are ill, involves getting the person to look fixedly at an object and deeply breathe in and out, meanwhile counting, as in "In 2, 3, 4—Out, 2, 3, 4." Another technique is to have the person blow bubbles,

as, for example, through a straw into a glass of water. Blowing bubbles usually works well with children. In addition, breath control is an essential component of Yoga, and a number of rhythmic breathing exercises can be found in any good book on Yoga.

For the person with ongoing pain, distraction is also often useful. If a person does not have diversional activities, he becomes much preoccupied with himself. Mild discomforts that might otherwise not be noted assume major importance. Such activities as reading, watching television, and talking with other people are important for the ill person, to provide diversions that take his attention away from himself.

Relaxation Techniques.   The extent to which anxiety and fear are contributing factors in pain is difficult to determine. Both anxiety and fear intensity a person's reaction to pain; if these can be successfully reduced, the individual is relieved of much of his distress. Many techniques for relaxation are being taught these days, including meditation, Yoga, rhythmic breathing exercise, and biofeedback techniques. Other relaxing methods that have been found useful in pain relief are music and conscious suggestion.

Rhythmic Breathing Exercises.   One of the Yoga breathing exercises which is particularly effective in helping a person to relax is the Alternate Nostril Breath.[7] It is one exercise that can easily be done by patients who are in bed, and it can be taught very easily.

ALTERNATE NOSTRIL BREATH*

I. *Benefits:*
   The Alternate Nostril Breath—
   • has a marvellously calming effect on the *nervous system.*
   • helps to overcome *insomnia.*
   • *relaxes* and *refreshes* the body.
   • purifies the *bloodstream* and aerates the *lungs.*
   • soothes *headaches.*
   • improves *digestion* and *appetite.*
   • helps to free the mind of *anxiety and depression.*

II. *Technique:*
   1. Sit in a comfortably cross-legged position, back straight.
   2. Raise your RIGHT hand and place your ringfinger against your LEFT nostril, closing it off *(A).*

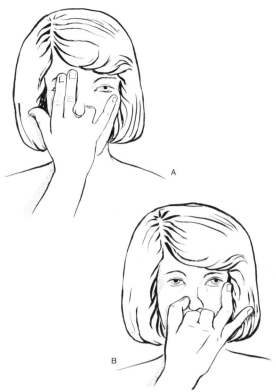

Alternate nostril breathing. (Redrawn from Zebroff, K.: *The ABC of Yoga.* Vancouver, B. C., Fforbez Enterprises, Ltd., 1971.)

   3. Inhale deeply and slowly through the RIGHT nostril to the count of four.
   4. Close off the RIGHT nostril with your thumb and retain the breath for a count of 1–4 seconds. *(B).*
   5. Open the LEFT nostril and exhale to the count of 4–8 seconds. The longer you make the exhalation, the better. Concentrate on completely emptying the lungs.
   6. Breathe in through the same LEFT nostril to the count of 4.
   7. Close off the nostril with the ringfinger again and hold to the count of 1–4 seconds.
   8. Exhale through the RIGHT nostril to the count of 4–8 seconds. This makes up one round.
   9. Repeat these rounds of alternate nostril breathing five more times, or up to ten minutes if you are concerned about insomnia.
   10. Practice a ratio of 4:4:8, if at all possible. Increase this to 8:4:8 eventually, then 8:8:8, after some months.

III. *Dos and Dont's:*
   DO NOT push yourself with the holding position or by increasing the ratio until you are comfortable doing so.
   DO make the breathing rhythmic, smooth and slow. You can work on making it inaudible eventually.
   DO practice the Alternate Nostril Breath when-

---

*Reprinted from Kareen Zebroff: *The ABC of Yoga.* Vancouver, B. C., Fforbez Enterprises, Ltd., 1971.

ever you need calming—if you are nervous, upset or irritable.

I cannot over-emphasize the importance of this particular breath. The body and mind are closely inter-related and one influences the other to a much greater extent than medicine admitted to for many years. As an all-round "soother" the Alternate Nostril Breath is incomparable.

Music. Music has, or course, been used from time immemorial to soothe and relax a person. The lullabies mothers sing to their infants and small children are intended to relax and put the child to sleep. Marketing people have been using soft music to soothe jangled nerves in their shopping centers for a number of years. Music has also been found to help nervous passengers to relax during the particularly worrying landing stages of an airline journey. So, it is no surprise that music is now being advocated as a pain reliever. Slow, quiet music is best, and it is helpful if the person is in a comfortable position and can close his eyes and try to imaging himself floating or drifting with the music.[6]

Conscious Suggestion. This technique is being used increasingly to help people to manage pain. It is basically a method of helping a person to relax and help himself. Affirmative suggestions are given by the nurse, who is careful not to appear to be giving orders but merely suggesting in a positive fashion, as in such statements as: "You want to relax, don't you?" and "You are going to relax, aren't you?" The calm, soothing voice of the nurse and her reassurances help to give the person a feeling of security. The use of positive suggestions, each one followed by a question that can only be answered with a "Yes," gets the person thinking positively, so that he is indeed able to relax.[8]

Hypnosis has also been used successfully to relieve pain in many patients, and sometimes "placebos" (which contain no drugs) are as effective as the administration of analgesics. In both hypnosis and placebo administration, *suggestion* is the key factor in relieving the patient's pain.

Cutaneous Stimulation. Stimulation of the skin and subcutaneous tissues by various means—by rubbing, by hot and cold applications, and by ointments—also has a long history of use in pain relief.

The pain-relieving actions of *heat and cold* are well known (see Chapter 19). In general, heat tends to relieve pain through increasing circulation in the part of the body to which it is applied. Hence, heat is often effective in the relief of muscular aches and pains, since the increased circulation helps to carry away metabolic waste products, which are thought to be a factor in causing muscular pain. A warm bath often helps to relieve aching muscles after a person has engaged in strenuous exercise. Cold has the opposite effect of heat—that is, it decreases peripheral circulation. In doing so, it helps to reduce swelling and therefore pressure on sensory nerve endings. An ice collar is frequently used to relieve pain following operations on the throat when the tissues are swollen and painful. Cold is also used sometimes as a local anesthetic agent. The intense cold in this case serves to deaden sensory nerve endings, thus preventing the transmission of pain impulses.

Therapeutic baths are also used to relieve pain. Sometimes the bath is a means of applying heat or cold to the body. Sometimes it is a vehicle for other agents, as, for example, the colloid baths that are frequently used for people with irritating skin conditions.

Massage has had a long history of use in the treatment of pain of muscular origin. The effect of massage is similar to that of heat in that it increases circulation to a part, thereby accelerating removal of the waste products of cellular metabolism.

Soothing balms in liquid or ointment form have long been used to assuage the pain in aching muscles and joints. Most of the ointments and liniments produce an immediate feeling of warmth (although some have a cooling effect), which may last for several hours. Many contain menthol, which appears to have a specific action in relieving pain, although the reason for this effect is not entirely clear. The warmth is produced by an increased blood supply in the area, so, to a certain extent, the effect is similar to that caused by the application of heat applications. It may be, too, that the menthol stimulates the release of endorphins that block the transmission of pain impulses. For whatever reason, menthol seems to be effective. Although used primarily for muscle and joint pain, it has also been found effective in treating headaches. Menthol ointments are also used in some parts of the world to relieve gas pains, the ointment being rubbed on the abdomen.[6]

When it is impossible to get at a painful area—a limb in a cast, for example, or an area covered by a dressing that cannot be removed—the skin in an opposite area can be stimulated (*contralateral stimulation*) to provide relief in the painful area. Any of the methods of cutaneous stimulation described above can be used.

Acupuncture. Acupuncture has been used for centuries in China for the treatment of various

These acupuncture charts show the traditional sites for insertion of acupuncture needles. (From Melzack, R.: *The Puzzle of Pain*. New York, Basic Books, Inc., 1973.)

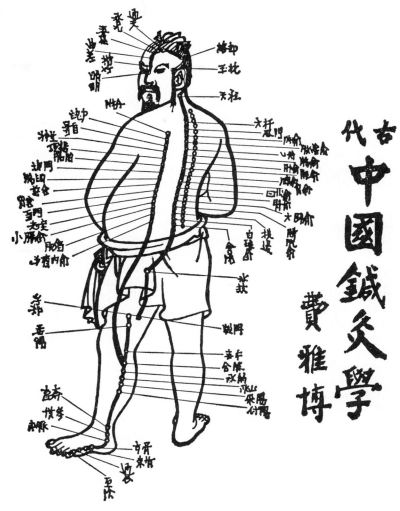

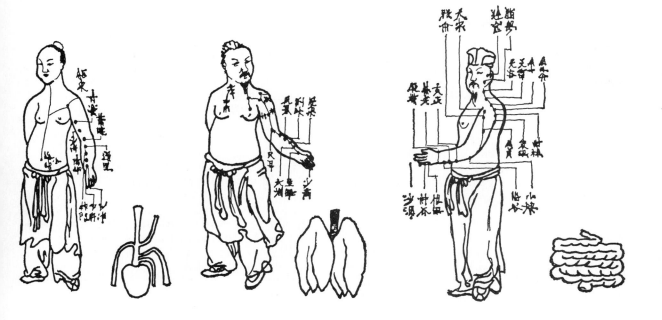

disorders, for the relief of pain, and, more recently, for surgical analgesia. During the past few years it has attracted the attention of Western medicine, and it is beginning to be utilized in some parts of North America as an alternative method of treating pain.

The technique of acupuncture consists of inserting long, fine needles into particular areas of the skin. Sometimes an electrical current is passed between two needles, but more commonly the needles are twirled continuously by hand. Traditional sites on the skin are used for the insertion of the needles; these sites are said to be associated with specific internal organs of the body, as indicated on the example of a typical acupuncture chart shown on page 461.

The physiological mechanisms involved in the relief of pain by acupuncture are not fully understood. However, the gate-control theory discussed earlier in this chapter offers a possible explanation. Melzack, in his book *The Puzzle of Pain*, suggests that acupuncture may be a special case of hyperstimulation analgesia.[2] In other words, the stimulation of particular nerves or tissues by the acupuncture needles results in increased input to the gate-control mechanism, causing the gate to close the pain impulses from selected areas of the body.

Medications. Then, too, there are the numerous *pharmacological agents* that are used for pain relief. These tend to fall into two groups: those that are "specifics" for certain conditions and those that have a general analgesic effect. Among the specifics are the muscle relaxants, such as meprobamate, which is used in conditions such as spastic paralysis, and phenylbutazone, which is a central nervous system depressant frequently prescribed for patients with arthritic conditions.

The principal drugs used as general analgesics include the narcotics, such as morphine, codeine, and their derivatives; synthetic compounds such as Demerol and Darvon; and the analgesic-antipyretic group of drugs, of which aspirin is by far the most widely used. Considerable controversy still exists over the physiological reason for the effectiveness of these drugs in pain relief. The narcotics, we know, have a depressant action on the central nervous system. Some experts believe that these drugs act on the corticothalamic pathways and the perceptive areas of the brain to cause a reduction in pain sensations. Others feel that the action of morphine and the other narcotics is principally that of mood alteration, so that the person remains aware of the pain, but his reaction to it is diminished. Morphine, its derivatives, and some of the stronger synthetic compounds, such as Demerol, are used in cases of severe pain; codeine is used for pain of lesser intensity. Tranquilizing drugs, such as Phenergan and chlorpromazine, are sometimes given at the same time as a narcotic. Their action appears to enhance the pain-relieving properties of the narcotic so that a smaller dosage of the analgesic may be used.

With regard to the analgesic-antipyretic group of drugs, most experts seem to agree that these agents in some way block the transmission of pain impulses, probably in the thalamic pathways, thus decreasing the perception of pain. Aspirin and other drugs of this group are used extensively for the relief of minor aches and pains.

The nurse's responsibility in the administration of analgesics is a crucial one. Sometimes prescriptions are written for analgesics to be given every 4 hours, or at other specified times (as, for example, is frequently the case with patients who have arthritic and rheumatic disorders). In most instances, however, the orders are written as *p.r.n.*, and the nurse must use her judgment as to the time of administration and the interval between medications. Many times the nurse is faced too with the decision of which of two or three analgesic orders to use for a patient. He may, for example, have morphine

Despite the warm hand and comforting manner of the nurse, this young man's pain persists anyway. Perhaps the medication will help.

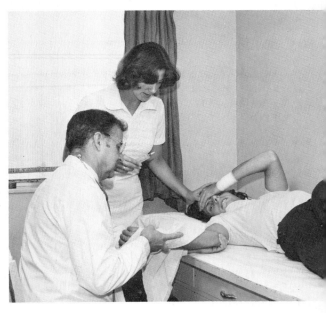

sulphate, Darvon, and aspirin all prescribed for pain relief. If the patient is having pain, the nurse must then decide on the medication to be used in this particular situation or whether, in fact, the patient may be made comfortable by measures other than drugs. In making this decision, the nurse is guided by her knowledge of the disease process the patient has, her understanding of the factors causing his pain, and her knowledge of the individual patient. A patient who is suffering from incurable cancer and is in the terminal stages of illness may require a strong narcotic to relieve his pain effectively. For the person who has a simple headache, aspirin may be sufficient to bring relief. Sometimes, changing the patient's position is all that is needed to make him more comfortable.

Measures to Help the Patient to Cope with Pain

One of the nurse's most important functions is the provision of psychological support for the patient in pain. Discussing the meaning pain holds for the patient is one way of doing this. Sometimes the nurse will find that it is not really pain that is bothering the patient but something else. He may be concerned with the results of his surgery, for instance, and view anything that he thinks is unusual as indicative that he has an incurable condition. Possibly the patient may be worried about his ability to tolerate pain, particularly if he has been raised with the Western ethic of stoicism.

Knowing what to expect in the way of pain often enables a person to prepare himself to cope with the situation; it also removes much of the fear of the unknown so that anxiety is lessened. Many diagnostic and therapeutic procedures are uncomfortable or even painful. If it is known that a patient is scheduled for an examination or treatment that is potentially painful, it is usually better to explain to the patient exactly what is going to be done, the nature of the pain he may experience, and what he can do to assist. If the individual understands also why the procedure is necessary, he is usually much better able to cooperate. Explanations of this sort can often help to change the individual's attitude toward the painful experience, since pain that is viewed as an aid in getting better is usually more tolerable than pain that is thought inflicted for reasons a person does not understand.

Even with children, telling them that a procedure is going to hurt a little, and what the hurt will be like, is much preferable to telling them that it is not going to hurt and then proceeding to inflict pain. The latter course of action can destroy a child's trust in health personnel. A factual explanation of exactly what is going to happen to them can usually eliminate much fear for both adults and children.

Reassuring the patient that pain will not be beyond his level of tolerance is sometimes advisable. "If it hurts too much, we will give you something to relieve the pain" is an example of words that can sometimes be used. Touch, for instance, placing a hand on the patient's arm, is often helpful when a patient is undergoing a painful procedure. The nurse should be careful in the use of touch, however. Some patients dislike it, particularly if they are striving to maintain their independence. Many, however, are grateful for a hand to hold when pain seems to much to bear alone.

Enabling the patient to retain a measure of control over the situation can also be helpful in minimizing the reaction to pain. "Tell me when it hurts and we will stop for a minute" is one way of doing this. Involving the patient in some part of the activity, such as holding a piece of the equipment, can help to make him feel a participating member of the health team rather than an object of its actions. Again, distraction can sometimes be used. If the patient is concentrating on taking deep breaths, for example, his attention will not be focused entirely on his pain.

After a painful experience is over, the nurse should make certain that the patient is settled comfortably. Evidence of the painful procedure, such as the dressing tray, should be removed as soon as possible. Some nurses have found that staying with the patient and allowing him to talk over the experience helps him to put it into perspective.

Helping the patient who suffers pain over a long period of time—for instance, the patient with a chronic disease condition—is frequently a challenge to nursing personnel. The nurse can often help to minimize his pain, if not always to completely alleviate it, by some of the measures discussed in previous sections. The nurse can also make certain that in her care of the patient she does not aggravate his pain. She can, for example, use gentleness when handling painful limbs and remove potential sources of pain and discomfort. It has been suggested, too, that helping the patient to find a meaning for his suffering can be of assistance to the patient in handling chronic pain. In this regard, many patients have found their spiritual counselor of considerable help and some have benefited from psychiatric counseling.

GUIDE TO ASSESSING PAIN

1. How old is the patient?

2. What words does the patient use to describe his pain?

3. Where does the patient feel pain? Can he describe its exact location?

4. How severe is the pain? Does its intensity vary?

5. When does the pain occur? How long does it last? Is it intermittent or steady?

6. Has the cause of the patient's pain been identified?

7. Is the patient aware of any factors that precipitate the pain? that aggravate it or relieve it?

8. What was the person doing when he first became aware of the pain?

9. Are there observable signs of pain—for example, evidence of muscular tension, protective posture, pallor, diaphoresis?

10. Are there signs that would lead you to suspect that the patient's pain has been sufficiently intense to cause a collapse of the body's adaptive mechanisms, such as a lowered blood pressure or weakened pulse?

11. Is the patient restless, irritable? Does he have difficulty in getting to sleep?

12. Are the patient's basic physiological needs being met?

13. Are there factors which might cause the patient to be anxious or fearful?

14. How much exertion can the patient tolerate without pain? Are there certain movements or activities which are painful?

15. Does he have to undergo any procedures which may be painful?

16. What measures have been prescribed for relief of the patient's pain?

GUIDE TO EVALUATING THE EFFECTIVENESS OF NURSING INTERVENTION

1. Does the patient state that he is more comfortable? Has the pain gone or lessened in intensity?

2. Does the patient appear more comfortable—that is, is he more relaxed or less restless and irritable?

3. Has the patient been able to get to sleep without difficulty? or to rest quietly?

4. Is he able to enjoy his usual activities?

STUDY SITUATION

Mrs. Jean Roberts is admitted to the hospital after an automobile accident in which she has possibly fractured her ribs. Mrs. Roberts' husband was also injured at the same time, and he is admitted to a nearby nursing unit. He has a fractured pelvis. Mrs. Roberts is 33 years old, has three small children at home and is in a great deal of pain upon admission. Her physician does not wish to bind her chest at this time. His orders include:

Demerol, 100 mg. I.M. q4h p.r.n.

Seconal, gr. 1½ q.h.s.

Up and about as desired
Food and fluids as desired
Chest x-rays as soon as possible

1. Describe the physiology of this patient's pain.

2. What factors would enter into this patient's perception of and reaction to pain?

3. How might this patient describe her pain?

4. What observation would indicate to the nurse that the patient has pain?

5. What should the nurse include in her recording about this patient's pain? Give an example of the recording, including subjective data, objective data, assessment, and plan.

6. What are the goals of nursing care of this patient?

7. What specific nursing intervention might help alleviate pain?

8. By what criteria can the nurse evaluate the success of the nursing care?

SUGGESTED READINGS

Coyle, N.: Analgesics at the Bedside. *American Journal of Nursing.* 79(9):1554–1557, September, 1979.

Fagerhaugh, S. Y., and Strauss, A.: How to Manage Your Patient's Pain . . . and How Not to. *Nursing '80,* 10(2):44–47, October, 1980.

Falconer, M. W., et al.: *The Drug, the Nurse, the Patient.* 6th ed. Philadelphia, W. B. Saunders Company, 1978, pp. 130–141.

McCaffery, M.: Understanding Your Patient's Pain. *Nursing '80,* 10(9):26–31, September, 1980.

McCaffery, M.: Patients Shouldn't Have to Suffer— Relieve Their Pain with Injectable Narcotics. *Nursing '80,* 10(10):34–39, October, 1980.

McCaffery, M.: Relieve Your Patient's Pain Fast and Effectively with Oral Analgesics. *Nursing '80,* 10(11):58–64, November, 1980.

McCaffery, M.: Relieving Pain with Noninvasive Techniques. *Nursing '80,* 10(12):55–57, December, 1980.

McGuire, L.: A Short, Simple Tool for Assessing Your Patient's Pain. *Nursing '81,* 11(3):48–49, March, 1981.

McGuire, L.: Managing Pain in the Young Patient. *Nursing '82,* 12(8):52, August, 1982.

Meissner, J. E.: McGill-Melzack Pain Questionnaire. *Nursing '80,* 10(1):50–51, January, 1980.

Panayotoff, K.: Managing Pain in the Elderly Patient. *Nursing '82,* 12(8):53, August, 1982.

Simonetti, D.: Prolapsed Mitral Valve: Living with Chest Pain. *American Journal of Nursing,* 80(8):1430–1432, August, 1980.

Steele, B. G.: Test Your Knowledge of Postoperative Pain Management. *Nursing '80,* 10(3):70–72, March, 1980.

Storlie, F.: Pointers for Assessing Pain. *Nursing '78,* 8(5):37–39, May, 1978.

West, B. A.: Understanding Endorphins: Our Natural Pain Relief System. *Nursing '81,* 11(2):50–53, February, 1981.

Wilson, R. W.: Endorphins. *American Journal of Nursing,* 81(4):722–725, April, 1981.

Wylie, L. (ed.): Achieving Pain Control in the Patient with Multiple Myeloma. *Nursing '79,* 9(11):34–39, November, 1979.

REFERENCES

1. Caplan, F. (ed.): *The First Twelve Months of Life.* New York, Bantam Books, 1978.

2. Melzack, R.: *The Puzzle of Pain.* New York, Basic Books, Inc., 1973.

3. West, B. A.: Understanding Endorphins: Our Natural Pain Relief System. *Nursing '81,* 11(2):50–53, February, 1981.

4. MacBryde, C. M., and Blacklow, R. S. (eds.): *Signs and Symptoms: Applied Pathologic Physiology and Clinical Interpretation.* 5th ed. Philadelphia, J. B. Lippincott Company, 1970.

5. Zborowski, M.: *People in Pain.* San Francisco, Jossey-Bass Inc., 1969.

6. McCaffery, M.: Relieving Pain with Noninvasive Techniques. *Nursing '80,* 10(12):55–57, December, 1980.

7. Zebroff, K.: *The ABC of Yoga.* Vancouver, B. C., Fforbez Enterprises, Ltd., 1971.

8. Holderby, R. A.: Conscious Suggestion: Using Talk to Manage Pain. *Nursing '81,* 11(5):44–46, May, 1981.

22

The Nurse Should Be Able to:

- Discuss sensory stimulation as a basic human need
- Explain briefly and in simple terms the process of sensory perception
- Discuss factors affecting sensory perception
- Discuss variations in sensory perception throughout the life cycle
- Assess the status of the patient's sensory abilities
- Identify common problems in sensory functioning
- Apply relevant principles in planning and evaluating nursing interventions
    a. to promote optimal sensory input for patients
    b. to help the patient to cope with a partial or complete sensory deficit
- Evaluate the effectiveness of nursing interventions

Section Two   ACTIVITY NEEDS

SENSORY NEEDS

CHAPTER 22

INTRODUCTION

Sensory stimulation is a basic human need. Psychologists and educators have long been aware of the need for adequate sensory stimulation to promote the optimal growth and development of children, but only in recent years has the subject received much attention in other areas of the health field, particularly for adults.

Yet, sensory stimulation is a vital component of our lives. Our sensory abilities of sight, hearing, smell, taste, and touch are the antennae that enable us to pick up signals that give us information about our environment. Without these abilities, we would not know what is going on in the world around us. Nor would we be able to communicate with other people, since communication involves both visual and auditory abilities, as well as abilities to symbolize, to write, and to make sounds. In discussions of sensory functioning, the ability to communicate is usually included because of the interrelationship of sensory functioning and communication.

The receiving and accurate interpretation of sensory input from the environment is essential for survival. The person who has lost the use of one of his senses is handicapped. One of his antennae is missing, so to speak, and he must pick up more stimuli from other sources to make up for it.

The person who is blind, for example, learns to distinguish sound with much more discrimination than the person whose sense of sight is intact. He also develops the sensitivity of his fingers to allow him to read Braille. But he may still require the help of another person or of a "seeing-eye" dog to protect him from hazards in the environment.

Similarly, the person who is deaf learns to "listen" to other people by reading their lips; if he is both deaf and mute (unable to speak), he may learn to talk in sign language. He also develops his sense of sight more keenly to interpret the meaning of nonverbal communications. But the deaf person is still at a disadvantage; he may not hear the horn of a car warning him to get out of the way when he is crossing the street.

Inability to communicate, either in speech or in writing, lessens a person's ability to make contact with other human beings and, hence, cuts off a major area of sensory stimulation. If speech is affected, the individual must either write his messages or depend on nonverbal means of communication. If the ability to write is lost, the person is more or less at the level of a child who has not yet learned to write.

Appetite is aroused by the sight and smell of food, but it is also dependent on direct stimulation of the taste buds. Thus, if the ability to taste is lost, a person's appetite diminishes, and he may take in insufficient nourishment to meet his body's requirements. Loss of the sense of smell lessens the pleasure of a cup of coffee, since the aroma of coffee contributes a great deal to its enjoyment. The loss of the sense of smell also entails other handicaps. A person may not be able to distinguish important odors, such as fumes. He may not, for example, smell the smoke of a fire, but must depend on his senses of sight and hearing to alert him to the danger.

If a person has lost the sense of touch in a part of his body, e.g., if his left arm and leg are paralyzed as a result of stroke, he is unable to tell if tissues in the affected arm and leg are being damaged. He cannot tell if a hot water bottle is burning his left foot, for instance. Loss of the sense of touch affects the ability to perceive pain, heat and cold, and pressure. It also affects a person's balance, since we use touch as a means of aligning ourselves with objects or persons in our immediate environment. We feel where we are sitting in a chair, for example, and shift ourselves around until we are comfortable. A person without the sense of touch is cut off from contact with other objects or human beings so far as the affected area is concerned. If his arm or hand is paralyzed, he is unable to feel the comfort of a soothing hand on his arm, or to feel the texture of a piece of silk in his hand.

Of course, a person can also suffer from too much sensory input. The excessive noise and constant barrage of stimuli from a variety of sources that seem to be a part of living in a large city these days can overload our sensory receiving mechanisms and result in problems in sensory functioning. One wonders, for example, about the possible damage done to the hearing abilities of people who frequent discotheques, since the noise emanating from them has often been measured at well above the safety limit for noise levels.

SENSORY PERCEPTION

The perception of sensory stimuli is a complex process, which has its origin in the five sense organs: the eyes, the ears, the skin, the nose, and the mouth. Receptors in the sense organs pick up stimuli from the environment and send this information along to the brain via distinct channels in the nervous system.* The information passes through several levels of increasing complexity in the brain, where it is modified, refined, and interpreted. This interpretation depends on a number of factors, such as the individual's state of well-being, his past experiences with stimuli of this sort, and the interrelationship of stimuli coming in from various sources. The result of this process, which takes less than a second of time, is known as *perception*.

In order to process sensory perception, the brain (in particular, the reticular formation) depends on a constant and varied barrage of stimuli from the environment. If the receptors are not picking up enough stimuli or are getting too much of the same stimuli, *adaptation* occurs, and the brain will no longer perceive the available stimuli. To illustrate this effect, the student might try sitting in a quiet, darkened room and staring at a luminous object. Gradually the object will seem to disappear until the student can no longer see it. Extreme concentration on any object or person will produce the same effect. This phenomenon has been known to be used by some cult leaders as a demonstration of their power over their followers. A lack of environmental stimulation will likewise result in a form of sensory adaptation. It is believed that, in this case, the brain will then focus on higher thought

*This is not so for the perception of pain, as we discussed in Chapter 21.

processes and tend to disregard the small amount of external stimulation that is availalble. Either situation—that is, too much of one stimulus or not enough stimuli altogether—results in sensory deprivation.

FACTORS AFFECTING SENSORY FUNCTIONING

There are two major sets of factors that affect sensory functioning:

1. Environmental factors. There may be either an undersupply or an excess of sensory stimuli in the environment.
2. Biological factors. Besides the physiological changes that occur throughout the life cycle, biological factors include (a) impairment of the sensory receptors themselves or the neural structures transmitting sensory impulses, and (b) impairment of the centers for processing sensory stimuli.

Environmental Factors

Inadequate Stimuli. People who have all of their sensory abilities intact are just as likely to suffer from a lack of sensory stimuli as are people with impairment of these abilities. The lack of stimulation may be in the physical environment, the psychosocial environment, or both. People with limited mobility, such as "shut-ins" at home, those confined to a wheelchair or a sickroom, or those whose ability to get around is limited in any way, are particularly vulnerable. Their opportunities for varying their surroundings and for meeting and talking with other people are seriously hampered. The potentialities for inadequate sensory stimulation are therefore greatly increased. People whose work or home environments are monotonous and lacking in stimulation may also suffer from sensory deprivation. The man who works on a assembly line, for example, and has few hobbies or after-work activities, and the housewife who stays home day after day with the same monotonous round of housework and who has no interests outside the home are both likely to suffer from sensory deprivation.

The problem of lack of stimulation is a very common one in people who are ill, particularly in the hospital setting. Profound disturbances caused by this form of sensory deprivation have been documented in studies on patients in isolation, in intensive care units, and in coronary care units, who have minimal contact with the outside world. Whether it is in the home or in a hospital, the normal sickroom is usually lacking in environmental stimuli. Noise is kept to a minimum, lights are low, and contact with family and friends is often restricted. In the hospital

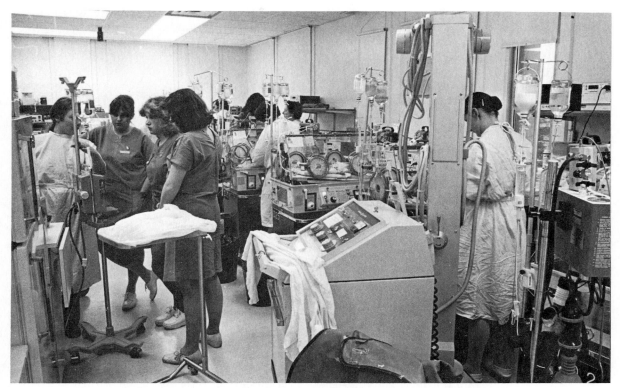

In the intensive care nursery, sensory overload is possible even in tiny babies.

setting, the walls are often bare and colors muted. All these factors were thought to act for the best interests of the patient, with the principal objective being to promote rest and comfort. Unfortunately, the reverse is often true.

Excess Stimuli. As we mentioned at the beginning of this chapter, a person may sometimes have an overabundance of sensory stimulation. This is not an uncommon problem in the sickroom or hospital setting. Although the atmosphere of the sickroom or the hospital is traditionally quiet and conducive to rest, often this is not the case. Many humorous articles have been written by patients about the disturbances of rest in a hospital, but the situation is not always amusing. The patient may be subjected to bright lights or disruptive noises, as, for example, those produced by the machinery used to provide life-giving assistance to him, such as a respirator or a renal dialysis (artificial kidney) machine. The noise of food carts being trundled along the hall can also be disturbing. The patient's rest may be constantly interrupted by members of the health team checking his vital signs or those of a roommate. Adequate rest and sleep are important in a person's physical and psychological well-being, as well as in his sensory perception; the specific effects of sleep deprivation are discussed more fully in Chapter 20.

Impairment of the Sense Organs

The sense organs and their accessory muscles, nerves, and blood supply must be intact for optimal sensory stimulation. Disease, injury, or a congenital defect can interfere with the receiving of adequate sensory input. The impairment may be temporary, or it may be permanent. A person recovering from eye surgery who has both eyes bandaged may be suffering only a temporary loss of vision, but it is a very distressing experience. While his eyes are bandaged, he must adjust to life as a blind person. The person with a permament sensory deficit must learn to adapt by making greater use of his remaining sensory abilities and learning to live with the deficit.

The loss of the sense of sight, of hearing, or of touch may mean a complete restructuring of a person's life. The person who loses some of his hearing may be able to use a hearing aid, but not all hearing problems can be helped by this means. The person who has lost any of the three senses just mentioned or his ability to speak loses at least some of his independence and, consequently, his self-esteem suffers as he finds he has to depend on others to do things he would normally do for himself.

Sensory impairment may be either partial or total. Partial loss of any of the senses can be almost as disturbing as total impairment. A per-

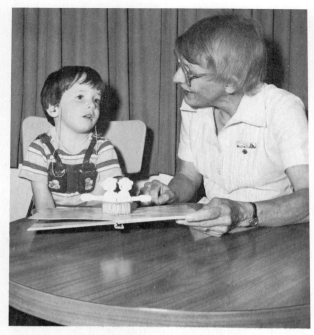

Hearing aids are helpful in many cases, but the patient may also need a great deal of teaching to learn to overcome a partial loss of hearing.

son recovering from an eye operation who has only one eye bandaged is .unable to perceive depth, which depends on focusing both eyes simultaneously. The individual who is "hard of hearing" often becomes very anxious and frustrated as he tries to catch what other people are saying. His social relationships may be impaired

Even the temporary loss of the sense of sight is a distressing experience.

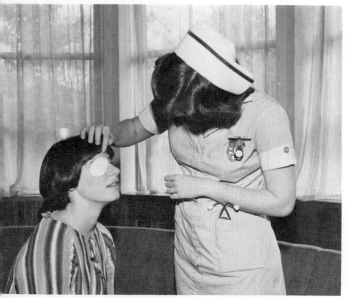

and he loses much in the way of sensory stimulation because of his difficulties in receiving spoken messages.

Distorted sensory perception can be equally distressing and potentially harmful to the individual. A person with distorted vision, for example, may stumble and fall as he tries to find where he should put his foot next. If you have ever walked through a "fun house" in an amusement park, you may remember how it feels to have your vision distorted in one of the convex or concave mirrors. This experience helps to give you some idea of the feelings of a person with distorted vision.

Impairment of the Centers for Processing Sensory Stimuli

Any factors that impair the functioning of centers in the brain that refine, modify, and interpret sensory input interfere with a person's sensory abilities. Diseases affecting mental processes, or damage to the brain itself resulting from disease processes or from injury, may cause disturbances in sensory functioning. Fever, for example, often distorts sensory perception: a very high fever may cause a person to have hallucinations. Hallucinations are something like dreams. They may be visual or auditory; the person may see persons or objects in his mind, or he may hear voices or other noises. Other senses, such as smell and touch, may also be involved, and sometimes several sensations may be experienced at the same time. When this occurs, the feeling that this is real, and not a dream, may be overpowering.[2]

A stroke (cerebrovascular accident) is a common cause of temporary or permanent impairment to brain tissues that interferes with sensory functioning. Paralysis often results from a stroke, and not infrequently there is interference with speech and hearing as well. Because the speech area in the brain is located in the dominant hemisphere, a stroke affecting this side of the brain may cause difficulties in speaking or aphasia (that is, a complete absence of the ability to speak). In people with heart problems, general circulation is impaired, and there may be interference with the blood supply to the brain. These people then may also experience disturbances in sensory functioning because of the inadequate oxygenation of brain tissues.

A person's level of consciousness affects both his ability to receive sensory input and his ability to process it. His antennae are turned down low, to pick up the analogy used at the beginning of the chapter, and the complicated mechanisms in the brain that process the sensory stimuli are functioning at less than optimal efficiency when the level of a person's consciousness is decreased.

Drugs that depress the central nervous system will decrease sensory functioning, since it is this system that carries information from the sensory receptors and also handles the processing of it. Many drugs are known to cause distortions in sensory perception. The hallucinogens, such as marijuana and LSD, cause a person to have hallucinations. Other drugs commonly used in the treatment of illness may also cause disturbances in sensory functioning, such as a blurring of vision, a ringing in the ears, or a distorted taste. These are side-effects, and are specific to each drug. When caring for patients on any type of medication therapy, the nurse should be aware of potential side-effects and be alert for their appearance in the patient.

A person's emotional state can also affect his sensory abilities. A happy person sees everything in a different light than when he is worried or depressed. The flowers have more color; other people look different, perhaps more friendly. The depressed individual, on the other hand, may be unaware of things in his immediate environment—his eyes just do not see them.

SENSORY FUNCTIONING THROUGHOUT THE LIFE CYCLE

Even before birth, the sensory antennae of the developing human being are beginning to function. The fetus responds to sounds of all kinds starting in the fifth month of gestation.[1] When he arrives in this world, the newborn has all of the essential sensory equipment, with most of the organs fairly well developed and ready to function. As we mentioned in Chapter 21, the newborn will withdraw from a painful stimulus, such as a pinprick. He will also turn toward a light, will respond to odors, and can detect visual patterns. His sense of smell is completely developed at birth. By the time the infant is 3 weeks old, he can imitate adult movements with the mouth. If the mother has not been sedated during delivery, the baby is likely to be very responsive and alert. If he is tired and hungry, however, he is capable of shutting out excessive stimulation and is less aware of outside stimulation.

From birth, infants are very sensitive to touch and pressure. Skin contact and warmth are the most powerful stimuli in the first few months. People often remark on the fact that "their" baby has very large eyes. In point of fact, all babies do; the eye of the newborn is three fourths the size of an adult's. During the first 12 months of life, the eye grows rapidly. This growth gradually slows down until the third year, when the eye reaches anatomical maturity. Visual matu-

rity is reached in the sixth year. Newborns do not cry with tears, the tear glands usually not being functional until the infant is two weeks old. Infants are aware of the relationship between sight and sound at a very early age, and by the time the child is ready to crawl, he is able to perceive depth. Screening for hearing defects can be done by the time an infant is 6 to 12 months old. Because the infant has taste buds all over his mouth, he tends to stuff his mouth as full as he can once he starts to feed himself. During infancy, it is important for the child to have a variety of sensory inputs. A lack of stimulation, as for example, in institutional care can result in depression and developmental delays.

The major change in sensory perception during the early years of childhood is the maturation of vision. The young child's eye is normally *hyperopic;* that is, a distant image will fall behind the retina, but because of the malleable lens the child's eyes accommodate for this easily. Sometimes this condition persists into adulthood. If the eye becomes too long during growth, the child will become *myopic,* that is, nearsighted. Such a child does not usually complain of poor vision, however, since he does not know anything else. With most children, vision usually improves up to the age of 5 years, when most have 20/20 vision. An annual vision screening is done in most school systems from kindergarten through the high school years. Periodic hearing screening is also done in most schools. This is important because a significant hearing loss is one of the most commonly overlooked serious handicaps in children.

By the time the individual reaches adolescence, there is a cessation of growth and a stabilization of sensory powers. As people grow older, their sensory functioning decreases. It takes more stimulation to whet the appetite, for example, because the sensory stimulation of taste is diminished (there are fewer taste buds functioning in the mouth). Yet older people, particularly those residing in institutions, are often given very bland meals. Of course, one has to consider other factors as well, such as the person's ability to chew food and any gastrointestinal problems he may have, but the monotony of institutional meals does not usually do much to encourage the intake of adequate nourishment by older people.

Vision also decreases as one grows older. As a person approaches middle age, he generally finds that he needs to wear glasses, even if he did not need them before. In old age, visual acuity is often impaired by cataracts or retinal degeneration. Most old people are farsighted, because of the loss of elasticity of the lens. The pupils are often small, and there may be white, ringlike deposits of cholesterol ester just inside the edge of the cornea. Eyeglasses are an important part of the older person's sensory equipment. Nurses should be especially careful to handle them gently and to make sure that the lenses are clean. Many publishers are now putting out an increasing number of books in large print, which many older patients greatly appreciate.

Hearing also becomes less acute as a person gets older. Men tend to lose the ability to hear high tones (such as women's voices), while women tend to lose the ability to hear low tones, such as men's voices. And this fact alone, it has been said, has saved many a marriage. The older person usually needs the radio or television volume set much louder than a younger person does. It is also often necessary to speak more loudly to him and to enunciate words distinctly.

Depth perception and position sense are two other sensory abilities that decrease with increasing age, rendering the older person more susceptible to falls. There are two basic factors operating here. First of all, there is the increased length of time required for sensory impulses to travel to the brain, and for motor impulses to travel from the brain to the periphery. Hence, reaction time is increased. Also, there are degenerative changes in the sensory organs themselves, which cause decreased vestibular functioning and lessened visual acuity.

Older people seem to burn themselves a lot. One of the reasons for this is that their response to temperature is decreased. It is usually the middle ranges of temperature that are not perceived accurately, and the older person can be easily burned by water that is just a little too hot, or a heating pad that has been turned up too high.

Stronger impulses are needed to stimulate all of the senses as a person get older. The ability to perceive light touch and vibration is often lost, and even deep pressure sensitivity is diminished. An example of the loss of deep pressure sense is the lessened response to the rectal reflex for evacuation of the bowel. As you will recall from Chapter 16, this reflex is activated by the perception of a feeling of fullness in the rectum.

COMMON PROBLEMS OF SENSORY FUNCTIONING

The most common sensory disturbances the nurse will encounter in patients are:

1. Sensory deprivation
2. Sensory overload
3. Sensory deficit, partial or complete

Sensory deprivation has been defined as "a lack or alteration of impulses conveyed from the sense organs to the reflex or higher centers of the brain. It may result from inadequate or monotonous stimuli (that is, sensory underload), poorly functioning sense receptors, or an inability to preceive environmental data."[3] When an individual is ill, his resistance to harmful stimuli and his energy level are considerably lowered; thus, the effects of sensory deprivation are bound to be more profound in the sick person. Florence Downs states that "realistic bodily concerns probably heighten an individual's susceptibility to (indeterminate sensory experiences) by intensifying environmental disruption and encouraging introspection."[4]

Sensory overload simply means the bombardment of an individual by too many stimuli at the same time.

Sensory deprivation and sensory overload are relative terms. What might be sensory deprivation for one person may be peace and tranquility for another. A person who comes from a large family may enjoy a quiet time by himself. He may, on the other hand, not find noise as disturbing as one who is used to a quiet household, and in fact may miss the stimulation of an active, busy home.

A *sensory deficit* is a lack or a deficiency in one of the sensory abilities. It may be partial, as for example impaired vision, or complete, as in total blindness.

ASSESSMENT

In order to identify problems a patient may be having with regard to sensory functioning, the nurse will find information about the following items helpful:

The patient's usual status with regard to sensory functioning
　His present status in this regard
　Health problems he may have
　The therapy he is receiving if he has a health problem
　His personality
　His usual lifestyle
　His normal environment
　His present environment

Sources of Information

From the nursing history and the nurse's initial clinical appraisal, the nurse can obtain information about the patient's usual and current status with regard to his sensory abilities. The report of the initial physical examination of the patient, and any tests done on specific sensory abilities, such as a hearing test, eye examination, and so forth, should be included in the patient's record, and the nurse can supplement the nursing data with this information. Similarly, information about the patient's health problems and the plan of therapy for these should also be available to the nurse from the physician's notations and doctors' orders on the record.

From these sources the nurse can usually identify long-standing sensory deficits or problems the patient has, and any that have occurred recently. She can also obtain information about corrective devices that the patient uses, such as eyeglasses or a hearing aid. In addition, it is helpful to find out the answers to such questions as: What is his mobility status? Is he confined to bed, for example? Does he use a cane? Does he need a wheelchair for getting about?

Through talking with the patient and with his family or friends (the significant others in his life), the nurse can usually learn something about the patient's basic personality structure to supplement information from the nursing history. Is this individual normally a quiet person? Or he is usually talkative? Is he gregarious and does he enjoy the company of other people? Or does he prefer the company of his family or of one or two close frineds? What are his usual activities during the day? What is his present environment like in comparison with his usual environment?

This is by no means an exhaustive list of questions the nurse might ask herself, but it may help her to think of other questions that might be useful in relation to this particular patient.

The nurse can further extend information about the patient's sensory abilities by her observations of the patient and his subjective reporting of changes that occur. The patient is the most reliable source of information about the functioning of his senses. Much of the information about these abilities must come from him. Because it is difficult to separate the subjective observations from the objective in this particular set of problems, the two have been combined in the discussion that follows. However, in notations on the chart, the nurse will record separately her own observations and the information the patient gives her.

Observing for Sensory Deprivation

Sensory deprivation has long been thought to be a problem requiring nursing intervention. Florence Nightingale herself was evidently concerned about this when she wrote:

It is an ever recurring wonder to see educated people who call themselves nurses, acting thus. They vary their own objects, their own employments, many times a day; and while nursing (!) some bedridden sufferer, they let him be there staring at a dead wall, without any change of object to enable him to vary his thoughts; and it never occurs to them at least to move his bed so that he can look out of the window.[6]

Much research has been carried out in recent years on sensory deprivation and its effects on the human organism. In psychology departments in many universities, this subject has come under close scrutiny. Health personnel are also focusing their attention on sensory deprivation as an area of concern, as exemplified in a study reported by Downs.[4] The purpose of this particular study was not to test the effects of sensory deprivation but to investigate the effects of bed rest as functions related to personality characteristics and varied auditory input. The subjects who participated in the study were healthy young adults between the ages of 18 and 35. The incidental findings of the study were astonishing. Subjects reported disturbances ranging from basic physical discomfort, space and time disorientation, sensory distortions, and difficulty in concentrating, to outright hallucinations. One woman experienced the sensation of her leg being detached from the rest of her body. Other subjects felt as though they were floating above the bed. As the subjects in this study were considered to be in an optimal state of physical and psychological well-being, one may well question what the effects of sensory deprivation might be on persons who are ill.

It is important for the nurse to be able to recognize the signs of possible sensory deprivation in her patients and to take steps to prevent this problem from occurring or to remedy the situation if it does occur. Cameron and co-workers list a continuum of behaviors manifested by the patient suffering from sensory deprivation: boredom, inactivity, slowness of thought, daydreaming, increased sleeping, thought disorganization, anxiety, panic, hallucinations.[3]

The person who is *bored* may also be *inactive*, or he may be overactive, usually with trivial or inappropriate occupations. He may annoy other patients or continually push his call button to summon staff members, usually for small requests that are unnecessary or that he could handle himself. Often he is irritable and tends to make mountains of molehills. If he is *inactive*, he may appear apathetic and just lie or sit in one place without seeming to respond to any form of stimulation.

A person experiencing *slowness of thought* may take considerable time to grasp even simple concepts, and there may be great lapses in his conversation as he tries to think of what he wants to say. His reaction time will be reduced and he may appear clumsy and awkward.

The *daydreaming* individual may sit for seemingly endless periods of time, happily absorbed in his thoughts and fantasies, ignoring what is going on around him. It may be difficult to rouse him from his reveries, and he may not know when he has taken a medication or that someone was talking with him. He may confuse reality with fantasy.

The person who *sleeps* for longer than usual periods of time may be bored and consider this an effective way to pass the time, or he may actually find it difficult to stay awake with no stimuli to arouse his nervous system.

The individual suffering from *thought disorganization* may find it difficult to remember what he was saying, or he may experience space and time disorientation. He may not know what time of day it is, which meal he has just eaten, or where he is. He may make inappropriate responses both in conversation and in his actions. For example, he may intend to put on his glasses, and instead remove his shoes or put on his dressing gown. He may experience distortions in sensory perception and, for instance, think he is eating fish when in fact he is eating fruit.

The person experiencing *anxiety* may feel that he is losing all faculties one by one or that he has a terrible brain disease affecting his sensory perception. He may become frightened and resort to the use of one of the defense mechanisms, as mentioned in Chapter 2.

Panic, as discussed in Chapter 30 is a severe state of anxiety. When an individual reaches the stage of panic where sensory disturbances are concerned, he may feel that he will be permanently blind, deaf, or paralyzed, or that he is going mad.

Downs places *hallucinations* at the extreme of her continuum.[4] A person suffering from hallucinations has lost all contact with reality. An explanation of the reason for hallucinations appearing in people who have experienced sensory deprivation is found in the following quotation from R. L. Gregory's book, *Eye and Brain:*

It seems that the brain is always spontaneously active, and that the activity is normally under the control of sensory signals. When these are cut off [as in an isolation chamber] the brain activity can run wild and instead of perception of the world, we become dominated by hallucinations which may be terrifying and dangerous, or merely irritating and amusing.[2]

Observing for Sensory Overload

The nurse should also be alert to factors in the patient's environment that may cause sensory overload, and she should be observant for signs of this in the patient. Ambulatory patients may suffer from an excess of sensory stimulation in their work or home environment, or in the sum of their daily activities. Everyone needs a quiet place in which to relax, to be free from the constant ringing of the telephone and from all the other noises and activities that form a part of the lifestyle of many active, busy people.

The busy mother with a houseful of noisy children may show signs and symptoms of stress, as may the harried executive whose phone is constantly ringing, and who goes immediately from one meeting to another. The noise of machines in a factory constitutes a real health hazard to employees, as does the constant noise of planes for people who work in airports. We are only beginning to realize both the physical and psychological effects of excessive sensory stimulation as stress factors contributing to illness.

People who are ill are particularly vulnerable to the effects of excessive stimulation. This, of course, has long been recognized. Rest and quiet are still considered the best therapy for many illnesses. In many instances the body will heal itself if it is not overwhelmed with the exigencies of the usual everyday activities. Indeed, illness is frequently the body's way of telling the individual that rest is needed.

We have already mentioned some of the sources of excessive sensory stimulation in people who are ill. The nurse should be alert to the factors that have been discussed as well as to excessive noise, interruptions of the patient's rest, too many people attending to the patient, or too many visitors, particularly for the person who is acutely ill.

People usually show signs of being tired from the effects of these. They may express their weariness verbally but often it is the nurse's responsibility to note if the patient's face looks tired and drawn, if his reactions are slowing down and every movement seems an effort, or if he is lying quietly in bed, trying to ignore the noise and what he views as widespread confusion around him.

Observing for Sensory Deficits

From her other sources of information, the nurse will be aware of existing sensory deficits, but she should be alert to pick up any that have not been identified, and also any that subsequently develop. Things to watch for in relation to specific sensory areas:

Visual: (1) Acuity, particularly lessened ability to see objects or persons. If the patient normally wears glasses, the nurse should also check to see if these are still suitable for him. Many times, people find that illness affects their sight, and the glasses they used to wear no longer help them. This may

PRINCIPLES RELEVANT TO SENSORY FUCTIONING

Nursing interventions are planned for patients with sensory disturbances in accordance with their specific problem, and are based on the individual's particular needs. It is helpful, however, to keep the following principles in mind.

1. Psychosocial equilibrium requires that individuals have adequate sensory stimulation.

2. Stimuli picked up by the sense organs provide the body with information about the external environment.

3. Integrity of the sense organs is essential for sensory perception.

4. Sensory perception can be distorted in persons who are ill.

5. Damage to brain tissues caused by disease processes or by injury can interfere with sensory perception.

6. Communication provides an important means of sensory stimulation.

7. All sensory receptors adapt, either partially or totally, to their various stimuli over a period of time.

8. The brain is active even in the absence of stimuli from the external environment.

9. Sensory perception diminishes as a person get older.

10. The length of time an impulse takes to travel to the brain increases with age.

11. Reaction time to environmental stimuli also increases with age.

---

be one reason the patient is not reading.

(2) Field of vision, particularly a decreased field; the patient may be unable to see things on either side of him without turning his head as well as he could previously.

(3) Unusual sensations, such as the perception of spots in front of the eyes, or black, grey, or sometimes other colored areas obscuring part of his vision in one or both eyes; or a ring or "halo" around objects.

Auditory: (1) Ability to distinguish voices, or to locate sounds.

(2) Unusual sensations, such as ringing or humming in the ears.

Olfactory: (1) Ability to distinguish odors.

(2) Unusual sensations, such as smelling an odor when there is no stimulus for it. In this regard, it should be noted that people sometimes experience the sensation of a specific odor just prior to a seizure (convulsion).

Gustatory: (1) Ability to discriminate sweet, sour, salty, and bitter tastes.

(2) Unusual sensations, such as a bitter or metallic taste in the mouth.

Tactile: (1) Ability to discriminate sharp, dull, light, and firm touch.

(2) Ability to perceive heat, cold, pain.

(3) Intactness of body image.

(4) Unusual sensations, such as prickling, a feeling of "pins and needles," and the like.

Speech: (1) The formation and perception of speech.

(2) Problems in phonation (ability to articulate words).

(3) Ability to understand and initiate speech.

GOALS FOR NURSING ACTION

The goals of nursing action for patients with actual or potential problems of disturbed sensory functioning depend on the nature of the problem. Regardless of whether they have problems or not, two goals are common for all patients:

1. To prevent sensory deprivation
·2. To prevent sensory overload

For people with sensory deprivation, the following goals would be applicable:

1. To restore adequate sensory input
2. To restore normal perception

For people with a temporary or permanent sensory deficit, the following would be applicable.

1. To assist the individual to adjust to his deficit

2. To ensure that the individual receives adequate stimulation via his remaining sense receptors.

For people with sensory overload the primary objective would be to lessen sensory input to an optimal level.

SPECIFIC NURSING INTERVENTIONS

Our sensory abilities function to provide us with information about our environment. The environment, then, is one of the principal factors to be considered in helping people with sensory disturbances. Other major factors that the nurse takes into consideration are the individual's reaction to disturbances in his sensory abilities and his needs in relation to learning to live with a deficit, if this is the problem.

Nursing interventions are considered in the light of their suitability for each individual's particular problem. The following possible approaches for nursing action are, therefore, outlined separately for each of the three common problems identified earlier in the chapter.

Sensory Deprivation

The logical approach to nursing action for the person who is suffering from sensory deprivation, or for those in whom this is a potential problem, is to ensure that the environment contains adequate stimuli to maintain or restore optimal sensory input. This implies a certain amount of environmental management on the nurse's part.

People in a home situation should be encouraged to vary both their physical and their psychosocial environment. The nurse may be able to make some suggestions in this regard, or to involve family and friends, or community organizations, to assist the individual if he is unable to do this for himself. Radio and television are great comforts to people who are unable to get out of their everyday environment, and they help to keep the individual in touch with the outside world. These can be supplemented with active participation in games, crafts, and other activities that keep them in contact with their environment. If the person is fond of reading, mobile libraries are available in many communities. A visit by a library staff member not only provides the person with new books and magazines to read, but also provides the stimulation of a new face and some conversation to relieve the monotony of the day.

People who deliver "Meals on Wheels" find that their clientele often look forward to the social aspects of the service as much as the actual meal. A number of service clubs, lodges, and other community groups visit shut-ins, and arrange for outings for senior citizens and handicapped persons. The nurse should be familiar with those services that are available in the community in which she works. Community centers and organizations such as the YWCA, YMCA, or YMHA, also provide activities for those who are ambulatory. Bridge clubs, arts and crafts classes, and a variety of courses, including academic subjects as well as other subjects such as gardening, swimming, and exercise classes, are among the many activities offered in a number of these centers.

For the person who is ill and in an institutional setting, the same types of approaches may be used. Volunteers and the resources of the community can help to provide the individual with sufficient change in both physical and psychosocial environment to ensure an adequate amount of sensory input.

Varying the patient's surroundings, even if it is just moving his bed so he can look out the window, as Florence Nightingale suggested, provides the individual with a different perspective.

For the person who must remain in an extended care facility, or one who is severely handicapped and confined at home, it is important to maintain their contact with reality. It is helpful to provide some devices to enable them to do this. The use of clocks and watches, calendars, fixed time schedules for meals, arts and crafts, physiotherapy classes and so forth, regular television or radio programs, and similar means help to keep the person oriented to time and place. Newspapers and magazines provide

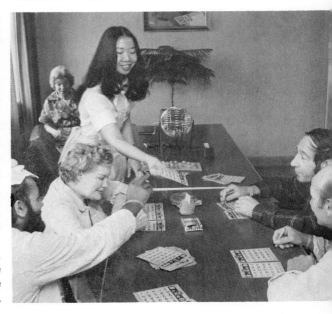

Active participation in games with other people provides a variety of sensory input that helps to keep an individual in touch with his environment.

a contact with what is going on in the world outside the agency setting.

The nurse may find brief explanations to the patient of nursing functions and treatments helpful, too, even if the activities are routine ones. They help to keep the person oriented as to where he is and what is being done for and to him. The nurse should not think that just because the patient does not respond that he does not hear. It is important to maintain auditory stimuli for the person who is seriously deprived of sensory input.

Nor should the nurse forget the therapeutic effects of touch as a means of communication. A number of articles have been written recently on this topic and the nurse will find reference to some of these in the suggested reading list at the end of the chapter. The "laying on of hands" that is so much a part of nursing has been shown to have definite therapeutic healing properties, from both a physical and a psychological point of view. The nurse's presence also means the patient has someone to talk to, and the different nurses coming on for different shifts help to provide a variation in people, which patients often find stimulating.

The nurse, then, functions both as a source of sensory input to the patient, and also as a resource person who can enlist the assistance of family, friends, visitors, and volunteers from community organizations to help the patient to receive adequate sensory stimulation. The nurse is frequently called upon to use her imagination to think of ways of getting people involved and providing the type of stimulation needed for a particular individual.

Sensory Overload

For the patient who is suffering from sensory overload, interventions that help to reduce the number of stimuli in the environment are indicated. In the community, the nurse may be able to help the individual to plan periods of rest in a busy day or to engage in activities that are relaxing for that individual. Physical exercise is often a good antidote for the person whose work keeps him in an office, a factory, or other enclosed surroundings. Some people need assistance in order to be able to rest and relax. Other people enjoy music or book reading or find a game of bridge relaxing. A change of stimuli is often as relaxing as a cessation of stimuli.

Some people need help in learning how to relax and clear their minds of stimuli activating them to do something. We discussed this topic in Chapter 21, and we will talk more about relaxation technique in Chapter 30.

We have already discussed some of the ways the nurse can help to reduce environmental stimuli for the ill person, at home or in hospital. In addition, it sometimes helps to explain things in the environment, the reason for all those tubes and machines that are surrounding the patient, the purpose of treatments, and the reason why other personnel come in to see the patient. Putting a structure to the sensory input helps a person to interpret stimuli meaningfully; he is not so apt to feel disoriented, and his anxiety is reduced.

Sensory Deficit

In helping a person to cope with either temporary or permanent impairment of any one of his sensory abilities, the nurse needs to be aware of the individual's reaction to it. Loss of sensory functioning has both physical and psychosocial ramifications. We have mentioned some of the psychosocial effects in our earlier discussions. If the person has suffered a permanent and total disability of one of the senses, he feels an acute sense of loss and will grieve. If the nurse is caring for someone who has recently experienced such a loss, she may find it helpful at this point to read Chapter 31 of this book on care of the terminally ill patient. This individual goes through the same process of grieving as the person described in Chapter 31.

With a partial or a temporary loss of sensory functioning, the person will probably be anxious and worried. Will he regain total functioning? What if he becomes totally blind, or deaf, or is permanently paralyzed? What if his speech never comes back? How is he going to cope with partial impairment? These are some of the spoken and unspoken questions the person asks.

The patient needs much psychological support in coping with his anxieties, even if he does not express them (see Chapter 30). He also needs assistance with handling his physical environment in such a way that the deficit does not interfere with daily activities.

The nurse should be alert to anticipate problems in this regard, and also be aware of tools that have been developed to assist the handicapped person with maintaining, or restoring, his physical independence. The nurse should, whenever possible, provide for the patient's needs before he has to ask for help, which threatens his self-esteem. Cutting up food for the person who is having problems with vision, or for the person who has the use of only one hand; anticipating the need for help in putting on a dressing gown, or slippers; moving furniture out of the way; these and similar activities are a few examples of actions the nurse can take. It should go without saying that things on the bedside table and the light cord, the hand signal, and things the patient needs are placed within easy reach. It is amazing how often nurses, busy with treatments or medications, forget these small details.

Many new utensils and mechanical devices are now available commercially, or ordinary ones can be adapted to assist people with such activities as eating, reading, getting in and out of bed, and moving about. These items eliminate problems for people who are blind, paralyzed, or otherwise handicapped in performing necessary activities or those that provide pleasure. The physical and occupational therapists are often helpful in making suggestions for increasing an individual's independence when he has lost the use of one of his sensory abilities.

Often people with sensory handicaps need the help of specialized health professionals, or the services available in specialized agencies, to enable them to learn to live with a sensory deficit. The nurse supports the work of people such as the physical, occupational, and speech therapists by following through on activities, such as exercises, suggested by them. The patient's increased independence is ensured when all nursing personnel are aware of the goals for the patient, and are consistent in their approach to the patient.

Rehabilitation centers offer tremendous help for people who are learning to live with a sensory deficit, such as blindness, deafness, and paralysis, and those who have lost the ability to speak. The nurse should, if possible, visit one of these centers early in her career to become aware of things that are available to help these patients cope with the daily activities of living. She may encounter people who require some of these in other nursing situations, such as an acute care setting where a person may be suffering a temporary loss of sensory functioning, or in a long-term care facility where she will probably meet people with multiple problems.

PLANNING AND EVALUATING THE EFFECTIVENESS OF SPECIFIC NURSING INTERVENTIONS

In planning the specific interventions to help each patient, the nurse needs to be explicit in the outcomes she expects from or hopes for in the patient. For example, for the person who remains in his room, sitting in his wheelchair most of the day, the anticipated outcome of the nurse's intervention might be to increase the number of hours he is out of his room each day, by setting definite criteria, such as 2 hours at first, perhaps increasing to 8 hours per day. Or, for the person who takes no initiative in going to arts and crafts, or other forms of activities, having him participate in these and take increasing responsibility for getting himself to arts and crafts (for example) would be worthwhile goals. For the person who is depressed or apathetic, even the patient's initiation of conversation would be a major achievement to be accomplished by nursing interventions. Having him feed himself or dress himself without help, and doing so on a regular basis, might be other goals the nurse considers important for the patient to attain. The general goals suggested earlier are helpful, but for planning specific interventions, the nurse will need to think of short-term goals that are realistic, attainable, and measurable for each patient.

If her goals have been explicitly stated, the nurse is able to evaluate the effectiveness of various interventions she has tried, and to try other alternatives if these have not been successful. It also helps the nurse to feel a sense of accomplishment when she notes the patient's progress and finds that goals are achieved, and she has been responsible in large part for their attainment. This aspect of nursing care is important for the nurse as well as the patient.

GUIDE TO ASSESSING SENSORY ABILITIES

1. Does the patient have long-standing deficits in regard to sensory functions, such as problems with vision, with hearing, with taste or smell, with speech communication? Is he paralyzed in any part of his body?

2. Does he normally use corrective devices for any sensory deficits he may have, such as eyeglasses, a hearing aid, or a cane, walker, or wheelchair (for the paralyzed individual), or does he need the help of another person to overcome a deficit in any of the sensory abilities?

3. What is the present status of his sensory abilities?

4. Does he have any health problem that might cause, or has caused, sensory disturbances?

5. Is there sufficient stimulation in his present environment? too much? How does his present environment compare with his usual one?

6. Is he receiving enough social stimulation to maintain adequate sensory input?

7. Does the individual show physical signs or behaviors indicative of sensory deprivation? of sensory overload?

8. What are this individual's usual personality characteristics?

9. What is his usual lifestyle?

STUDY SITUATION

Mr. Jones is a 75-year-old retired school principal who had a cerebrovascular accident (stroke) with resultant hemiplegia (left-sided) 9 months ago. Following the acute episode, he was admitted to a rehabilitation unit but did not progress as well as expected and was transferred to an extended care facility, where he has been ever since. His mental faculties appear unimpaired; his speech is intact; visual and auditory functioning are decreased. He has some movement in the left leg, but the arm is flaccid. He is helped into a wheelchair daily and can propel himself about a little. Mr. Jones' wife died 2 years ago; two of his four adult children (a son and a daughter) live in town—the other two sons at a considerable distance—and both visit frequently, as do their children.

Prior to his disability, Mr. Jones was active in the local community center, played golf regularly, and liked to travel.

On the ward, he spends most of his time in his room, staring out of the window; he does not go to the TV room and has given up reading newspapers because he says he can read nothing but the headlines. He can never remember if visitors have been in or not. He has his radio on most of the time, but keeps it on low because other patients were complaining about it.

What can the nurse do to help Mr. Jones?

SUGGESTED READINGS

Ashworth, P.: Sensory Deprivation . . . The Acutely Ill. *Nursing Times*, February 15, 1979.

Boyd-Monk, H.: Examining the External Eye. Part 1. *Nursing '80*, 10(5):58–63, May, 1980.

Boyd-Monk, H.: Examining the External Eye. Part 2. *Nursing '80*, 10(6):58–63, June, 1980.

Bozian, M. W., and Clark, H. M.: Counteracting Sensory Changes in the Aging. *American Journal of Nursing*, 80(3):473–477, March, 1980.

Crow, R.: Sensory Deprivation in Children. *Nursing Times*, February 8, 1979.

Fenwick, A., et al.: Traumatic Blindness: A Flexible Approach for Helping a Blind Adolescent. *Nursing '79*, 9(1):36–41, January, 1979.

How to Test Your Patient's Hearing Acuity. *Nursing '80*, 10(7):60–61, July, 1980.

Kratz, C. R.: Sensory Deprivation in the Elderly. *Nursing Times*, February 22, 1979.

Krieger, D.: Therapeutic Touch: The Imprimatur of Nursing. *American Journal of Nursing*, 75:784, May, 1975.

Lindenmuth, J. E., et al.: Sensory Overload: An Approach to Nursing Care. *American Journal of Nursing*, 80(8):1456–1458, August, 1980.

Reynolds, B. J.: Suddenly Blind at 80. *Nursing '79*, 9(7):46–49, July, 1979.

Stern, E. J.: Helping the Person with Low Vision. *American Journal of Nursing*, 80(10):1788–1790, October, 1980.

Tobiason, S. B.: Touching is for Everyone. *American Journal of Nursing*, 81:728–730, April, 1981.

Wahl, P. R.: Psychosocial Implications of Disorientation in the Elderly. *Nursing Clinics of North America*, 11:145–156, March, 1976.

REFERENCES

1. Caplan, F., and Caplan, T.: *The Second Twelve Months of Life*. New York, Grosset and Dunlap, 1979.
2. Gregory, R. L.: *Eye and Brain*. 2nd ed. New York, McGraw-Hill, 1973.
3. Cameron, C. F., et al.: When Sensory Deprivation Occurs. *Canadian Nurse*, 68:32–34, November, 1972.
4. Downs, F. S.: Bed Rest and Sensory Disturbances. *American Journal of Nursing*, 74:434–438, March, 1974.
5. Nightingale, F.: *Notes on Nursing*. New York, Appleton, 1946.

23

The Nurse Should Be Able to:

- Discuss the importance of mobility in a person's life
- Compare and contrast the dangers of bed rest and the benefits of exercise, relating these to the sick person and the well individual
- Explain the major functions of bones, muscles, joints, nerves, and their blood supply in body movement
- Discuss factors interfering with motor functioning
- Discuss the development and gradual decline of motor abilities throughout the life cycle
- Assess an individual's motor abilities
- Identify potential or actual problems in the patient's motor abilities
- Establish priorities for nursing action
- Apply relevant principles in planning and implementing nursing interventions
  a. to promote the patient's optimal motor functioning
  b. to prevent problems in motor functioning from developing
  c. to restore optimal motor functioning in patients whose abilities have been lessened by illness
  d. to assist patients whose mobility is limited with the activities of daily living
- Evaluate the effectiveness of nursing interventions

480

MOVEMENT AND EXERCISE NEEDS

CHAPTER 23

INTRODUCTION

All living creatures move. The lusty cry and accompanying body movements of the newborn indicate to the doctor or midwife that the child is indeed alive. The cessation of all movement is the first observable sign of death. Movement is such a vital part of our lives that permanent loss of the ability to move any part of the body is one of the major tragedies that can occur in a person's life. Loss of mobility lessens the concept a person has of himself. His body image is affected and he thinks of himself as less a person than he was—he is less than "whole." Independence is threatened and, if the immobility affects one or more of the principal locomotor parts of the body, the threat to independence assumes major proportions. The individual's opportunities for communication are also jeopardized if he cannot move around, and sensory deprivation becomes a real possibility. Communication itself depends on motor abilities for speaking, writing, and using nonverbal "body language" to send messages to other people.

The ability to move enables the infant to explore first himself and then his surroundings. Infants deprived of sufficient opportunities for movement, for any reason, do not develop as well physically, intellectually, or psychosocially as those who are free to move. One has only to think of the ancient Chinese custom, which prevailed until comparatively recent times, of binding the feet of female babies to keep them small—and the hobbling gait that resulted–to appreciate the importance of movement in physical growth.

Intellectual development depends to a large extent on the child's exposure to an ever-widening world. A child who has never seen an airplane and perhaps not even a bird, has difficulty understanding the concept of flying. Children whose mobility is restricted because of illness or economic reasons (whose parents cannot afford to take them to the zoo and other cultural places) do not have the same opportunities to expand their intellectual horizons. This was one of the principal reasons behind the Head Start programs in the United States for socially disadvantaged children, who were often judged intellectually inferior to children who had had greater opportunities. Intelligence, as measured on standard IQ tests, has very often been substantially increased in children who have participated in Head Start programs.

All systems in the body function more efficiently when they are active. Disuse of the neuromuscular system quickly leads to degeneration and subsequent loss of functioning. If muscles are immobilized, the process of degeneration begins almost immediately. It has been estimated that the strength and tone of immobilized muscles may decrease by as much as 5 per cent per day in the absence of any contraction of the muscle.[1]

The process of degeneration in muscles occurs very quickly. The restoration of muscle strength and tone, on the other hand, is a very slow process that may take months or years to accomplish. In this case, then, prevention is by far the better part of cure. Nurses caring for patients during the acute stage of illnesses requiring more than a few days of bed rest have a responsibility to do everything possible to prevent degeneration of unused muscles and the development of complications that will limit the person's mobility or prolong his recovery and restoration to health.

BED REST, EXERCISE, AND THEIR IMPLICATIONS

The Dangers of Bed Rest

The dangers of prolonged bed rest have been well documented in numerous study reports, books, and articles in both the nursing and medical literature over the past 30 or 40 years. The custom of early ambulation of patients following surgery, childbirth, and acute illness was introduced just after World War II. The results have been phenomenal in preventing complications and hastening patients' recovery.

Among the adverse effects of lengthy bed rest that have been noted are: a slowing down of the basal metabolic rate; a decrease in muscle strength, tone, and size; postural changes; constipation; increased vulnerability to pulmonary and urinary tract infections; circulatory problems, such as thrombosis (the development of a clot in the blood stream) and embolus (which occurs when the clot becomes detached and travels through the blood stream until it comes to a vessel too small for it to pass through, where it lodges). The degenerative process affects bone and skin tissues as well.

The pulse rate increases, as the heart works harder in an attempt to cope with the extra amount of blood "dumped" into the general circulation from the legs when the body is lying down. There is increased excretion of calcium, nitrogen, and phosphorus, and the individual may suffer severe depletion of these elements. The person usually develops feelings of anxiety and frequently hostility as a result of disturbed functioning of physical and mental activity, as well as disruption of his sleep patterns.

The Benefits of Exercise

Exercise, in comparison, increases the efficiency of functioning of all body processes. The physiological, psychological, and social benefits of exercise have been receiving increasing attention in recent years. The predominantly sedentary way of life of so many North Americans has been viewed as a major factor contributing to many of the illnesses with which we are plagued, such as coronary heart disease (the leading cause of death in North America), hypertension, diabetes, and obesity.

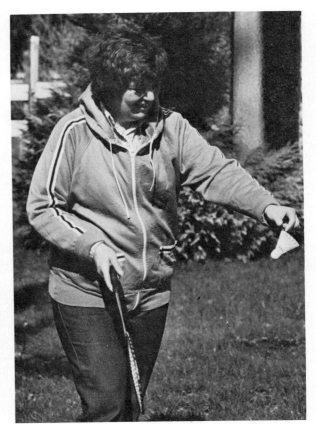

Sports, organized or just for fun, are an important means of exercise, promoting muscle tone and coordination.

Many studies have been undertaken in the United States, Canada, and a number of other countries, to determine the exact physiological changes that result from a regular exercise program. Among those that have been found are: increased muscle strength, tone, and size; increased efficiency of the heart; increased work tolerance; increased pulmonary efficiency; improved digestion; better mental alertness; improved sleep patterns; increased hemoglobin levels in the blood; decreased blood pressure; decreased deposits of fatty tissue; and decreased cholesterol levels in the blood.[2] It has been demonstrated that exercise following a fatty meal will help to clear the blood of excessive cholesterol, and thus increase fat tolerance.

Implications for the Sick and the Well

The documented dangers of bed rest and benefits of exercise have implications both for the prevention of illness and for the restoration to health following illness. Physically fit people are less vulnerable to such illnesses as heart problems, hypertension, obesity, and diabetes in that the "risk factors" that predispose people to these disorders are lessened. There is evidence to support the belief that their chances for survival following a heart attack are also better. They usually recover more quickly from infections than those who are physically unfit. Lest you think that it is necessary to undertake a strenuous athletic program to achieve these benefits, it has been demonstrated that a 6-week program of three half hour sessions per week, at such activities as swimming, jogging, cycling, or calisthenics, followed by a once or twice a week maintenance program, will significantly improve fitness in all aspects of physiological functioning enumerated in the previous section.[2]

Rest and enforced immobility are needed for recovery from many illnesses. An injured part of the body must be put to rest to prevent further injury while the tissues repair themselves. Following a heart attack, for example, it is important that the heart be relieved of as much work as possible so that the process of tissue repair can take place with no more strain on the heart than is absolutely necessary Similarly, broken bones and torn ligaments must be immobilized to allow the bone tissues or ligament fibers to knit sufficiently to withstand the normal wear and tear they receive in the course of daily activities.

Many other illnesses also require lengthy periods of rest. Some disorders result in partial or total loss of mobility—e.g., arthritis (inflammation of the joints, which often results in limited mobility for the individual) and paralysis, which can cause total immobility of half or more of the body.

Any person who is on bed rest for more than a few days, or whose mobility is limited in any way, requires exercise to those parts of the body that are not immobilized of necessity. These days, even cardiac patients are being started on exercise programs at an early stage of their recovery, and gradually increasing exercise is a part of their therapy. People who have had a myocardial infarction are even receiving training in marathon running in some parts of the country. For people with most illnesses exercise is started almost immediately after the crisis stage is over. The new postoperative patient is out of bed and walking (with help) down the hall, within a few hours following surgery, in some cases. He may have to carry his intravenous infusion apparatus with him, or his drainage tubes and bottles, but walk he must.

People who cannot get out of bed must have their exercise in bed, in the form of active or passive range of motion exercises (and others) as tolerated. This is now an accepted nursing responsibility that is carried out on all patients unless there are contraindications. How to help patients with range of motion exercises will be discussed in a later section of this chapter.

NORMAL MOTOR FUNCTIONING

The principal systems involved in body movements are the skeletal system, the muscular system, and the nervous system. The circulatory system is also involved in that it provides nourishment to the tissues of these systems. If circulation to any part of the body is impaired, degeneration of the tissues in the area begins, since the body cells cannot live without adequate nourishment. However, it is the bones, the nerves, and the muscles that make movement possible.

The bones of the skeletal system have two functions in movement—they provide an attachment for muscles and ligaments, and they act as levers. The *proximal* end of a muscle is attached to a less movable bone, such as the scapula in the shoulder. This point of attachment is called the *origin of the muscle*. The *distal* end of the muscle is attached to a freely movable bone, such as the humerus in the upper arm. This point is called the *insertion* of the muscle.

"Lever" is a term taken from the physical sciences, meaning a rigid bar that revolves

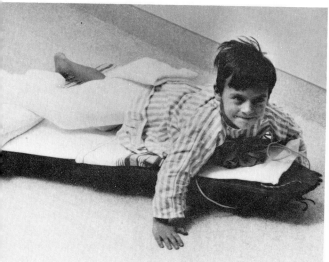

Use of a skateboard allows this child to exercise other parts of his body while his leg is immobilized by a hip spica cast. (Courtesy Canadian Nurses Association, Helen K. Mussallem Library.)

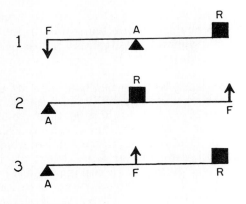

F = Force
A = Axis or fulcrum
R = Resistance or weight

Three types of levers.

acoscapular muscles. To move the thigh alone involves all the gluteus muscles, as well as the adductor muscles.

The spinal nerves are directly involved in trunk and limb movements. Each spinal nerve has an anterior and a posterior root in the spinal column. The anterior root conducts impulses to the muscles from the central nervous system. The posterior root conducts messages from the sensory receptors to the central nervous system.

Almost all patterns of movement can be initiated by the spinal cord alone. Balance and the progression, coordination, and purposefulness of movement, however, require participation of progressively higher levels in the brain. Motor areas located in the frontal lobes of the cerebral cortex serve as the "master control" for directing and controlling specific movement in various parts of the body.[3]

Types of Movement

The body has six large movable parts: the head, the trunk, the two arms, and the two legs. It also has smaller movable parts, such as the hand, fingers, feet, and toes, which form part of a larger part but may move independently of it. You can move a hand without moving the rest of the arm, for example, or finger independently of any other part of the body.

These body parts are capable of various kinds of movements:

• *Abduction:* Movement away from the central axis (midline) of the body.

• *Adduction:* Movement toward the central axis (midline) of the body.

Flexion: The act of bending; the angle between the two moving parts is decreased.

Extension: The act of straightening; the angle between the two moving parts is increased.

Hyperextension: Extension beyond the normal range of motion—for example, in bending the head back toward the spine.

Gliding: Movement in one plane, as in sliding.

Rotation: Turning in a circular motion around a fixed axis.

Circumduction: Circular motion of a limb or part when the limb or part forms part of a cone, as in swinging the arm in a circular motion.

• *Pronation:* Turning down toward the ground.

• *Supination:* Turning upward (the opposite of pronation).

Inversion: Turning inward towards the body.

Eversion: Turning outward away from the body.

These movements are illustrated on pages 485 and 486.

around a fixed axis called a fulcrum. The simplest example of a lever is a teeter-totter or seesaw. Two children of equal weight can balance on a teeter-totter that is resting on a fixed point or axis, if they are equidistant from the middle. If one child exerts force, by pushing down, or moves his weight further backwards, his end of the board will move towards the ground, assisted by the pull of gravity. To raise his end of the board and bring down his partner, he must exert force to push upwards against the force of gravity, which is resisting his movement. Using the board as a lever, however, he is able to lift the weight of the other child off the ground—to a considerable height, if you stop to think about it—a feat he could not accomplish if he tried to do it while standing on the ground and trying to lift him in his arms.

An axis need not always be in the center of a lever. Three different types of levers are shown in the figure above.

The muscles contract to produce motion. Muscles for movement are always in pairs, one on either side of a bone or joint, and have opposing functions; as one contracts, the other extends (stretches) to cause the bone to move in a certain direction. The action is similar to that involved in the manipulation of a puppet by strings: you shorten one string and lengthen another to make the puppet move in the direction you want it to go.

Muscles also tend to work in groups rather than in single pairs. Breathing, for example, requires the coordinated activity of a number of muscles, including the intercostals, the diaphragm, and the sternocleidomastoid muscles, the scalenes, the thoracohumeral, and the thor-

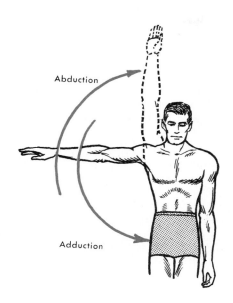

Abduction

Adduction

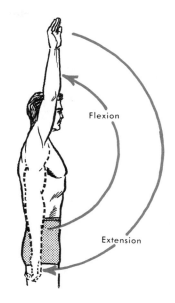

Flexion

Extension

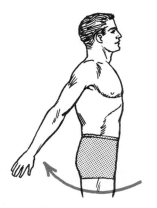

Hyperextension

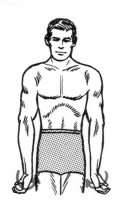

Inward rotation

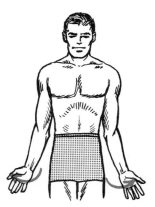

Outward rotation

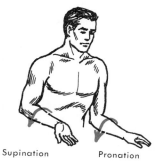

Supination   Pronation

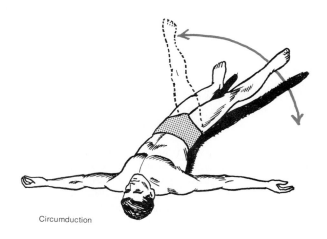

Circumduction

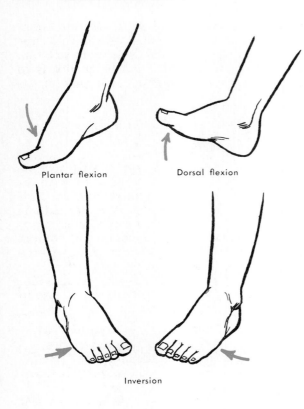

Plantar flexion   Dorsal flexion

Inversion

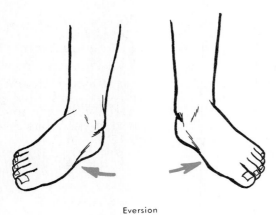

Eversion

Types of Joints

The various types of movements are made possible by the *joints*, which connect one bone to another. The body does have some joints that are immovable, such as those connecting the bones in the skull, but the major purpose of the joints is to serve as hinges to enable the body to move. Each movable joint is constructed to make possible a certain type of movement, and each has a circumscribed range.

The body has six types of movable joints.

Hinge: This is a uniaxial joint that permits flexion and extension. An example of a hinge joint is the knee.

Pivot: This is also a uniaxial joint. It permits rotation. An example is the atlantoaxial joint (between the first cervical vertebra and the base of the skull).

Condyloid: This is a biaxial joint. It permits flexion, extension, abduction, and adduction. A combination of these four movements is called circumduction. The wrist is a condyloid joint.

Saddle: This is another biaxial joint. It permits flexion, extension, abduction, adduction, and circumduction. An example is the thumb.

Ball and socket: This type of joint is polyaxial. Movements permitted include flexion, extension, abduction, adduction, circumduction, and rotation. The hip joint is a ball and socket joint.

Gliding: This a *plane* joint and permits gliding movements. An example is the acromioclavicular joint of the shoulder.

Planes of the Body

Body movements are often described in relation to *planes*, another term from the physical sciences, which means that when the body is in a standing position, as shown in the figure above, the *sagittal plane* divides it into right

Sagittal, frontal, and transverse planes of the body.

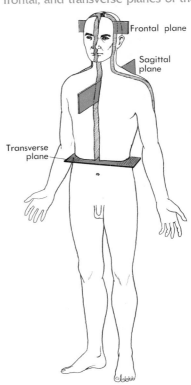

Frontal plane

Sagittal plane

Transverse plane

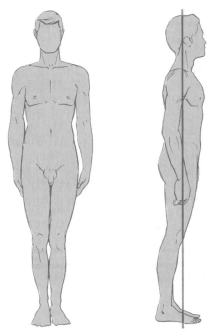

The anatomical position.

and left sections, the *frontal plane* into dorsal and ventral sections, and the *transverse plane* into upper and lower sections.

This figure shows the body in good anatomical position—that is, the alignment of body parts is balanced, and their weight is also balanced. In the anatomical position, the individual stands with his hands at his sides, thumbs adducted, and hands supinated. The head is erect; the spine, pelvis, legs, and feet are in good alignment with the head. The feet are slightly apart and directed forward, and the knees and fingers are slightly flexed.

Movement of the body is much easier when the body parts are in good alignment, when the weight of the body is evenly balanced, and when the feet are set a little farther apart (about one foot apart) than in the anatomical position. Setting the feet this far apart provides the body with a wider base of support for its weight than the normal standing posture does.

The center of weight (center of mass or gravity) in the body is located in the pelvis at approximately the level of the second sacral vertebra. The line of gravity is an imaginary straight line that passes from the top of an object through its center of gravity to form a right angle with the ground.

When the body is erect, in good anatomical position, the line of gravity falls in the frontal plane downward behind the ear, through the center of gravity in the pelvis, and slightly in front of the knee and ankle joints, to the middle of the body's base of support, so that the line is perpendicular to the ground, as shown in the figure on this page. The body is more stable in this position because its line of gravity is in direct line with the gravitational pull of the earth.

Motor Abilities Needed for Activities of Daily Living

The ability to make parts of the body move and to control these movements enables an individual to develop the motor skills needed for the activities of daily living. A motor skill is used here to mean a series of coordinated movements. It also permits the development of more highly refined motor skills, such as playing the piano, playing tennis, dancing, and so forth.

The basic motor skills needed for the activities of daily living are those that are learned early in life:

1. Lifting the head when lying on the back
2. Grasping an object in the hand
3. Raising an object to the mouth
4. Turning over onto one side or the other from a back-lying position
5. Rolling over, from back to abdomen and the reverse
6. Sitting up from a back-lying position
7. Standing up and sitting down
8. Transferring from one place to another
9. Walking

Control over the bodily processes of elimination, which also is essential to daily living, involves control over muscular functioning. Problems in relation to these processes are discussed in Chapters 15 and 16.

MOTOR FUNCTIONING THROUGHOUT THE LIFE CYCLE

During late pregnancy, there is a general relaxation of all body ligaments, particularly those involving the pelvic bones and the back. The woman's center of gravity is moved backwards by the enlarging uterus, and this tends to throw her off balance. She usually feels awkward in her movements, being hindered by her increasing bulk as well as her protruding abdomen. A woman needs exercise throughout pregnancy to keep herself in good physical condition generally, and specifically to aid in circulation, to strengthen the muscles used in expulsion of the baby, and to learn relaxing techniques. The relaxing techniques are helpful in making labor and delivery easier for the woman; there is also a need to learn to relax specific muscles used in delivery, such as the pelvic and perineal diaphragms.

After delivery, exercises are needed to strengthen the abdominal muscles and the muscles of the pelvic floor, which have been stretched during labor and delivery. Most prenatal programs include both pre- and postnatal exercises, as well as teaching women relaxing techniques.

Expectant parents are usually excited when the mother first feels the baby kick in her womb. The event is called "quickening" and usually occurs during the fourth or fifth month of gestation. The infant continues to move until just before birth, when the head becomes engaged in the birth canal.

After birth, the newborn's movements are mainly random. He has poor motor control at first, because most of his movements are reflex actions.

Some infants are much more active than others and some acquire motor skills at an earlier age than others do. Babies are highly individualistic in this regard. However, it can be very traumatic to a new mother when her year-old-child is still not walking while the neighbor's child has been running around since he was 9 months of age. It helps if the nurse can reassure the mother that her child is just as normal as the neighbor's. A chart of development for the first year of life (shown below) identifies the average age in months when specific achievements are attained by 95 per cent of normal infants. The chart is helpful in reassuring mothers and is also useful in identifying children who are not developing at a normal rate.

During the first year of life, the major accomplishments in motor skills are learning to walk

Average age for the achievements selected and zone in which 95 per cent of observations fell in a group of 215 normal infants. (From Johnson, T. R., and Moore, W. M.: *Children Are Different: Developmental Physiology.* Ross Laboratories, Columbus, Ohio, 1978, p. 33.)

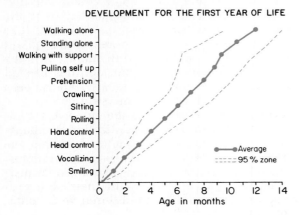

DEVELOPMENT FOR THE FIRST YEAR OF LIFE

and learning to use the hands as tools (prehensile skill). These skills depend on physical maturation, although it is generally believed that a stimulating environment can accelerate motor development. A passive infant may need stimulation to exercise, as, for example, brightly colored objects suspended above the crib within the infant's reach, or a "Jolly-jumper" to encourage the infant to exercise his legs. During infancy, the bones are soft and pliant and the pelvis is usually tilted forward. The back is rounded when the baby is sitting. Because his head is large in comparison with his body, balance is difficult. Hence, the baby often falls over when he is first learning to sit and totters in his first attempts at walking.

During childhood, the extremities grow faster than the trunk, the pelvis straightens, and a convex spinal curvature develops. The toddler usually toes out, the older preschooler may toe in when walking. Children delight in activities that use their large muscles, such as running, hopping, jumping, and the like. By the time a child is 6 years of age, he has usually acquired rudimentary motor skills that enable him to get about on skates, to ride a two-wheel bicycle, and to swim. By the time he is 11, the child has gained control of his motor skills to the extent that he appears graceful and coordinated in his movements. The development of fine motor skills usually lag behind gross motor skills. Girls as a general rule have much better dexterity with their fingers and hands than boys do. Hence, their writing is better in school, and their drawings are usually neater.

Adolescence is characterized by a rapid growth spurt, and, for a while, the child looks as if he is all arms and legs. His hands and feet grow rapidly in length, his pelvic and shoulder diameters increase, and his head circumference gets larger. He also attains an adult posture. With all of this growth going on, the individual often looks and feels awkward as he learns to adjust to his new body size. The adolescent usually has a lot of excess energy, which needs to be channeled constructively. This is the time for outdoor sports and active physical exercise to wear off the tremendous amount of energy that adolescent boys in particular seem to have.

It is during the late teens that an individual reaches his peak insofar as athletic performance is concerned. By the time he is a young adult, his physical performance involving strength and endurance is beginning to decline. If the individual continues to put excessive demands on his musculoskeletal system to reach the levels he did before, he is likely to suffer injury and inflammatory conditions. Traumatic injuries, for example fractures caused by skiing accidents, are common. Inflammation of the deep surface

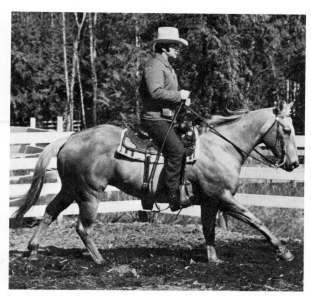

Exercise is important in daily life. This person gets the double benefit of fresh air and exercise.

of the kneecap is another common exercise-related problem.

During the middle years, there is a progressive decrease in bone density and mass, and accidents that previously would have caused only minor injuries may now result in fractures. As a person gets older, he gradually loses height, because of a gradual decompression of the vertebrae. The regenerative capacity of articular cartilage is also diminished, and the cumulative effect of injuries ot the joints (such as the inflammatory conditions of the knees we mentioned above) may lead to arthritis. The frequency of joint disease increases with age. Most people do not participate in active sports to the same extent they did in their youth, and a more sedentary lifestyle often leads to a "middle-age spread." A person's functional aerobic capacity also diminishes with age because his heart and his lungs are not as efficient. Regular exercise is important for several reasons: (1) to improve a person's functional aerobic capacity, (2) to reduce the risk factors that can lead to coronary artery disease (such as overweight and cholesterol accumulation in the blood stream). and (3) to maintain joint flexibility.

People over the age of 65 years are usually an inch or so shorter then they were in their youth. This is because of the thinning and, sometimes, anterior wedging and collapse of the intervertebral discs, in addition to the previously mentioned compression of the vertebral bodies themselves. There is usually also a loss of cartilage in the large joints and a proliferation of adjacent bone. Women, in particular, are vulnerable to osteoporosis (see Chapter 14). The reflexes that minimize sway in the erect posture become sluggish and blunted, and deep tendon reflexes are often diminished or absent. There is a gradual, progressive loss of muscle bulk and strength. Often, there is a limited range of motion in the neck. The changes that are taking place in the musculoskeletal system and the changes taking place in the nervous system (see Chapter 22) combine to make walking and other coordinated movements more difficult. Exercises to promote joint flexibility and to improve circulation are particularly important for the older person.

exersis: ↑O₂ ↓ health risk, ↑ joint flex.

FACTORS INTERFERING WITH MOTOR FUNCTIONING

The ability of the body to move its various movable parts and to control these movements so that they are performed in a coordinated fashion depends on the integrity of the muscles, the bones, the joints, the nerves innervating these structures, and the circulation nourishing them. Injury, disease, or congenital problems affecting the bones, muscles, joints, or their collateral nerve or blood supply may, then, cause impairment of motor functioning.

Even a minor injury, such as a sprained ankle, which damages muscles and ligaments in that area, will limit a person's ability to walk until the muscle fibers and ligaments have healed. Fracture of a bone limits the ability to move the part of the body in which the fracture is located. People who are injured in car accidents, severe falls, or other types of accidents may sustain injury to the spinal cord. Because the cord is essential in the transmission of nerve impulses to and from the area in the brain controlling motor function, all movements below the site of the injury may be cut off. The person may be paralyzed from the waist down (*paraplegic*), if the injury is located at that level, or from the neck down (*quadriplegic*), if the injury is in the cervical region.

A stroke is the result of a cerebrovascular accident. This problem frequently impairs the blood supply to motor areas in the frontal lobe of the brain of one hemisphere, with resultant loss of motor functioning on one side of the body (*hemiplegia*). The motor abilities needed for speech may also be impaired if the accident is in the dominant half of the brain.

Congenital abnormalities are one of the common troubles causing hospitalization in infants and small children. Many children whom the nurse will encounter on the pediatric units of hospitals are there for repair of congenital malformations that interfere with their ability to walk, as, for example, the children with "clubfoot," or a "congenital hip."

Contractures of muscles controlling movement of the joints of the body, at the wrist or ankle joints for example, will also cause limitations in mobility. These contractures frequently result from the hand or the foot not being supported in good anatomical position when the person was immobilized for another reason. It should be noted here that these contractures require intensive therapy, over a prolonged period of time, to correct. Briefly, the hand should be supported in a straight line with the lower part of the arm and the fingers slightly flexed. The foot should be at a right angle to the lower part of the leg, in walking position if the person were standing up. (These topics are discussed further in Chapter 20.)

Serious illness of any kind lessens an individual's muscular strength and tone. The individual may be completely helpless and unable to lift his head, to move himself in bed, or to turn himself onto his side. Or he may be semi-helpless, that is, requiring assistance to be able to do these activities and to sit himself up in bed. Surgical patients are usually restricted in their movements because of pain in the operative area and the need to avoid movements that could cause a freshly sutured wound to break open.

Restrictions are put on a patient's movements as soon as he is placed on bed rest for any reason in any type of illness, as we noted earlier in the chapter. The individual may have limitations placed on his mobility for therapeutic reasons, even if he is not confined to bed, as, for example, the person with a sprained ankle, or one with a "wry neck" (torticollis), which is a not uncommon occurrence in people who have been involved in automobile accidents.

A person who is isolated because of infectious precautions also has his mobility restricted (see Chapter 26).

The movements of some patients may be curtailed by the use of restraints if it is in their best interests to do so (for example, if they are confused and may hurt themselves trying to get out of bed (see Chapter 24).

Some people may be restricted in their mobility because of other disabilities that limit their ability to get around without help, as, for example, a blind or deaf person. Others may be restricted because of their environment. People who reside in nursing homes, for example, may have limited opportunities to move about, and usually they have physical mobility problems as well. Children from disadvantaged homes, as we mentioned at the beginning of the chapter, may also be limited in mobility because of economic circumstances.

Some people, of course, limit their own mobility; probably we all know people whose only movement are from the house to their car, from the car to the office, and home again, where they sit for the rest of the evening.

COMMON PROBLEMS IN MOTOR FUNCTIONING

People whose motor abilities are impaired because of illness or injury often need help to perform the daily activities of living. Among the common problems with which they may need the nurse's help are inability or limited ability to raise the head; to grasp objects; to move themselves in bed; to turn on their side or to turn over; to raise the buttocks when lying flat, or when sitting up (necessary for use of the bedpan); to sit up; to stand; to transfer, as from the bed to a chair, or the reverse; or to walk.

The problem of maintaining the functional ability of unused muscles and preventing their degeneration is common to all patients on prolonged bed rest, and to those whose muscles are not being used for any reason. Maintaining optimal functional ability in muscles is common also to many who are otherwise well, but whose mobility is restricted either voluntarily or because of circumstances beyond their control.

Because the degenerative process affects the skin, as well as muscles and bone, in persons on bed rest and those whose motor abilities are impaired, there are problems in maintaining the skin in good condition (this is further discussed in Chapter 25). The maintenance of nutritional status is also a problem in patients on bed rest because of excessive losses of protein, calcium, and nitrogen (see Chapter 14). Maintaining psychosocial equilibrium is another problem commonly seen in patients with limited mobility. Anxiety and sensory deprivation are other potential problems, as we discussed in Chapters 22 and 30.

The patient's safety may also be of concern, because the person who is not able to move about well cannot protect himself from environmental hazards (see Chapter 24). Potential problems with regard to infections will also exist, because of the patient's possibly poor nutritional status or poor skin condition (see Chapter 26).

ASSESSMENT

In assessing a patient's motor status when developing a plan of care for him, the nurse needs information about his usual motor abilities and his present status with regard to these abilities (see Chapter 9). She also needs information about any recent health problems he has had in addition to his current problems. If the patient has, or recently had, a health problem, she should be aware of the physician's diagnostic and therapeutic plans of care for the patient. She needs to know, for example, if other health workers, such as the physical therapist or the occupational therapist are involved in helping the patient. She needs to be aware of any restrictions that have been placed on the patient's mobility, such as bed rest or no exercise.

She should also be aware of the patient's potential prognosis. It should be noted, however, that it is often difficult to predict the patient's chances of regaining motor functioning that has been impaired by illness, such as stroke or spinal injury. Recovery is often slow, and in some cases, may take years to accomplish. One should never give up simply because a tentative prognosis is not hopeful.

Much of the information needed is available from the patient's record, the nursing history, the initial clinical appraisal form, the physician's notations on the record, and reports of assessments done by other health professionas. If a physical therapist has been called in, he or she usually does a thorough assessment of the patient's motor functional abilities. When a patient has disturbances of motor functioning, specialist physicians, such as the neurologist and the physiatrist, are frequently consulted by the attending physician, and their reports should also be on the patient's record.

The patient's family are often very helpful in providing information about the patient's abilities with regard to motor functioning.

The nurse's observations and the patient's subjective observations are both important in the initial and continuous assessments of his motor status. Sensory functioning and motor functioning are usually closely interrelated, and often the patient's ability to feel pressure is the first sign of a return of functioning ability in a limb. The patient, the nurse, or a member of the patient's family may be the first to notice this in the patient. The nurse must be alert to signs of increased muscle tension, or of movement in flaccid muscles, when she is doing passive range of motion exercises for the patient, and note these on the record.

PRIORITIES FOR NURSING ACTION

In establishing priorities for nursing action for limited mobility, the nurse takes into account two sets of problems. For the individual whose mobility is curtailed, the overwhelming priority is the preventive aspect of making sure that those unused muscles whose movement is not contraindicated for therapeutic reasons receive sufficient exercise to prevent their deterioration.

When patients cannot move themselves and need the nurse's help to move, assistance in the daily activities of living ranks high on the nurse's list of priorities. The patient who cannot feed himself should not be left until his food is cold. Patients who need help in turning must be turned at scheduled times, or serious skin problems may result. The individual who needs the nurse's help to use the bedpan or a urinal needs it immediately, not half an hour from now. The person who needs assistance in getting up, getting in or out of bed, or getting in or out of the wheelchair likewise should not be left waiting for lengthy periods to be helped with these activities.

The nurse uses judgment, then, in scheduling her activities to ensure that patients who have problems in meeting their basic physiological needs are given the needed assistance at the time they need it. The nurse must also be sufficiently flexible to interrupt other activities that can be deferred to assist patients who need immediate assistance with the basic needs. Recording, for example, can be interrupted when the nurse sees a patient's signal light go on. The ignoring of or slow response to their signals for help is one of the most common complaints patients have when they are ill in the hospital.

PRINCIPLES RELEVANT TO THE CARE OF PATIENTS WITH PROBLEMS IN MOTOR FUNCTIONING

The principles relevant to the care of patients with problems in motor functioning may be divided into two categories: those relating to exercise needed to prevent muscular degeneration, or to improve muscular strength and tone; and those relating to helping people who are unable to help themselves in moving. The specific nursing interventions that the nurse considers when developing a nursing care plan for patients with these problems may also be divided into two groups of activities. Thus, we will consider each set of principles as they relate to specific nursing interventions.

GOALS FOR NURSING ACTION

The goals of nursing action for patients who have existing or potential problems in motor functioning abilities are directed towards:

1. Maintenance of strength and tone in unused muscles whose movement is not contrain-

dicated by the nature of health problem(s) they may have

2. Prevention of degeneration of these muscles

3. Prevention of contractures that could hinder the mobility of joints

4. Restoration, insofar as possible, of strength and tone of muscles so impaired

5. Promotion of optimal strength and tone of muscles

6. Prevention of deterioration of the patient's other functional abilities as a result of limited mobility

7. Retention or regaining of independence in the activities of daily living insofar as this is possible

Note: Goal number 6 is discussed in other chapters concerned with specific functional abilities.

NURSING INTERVENTIONS FOR EXERCISE

There are very few patients for whom all exercise is contraindicated. The physician generally orders the degree of activity for patients in an inpatient health agency, that is, whether he is to be comfined to bed, have bathroom privileges, and so on. The patient who has a specific need for remedial exercises—for example, the patient with a paralyzed arm—is often guided in his exercise by the physical therapist and the nurse. For many patients, exercise is part of their nursing care and most of the guidance they receive is provided by the nurse. It is an important independent nursing function to assess the patient's exercise needs and provide for suitable exercise within existing limitations and contraindications.

Patients who remain in bed for a prolonged period are prone to develop complications as a result of their inactivity, as we mentioned earlier. Exercise helps maintain and create good muscle tone and prevent atrophy. For the person in bed, this means that the strength of his muscles is maintained or developed in readiness for greater activity. Exercise also helps in the elimination of waste products from the muscles. The contraction of muscles increases circulation and the removal of wastes from the body. Increased circulation is particularly important for the person who remains in bed. Stasis of blood is a predisposing factor in the formation of clots, which can lead to serious complications.

The increased basal metabolic rate that results from exercise increases the body's need for oxygen. This in turn results in an increase in both the rate and depth of respirations, thus improving lung aeration and helping to prevent infectious processes in the lungs, which occur as a result of inactive lung areas and stagnant secretions. Improved blood circulation also increases the delivery of oxygen and nutrients to tissues, thus maintaining their health and preventing deterioration and ulcer formation.

Contracture of the muscles and stiffening of the joints are other unfortunate side effects of prolonged inactivity. By putting joints through their full range of motion, these can often be avoided.

Kinds of Exercise

Basically, there are three types of exercise:

1. *Passive exercise.* In passive exercise the body part is moved by someone other than the patient. In passive exercise, the muscles do not actively contract. This type of exercise helps to prevent contractures, but it does not increase muscle strength and tone.

2. *Isometric exercise.* This is a form of active

PRINCIPLES RELEVANT TO EXERCISE PROGRAMS FOR PATIENTS

1. The process of degeneration starts almost immediately when muscles are unused.

2. The process of degeneration involves bone and skin tissues as well as muscle tissue.

3. All joints have a circumscribed range of motion.

4. Passive exercise of the body's movable parts through their full range of motion prevents the development of contractures that can interfere with joint mobility.

5. Active contraction of muscles is required to maintain and improve their strength and tone.

6. Active contraction of muscles on one side of the body causes the corresponding muscles on the other side of the body to contract.

7. Exercise has beneficial effects on all body systems.

exercise in which the patient consciously increases the tension of his muscles, but there is neither joint movement nor is there change in the length of the muscle. This type of exercise, sometimes referred to as "muscle-setting exercises," can help considerably in maintaining or improving muscle strength and tone.

3. *Isotonic exercise.* This, too, is a form of active exercise. In this type, the patient supplies the energy to actively exercise his muscles and move the limb or other body part. In isotonic exercise, the muscle actively contracts or shortens, causing the limb to move. Isotonic exercises increase muscle strength and tone and help joint mobility.

Regardless of the kind of exercise the patient is to have, the nurse must see that he avoids fatigue.

Exercises are planned as a regular part of her nursing activities. During the bed bath, for example, the nurse has an excellent opportunity to move the patient's limbs through their full range of motion. The patient is encouraged to exercise actively those muscles that he is permitted to use. The nurse passively exercises those he cannot. Patients can learn to do isometric exercises on their own while they are otherwise inactive in bed, and can supplement programs of regular isotonic exercise by this means.

Regular isotonic exercise is often prescribed as part of the patient's therapy. He may go to the physiotherapy department for this, or the physical therapist may come to the nursing unit. If a program of regular exercise is not undertaken by another health worker for patients, the nurse institutes a program for all patients for whom active exercise is not contraindicated. Both individual and group exercises are used.

Group exercises are helpful from a social point of view (increasing sensory stimulation), as well as having physically therapeutic benefits. There is greater motivation to put forth more effort in a group when everyone is doing the same thing. In many agencies, group physiotherapy classes are organized by the physical therapy department, but there is no reason why a nurse cannot organize these on a nursing unit. It is frequently done on some obstetrical units to assist patients to regain lost muscle tone resulting from pregnancy and childbirth.

Occupational therapy is often used to supplement physical therapy to assist people in maintaining or regaining muscular strength and preventing loss of joint mobility.

Range of Motion. When a patient is exercising, his joints should go through their full range of motion. For example, the normal shoulder and upper arm movements are flexion, extension, hyperextension, abduction, adduction, circumduction, inward rotation, and outward rotation. The chief muscles involved in these movements are the deltoid (abducts the upper arm), pectoralis major (flexes and adducts the upper arm), trapezius (raises and lowers the shoulders), latissimus dorsi (extends and adducts the upper arm), and serratus anterior (pulls the shoulder forward).

Hand and finger exercises are often a part of a patient's therapy. Flexing, abducting, extending, and adducting the hand, as well as flexing and extending the joints of the fingers, are exercises commonly carried out by patients who have some functional impairment as a result of a stroke. It is particularly important to exercise the thumb. The ability of man to bring the thumb in opposition to the tip and base of the fingers is a key factor in using the hands. It permits the individual to hold a pencil and write, and to hold a fork and eat, or to do any number of ordinary activities.

The knees and the elbows can be flexed and extended. The biceps, quadriceps, and hamstring muscles are active in these movements. The forearm can be supinated and pronated. The four principal muscles that move the forearm are the biceps brachii (flexes and supinates), brachialis (flexes and pronates), triceps brachii (extends), and pronator quadratus (pronates).

Thigh movement involves the gluteus muscles and the adductor muscles. The gluteus muscles (maximus, medius, and minimus) extend, rotate, and abduct the thigh. The adductor muscles adduct the thigh and adduct and flex the leg. Flexion, extension, abduction, adduction, and inward and outward rotation from the hip are usually possible. Circumduction of the hip involves all the movements of the hip. Most hip movements involve movement of the pelvis as well.

Movements of the feet and toes are also important. The ankle is a hinged joint that permits plantar flexion and dorsiflexion. Inversion and eversion of the feet take place in the gliding joints. The joints of the toes permit flexion, extension, abduction, and adduction.

Normally the vertebral joints permit flexion, extension, lateral flexion, and rotation of the cervical spine and trunk. The rectus abdominus, the external and internal oblique muscles, and the sacrospinal muscle are involved in these movements.

The degree to which people can tolerate exercise varies considerably. A patient should avoid fatigue and pain while exercising. Joints need to be exercised to their full range of motion,

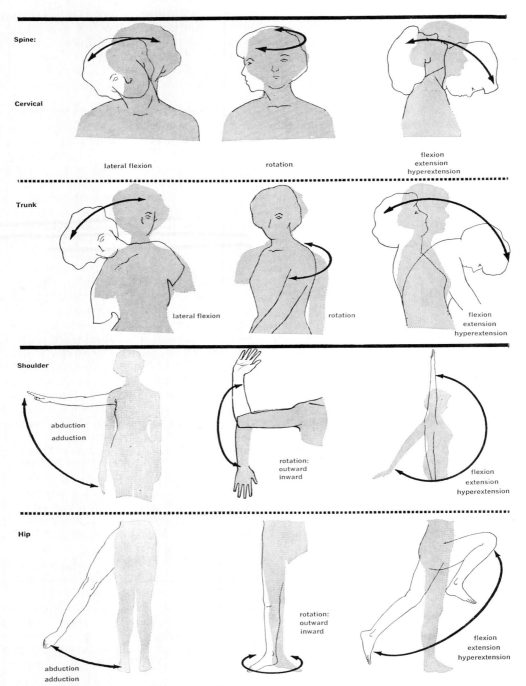

From Kelly, M. M.; Exercises for Bedfast Patients. © October, 1966, The American Journal of Nursing Company. Reproduced with permission from *The American Journal of Nursing,* Vol. 66, No. 10.

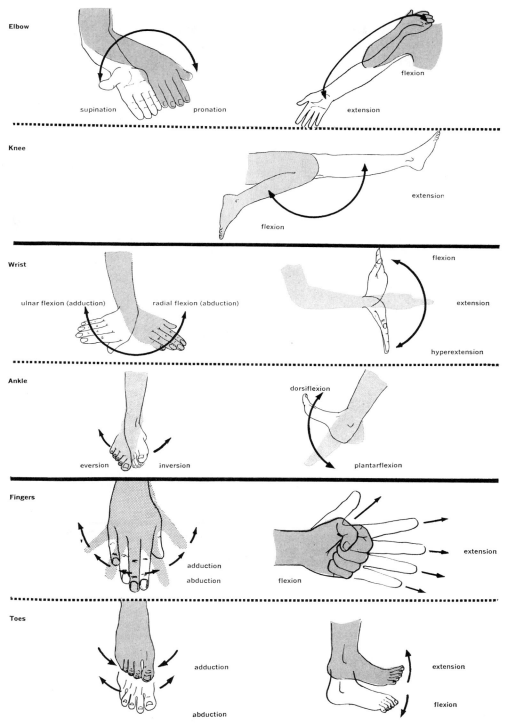

From Kelly, M. M.: Exercises for Bedfast Patients. © October, 1966, The American Journal of Nursing Company. Reproduced with permission from *The American Journal of Nursing*, Vol. 66, No. 10.

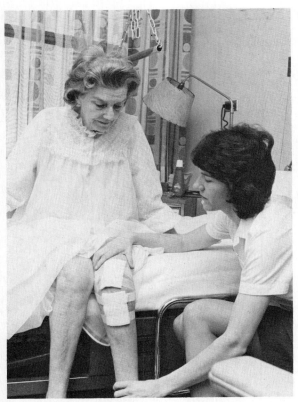

Regaining movement in an injured joint requires gradually increasing exercise.

but the nurse should not force movement when it is painful to the patient or when she meets resistance.

Exercises in Preparation for Walking. Everything should be done to help the patient to maintain strength and tone in muscles that are needed for walking, or to regain these if they have deteriorated because of illness. Patients who may have to use a walker, crutches, or a cane need to gain additional strength in their hand, arm, and shoulder muscles because much of the weight of their body must be supported by these muscles when using such aids. All patients need their leg and abdominal muscles strengthened in preparation for walking. If active isotonic exercises are not contraindicated, the patient should be encouraged to do these while in bed.

Active exercises for patients requiring additional strength in their arms and shoulders in preparation for crutch or walker-assisted ambulation include push-ups (lying on the abdomen with the hands under the shoulders and pushing the head and upper half of the trunk up, taking the weight on the hands), and sit-ups (pulling oneself to a sitting position from lying down). A

trapeze supported from an overbed frame is often used to assist patients to pull themselves to a sitting position if they are unable to manage it themselves. Another exercise for strengthening hand, arm, and shoulder muscles is to have the patient lie flat in bed, reach his arms up to grasp the head of the bed, and pull himself up in the bed.

If isotonic exercises are not feasible, isometric exercises can be used. It is possible to develop almost as full an extent of muscular tension in muscles by exercising them isometrically as isotonically. In isometric exercises the individual alternately tenses and relaxes muscles without moving joints. The muscle does not move outwardly, and no work is performed. Hence, this type of exercise is useful for people who do not have sufficient strength to do active range of motion exercises, or it can supplement them. Isometric exercises are also useful for patients in whom active isotonic exercise is contraindicated.

For increasing muscular strength, even a one second maximal contraction done isometrically once a day is effective. Muscle strength can be increased more quickly if the maximal contractions are increased to five per day, each lasting six seconds.

[These are] particularly useful for maintaining the tone of postural muscles of the buttocks, abdomen, and thighs. The patient can set the quadriceps, gluteal, and abdominal muscles separately, or he may set all of them simultaneously by lying supine with legs extended and hands at his sides, then lifting his buttocks off the bed, bearing his weight on shoulders and heels.[1]

Exercises for the Ambulatory. All ambulatory patients should be encouraged to participate in a regular exercise program, unless there are health reasons which preclude this. Exercises are planned to suit each person's needs and his motor abilities, taking into consideration his age, sex, degree of mobility, and limitations imposed by chronic or current health problems, and his interests. The individual who starts on an exercise program should always have a complete physical examination first to make sure there are no contraindications to exercise, as well as to find out if there are any limitations on the type or amount of exercise that should be planned.

The program may be planned for the patient to do either at home or outside the home. Many community organizations offer a graded series of exercise classes to assist people in maintaining or regaining optimal physical fitness. Exercises for the elderly have become a regular feature of many of these programs. Exercise

✓PRINCIPLES UNDERLYING BODY MECHANICS

1. **Large muscles fatigue less quickly than small muscles.**
2. **Muscles are always in slight contraction.**
3. **The stability of an object is always greater when there is a wide base of support and a low center of gravity, and when the line of gravity is perpendicular to the ground and falls within the base of support.**
4. **The amount of effort required to move a body depends upon the resistance of the body as well as on the gravitational pull.**
5. **The force required to maintain body balance is greatest when the line of gravity is farthest from the center of the base of support.**
6. **Changes in activity and position help to maintain muscle tone and avoid fatigue.**
7. **The friction between an object and the surface on which the object is moved affects the amount of work needed to move the object.**
8. **Pulling or sliding an object requires less effort than lifting it, because lifting necessitates moving against the force of gravity.**
9. **Using one's own weight to counteract a patient's weight requires less energy in movement.**

---

programs can be found to accommodate all age groups and to cater to virtually all interests, such as hiking, swimming, and other sports, as well as simple calisthenics.

For people in good health, a regular program of isotonic (also called "dynamic") exercise is usually recommended. According to the American Heart Association, the program should include physical activity that is "rhythmic, repetitive, involves motion and the use of large muscles, and challenges the cardiovascular system."[4] It should be carried out at least 3 times per week, preferably on alternate days.

All exercise sessions should start with a "warm-up" period of exercises that gradually increase respiration, circulation, and body temperature and stretch muscles. The warm-up is followed by a "conditioning" period of more vigorous activity designed to challenge the cardiovascular system by significantly increasing blood flow to the working muscles over an

extended period of time. Such activities might include walking, hiking, jogging, running, swimming, dancing, vigorous calisthenics, or active games and sports. It is important that the intensity of the activity is moderate, not exhaustive. A person's exercise tolerance should be built up gradually, through regular sessions of gradually increasing intensity, rather than in intermittent spurts—and never carried to the point of exhaustion.

Following the exercise period, a gradual "cooling down" is recommended. This should involve slower movements, such as relaxing exercises or simply walking around for a few minutes to allow the body time to adjust to a lessened physical demand.

The American Heart Association has an excellent pamphlet that elaborates on the points made above and includes the "exercise check list" shown on this page.

EXERCISE CHECKLIST

☐ Check with your doctor
☐ Pick activities which are rhythmic, repetitive and which challenge the circulatory system, at an intensity that is appropriate for **you.**
☐ Pick activities which you enjoy, which are suited to your needs, and which can be done year-round.
☐ Wear clothing appropriate for the exercise—consider the temperature, humidity, proper footwear and comfortable clothes.
☐ Remember your warm-up and cool-down periods.
☐ Follow the program regularly, at least 3 times per week, preferably not on consecutive days.
☐ **Enjoy!**

From American Heart Association: "E" is for Exercise. Dallas, Texas, American Heart Association, 1977.

NURSING INTERVENTIONS FOR HELPING PATIENTS TO MOVE

A knowledge of the principles of body movement and skill in their application are important to both the patient and the nurse.

It is important that the nurse use her body in a way which not only avoids muscle strain but also uses energy efficiently. The practice of good body mechanics is not restricted to nursing care; it is integral to healthy living for all people. In health and in illness, good posture and efficient body movement are essential both therapeutically and aesthetically.

Once a person has a knowledge of the principles underlying body mechanics, he should put them into practice in order to establish good habit patterns of body movement. As these patterns are established, movements become smooth and place a minimum of strain upon the body muscles. The nurse will find that she can help patients to move more easily, and the patient will be more comfortable.

Understanding of these principles, and of their application in the correct use of the nurse's muscular energy and weight, will contribute greatly to ease of nurse-patient physical interactions and reduce the likelihood of injury to either party.

1. *Large muscles fatigue less quickly than small muscles.* Using a group of large muscles places less strain on the body than using a group of smaller muscles or a single muscle. For example, less strain results when a heavy object is raised by flexing the knees rather than by bending from the waist. The former movement utilizes the large gluteal and femoral muscles, whereas the latter utilizes the smaller muscles such as the sacrospinal muscle of the back.

2. *Muscles are always in slight contraction.* This condition is called *muscle tone.* If the nurse prepares her muscles for action prior to activity, she will protect her ligaments and muscles from strain and injury. For example, she will be better prepared to lift a heavy object if she first contracts the muscles of her abdomen and pelvis and the gluteal muscles of the buttocks.

3. *The stability of an object is greater when there is a wide base of support and a low center of gravity, and when the line of gravity is perpendicular to the ground and falls within the base of support.* In her motions the nurse can assume a broad stance and bend her knees rather than bend at the waist. This practice keeps the vertical line of her center of gravity within her base of support, thus providing her with greater stability. For example, in helping a patient to move, the nurse's position is more stable and she is therefore better able to maintain her balance if she stands with her feet apart and bends her body at the knees rather than at the waist.

4. *The amount of effort required to move a body depends upon the resistance of the body as well as the gravitational pull.* By utilizing the pull of gravity rather than working against it, the nurse can reduce the amount of effort required in movement. For example, it is easier to lift a patient up in bed when he is lying flat and his center of gravity has been shifted toward the foot of the bed than it is when he is in a sitting position in which the resistance of the body to movement is much greater.

5. *The force required to maintain body balance is greatest when the line of gravity is farthest from the center of the base of support.* Therefore, the person who holds a weight close to his body uses less effort than the person who holds the weight in his extended arms. For example, when moving a patient from a bed to a stretcher, it is easier for the lifters if they hold the patient's body close to their own.

6. *Changes in activity and position help to maintain muscle tone and avoid fatigue.* If a person changes his position even slightly while he is carrying out a task, and if he changes his activity from time to time, he will maintain better muscle tone and avoid undue fatigue.

7. *The friction between an object and the surface upon which the object is moved affects the amount of work needed to move the object.* Friction is a force that opposes motion. The smoothest surfaces create the least friction; consequently less energy is needed to move objects on smooth surfaces. The nurse can apply this principle when a patient changes his position in bed by providing a smooth foundation upon which the patient can move.

8. *Pulling or sliding an object requires less effort than lifting it, because lifting necessitates moving against the force of gravity.* If, for example, the nurse lowers the head of a patient's bed before she helps him to move up in the bed, less effort is required than when the head of the bed is raised.

9. *Using one's own weight to counteract a patient's weight requires less energy in movement.* If a nurse uses her own weight to pull or push a patient, her weight increases the force applied to the movement.

Lifting the Patient and Helping Him to Move

Often the nurse is called upon to help a patient to move or to change his position. Gentle, sure motion on the nurse's part, based on her knowledge of body mechanics, not only helps patients to move easily but also gives them a sense of confidence in the nurse. Some patients, unable to move by themselves, are completely dependent upon the nurse for their changes in position and their exercise. The nurse is frequently called on to assist her patients to make the movements described in this section. It should be noted that there are various methods of performing each movement. The techniques and illustrations used here present one way of doing them.

Helping the Patient Move to the Side of the Bed. The nurse may be called upon to help a patient who is lying on his back (dorsal recumbent position) to move to the side of the bed, as when she is planning to change his surgical dressing. To lift the patient would require a great deal of effort upon the nurse's part, possibly putting unnecessary strain on her muscles as well as upon the patient. The patient can be helped to move more easily, however, if the nurse uses her own weight as a force to counteract the patient's weight and her arms to connect her with the patient so that they move as one.

1. The nurse stands facing the patient at the side of the bed toward which she wishes the patient to move.

2. She assumes a broad stance with one leg forward of the other and with her knees and hips flexed in order to bring her arms to the level of the bed.

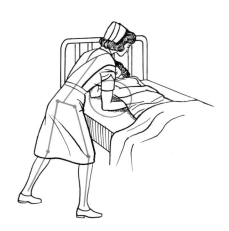

3. The nurse places one arm under the shoulders and neck of the patient and the other arm under the patient's buttocks.

4. She shifts her body weight from her front foot to her back foot as she rocks backward to a crouched position, bringing the patient toward her to the side of the bed. The nurse's hips come downward as she rocks backward. The patient should be pulled rather than lifted in this procedure.

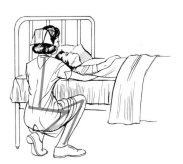

Care should be taken not to pull the patient off the side of the bed. If the patient is unable to move the arm that is nearer the nurse, it should be placed across the patient's chest so that it will not hinder movement or be injured. In moving a patient in this manner, the nurse should feel no strain across her shoulders; it is her own weight that supplies the power to move the patient.

Raising the Shoulders of the Helpless Patient. Some patients are unable to raise their shoulders, even for a short time. When the nurse finds it necessary to raise such a patient, as when changing the pillows, she should proceed as follows:

1. The nurse stands at the side of the bed and faces the patient's head. She assumes a wide stance with her foot that is next to the bed behind the other foot.

2. She passes her arm that is farther from the patient over the patient's near shoulder, and rests her hand between the patient's shoulder blades.

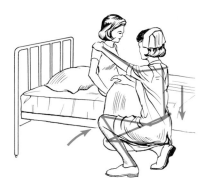

3. In order to raise the patient the nurse rocks backward, shifting her weight from her forward foot to her rear foot, her hips coming straight down in this motion.

The nurse can either guide the patient with her free arm or use it for balance. Again it is the nurse's weight that counteracts the patient's weight.

Raising the Shoulders of the Semihelpless Patient. The semihelpless patient can move to some extent; however, he needs considerable support in most of his movements. In order to help the semihelpless patient raise his shoulders, the nurse uses her own arm as a lever and her elbow as the fulcrum.

1. The nurse stands at one side, facing the head of the patient's bed. Her foot next to the

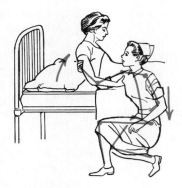

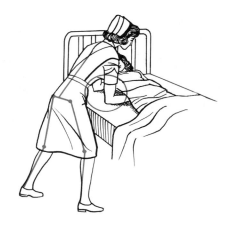

bed is to the rear and the other foot is forward. This position provides a wide base of support.

2. She bends her knees to bring her arm that is next to the bed down to a level with the surface of the bed.

3. With her elbow on the patient's bed the nurse grasps the posterior aspect of the patient's arm above the elbow, and the patient grasps the nurse's arm in the same manner and pushes with the other hand.

4. The nurse then rocks backward, shifting her weight from her forward foot to her rear foot and bringing her hips downward. Her elbow remains on the bed and acts as the fulcrum of the lever.

Moving the Helpless Patient Up in Bed. Helpless patients are best assisted to move up in bed by two persons rather than one; however, one nurse can help a patient to move up in bed by moving him diagonally toward the side of the bed. By moving the patient in sections and by using her own weight to counteract the patient's weight, the nurse can safely move the helpless patient up in bed. This is most easily done if the head of the bed is lowered; then the nurse is not working directly against the force of gravity.

1. The nurse stands at the side of the patient's bed and faces the far corner of the foot of the bed. She places one foot behind the other, assuming a broad stance.

2. She flexes her knees so that her arms are level with the bed and puts her arms under the patient. One arm is placed under the patient's head and shoulders, one arm under the small of his back.

3. The nurse rocks forward, then shifts her weight from her forward foot to her rear foot, her hips coming downward. The patient will slide diagonally across the bed toward the head and side of the bed.

4. This is repeated for the trunk and leg the patient. (See the procedure for moving patient to the side of the bed.)

5. The nurse then goes to the other side of the bed and repeats steps 1 to 3. She continues this process until the patient is satisfactorily positioned.

Moving the Semihelpless Patient Up in Bed. This movement is facilitated if the patient can assist by flexing his knees and pushing with his legs. In assisting the patient to make this movement, the nurse should take precautions that his head does not hit the top of the bed. Thus the nurse can lower the head of the bed and put the patient's pillow at the head of the bed, where it can act as a pad. Helping the patient move up in bed can be done by one or two nurses; in the latter instance one nurse stands at each side of the patient's bed. The procedure for one nurse is described here.

1. The patient flexes his knees, bringing his heels up toward his buttocks.

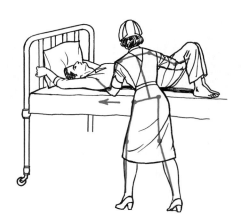

2. The nurse stands at the side of the bed, turned slightly toward the patient's head. One foot is a step in front of the other, the foot that is closer to the bed being to the rear; her feet are directed toward the head of the bed.

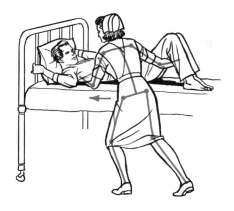

4. As the nurse shifts her weight from her forward leg to her rear leg, the patient is turned toward her. The nurse's hips come downward during this motion.

5. The patient is stopped by the nurse's elbows, which come to rest on the mattress at the edge of the bed.

Helping the Semihelpless Patient Raise the Buttocks. In this motion the nurse's arm acts as the lever, her elbow as the fulcrum.

1. The patient flexes her knees and brings her heels toward her buttocks. She is then ready to assist by pushing when the nurse tells her to do so.

2. The nurse faces the side of the bed and stands opposite the patient's buttocks. She assumes a broad stance.

3. With her knees flexed to bring her arms to the level of the bed, the nurse places one hand under the sacral area of the patient, her elbow resting firmly on the foundation of the bed.

4. The patient is instructed to raise her hips.

5. As she does so, the nurse comes to a crouching position by bending her knees, while her arm acts as a lever to help support the patient's buttocks. The nurse's hips come straight down in this action. While the nurse supports the patient in this position she can use her free hand to place a bed pan under the patient or to massage the sacral area.

3. The nurse places one arm under the patient's shoulders and one arm under his buttocks. Her knees are flexed to bring her arms to the level of the surface of the bed.

4. The patient places his chin on his chest and pushes with his feet as the nurse shifts her weight from her rear foot to her forward foot. By grasping the head of the bed with his hands, the patient can help pull his own weight.

Helping the Patient Turn on His Side. When a patient needs help in order to turn on his side, the nurse must take particular care that the patient does not fall off the bed. She can control his turning by placing her elbows on the bed as a brace to stop his roll.

1. The nurse stands on the side of the bed toward which the patient is to be turned. The patient places his far arm across his chest and his far leg over his near leg. The nurse checks that the patient's near arm is lateral to, and away from, his body so that he does not roll upon it.

2. The nurse stands opposite the patient's waist and faces the side of the bed with one foot a step in front of the other.

3. She places one hand on the patient's far shoulder and one hand on his far hip.

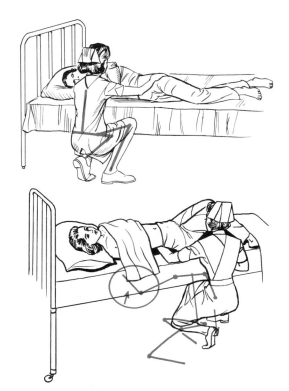

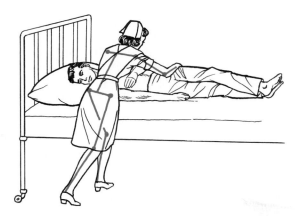

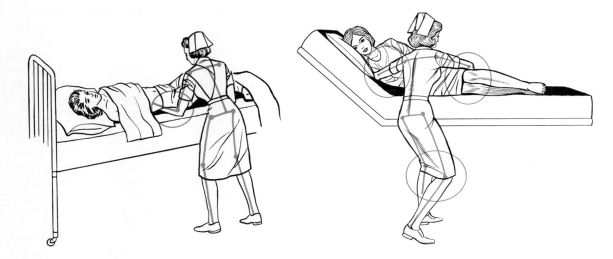

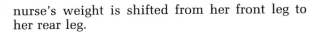

Assisting the Patient to a Sitting Position on the Side of the Bed. 1. The patient turns on her side toward the edge of the bed upon which she wishes to sit. (See the procedure for helping the patient turn on her side.)

2. After ensuring that the patient will not fall off the bed, the nurse raises the head of the bed.

3. Facing the far bottom corner of the bed, the nurse supports the shoulders of the patient with one arm, while with the other she helps the patient to extend her lower legs over the side of the bed. She assumes a broad stance, with her foot that is toward the bottom of the bed being to the rear of the other foot.

4. The patient is brought to a natural sitting position on the edge of the bed when the nurse, still supporting the patient's shoulders and legs, pivots her body in such a manner that the patient's lower legs are swung downward. The

nurse's weight is shifted from her front leg to her rear leg.

Assisting the Patient to Get Out of Bed and Into a Chair. In this procedure the bed should be at a height from which the patient can step naturally to the floor. If the bed cannot be lowered sufficiently, the nurse should obtain a footstool for the patient. The footstool must be stable and have a surface upon which the patient is unlikely to slip. Also, it is advisable for the patient to wear low-heeled shoes rather than loose slippers. The shoes enable the patient to walk comfortably and provide support, but are not as likely to slip.

1. The patient assumes a sitting position on the edge of the bed and puts on shoes and dressing gown.

2. A chair is placed at the side of the bed with its back toward the foot of the bed.

3. The nurse stands facing the patient; her foot that is closer to the chair is a step in front of the other, to give her a wide base of support.

4. The patient places her hands upon the nurse's shoulders, and the nurse grasps the patient's waist.

5. The patient steps to the floor, and the nurse flexes her knees so that her forward knee is against the patient's knee. This prevents the patient's knee from bending involuntarily. *Note:* If the patient has to step onto a footstool before standing on the floor, it is almost impossible to give knee support.

6. The nurse turns with the patient while maintaining her wide base of support. She bends her knees as the patient sits in the chair.

Lifting the Patient From a Bed to a Stretcher (Three Man Carry). To move a patient who

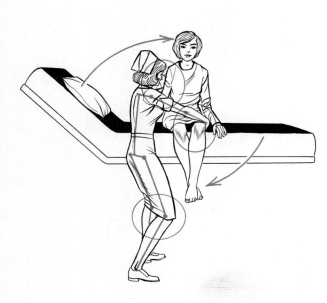

must remain in the horizontal position from one place to another—for example, from a bed to a stretcher—three persons are usually needed. The tallest person should take the top third of the patient, because he probably has the longest reach and can most easily support the patient's head and shoulders. The shoulders are the heaviest part of the body in men. The second person supports the middle third of the patient, usually the heaviest part in women. He will be helped if the first and third persons put their arms beside his. The shortest person supports the patient's legs.

Before the patient is moved, a stretcher is placed at right angles to the bed, with the head of the stretcher almost touching the foot of the bed. The stretcher wheels should be locked. To coordinate their movements, the three persons must work by counting off numbers; the person who takes the head of the patient calls the numbers.

1. The three who are to move the patient face the side of the patient's bed. Each assumes a broad stance, with his foot that is toward the stretcher being foward.

2. At the call of "one," the three bend their knees and place their arms under the patient. The first person places one arm under the neck and shoulders and the other arm under the small of the patient's back. The middle person places one arm under the small of the patient's back and the other arm under his hips. The person at the foot of the bed places one arm under the patient's hips and the other arm under the patient's legs.

3. At the call of "two" the patient is turned toward those who are lifting him. This is accompanied by rolling the patient toward the lifters. The patient's arms should not be allowed to dangle freely. The lifters hold him close to their bodies in order to avoid back strain.

4. At the call of "three," they rise, step back (with the forward foot), and walk in unison to the stretcher.

5. At the call of "four," they bend their knees and rest their elbows on the stretcher.

6. At the call of "five," each lifter extends his arms so that the patient rolls to his back at the middle of the stretcher. Protection is needed at the far side of the stretcher to prevent the patient from rolling off.

7. At the call of "six," each lifter withdraws his arms.

In lifting the patient, the lifters should hold the patient close to their bodies. It is also important to lift and lower the patient with an easy, smooth motion in order not to jar or frighten him.

Some Devices for Assisting the Patient to Move

The Liftsheet. A liftsheet, or full sheet folded in half, placed under a helpless patient is a useful aid in moving him in many situations. The liftsheet should extend from the patient's arm level to the bottom of the buttocks.

At least two nurses are needed to move a patient by this means. One nurse stands at each side of the patient, grasps the liftsheet firmly near the patient, and moves the patient and liftsheet to the desired position—up in the bed or toward the side, for example.

To turn a patient on his side, his arms and legs are first positioned safely (see page 501). The nurse then reaches over the patient, grasps the liftsheet on the far side, and pulls it toward her in such a way that the patient rolls on his side toward the nurse. Again the nurse should take precautions to ensure that the patient does not roll off the side of the bed.

Mechanical Devices. There are several mechanical devices available for moving a patient. One is the hydraulic lift, which can elevate a person and move him—from his bed to a stretcher, for example. Some models have heavy canvas supports which fit under the patient's buttocks and behind his back to provide support. These lifts can be used to assist a patient in and out of the bathtub and in and out of bed. A note of caution: Some models can tip quite easily. It is important to have sufficient help to carry out the procedure safely—to watch both the lift and the patient.

Ambulation

It is often necessary for patients to relearn to walk, often with the aid of crutches, braces, or canes. This is usually the responsibility of the physical therapy department, but there are some situations in which it is necessary for the nurse to assist the patient.

The patient may be learning to walk again following an extended period of bed rest. Preparing the patient for this task involves both psychological and physical measures. The nurse can help the patient to gain confidence in his ability to walk again. Often her encouragement and her faith in his ability can bolster his. If an appropriate exercise program has been maintained throughout his illness, the task is easier. Before attempting to stand, it is important for the patient to learn to maintain good trunk balance first in a sitting position, then in a standing position, before he attempts to walk.

When he can maintain a standing position and feels confident in his balance, a few steps should be tried. Since good balance is essential and the patient must feel steady on his feet, it is important that he wear shoes with good support rather than slippers when he is standing or walking. The patient should not be allowed to become fatigued and should attempt only short distances at first. The nurse can help to promote the patient's feelings of self-confidence by helping him to set small goals for each day's activity and acknowledging his accomplishment of these goals.

Most patients who are learning to walk again following a lengthy period of bed rest require physical support when they are first starting. There are several ways the nurse can provide this support. The nurse can place the arm that is nearer the patient under his arm at the elbow and grasp his hand in hers. She synchronizes her steps with his, moving her inside foot forward at the same time as he moves his inside foot.

Another method is to grasp the patient's left hand in her left hand, and encircle his waist with her right hand. Again, the walking is synchronized to provide as wide a base of support as possible.

The patient can also be supported by being held at the waist from the rear. This can be accomplished with a towel folded lengthwise and encircling the patient's waist. There are also special belts designed for this purpose. Such support helps the patient to maintain his balance and keep his center of gravity within his base of support. If the patient requires more support than this, it is advisable for the nurse to have a second person to assist him.

In some situations, however, the nurse may have to assist a person with weakness on one side of the body to walk, with no second person to assist. There appears to be a great deal of controversy over whether the nurse should be on the patient's unaffected side, or his weak side, to provide best support. Some physical therapists advocate one position, others the opposite. Before attempting to assist the patient, the nurse should find out which position is recommended in the agency in which she is working and use it. We will describe both.

If the nurse is standing at the patient's weak side, she puts her arm that is nearest to the patient under his, grasping the inside of his upper arm. With her far arm, then, she reaches over and takes hold of the patient's lower arm or hand. In this position, she can also provide support with her leg to the patient's weakened one if necessary, thus providing maximum support for the affected side.

The second method is for the nurse to support the patient on his unaffected side. The patient puts his good arm around the nurse's shoulder and clasps her hand. The nurse puts her other arm around the patient's waist. Together, they step forward, the patient using his weak foot first and the nurse her opposite foot to provide as wide a base of support as possible.

For hemiplegic gait training or ambulation training, however, the patient is encouraged to take some weight, and eventually as much weight as possible, on his affected side. During the rehabilitation phase, it is important that the nurse consult with the physical therapist regarding the walking pattern being taught to the patient and the best method of assisting him.

Braces give support to a particularly weak leg. In the past braces were made of heavy material with sufficient rigidity to hold the limb in place and provide it with support. A new type of lightweight inflatable brace has been developed recently which should prove very useful for patients who need the legs supported for walking without the extra weight. There are also a variety of walkers available which provide support for a person while he is walking. When a patient uses a walker, much of his weight is borne by his hands and arms as he pushes the walker forward.

Some patients find it necessary to use crutches for a period of time. There are many kinds available: underarm, elbow extension, and Lofstrand crutches, for example. Sometimes the

The use of a walker is part of the retraining program for many people whose mobility has been affected by illness.

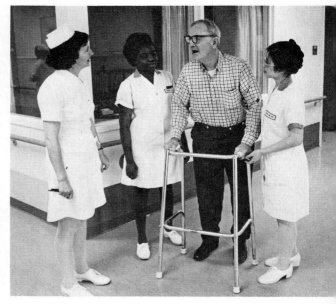

nurse measures a patient for crutches and helps him learn to walk with them. Several methods are used to measure a person for an underarm crutch. One method is to measure the distance from the patient's axilla to the heel of his foot while he is in bed. To this distance, 2 inches is added. A second method is to measure from the anterior fold of the axilla to a point 6 inches lateral to the heel. When crutches are of appropriate length, the hand bar permits slight flexion of the elbow, and the weight is borne by the hand and arms rather than at the axilla. The nerves in the axilla are not protected against pressure except by a layer of fat, which is compressible. If weight is borne on the axilla, the pressure may result in nerve damage and possibly paralysis. For this reason the top of the crutch should be 2 inches below the axilla and should not be padded initially.

Gaits. There are seven basic crutch gaits:

Two Point Crutch Gait. This gait has the following sequence: right crutch and left foot simultaneously; left crutch and right foot simultaneously.

Three Point Crutch Gait. This gait has the following sequence: both crutches and the weaker limb; then the stronger limb.

Four Point Crutch Gait. This gait has the following sequence: right crutch, left foot, left crutch, right foot. This is a particularly safe gait because there are always three points of support on the floor at one time.

Tripod Gaits. There are two tripod gaits: in one, the patient puts the crutches forward simultaneously and then drags his body forward; in the other, he puts his crutches forward one at a time, and then drags his body forward.

Swing Gaits. There are two swing gaits: in one, the patient puts his crutches forward and then swings his body up to his crutches; in the other, he swings his body beyond them.

The advantage of possessing skill in more than one gait is twofold: the patient can use a slow or fast gait as he wishes and, since each gait requires a different combination of muscles, he can change gaits when he becomes fatigued.

Before a person uses crutches he would be wise to strengthen the muscles he will need, particularly the shoulder depressors (trapezius), triceps, and the latissimus dorsi muscles. These can be strengthened by simple exercises that the patient can carry out in bed, as mentioned earlier.

PLANNING AND EVALUATING SPECIFIC NURSING INTERVENTIONS

Nursing interventions are planned to suit each individual patient, his problems, and his needs. It is again helpful to set specific targets to be accomplished by nursing action and then to decide on the appropriate interventions to accomplish these objectives. The patient and his family should be involved in the establishment of expected outcomes and in the selection of the interventions to be used, and should participate in the implementation of exercise programs as much as possible. The nurse works closely with the physical therapist and the occupational therapist in planning appropriate exercises that are consistent with the physician's plan of care for the patient. The prevention of muscle deterioration and the maintenance and improvement of muscle strength and tone in patients whose mobility is limited require the intensive effort of all concerned.

The process of recovery for people who have lost partially or completely one or more of their motor abilities is often a long one. Short-term goals are therefore very important. The achievement of each small step of progress is something to work toward and provides the nurse, the patient, and his family with motivation to work towards further goals. The outcomes of nursing interventions, such as range of motion exercises, might include, for example, that the patient be able to put his arm or leg (or a smaller appendage, such as a hand or a foot) through a more complete range of motion and that he accomplish this feat daily (or twice a day). Specifics should be included as to what his range of motion was at the start and what the expected outcome will be at the end of a given period. The expected outcomes of passive exercises done by the nurse would be the prevention of contractures that could hinder joint mobility, such as in the wrist, the ankle, the shoulder, the knee, and so forth.

For the patient who needs help in moving, the expected outcomes would be related to the various activities and functional abilities. For example, helping the patient to turn might be related to maintaining the status of his skin, his respiratory functioning, or his circulatory status, and to the prevention of complications with regard to these abilities. Assisting the patient to use the bedpan or urinal would be related to the maintenance of adequate elimination.

For the patient who needs help in sitting up, or in learning to move from bed to chair and the reverse, or in learning to walk again, the nursing interventions are directly related to motor functioning and increasing the patient's independence in carrying out the activities of daily living. Again, outcomes should be established on a short-term basis, with explicit details as to what is to be accommplished in a given period of time. An example could be the patient's being able to pull himself up to a sitting position using a trapeze in bed, and doing it so many times a day. Or, the patient is able to sit or maintain himself in an upright position while sitting for gradually increasing specific periods of time.

It should be noted that the road to recovery is not always a smooth one. Patients need encouragement and support when temporary setbacks occur in their progress. A major nursing responsibility is providing the support the patient needs, both physically and psychologically.

If the expected outcomes of her nursing interventions have been sufficiently explicit, the process of evaluating the effectiveness of these becomes relatively simple. Have the expected outcomes been achieved? Is the patient's range of motion extended? Can he do more of the exercises himself? Does he carry out isometric exercises on his own the prescribed number of times as stated in the goals? Is he able to sustain the contraction for one second, or for the number of seconds specified as his target goal?

The nurse also keeps in mind the long-range goals of nursing action. Have unused muscles whose movement is not contraindicated been maintained in strength and tone? Has the process of degeneration been prevented in these muscles? Have contractures that could interfere with joint mobility been prevented? Has joint mobility been maintained? Have muscular strength and tone been improved? Has the patient regained independence in carrying out activities of daily living? Or is he making progress towards this? What progress has he made towards this goal? If the patient requires help in moving to carry out these activities, has he received this help when he needed it and in such a way as to enable him to maintain his other functional abilities? Is there optimal functioning of his other abilities?

GUIDE TO ASSESSING MOTOR FUNCTIONING ABILITIES

1. Is the patient able to walk normally? Or does he need aids for mobility, such as a cane, crutches, a walker, a wheelchair, another person, or a stretcher?

2. Does he have limitations in mobility due to chronic health problems, as, for example, paralysis, weakness, difficulty of movement in one or more limbs or other part of the body? Has he had an amputation?

3. How does his present motor status compare with his usual status?

4. Does he have any current health problems that may be interfering, or could interfere, with his motor functioning abilities? Or, has he had any recently?

5. What is the patient's response to activity?

6. Does the patient need help with raising his head and shoulders? With moving in bed? With turning? With sitting up? With using the bedpan or urinal? With standing? With transferring from the bed to a chair and the reverse? With walking?

7. What are the physician's diagnostic and therapeutic plans of care for this patient?

8. Have reports been received on diagnostic tests or examinations done on this patient? If so, how do these affect the planning of nursing care for this individual?

9. Have restrictions been placed on the patient's mobility? On exercises he can perform?

10. Is the physical therapist involved in helping this patient? The occupational therapist? What are their plans for the patient? How can you help with these plans?

11. Can the patient do these exercises himself?

12. Can the patient's family help the patient in carrying out exercise activities?

Mr. George Ellis, age 28, had his foot crushed in a logging accident 3 days ago. He works as a scaler for a large forest products company. Following surgery to repair the soft tissue damage, the physician has encased the foot in a cast. He has ordered that Mr. Ellis remain in bed for an unspecified period of time. He has told Mr. Ellis that when he is allowed up, he must learn to walk with crutches or use a wheelchair to get around in. Mr. Ellis is a healthy, active individual, and objects strongly to being confined to bed. He says he is not going to use a wheelchair if he can help it. He wants to know if there is anything he can do while in bed that will help him when he is allowed up from bed.

1. What information would you need to help you in planning Mr. Ellis's care?
2. What sources would you use to obtain this information?
3. What problems might Mr. Ellis have in addition to his mobility?
4. What other health professionals might be involved in Mr. Ellis's care?
5. What factors would you take into consideration in planning Mr. Ellis's care?
6. What exercises might Mr. Ellis do on his own to prevent the deterioration of muscular strength and tone? To prepare himself for using crutches?
7. What other help would Mr. Ellis require in carrying out daily living activities?

SUGGESTED READINGS

Brassell, M. P. (consultant): Teaching Patients to Cope with Polymyalgia Rheumatica. Nursing '78, 8(5):14–16, May, 1978.

Cohen, S.: Programmed instruction—Patient Assessment: Examining Joints of the Upper and Lower Extremities. American Journal of Nursing, 81(4):763–786, April, 1981.

Dehn, M.: Rehabilitation of the Cardiac Patient. The Effects of Exercise. American Journal of Nursing, 80(3):435–439, March, 1980.

Farrell, J.: Caring for the Laminectomy Patient: How to Strengthen Your Support. Nursing '78, 8(5):65–69, May, 1978.

Frankel, L. J., and Byrd, B.: Exercise to Help the Elderly—To Live Longer, Stay Healthier, and Be Happier. Nursing, '77, 7(12):58–63, December, 1977.

Drapeau, J., and Prave, M.: Getting Back into Good Posture: How to Erase Your Lumbar Aches. Nursing '75, 5(9):63–65, September, 1975.

Hoepfel-Harris, J. A.: Improving Compliance with an Exercise Program. American Journal of Nursing, 80(3):444–445, March, 1980.

How to Negotiate the Ups and Downs, Ins and Outs of Body Alignment. Nursing '74, 4(10):46–51, October, 1974.

Krafchik, H.: Fitness for 39¢. Canadian Nurse, 71:45, August, 1975.

Sivarajan, E. S., and Halpenny, C. J.: Exercise Testing. American Journal of Nursing, 79(12):2162–2170, December, 1979.

Wilson, R. L.: An Introduction to Yoga. American Journal of Nursing, 76:261–263, February, 1976.

Winslow, E. H., and Weber, T. M.: Rehabilitation of the Cardiac Patient. Progressive Exercise to Combat the Hazards of Bed Rest. American Journal of Nursing, 80(3):440–443, March, 1980.

Young, C., Sr.: Exercise: How to Use It to Decrease Complications in Immobilized Patients. Nursing '75, 5(3):81–82, March, 1975.

Ziegler, J. C.: Physical Reconditioning—Rx for the Convalescent Patient. Nursing '80, 10(8):21–23, August, 1980.

REFERENCES

1. Brower, P., and Hicks, D.: Maintaining Muscle Function in Patients on Bed Rest. American Journal of Nursing, 72:1250–1253, July, 1972.
2. Mathews, D. K., and Fox, E. L.: The Physiological Basis of Physical Education and Athletics. 2nd ed. Philadelphia, W. B. Saunders Company, 1976.
3. Guyton, A. C.: Basic Human Physiology and Mechanisms of Disease. 3rd ed. Philadelphia, W. B. Saunders Company, 1982.
4. American Heart Association: "E" Is for Exercise. Dallas, Texas, American Heart Association, 1977.

24

The Nurse Should Be Able to:

- Discuss the nurse's role in protecting against environmental hazards
- Identify factors affecting a person's ability to protect himself from environmental hazards
- Discuss particular safety needs at different stages in the life cycle
- Identify existing and potential hazards in the environment of sick people
- Apply relevant principles in selecting, planning, and implementing safety precautions for ill persons
- Take appropriate action to protect the safety of ill persons in case of fire
- Evaluate the effectiveness of nursing interventions

Section Three PROTECTION AND SAFETY NEEDS

SAFETY NEEDS

CHAPTER 24

INTRODUCTION

Accidents are listed among the five leading causes of death each year in North America. They are the principal cause of death among children and young adults and a major cause of hospitalization in people of all ages. Accidents are usually related to hazards in the environment.

As with so many other aspects of her role today, the nurse's responsibilities with regard to environmental safety are rapidly expanding. In the past, the nurse thought only in terms of protecting the sick person from hazards in his immediate environment. Today, however, nurses, as informed and knowledgeable health professionals, are concerned with health hazards in the communities in which they live and work. They are taking action and making their voices heard, both individually and collectively through their professional associations, to make the environment more conducive to healthy living. Local, state (provincial), and national nursing associations are expressing their concerns about air pollution, the pollution of our rivers, lakes, and coastal waters, highway safety, the safety of our water, milk, and food supplies, the safety of drugs and cosmetics, and the presence of disease-carrying animals, insects, and other potential sources of infection that are adversely affecting health. They are issuing statements and petitioning municipal, state, and provincial authorities to take action to eliminate environmental hazards to health, as well as actively participating in community action themselves to detect, minimize, or eliminate these hazards.

Our international nursing association has strongly urged nurses to participate in actions to safeguard the human environment. The following statement is pertinent for all nurses:

The Council of National Representatives (CNR) of the International Council of Nurses, meeting in August 1975, adopted a policy statement which outlines the role that nurses can play in protecting and improving the environment and thereby contribute to better health for all people. The ICN Policy Statement reads as follows:

"The preservation and improvement of the human environment has become a major goal of man's action for his survival and well-being. The vastness and urgency of the task places on every individual and every professional group the responsibility to participate in the efforts to safeguard man's environment, to conserve the world's resources, to study how their use affects man and how adverse effects can be avoided.

"The nurse's role is to:—help detect ill-effects of the environment on the health of man, and vice-versa;

—be informed and apply knowledge in daily work with individuals, families and/or community groups as to the data available on potentially harmful chemicals, radioactive waste problems, latest health hazards and ways to prevent and/or reduce them;

—be informed and teach preventive measures about health hazards due to environmental factors as well as about conservation of environmental resources to the individual, families and/or community groups;

—work with health authorities in pointing out health care aspects and health hazards in existing human settlements and in the planning of new ones;

—assist communities in their action on environmental health problems;

—participate in research providing data for early warning and prevention of deleterious effects of the various environmental agents to which man is increasingly exposed; and research conducive to dis-

sensory, consciousness, anxiety, mental state, mobility, state of health

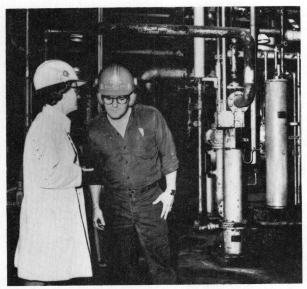

Environmental hazards at the workplace are a concern of community and occupational health nurses. Like the worker, the nurse visiting this power plant wears a protective helmet and safety glasses. The worker, who may be exposed to noise from machinery for several hours a day, must also have protection for his ears. (Photo by Suzanne Emond, Toronto, Ontario. Courtesy Canadian Nurses Association, Helen K. Mussalem Library.)

cover ways and means of improving living and working conditions."[1]

In courses in community health nursing, which are being incorporated into virtually all nursing education programs today, the student will increase her knowledge of environmental hazards in the community at large and will develop skills in identifying and taking appropriate nursing action concerning these. We will, therefore, concentrate in this chapter on the nurse's responsibilities in regard to protecting the safety of persons who are handicapped in their abilities to protect themselves because of illness or infirmity.

FACTORS AFFECTING A PERSON'S ABILITY TO PROTECT HIMSELF

In Chapter 22, we discussed the fact that our sensory receptors provide us with information about the surrounding environment. It is through our abilities to see with our eyes, hear with our ears, smell with our noses, taste with the taste buds in our mouths, and feel through touching that we are alerted to dangers in our environment. Impairment of any of the sensory receptors, of the neural pathways carrying sensory impulses to and through the central nervous system, or of the ability to interpret these impulses results in lessened ability to sense harm-

ful, or potentially harmful, factors in the environment.

The person with limited vision may not see the footstool that he is about to trip over. The person who is hard of hearing may not hear the warning call to watch his step. Someone who has lost his sense of smell may not be aware of the odor of escaping gas from the kitchen stove. Loss of the ability to taste prevents one from detecting the slightly "off" flavor of food that has been improperly preserved. A person who cannot feel does not receive the warning signal that he should remove himself from a seat too close to the fire.

If a person's mental faculties are clouded, or impaired for any reason, his sensory perception is diminished, as is his ability to interpret stimuli. The perceptual abilities of the person suffering from sleep deprivation are usually diminished, or his perception may be distorted (see Chapter 21). A person who is merely drowsy is a hazard when he is driving on the highway, because his sensory abilities are dulled; he may not see the car approaching on his side of the road. His own car may veer suddenly because his sense of touch is impaired; he does not perceive the infinitesimal shift in the steering wheel that tells him that he is not on his proper course. It may also take him longer than usual to realize that he is dangerously close to the edge of the road or in the wrong lane. Alcohol and drugs, which are central nervous system depressants, have the same effect of dulling the senses.

In fact, any alteration in a person's state of consciousness will affect his ability to perceive sensory stimuli, to interpret them, and to react appropriately. The confused or disoriented individual may mistake the door leading to the stairs for the door to the bathroom. Thinking that he is at home, he may also try to get out of a hospital bed to go to the bathroom, and climb over the bed rails to do so. The person who is roused out of a sound sleep, as we mentioned earlier (see Chapter 20), is often confused and disoriented. Older people may become excited and confused by medications given to help them get to sleep (see Chapter 20).

Anxiety and other emotional states may also affect a person's perception of harmful stimuli in the environment, his interpretation of these, and his ability to react to them. Mild anxiety increases perceptual awareness, but increased levels of anxiety progressively decrease it (see Chapter 30). A person can attend to only so many stimuli at one time, and if other stimuli are of more importance, a person may not be alert to potential dangers in his environment. The person whose thoughts are turned inward or fixed on one object, or who is lost in reverie, may bump into objects because he does not see them, step off the curb without looking, or do any one of a number of things that endanger life and limb. The stereotypes of the absent-minded professor and the person in love exemplify this problem.

Then, too, there is the phenomenon of adaptation to sensory stimuli, which can also provide hazards (Chapter 22). The smell of leaking gas may be so insidious that a person becomes accustomed to it or is never even consciously aware of it. The sense of smell is one that adapts very quickly, it seems. The nurse should keep this in mind in relation to offensive odors on the nursing unit. It is sometimes helpful to breathe fresh air for a change; then one's nose will be able to pick up the stimulus again.

Distorted sensory perception can also cause problems in relation to safety, as discussed in Chapter 22.

The individual's ability to respond to stimuli must also be considered. The brain must be functioning sufficiently well to make decisions and to initiate appropriate action in response to sensory stimuli. Some of our actions are reflexes that are initiated in the spinal cord; for example, the withdrawal of the hand from a hot stove becomes an almost instinctive reaction that is a learned cord reflex. A cord reflex can be developed in the bladder of a paralyzed patient to enable him to control his voiding when neural pathways to and from the brain itself have been sufficiently impaired to cut off voluntary control by the cerebral cortex.

Most actions, however, are initiated and controlled by higher centers of the brain (see Chapter 23); an example is the ability of a person to move himself out of the way of approaching danger. If the ability to initiate, coordinate, and carry out motor actions is impaired for whatever reason, the person's ability to protect himself from environmental hazards is decreased. The sleepy driver we mentioned may not be sufficiently alert to turn his steering wheel fast enough to get himself back on course before he goes over the edge of the road or runs into an approaching car. His reaction time is slowed. Alcohol is well known for its effect of slowing a person's reactions, thus making the person who has been drinking a potential hazard both to himself and to others. The relationship between alcohol consumption and a substantial proportion of motor vehicle accidents, fires, and other types of accidents was mentioned in Chapter 4. This lifestyle factor is a definite health hazard.

Communities, in trying to cut down the amount of carnage on the highways, are passing increasingly stringent regulations about drinking and driving. The situation is particularly serious over the Christmas holiday season, when parties contribute to the number of drinking drivers on the road and hazardous winter driving conditions make driving with impaired senses particularly dangerous. At the beginning of December, some cities establish roadblocks to check all drivers for the effects of alcohol, with the police having the power to suspend a person's license on the spot if he is found to be inebriated. The roadblocks have proved to be a good preventive measure.

Injury or illness affecting the specific areas of the brain initiating and controlling movement, or the neural pathways transmitting motor impulses, will also limit a person's safeguarding abilities. People who have lessened mental faculties because of congenital problems, such as the mentally retarded or those with cerebral palsy (a motor disorder from non-progressive brain damage), are hampered in their abilities to protect themselves.

Anyone who has lessened motor abilities of any kind, or who has had restrictions placed on his mobility, is at a disadvantage when it comes to protecting himself from environment hazards. The person in a wheelchair, for example, is severely handicapped. He cannot move as quickly as a person on two feet, and he is hampered by having to maneuver the chair around obstacles or out of the way of dangerous objects. One who cannot grasp objects or move his arm or leg with normal agility and speed is disadvantaged insofar as his protective abilities are concerned.

The sick person is particularly prone to accidents and injury because of the nature of illness itself. He is often physically weak and impaired in his ability to carry out normal daily activities. As a result, he may fall while walking or easily lose his balance on an uneven surface. The protective senses of the sick person (as, for example, his sight) may be so impaired that he cannot perceive dangers to himself. Moreover, the anxiety that goes along with illness may interfere with his perceptual abilities and his capacity to concentrate, as well as his ability to make judgments, and thus expose him to injury. Many people who are ill suffer temporary or prolonged periods in which there is an altered state of consciousness. The preoperative patient who is under sedation, the postoperative patient recovering from anesthesia, the person with a severe head injury, and the unconscious patient all have their sensory perceptual abilities decreased, as well as their abilities to respond to environmental stimuli and to make decisions based on good judgment.

In many illnesses, a person is rendered helpless or semihelpless by the nature of his illness. He must then depend on other people to protect him from environmental hazards. In some instances, it is necessary to restrain a person in his movements to protect him from his own actions, which may cause him injury. Restraining a confused or disoriented person often distresses him, however, and he may fight against the restraints, creating additional safety problems.

Sometimes therapy that is prescribed makes the person more vulnerable to accidents or injury, or has inherent hazards in itself. Medication therapy carries with it many potential hazards, such as adverse reactions or the possibility that the wrong patient will get the medication. Radiation therapy also has its hazards. The very act of penetrating the skin surfaces for surgery renders a person more vulnerable to infection and causes physiologic stress, which makes the individual more susceptible to other disturbances of body functioning, such as fluid and electrolyte imbalance—to mention only one.

PROTECTION AND SAFETY NEEDS THROUGHOUT THE LIFE CYCLE

The expectant mother must be protected against potential injury, not only for her own sake but also for that of the new life growing within her body. The fetus is protected, to the extent that nature is able to do so, by its cushion of amniotic fluid within the uterus. Trauma to the mother may, however, dislodge the placenta from its attachment to the uterine wall, causing a miscarriage or premature labor, depending on the stage of development, or it may cause malformation of the fetus. Pregnant women are generally advised not to participate in sports that cause jolting, such as horseback riding, although swimming and most other sports are not contraindicated. Indeed, as we mentioned in Chapter 23, exercise in moderation is important to the health of both mother and baby.

The young infant must also be protected. The newborn has very limited ability to protect himself (see Chapter 22) and is highly dependent on the people who are caring for him to keep his environment safe for him. As he grows and develops he will learn to avoid certain hazards in the environment, since it is through education and trial and error that an individual learns to identify harmful and potentially harmful situations and to protect himself from harm. Accidents often occur because an infant makes a developmental advance for which the parent is not prepared. Although he may appear to his mother to be perfectly safe lying on his back, the 6-month-old infant may pull himself to a sitting position and, because his balance is still

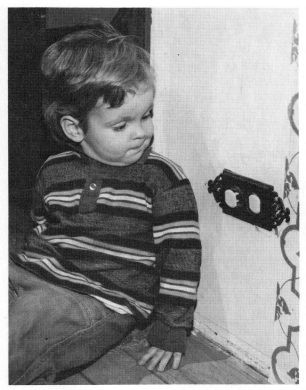

The use of safety covers on electrical outlets is one way to protect the young child from harm that he might suffer since he has no sense of danger.

not very good, may tumble out of his carriage or off his bed.

The very young child has no sense of danger. It is only as the world he knows by experience enlarges that he is able to interpret the meaning of potentially harmful stimuli that he perceives. He plays with matches and is fascinated by the flame. Until he burns himself, however, or unless mother is sufficiently impressive in her admonishments, he does not perceive matches as dangerous objects. Similarly, he cannot read the warning label that tells him that the cleaning fluid is poisonous, and he may drink it. He may lick the chipping paint on his crib, or on a windowsill, and suffer from lead poisoning, if the paint is one that contains lead. Some children suffer from *pica*, the eating of unnatural substances. These children must be supervised especially carefully, and potentially harmful substances must be kept out of their reach. The table on page 513 lists typical accidents, normal behavior characteristics contributing to them, and precautions to safeguard against them, for children in their first and second years of life.

The growing child is most vulnerable to accidents when he is participating in newly acquired activities and when exercising newly won free-

ACCIDENT PREVENTION IN INFANCY

Typical Accidents	Normal Behavior Characteristics	Precautions
First Year		
Falls	After several months of age can squirm and roll, and later creeps and pulls self erect	Do not leave alone on tables or on any surface from which falls can occur Keep crib sides up
Inhalation of foreign objects Poisoning	Places anything and everything in mouth	Keep small objects and harmful substances out of reach
Drowning	Helpless in water	Do not leave alone in tub of water
Second Year		
Falls	Able to roam about in erect posture Goes up and down stairs	Keep screens in windows Place gate at top of stairs
Shocks	Has great curiosity	Cover unused electrical outlets; keep electric cords out of easy reach
Motor vehicles	Has great curiosity	Keep in enclosed space when outdoors and not in company of an adult
Ingestion of poisonous substances	Puts almost everything in mouth	Keep medicines, household poisons, and small sharp objects out of sight and reach
Burns	Has great curiosity	Keep handles of pots and pans on stove out of reach and containers of hot foods away from edge of table
Drowning	Helpless in water	Protect from water in tub and in pools

From Robinson, N. M.: Common Problems of Infancy. In Smith, D. W., et al.: *The Biologic Ages of Man*. 2nd ed. Philadelphia, W. B. Saunders Company, 1978. Adapted from Shaffer, T. E.: Symposium on Clinical Advances: Accident Prevention. *Pediatric Clinics of North America*, 1:421–432, May, 1954.

dom. A 4-year-old may be given permission to visit a friend up the block but, while doing so, he may dart out into the street to retrieve a ball that has bounced out of his reach. The child who is just learning to ride a bicycle may not be able to stop it and may ride out on the road and into the pathway of an oncoming automobile.

Laws have been passed in both the United States and Canada to protect children from some of the more common types of accidents. Children's clothes must be made from non-inflammable material, for example. Drugs must be sold in childproof containers, and poisonous products must be clearly labeled as such. There is a national network of poison control centers in the United States and a poison control center in every major city in Canada (see Chapter 28). The most effective form of accident prevention, however, is supervision and environmental control of potentially harmful factors. The modeling of safe behaviors by parents is by far the most effective form of teaching. If father takes a child's hand and darts across a busy street in the middle of the block, his son is likely to do the same thing when he is on his own. If, on the other hand, father walks to the corner, presses the walk signal button, and waits for the signal to change before crossing, this is the behavior the child is most likely to learn.

By pre-adolescence, prevention has largely become a matter of self-discipline. Some children are accident-prone, however, and always seem to suffer from more cuts, bruises, and scrapes than their brothers and sisters. The tendency often persists into adulthood. Some people may drive a car for 20 years without an accident, while others have one accident after another. It is believed that emotional disturbances underlie the trait of being accident-prone. Tension of any kind is likely to make an individual more susceptible to accidents by impairing his critical functions and exhausting his defenses.

A person who has a history of being accident-prone will need extra safety precautions when he is ill. The nurse's alert observation of potential hazards in the environment is an important measure in preventing accidents, as is the provision of adequate support to the patient—when he needs help with walking, for example. Efforts to minimize anxiety should also be made. Sometimes accident-prone people need psychiatric assistance to learn to cope with their problems.

Insurance statistics repeatedly point up the disproportionately large number of automobile

514 MEETING BASIC NEEDS

accidents involving young male drivers. Risk-taking behavior is common among young adults, (more so among males) because they tend to view their bodies as indestructible. Many, though not all, will drive their cars at high speeds, take the steepest trail down the mountain when skiing, and generally operate under the philosophy that "it can't happen to me." Many young adults have unrealistic perceptions also about their physical capabilities and will push themselves to the limit of their endurance. "Shin splints" (periostitis or inflammation of the periosteum) is a common problem that results from excessive demands being put on the musculoskeletal system. Much trauma is related to sports, although the largest percentage of injuries to young adults still results from automobile and motorcycle accidents.

In adulthood, most automobile accidents are related to the use of alcohol. The trauma resulting from motor vehicle accidents usually gives rise to musculoskeletal problems such as fractures, head injuries, and torn ligaments. Repetitive trauma may result in painful inflammatory lesions of the periarticular structures. Because bone mass declines in a linear fashion in middle age, injuries to the joints that would affect ligaments in young adults cause fractures in middle aged adults.

As a person gets older, his sensory abilities diminish. His vision is not as good as it used to be. His hearing, too, is not quite as sharp, and sometimes may be considerably decreased. The sensory receptors for smell in the nose are often damaged in accidents when people have any kind of a head injury and, in any case, are usually diminished with age. Atrophy of the taste buds is one of the unfortunate aspects of getting older, and even the receptors for touch lose their acuteness with the changes that occur in the aging skin. The older person, then, like the young child, is very vulnerable to environmental hazards, but for a different reason. In the case of the elderly, their "early warning system" in the sensory receptors is not as efficient, and their responses to environmental hazards that are perceived are slower and not as effective. Vestibular function declines, and there is an increased risk of falling. The loss of vision is a major factor in accidents, as is absent-mindedness, and traffic accidents involving elderly pedestrians are common.

mishap."[2] Almost all accidents that occur could have been prevented if the person or persons involved had thought more carefully about their actions, used protective equipment, taken recognized safety precautions, or thought about their own safety and that of others.

The most common types of accidents occurring at home, at work, in school, in hospitals, and elsewhere are those due to:

1. Falls and other injuries caused by mechanical objects in the environment
2. Fire and other types of thermal injuries
3. Chemical injuries

A hospital is generally thought of as a place where the sick and injured come for care; it is seldom thought of as a place where people are injured. Yet, the number of accidental happenings in hospitals is extraordinarily high compared with those in most industries.

The problems of safety in health agencies concerned with caring for the sick and the injured are multiple. There are three groups of people to consider: the patients, who require additional protection because they are ill; the staff, who because of the nature of their work are vulnerable to many types of accidental injury (such as back strain, from lifting heavy patients incorrectly, and infections); and the visitors, who are usually anxious and worried about the person they have come to see.

A hospital is a busy place, and is usually fraught with tension and stress. It must function as a hotel, and the staff members have all the responsibilities of an innkeeper for the safety of the guests. There is usually a large mechanical plant with heavy equipment that keeps the establishment running. Food service is part of the daily activities, and safety in good preparation, handling, and serving must be considered. Diagnostic procedures for patients are often hazardous from the point of view of possible chemical and mechanical injuries to patients and staff, as well as being potential sources of infection. In addition, there is the ever-present threat of fire, the hospital administrator's nightmare, which could be a major catastrophe since the majority of the resident population are weakened by illness or otherwise limited in mobility. Thus, the hospital atmosphere itself is a contributing factor in the likelihood of accidents occurring.

COMMON SAFETY PROBLEMS

An accident has been defined as "anything that occurs unexpectedly and unintentionally" or "an unexpected and undesirable event: a

ASSESSMENT

The nurse's assessment of problems in protecting patients, visitors, and staff from environmental hazards involves two sets of activities:

must be aware of : age, sensory perception, state of health, mobil:

1. Assessment of factors interfering with the patient's ability to take adequate precautions to protect himself

2. Assessment of potential hazards in the environment which could be harmful to patients, visitors, or staff

We will discuss the second aspect of the assessment when we cover specific nursing interventions to assist in preventing mechanical, chemical, and thermal injuries, and will concentrate here on assessing the patient's ability to protect himself.

In her assessment, the nurse needs to be aware of both the patient's age and the integrity of his sensory abilities. She should be alert to any sensory deficits he has, such as impairment or loss of sight, hearing, smell, taste, or touch. She also needs information about any restrictions that have been put on his mobility, such as bed rest, position restrictions, or immobilization of a part (as with a cast or traction apparatus). She should be aware of any aids he requires for mobility (a cane, a walker, or a wheelchair, for example).

She also needs information about his general state of health, the nature of any health problems he has, and the physician's plan of diagnostic and therapeutic care. She should know if the patient is helpless, or semihelpless, or whether the nature of his illness may cause loss of strength, impairment of sensory or motor functioning, or short or prolonged periods of altered state of consciousness. Is he to have surgery, for example, with its attendant preoperative and postoperative periods when the patient's mental faculties may be lessened by sedation or anesthesia? She should be aware of diagnostic procedures being performed that may involve the use of potentially hazardous equipment, potentially harmful reactions, and the possibility of infection. She also needs information about medications the patient is receiving and the nature of other treatments planned for the patient. Is he receiving medications that may diminish his ability to perceive and respond to harmful stimuli, such as analgesics for pain? May his medications cause him to be confused? Is he having treatments, such as oxygen therapy, that require extra safety precautions?

We have said that all patients are anxious, and the nurse should be particularly watchful for evidence of this in the patient. She should also note the level of anxiety the patient is showing. The emotionally upset person (patient, visitor, or staff member) may rush blindly into danger. A person who is worried, preoccupied, or emotionally distressed is often less able to make judgments that are in the best interests of his physical or mental health. These patients require extra vigilance from the nursing staff. The nurse also needs to know if the patient is an accident-prone individual.

The nurse can obtain much of the information she needs from the nursing history and clinical appraisal concerning the patient's usual status and current status at the time of admission with regard to sensory and motor abilities, state of comfort, rest, and sleep, and emotional and mental state. The patient's status changes constantly, however, and the nurse must rely on her own observations and her own judgment regarding safety precautions that need to be taken.

The patient's record is, of course, the most reliable source of information about diagnostic procedures, medications, and other therapeutic measures in the patient's overall plan of care. The nurse supplements this information by increasing her own knowledge about medications, tests and examinations, and treatments by asking knowledgeable people, such as the physician, her nursing instructor, the nursing team leader, or the head nurse, and by reading up on these matters in her texts and in the library.

The patient's subjective observations are also very helpful to the nurse. He may say that he cannot reach the things on his bedside table, for example, or that he is weak or feels dizzy when sitting up, or standing, or trying to walk. He can alert the nurse to things that are causing him pain or discomfort so that she can take appropriate action to remove the cause. For example, his arm may be in the wrong position under him. The astute observant nurse should be aware of this, but patients can be very helpful in assisting the nurse to adjust his position to the most comfortable and safe one for him. The patient is often aware when his mental faculties are impaired—he may say that he just cannot think clearly, or that everything seems to be fuzzy.

The patient's family or significant others often alert the nurse to dangerous situations for the patient. Many agencies permit family members to stay with confused or sedated patients, if they wish to do so, and this can be of great assistance to the nurse. She must be careful, however, that the family member knows what to do in helping the patient or will call the nurse if he needs additional help. The nurse does not neglect her responsibilities in watching over the patient's safety because a family member is with him.

Again, nothing substitutes for the nurse's own observations. She must be alert to all factors interfering with the patient's protective abilities and to all factors in the environment that have the potentiality for causing him harm.

PRINCIPLES RELEVANT TO PATIENT SAFETY

1. **Normally functioning body senses inform the individual about hazards in his environment.**
2. **A person's age affects his ability to perceive and interpret sensory stimuli from the environment and his ability to take effective action to protect himself from harmful stimuli.**
3. **Familiarity with the environment makes it less hazardous.**
4. **A person's ability to protect himself is affected by his sensory status, his mental status, his emotional status, his mobility status, and his status of comfort, rest, and sleep.**
5. **Illness renders a person more vulnerable to accidents and injury.**
6. **Diagnostic and therapeutic measures have inherent potential for causing a patient harm, in addition to aiding in the resolution of his health problems.**

PRIORITIES FOR PATIENT SAFETY

Safety and security needs were designated by Maslow as the second most important in his hierarchy of human needs, and assigned to third place by Kalish in his modification of the Maslow hierarchy (see Chapter 13). Regardless of whether one considers them second or third on a priority listing, however, safety needs are among the most basic of all human needs. Safety is important for all people, but especially to those who are ill. The protective aspects of the nurse's role are among the most important of all her functions, and the nurse incorporates the patient's safety as the number one priority in all aspects of patient care.

Assuring the safety of patients when a fire occurs takes precedence over all other nursing responsibilities. The nurse must know the procedure used in the event of fire in the agency in which she is working, understand how to use the equipment for controlling fire, and know her responsibilities with regard to patient safety. She must be ever alert to potential fire hazards and take action to see that the danger is eliminated, if possible, or minimized if it can't be eliminated.

GOALS FOR NURSING ACTION

The goal of nursing action in regard to patient safety is the prevention of accidental injury to the patient.

SPECIFIC NURSING INTERVENTIONS

In nursing, a knowledge of safe nursing practices is essential. This involves not only a sound knowledge of the nursing and allied sciences, but also a knowledge of preventive nursing measures. To recognize circumstances that could result in an accident and to intervene effectively are essential. The nurse therefore needs to be alert to any activity that could cause injury and to evidence of anything that could cause accident. Her observations should encompass the patient's total environment, in which she can look for such hazards as dangling electric cords, misplaced footstools, and slippery floors—in short, any situation that could result in an accident.

General considerations of environmental factors include arranging everything for the patient's maximal comfort and convenience, as well as that of his family, other visitors, and the staff. The equipment used in hospitals is generally portable, so that it can be moved easily to a more convenient position or location. Hospitals try to obtain equipment that is also quiet, durable, simple to operate, and easily repaired. More and more facilities are being built into the patient's unit so that they are easier to use and always conveniently at hand, and as a result there are fewer hazardous objects in and around the patient's bed.

The patient's unit and the nursing unit itself should be kept as free of clutter as possible. When giving care to a patient, the nurse always makes sure that she has a clear space in which to work, that she can see what she is doing, and that she is able to practice good body mechanics in any lifting and moving that is involved. It is awkward to work over side rails, for example, or to have to reach around objects to get at things she needs.

All accidents—that is, all events that have resulted or could have resulted in injury to a patient, a visitor, or a staff member are reported so that remedial measures may be instituted. For example, if a patient receives an incorrect medication, notifying the nursing supervisor or the physician permits the initiation of measures to prevent a recurrence of this error or to remedy the effects of the incorrect medication.

Another purpose of reporting accidents is to guide the safety committee of an agency in its preventive program. The findings of these committees can be used as the bases for changes in medical and nursing practices and as indications of the need for the education of patients and personnel.

The Prevention of Accidents of a Mechanical Nature

Among the most frequently occurring types of *mechanical* accidents are falls. Falls from beds, from chairs, while walking, or while getting into or out of a bathtub are not uncommon occurrences but are often preventable. A person who is weakened by illness can lose his balance and fall while simply leaning toward a table that is out of reach. Nurses can prevent many accidents of this kind by being alert to potentially dangerous situations and remedying them. For example, beds that can be raised or lowered can be left in the low position when the nurse is not present. At this level the patient will be able to get in and out of bed more safely. Also, patients who have been in bed for several days or who are weakened by illness can be helped to recognize their need for assistance in getting about.

Slippery floors can be dangerous to people in any situation, not only to patients. To minimize this danger non-slippery materials are used on the floor surfaces of hospitals. Also, since any material spilled on a floor is likely to make it slippery, it should be mopped up before someone slips on it. Floors should be washed and polished at a time when there is little traffic upon them, and signs should be prominently placed to notify people that the floor is wet and slippery.

Untidiness can also contribute to accidents. People can trip over electric cords, footstools, bed gatches, and equipment that is left on the floor. Walkways, such as areas from patient's beds to bathrooms, can be particularly hazardous when they are not kept clear. Patients have fallen from their beds while reaching for articles on their bedside tables or while looking for a misplaced call light. The nurse can help the patient to arrange these items so that they are within easy reach.

Other possible causes of falls are movable wheelchairs or stretchers. So often, just as a patient is about to sit in a wheelchair, it moves out of place. Most movable equipment is furnished with locks for the wheels. These locks should be set when the equipment is to be used and released only after the patient is secure.

When a patient first becomes ambulatory after a period of time in bed, he often requires some physical support (see Chapter 23). Many hospitals and other health agencies have rails in the halls to guide and support patients while they are walking. These, as well as rubber treads on stairs, can prevent many falls.

A procedure that poses a threat chiefly to people working within the hospital is the discarding of broken glass and sharp instruments. Most institutions have special containers for glass, razor blades, and the like in order that they can be disposed of separately from other materials. In this way there is less danger of injuring hospital personnel. It is the policy of many hospitals that an employee who is injured at work should report to the employees' health clinic or to a physician for care. In addition, a written report is usually required.

Safety Devices. In her concern for her patient's safety, the nurse may employ specific safety devices. There are dangers involved in the use of many of these devices, however. Disoriented patients may become dangerously entangled in restraints, for example, or a safety device may make the patient unable to move in case of a fire. Many safety devices, therefore, should not be used unless absolutely necessary. In most institutions devices are used either upon the request of the attending physician, or when, in the judgment of the nurse, they become necessary. Policies vary from place to place, however, and the nurse should be familiar with the practice in the institution in which she works. The student should always check with the team leader or with her teacher before using safety devices for patients.

Side Rails. Side rails on beds can stop the patient from rolling off the bed. They do not deter the patient from climbing out; rather, they serve merely as reminders to the patient that he is in bed and should exercise care. Most hospitals have policies regarding the use of side rails. Frequently they are required on the beds of patients who are blind, unconscious, or sedated, or who have muscular disabilities or seizures. Some hospitals require that the beds of all patients over the age of 70 years have side rails. A number of hospitals have adopted a policy of using side rails on the beds of all patients, particularly at night.

It is important when side rails are in use that both rails be up. For example, even when the

RIVERSIDE HOSPITAL OF OTTAWA
CASUALITY OR COMPLAINT REPORT
DETAILS OF CASUALTY OR COMPLAINT
casualty complaint

NOV 4 82

BLACK   GRACE   SP 1242
451 TOLL RD   OTT 234-7566-600
BLACK   GEORGE   HUS
SAME
8.30.82 1PM F 36 M SURG   RC
      420   1

Date of Casualty
or complaint ___Sept 2/82___

Time of Casualty
or Complaint ___7³⁰___ A.M. / P.M.

Examined by Doctor (name) ___White___

Date of Examination ___Sept 2/82___ Time ___8¹⁵___ A.M. / P.M.

Attending Doctor Notified   Yes ✔ No. ☐

On entering Mrs Black's room (212) I found her sitting on the floor between her bed and an armchair. She stated she had wanted to go to the bathroom and felt dizzy on getting OOB. She didn't want to fall so she sat on the floor and grabbed the foot of the bed c̄ her left hand. She is complaining of left wrist being sore — no signs of swelling or bruising. Patient is allowed up and about as desired. She received no sedation at any since bedtime. Call-bell attached to pillow & bed lowered to floor. Supervisor & doctor notified.

Ward ___4N___ Date ___Sept 2nd.___ 19 _82_   Signature ___W Stratton, Reg N.___

REPORT OF INVESTIGATION

No evidence of Nursing neglect — patient allowed to be up and about without assistance

Date ___Sept 2___ 19_82_   Signature of Investigator ___E Able___   Position ___Supervisor___

NOTE: SEND THIS FORM, WHEN COMPLETED, TO NURSING
       OFFICE IMMEDIATELY

2-8750

(Courtesy of Riverside Hospital of Ottawa.)

(Courtesy of Riverside Hospital of Ottawa.)

patient's bed is against the wall both rails should be used; the wall does not serve as a good replacement for the rail. When caring for the patient whose bed has side rails, the nurse normally takes down the side rail on the side at which she is working. She should go no farther than an arm's length from that side of the bed without returning the side rail to its "up" position. Many patients dislike the use of side rails; they may find them an embarrassing reminder of their childhood crib. Some people are fearful of them, while to others side rails signify a loss

RIVERSIDE HOSPITAL OF OTTAWA

DOCTORS CASUALITY REPORT

NOV 4 82

BLACK   GRACE   SP 1242
451 TOLL RD   OTT 234-7566-600
BLACK   GEORGE   HUS
SAME
8.30.82 1PM F 36 M SURG   RC
      420   1

Date of Casualty *Sept 2/82* TIME *7³⁰* AM

Date of Examination *Sept 2/82* TIME *8¹⁵* AM

NATURE OF CASUALITY:

Patient apparently tried to go to the washroom and felt dizzy when she got up - slipped to the floor.

PHYSICAL FINDINGS ON EXAMINATION OF PATIENT

- No signs of swelling a discoloration
- Complaining of left wrist being sore

DATE OF X-RAY EXAMINATION *Sept 2/82* TIME *10²⁵* (A.M) P.M.

X-RAY FINDINGS: *NIL*

Ward *4N* Date *Sept 2/82* _____ M.D.

(To be filled out by the Doctor and forwarded to the Office of the Administrator of the Department of Nursing, immediately on completion.

To be filled on patient's chart on discharge.

(Courtesy of Riverside Hospital of Ottawa.)

(Courtesy of Riverside Hospital of Ottawa.)

of independence and control over their situation. An explanation of the purpose for using side rails often helps such patients to accept them. Generally side rails will not keep a patient in bed against his will; if a patient needs restraining, a safety jacket should be used.

Safety Jackets and Posey Belts.

Patients who are confused sometimes try to climb over the side rails of the bed. They are frequently unaware of their surroundings; they just want to leave the bed. These patients can often be restrained comfortably in bed by means of a safety jacket or Posey belt. The jacket is an inconspicuous sleeveless garment which has long crossover ties in front or in back that can be attached to the frame on either side of the bed. The ties are secured to the frame out of the reach of the patient. Some safety jackets can also be used to hold patients securely upright in wheelchairs.

The Posey belt performs the same function as the jacket. It is secured around the patient's body, and ties are attached to the bed frame. Both the safety jacket and the Posey belt allow the patient to move relatively freely in bed, yet restrain him from climbing over the siderails and possibly falling to the floor.

Arm and Leg Restraints.

Occasionally it is necessary to apply arm or leg restraints to patients in bed. Generally this is an undesirable nursing care measure because it limits a patient's movements, and this in turn often causes anxiety, increasing restlessness and subsequent fatigue. It is a particularly dangerous practice to restrain only one side of the body (as, for ex-

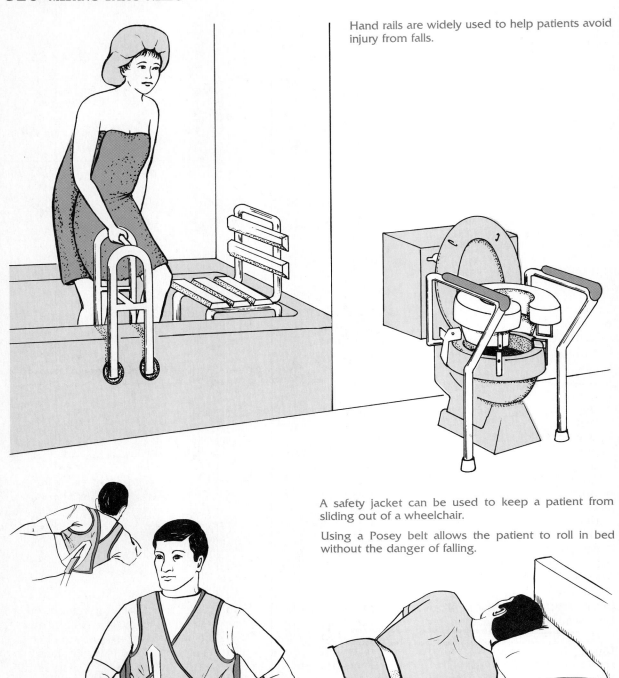

Hand rails are widely used to help patients avoid injury from falls.

A safety jacket can be used to keep a patient from sliding out of a wheelchair.

Using a Posey belt allows the patient to roll in bed without the danger of falling.

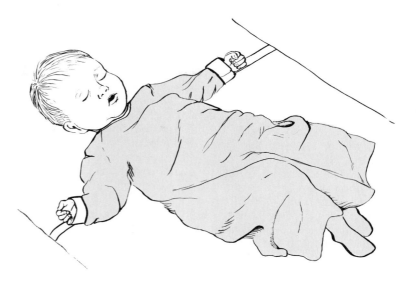

Limb holders are often used for patients too young to understand that they must limit their movements.

ample, the right arm and leg). This practice tends to increase the patient's restlessness, and he may injure himself as he tries to move the arm and leg that are restrained. If only two limbs are restrained, they should be opposite limbs. Few patients like to be tied down, regardless of how irrational they are. Their reaction is usually to struggle against whatever is hampering their movement and they may become quite agitated. Injury to the tissues of the wrists and ankles may result from the friction engendered by rubbing against the restraints. Occasionally, leather restraints may be used. Many agencies will not permit their use except on a doctor's order. There is a greater possibility of both adverse patient reaction to leather restraints and injury to the patient from them.

An arm restraint may be prescribed during an intravenous infusion. Its chief purpose in this instance is to remind the patient to keep his arm immobilized during the treatment.

Arms and legs should not be restrained any longer than is absolutely necessary, and at least every 4 hours the restraints are loosened and the limbs are exercised. There is a danger that a patient's circulation may be restricted if a restraint is tight or if a limb is restrained in an abnormal position. In some agencies a washcloth or other soft cloth may be used to pad the skin under the restraint. A knot over the pad serves to keep the restraint from being too tight. Absorbent cotton should never be used because it has a tendency to flatten out and form into lumps. At any sign of blueness, pallor, or cold, or if the patient complains of tingling sensations in the extremity, the restraint is loosened and circulation restored by exercise and massage. A limb is best restrained in a slightly flexed position.

Mittens. Mittens are indicated for patients who are confused or semiconscious and may pull at their dressings and tubes. The mittens are often used, for example, for a patient with a head injury or for a patient who is confused following a stroke. They have the advantage of not permitting the patient to grasp such objects as dressings, tubing, or bed rails, but they do not limit movement. A mitten is like a soft boxing glove that pads the patient's hand. Commercial mittens are available, or mittens may be made

Mittens can be used to keep the patient from pulling off dressings or pulling intravenous tubes out of place.

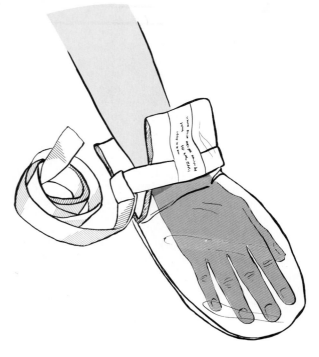

using dressing pads, gauze bandage, and adhesive tape. One method of making mittens is as follows:

Before applying a mitten the patient's hand is placed in a naturally flexed position. This allows unrestricted circulation and places little strain upon muscles. A soft rolled dressing is grasped by the patient so that his thumb approximates his fingers. The soft pad permits the patient to flex his hand while the mitten is in place. All skin surfaces are separated to avoid irritation. The patient's wrist is padded with a dressing to avoid rubbing bony prominences.

Two dressings are then placed over the patient's hand; one medial to lateral, one dorsal to ventral. Large 8 by 16 inch (20 by 40 cm.) dressings are suggested. These are secured by a gauze bandage applied in figure-eight patterns (Chapter 27).

To secure the dressings a stockinette is fitted over the hand and secured by adhesive tape just beyond the wrist pad. A double fold of stockinette open at one end suffices.

Mittens need to be removed at least once every 24 hours. At this time the patient washes his hands and exercises them, or the nurse may do this for him. Mittens should not be so tight as to impede circulation, but they must be secure and pad the patient's hands well.

The Prevention of Accidents Involving Chemicals

Accidents involving chemicals generally result from the incorrect use of pharmaceutical preparations. Physicians and nurses are well aware of the dangers incurred through errors in the administration of medications. Many institutions have special policies and rules that are designed to prevent errors of this nature. Thus, medicines are generally kept in locked cupboards in special areas away from patients and busy nursing-unit offices. Medicines for topical use are separated from medicines administered orally or parenterally. Drugs that are poisonous are well marked. Usually narcotics such as codeine and morphine are kept in a separate double-locked cupboard and counted at the end of each nursing shift, and the tally is recorded in a special book. Medicines that are provided for use at home are labeled with complete instructions as to dosage and frequency of administration. It is common practice for the name of the drug to be included on the label of medications for home use so that the patient will not inadvertently take the wrong drug or one to which they are allergic.

It is common practice for medications that a patient brings in with him from home to be picked up by the nurse who admits him to the nursing unit. The nurse should ascertain the nature of the drugs contained in these medications. She should also notify the attending physician of any medications the patient is using that were prescribed by another doctor. For example, the patient may be under the care of a surgeon while in the hospital and yet have an eye condition for which his ophthalmologist has prescribed twice daily eye drops. The attending physician (in this case, the surgeon) should be alerted to the medication the patient is receiving for his eye condition.

In addition to these generally accepted practices, many agencies require that the nurse have her computations of doses checked by another nurse before the drug is actually prepared. In this way any errors in arithmetic are found before a patient can be harmed. Most hospital pharmacies try to provide nurses with the exact dosage ordered by the physician in order that arithmetical calculations and the division of prepared medicines can be avoided.

Many hospitals now use drugs that are packaged in individual dosages. This practice makes the administration of medications both easier and safer; there is less chance of error. In an increasing number of agencies, medications are delivered from the pharmacy directly to the patient's room, where they are administered by the nurse. This practice helps to reduce the possibility of giving a medication to the wrong patient, another potential hazard in the administration of medications.

Specific orders by the physician help to avoid errors due to ambiguity and misinterpretation. This does not mean that a nurse does not require a thorough knowledge of the pharmaceutical preparation that she is administering. She needs this knowledge in order to protect the patient from harm, to make intelligent observations, and to give intelligent nursing care.

If an error is made in the administration of a medicine, it should be reported immediately to the nursing supervisor and to the patient's physician. In this way steps can be taken to protect the patient from injury. Hospitals usually require that a written account of the error be submitted subsequently. The nurse's responsibilities in the administration of medications are further discussed in Chapter 28.

The Prevention of Injuries from Fire and Other Thermal Accidents

Thermal accidents involve the presence of harmful levels of heat or cold. The most common sources of thermal injuries are fire, hot appliances, or any electrical circuit that is functioning improperly. It is generally a hospital policy that electrical appliances be regularly checked and adequately maintained in order to prevent injury. As an added precaution, patients are often required to have their radios, electric razors, and other appliances checked by the hospital maintenance staff before they use them in hospital. Hot water bottles, heating pads, and infrared lamps are also possible sources of thermal injury. Heat that is applied to a patient is generally regulated well within the safety limits for that patient.

Fire is a constant threat in institutions. Even though modern construction materials have lessened the danger of the actual building catching fire, there are many materials within a hospital that are highly combustible. Oxygen, for example, supports combustion, and substances such as ether are highly inflammable.

For a fire to start there must be three elements present: a combustible material, heat, and oxygen. A *combustible* material is anything that will burn. Among the most common materials involved in hospital fires are: paper, as in wastebasket or garbage chute fires; textiles, such as patient's bedding or oily rags; flammable liquids, such as ether or other liquid gases (for example, those used as anesthetic agents); and electrical equipment. Heat sufficient to ignite the combustible material may come from such sources as a lighted match, a live cigarette, a spark, or friction. There is usually enough oxygen in the atmosphere to support combustion if the other two elements are present. Fire prevention is usually directed, therefore, toward controlling the first two elements, that is, the combustible materials and heat; fire extinguishing measures toward the reduction of heat (as by water cooling) and the exclusion of oxygen.

Fire Prevention. Most hospitals have active programs in fire prevention. Education of the patients, the personnel and the public in safe practices is an essential part of such programs. Some of the areas that are included in the fire control programs of hospitals are discussed in the following paragraphs. One of the most common causes of fire is carelessness with cigarette smoking. In many health agencies smoking is prohibited except in designated areas or when authorized by the patient's physician.

Smoking Regulations. Usually smoking is prohibited in certain areas of the hospital, and these areas are well marked. The no smoking rule is enforced within 12 feet of equipment for administering oxygen, in operating rooms where combustible gases are used, and in places where combustible materials are stored.

Patients who do smoke require ashtrays that do not easily tip and that are so constructed that if a cigarette is left burning it will fall into the ashtray. Some patients—for instance, those who are confused or under the influence of a sedative or hypnotic drug—should not smoke unattended. It may be necessary to keep matches and cigarettes locked in a cupboard if the patient is confused.

Scrupulous Housekeeping. Thorough housekeeping and adequate maintenance of equipment lessen the likelihood of fires. Oily rags, paints, and solvents are stored carefully in a special area so as to prevent spontaneous combustion.

Adequate Storage and Distribution of Volatile Liquids and Gases. Generally large quantities of ether should not be kept in patient areas because of the danger of fire. *Volatile* gases and liquids (those that are easily turned into vapor) are distributed to the various areas of the agency under strict control and all the necessary fire precautions are observed.

Fire Prevention and Fire Extinguishing. In an active fire prevention program all employees must be educated in fire prevention and fire extinguishing.

Types of Fires and Fire Extinguishers. Fires have been categorized into four major classes, based on the type of material that is burning. Class A fires are those involving paper, cloth, wood, and similar solid combustible materials; Class B, flammable liquids and gases; Class C, electrical equipment; and Class D, metals.[3]

Fire extinguishers are simply containers for an agent, such as water or chemicals, with which to put out a fire. The agent acts by one of the following methods:

1. Cooling the burning substance below its ignition temperature
2. Cutting off the supply of oxygen
3. Cutting off the supply of fuel
4. Some combination of the above

Many kinds of extinguisher are available for home, institutional and industrial use. They come in dry chemical, foam, carbon dioxide, water, or halon types. It is important that the right type of extinguisher be used to fight a fire. Some are dangerous when used on the wrong type of fire, as, for example, a water extinguisher (for Class A fires) on a grease (Class B) or an electrical (Class C) fire. It is becoming common practice to label fire extinguishers with picture symbols that identify the type(s) of fire on which they should and should not be used.

The nurse needs to know the types of fire extinguishers used in the agency in which she works, and how to operate these. The four basic steps in using most types of extinguishers are illustrated below.

It is important to read the directions on the extinguisher for variations.

Fire extinguishers must be accessible to personnel. Generally they are kept in obvious places in all patient and service areas. The kind of extinguisher that is placed in a specific area depends upon the type of fire most likely to occur there. Part of a safety program is the regular inspection and maintenance of fire extinguishers.

In addition to having fire extinguishers, nursing units and other departments of a hospital are usually equipped with fire hoses, and personnel are instructed in their use. In the event of a small fire, it may be easier and quicker to use material near at hand, for example, to smother the fire with a blanket or mattress pad, or to pour a pitcher of cold water over it.

The Nurse's Responsibilities in the Event of Fire. If a fire does occur in a nursing unit, the nurse should make sure that the following steps are carried out:

1. Remove patients from the immediate danger area
2. Report the fire
3. Shut off the fire area and decrease the ventilation to the area
4. Employ available extinguishing equipment

In some health agencies it is accepted practice to telephone the fire department, directly reporting the exact location of the fire. Other agencies have a fire alarm system that when set off causes an alarm to ring in the fire station. A third method of reporting a fire is to telephone the operator at the central hospital exchange, who then notifies the fire department. When reporting a fire, it is important that the nurse must be familiar with the locations of the fire alarm pull stations in her unit.

The Removal of Patients. When a fire occurs, the nurse in charge of the nursing unit assumes responsibility for directing the activities of the hospital personnel until the firemen arrive. All fire doors should be closed. Patients in immediate danger must be moved to safety quickly. Generally, ambulatory patients are assisted in walking to safety. In moving immobilized patients, the entire bed is wheeled to a safe area. When it is not feasible to move the entire bed, a portable stretcher can be employed to move immobilized patients. The nurse may occasionally find it necessary to carry a patient in order to remove him from danger. Six basic carries are:

Cradle. This technique is used for people who are light in weight and for children. The nurse lifts the person by passing one of her arms beneath his two knees and the other around his back.

Pack strap carry. With the patient in a sitting position in bed, the nurse faces the patient and grasps the patient's wrists, the right wrist in the left and the left wrist in the right hand. The nurse then pivots and slips under the patient's arm so that the patient's chest is against her shoulders and the patient's arms are crossed on the nurse's chest. With one leg forward for balance the nurse then rolls the patient off the bed and on to her back.

"Piggy-back" carry. If the patient is conscious and able to give some help, the familiar "piggy-back" carry can be used. The patient sits at the edge of the bed, and the nurse stands in front of him with her back to him. The patient reaches

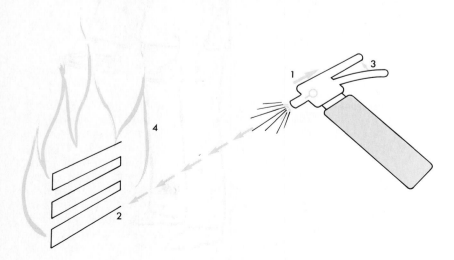

Most fire extinguishers are operated by the following four steps: (1) Pull the pin. This may involve releasing a lock latch, pressing a puncture lever, inversion, or other motion. (2) Aim the nozzle at the base of the fire. (3) Squeeze (or press) the handle. (4) Sweep from side to side at the base of the fire until the contents of the extinguisher are discharged. However, some extinguishers are operated slightly differently. The nurse should be familiar with the extinguishers available in the health agency where she works.

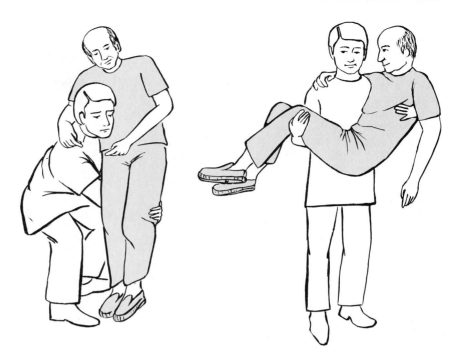

Position for the cradle carry.

Position for the "piggy-back" carry.

Position for the pack strap carry.

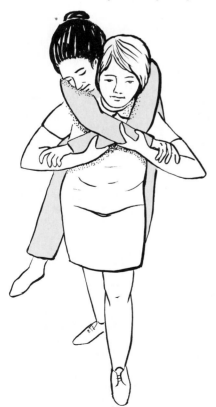

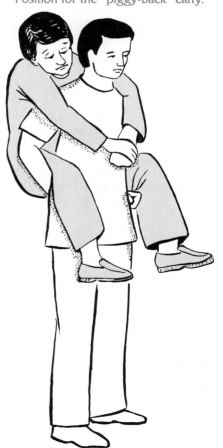

over the nurse's shoulders and holds his hands together in front of her. The nurse then grasps the backs of the patient's legs, slightly above the knees, which allows her to support the weight of the patient in an easier position for carrying than the pack strap carry affords.

Hip carry. The patient lies on her side near the edge of the bed. The nurse faces the head of the bed and puts her arm that is nearest the patient around the patient's back and under the armpit. She then turns so that her hips are against the patient's abdomen and puts her other arm around the patient's thighs and under her knees. The patient is then drawn up on the nurse's hip and the nurse carries her from the bedside.

Swing carry by two nurses. One nurse stands on each side of the patient. The patient's arms are extended around the nurses' shoulders and each nurse grasps one of the patient's wrists with the arm that is farthest from the patient. Each nurse then reaches behind the patient's back with her free arm (nearest the patient) and grasps the other nurse's shoulder. The patient's wrists are then released. Each nurse reaches under the patient's knees and grasps the other's

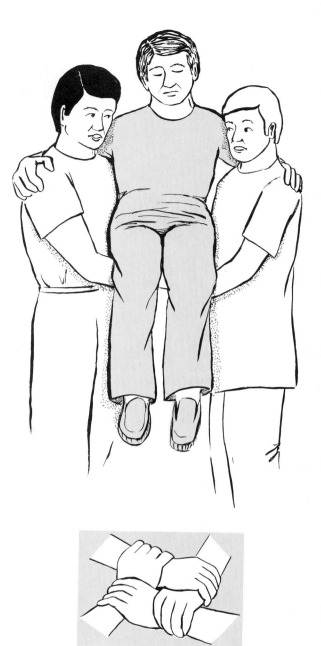

Position for the swing carry.

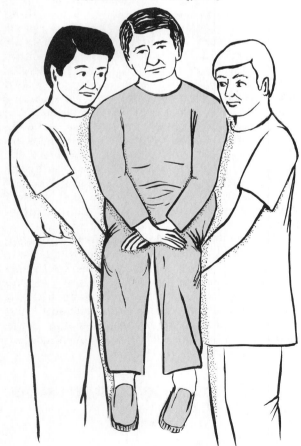

Position for the four-handed seat, with a close view of how the hands are held.

wrist. The patient is then in a sitting position between the nurses. This carry is sometimes called a two-handed seat. A variation of this technique is the four-handed seat, which is used for patients who are able to sit up without support.

Three man carry (see Chapter 23).

As part of any fire prevention and fire extinguishment program, all agency personnel require information about specific policy and practice. Demonstrations in the use of fire equipment, practice in moving patients, and a knowledge of the established practice to be followed upon the discovery of a fire are important. It is only through a continuous in-service educational program in fire prevention and extinguishing methods that the safety of all is safeguarded.

Safety Programs

A safety program is an endeavor to control the physical environment in such a manner that accidents can be prevented. In order to be effective, a program must involve all the people who are concerned with the agency. Many hospitals have safety committees whose job it is to plan a safety program for the institution. Nurses are frequently members of these committees.

The committee's function is to conduct a continual analysis of the kind of accidents that occur in the hospital and their causes. On the basis of this analysis an active program is developed. Continual assessment of hospital practices and continual education of employees are important. Another part of a safety program is the regular inspection of agency facilities; for example, fire extinguishers are checked as often as recommended by the manufacturer. To be effective, a safety program must motivate all employees to accomplish the purpose of the program, for it is only through the active cooperation of all the people in an agency that accidents can be prevented.

PLANNING AND EVALUATING SAFETY MEASURES

Adequate precautions for the patient's safety are an integral component of all nursing measures and of all nursing care planning. Additional safety precautions are needed when the patient is very young or very old, when his perceptual abilities are lessened for any reason, or his ability to react to harmful stimuli is decreased, when potentially harmful equipment is being used in his care, and when he is an accident-prone individual.

All patients have learning needs in relation to protecting their own safety while in the agency, and these are included in the nursing care plan.

A good orientation to the physical layout of the nursing unit and the equipment in his immediate surroundings is essential. He also needs to know how to call for assistance if he needs it (and his call bell must be placed within easy reach). He needs to know how to use the various pieces of equipment that are in and around his bed, and be alerted in regard to safety precautions in their use. An explanation of all safety measures is important to ensure his cooperation, as, for example, an explanation of why the side rails are put up on the bed at night, or, when he is sedated, why it is important not to smoke when oxygen equipment is in use. Each nursing measure, each diagnostic test or examination done, and each therapeutic measure undertaken has important safety precautions that the patient needs to be aware of to protect him from harm. When the patient is unable to protect himself, it is the nurse's responsibility to do it for him.

The expected outcomes of nursing interventions with regard to patient safety are usually expressed in terms of prevention of the undesirable event. Usually the potential problem, such as "the patient may fall from the bed," is stated and expected outcome is written simply as "prevent."

Potential safety problems almost always result from another problem the patient has, or from the nature of the diagnostic or therapeutic plans of care for him. The patient's safety may be jeopardized, for example, when he is under sedation for pain relief. The basic problem is pain; that the patient may fall from the bed when sedated is a potential problem resulting from the nature of his therapy. Evaluation of the effectiveness of nursing interventions is the absence of accidents. If the potential problems are stated explicitly, the nurse can evaluate the success of her interventions, in this case by the fact that the patient did not "fall from the bed," or did not "burn himself or set the bed on fire," if he is a smoker and these are potential problems.

The patient's condition is subject to constant change. It is therefore necessary for the nurse to continuously reassess his abilities to protect himself from environmental hazards and modify her nursing care plans in accordance with his changed status. She must also be constantly alert to new dangers in the environment that could harm the patient, herself, visitors, or other staff.

GUIDE TO ASSESSING SAFETY NEEDS

1. How old is the patient?
2. Is the patient alert, conscious and in full command of his mental faculties?

3. Does he require additional safety precautions because of his age, his physical condition, or his mental state?

4. Is the patient receiving medications that impair his senses?

5. Does the patient require restraints of any sort?

6. Does he smoke?

7. Is electrical equipment in use in the patient's room? Does the patient have electrical appliances at his bedside?

8. Is heat or cold used as a therapeutic agent in the care of this patient?

9. Is the patient on oxygen therapy?

10. Are there any information or safety practices which can help the patient to avoid injury or accident?

11. Is the patient comfortable?

12. Can he reach everything he needs?

13. Is his call signal within easy reach?

14. Is he safe from mechanical injury, such as that resulting from falls?

15. Is he being protected from burns, as for example from a heating pad or a hot water bottle?

16. What precautions are taken to ensure that medications are given safely?

STUDY SITUATION

Mrs. R. Ross, who is 73 years old, is in the hospital because she has a fractured femur. The physician has ordered that she sit in a chair for 15 minutes twice a day. Mrs. Ross walks with considerable difficulty and requires support.

1. What factors should the nurse be aware of in providing a safe environment for Mrs. Ross?

2. List six specific measures that the nurse should take to prevent mechanical injury to Mrs. Ross.

3. If there is a fire in this patient's room, what should the nurse do? How should this patient be moved?

4. By what criteria can the safety of Mrs. Ross's environment be evaluated?

SUGGESTED READINGS

Carmack, B. J.: Fighting Fire: Your Role in Hospital Fire Safety. Nursing '81, 11(8):61–63, August, 1981.

Cooper, S.: Common Concern: Accidents and Older Adults. Geriatric Nursing, 2:287–290, July-August, 1981.

Feyock, M. W.: A Do-it-yourself Restraint That Works. Nursing '75, 5(1):18, January, 1975.

Hefferin, E. A., et al.: Analyzing Nursing's Work-related Injuries. American Journal of Nursing, 76:924–927, June, 1976.

Kukuk, H. M.: Safe Precautions: Protecting Your Patients and Yourself. Nursing '76, Part I, 6(5):45–51, May, 1976; Part II, 6(6):49, June, 1976; Part III, 6(7):45–49, July, 1976.

Misik, I.: About Using Restraints—With Restraint. Nursing '81, 11(8):50–55, August, 1981.

Mylrea, K. C., et al.: Electricity and Electrical Safety in the Hospital. Nursing '76, 6(1):52–59, January, 1976.

Phegley, D., et al.: Improving Fire Safety with Posted Procedures. Nursing '76, 6(7):18, July, 1976.

Roth, H., et al.: Electrical Safety in Health Care Facilities. New York, Academic Press, 1975.

Witte, N. S.: Why the Elderly Fall. American Journal of Nursing, 79:1950–1952, November, 1979.

REFERENCES

1. Registered Nurses Association of Ontario: *RNAO News,* 32:19, January-February, 1976.
2. *The American Heritage Dictionary of the English Language.* New College Edition. Boston, Houghton Mifflin Company, 1976.
3. National Fire Protection Association: "This Is Your ABCD's of Portable Fire Extinguishers" (pamphlet). Boston, National Fire Protection Association, 1976.

25

The Nurse Should Be Able to:

- Discuss the importance of good personal hygiene to optimal health
- Briefly explain the basic anatomy and physiology of the skin, its appendages, the teeth, and the mouth
- Identify factors that may contribute to impairing the status of an individual's skin and its appendages, his teeth, and his mouth
- Discuss specific hygiene needs at various stages in the life cycle
- Identify common problems patients have in meeting their hygiene needs
- Identify and intervene appropriately in situations requiring immediate nursing action to meet the patient's hygiene needs
- Apply relevant principles in planning and implementing nursing interventions
    a. To promote good hygiene in patients in respect to bathing, mouth care, and care of the nails and hair
    b. To maintain the integrity of the patient's skin
    c. To maintain the skin and its appendages, the teeth and soft tissues in the oral cavity in good condition
- Evaluate the effectiveness of nursing interventions

HYGIENE NEEDS

CHAPTER 25

INTRODUCTION

Hygiene is the science of health and its preservation. The term also refers to practices that are conducive to good health. Good personal hygiene is important to a person's general health.

Good personal hygiene usually means those measures a person takes to keep his skin and its appendages (his hair, fingernails, and toenails) and his teeth and mouth clean and in good condition. The healthy unbroken skin is the body's first line of defense against infection and against injury to underlying tissues. The skin is also important to the regulation of body temperature. In addition, it serves as one means for the excretion of body wastes. Healthy teeth and gums are essential for maintaining nutritional status. Decayed teeth and poor condition of the oral cavity are potential sources of infection as well as sources of discomfort and pain for the individual.

Bathing and personal grooming are important rituals in every culture. In our cleanliness-conscious North American society, most children are taught to wash their hands before meals, after voiding or having a bowel movement, and at other times when their hands are dirty. Washing the hands and face and cleaning the teeth the first thing in the morning and again before retiring are habits many people acquire at an early age. With the increased emphasis on dental health these days, many people also brush their teeth after every meal.

Looking after one's personal hygiene and grooming are important independent functions both for children (once they have learned to do this themselves) and for adults. When an individual is ill, he must often depend on others to help him with personal hygiene that he is no longer able to take care of himself. This, of course, threatens a person's self-esteem. Having someone else wash your hands and face and look after the very personal aspects of hygiene is demeaning, and most people find it embarrassing. They often hesitate to ask for help and their mental distress in having to ask adds to their physical discomfort.

It also puts the nurse somewhat in the role of substitute mother, a situation that is sometimes difficult for young students. It will help both the nurse and the patient to feel more comfortable if the nurse can anticipate the patient's needs and provide help in a competent, matter-of-fact manner before it is requested, acknowledging the patient's feelings and not treating him like a child.

The person who is ill has a lowered resistance to infection. Consequently, the presence of pathogenic bacteria in his environment poses a constant threat of infection. Helping the patient to keep clean by removing dirt, excretory products, and secretions eliminates many substances in which these bacteria flourish. In addition, hygienic measures help the patients to feel more comfortable and relaxed. Most people feel better when they are fresh and clean, and many who have been unable to rest will sleep soundly after a relaxing bath.

People who are ill are frequently concerned about unpleasant odors. Excessive perspiration and the presence of bacteria in the mouth and on the skin are common causes of such odors. Bad breath (halitosis) is most frequently caused by bacteria and old food particles in the mouth. Good oral hygiene usually eliminates this source of unpleasantness.

Another reason that good personal hygiene is desirable for the sick person is that a clean, refreshed feeling helps his morale. Generally, a well-groomed appearance is indicative of good mental health. The nurse often observes that a patient who is very ill does not care about grooming; once he begins to feel better, he often suggests to the nurse that he shave. Similarly, a female patient who is beginning to feel better

↓ self-esteem, embarrassing,
↑ therapeutic, ↑ morale, — infection

may ask for her cosmetics. Such requests are usually a sign that a person is feeling better, and that he is more aware of his immediate environment.

ANATOMY AND PHYSIOLOGY WITH RESPECT TO HYGIENE

The skin is composed of two main layers, the outer, thinner layer or epidermis, and the inner, thicker layer or dermis. Underlying these layers is subcutaneous tissue and adipose tissue. The epidermis itself has four layers on most areas of the body except the palms of the hands and the soles of the feet, where there are five. The outermost, horny later of epidermis continually flakes off. This horny layer is particularly thick on elderly people.

The nails of the fingers and toes are composed of epidermal cells that have been converted to *keratin*. Epithelial cells lie under the crescent of each nail, and it is from these cells that the epidermal cells of the nails grow. The mucous membrane, which is also composed of epithelial tissue, lines the body cavities and passageways. For example, mucous membrane lines the digestive tract, the respiratory passages, and the genitourinary tract.

Hair is the term applied to the threadlike appendages of the skin that are in particular abundance on the scalp and the pubic and axillary areas of the body. The term is also frequently used to refer to the aggregate of hair in the scalp. Each hair is composed of a long, cylindrical shaft and a root that is embedded in a depression, called a hair follicle, which penetrates the epidermis to the subcutaneous tissues. The hair receives its nourishment from the blood supplying the skin tissues through the root. *Dandruff* is the term used for the dry, scaly material that is normally shed from the skin of the scalp.

There are three kinds of skin glands in the body. The *sebaceous glands* secrete oil and are present wherever there is hair. The oil (sebum) keeps the hair supple and pliable. A second type of gland is the sweat gland. These are most numerous in the axilla, on the palms of the hands and the soles of the feet, and on the forehead. Their function is to help maintain body temperature and to excrete waste products. Sweat from these glands has a distinctive odor, which is distasteful to some people of Western cultures. The *ceruminous glands*, located in the external ear canal, secrete cerumen (wax). Some people accumulate a large amount of cerumen in their ears, and this can impair hearing. In

such cases, the excessive wax can be removed by cleansing with a syringe, a technique that many nurses learn to do in more senior courses.

The *mouth* is the anterior opening of the alimentary canal. It is lined with mucous membrane and contains three important anatomical structures, the tongue, the teeth, and the gums. The tongue is a movable muscular organ and is an important sensory receptor. It also assists in the acts of chewing (*mastication*), swallowing, and sound articulation. The teeth are small, hard structures set in the jaw that are essential for the chewing of food. Each tooth has a crown and a root or roots. The tooth is solid except for the inner soft pulp cavity. The crown is covered with a hard inorganic substance called *enamel*, which protects the soft structures beneath it. The root is protected by *cementum*, which is true bone. The teeth protrude up through the gums (*gingivae*), which are made up of mucous membrane with supporting fibrous tissue. The hard portion of the gum is firm, dense, normally pink in color, stippled, and tightly attached to the teeth, the periosteum, and the bone of the jaws. A soft portion of the gums protrudes upward in the spaces between teeth.

FACTORS AFFECTING THE SKIN, ITS APPENDAGES, THE TEETH, AND THE MOUTH

Each person's skin is different. Just as each individual is unique in other aspects of his biological being, so, too, is his skin unique. There are individual differences in texture, pigmentation, thickness of the skin tissues, the amount of subcutaneous fat, susceptibility to bruising, and ability to tolerate heat, cold, and exposure to the sun's rays. There are also variations in hair texture, color, and thickness, whether the hair curls or not, and the rapidity with which it grows. Variations also occur, of course, in the teeth, the mucous membranes, and the nails. Each person has inherited a different set of genetic factors that determine the nature of these parts of his anatomy, and these have been influenced by his environment, his lifestyle, and the health care he has received.

The skin is nourished by nutrients delivered by the blood. Since the skin itself has limited absorbent ability, the nutrient creams that are so widely advertised on television and in magazines have only a limited value in promoting skin health. If food and fluid intake is interfered with, the skin will very likely show some ill effects. If fluid intake is insufficient, the patient becomes dehydrated, and his skin appears dry and loose, a condition called *poor tissue turgor*. The skin of a patient who has suffered prolonged nutrient insufficiency heals very slowly after injury.

Exercise, as we mentioned in Chapter 23, also affects the health of the skin and its appendages. Exercise improves circulation in general and helps to bring a nourishing supply of blood to the surface tissues; it also aids in the elimination of waste products, both through the skin and through other excretory routes.

The weather also affects the skin. In cold weather, the skin often becomes dry and chapped, and, if the internal environment is dry also (as in many homes and apartment buildings with central heating), this contributes to the drying out of the skin tissues. You have no doubt found that it is necessary to use skin creams and hand lotions more frequently in cold weather. Very warm weather can also be hard on the skin. A person perspires much more than usual in hot weather, and frequent bathing is needed to rid the skin surface of bodily wastes excreted through this route. Sunshine is an important factor in the health of the skin, but overexposure to the hot sun has a "weathering" effect on the skin and can be as harmful as too little sun.

The health of the skin and its appendages is also affected by a person's hygiene habits.

Hygienic practices vary widely among individuals. These differences are accounted for by cultural patterns and home education, as well as by individual idiosyncrasies. Some people, for example, are accustomed to bathing daily, others once a week. Not every patient needs a bath every day, and indeed for some patients a complete bath daily may be harmful. This is particularly true of the elderly, whose skin tends to be thinner, drier, and less elastic than the young person's.

Then, too, some people are not aware of the beneficial effects of keeping the skin clean to prevent infection, and to rid the body of the waste products excreted through this route, nor of the importance to their health of maintaining their teeth and mouth in good condition. One also encounters people in whose value system these things simply are not important. We sometimes forget, too, that hygiene is more difficult when the facilities for maintaining good practices of cleanliness are not available or are difficult to obtain. People who live in poor, crowded, or unsanitary conditions often do not have the opportunity to practice good personal hygiene even if they would like to do so. The person who has to cut a hole in the ice to obtain water in the wintertime, or the one who has to share a bathroom with a dozen other people (or more sometimes) may not make a practice of bathing as often as some other people do. Teeth are frequently neglected because the individual cannot afford to go to the dentist, and sometimes diet is also poor and contributes to dental caries.

A person's general health status is also very important, both in relation to the person's ability to maintain his own hygiene and with respect to the effect of health problems on the skin and its appendages. Poor health, for whatever reason, is usually reflected in the condition of the skin. The ill person is more susceptible to infection, and illness renders a person more vulnerable to malnourishment, to gastrointestinal problems, and to other disturbances of body functioning that can affect the condition of the skin. There are also many types of disorders specifically affecting the skin, in addition to the common acne that plagues so many teenagers. The students will learn about a number of these skin problems in her courses on medical-surgical nursing.

Drugs and other forms of therapy may cause reactions in a person's skin and its appendages. Drugs not infrequently cause an allergic skin reaction (see page 538). Radiation therapy, which is used extensively in treating patients with cancer, is one example of a form of therapy that may affect the skin. Because the irradiation must penetrate the skin to reach and destroy cells in the part being treated, the skin and its underlying tissues may also suffer damage. The nurse should be alert to redness, sloughing of the skin, and spider-like spots under the skin (these result from damage to the small capillaries underlying the skin surface) in patients on any form of radiation therapy.

Perhaps of most concern to the beginning student, who will be looking after ill people in a hospital or other institutional setting, are the people who need help to maintain the integrity of the skin and to carry out their personal hygiene. This is affected by the individual's motor abilities and the degree to which he is rendered helpless by his illness, as well as the nature of his illness. Fever, for example, usually causes increased perspiration, which is uncomfortable for the individual. Irritating drainage seeping onto the skin from surgical or other wounds can cause problems in the surrounding skin area. Incontinence of urine or feces is a major factor in skin breakdown in the vulnerable sacral area. This area is already predisposed to tissue breakdown in the ill person because the sacrum bears most of the weight of patients who are in bed. It is also subject to a considerable amount of friction from rubbing on the bed linen. We mentioned in Chapter 23 that friction is caused by the rubbing together of two irregular surfaces—in this case, the body surface rubbing against the bedsheets. Wrinkled sheets, crumbs in the bed, and the like increase the irregularity of the sheet surface and hence increase the friction. A smooth, firm foundation on the bed helps to lessen this friction and thus is an aid in preventing tissue breakdown.

The skin also needs to be kept dry. Wetness of the bed linen also contributes to the possibilities for tissue breakdown.

HYGIENE NEEDS THROUGHOUT THE LIFE CYCLE

One of the first changes in her body that a pregnant woman notices is increased pigmentation of the nipples and areola of her breasts. They become dark in color. Often, too, *striae* (stretch marks) and accentuated venous patterns appear over the breasts as they enlarge and prepare for their function of nourishing the infant. The tendinous middle line of the abdomen also shows increased pigmentation (*linea nigra*) and stretch marks usually appear on the abdomen. As the pregnancy progresses, there is often an increase in vascular spider-like spots, particularly on the legs, and *palmar erythema* (reddened areas on the palms of the hands) is also common. The increase in a woman's total blood volume and her red blood cell count during pregnancy account for a number of these changes. The gums often become soft and *hyperemic*, that is, filled with more blood than usual. They are sensitive and tend to bleed easily, even with the mild trauma of brushing or flossing. Some women develop small, vascular swellings on the gums. These are called the *epulides of pregnancy,* epulis being a nonspecific term that is applied to any growth on the gums.

A daily bath or shower is usually recommended for pregnant women, with particular care taken, especially during late pregnancy, to avoid slipping in the tub. The pregnant woman's balance is impaired and she is more likely to fall than the normal non-pregnant woman of the same age. The jarring of her body in a fall could cause injury to the fetus, or could start the woman into premature labor (see Chapter 24).

Hygiene is important during labor, particularly if the labor is prolonged. Most women like to brush their hair, and facilities for washing their hands and faces and for sponging of their body should be available. If the woman is not able to wash herself, the nurse should be alert to her need and assist the patient. After delivery, the mother will appreciate the opportunity to cleanse herself, to wash her hands and face, to comb or brush her hair, and to put on some lipstick. During the postpartum period, a shower is usually recommended, rather than a tub bath, until the genital area has had time to heal. Sometimes, warm sitz baths are ordered to relieve the discomfort from perineal stitches. An infrared lamp is also used sometimes to promote perineal healing.

The new mother requires special care to the perineal area (see Chapter 29). Nursing mothers also require special care to the breasts. This generally includes cleansing before and after each feeding and, often, an application of emollient cream to prevent cracking of the nipples. An infrared lamp, an antibiotic ointment, and tincture of benzoin are the traditional treatments used for cracked nipples, and these are still very effective.

The newborn's skin is usually red, wrinkled and covered with *vernix,* a white sticky coating that has protected the skin in utero. Some newborns are also covered with a downy hair called *lanugo;* premature babies almost always have this additional protective coating. The eyes are usually red and swollen from the silver nitrate drops that have been put into them in the delivery room to prevent the development of ophthalmia neonatorum, a gonococcal infection of the eye that can result in blindness. Some newborns have tiny white pimples on the face, but these usually disappear within a few days. Sometimes the newborn will develop a blister in the center of his lips; this is from sucking and will disappear on its own.

An infant's skin is less resistant to injury and infection than an adult's skin. Therefore, his skin should be handled particularly carefully to prevent injury. Often infants need special soaps and lotions that are mild and nonirritating. Generally, soap is not needed in bathing the very young infant. Most babies love a bath when they are a few weeks old, but at first some do not—possibly because there is too much freedom of movement and they do not feel secure. Such babies can be bathed on the lap and dipped in the tub for a quick rinse. The infant's skin is very sensitive to heat and cold. The water should be at body temperature (it should feel comfortable on the inside of your wrist). After bathing, the infant should be wrapped in a towel immediately. The hair and the head should be washed and dried separately because most heat is lost through the head. It is important that the room in which the infant is bathed also be kept warm so the baby does not get chilled. The nails of infants must be kept short so that the infant does not scratch himself.

Diaper rash is probably the most common skin

problem with infants, because of their very sensitive skin. Frequent diapering is essential to combat this problem. The skin in the genital area should always be cleansed and a mild ointment or petrolatum applied before a fresh diaper is put on. Often, getting the infant to take more water will help the problem, because it dilutes the urine and makes it less irritating.

Two common problems of infancy are *cradle cap* and *thrush*. Cradle cap is an oily, yellowish crust that develops on the scalp of some infants, particularly in those who are breast fed. It is caused by an excessive amount of secretion from the sebaceous glands of the scalp. Applications of a mild oil (such as mineral oil) or a bland ointment, and frequent shampoos, will usually remove the crust within a few days. Thrush is a mild fungal infection of the mouth. Having the baby drink approximately a half ounce of sterile water after a milk feeding helps to prevent this problem.

Most children are taught basic hygiene measures in the home. By the time children are of school age, these have usually become ingrained habits. Teachers and the school nurse, however, often need to reinforce the early home teaching.

Because they are just developing their motor skills, and because their play is usually vigorous, most children suffer an untold number of cuts, bruises, and scrapes during the preschool and primary school period. The school nurse—and mothers—should keep a good supply of a mild disinfectant and simple bandage materials on hand to protect the childhood wounds from becoming infected. Another common skin problem of childhood is allergic eczema, which can be very distressing for both the child and his parents. Medical guidance is important in caring for the child with this problem. The child who

has a problem with enuresis should have a morning shower or bath, so that the child is not sent off to school or to play with the odor of urine on his body, an unpleasant reminder of his problem.

The adolescent's skin is often a source of embarrassment to him. Acne is a common problem in many teenagers. Hormonal changes occurring at this stage of the life cycle, blockage of the excretions of the sebaceous glands onto the skin surface, and possibly bacterial infection are thought to be factors in teenage acne. Cleanliness and a good diet are of the utmost importance during this period to prevent secondary infections from acne. Severe acne requires medical attention.

Adolescents are usually very concerned about their personal appearance and their hygiene. This is the time when sweating from the axilla commences, and the teen-ager is usually very self-conscious about the odor of perspiration. Teen-agers are noted for spending long periods of time in the bathroom bathing and grooming themselves, often to the annoyance of other family members.

As a person advances in age, two kinds of skin change take place. First, there is wrinkling, sagging, and increased pigmentation due to exposure to sunlight. Secondly, there is a general thinning of the skin accompanied by increased dryness and inelasticity. This aging takes place in the epidermis and dermis and in the subcutaneous fat. The epidermis is generally thinned and flattened, and sometimes there is an increased growth of the outer layer of the epidermis. A decrease in oil secretions leads to increased dryness and scaliness, and as a result, older people tolerate soap less well than younger adults. If the elderly person bathes too fre-

Good oral hygiene begins at an early age. Brushing should begin as soon as the teeth appear.

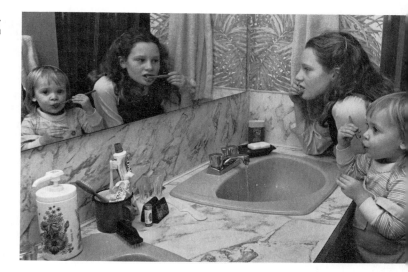

quently, his skin will become very dry. Oily liquids and skin creams are often better for the elderly patient than too much soap and water or alcohol rubs.

The aging process also takes its toll on the hair, the nails, the teeth, and other structures in the mouth. Hair often becomes thin and loses its texture (this does not always occur, of course—one comes across many older persons whose hair has retained its color, thickness, and vitality). The mucous membranes lining the mouth become thinner and more fragile with age. The fingernails and toenails become tougher and more difficult to cut. A very large proportion of older people in North America have lost all or most of their teeth. It is hoped that with better dental care for children, and throughout life, this situation will improve in the future.

COMMON PROBLEMS

• Probably the most common problem the nurse encounters in looking after ill people is the inability to maintain their own hygiene. The patient may be completely dependent on other people to bathe him, to clean his teeth, to comb his hair, and to cut his fingernails and toenails, or he may need assistance with some (or all) aspects of only one or a few of these. The nurse must put herself in his place and think of the things that need to be done to ensure that his hygiene is maintained the way he would wish and in a manner that is conducive to good health.

Problems resulting from the patient's inability to maintain his own hygiene are numerous. The skin, the hair, and the teeth may become dirty, and offensive odors from his own body may cause him discomfort, both physical and mental. Ingrown nails frequently result from uncut toenails, and may even interfere with the person's ability to walk. If skin care is neglected or carried out inadequately, pressure areas are likely to develop and the skin may break down, causing the patient considerable discomfort and pain, rendering him more vulnerable to infection, and causing the nursing staff untold hours and effort to restore the skin to a healthy condition.

If the patient has been unable to look after his own oral hygiene and has not been assisted with it, the teeth and the mucous membranes lining the mouth soon show evidence of this. The nurse will probably see many patients in whom the poor condition of the mouth has become an existing rather than a potential problem, not necessarily because of poor nursing care, but because these patients did not get help in time.

A common problem nurses may encounter in the mouths of patients is *gingivitis,* that is, inflammation of the gums. When oral hygiene is not carried out adequately, a film of mucus and bacteria (*plaque*) and *calculus* (tartar) accumulate on the surface of the teeth and particles of food gather around the teeth and in the crevices of the gums. Normally, these substances are removed by brushing the teeth and rinsing the mouth. When this is not done, the substances accumulate and become a source of mechanical irritation. The tissues of the gums become swollen and inflamed and may separate from the teeth.

Gingivitis not only is uncomfortable for the patient, it also leads to poor nutrition and is a potential source of infection—e.g., in the parotid glands and the gastrointestinal and respiratory tracts. When oral hygiene is neglected the teeth and the tongue also suffer. Decay of the teeth (caries) may result; this problem requires the assistance of dental health professionals. The tongue becomes coated with a thick, furry substance that is often referred to as *sordes.* This adds to the patient's discomfort and diminishes the ability of the taste buds to receive stimuli, contributing to the potential problem of malnourishment.[1]

One of the common problems affecting the hair is excessive dandruff. Small flakes of the outer layer of the skin are continuously being sloughed off from all skin surfaces. Excessive dryness of the scalp results in excessive dandruff. Normally, dandruff is removed by combing, brushing, and washing the hair. These procedures also help to remove the accumulation of excess sebum, the oily secretion of the sebaceous glands that keeps the hair supple and pliable. People whose hair is oily owing to the excessive secretions of sebum need to shampoo their hair frequently to remove the oil. If there are breaks in the skin surface, infection may develop. Thus, people who have an irritation of the scalp should be referred to the physician for investigation into their problem.

The nurse may encounter patients whose hair and body are infested with lice or some other vermin. This problem is not as uncommon as one would like to think, particularly in persons who, for one reason or another, have neglected their personal hygiene. Head lice are a frequent problem in schools, where the infestation is quickly spread from one child to another.

Some patients may need help in acquiring good hygiene habits. The nurse serves as a role model as well as a teacher in this regard. If she is careful to wash her hands before and after caring for the patient, maintains good personal standards herself regarding cleanliness and good grooming, and is meticulous in adhering to techniques that have been developed to prevent infection, she presents an excellent role model for the patient. Patients notice all of these things, and their opinions of the care they receive are often based on such criteria as these.

ASSESSMENT

The nurse's assessment of the status of the patient's skin, hair, nails, teeth, and mouth is based principally on her objective observations. She looks at the condition of the skin and the hair; she examines the fingernails and toenails; she opens the patient's mouth, or has him open it, and observes the condition of the teeth, the gums, and the soft tissues in the oral cavity (see Chapter 9).

She also takes into consideration the patient's motor abilities; is he able to carry out his own hygiene? Does he need help with this? She assesses his nutritional status and considers the possibility that other health problems may be affecting the condition of his skin. She also considers the effect of age on the individual's skin, hair, and nails and on the condition of his teeth and mouth. She notes the therapeutic care plans for the individual. Is he going to have to remain in bed for a long period? Are there restrictions on his position in bed? Is he receiving medications that may be causing problems with his skin condition? Are there necessary treatments that could potentially cause skin irritation or damage to skin tissues? Is the patient incontinent? Is he perspiring profusely? These are some of the questions the nurse asks herself.

The nurse also needs information about the individual's usual hygiene habits (see Chapter 8), and his attitude toward cleanliness and grooming. Are these important to him?

The nurse can obtain much information about the patient's usual hygiene practices from the nursing history, and about the current status of his skin, hair, nails, teeth, and mouth from the initial clinical appraisal. Information about the patient's motor and nutritional status should also be available from these sources. None of this information, however, substitutes for the nurse's own observations.

Information about the patient's past and current health problems, and the therapeutic plan of care for him, will be found on the patient's record. From this source the nurse can obtain data on medications prescribed for the patient and restrictions on his mobility, as well as on the nature of his illness and treatments prescribed for him.

The nurse often contacts nursing personnel about the status of the patient's skin and appendages, such as other nurses, nursing orderlies, or attendants. Observations made by the nurse herself in her assessment, and those made by other members of the nursing team, should always be communicated both orally and in writing to all other nursing personnel caring for the patient. The first sign of redness over bony prominences or of breaks in the skin should be reported promptly so that adequate steps can be taken to prevent deterioration of the skin tissues.

The patient is also, of course, a good source of information about the condition of his skin, provided that he is able to communicate. Pain is one of the body's warning signs that tissues are being damaged. Discomfort (which may increase to actual pain), heat (which the patient may describe as a warm feeling or a burning sensation), and redness (as noted above) in any area of the body are all early warning signs of potential tissue breakdown. The patient may be the first one to notice some of these signs.

The nurse also learns from the patient the details of his particular preferences and habits with respect to hygiene and personal grooming. Each person has his own idiosyncrasies about the way he likes to take his bath, the times to clean his teeth, the kind of soap to use, the way to comb his hair, and many other small details of bathing and grooming. Attention to these small details can contribute immeasurably to the patient's feelings of comfort and well-being.

The patient's family (or significant others in

Oral assessment is an important aspect of the care of hospitalized patients.

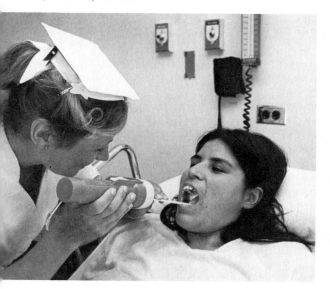

his life) can often help the nurse to learn about the patient's usual habits and preferences in regard to hygiene and grooming. They are also usually very observant of the condition of the patient's skin (they worry about him) and are also often very helpful in assisting patients with many details of personal hygiene and grooming. They may like to take care of helping the male patient with shaving, for example, or to fix the hair of the female patient. This gives family members a feeling that they, too, are doing something for the patient, which helps to assuage some of the helplessness they often feel as visitors, and possibly some guilt feelings they may have about having to turn over the care of their loved one to someone else.

Older people, however, are sometimes reluctant to have their children do things for them; it is a reversal of roles that is sometimes very difficult to accept.

PRIORITIES FOR NURSING ACTION

One particular skin problem to which nurses should be alert from the beginning of their course is the allergic skin reaction, which may occur as a result of a reaction to certain drugs. Penicillin is perhaps the most outstanding culprit for causing allergic reactions, but many other drugs do too. The nurse should watch for skin eruptions, lesions, reddened or weeping areas on the skin, or sloughing of the skin tissues, and report these promptly so that they can be investigated and treatment initiated early.

Allergies may be due to a number of causes other than drugs, such as specific foods, dust, and many other things, but the possibility of a drug reaction must always be kept in mind. This underscores the need for the nurse to be aware of the possible side-effects of drugs she is administering to the patient.

Patients who need help in carrying out hygiene measures are the nurse's most important priority. Serious problems can develop if basic skin care and oral hygiene are not attended to on a regular, planned schedule. As with problems in mobility, *prevention* is the priority. Deterioration of the condition of the patient's skin and the condition of his mouth can develop very rapidly, sometimes with little forewarning. Repair of the damage is a slow process that entails much discomfort and suffering on the patient's part and much work on the nurses' part—work that could have been avoided if simple precautionary measures had been taken.

GOALS FOR NURSING ACTION

The goals of nursing action with regard to the patient's hygiene are basically four:

1. To maintain good hygiene in respect to bathing, mouth care, and the care of nails and hair
2. To maintain the integrity of the skin
3. To maintain the skin tissues in good condition
4. To maintain the teeth and soft tissues in the oral cavity in good condition

PRINCIPLES RELEVANT TO HYGIENE

1. The intact skin is the body's first line of defense against infection and against injury.
2. Individual differences exist in the nature of the skin and its appendages.
3. Changes occur throughout the life span in the skin, the mucous membranes, the hair, the nails, and the teeth.
4. The health of the skin and mucous membranes is highly dependent on adequate nourishment, fluid intake, and exercise.
5. A person's general health affects both the status of his skin and appendages, teeth, and mouth, and his ability to look after his own hygiene.
6. Hygiene practices are learned.
7. Hygienic practices vary with cultural norms, personal idiosyncrasies and values, and the ability to maintain good habits of cleanliness and grooming.
8. The ability to look after one's own hygiene is an important independent function in older children and adults.
9. The skin and its appendages may be affected by drugs and other forms of therapeutic treatment.

SPECIFIC NURSING INTERVENTIONS

A regular schedule of basic hygiene measures for all patients is established on most nursing units in inpatient health agencies. These usually include morning and evening care, and a daily bath. For patients requiring additional skin and mouth care, interventions are planned on an individual basis as part of their total nursing care plan.

General Morning Care

Before breakfast is served, patients are usually awakened. They are offered a bedpan or urinal, or assisted to the bathroom if they can get up. Each patient who must remain in bed is provided with the necessary materials for washing his hands and face and for mouth care, and assisted with these activities if he requires help. The patient is then helped to prepare for his meal—that is, his bed is straightened, he is assisted to the most comfortable position for eating, and a place is prepared for his tray.

General Evening Care

The evening care routine is somewhat similar in that the patient is offered a bedpan or urinal (or assisted to the bathroom), and is given the opportunity to wash his hands and face and

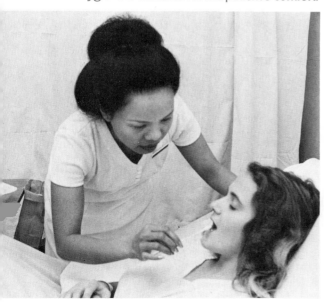

Good oral hygiene is essential for the patient's comfort.

clean his teeth. In many agencies, the bed patient's back is washed and a back massage is given as part of the evening routine. As we mentioned in Chapter 20, a back massage is beneficial for all patients prior to bedtime, not just those who are confined to bed. The nurse makes sure that the foundation of the patient's bed is clean and free from wrinkles, crumbs, and so forth. The bottom sheet and drawsheet (if one is used) are tightened, and top bedclothes straightened and tucked in. If the patient needs an extra blanket, this is put in place. The patient's bed is placed in the position the patient finds most comfortable for sleeping (unless otherwise specified), he is assisted to his most comfortable position, and his pillows are fluffed and arranged to his preference. Side rails, if they are needed, are put up on *both* sides of the bed. The call signal is put within easy reach, and any other items the patient feels he wants near at hand, such as a clock, his jug of water, and a glass are placed within easy reach on his bedside table.

Mouth Care

Oral care includes regular care by dental professionals as well as adequate cleansing of the teeth. Brushing the teeth removes food particles that provide a likely medium for bacterial growth. Brushing also massages the gums and stimulates circulation. It helps to keep the tongue, mucous membranes lining the mouth, and the lips moist as well as clean. A clean, fresh taste in the mouth is important in the desire for and the enjoyment of food. Thus, good oral hygiene helps to promote good nutritional status.

Most people brush their teeth at least twice a day, in the morning and before going to bed. Many dentists advocate brushing the teeth after every meal or at least rinsing the mouth after food is taken. These measures help to prevent the accumulation of food particles on and between the teeth, which predisposes to dental caries. Patients usually bring their own toothbrushes and their own dentifrice with them to hospital. If they do not, they should be provided with a brush and toothpaste or other substance to use. A mixture of salt and sodium bicarbonate flavored with peppermint has been recommended as an unexpensive and effective substitute for toothpaste.[1] Many agencies now have disposable toothbrushes for patients to use.

If a patient cannot brush his teeth himself the nurse assists him. It has been recommended that in brushing teeth the brush should be moved from the gum to the crown of the tooth. This motion is carried out on both the inner and outer aspects of the teeth. The procedure is easier if the lips are pulled back with one hand and the brush is held in the other.[1] This is just one method. Currently, there is much debate over how the teeth should be brushed.

Mouth care is also essential for patients with artificial dentures. Usually the patient with dentures prefers to take them out and clean them himself with a dentrifrice and water, then to rinse his mouth before reinserting the dentures. A mouthwash is often refreshing to these patients. If a person cannot remove his own dentures, the nurse can remove and clean them for him. Care should be taken in removing dentures, in handling them while cleaning, and in storing them. Dentures are expensive articles. Their replacement takes time, and the person who wears them is uncomfortable without them. He cannot eat anything that has to be chewed, he finds speech difficult, and he often is embarrassed to be seen without a full complement of teeth.

In removing dentures, it is usually easier to remove the upper plate first, grasping it between thumb and forefinger and wiggling it slightly to break the vacuum that holds it to the roof of the mouth. It is placed in a container, and the lower plate is then removed. This plate usually slides out easily but may be difficult to remove if the person uses a dental adherent substance. If it does not come out easily it can be loosened by lifting up the lower edge and gently wriggling it. For washing, it is safer to put the plates in a basin full of water than to wash them under the tap. The plates are often slippery and hard to hold. They can easily fall from the nurse's hands while being washed. Sinks are made of hard substances, and the dentures can be damaged if they slip out of the nurse's hands. The teeth should be brushed with a dentifrice and rinsed with cold water. Care should be taken not to use water that is too hot on dentures; they may crack or become misshapen. Since many people remove them at night, a container should be provided for the safe storage of dentures when they are not in use. Agencies often have a special container for this purpose; it should be labeled with the patient's name, hospital, and bed number. Dentures are among the most frequently lost articles in a hospital, and precautions should be taken for safeguarding them.

Patients whose food and fluid intake is restricted, either because of NPO orders or because they are unable to eat and drink sufficiently (as, for example, very weak patients and those who are unconscious), require mouth care at frequent intervals (q4h and as indicated is usually rec-

ommended) to keep the tongue, teeth, gums, and mucous membranes lining the oral cavity clean, moist, and in good condition, and to keep the lips from drying out and cracking. If the patient is able to use it, chewing gum is helpful in stimulating the secretion of the salivary glands and keeping the mouth moist. Rinsing the mouth is another means of providing moisture without violating imposed restrictions. Sometimes the patient is permitted to suck ice chips, but permission for the patient to do so must be obtained from the physician.

If ordinary oral hygiene is not feasible, the mouth and teeth must be cleaned by other means. Although cotton-tipped applicators soaked in a glycerine and lemon solution have traditionally been used for this purpose, it is now held by some authorities that the teeth *must be brushed* for the cleansing to be adequate and for gingivitis to be prevented. Rinsing of the mouth before brushing helps to remove food particles that have accumulated; rinsing after brushing is essential. If the patient is unable to

For the patient who cannot rinse her mouth, an Asepto syringe can be used to help remove food debris. And for the person who cannot expectorate, suction is used. (From Marie Reitz and Wilma Pope: Mouth Care. © October, 1973. The American Journal of Nursing Company. Reproduced with permission from *The American Journal of Nursing*, Vol. 73, No. 10.)

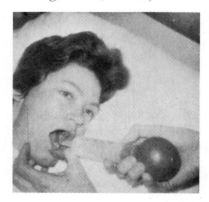

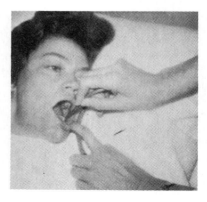

do this himself, an Asepto syringe may be used. If the person cannot spit out the material, it must be removed by suction, so that is is not aspirated into the respiratory tract.

In some agencies, gauze sponges may be wrapped around a tongue depressor and used for cleaning the mouth. Both the cotton-tipped applicators and the tongue depressors are hazardous when used with patients who may chew on them or bite off the end that is in the mouth. There is also the danger of injuring the delicate mucous membranes if hard objects are used for cleansing inside the mouth. Sometimes gauze is wrapped around the fingers to clean the mouth, and this lessens the danger of injuring tissues. Great care must always be taken in cleansing the mouth of a patient to avoid injuring the mucous membranes.

Petrolatum substances sold commercially for chapped or dry lips can be used to lubricate the lips.

The Patient's Bath

Bathing has several purposes: It cleanses, promotes comfort, stimulates blood circulation, and affords an opportunity to exercise. When a nurse assists a patient to bathe, she has an opportunity to incorporate the teaching of desirable hygienic measures and other health teaching as needed. In addition, she has an opportunity to assess the status of his skin and appendages, his motor status, and his nutritional, circulatory, and respiratory status. She may also observe his status in relation to comfort, rest, and sleep. For example, during the bath is a good time to observe the condition of the patient's skin, nails, and hair and to note such factors as the presence of edema, the quality of respirations, and any difficulty or pain the patient has on moving.

It is also a good time to assess the patient's mental and emotional status. Many patients find it much easier to talk to the nurse when she is assisting them with their bath than at other times. It has been suggested that the reason for this is that the act of giving physical care is perceived by many patients as caring about them.[2] Thus, the bath provides an excellent opportunity for the nurse to establish rapport with the patient and facilitate communication between patient and nurse.

The hospital patient may have a bed bath, a tub bath, or a shower. The type of bath that a person can have is often prescribed. The decision is based not only on the amount of activity involved but also on the specific problems of the individual. For example, a patient who has had a recent abdominal operation will probably not have a tub bath or shower until his incision is healed, because of the danger of getting it wet and contaminated. Both the tub bath and the shower require more activity on the part of the patient than a bath in bed.

In the bed bath, the nurse may give the entire bath to the patient, or the patient may participate within the limits of his physical condition. Patients usually prefer to help themselves as much as possible and should be encouraged to do so. This provides an opportunity to exercise muscles and stimulate blood circulation, and gives the patient a feeling of accomplishment and increasing independence.

It is believed by many, however, that the nurse should be careful to retain some aspects of assisting the patient with personal hygiene. If she does not, she loses a valuable time for free and spontaneous talk with the patient, for which other opportunities must be found.[2]

Not all patients require a bath every day while they are in the hospital; nor is it necessary for all patients to receive a bath in the morning. For the patient who tires very easily or who is very ill, the bath may be contraindicated. The older person's skin will often become overly dry if he bathes too frequently. For these people as well as for other patients who do not require complete bed baths, a partial bath is indicated. This includes washing the patient's hands, back, axillae, and perineal area, as well as providing for oral hygiene and massaging bony prominences. The nurse makes these judgments based upon the needs of the patient and her assessment of the situation.

The Bed Bath. The equipment required for the bed bath includes bath towels, wash cloths, a water basin, and soap. A bath blanket is also required to cover the patient so as to avoid embarrassing exposure and to keep him warm. The kind of soap used will depend largely on the individual needs of the patient and on the policy of the health agency. Some institutions permit patients to use their own soap; others prefer that the patient use the soap provided by the agency. Many agencies have their own particular procedure for giving a patient a bed bath. One suggestion is as follows:

1. Offer the patient a bedpan or urinal
2. Provide for oral hygiene
3. Remove the upper bedclothes
4. Cover the patient with a bath blanket
5. Bathe the patient
6. Cut fingernails and toenails if needed
7. Remake the bed

Guiding Principles for the Bed Bath

Heat is conveyed from the body by the convection of air currents. Care should be taken not to expose the body surface unduly. Drafts are to be avoided and the patient should be kept warm during his bath. The nurse can close the windows of the patient's room if it is cool outside or if there is any danger of a draft. The bed unit is screened for privacy, the patient's spread and blanket are removed, and a bath blanket is placed over the patient. The top sheet is then slipped out from under the bath blanket to prevent exposing the patient unnecessarily. The patient then removes his gown. Dirty linen should be placed in a container (dirty linen hamper) as soon as possible after it is removed from the bed. Agency procedures vary in this regard, but it is generally accepted that bed linen is a potential source of infection, and suitable precautions are taken in handling it.

People differ in their tolerance of heat. Most patients require bath water between 110 and 115° F (43.3 to 46.1° C). Water at this temperature is comfortable to most patients and it does not injure skin or mucous membranes. Water at 120° F (48.9° C) in the basin will cool to the safe temperature range by the time it comes in contact with the patient's skin. The nurse collects the equipment and takes it to the patient's bedside before she gets the water so that the water does not cool too much before it is used. It may be necessary to add additional hot water during the procedure, or to change the water. Patients who are particularly sensitive to heat may require cooler water.

The skin is sometimes irritated by the chemical composition of certain soaps. Soap can be irritating to a patient's skin and particularly to his eyes. Therefore patients are often advised not to use soap on their faces.

Long smooth strokes on the arms and legs that are directed from the distal to the proximal increase the rate of venous flow. Distal means farther from the point of attachment; proximal means closer to the point of attachment. For example, the hand is distal to the elbow.

Moving the body joints through their full range of motion helps to prevent loss of muscle tone and improves circulation. The nurse can use the bed bath as an opportunity to help the patient to put his joints through their full range of motion (see Chapter 23).

The following order is suggested for bathing the patient:

1. Eyes—inner to outer canthus (no soap)
2. Face
3. Arms, hands, and axilla
4. Chest and breasts
5. Abdomen
6. Legs
7. Back and buttocks
8. Perineal area
9. Rectal area

When bathing the patient, the nurse folds the wash cloth in such a way that the corners are folded on the palm of the hand to form a pad.

Only the area being washed should be exposed. This lessens the patient's embarrassment and helps him keep warm. Each area of the skin is dried immediately after it has been washed and rinsed and before the next area of the body is exposed.

If the patient soaks his hands and feet in the basin of water he will feel more refreshed. This practice also serves to soften the patient's nails so that they can be easily cut and cleaned. The pan of water should not be too full or the water may spill when the hands or feet are immersed. Washing the patient's back is best done with the patient lying on his abdomen. If this is impossible the patient can turn to one side while the nurse washes the other side of his back and then can reverse his position. A back massage is given after the back is washed and dried.

The nurse should take special care to wash, rinse, and dry well the creases in the patient's skin and to massage bony prominences. These areas are particularly prone to irritation. The body skin creases become excoriated if they remain moist; the bony prominences are irritated by constant friction and pressure against the bedclothes. *Excoriation* is the superficial loss of skin substance. Also, the areas that bear the weight of the patient while he is in bed are prone to irritation.

The patient's skin is then dried well. Skin that remains wet over a long period is uncomfortable and becomes irritated.

Usually patients prefer to wash the genital areas themselves, if they are able to do so. If, however, they are not able, the nurse does this for them. In some agencies, when the patient is male and the nurse female, the nursing orderly is asked to assist the patient. In some situations, however, the nurse may have to undertake this part of the bath for the male patient. In doing so, the nurse uses a washcloth or towel to hold the genitals while she washes between the folds of the body with another washcloth. The genitals are washed as with other parts of the body, rinsed, and dried.

The Tub Bath. Tub baths are taken for hygienic and therapeutic reasons. The physician may order a therapeutic bath for some patients as, for example, sitz baths for the patient who has had rectal surgery. Patients with skin diseases often have oatmeal or medicated baths. Various types of therapeutic baths were discussed in Chapter 19. Aside from these therapeutic measures, a tub bath is most often a hygienic measure enjoyed by most people.

Bathtubs in hospitals frequently have rails, or the adjacent wall is equipped with handles to help the patient climb in and out of the tub. Most tubs also now have safety strips on the bottom which help to prevent slipping. No sick person should lock himself into the bathroom unattended; he may require help. The nurse or attendant should know when a patient is bathing, and often it is wise to check that he is all right. If a patient is out of bed for the first time after even a few days of bed rest, it is generally unwise to leave him alone in the bath. An attendant can stay just outside the curtains if the patient prefers privacy.

The bathtub is filled one-third full of water. Unless otherwise ordered, the water is drawn at 105° F (40.5° C), a comfortable and safe temperature for most people. The length of time that a person bathes depends upon his endurance and strength. If the bath is too lengthy, it may fatigue him unnecessarily. A very hot bath will cause the blood to be diverted away from the vital centers of the brain to the surface areas of the body. As a result he may feel faint and lose consciousness.

Getting into and out of the bathtub is often a difficult maneuver, and the patient may need assistance from the nurse. Usually it is easier if the patient first sits on the edge of the tub with his feet inside the tub, then reaches over to grasp the rail on the other side and gradually eases himself down. In helping the patient out of the tub, it is a good practice to let the water out before the patient attempts to stand up. There are many mechanical devices available today for assisting with the tub bath procedures. A mechanical lift (or hoist), for example, can be used in either hospital or home situations. The use of a shower stool, so that the patient can sit while having a shower, is another solution to this problem.

Decubitus Ulcers

Decubitus ulcers (bedsores, pressure sores) are areas from which the skin has sloughed. These sores may develop in persons who are ill in bed for a long period of time, especially if the patient is unable to move about freely, or they may occur in people who sit in wheelchairs for several hours at a time. They occur as a result of prolonged pressure on one part of the body with resultant loss of circulation to the area and subsequent tissue destruction. Although decubitus ulcers may occur in any patient, if there is sufficient pressure on one area to cause ischemia, they are seen most frequently in individuals with poor nutritional status, especially if there is a negative nitrogen balance. They are most often seen on the bony prominences of the body. If decubitus ulcers are not treated, they quickly increase in size and become very painful. Secondary infection often complicates the picture.

The conditions that predispose to decubitus ulcers include continuous pressure on one area, dampness, a break in the skin surface, poor nutrition, dehydration, poor blood circulation, thinness (bony prominences unprotected by adipose tissue), and the presence of pathogenic bacteria. Early signs of a decubitus ulcer include redness and tenderness of an area. The patient usually complains of a burning sensation. Other early warning signs include coldness of an area and the presence of edema. Unless special measures are taken at this time to relieve pressure and increase local tissue nourishment, a break in the patient's skin usually follows. The sore then increases in depth and the tissue gradually sloughs off. Decubitus ulcers are difficult to cure; some require surgical intervention. Consequently, preventive measures are always indicated.

There are many nursing care measures that can be employed in order to prevent decubitus ulcers. Frequent changes in position to rotate the weight-bearing areas relieve pressure on any single group of bony prominences. The normal healthy individual shifts his body position every few minutes. For the patient who is unable to do this himself, it is the nurse's responsibility to see that his position is changed. A regular schedule should be set up for turning the patient as often as necessary to keep the skin in good condition. Usual recommendations are every 2 hours and as needed.

Massage and exercise stimulate circulation and thus improve the nourishment to the cells of the skin. Keeping the skin dry and clean inhibits the growth of disease-producing bacteria and prevents skin from becoming excoriated; body secretions and excreta are particularly irritating to a patient's skin. The nurse should take particular care that a patient's linen and dressings are dry and clean. In areas where secretions cannot be prevented, protective oint-

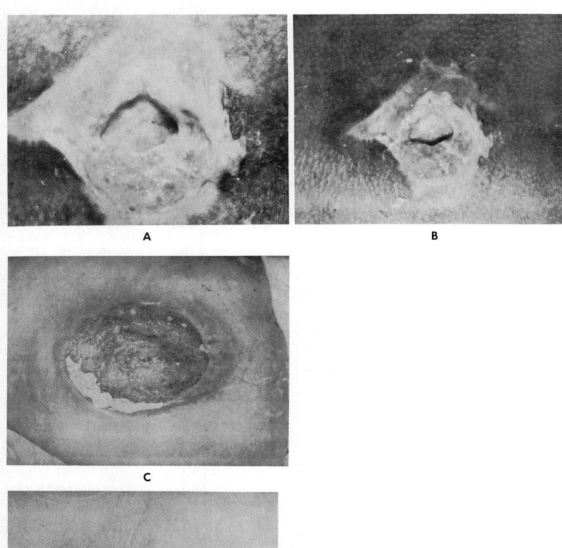

A, A decubitus ulcer, on a hip, which needs to be packed with benzoyl, 20 per cent lotion. B, The same decubitus ulcer as in A, after 4 weeks of treatment with benzoyl lotion. C, Severe decubitus ulcer on buttocks area. Note packing in lower left area of the ulcer. D, Same decubitus ulcer as in C. This ulcer completely healed after treatment. (Reprinted with permision from The Canadian Nurse, Vol. 69, No. 10, October 1973.)

ments, such as zinc oxide or petrolatum, can be used to prevent excessive irritation.

Another preventive measure for decubitus ulcers is the use of devices to relieve pressure on specific areas of the patient's body. An overbed cradle will keep bedclothes off the patient, and other aids such as alternating pressure mattresses, oscillating beds, and fluidized air or water mattresses may also be used. Many hospitals use a special bed frame, which permits the patient to be turned easily. Another measure that has been found helpful in the prevention of decubitus ulcers is the use of sheepskin under pressure areas. It is considered preferable to use the whole skin, but small pads have been found effective in protecting areas such as the heels or elbows of the patient.[3] These woolskins are being used extensively in many hospitals and nursing homes. They are particularly helpful in home situations where expensive mechanical devices may not be available.

Attention to the patient's nutritional status is essential. Since decubitus ulcers occur most frequently in patients with a negative nitrogen balance, the protein intake should be increased. Foods that contain complete proteins, such as eggs, milk, and meat, are recommended. The proteins are needed for the regeneration of body tissue. Usually, supplementary amounts of vitamin C are prescribed also because of the role of this vitamin in the healing process. Care must be taken also that an adequate fluid intake is maintained. Dehydration results in poor tissue turgor, which is another predisposing factor in the development of decubitus ulcers.

When a decubitus ulcer develops, the nurse faces a challenge in curative nursing care. The outside area of the decubitus ulcer is often less extensive than the inside area. The preventive measures just mentioned can be employed therapeutically and, in addition, the application of dry heat, such as that from an infrared lamp, increases circulation to the area and dries secretions. The latter measure is generally ordered by the physician. Decubitus ulcers are prone to infection by bacteria; the moist, poorly nourished tissue provides a good medium for the growth of pathogenic bacteria. The use of aseptic technique in the care of an infected ulcer prevents secondary infection and the transfer of bacteria to other areas of the body and to other patients.

A therapeutic regimen for the care of the patient who has a decubitus ulcer is planned. Antiseptic solutions, soap and water, and antibiotic creams have all been advocated at one time or another. Sometimes it is necessary to graft skin over a decubitus ulcer. Ulcers are very difficult to cure; the best nursing care is prevention.

Hair Care

Care of the patient's hair is important to both his grooming and his sense of well-being. As part of the daily toilet each patient's hair needs to be brushed and combed. Thorough brushing stimulates circulation to the scalp and improves the nourishment of the epithelium. Most patients can attend to this themselves, but the nurse may have to assume the responsibility for the aged or very ill patient.

The nurse, by seeing to daily care of the hair, can ensure that the patient's hair does not become matted. Often, long hair is braided so that it will stay neatly in place and make the patient feel more comfortable. Patients who are in the hospital for some length of time may want a shampoo. Permission for this may have to be obtained from the physician in some agencies. For the patient who is out of bed a shampoo is no problem. The sink in his room or the shower bath affords facilities for hair washing.

If a patient must remain in bed, however, the shampoo is given while he is in bed or on a stretcher. If a stretcher is used, it is best to move the patient to a sink and support his head on the edge of the sink. If it is necessary for the patient to remain in bed, then the nurse can use a folded plastic sheet or a specially constructed waterproof pad to direct the water from the patient's hair into a pail. The nurse uses pitchers of water, taking precautions to keep the patient's bed dry. The patient's hair needs to be dried quickly after the shampoo in order to avoid chilling. Most hospitals have hair dryers for this purpose. Many brands of dry shampoo are now available, and these may be used for patients whose condition contraindicates a regular shampoo.

Today many large hospitals have hairdressing and barber services for patients. Often the patient will request the services of the barber or the hairdresser, and the nurse then makes arrangements. The nurse is usually responsible for telling the patient what services are available and what charges are made for them.

Shaving. Male patients usually feel better when they are shaved. If the male patient cannot shave himself, the nurse may be asked to do this for him. If the patient has an electric razor this is no problem, but a safety razor requires more skill. Very warm water is needed to give an adequate shave. After the skin has been lathered with shaving soap, the skin is held tautly and the razor is drawn over the skin in short strokes. The nurse will find that the safest way to shave the patient is to stretch the skin over the bone in a particular area and then to shave in the direction in which the hair is growing. Areas around the mouth and nose are particularly sensitive; in these areas the nurse's motions need to be firm but gentle. After the patient has been shaved he will likely prefer a shaving lotion for his skin. Most shaving lotions are refreshing and have a slightly antiseptic effect.

After a shave, the male patient will not only look better but he will also in all probability feel better. Relatives are often reassured when the male patient is well groomed, chiefly because this is the way they are accustomed to seeing him.

Many women are accustomed to shaving the hair in the axilla and to removing superfluous hair from their faces and legs. Opportunity should be provided for them to maintain these practices while they are ill if they so desire. Women are usually particularly sensitive about unwanted hairs on the chin and upper lip. A number of good depilatory creams are available. These preparations should be used with caution, however, because they are irritating to the skin and many people cannot tolerate them. Tweezers may be used instead to remove facial hairs.

Nail Care

Care of the nails is another area of grooming that most patients can attend to themselves. For the very ill patient or the patient who has difficulty in moving, however, nail care may be the nurse's responsibility. Often nail polish is not advised for a patient because the physician or the nurse may want to check the color of the tissue underneath the nails. This is particularly true for patients who are to undergo surgery. Most hospitals prohibit the use of colored nail polish for these patients.

The responsibility for cleaning and trimming the nails of patients who are unable to do this themselves usually falls to the nurse. Toenails are cut straight across, fingernails in an oval shape. Many people prefer that their fingernails be filed rather than cut so that they can be shaped attractively. For patients who are particularly prone to infection—for example, patients with diabetes mellitus or circulatory problems— it is advisable that the nurse not cut the toenails herself for fear of injuring the skin or cuticle around the nail.

To prevent hangnails, it is best to keep the cuticle of the nail pushed well back and lubricated with oil. Some patients have very hard fingernails and horny toenails. If the patient soaks his feet for 10 to 15 minutes in warm water, the nails will soften sufficiently so that they can be cut with nail cutters. Special nail clippers are available that are particularly helpful in cutting thick toenails. If the nails are too thick and difficult to cut, the services of a *podiatrist* (foot specialist) should be obtained.

Eye Care

Nursing care also involves the care of the eyes. On occasion the nurse will be called on to help a patient to care for his eyes when they have become irritated or infected. The physician usually orders a special solution to cleanse the eyes. Tap water or normal saline is also used. With absorbent cotton dipped in the solution, the eye is wiped from the inner canthus to the outer canthus. The nurse uses a clean piece of cotton each time she wipes the eye. Water or normal saline will soften crusts so they are easily removed. The motion from the inner to the outer canthus washes the discharge away from the nasal lacrimal duct, which is located on the inner aspect of the orbit of the eye.

Unconscious patients require special attention to protect their eyes from damage. The upper and lower lids should be kept clean and free from discharge. The lids should be closed when the patient is being turned to prevent scratching of the cornea.

Patients' glasses, contact lenses, and other prostheses should be looked after carefully and the patient assisted with their care if he is unable to care for them.

Care of Patients with Pediculosis

Occasionally a patient will be found to have pediculosis (infestation with lice). His care involves killing and removing all the pediculi (lice) and their eggs (nits) that have infested the skin, hair, and clothing. There are three main types of pediculosis: pediculosis capitis or infestation of the scalp with lice, pediculosis corporis or infestation with body lice, and pediculosis pubis or infestation of the pubic hair with lice. There are several methods of ridding patients of pediculi. For body lice, the patient's clothing is removed for washing or cleaning and the patient is usually given a cleansing bath, and then drugs are applied. In the case of head lice, or if the body lice have infected the scalp,

Kwell shampoo is often used for treatment. A number of new drugs are available that are effective with only one application. *Para*, for example, is a spray that can be applied easily. It is left on for a half hour and then washed off the hair by means of an ordinary shampoo or bath. A second treatment a week later is recommended. Infested patients are often separated from other patients for 24 hours after treatment has been initiated to avoid spreading the pediculi. The treatment is repeated until pediculi cannot be found on the patient.

Pediculi are spread by direct contact and through vehicles such as clothing, eating utensils, and combs. Pediculi are usually found in environments where poor hygienic measures are practiced.

PLANNING AND EVALUATING SPECIFIC NURSING INTERVENTIONS

Nursing interventions to ensure that the patient's skin and its appendages, hair, fingernails and toenails, and teeth and mouth are kept clean and in good condition are planned as an essential part of the nursing care of every patient. Basic hygiene measures are normally a part of the nursing care plans for all patients on the nursing units of inpatient agencies. If the patient requires help in carrying out these measures, or if these need to be modified in any way, this is drawn to the attention of all nursing personnel through notations on the patient's nursing care plan. A regular schedule outlining specific instructions is developed for those patients requiring additional skin or mouth care. A flow sheet may be helpful in this regard, in addition to incorporating the directions on the care plan. When writing the schedule out, space should be left for the initialing of each intervention as it is done, to ensure that the required care is carried out as planned. The nurse notes her observations in the progress notes of the patient's record.

For patients who need help in acquiring good hygiene habits, a teaching plan is incorporated into the nursing care plan. Much of the teaching may be done while carrying out specific nursing interventions, such as in the bed bath. Because personal hygiene is a very personal matter, tact is needed in this teaching, and care taken that the patient's self-esteem is protected in the process. Putting the teaching in terms of promoting optimal health and including an explanation of the reasons for the development and maintenance of good hygiene practices help to put the teaching on a more objective, less personal basis.

The expected outcomes of nursing interventions are often expressed in terms of prevention of potential problems, and specific criteria are given concerning the state of the skin and its appendages, or the oral cavity, that is to be maintained or restored. An expected outcome for the potential problem of poor mouth condition might be that the patient's lips and tongue are moist and normal tissue turgor of the mucous membranes is maintained at all times.

Successful nursing interventions are evidenced in the healthy state of the patient's skin, hair, nails, and mouth. Continuous reassessment of the status of all of these is required. The poor condition of any is a sad reflection on the nursing care the patient has received.

GUIDE TO ASSESSING THE STATUS OF THE SKIN, ITS APPENDAGES, THE TEETH, AND THE MOUTH

1. What is the condition of the patient's skin, hair, teeth, and nails? Is the skin clear, intact, warm to the touch? Did you notice any abnormalities with regard to color, blemishes, temperature, breaks in the integrity of the skin, poor tissue turgor? Is the hair clean, well-groomed, and in good condition? Are the nails clean and in good condition?

2. What did you observe about the patient's lips, tongue, gums, and teeth? Did you notice any abnormalities such as dryness or cracking of the lips? a furry coating on the tongue? a film on the teeth, or tartar? food particles and mucus in the mouth or around the teeth? Are the mucous membranes pink, or are they red and inflamed? Are the gums swollen and inflamed? receding from the teeth? Is there any bleeding in the mouth? Are the teeth in good condition? Are there missing teeth? caries? Does the patient wear dentures?

3. What are the patient's usual habits with regard to hygiene practices?

4. Does the patient need help in maintaining his hygiene? What is his motor status in this regard? Is he weak, helpless, or unconscious?

5. Does he have a health problem(s) that may be affecting the status of his skin and appendages? that interferes with his ability to maintain his own hygiene?

6. Is he receiving medications or other therapy that may affect the status of the skin or its appendages?

7. Does he require additional skin or mouth care over and above the usual hygiene measures?

8. How old is the patient?

9. Are there any signs of body or head lice?

STUDY SITUATION

Mr. Charles Rose, who was admitted to hospital yesterday for investigative procedures, has been assigned to your care. He is a 32-year-old bachelor and has been working on a trapline in the north woods for the past 2 years. He lives alone in a remote cabin, coming into town only occasionally to replenish his supplies, which consist mainly of canned and dried foods. The cabin does not have electricity or running water; it is heated by a wood stove and Mr. Rose has to fetch his water from a stream a quarter of a mile away.

He spends several days at a time out in the woods inspecting his lines, with only his dog for company. He tells you he hit his head 2 or 3 weeks ago on a fallen tree trunk when he was straightening up after looking at a trap. He hasn't been feeling too well since, and has had headaches of increasing severity, so he went to the doctor in town, who admitted him to the hospital. You notice that Mr. Rose is thin, his skin is dry, and he has some lesions on his arms and legs; his long hair is matted, his nails are dirty and chipped, and his teeth and fingers are stained with nicotine. The physician has ordered bed rest for Mr. Rose.

1. What problems can you identify relative to Mr. Rose's hygiene? to the status of his skin, its appendages, and the teeth?

2. What factors do you think contributed to these problems?

3. What principles would assist you in planning hygiene measures for Mr. Rose?

4. What specific nursing interventions would you plan?

5. What would be the expected outcomes of these interventions?

Mr. Rose's condition deteriorates over the next few days; he appears to be very weak and drowsy. The physician and a neurosurgeon who has been called in are contemplating surgery.

6. What additional nursing interventions would you plan for Mr. Rose with regard to hygiene?

7. How would you evaluate the effectiveness of your interventions?

SUGGESTED READINGS

Cameron, G.: Pressures Sores: What to Do When Prevention Fails. *Nursing '79,* 9(1):42–47, January, 1979.

Gannon, E. P., and Kadezabek, E.: Giving Your Patients Meticulous Mouth Care. *Nursing '80,* 10(3):14–20, March, 1980.

Hyland, D. B., and Kirkland, V. J.: Infrared Therapy for Skin Ulcers. *American Journal of Nursing,* 80(1):1800–1801, October, 1980.

Meissner, J. E.: A Simple Guide for Assessing Oral Health. *Nursing '80,* 10(4):24–25, April, 1980.

Meissner, J. E.: Which Patient on Your Unit Might

Get a Pressure Sore? *Nursing '80, 10*(6):64–65, June, 1980.

Mikulic, M. A.: Treatment of Pressure Ulcers. *American Journal of Nursing, 80*(6):1125–1129, June, 1980.

Ostchega, Y.: Preventing. . . and Treating . . . Cancer Chemotherapy's Oral Complications. *Nursing '80, 10*(8):47–53, August, 1980.

Schweiger, J. L., et al.: Oral Assessment: How to Do It. *American Journal of Nursing, 80*(4):654–657, April, 1980.

Uhler, D. M.: Common Skin Changes in the Elderly. *American Journal of Nursing, 78*(8):1342–1344, August, 1978.

REFERENCES

1. Reitz, M., and Pope, W.: Mouth Care. *American Journal of Nursing, 73*:1728–1730, October, 1973.
2. Davis, E. D.: Giving a Bath? *American Journal of Nursing, 70*:2366–2367, November, 1970.
3. Brownlowe, M. A., et al.: New Washable Woolskins. *American Journal of Nursing, 70*:2368–2370, November, 1970.

26

The Nurse Should Be Able to:

- Explain the importance to health of preventing and controlling infection
- Briefly explain the infectious process, including common pathogens infecting man, the cycle of infection, and the body's reactions to infection
- Discuss common sources of infection in health agencies and ways infection is spread in these agencies
- Discuss specific needs of people at various stages of the life cycle in regard to preventing infections
- Identify people who are particularly at risk to infection
- Assess a patient for potential or actual problems of infection
- Identify potential or actual problems of infection in patients
- Apply relevant principles in planning and implementing nursing interventions
    a. to prevent infection
    b. to control infection
- Evaluate the effectiveness of nursing interventions to prevent and control infection

THE PREVENTION AND CONTROL OF INFECTION

CHAPTER

26

INTRODUCTION

In Chapter 4, when we discussed health problems, we pointed out that the control of infectious diseases has been one of the principal reasons for the dramatic reduction in infant and child mortality, and the consequent lengthening of the life span in the developed countries of the world. Four major factors have contributed to this achievement: the development and widespread use of specific immunizations against many of the common communicable diseases; the discovery and widespread use of antimicrobial agents (such as the antibiotics); the application of basic sanitary measures to protect the safety of water, milk, and food supplies, along with the disposal of garbage and sewage; and the overall raising of standards of living, with its resultant improvement in the general health of people (from better nutrition, better housing, and the like).

The infectious diseases are certainly a much greater health problem in developing countries than in developed ones, but we have by no means eliminated all illnesses caused by infections in the Western world. The respiratory infections continue to be an important cause of death and of acute illness throughout the life span of the peoples of North America. Gastrointestinal infections are one of the most common causes of short-term illness. The sexually transmitted diseases have attained epidemic proportions in the past few years, and such diseases as chickenpox and hepatitis are still prevalent. Institution-acquired infections (called *nosocomial infections*) continue to plague hospitals throughout the United States and Canada.

The prevention and control of infection is one of the principal concerns of all health personnel, whether they work in ambulatory care settings in the community or in inpatient facilities for the care of the sick. The most common causes of infection are microorganisms. Wherever there are sick people, microorganisms that are capable of producing infection pose a constant and serious threat, since the average patient is highly susceptible to infection as a result of his generalized debility. Moreover, since some patients have particularly serious infections, their close proximity to other patients produces situations conducive to the transfer of microorganisms.

Microorganisms capable of producing infection are found in the air, on the floors, on equipment and furniture, and on articles that have come in contact with a person who has an infection, as well as on the skin and mucous membranes, and in the expired air, secretions, and excretions of the person himself. They can be spread through the air and by such things as linen, dishes, and even a nurse's hands. Health personnel sometimes unknowingly act as carriers of microorganisms. When handwashing techniques break down, for example, microorganisms are passed on to others. In spite of stringent cleaning practices, health agency personnel are continually working in an evironment that harbors many varieties of organisms. Every once in a while a particularly virulent organism is introduced, and a worker with an open cut or lowered body resistance becomes infected. An unbalanced diet, fatigue, scratches, cuts, or other wounds may predispose any person to infection.

In order to understand the rationale behind nursing measures taken to protect patients and staff from infections, it is important to keep in mind the sources, methods of transfer, and modes of spread of microorganisms. In her courses in microbiology and anatomy and physiology, the student will have gained a good base of knowledge about the infectious process and the body's reactions to it. In subsequent courses in medical surgical nursing, she will increase her knowledge of specific communicable diseases. We will, therefore, confine ourselves here to a brief review of the infectious process and the body's reactions to it, in order to provide a framework for discussion of the care of patients with existing or potential problems of infections.

THE INFECTIOUS PROCESS

Infection is the invasion and multiplication of microorganisms in body tissues. The agent causing the infection is called a *pathogen*.

Common Pathogens

Common agents causing infections in man are the pathogenic bacteria, some protozoa, fungi, viruses, and helminths.

The *pathogenic bacteria* include those that are true pathogens—that is, they are virulent microorganisms capable of invading healthy tissue, as, for example, some species of *Salmonella*, which can cause an acute form of gastroenteritis; the parasitic bacteria, which are opportunists—that is, they do not usually invade body tissue but will do so if given the opportunity, as, for example, some of the streptococci and staphylococci, which can cause wound infections; and those bacteria that do not invade body tissue but produce toxins capable of producing disease, such as *Clostridium tetani*, which is the causative agent of tetanus.

Protozoa are single-celled animals; some varieties cause disease in man; an example is *Entamoeba histolytica*, which causes the intestinal infection of amebiasis.

Fungus infections include those caused by yeasts and molds, such as ring worm and athlete's foot, which are caused by cutaneous mycoses.

Many of the common communicable diseases are *virus infections*; measles, mumps, chickenpox, infectious hepatitis, and smallpox are all viral infections.

The *helminths* are worms; some are common parasites in humans, as for example, the pinworms often found in children.

The Cycle of Infection

The *cycle of infection* is best visualized as a circle. There must first of all be an *infectious*

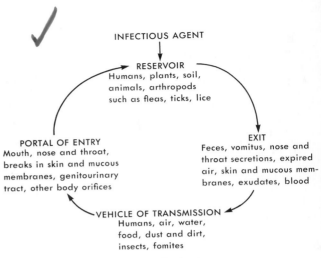

INFECTIOUS AGENT

RESERVOIR
Humans, plants, soil, animals, arthropods such as fleas, ticks, lice

PORTAL OF ENTRY
Mouth, nose and throat, breaks in skin and mucous membranes, genitourinary tract, other body orifices

EXIT
Feces, vomitus, nose and throat secretions, expired air, skin and mucous membranes, exudates, blood

VEHICLE OF TRANSMISSION
Humans, air, water, food, dust and dirt, insects, fomites

The Cycle of Infection.

agent, such as one of those organisms we have mentioned above. The agent must have a place (*reservoir*) in which it grows and multiplies. It leaves the reservoir by an exit route, and utilizes a means of travel, or a *vehicle of transmission*. By using this vehicle, it gains entrance through a *portal of entry* to the body of a *susceptible human being*, who then becomes its *host* and constitutes a potential reservoir to start the cycle again.

Common *reservoirs* for infectious agents causing disease in man are: human beings, animals, plants, the soil, and arthropods, such as mosquitoes, fleas, ticks, and lice.

Exit routes whereby the infectious agent leaves its reservoir are usually the respiratory tract, the gastrointestinal tract, the skin or mucous membranes, the blood, or the secretions or excretions of the individual. No portal of exit is required for organisms harboring in the soil.

Vehicles of transmission for infectious agents include:

1. *Air*. For example, *Mycobacterium tuberculosis* frequently adheres to dust or other small particles and is subsequently carried by air currents.

2. *Water*. For example, *Vibrio comma*, which causes cholera, may be carried in fecally contaminated water.

3. *Food*. For example, some strains of *Staphylococcus*, which is the causative agent of gastroenteritis, may be transmitted by improperly refrigerated food.

4. *Dust and dirt*. For example, *Clostridium tetani*, which causes tetanus, may be carried by soil, dust, and human or animal feces.

5. *Insects*. For example, flies pick up pathogens from open garbage and sewage and carry them to food and drink.

6. *Inanimate objects* (called *fomites*). For ex-

ample, the spirochete *Borrelia vincentii*, which causes Vincent's angina or "trench mouth," may be transmitted via poorly washed dishes (it often harbors in cracks of cups and dishes).

Endogenous contact is a mode of transmission of infection from one area of the body to another in the same person, as from an infected wound to a scratch on the skin.

Person to person contact is a common mode of transmitting infection. It may be direct, as by kissing or sexual contact, or through touching infected parts of the body or discharges such as exudates from an infected wound. People may also infect one another through *droplet infection,* that is, the spray of droplets from the nose and mouth onto the skin or mucous membranes of another (as, for example, in the common cold). Person to person contact may also be indirect; for example, organisms may be transferred from one patient to another via the nurse's hands if she does not wash them adequately before and after giving patient care.

Portals of entry whereby infectious agents gain access to the body of a susceptible human being are, in many instances, the same as those by which the agents left the host reservoir, that is: the *gastrointestinal tract,* usually via the mouth in food or drink; the *respiratory tract,* in inspired air; the *skin and mucous membranes,* usually through breaks in these tissues; and the *genitourinary tract,* usually through the external openings, whence the infection travels up the tract via its mucous membrane lining.

The portals of entry to the human body and exit routes from the body used by different infectious agents vary, as do their capacities to live outside their original reservoirs. The method of transfer for each infectious agent depends on the specific portal of entry, exit route, and ability to live outside its reservoir. In order to plan adequate precautionary measures to prevent and control infection, then, it is important that the specific causative agent of the infection be identified.

The Body's Reaction to Infectious Agents

The human organism is equipped with various mechanisms that help to prevent the invasion of body tissues by infectious agents and to control their growth and multiplication in the body if they do get past the first lines of defense.

Innate Immunity. The body has an *innate immunity*—that is, built-in mechanisms to ward off diseases through such factors as:

1. The skin's resistance to microbial invasion

2. The ability of the acid digestive juices and digestive enzymes to destroy ingested bacteria and other organisms

3. The ability of the white blood cells and the reticuloendothelial system to destroy microorganisms and toxins

4. The ability of certain chemical compounds in the blood to attach themselves to infectious agents or their toxins and destroy them

Acquired Immunity. The body also has the ability to develop specific resistance to various infectious agents or their toxins. In response to an infectious agent that has penetrated the first lines of defense, the lymph tissues develop *specific antibodies,* which are specialized protein molecules, and *sensitized leukocytes;* both of these are capable of attacking and destroying the antigen (any substance capable of producing antibody formation; this reaction is believed to be a response to large protein molecules or polysaccharides in the infectious agent or its toxin) in its host.

Active immunity may be acquired by a person in response to actual invasion by an infectious agent; if a person has measles in childhood, for example, he is usually immune to it for the rest of his life. Active immunity may also be acquired artificially by the injection into the body of (1) attenuated organisms—that is, live organisms that have been processed so they will no longer cause the disease but still carry the specific antigen (smallpox vaccination is an example); (2) dead organisms that still have their

Immunization programs have helped to lessen the number of deaths from infectious diseases.

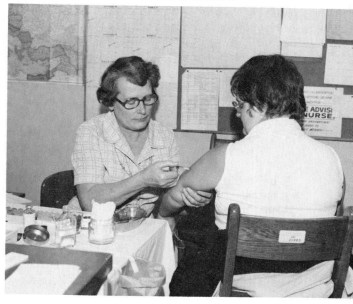

chemical antigens (as in typhoid fever inoculations); or (3) treated toxins whose toxic nature has been destroyed but that still retain their antigenic properties (as, for example, tetanus inoculation).

Passive immunity may be conferred by the administration of preformed antibodies or specifically sensitized leukocyte cells in the form of immune serum globulins, antitoxins, or antiserums.

Other Responses of the Body to Infection. As we discussed briefly in Chapter 2, the body has both a generalized reaction to stress (the General Adaptation Syndrome or G. A. S.) and a localized reaction that occurs at the site of stress (the Local Adaptation Syndrome). The early *general reaction* of the body to the stress of invasion by infectious agents is the same as the "just feeling sick" phenomenon described by Selye. This usually includes headache, malaise, a feeling of tiredness, slight elevation in temperature, and loss of appetite (sometimes followed by nausea and vomiting). In response to infectious agents there is usually a swelling of the lymph nodes as well.

It is in the second stage of the syndrome that the signs and symptoms of the specific infectious disease usually appear; an example of this is the typical vesicular rash seen in chickenpox.

The *localized reaction* that occurs at the site of injury or invasion represents the body's attempt to wall off the invader and destroy it before it can travel further to other parts of the body.

Inflammation is the localized protective response that is the body's reaction to injury or destruction of tissues, whether caused by the invasion of infectious agents, or by chemical, thermal, or physical means.

When body tissues are damaged, an increased supply of blood is always diverted to the area and certain substances are released by the injured cells to promote the repair and regeneration of the tissues. Among these substances are *leukotaxine* and *histamine*. Leukotaxine draws white blood cells to the area, where they help to destroy and remove foreign substances such as bacteria and decaying tissue cells. Histamine, along with other substances, increases permeability of the capillary walls, which allows the fluids, proteins, and white blood cells to move into the area. The clotting mechanism is also activated, so that the fluids clot and serve to "wall off" the injured areas.

Typically, there are five observable results from the inflammatory process: heat, redness, pain, swelling, and limitation of function. The redness is due to the local dilation of blood vessels and consequent increase in the supply of blood to the part. The warmth of the area is also the result of the increased blood supply. The swelling results from the exudative process, in which serum and leukocytes leave the blood stream to invade the area. The pain is believed to result from the stimulation of pain receptors in the area by certain substances released by the damaged cells and possibly also by the pressure of accumulated fluid (see Chapter 20). Limitation of function is usually due to the swelling and the pain.

Factors Affecting an Individual's Susceptibility to Infection

A person's resistance to infection is much better when he is in good general health. As we have mentioned in previous chapters, good nutrition, adequate exercise, a sufficient amount of rest and sleep, and good hygiene practices all contribute to increasing the body's ability to fight off infections. To supplement this general type of resistance, immunization is an effective method of preventing many communicable diseases, such as whooping cough, smallpox, measles, tetanus, typhoid fever, poliomyelitis, and many other formerly common infectious diseases.

Infants and small children are particularly vulnerable to infections, as are the very old. So, too, are sick people, as we mentioned earlier, because of their general debility. People with cuts or lesions in the skin (such as the surgical patient, or anyone with a wound of any kind) have an obvious portal of entry for infectious agents. Individuals who have been exposed to infectious diseases and have not been adequately immunized are also on the list of those "at risk" of infections.

If any of these individuals are malnourished, do not have optimal strength and tone in their muscles, are tired, or have not maintained good hygiene practices, their vulnerability to infection is increased.

COMMON SOURCES OF INFECTION AND TRANSMISSION MODES IN HEALTH AGENCIES

In the introduction to this chapter, we mentioned that institution-acquired infections continue to be a problem in hospitals in the United States and Canada (and in many other countries, too). The nurse should be aware, then, of common sources of infection and some of the ways infection is spread in health agencies.

The most important reservoir of organisms within a health agency is probably the patients themselves. Usually, every patient who comes into a hospital or other inpatient facility is observed for any sign of infection: any boils, fever, septic wounds and the like are reported for further investigation. In most hospitals, the charge nurse has the authority to order precautionary techniques for a patient if she suspects that he harbors pathogenic organisms which could be spread to other patients and the staff.

A routine measure for most newly admitted patients in a clinic, nursing home, or hospital is the chest x-ray. The intent of the x-ray is to detect pulmonary tuberculosis. This is considered particularly important diagnostically for elderly patients. Serological tests for syphilis are done also on all newly admitted patients in many agencies. With the alarming increase of venereal disease among the population in recent years, this is another important diagnostic measure.

As mentioned earlier, people working in a health agency can also be reservoirs of infection. Any person with a fever, diarrhea, nausea, and most certainly, a cold, may be spreading infectious organisms. This is particularly serious in the operating room, the nursery, and the intensive care and coronary units, where infection seriously threatens the safety of patients and where the transmission rate is high.

Patients' visitors can also transmit infections, although normally the length of their period of contact is minimal in comparison with that of personnel. Food, vermin, and dirt also transmit disease, but they are an unlikely source in a modern institution. Hospital dust is probably heavily laden with pathogenic organisms. However, dryness inhibits their growth, and most hospitals have housekeeping policies that eliminate unnecessary moisture and maintain a high standard of cleanliness.

Among the common sources of infection in hospitals and other inpatient facilities for the care of the sick are:

1. Nose and throat secretions and the expired air of people with respiratory infections.
2. Vomitus and feces (feces more than vomitus, since microorganisms do not flourish well in the stomach)
3. Urine from patients with genitourinary tract infections
4. Discharges from body orifices
5. Exudates from infected wounds or skin lesions

6. Equipment used in the care of patients with infections
7. Bed linen and personal linen used by patients with infections

Common Vehicles for the Transmission of Infection in Health Agencies

The most common means by which infection is spread in health agencies are:

1. *Personal contact.* One child with measles, for example, may give measles to a whole ward of children. A nurse with a cold may give the cold to all her patients.
2. *Aerial routes. Staphylococcus aureus,* which has been the cause of so many hospital infections, is air-borne. The organisms are often transferred by droplet infection from the nose and throat passages of carriers; they may also travel quickly from one place to another by attaching themselves to dust particles in the air. *Staphylococcus aureus* organisms in large quantity have frequently been found on patients' bedding. The nurse must take particular care, therefore, when changing the bed linen, not to shake sheets and blankets. Used linen should be put into a hamper (preferably a closed one) as soon as possible after removal from the patient's bed.
3. *Animals and insects.* Rats and mice may be a concern in some agencies. They spread *Salmonella* and *Shigella* organisms, among others. Flies also are well-known carriers of microorganisms. Windows in a health agency should always be screened. This is not usually a problem in modern hospitals but may be in a neighborhood health center or a remote nursing station.
4. *Fomites.* Inanimate objects, such as needles and syringes, are possible sources of infection in health agencies. A number of cases of infectious hepatitis, for example, have been traced directly to contaminated needles or intravenous equipment which has been inadequately cleaned and sterilized. The use of disposable equipment has reduced this hazard, but in agencies where needles, syringes, and infusion or drainage sets are reused, cleaning and sterilizing standards must be scrupulously enforced.
5. *Food and drink.* Impure water and contaminated food are known to cause outbreaks of such diseases as cholera, typhoid fever, and infectious hepatitis. Although regulations to safeguard the water supply are stringent in most parts of the United States and Canada, there are still remote areas where this is a problem. Con-

tamination of food by workers who are carriers of disease (as, for example, the well-known cases of typhoid carriers), is another concern of all institutions, hotels, restaurants, and other eating places.

6. *Endogenous spread*. Spreading of organisms from one area of a person's body to another, as from the skin to an open wound, is also common. The maintenance of strict aseptic technique, is important to prevent the endogenous spread of organisms.

INFECTION CONTROL NEEDS THROUGHOUT THE LIFE CYCLE

Pregnant women are usually tested for gonorrhea, for syphilis, and for immunity to rubella, because all three of these communicable diseases can seriously affect the health of the unborn infant. Both rubella (during the first trimester) and syphilis cause damage to the fetus in utero, the organisms being transmitted via the mother's bloodstream to that of the infant. Aftereffects, such as deafness and mental deficiency, may show up in the infant after birth. Gonorrhea is usually picked up by the infant during its passage through the birth canal and may result in a gonorrheal infection of the eyes of the newborn. Drops of silver nitrate are routinely placed in the eyes of newborns to prevent this infection. During its early stages, the fetus provides an excellent medium for the growth of many viral agents. These tend to cause widespread fetal disease that can result in abnormalities such as missing cells or incomplete development.

The pregnant woman, then, needs to be protected as much as possible from viral infections such as colds, influenza, and the like. The woman is also highly vulnerable to urinary tract infections because of the increased tendency toward stasis of urine in the bladder and increased bacteriuria in pregnancy. If infection travels up the urinary tract to the kidneys, it may cause high fever and severe systemic reactions and can start the woman into premature labor.

The neonatal period is probably the most dangerous time of life for any individual. Infections occur more often at this time than at any other age. The newborn produces little or no immunoglobulin on its own; its passive immunity is limited to that which it has received from the mother. Newborns are very susceptible to gram-negative bacilli (two examples of these are the *Neisseria gonorrhea* organism and the Salmonella group), the group B beta-hemolytic streptococci, and *Staphylococcus aureus*. They are particularly vulnerable, then, to infections that may be present in health agencies, such as the nosocomial infections caused by *Staphylococcus aureus*, to infections that may be transferred from a sick infant to a well one, as for example dysentery caused by *Salmonella*, and to infections that may be harbored by staff, as in the case of a person with a developing "strep throat." It behooves nursing personnel working in newborn nurseries, then, to be meticulous in their technique and to make sure that they are free from infection themselves in order to protect the infants entrusted to their care.

Breast milk provides the infant with immunity to many infections (see Chapter 14), but the newborn's inflammatory response is not well developed and he localizes infections poorly. An infection caused by a contaminated needle may then become a generalized infection rather than being localized and walled off at the site.

The widespread immunization of infants and children has drastically reduced the incidence of diseases such as measles, mumps, rubella, diphtheria, and whooping cough (pertussis), and even tetanus and polio, over the past few decades. Parents today have not experienced the tragic epidemics that used to sweep the country and ended in the deaths of so many infants and children not too many years ago. Many people have, as a result, become unconcerned about the need for immunization. Yet, children are just as vulnerable to these diseases today as they were before the vaccines were developed. The nurse who is counseling young mothers is in an excellent position to advise on the needed immunizations for children at different ages. Schedules of recommended immunizations are prepared by such organizations as the Committee on Infectious Diseases of the American Academy of Pediatrics and state and provincial departments of health. These schedules are revised periodically and the recommendations vary slightly from one place to another. The nurse is well advised to consult the current schedule recommended by her local department of health before advising parents. The recommended immunization schedule put out by the Ontario Council of Health in 1977 is shown on page 557.

Among the most common infections infants develop is the acute respiratory disease—the common cold. The infection may progress into an inflammation of the bronchioles, causing bronchitis. Inflammation can also block the eustachian tube, causing an infection in the middle ear, otitis media. If untreated, the latter can cause significant hearing impairment in a child. Influenza infections are also common in infants

RECOMMENDED IMMUNIZATION SCHEDULE

Age	Diphtheria Toxoid	Pertussis Vaccine	Tetanus Toxoid	Salk Polio Vaccine	Measles Vaccine	Mumps Vacinine	Rubella Vaccine
2 months	●	●	●	●			
4 months	●	●	●	●			
6 months	●	●	●	●			
12 months to puberty					●	●	●
16–18 months	●	●	●	●			
4–6 years (school entry)	●	●	●	●			
11–12 years	●			●			
16–18 years (school leaving)	●			●			
	Diphtheria and tetanus toxoid combined with pertussis and purified poliomyelitis vaccines are usually administered in combined form (DPT Polio).				Combined measles, mumps and rubella vaccine is usually administered as a single injection and should be given as soon as possible after the first birthday.		

Ontario Council of Health, 1977. Reprinted courtesy of Ontario Council of Health, 700 Bay Street, Toronto, Ontario, M5G 1Z6.

from 6 months to 2 years of age. Potential complications, such as pneumonia and meningitis, pose a serious threat to the infant's health.

Infection is still the second most frequent cause of death in young children, and the fourth in older children. Young children succumb very easily to colds, intestinal infections, and the common contagious diseases. Smaller children, of course, suffer more quickly from dehydration when they have a fever, are not eating well, or are losing fluids from the gastrointestinal tract with vomiting and diarrhea. Children build up their immunity to the common pathogens in their environment upon exposure to them. As soon as they have started off to a day care center, nursery school, or kindergarten, where they have more social contacts, they seem to come down with one thing after another. The oldest child in a family usually catches everything that is going around at school and brings it home to his younger brothers and sisters, who thus develop their immunity at an earlier age. Regular immunization boosters are usually given at age 4 to 6 years (school entry), at 11 to 12 years, and at 16 to 18 years (when leaving school).

Among the more common infections of childhood, now that the communicable diseases are no longer the scourge they once were, are otitis media, the streptococcal infections (which can cause scarlet fever and lead to rheumatic fever), and urinary tract infections (which are usually caused by fecal flora and are more common in girls than in boys).

Adolescents are susceptible to all types of viral and bacterial infections. Effective immunization has reduced the number of cases of the childhood diseases, so that it is rare for a teenager to come down with measles, mumps, or other contagious diseases these days. Another disease that seems to attack adolescents particularly is infectious mononucleosis, a viral infection that has a low communicability and is transmitted by droplet infection. In young adulthood, acute appendicitis is still a commonly occurring infection problem. The occurrence of viral hepatitis reaches its peak in the 20- to 24-year-old group, predominantly among urban white males. Among young women, urinary tract infections are common. Many young adults develop immunological disorders such as allergic rhinitis (hayfever) and sinusitis, which reach their peak incidence in this age group. Eczema and asthma are also common, and arthritis begins to show up as a major problem.

During the middle years, the viral infections, especially those affecting the respiratory tract, are common. Most individuals have built up sufficient immunity by this stage of their life, however, to ward off the more serious complications of these infections. Bacterial infections are not usually a severe problem, unless the individual's defense mechanisms have been weakened by other stressors. Alcoholics and those who have disorders such as cancer, for example, seem to be much more vulnerable to infections than most other middle-aged adults. Allergies causing hay fever or bronchial asthma and drug allergies may emerge or become more severe during middle age.

Among the older age group, the respiratory tract is the principal site of serious viral infections. Pneumonia is common, and influenza is often fatal, particularly if the individual has existing cardiopulmonary problems such as heart disease or chronic bronchitis. Older people are also prone to urinary tract infections, which is often related to two factors: Most do not drink enough fluids, and there is a general slowing down of all bodily processes, with more of a tendency toward stasis of urine in the bladder. Diminishing skin integrity increases the risk of infection for the older person. With aging, there is also a decline in the efficiency of a person's immune response to infectious agents. Neoplastic disorders (such as cancer) tend to reduce it further. Treatment of disorders by drugs that suppress the immune reaction, as for example chemotherapy, which is often used in treating cancer, may further impair resistance to infection.

ASSESSMENT

Every patient in a health agency has a potential problem of infection, as does every health worker. The nurse must be alert to watch for infections in those who are particularly "at risk": (1) the very young; (2) the very old; (3) people who are generally debilitated, e.g., malnourished, tired, or weak; (4) those who have not maintained good hygiene practices; and (5) those who have been exposed to infectious disease.

From the nursing history and the initial clinical appraisal, the nurse can obtain information about the general health status of the patient, i.e., current state of functional abilities and state of health at the time of admission to the agency. This information is supplemented by data about the patient's past and current health problems, and the physician's diagnostic and therapeutic plans of care, as found in the patient's record. Laboratory tests and x-ray reports are also very helpful, if they have been done.

In many health agencies, all new patients undergo chest x-rays and serologic tests for syphilis. Other laboratory tests may be ordered to identify the specific agent causing an infection. The nurse must be alert for medical orders that place the patient on infection precautionary status or that require special handling of urine, feces, or other bodily excretions or secretions, or of wounds.

Ultimately, the nurse's observations of the patient are of prime importance in identifying infections. She watches for signs and symptoms of the body's general and local responses to invasion. The vital signs—temperature, pulse, and respirations—are particularly helpful observations in early detection of infection in the patient. His complaints of tiredness, headache, or loss of appetite, or that he generally is not feeling well, are also among the early warning signs the nurse should watch for as possible indications of a generalized reaction to infection. If a patient complains of any of these it is always wise to check his temperature, pulse, and respirations to see if they are elevated. The patient's subjective observations and the nurse's objective findings are both reported promptly.

The patient may be able to tell the nurse about localized symptoms, too, such as pain, warmth in the area, and loss of function. Combined with her observations of redness and swelling (she may also observe the patient's reactions indicating pain, feel the warmth of the area, and observe limitation of movement), these would certainly lead her to suspect a localized infection.

She should also be alert to secretions from the nose and throat, coughing, sneezing, or the expectoration of sputum by a patient. Exudates from wounds or other breaks in the skin, or from any of the body orifices, should also warn her of the possibility of infection, as would any vomiting or diarrhea.

The patient and his immunization record are usually the best sources of information about prior exposure to infectious diseases. In some agencies, this information is included in the data gathered during the nursing history. If the patient is a child, a very ill adult, or unable to communicate, the family would be the best source of information on this point.

COMMON PROBLEMS

Potential or actual infections are the basic problems in this instance. A known or suspected infection brings with it additional problems, such as control of the spread of infection to other patients, to visitors, and to staff. The patient who is placed on special precautionary measures because he has, or is suspected to have, an infection, will have increased anxiety as well as potential problems of sensory deprivation and feelings of isolation. He will no doubt be worried about the cause of the infection, about spreading it to other people, about the seriousness of the infection, and about what it means. He is usually set apart from others physically, as, for example, by being placed in a private room, or by having his unit demarcated by signs that advise staff, visitors, and other patients that he is "infected." He has to learn how to prevent the spread of his infection to others. The patient's family and other visitors need to learn the reason for the precautionary measures and the various other measures they need to take to protect themselves and others.

PRIORITIES FOR NURSING ACTION

If a patient is suspected of having an infection—that is, if the nurse observes signs of localized or general infection in the patient, she reports these promptly to the physician so that appropriate diagnosis and therapy can be initiated and precautionary measures started. In many agencies, as mentioned earlier, the head

✓ PRINCIPLES RELEVANT TO THE PREVENTION AND CONTROL OF INFECTION

1. Of the many varieties of microorganisms, only a few are true pathogens.
2. Many microorganisms normally present in the environment and in the body are opportunists and will become infectious agents if given the chance to do so.
3. The integrity of the skin and mucous membranes is the body's first line of defense against invasion by infectious agents.
4. A person's resistance to infection is lessened when he is very young or very old, when his health status is poor, when hygiene is neglected, and when he has not been adequately immunized against infectious diseases.
5. Infectious agents may be transported by a number of different routes to a susceptible human being.
6. The modes of transfer of infectious agents vary depending on their usual portal of entry, exit route, and ability to live outside their reservoir.
7. Some individuals carry infectious agents but do not themselves show clinical signs and symptoms of the infection.
8. Infectious agents may be destroyed by sufficient heat, by chemical agents, and by other known means.

nurse has authority to institute these measures based on her own judgment, to safeguard other patients, visitors, and staff from acquiring the infection. Some organisms are particularly virulent, and even their suspected presence constitutes an emergency situation. *Bacillus anthracis*, which causes anthrax, for example, is very virulent. A person suspected of having anthrax is isolated immediately and the room in which he was examined is thoroughly disinfected before being used again.

GOALS FOR NURSING ACTION

The basic goals of nursing action in regard to infection are threefold:
1. To prevent infection
2. To control infection
3. To ensure the patient's comfort, safety, and psychosocial well-being when he is placed on precautionary measures for infection

SPECIFIC NURSING INTERVENTIONS

Cleaning Methods, Disinfection, and Sterilization Techniques

Clean equipment is essential to safe patient care. Many hospitals have a central supply department where all equipment is cleaned and prepared for use. The availability of disposable equipment has contributed greatly to patient safety and has also lessened the amount of time spent by nurses in cleaning and sterilizing equipment. In spite of the increasing use of disposables and the current practice of employing other personnel to clean and prepare equip-

Many health agencies have separated departments in which supplies and equipment are prepared for use. The nurse selects a sterile dressing tray from the central supply cart which has been brought to the service room of a nursing unit.

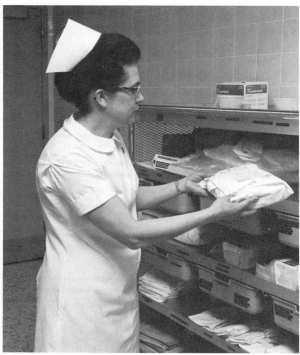

ment and supplies, the nurse is nonetheless well advised to be familiar with standard cleaning methods and disinfection and sterilization techniques to ensure the safety of her patients.

Cleaning Methods. Articles are referred to as *clean* when they are free from disease-producing organisms (pathogens). Dirty or contaminated materials harbor pathogens. An article is said to be *sterile* when it is free of all microorganisms, and unsterile when there are any living organisms on it.

Most utility rooms have a "clean" area and a "dirty" area. The clean area is used for the storage of sterile and clean supplies and the preparation of treatment trays. The dirty area is used for washing and cleaning trays and equipment and for storing used equipment prior to its return to the central supply (or other) department.

A basic cleaning procedure that is applicable to most equipment is the following:

1. Rinse the article in cold water in order to remove any organic material. Heat coagulates protein and thus tends to make blood and pus stick to equipment.
2. Wash the article in soap and hot water. The emulsifying power of the soap, as well as its surface action, facilitates the removal of dirt. The water helps wash the dirt away.
3. Cleanse with an abrasive when necessary.
4. Rinse well with hot water and then dry.
5. Sterilize or disinfect as necessary.

A stiff brush helps in cleaning many types of equipment; it makes it easier to reach crevices and corners. There are specially constructed brushes for cleaning the lumina of test tubes, tubing, and the like.

Disinfection and Antisepsis. Disinfection and antisepsis are processes by which disease-inducing organisms are killed or their growth is prevented. A *disinfectant* is an agent, usually chemical, that kills many forms of pathogenic microorganisms but not necessarily the more resistant forms, such as spores. An *antiseptic* prevents the growth and activity of microorganisms but does not necessarily destroy them. Disinfectants are commonly used to destroy pathogens on inanimate objects such as scalpels, whereas antiseptics are used on people's wounds or skin. A substance is also spoken of as *bactericidal* if it kills bacteria and *bacteriostatic* if it merely prevents their growth.

Many disinfectants and antiseptics are available commercially. When choosing a disinfectant, five factors are considered:

1. The disinfectant should kill the pathogens within a reasonable time
2. The disinfectant should not be readily neutralized by proteins, soaps, or detergents
3. The disinfectant should not be harmful to the material on which it is to be used
4. The disinfectant should not be harmful to the human skin
5. The disinfectant should be stable in solution

The choice of the disinfectant for a specific purpose is best made after tests have been made of their conformity to these criteria.

Sterilization. Sterilization refers to the killing of all forms of bacteria, spores, fungi, and viruses. It can be accomplished by heat or chemicals. The autoclave is considered to be the most effective method of sterilizing hospital supplies. Generally, it is thought that steam at a pressure 15 to 17 pounds per square inch and at a temperature of 250 to 254°F (121 to 123°C) for 30 minutes is effective in sterilizing supplies. Prior to autoclaving, the equipment to be sterilized is washed and wrapped in such a way that it will remain protected after it is removed from the autoclave. A piece of autoclave tape, which indicates when the sterilization is completed, is often put on a package before it is sterilized. One type of tape has white lines that turn dark during the process to indicate that the equipment has been sterilized. Glass indicators are also available for this purpose. A chemical inside the glass changes color upon autoclaving.

When the nurse loads the autoclave for sterilization certain guides are best followed:

1. Place equipment in the autoclave in such a manner that steam circulates freely around each item
2. Turn bowls and other vessels on their sides so that water will not collect in them
3. Separate rubber surfaces so that they will not stick together as a result of the extreme heat
4. Check to be sure that the autoclave is set to sterilize the specific equipment

Boiling is another method of rendering articles free of microorganisms. It is believed that boiling for 10 to 20 minutes will destroy all pathogens with the exception of spores and the virus of infectious hepatitis. The article to be sterilized must be completely submerged in water during the entire time, the boiling time being counted after the water comes to a full boil.

Dry heat is sometimes used to sterilize supplies. Heating most objects for two hours at 340°F (171°C) has been found to be effective for sterilization, but petrolatum and oils require a higher temperature or more prolonged exposure to heat. In the home, an oven can be used to sterilize materials.

Chemical sterilization necessitates the submerging of the object in a sterilizing solution for a specified period of time. Many pharmaceutical preparations are available for this purpose; the choice depends upon the article to be sterilized and the kind of microorganism present. The object is soaked for the specified time before it is considered sterile.

Gas sterilization with ethylene oxide has also been found effective in many situations. According to research reports, all microorganisms subjected to a temperature above 110°F (43.3°C), a relatively high humidity, and a concentration of ethylene oxide of 440 mg. per liter have been destroyed. Ethylene oxide sterilization has been widely used for plastics, rubber, and fabrics. Its effectiveness, however, is reduced in the presence of biological products such as blood. The Environmental Protection Agency in the United States has been considering banning the use of ethylene oxide because it is a very toxic substance.

Exposure of articles to direct sunlight for a period of 6 to 8 hours is also considered an effective method of disinfection. It may be used in some areas for articles that are difficult to disinfect by other means—as, for example, rubber drawsheets.

Asepsis

The term *asepsis* refers to the absence of all disease-producing organisms. Both medical and surgical asepsis are practiced in patient care. *Medical asepsis* comprises those practices that are carried out in order to keep microorganisms within a given area. For example, if a patient has active tuberculosis, the patient and any articles with which he has had contact are considered to be contaminated with *Mycobacterium tuberculosis* and are therefore able to pass on the infection. In medical aseptic practices microorganisms are kept within a well-defined area, and any articles or materials removed from this area are immediately rendered free of bacteria so that they cannot transfer the infection.

Surgical asepsis refers to practices carried out in order to keep an area free of organisms. It is just the opposite of medical asepsis in that surgical aseptic practices are designed to keep organisms *out of* a defined area. Thus, an operative wound is kept surgically aseptic.

Handwashing

Handwashing is an important measure in preventing the spread of microorganisms. Good aseptic technique involves limiting the transfer of organisms from one person to another. The nurse's hands should be washed before and after contact with a patient. The "before" wash is to avoid carrying microorganisms to the patient from someone or something else. The "after" wash is to minimize the spread of microorganisms to other people, particularly other patients. A 15-second (or longer) wash is suggested by the Centers for Disease Control before and after routine nursing care. In handwashing, both mechanical and chemical means are used to remove and destroy organisms. The running water mechanically washes away organisms, while soaps emulsify foreign matter and lower surface tension, thus facilitating the removal of oils, greases, and dirt.

For cleansing after contact with a person or an object such as a sputum cup, which harbors pathogenic organisms, it is recommended that a longer wash be done with an alkaline detergent or a bar of ordinary soap. In surgical asepsis, handwashing is indicated prior to working with sterile equipment in order to render the hands as free as possible from bacteria. In either medical or surgical asepsis it is advantageous to wash one's hands at a deep sink where the water can be regulated by a foot or leg control. One procedure for the handwash is as follows:

1. Roll up sleeves above elbows and remove watch.
2. Clean the fingernails as necessary. Disposable sticks are often provided for this purpose.
3. Wash hands and arms to the elbow thoroughly with soap and warm water. Wash in continuously running water, using a rotary motion and taking care to clean the interdigital spaces.
   a. In surgical asepsis, always hold the hands higher than the elbows so that water will flow from the cleanest to the dirtiest area. A surgical scrub brush is sometimes used, although the danger of creating abrasions on the skin needs to be considered.
   b. In medical asepsis, hold hands lower than the elbows while washing in order to prevent microorganisms from contaminating the arms.
4. Rinse hands and arms, allowing water to flow freely.
5. Repeat steps 3 and 4.
6. Dry hands thoroughly with paper towels or a fresh clean towel. Many agencies now use hot

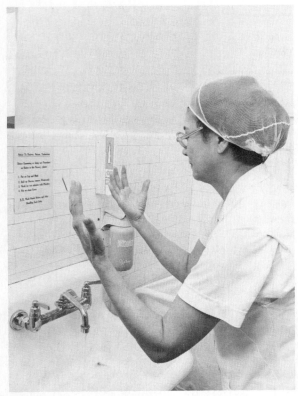

The hands are held higher than the elbows during a surgical asepsis handwash so that the water will flow from the hands to the elbows, i.e., from the cleanest to the dirtiest areas.

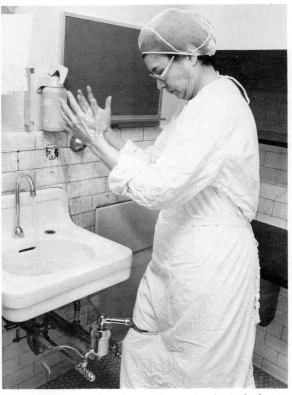

The taps are considered grossly contaminated; therefore, most sinks in health agencies are equipped with foot or leg controls to turn off the water after the handwash.

air hand driers, which eliminates the use of paper or cloth towels. During the drying process the hands and arms are held higher than the elbows, whichever method of drying is used.

When washing her hands, the nurse should take precautions to protect her uniform from getting wet. She should stand so that her uniform does not touch the wash basin and should hold her hands and arms away from her body when she is drying them. For turning off water at a sink that does not have foot or leg controls, a dry towel is used to handle the taps; they are considered grossly contaminated. The basin is considered contaminated also. If a break in technique occurs—for example, if the nurse accidentally touches the side of the basin during or after the handwash—the wash should be repeated from the beginning. It is important that the nurse keep the skin on her hands in good condition. Hand lotions or creams should be used frequently.

In caring for patients with some infections, it is often advisable to wear rubber gloves in han-

dling excreta or in giving direct care. The method of putting on sterile gloves is discussed in Chapter 27.

Masking

Masks are used in a variety of situations. Their general purpose is to limit the spread of micro-

Masks are worn to filter both inspired and expired air. (From Wood, L. A., and Rambo, B. J., eds.: *Nursing Skills for Allied Health Services.* 2nd ed. Vol. 3. Philadelphia, W. B. Saunders Co., 1980.)

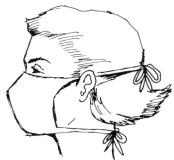

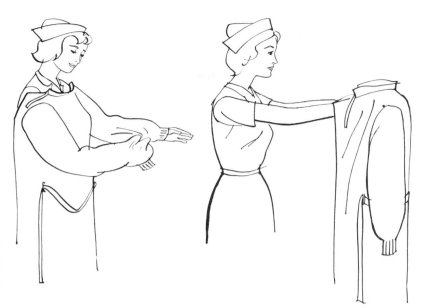

When taking off a contaminated gown that is to be discarded, the nurse keeps her "dirty" hands and the contaminated side of the gown away from her.

organisms. Putting a mask over one's mouth and nose serves to filter both inspired and expired air. In some situations visitors and patients wear masks—for example, to protect an open wound.

Masks may be made of cotton, gauze, or glass fiber, although disposable paper masks are increasingly being used. Generally a mask should be worn only once, then discarded. It is a violation of technique to hang a mask around one's neck when it is not in use. Masks are changed

When reusing a contaminated gown, the nurse slips her clean hands inside without contaminating herself with the gown.

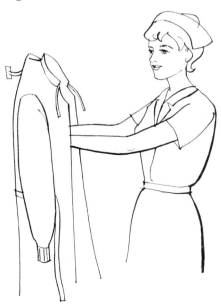

when they become wet, since moisture facilitates the passage of bacteria through the mask.

In surgical asepsis, masks are generally worn by personnel to keep equipment sterile or a wound free from microorganisms. It is inadvisable to cough or to sneeze while masked, and one talks only when necessary. Although the mask acts as a barrier, bacteria can escape around the sides of the mask and through the material itself, particularly during forceful respirations. Masks should be changed frequently. Although the length of time a mask is effective has not been precisely determined, it is recommended that it be worn no longer than 20 minutes.

When doing dressings or other treatments for a number of patients, the nurse should don a new mask each time she begins to treat a different patient.

Policies on the use of masks in medical asepsis vary from place to place. It is sometimes indicated for hospital personnel to wear masks in order to protect themselves from the pathogenic organisms of patients.

Gowning

Gowning is indicated if there is any possibility that the nurse may contaminate her uniform while she is attending a patient with an infection. The gown is long enough to cover a dress completely or a pantsuit to below the knees. Generally it is not worn outside the boundaries of the patient's unit.

The simplest and safest practice is to use a clean gown each time it is necessary to protect one's uniform. When the gown is taken off it is discarded in a container within the patient's unit. Care is taken that the outside of the gown, which is contaminated, does not touch the nurse's uniform. The nurse washes after she has discarded her gown.

If it is not possible to use a clean gown each time, then the nurse removes the gown *after* she has washed. When she takes it off she hangs it in such a way that the clean side is protected from contamination and the gown can be safely and easily put on later. The neck ties are kept against the clean side so that they do not become contaminated. The next time the nurse uses this gown, she picks it up by the clean side and ties the neck ties before she contaminates her hands on the outer side of the gown.

For visitors' use, many agencies now provide disposable gowns. These are used once and thrown away.

Infection Precautions

In situations in which the presence of pathogens is suspected or has been proved, medical aseptic practices are observed in order to control their spread and contribute to their destruction. Such medical aseptic practices are called infection precautions. The very word "isolation" describes what can happen to a patient who has an infection. It has been observed that hospital personnel and other patients tend to actually isolate such patients, who then become lonely and feel that they are nuisances. In many instances the words "dirty," "contaminated," and "isolated" have a moral significance for the patient, causing him to feel unworthy and unaccepted. Patients for whom barrier technique is necessary should not be psychologically isolated from others; indeed, physical isolation is often unnecessary when proper precautions are taken. The importance of explanations and support is paramount for these patients; consequently, the nurse needs to understand both her own attitudes and the practices that contribute to her own safety and that of the patient. The exact technique employed in a particular situation depends upon the portal of exit, the method of transfer, and the portal of entry of the particular pathogen (see Chapter 27).

Terms you may hear used in connection with infection precautions are barrier technique and reverse barrier technique. In *barrier technique,* mechanical barriers are established to confine the organisms within a given area. The boundaries in a hospital or at home can be the patient's unit or a single room, but all equipment within the designated area is considered contaminated. Barrier technique has the psychological advantage of reminding people of the existence of the pathogenic organisms and the physical advantage of a separate room, which decreases the transfer of organisms by air.

In *reverse barrier technique,* the patient is protected from pathogens in the environment. Instead of keeping pathogens within a defined area, as in barrier technique, the organisms are kept outside the defined area. This is done in a variety of ways, one of which is to place a plastic enclosure around the patient. All air reaching the patient is filtered, and all equipment entering the enclosed area is free of pathogens. Reverse barrier technique is used for patients who are particularly susceptible to infections, for example, people who have severe burns or leukemia. Since these patients do not have normal resistance to pathogenic microorganisms, they are protected within barriers that permit an aseptic environment to be established.

Care of Equipment and Supplies. The increasing use of disposable equipment and supplies has simplified the practice of barrier technique. The wide range of disposables currently available includes dishes, cutlery, medicine cups, syringes, needles, treatment trays, gloves, intravenous sets, drainage sets, bedpans, and bedpan covers. When these articles are used for a patient who requires barrier-technique nursing, concurrent disinfection is considerably easier. There are still some aspects of patient care, however, for which disposables are not applicable. Disposables are also costly and may not be used in all situations. The nurse should, therefore, be familiar with measures that may be used in concurrent and terminal disinfection to control the spread of microorganisms.

Concurrent disinfection refers to the ongoing measures taken to control the spread of infection while the patient is considered infectious. Pathogenic organisms are destroyed continually while the patient requires barrier technique. Measures for concurrent disinfection are detailed later in this section. *Terminal disinfection* comprises those measures that destroy pathogenic organisms after a patient leaves an examining room or a hospital or when he no longer requires barrier technique. In terminal disinfection all equipment within the patient's room is rendered free of pathogenic organisms by appropriate means; for example, the walls and floor are washed with a disinfectant, and linen is wrapped and sent to the laundry to be disinfected. If the patient is to remain in the hospital, he usually takes a shower and then goes to another bed unit with clean equipment. The tub or shower is also cleaned with a disinfectant after use.

Equipment. All equipment used for a patient who has an infection is rendered clean immediately after it is taken from the patient's unit. Equipment such as glass medicine containers, artery forceps, and stainless steel bowls can be autoclaved and thus rendered safe easily and quickly. Many hospitals place such equipment in two heavy paper bags in such a way that the outer bag remains clean. The bag is marked "infectious" and is then autoclaved. If equipment is wet the inner bag should be made of waxed paper in order to contain the moisture and the organisms.

If equipment cannot be rendered safe by autoclaving, it can be exposed to ultraviolet light or soaked in or wiped with a disinfectant solution. Gas sterilization may also be used for some articles. The exact method depends upon the organism of infection and the type of equipment available.

Laundry. Linen bags are generally placed in the patient's unit to hold contaminated linen. When linen has accumulated in the bag, a designated person brings in a clean linen bag, and the contaminated bag is placed in it carefully in

Concurrent disinfection includes the safe disposal of contaminated linen. These nurses are using a "double bagging" technique for the linen which has been taken from the patient's room.

In many agencies contaminated equipment is placed in two heavy paper bags in such a way that the outer bag remains clean.

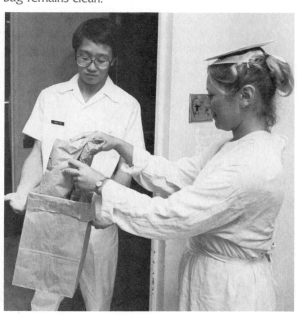

order to avoid contaminating the outside of the clean bag. In this way the linen can be transported without danger of contaminating other personnel or equipment. The outer bag is marked "infectious."

The washing methods used in most hospital laundries render most contaminated materials clean. If it is necessary to take special precautions, as with spore-forming bacteria, linen is usually autoclaved prior to laundering.

Dishes. After a patient who has an infection has eaten, his dishes are removed to the bathroom, where the uneaten foods and fluids are disposed of (in the same manner as excreta; see following section); the dishes are then either replaced on the tray and taken to the dishwasher or they are doubled-bagged and autoclaved prior to washing. Many health agencies have automatic dishwashers that render dishes free of pathogens.

If an autoclave or dishwasher is not available, dishes can be boiled after they have been rinsed or they can be soaked in a disinfectant solution. The latter method is the least desirable, because of the difficulty of immersing the dishes completely and because of the errors that can occur. For example, organic material left on dishes can protect pathogens sufficiently for them to remain active after the normal soaking time.

Disposal of Excreta. Most contaminated excreta can be safely disposed of in the general sewage, where it is subsequently rendered harmless by the sewage treatment facilities of the community. In areas where the treatment of sewage is not considered satisfactory for a particular infectious organism, excreta must be rendered safe before disposal into the sewage system. One method of doing this is to treat the excreta with a prescribed disinfectant, such as chloride of lime, for the time necessary to destroy the pathogens.

Patient Teaching in Infection Precautions. Patients for whom infection precautions are being maintained have special needs for emotional support. They are frequently physically isolated from other patients, and the hospital staff tends to ignore them, to "leave them until the last." Some patients attach a moral significance to their disease; they feel unworthy and think they are creating extra work for the nurse. If a nurse hesitates in full view of the patient before she enters his room and if she puts on a gown reluctantly or as if it is a bothersome duty, she will only enhance his feeling of unworthiness and lowered self-esteem.

Often a patient will want some recreational activity. Such activities should be designed so that they do not interfere with barrier technique, yet still meet the patient's needs. Materials such as magazines or woodcraft sets can be made safe after they are removed from the contaminated area. Magazines can usually be destroyed, and wood can be sterilized. With a little ingenuity the nurse can usually provide materials that can be either destroyed or sterilized after they have been used.

The explanations provided to a patient who requires infection precautions are crucial to his care. Most people want to participate in their own therapy; moreover, the success of medical asepsis is largely dependent upon the patient's willingness to help. The nurse is guided in her explanations by the needs of the patient to understand the reason for the various precautionary measures, the possible causes of the infection, what it means in terms of his health problem, and how he can help in measures to protect himself from further infection and to help prevent others from acquiring it. The spread of pathogens from the respiratory tract of patients is thought to be best controlled by teaching safe hygiene practices, which include frequent handwashing under running water. A patient with a pulmonary infection is taught to use several thicknesses of paper handkerchief to cover his nose and mouth when he sneezes or coughs. Also, covered, waterproof containers are provided for sputum. Facilities are also made available for the adequate disposal of paper handkerchiefs and sputum containers after they have been used.

The nurse needs to understand what an infection means to the patient. Frequently a patient acquires an infection as a complication of another disorder after admission to the hospital. Such a complication means a lengthened hos-

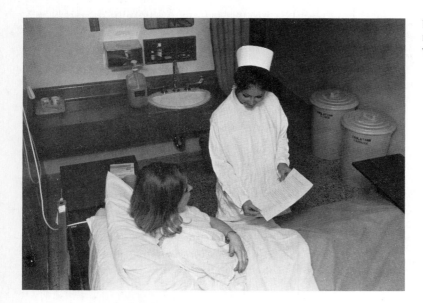

Patients for whom barrier technique is required need an explanation of the various measures involved.

pital stay, increased financial cost, and perhaps a real threat to life. Some patients react to these stresses with aggression and hostility directed toward the hospital in general or perhaps toward the nursing staff and the doctors. The nurse can offer support by providing an accepting environment in which the patient feels free to work through his feelings. She can also instruct patients in the possible sources of infections. For example, some people acquire infections because of the manner in which they carry out their daily activities, and some find it difficult to see how faulty hygienic practices could be contributing factors.

The patient with an infection or a communicable disease usually has other problems requiring nursing intervention. Many of these, for example, those associated with fever and wounds, are discussed in other chapters in this text.

PLANNING AND EVALUATING NURSING INTERVENTIONS

The prevention of infection is an integral component of the planning and implementation of all nursing action, whether directly or indirectly concerned with patient care. Adherence to good standards of cleaning and to tested methods of disinfection and sterilization is vital to the prevention and control of infection in a health agency. Adequate handwashing before and after giving patient care to each patient is perhaps *the* most important means of preventing the spread of infection from one patient to another. Combined with strict adherence to good technique and good housekeeping practices, agency-based infections (and all others) can be kept to a minimum, if not completely eliminated.

When patients have a known infection or one is suspected, appropriate precautionary measures are initiated. The specific precautions taken depend on the nature of the infection, the portal of entry of the infectious agent, its exit route from the body, and its mode of transfer. Full barrier technique may be indicated in some cases; in others, precautions with respect to some aspects of care (as, for example, skin and wound care or care with regard to excreta) may be indicated. The United States Centers for Disease Control have developed a set of recommended precautions for hospital use in the care of patients with specific diseases or conditions. These are shown on pages 568–569. Many hospitals are now using these recommendations as guidelines. However, the specific precautions taken tend to vary according to the policies of the agency, and the nurse needs to be aware of those of the agency in which she is working.

A planned teaching program for the patient, his family, and other visitors is incorporated into the nursing care plan of all patients who are placed on precautionary measures for infections. Evaluation of the effectiveness of the teaching program lies in the acceptance by patient, his family, and other visitors of the need for these precautions, and their understanding of these through their demonstrated careful maintenance of the techniques and procedures recommended.

Some questions the nurse might ask herself to evaluate the effectiveness of her teaching are:

1. Is the technique keeping the organisms within defined areas? How would you know?
2. Are other people in the environment free of the infection?
3. Does the patient have the knowledge and skills he requires to prevent the spread of his infection and to participate actively in his care insofar as he is able?
4. Does he have misconceptions about his infection?
5. Does the patient indicate in any way that he feels isolated? For example, does he complain verbally or show signs of depression?
6. Does he have the contact he wishes with his family, hospital personnel, and other patients without endangering their health?
7. Does he get exercise adequate to meet his needs?
8. Does he demonstrate an active interest in and is he encouraged to participate in his care insofar as he is able?
9. Does he have diversionary materials that interest him?
10. Do the people in the environment know and take the appropriate precautions to prevent their infection?

Evaluation of the effectiveness of nursing intervention is also measured by absence of the infection in other patients, in visitors, and in staff. Many agencies have an infection committee who keep a record of infections in patients in the agency. It is only through the accurate recording and maintenance of statistical records over a period of time that the effectiveness of infection control can be evaluated. Nurses must report signs of infection in a patient promptly. In some agencies nurses must complete an unusual occurrence form on every patient with an infection to facilitate the investigation and follow-up of cases, to evaluate the effectiveness of current practices, and to institute new measures as needed to prevent and control infection.

✓

STRICT ISOLATION

Strict Isolation Precautions

*Visitors—Report to Nurses' Station
Before Entering Room*

1. Private Room—*necessary;*
   door must be kept closed.
2. Gowns—must be worn by all persons entering room.
3. Masks—must be worn by all persons entering room.
4. Hands—must be washed on entering and leaving room.
5. Gloves—must be worn by all persons entering room.
6. Other articles—must be discarded, or wrapped before being sent to Central Supply for disinfection or sterilization.

Diseases Requiring Strict Isolation*

Anthrax, inhalation
Burn wound, major, infected with *Staphylococcus aureus* or group A streptococcus
Congenital rubella syndrome
Diphtheria (pharyngeal or cutaneous)
Disseminated neonatal *Herpesvirus hominis* (herpes simplex)
Herpes zoster, disseminated
Lassa fever
Marburg virus disease
Plague, pneumonic
Pneumonia, *Staphylococcus aureus* or group A streptococcus
Rabies
Skin infection, major, infected with *Staphylococcus aureus* or Group A streptococcus
Smallpox
Vaccinia (generalized, progressive or eczema vaccinatum)
Varicella (chickenpox)

RESPIRATORY ISOLATION

Respiratory Isolation Precautions

*Visitors—Report to Nurses' Station
Before Entering Room*

1. Private Room—*necessary;*
   door must be kept closed.
2. Gowns—not necessary.
3. Masks—must be worn by any person entering room unless that person is not susceptible to the disease.
4. Hands—must be washed on entering and leaving room.
5. Gloves—not necessary.
6. Other articles—those contaminated with secretions must be disinfected.

Diseases Requiring Respiratory Isolation*

Measles (rubeola)
Meningococcal meningitis
Meningococcemia
Mumps
Pertussis (whooping cough)
Rubella (German measles)
Tuberculosis, pulmonary (including tuberculosis of the respiratory tract)—suspected or sputum-positive (smear)

ENTERIC PRECAUTIONS

Enteric Precautions

*Visitors—Report to Nurses' Station
Before Entering Room*

1. Private Room—*necessary for children only.*
2. Gowns—must be worn by all persons having direct contact with patient.
3. Masks—not necessary.
4. Hands—must be washed on entering and leaving room.
5. Gloves—must be worn by all persons having direct contact with patient or with articles contaminated with fecal material.
6. Other articles—special precautions necessary for articles contaminated with urine and feces. Articles must be disinfected or discarded.

Diseses Requiring Enteric Precautions*

Cholera
Diarrhea, when acute, with suspected infectious etiology
Enterocolitis, staphylococcal
Gastroenteritis caused by
    Enteropathogenic or enterotoxic *Escherichia coli*
    Salmonella species
    Shigella species
    Yersinia enterocolitica
Hepatitis, viral, type A, B, or unspecified
Typhoid fever *(Salmonella typhi)*

*See *Isolation Techniques for Use in Hospitals* for details and recommended duration of isolation.
Source: Center for Disease Control, U.S. Dept. of Health, Education, and Welfare, *Isolation Techniques for Use in Hospitals*, 2nd ed., Washington, D.C., 1975.

PROTECTIVE ISOLATION

Protective Isolation Precautions

Visitors—Report to Nurses' Station Before Entering Room

1. Private Room—*necessary;* door must be kept closed.
2. Gowns—must be worn by all persons entering room.
3. Masks—must be worn by all persons entering room.
4. Hands—must be washed on entering and leaving room.
5. Gloves—must be worn by all persons having direct contact with patient.
6. Other articles—see manual text.

Conditions That May Require Protective Isolation*

Agranulocytosis
Dermatitis: noninfected vesicular, bullous, or eczematous disease when severe and extensive
Extensive, noninfected burns in certain patients
Lymphomas and leukemia in certain patients (especially in the late stages of Hodgkin's disease and acute leukemia)

WOUND AND SKIN PRECAUTIONS

Wound and Skin Precautions

Visitors—Report to Nurses' Station Before Entering Room

1. Private Room—desirable.
2. Gowns—must be worn by all persons having direct contact with patient.
3. Masks—not necessary except during dressing changes.
4. Hands—must be washed on entering and leaving room.
5. Gloves—must be worn by all persons having direct contact with infected area.
6. Other articles—special precautions necessary for instruments, dressing and linen.

NOTE: See manual for special techniques when changing dressings.

Conditions Requiring Wound and Skin Precautions*

Burns that are infected, except those infected with *Staphylococcus aureus* or group A streptococcus that are not covered or not adequately contained by dressings (*see* Strict Isolation)
Gas gangrene (due to *Clostridium perfringens*)
Herpes zoster, localized
Melioidosis, extrapulmonary with draining sinuses
Plague, bubonic
Puerperal sepsis—group A streptococcus, vaginal discharge
Wound and skin infections that are not covered by dressings or that have copious purulent drainage that is not contained by dressings, except those infected with *Staphylococcus aureus* or group A streptococcus, which require Strict Isolation
Wound and skin infections that are covered by dressings and the discharge is adequately contained, including those infected with *Staphylococcus aureus* or group A streptococcus. Minor wound infections, such as stitch abscesses, need only Secretion Precautions

*See *Isolation Techniques for Use in Hospitals* for details and recommended duration of isolation.
Source: Center for Disease Control, U.S. Dept. of Health, Education, and Welfare, *Isolation Techniques for Use in Hospitals*, 2nd ed., Washington, D.C., 1975.

GUIDE TO ASSESSING THE PATIENT FOR EXISTING AND POTENTIAL PROBLEMS OF INFECTION

1. Is the patient very young? very old? malnourished? tired? weak? generally debilitated?

2. Is there evidence that he has maintained good hygiene practices? Does he need help to maintain them now?

3. Does he have any breaks in the skin or observable mucous membranes? Does he have lesions on the skin? Has he had wounds of any sort? Is he going to have, or has he had, surgery?

4. Has he been exposed to any infectious diseases?

5. Has he been immunized against communicable disease? If so, what immunization has he had and when were they done?

6. Does he have a health problem(s) or has he had one that reveals a history of infection, causes a present infection, or would make the person more susceptible to infection?

7. Have diagnostic tests for any infectious agents been done? If so, what do the reports indicate?

8. Is the patient showing generalized signs of infection? signs of inflammation?

9. Is the patient coughing, sneezing, or bringing up sputum? Are there secretions from his nose and mouth?

10. Are there exudates from wound or skin lesions? from any of the body orifices?

11. If the patient is on precautionary measures for infection, why have these been ordered? What types of precautions are being taken?

12. Has the causative agent been identified? If so, what are its usual portal of entry, mode of spread, and exit route?

13. What special precautions are indicated to prevent the spread of the patient's infection?

14. If the patient is on infection precautions, what knowledge and skills does he need to protect himself and others?

15. What measures can you take to minimize his anxiety and prevent sensory deprivation and feelings of isolation?

STUDY SITUATION

Mrs. R. Jackson is admitted to a hospital for an operation to remove an ulcer on her left leg. Three days after her surgery, Mrs. Jackson's wound appears reddened and has a purulent discharge. A wound culture has been ordered to identify the infecting organism. Infection precautions are being taken.

Mrs. Jackson, who is 54 years old, is in a room that has four beds and a shared bathroom. Her physician suggests that she move to a private room on the same floor where she will have her own bathroom.

1. What specific precautions should be taken?

2. What factors would you consider prior to explaining these precautions to this patient?

3. What should you include in your suggestion to Mrs. Jackson that she move to single room?

4. Why might she not want to move?

5. Why would it be advantageous for the patient to move?

6. The infecting organism is found to be *Staphylococcus aureus*. What do you need to know about this organism in order to establish a safe environment?

7. Mrs. Jackson's wound is dressed at least twice a day. After this measure what is done with the (a) old dressing, (b) linen drapes, (c) artery forceps, and (d) unused disinfectant?

8. "The safety of an environment is related to the number of pathogenic organisms in it." What measures in medical asepsis are based on this principle?

SUGGESTED READINGS

Brandt, S. L., and Benner, P.: Infection Control in Hospitals. What Are the Challenges. *American Journal of Nursing*, 80(3):432–434, March, 1980.

Can Handwashing Practices Be Changed? *American Journal of Nursing*, 80(1):80, January, 1980.

Castle, M.: Isolation: Precise Procedure for Better Protection. *Nursing '75*, 5(5):50–57, May, 1975.

Jacob, S. W., et al.: *Structure and Function in Man*. 5th ed. Philadelphia, W. B. Saunders Company, 1982, Chapter 12.

Mackey, C. L., and Hopefl, A. W.: Keeping Infections Down When Risks Go Up. *Nursing '80*, 10(6):17–21, June, 1980.

Meth, I. M.: Electrical Safety in the Hospital. *American Journal of Nursing*, 80(7):1344–1348, July, 1980.

Nadolny, M. D.: Infection Control in Hospitals. What Does the Infection Control Nurse Do? *American Journal of Nursing*, 80(3):430–431, March, 1980.

Pilgrim, M. C.: Are You Infecting Your Patients? *Journal of Practical Nursing*, 31:18–21, April, 1981.

Selekman, J.: Immunization: What's It All About? *American Journal of Nursing*, 80(8):1440–1441, August, 1980.

27

The Nurse Should Be Able to:

- Explain how surgery affects an individual's basic needs
- Describe the process of wound healing
- Identify factors making surgery more hazardous for a specific individual, both generally and in regard to wound healing
- Identify common problems that the surgical patient may encounter
- Identify situations in the pre- or postoperative care of patients that require prompt medical or nursing intervention
- Take appropriate action in these situations
- Utilize relevant principles in the care of the surgical patient pre- and postoperatively
- Demonstrate beginning skill in carrying out the following interventions:
   Immediate preoperative care
   Preparation of the skin for surgery
   Immediate postoperative care
   Continuing postoperative care
   Changing a sterile dressing
   Applying binders
   Bandaging specific areas of the body
- Accurately document her observations of the surgical patient and specific interventions she has carried out in his care
- Evaluate the effectiveness of her nursing interventions

PRE- AND POSTOPERATIVE CARE

CHAPTER 27

INTRODUCTION

In the early 1800's wound infection was so common that as many as 80 per cent of all wounds became septic. Surgery was hazardous, and limited to measures that were essential to saving a person's life, such as setting a broken bone, removing gunshot from the flesh, or amputating a smashed limb, and to minor procedures such as removing an aching tooth, incising an abscess, or draining an infected wound. A lack of cleanliness in carrying out procedures and in dressing wounds was a major factor in the high rate of infection. The nineteenth century was noted for developments in cleanliness, such as the use of disinfectants and aseptic techniques, that rendered surgery a less hazardous undertaking. Today, we are still refining the procedures, although the safety factor has been reinforced by the use of chemotherapeutic agents and antibiotics. The utilization of disposable materials, better procedures for sterilization of equipment, and cleaner and better-ventilated operating theatres have all contributed to making postsurgical infection rare today. There are still the dangers, though, with our present heavy reliance on antibiotics, that techniques will be relaxed and that antibiotic-resistant strains of bacteria will develop, causing us to be faced once again with massive problems of infection.

The calamitous outbreak of *Staphylococcus aureus* infections that spread through hospitals during the 1960's was a forceful reminder that standards of cleanliness and good technique must be maintained at all times in carrying out surgical procedures.[1]

Most health agencies now have an infection control committee, and a committee that reviews surgical operations conducted in the agency to develop and maintain rigorous standards in its operating rooms and on nursing units that provide pre- and postoperative care for patients.

Each agency has its own specific procedures on measures to be included in preoperative teaching and postoperative follow-through, in preparation of the skin for surgery, on measures to be taken immediately before the patient goes to the operating room and after the patient's return to his nursing unit.

Possibly no other single aspect of health care has elicited so much controversy over the years as the best method to care for wounds. Although the process of wound healing has been well known and well documented in the literature for many years, there is still no single standardized method of caring for a wound during the process of healing.

The techniques for wound dressing vary from one agency to another, with each agency hoping by its techniques to eliminate all possible sources of wound contamination. The nurse must use all possible care in maintaining good technique in the dressing of all wounds. She is guided in the techniques she uses by the procedures that are recommended by the agency in which she is working. The techniques suggested in this chapter provide general guidelines, utilizing basic principles, to provide good safe care to the surgical patient during the pre- and postoperative period.

The goals of nursing action in the care of pre- and postoperative patients are to make the surgical experience as safe and as comfortable as possible for the patient; to prevent, insofar as it is within the nurse's province to do so, the development of postoperative complications; and to help the patient to cope with the stress of surgery.

TYPES OF SURGICAL INTERVENTION

Surgery involves the deliberate and planned alteration of a person's anatomical structures in

573

order to arrest a pathological process, alleviate it, or eradicate it. It may be done on an *urgent* or *emergency* basis if the condition is seriously threatening a person's health. A person who is hemorrhaging or has acute appendicitis, for example, requires surgery immediately. On the other hand, a condition that could be helped by surgical intervention but is not causing the individual a great deal of pain or serious dysfunction may be treated by elective surgery. The operation in this case would be scheduled for a time and place convenient to both patient and surgeon.

Some health problems are aesthetic in nature and, although not necessary for a person's physical health, surgery may be important for his self-esteem and be requested by the patient. This type of surgical intervention is designated *optional* surgery. One example is plastic surgery for beautification purposes, such as shortening a nose that the person feels is too long, or lifting a sagging chin.

Surgery may also be designated as *major* or *minor*, depending on the hazards involved and the physiological effects of the procedure on the body. For example, removal of an ingrown toenail and the incision and drainage of a carbuncle (boil) are considered minor surgery. These procedures are often performed in a physican's office, an outpatient clinic, or other ambulatory setting. A hysterectomy (removal of the uterus), on the other hand, is considered a major surgical procedure and would be performed in an operating room.

The terms *curative* and *palliative* are also used to describe surgery. Curative surgery is intended to arrest a pathological process by removing the cause. Palliative surgery is done to lessen the distressing symptoms of a pathological process without removing the cause. A person may have obstructive jaundice, for example, which may be caused by stones in the biliary system or by malignancy. If, on opening the abdomen, the surgeon finds stones blocking the biliary tract, he will remove them. This procedure would be curative surgery. If, however, he finds that there is a large tumor of the pancreas interfering with the passage of bile from the gall bladder to the intestines, and the tumor is too large to be removed, he might simply create a bypass from the biliary tree to the intestines to circumvent the obstruction. This procedure would be a case of palliative surgery. The obstructive jaundice would be ameliorated, but the cause of the problem would remain.

Some types of surgery are readily evident to the patient. These are the *external* procedures,

which involve surface structures of the body. An example is the removal of a breast (mastectomy). The patient can see and feel what has been done. With *internal* procedures, where deeper structures are concerned, such as the removal of an inflamed appendix, the nature of the operative procedure is not so readily evident.[2]

Surgery may also be categorized on the basis of the nature of the procedure undertaken, as *constructive, reconstructive,* or *ablative* surgery. *Constructive surgery* involves the building or correction of a body part to improve function or appearance. A child who is born with a congenital defect, such as a missing nose, might have one constructed in plastic surgery. *Reconstructive surgery,* as the name suggests, is performed to repair damage to appearance or functioning caused by trauma or disease in a previously intact anatomical structure. *Ablative surgery* involves the removal of a diseased or damaged organ as, for example, cholecystectomy to remove a diseased gallbladder.[2]

EFFECTS OF SURGERY ON BASIC NEEDS

Surgery constitutes an assault on the body that affects the individual's ability to meet all of his basic needs. Some bodily functions are more disturbed than others, as you will note as we discuss the effects of surgery on the basic needs we have talked about in previous chapters and some of those we will be considering in later chapters.

Oxygen Needs

Oxygen needs are primary and must be a priority concern of all health personnel caring for the patient. During general anesthesia, the central nervous system is depressed and musculature relaxed. The anesthetic and the insertion of an artificial airway are both irritating and cause an increase in the secretion of mucus in the throat. There is, however, a lack of muscle tone to expel the mucus and any other debris that collects. When he is under the influence of a general anesthetic, the patient is unable to keep his tongue from falling back and occluding the airway. During surgery, his breathing is assisted by the insertion of an artificial airway. When he is recovering from the anesthetic, care must be taken to ensure that the airway is clear, and the patient must be assisted to rid himself of excess mucus in the throat and lungs.

Postoperatively, movement is usually restricted, and secretions and other debris tend to collect in the respiratory tract. The patient must be encouraged, and assisted as necessary, to use deep breathing, and change positions to prevent the stasis of fluids in the lungs.

Temperature Regulation

Many general anesthetics cause vasodilation and a resultant loss of body temperature during the intraoperative period. The effect of the vasodilation is compounded by surgical exposure. As a result, the immediate postoperative body reaction is shivering. The shivering requires an increased metabolism. Increased metabolism is also required for tissue repair, and body temperature is usually slightly elevated in the early postoperative period. This is generally considered to be a good sign that the body's recuperative mechanisms are functioning. A marked elevation of temperature, however, should alert the nurse to the possibility of infection, which causes the body's metabolism to be greatly speeded up in efforts to combat the invading pathogens.

Fluid and Electrolyte Needs ✓

Surgery always results in a loss of fluids from the body, from the blood vessels, from the interstitial spaces, and from cells as tissues are cut through during the surgical procedure. The body's water-conserving mechanisms are called into play (see Chapter 16), and characteristically both water and sodium are retained postoperatively. With surgery, there is also a loss of potassium, as large amounts are released from damaged cells and excreted in the urine. It is important to remember that levels of potassium can become dangerously low before the loss shows up on laboratory tests. Muscle activity can be seriously impaired if the potassium loss is excessive.

Following major surgery, there is usually a disturbance of the body's acid-base balance, with a tendency towards alkalosis. This may be caused by a number of factors. There is a decrease in the ability of the kidneys to excrete sodium bicarbonate, which results in a more acid urine. The retention of sodium and increased loss of potassium appear to reinforce this tendency. Hyperventilation in the early postoperative period also contributes to the acid loss, as carbonic acid (in the form of carbon dioxide and water) is expired from the lungs. If the patient is on nasogastric suctioning following surgery, there is further depletion of acid from the gastric secretions, and this aggravates the tendency towards alkalosis.[2]

Nutritional Needs

All types of injury to the body, including surgery, result in an increased metabolic rate, as the body mobilizes its forces to repair the damaged tissue. Tissue protein, especially that in the skeletal muscles, is metabolized as an energy source, with excess nitrogen being excreted in the urine. There is also a breakdown of fat, which becomes a major source of energy in the immediate postoperative period.

At the same time that nutritional needs are increased to keep up with the increased metabolic rate, there is a decrease in food and fluid intake. Most surgical patients are allowed nothing by mouth for several hours prior to surgery, and are unable to tolerate food and fluids for varying lengths of time postoperatively. In addition, some anesthetic agents cause nausea and vomiting, which depletes the individual's nutritional reserves. Frequently, the person's nutritional needs must be met by other than oral means. Usually, intravenous fluids are ordered until the person is able to tolerate a sufficient amount of nourishment by mouth to meet his nutritional needs.

Elimination Needs ✓

The loss of body fluids during surgery stimulates secretion of the antidiuretic hormone to directly reduce urinary output to lessen the loss of water from the body. The retention of sodium also helps to hold fluid in body tissues, further contributing to a decreased output of urine. A relative oliguria is thus common in postsurgical patients for the first 2 to 3 days.

Elimination from the gastrointestinal tract is also disturbed by surgery. There is, first of all, a lack of solid food intake in preparation for surgery and, usually, for a few days postoperatively, so that there is insufficient bulk to stimulate the bowel. The restrictions imposed on activity following surgery also contribute to a sluggish bowel.

Then, too, central nervous system depressants used in anesthesia and as analgesics depress neuromuscular functioning generally, causing a slowing down of the functioning of both bladder and bowels. An *atonic bladder* may result in a patient's inability to void—a not uncommon occurrence in the immediate postoperative period. A *paralytic* or *adynamic ileus* (obstruction of the intestines resulting from an inhibition of motility of the gastrointestinal tract) is also a fairly common occurrence following major surgery, especially if the peritoneum has been perforated, and may persist for a short period (1 to 3 days). A postoperative atonic bladder and decreased gastrointestinal motility occur more frequently when these organs have been manipulated during the surgical procedure.

Comfort, Rest and Sleep Needs

Because of the trauma to body tissues, the patient usually experiences pain following surgery. The pain disturbs his comfort and may interfere with his rest and sleep. The intensity of the pain varies considerably with the extent of his surgery, the location of the incision, and the organs or other parts of the body involved. If there has been tissue damage in any part of the body that is important in mobility, any movement is likely to cause pain. Then, too, some structures of the body are more richly endowed with sensory receptors than others, and the person feels more pain if these structures are involved (see Chapter 21).

Movement and Exercise Needs

The surgical patient is usually limited in his mobility, often for a number of reasons. During the operative phase, if he has a general anesthetic, he will be unconscious and unable to move. With a spinal anesthetic, the person is likewise unable to move any part of the body below the site of injection of the anesthetic. Even a local anesthetic causes immobility in and around the area that is being manipulated by the surgeon. Postoperatively, pain is a major factor limiting a person's mobility. Damaged tissue requires a considerable amount of time to repair itself, and the pain in and around the operative area is a good reminder to the individual not to put too much strain on healing tissues. He can feel the strain on tissues in the operative area when he turns in bed or tries to sit up, to get out of bed, or to walk after he has had surgery. Most people do not realize the extent to which the abdominal muscles are involved in respiration until they try to ventilate their lungs fully or cough after surgery, and feel the pull on muscles in the area of an abdominal incision. With some types of surgery, it is often necessary to immobilize a limb or other part of the body to allow time for the tissues to heal. The immobility may be achieved by enclosing the part in a cast, or attaching it to various pieces of equipment. These procedures severely curtail a person's movements. Often, surgical patients are receiving nourishment by intravenous infusion, which limits their movement, or they may have various tubes and drains that are hooked up to other pieces of equipment and hamper freedom of movement. Immobility can cause all sorts of problems, such as congestion in the lungs and a slowing down of circulation, as well as a loss of muscle tone through disuse. Slowing of circulation makes the individual more vulnerable to clot formation in the blood vessels, with the potential risk of emboli to the lungs, heart, or other vital organs. There is also a depletion of protein from the muscles and calcium from the bones of immobilized patients, which further interferes with mobility.

Sensory Needs

Surgery could not have developed to the extent that it has without the discovery and widespread used of anesthetic agents to render a person insensitive to the pain of cutting through and manipulating body flesh. The general anesthetics depress all sensation, and the person is maintained in an unconscious state for the length of time the surgery takes. Other types of anesthetic agents depress sensation in the specific area of the body being operated on; spinal anesthetics eliminate sensation in the part of the body below the insertion site in the spinal column, whereas local anesthetics depress neural activity in the specific area that is to be incised.

Sensory perception is also dulled by the administration of sedatives and analgesics, both preoperatively and postoperatively. These drugs sometimes result in confusion, poor defense responses, and imbalance in patients.

Protection and Safety Needs

While the patient is under the influence of medications or anesthetic agents that dull or distort sensory perception, he is not able to look after his own safety needs. It is necessary, then, for all health personnel (nurses particularly, since they are the ones most often with him) to assume the responsibility for protecting him from all hazards. We discussed the safeguarding of the unconscious patient, the confused patient and the individual with disturbed sensory functioning in Chapters 21 and 23. You will probably want to refer to these chapters when you are preparing to care for surgical patients both pre- and postoperatively, as well as during the intra-operative stage.

One of the most important needs for all persons undergoing surgery is protection from infection. Cutting through the skin penetrates the body's first line of defense, and provides a ready access to deeper tissues for infectious agents. The surgical patient is already vulnerable to disease processes because his physical resources have been weakened by the trauma of surgery, frequently in addition to the stress of an injury or illness that made surgery necessary. A major stress reaction has been evoked, and the body may simply not be able to cope with the additional stress of invasion by infectious agents.

Security and Self-Esteem Needs

Surgery almost invariably poses a threat to the person's security and jeopardizes his self-esteem. Anxiety is a common companion to surgery. A person worries that he may die on the operating table; that he may be mutilated or disfigured by the surgery; that the surgeon will find evidence of a malignancy, or worse, still, one too large to remove; or that there are more deep-seated problems than seem evident; he may be anxious because he is going into a situation that is unknown to him, and he will be cut off from his family and friends. Postoperatively there are other worries. Will he be able to breathe without the ventilator? move without pain? void when they remove the catheter? get his bowels moving again? walk the length of the corridor? When will he be able to go home? go back to work? drive his car? Will he look any different?

The person coming into a hospital for surgery finds it very dehumanizing to be labeled with an arm band, stripped of all his own clothes, garbed in a hospital gown, jabbed with needles, and suddenly be totally dependent on other people as he feels himself losing control of his body. The presence of someone who treats him as a person, who is kind, considerate, and gentle, is very important to the surgical patient's security. It is usually the nurses who provide the constant care and comfort and are the main source of reassurance for the surgical patient.

An excerpt from the book *Heartsounds*, the story of one physician's experience with a serious illness that necessitated surgery, seems particularly pertinent here.

Who would have believed . . . that the nurses were so much more important to sick people than the doctors were? As a doctor, he had always thought of the nurse . . . as an executive secretary. . . . But, now that he was a patient, he could see that nurses were . . . his lifelines.[3]

THE PROCESS OF HEALING

A wound, by definition, involves damage to body tissues. Whenever tissue damage occurs, the localized response of the body is the process of inflammation, which is described in Chapter 26. The early part of wound healing, then, shows evidence of this process. The student will note many similarities between the following outline of the process of wound healing and the description of inflammation.

The process of wound healing can be divided into three phases: the *lag phase*, the *fibroplasia phase*, and the *phase of contraction*.

In the lag phase, as a result of the injury to the cells, the capillaries become dilated in the injured area. The volume of blood in the area is increased, but the speed of the flow of blood is slowed. The blood brings leukocytes and plasma, which form an exudate in the injured area. At this time, the injured cells disintegrate and there is some swelling because of the plugging of the lymphatics by fibrin. During this phase, the wound is usually covered lightly by a scab or fibrin network, which is later absorbed.

In the fibroplasia phase there is an ingrowth of new capillaries and lymphatic endothelial buds in the wounded area. Fibroplasia results in the formation of *granulation tissue* (a connective tissue); subsequently there is *epithelization (keratinization)*. The wound appears pink, owing to the new capillaries in the granulation tissue, and the area is soft and tender.

In the third phase, that of contraction, there is *cicatrization* or scar formation by the fibroblasts after the cessation of fibroplasia. The capillaries and lymphatic endothelial buds in the new tissue disappear, and the scar then shrinks.

Open wounds require the formation of more granulation tissue, fibrous tissue, and epithelial tissue than closed wounds. During the first 5 or 6 days there is little strength in a healing wound; it is usually held together by sutures at this point. During the next 10 days, however, the tissue becomes stronger and better able to withstand tension.

Types of Healing

Healing by First Intention. In healing by first intention the sutured wound heals without infection or separation at the edges. There is minimal granulation tissue present, and thus a small scar results. In most surgical incisions, the edges of the wound are sutured closely together and healing occurs by first intention.

Healing by Second Intention (Healing by Granulation). In this type of healing, there is a closure of the wound by granulation tissue, which forms from the base of the wound and both sides toward the surface. It usually occurs when there is infection or excessive loss of tissue. Sometimes, a wound may initially be left open and later sutured, or it may break open after an original suturing and have to be resutured. There is considerable granulation tissue formed in either case. Healing takes longer because a large area must be filled with granulation tissue. This process usually results in a large and irregular scar, which may later shrink and contract surrounding tissue.

FACTORS AFFECTING AN INDIVIDUAL'S ABILITY TO COPE WITH SURGERY

General Factors

Surgery involves an invasion of the body tissues and is always fraught with danger for the individual undergoing it. Some persons are, for one reason or another, more vulnerable to untoward reactions than others. The principal factors affecting surgical risk are:

Age. The very young and the elderly are more at risk than others in the age spectrum. Before the age of 6 months, the child's circulation and renal function are not developed sufficiently to permit him to cope adequately with the stress of surgery. In the elderly, circulation is often impaired by arteriosclerosis and limited cardiac functioning. The elderly person's energy reserves are low and, often, his hydration and nutritional status are poor. In addition, the older individual is often more sensitive to medication than the younger person is, and may react badly to sedatives, analgesics, and anesthetic agents.

Normal changes of aging that affect the older individual's ability to tolerate surgery include: (1) decreased intracellular fluid, which increases vulnerability to fluid imbalances; (2) decreased amount of subcutaneous tissue, which increases vulnerability to a loss of body temperature and decreases resistance to trauma; and (3) changes in muscle tissue of the heart and lungs, which increases vulnerability to cardiac and respiratory dysfunction.

General Health. People in poor health generally are greater surgical risks than those who are physically fit. Particularly vulnerable to problems are those with respiratory tract infections, with cardiovascular diseases, those with abnormal blood coagulant patterns, and those with certain metabolic disorders such as diabetes and ones causing vascular insufficiency.

Mental Health. People who are extremely anxious are poor surgical risks. The person may not be able to cope with the additional stress of a surgical procedure.

Use of Medications. Drugs such as anticoagulants, tranquilizers, and other central nervous system depressants can have adverse effects on people undergoing surgery.

Extent of Surgery. It stands to reason that the more body tissue is involved in a surgical procedure, the greater is the risk of shock, infection, and other complications. People who have to undergo two or more surgical operations close together in time are also more at risk. Surgery is a major trauma, and the body requires time to recover from one assault before another is imposed on it.[2]

Factors Affecting Wound Healing

Many factors affect the speed and the character of the healing process. Some of the principal factors include:

Extent of the Injury. The process of repair and regeneration is naturally longer when tissue damage is extensive.

Age. Healing is more rapid in children than in adults. It is particularly slow in elderly people, because of a number of factors. These include a lessened efficiency of the circulatory, renal, respiratory, muscular, and sensory systems, and an increased likelihood of poor nutritional status.

Nutritional Status. An individual's nutritional status has a considerable effect on the healing process. Protein is necessary for the formation of new tissue. Protein deficiencies retard vascularization, lymphatic formation, fibroplastic proliferation, collagen synthesis, and wound remodeling. Carbohydrates and fats are needed for cellular energy. Vitamin C is involved in the maturation of collagen fibers during the later stages of healing. Vitamin K deficiencies may cause bleeding and resultant hematomas, which interfere with wound healing. Although a poorly understood mechanism, B-complex vitamins are necessary for protein, fat, and carbohydrate metabolism. In obese patients, there is a greater incidence of wound complications, such as incisional hernias, infection, and dehiscence (the breaking open of a wound).

Diabetes. Diabetes is one of the most common metabolic disorders. It causes disturbances in carbohydrate, protein, and fat metabolism that render the diabetic patient more vulnerable to the effects of surgery. Delay in wound healing and infection are common problems. When infection occurs in a diabetic, it is usually more severe and lasts longer. Postoperative nursing care is directed toward scrupulous aseptic technique in caring for the wound to prevent infection, and to the maintenance of blood sugar levels. Insufficient insulin in the body will also seriously compromise healing.

Infection. Infectious processes result in tissue destruction and, hence, delay the healing process. The presence of a foreign body in a wound also interferes with healing and is a potential source of infection.

Adequacy of Blood Supply. Blood supplies the products used in healing, and provides the mechanisms for combating infection. Hence, any factor that restricts circulation to a wound area interferes with healing and renders the area more vulnerable to infection. Although there is some evidence that a small amount of edema enhances fibroplasia, gross edema hinders healing by inhibiting the transport of substances needed for healing to the area. Restrictive bandages will also impede circulation, as will damaged arteries in and around the wound area. Healing is also slowed in persons with anemia and with blood disorders that cause vascular insufficiency, such as *atherosclerosis*, in which there is an accumulation of fatty deposits in the walls of large and medium-sized arteries.

Immunosuppression. The immune system of the body provides an environment for wounded tissue that is conducive to regeneration and repair; an example of this is the effect of the inflammatory response in promoting phagocytosis. An individual's normal immune response may be artificially prevented, or diminished, by irradiation, or by the administration of antimetabolites, antilymphocyte serum, or specific antibodies. The immunosuppressed patient has special problems in regard to wound healing. The nurse must protect vulnerable tissues, such as the surgical wound, from pathogenic organisms and must recognize the subtle signs of infection in the immunosuppressed patient.

Radiation Therapy. Healing is slowed in the surgical patient who has undergone radiation therapy, not only because of immunosuppression but also because there has already been extensive tissue damage in the organ or part of the body treated. If a patient is irradiated before surgery, the ideal operative time is considered to be 4 to 6 weeks after the therapy is completed. This is because the tissues are in the proliferative phase of healing before fibrosis and vascular narrowing occur. Complications in wound healing are common with the irradiated patient. These include delayed healing, dehiscence, and fistulas. It is important for the nurse to remember that irradiated tissues are more *friable*, that is, more easily pulverized or crumbled, than normal tissues and therefore require very gentle handling.

COMMON PROBLEMS

A knowledge of the effects of surgery on a person's ability to meet his basic needs helps the nurse to identify common problems that are likely to interfere with need fulfillment in the surgical patient. A knowledge of the common problems, in turn, enables the nurse to select appropriate pre- and postoperative measures to prevent, minimize, or alleviate these problems, insofar as it is within her province to do so, or to obtain the help of other health professionals to assist the patient when necessary.

In more senior nursing courses, the specific problems of patients with different types of surgery will be covered. In this chapter, we will concentrate on potential and actual problems that are common to all patients undergoing surgery. You will note as we review these problems and discuss assessment for them and general nursing approaches to resolve them that three very important aspects of the nursing role are stressed. These are the teaching aspects, the caring aspects, and vigilant, directed, and purposeful observation.

In reading through the previous section on the effects of surgery on an individual's ability to meet his basic needs, you have probably already noted a number of problems. These include:

1. Difficulties in breathing
2. Other disturbed vital signs
3. Fluid and electrolyte imbalances
4. Inadequate nutrition
5. Difficulties in voiding
6. Disturbed bowel functioning
7. Decreased mobility
8. Infection
9. Pain

10. Disturbed sensory functioning
11. Altered mental functioning
12. Anxiety or depression
13. Lessened capacity for self-protection

ASSESSMENT

In her preoperative assessment of the surgical patient, the nurse needs to be aware of the basic nature of the patient's health problem. She should also be aware of the type of surgical intervention that is planned and, if possible, the nature of the anesthetic agent to be used, e.g., general, spinal, or local. She also needs information regarding the patient's age and his general health status. Much of this information is usually available to the nurse from the initial clinical appraisal that has been done on the patient.

In the usual course of events prior to a patient's admission for non-emergency surgery, the individual will have had a complete physical examination by his own general practitioner before being referred to a surgeon. Before scheduling surgery, the surgeon completes a thorough investigation to determine insofar as possible the nature of the patient's problem and possible causes of it. A brief history of the patient and the presurgical findings of the surgeon, the possible cause of the problem, and the nature of the anticipated surgery will be documented in the medical history on the patient's record. Some health agencies request the individual to report on an outpatient base for laboratory tests a few days before admission. Tests such as urinalysis, chest x-ray, electrocardiogram (usually done routinely on all persons over the age of 35 or 40 years, depending on the policy of the health agency) and blood tests are usually included in the preliminary studies so that the surgeon is aware of existing or potential problems before the person is admitted. If the findings are abnormal, the surgeon will use his judgment to decide whether the pending operation should be performed, postponed, or canceled entirely.

When a patient is admitted to a health agency for surgery, basic demographic and social data are gathered in the admitting office, and the completed admission form is forwarded to the nursing unit. The nurse admitting the patient to the unit, or one assigned to his care, will take a nursing history. The resident physician on the service, or an intern who is receiving experience in surgery, will undertake a physical examination of the patient. Sometimes months intervene between the surgeon's initial assessment of the patient and the date of his admission to the agency. Sometimes the interval is short. The resident's (or intern's) examination of the patient helps to substantiate the surgeon's initial findings and to determine if the patient's condition has worsened in the meantime, or if other problems have developed.

The anesthesiologist also visits the patient the evening before surgery, and his notations on the patient's condition are incorporated into the medical record. It is he who usually orders the preoperative sedation for the patient, and the nurse will find these orders on the doctor's order sheet of the record.

Additionally, in many agencies, the operating room nurse visits the patient preoperatively to assess the patient and to plan for intraoperative care. A report of the events that take place in the operating room, including the anesthetic records, the operating room nurse's notes, and a description of the surgical procedures, is also incorporated into the record. The record accompanies the patient to the postanesthetic recovery room, where the patient is closely monitored for several hours after surgery. As events take place in that area, they are documented and incorporated into the record, which is sent with the patient to the nursing unit. There will also be postoperative orders written on the doctor's order sheet when the patient returns to the nursing unit.

Assessing for Specific Problems

1. Difficulties in Breathing. Preoperatively, it is important for the nurse to assess the status of the patient's respiratory functioning carefully. She should have good baseline data with which to compare her postoperative observations regarding the rate and character of respirations. She should know of any existing respiratory problems the person has, such as chronic obstructive lung disorders. Particular signs to look for include: coughing, wheezing, shortness of breath, orthopnea, ankle edema, cyanosis, clubbing of fingers, history of excessive smoking, asthma, chest pain on exertion, and barrel chest. If one or more of these signs or symptoms are encountered, the nurse should be on guard for postoperative cardiorespiratory difficulties. Signs or symptoms of a cold or other respiratory infection, however minor, should be recorded and reported. These should be documented carefully for the benefit of others who look after the patient.

There is always a potential problem of respiratory difficulties with any type of surgery involving general anesthesia; therefore, if the person has an acute infection, even of a transitory or minor nature, surgery may be delayed. In some agencies, a chest x-ray is done routinely on all preoperative patients, or even as part of the admission procedure for all patients. As we mentioned earlier, it may be done just prior to admission or after the person is admitted. The nurse caring for the patient preoperatively should check to see if a chest x-ray has been performed and, if so, note the results to aid in her own assessment. Deep breathing exercises are usually taught preoperatively to the patient to assist in preventing postoperative respiratory complications. During her teaching the nurse has a good opportunity to assess the patient's respiratory functioning.

Postoperatively, it is very important for the nurse to check on the patient's breathing and skin color frequently to identify incipient problems and take steps to correct them before they assume major proportions. In caring for a patient who is recovering from anesthesia or a postoperative patient who is partially or completely immobilized, it is important to make sure that the patient is positioned so that the tongue does not occlude the airway and so that secretions and vomitus can drain from the mouth rather than being aspirated. The nurse has a responsibility to encourage and assist the patient to change position at frequent intervals postoperatively to prevent the accumulation of secretions and debris in the respiratory tract. Particular signs of distress to watch for are the characteristic rasping sound made by a person whose airway is partially blocked, the signs of wet or noisy breathing, the use of accessory muscles in breathing, and changes in the patient's color. In monitoring his practice of the deep breathing exercises he was taught preoperatively, the nurse should be alert to evidence of pain the patient feels in trying to breathe deeply or cough, because the discomfort may cause him to neglect to carry out the exercises on his own. The nurse may need to support the patient's incision at first, and to teach him to support it himself in order to make deep breathing and coughing easier. A small pillow may be helpful in this regard, as we mentioned in Chapter 18.

2. Other Disturbed Vital Signs. Preoperative assessment of the patient's other vital signs is also an important part of the nurse's general assessment. Not only is the nurse obtaining baseline data to assess these signs postoperatively, she is also looking for deviations that indicate the patient is not in good general health—which may require the postponement of surgery. An elevated temperature, irregular heart beat, or abnormal blood pressure findings are vitally important to document and to report so that the surgeon, the anesthesiologist, and others involved in his care are all aware.

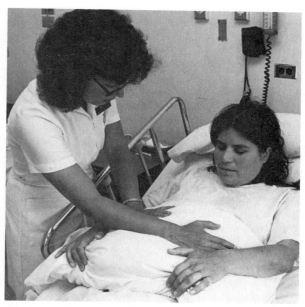

The nurse holds a pillow against the postoperative patient's abdomen to assist her in coughing.

Immediately following surgery, when the patient is returning to consciousness following general anesthetic, the vital signs of pulse, respiration, and blood pressure are checked at frequent intervals. A flowsheet is usually kept at the patient's bedside for the nurse's notations on a 15-minute (or more frequent) basis until the vital signs are stabilized. In most health agencies, the patient is kept in a postanesthetic recovery room until his vital signs are stabilized. When the patient returns to the nursing unit, the nurse who receives him checks his state of consciousness and his vital signs.

For the first 48 hours, temperature, pulse, and respiration are usually checked every 4 hours, and blood pressure according to the physician's order. If the nurse is concerned about the patient, she will want to check the vital signs more frequently. If she has any reason to suspect that the patient is going into shock, or if he seems feverish, she will want to check the vital signs at once in order to assess the need for nursing or medical intervention.

3. Fluid and Electrolyte Imbalances. Shock and hemorrhage are always potential problems in patients who have undergone major or even minor surgery. The nurse must, then, be particularly watchful for signs or symptoms indicative of these problems. An assessment of the patient's blood volume is done preoperatively by means of tests that include a red blood cell count, and hematocrit or hemoglobin determination. Tests are also usually carried out to assess electrolyte balance. A cross-match is also done, in case transfusions are needed. Blood is routinely given to patients undergoing many types of surgery. If the patient is anemic, blood may be given preoperatively, as well as during surgery and postoperatively. The patient's preoperative blood sample is also a test for clotting (prothrombin) time, to identify potential problems in bleeding. In order to maintain fluid volume and offset the anticipated loss during surgery, intravenous infusions are also almost routinely given during and following surgery. Bleeding in the surgical patient may result from the rupture of small surface blood vessels, or from trauma to larger, deeper-lying ones. It may be caused by spontaneous rupture of a vessel that has been weakened in the process of trauma, by the giving way of sutures that have been used to repair damaged vessels, or by problems in the clotting mechanism resulting from a lack of certain clotting factors in the blood.

The presence of bright red blood on dressings from a wound that is healing is always a warning to the nurse of the possibility of hemorrhage, and it should be reported promptly. The beginning nurse should always ask her team leader or instructor to check a wound when she observes fresh red blood on a dressing. If, in the senior nurse's opinion, the situation is serious, the physician is alerted immediately and the wound is checked frequently (every 15 to 20 minutes) to see if the bleeding is increasing. If bleeding becomes excessive, the patient may show signs of shock, which occurs whenever there is any major trauma to the body. Evidence of shock is observed in changes in the vital signs, such as falling blood pressure, a rapid weak pulse, pallor, cold and clammy skin, weakness, and restlessness. (The subject of shock was discussed in more detail in Chapter 16.) If the nurse detects any of these signs in the patient, the team leader should be alerted at once so that prompt intervention can be initiated.

Dehydration and edema are also among the common potential problems in surgical patients. Preoperatively, the patient's hydration status should be carefully assessed. In this regard, the patient's weight is important, as well as his nutritional status and the status of his skin and appendages (see Chapter 16). In many agencies, taking the patient's weight and height is part of the standard preoperative measures for all surgical patients. Postoperatively, it is important to monitor the patient's intake and output, and to watch closely for signs of dehydration in the patient. During the postoperative period when the patient is receiving nothing by mouth, it is particularly important to continually monitor his oral status, noting the condition of the tongue

and mucous membranes in the oral cavity and watching the lips especially for signs of dryness (see Chapter 16). Equally important is to watch for signs of edema around the incision site, in the tissues around the site of an intravenous infusion, and in dependent areas of the body generally.

With regard to electrolyte imbalances, we mentioned that there is generally a retention of sodium and loss of potassium with major surgery. Preoperatively, it is important to know if the patient is in a state of normal electrolyte balance. This information should be available to the nurse from the preoperative laboratory reports on all patients undergoing major surgery. Postoperatively, she will probably note in the urinalysis reports an increase in the urine sodium as well as a lessened amount of urine output. An important set of signs to watch for in the postoperative patient are those indicating excessive potassium deficit. The early signs include a general malaise, anorexia, and gas in the intestinal tract. The muscles become soft and the person may have tremors and may become disoriented. The nurse, then, should monitor the condition of the patient's muscles for signs of flaccidity. She should also be alert to signs of agitation, such as the patient's plucking at the bedclothes, and for signs of disorientation or confusion. If the potassium deficit is severe, muscles in the arms and legs may become flaccid, and there may be paresthesia. A heart block, cardiac arrest, or both can occur with severe potassium depletion.[4] The nurse should also be watchful for disturbances in the acid-base balance as these are evidenced by physical signs and symptoms and by laboratory findings (see Chapter 16).

Other circulatory disturbances can occur. One of the most common in surgical patients is the development of an *embolus*. Emboli are clots in the blood that have broken off and travel through the circulatory system until they reach a point where the vessel is too small for them to pass through. They then lodge in the vessel, blocking the passage and cutting off circulation to, or from, the tissues supplied by the artery or drained by the vein. Pulmonary embolism is a potential hazard for surgical patients.

Preoperatively, an assessment of the patient's circulatory status is essential. Existing problems such as diabetes, chronic heart conditions, varicose veins, or circulatory disorders causing cold extremities and poor circulation should be noted and recorded, as contributing factors in a person's vulnerability to clot formation following surgery. Postoperatively, one of the best measures to prevent clot formation is to get the patient mobile as quickly as possible. In some

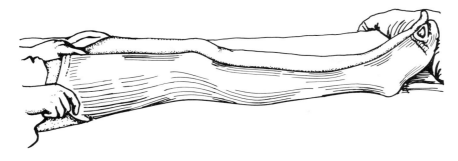

Antiembolism stockings force blood out of smaller blood vessels into the deep veins and also prevent pooling of blood in the legs. The stockings are removed several times a day to check the color of the skin, and toenail color can be checked more frequently through the opening in the stocking at the toes, to assure that the stockings are not exerting too much pressure and reducing circulation to the legs.

agencies antiembolism stockings are put on all patients who have undergone major surgical procedures. Frequent turning and passive exercises are needed for the patient whose condition does not warrant early ambulation. The nurse also needs to be observant for signs of *phlebitis* (inflammation of the veins), which is predisposing to clot formation. A common site for phlebitis is the thigh. Characteristic signs are redness, edema, pain, and warmth in the area. If the patient complains of any of these, the area should be carefully assessed by the nurse. Her observations should be documented accurately and reported immediately so that action can be taken to alert the patient's physician to the problem. It is very important in this instance for the nurse not to rub the affected area. If a clot has already formed, rubbing may cause it to become detached and start to travel through the circulatory system.

4. Inadequate Nutrition. Preoperatively, it is important to have good baseline data on a person's nutritional status, as well as his preferences in regard to food and fluids. Special dietary needs, as for example a low sodium diet or a diabetic diet, should be documented and the information passed along to the dietary department. In the immediate preoperative period, it is important for the nurse to see that the patient has nothing to eat or drink, in order to minimize the possibility of vomiting and aspiration of vomitus on induction of anesthesia or when the patient is coming out of anesthesia. Postoperatively, intravenous fluids are usually ordered for the first while. Then, the patient is gradually started on clear fluids, with the diet modified as the patient's tolerance for food and fluids increases. Some patients are on nasogastric feedings postoperatively. Some are maintained on nothing by mouth for a lengthy period of time,

in which case total parenteral nutrition may be required. The nurse's responsibilities include the monitoring of intravenous infusions and giving nasogastric feedings if these have been ordered. The nurse should observe the patient's food and fluid intake and encourage the patient to increase these gradually as his tolerance improves. A careful record of the patient's intake and output must be maintained. It is very important also for the nurse to watch for incipient signs of nausea and vomiting (see Chapter 14) particularly in a person who is recovering from anesthetic, is under sedation, or has limited mobility. The aspiration of vomitus is a major hazard in surgical patients, and it is a nursing responsibility to prevent this.

5. Difficulties in Voiding. Unless emergency surgery is being performed, the nurse usually has an opportunity to gather baseline data about the patient's normal voiding pattern and any problems he currently has, or has had recently, in urinary functioning. This information is usually picked up in the nursing history. If there is a long-standing problem, it will probably have been investigated prior to surgery, and the nurse will find information concerning it on the medical history of the patient.

A routine urinalysis is always done preoperatively, unless surgery is so urgently required that there is not time to obtain a urine sample. The nurse who is caring for the patient is usually responsible for collecting the sample and sending it to the laboratory. She should always check to see if it has been done, in any case, and should note the results for her baseline data about the patient. If there is abnormality in the test results—the presence of sugar in the urine is particularly important in that it may be indicative of a diabetic condition—this fact should be drawn to the surgeon's and the anesthetist's attention. Immediately preoperatively it is important for the nurse to observe the condition of the patient's bladder. The bladder should be empty before the patient is sent to the operating room. The nurse should see that the patient voids and also assess the patient's abdomen for possible bladder distention (see Chapter 15). A distended bladder can aggravate a potentially atonic condition postoperatively. There is also the danger of the bladder emptying reflexly when muscles are relaxed during anesthesia.

Postoperatively, it is important to monitor voiding closely. Both time and volume should be noted. The nurse should, again, check the patient's urinary output upon his return from the operating room with a catheter in situ, which must be monitored.

6. Disturbed Bowel Functioning. In the nursing history, the nurse collects information about the patient's normal bowel patterns and any long-standing or recent problems he has, as well as aids he may use to assist in regulating his bowels. The lower bowel and the rectum are usually cleared of stool by giving the person a preoperative enema. Sometimes, laxatives are given the evening before surgery as an alternative to an enema. These measures may be omitted if surgery is being performed on a very urgent basis. The nurse's observations of the results are recorded in the nurses' notes.

Postoperatively, the physician usually waits until there is a return of normal bowel sounds before permitting the patient to have solid foods. Frequently, it is a nursing responsibility to listen for bowel sounds with a stethoscope. The patient's ability to pass gas by rectum is an important observation for the nurse to make and record. Many surgical patients are distressed by the accumulation of gas in the intestines, and the nurse should assess the abdomen for distention indicating that this is occurring. Abdominal distention is minimized in the patient who has a nasogastric tube in place. If the patient has distention, a rectal tube is often inserted to aid in relieving the problem. The first passage of feces postoperatively is important to note; the patient may need laxatives or an enema to aid in evacuation of the bowel because of the slowing up of bowel functioning. The nurse should also monitor fluid intake in this regard, since an insufficient fluid intake will contribute to difficulties in passing stool. She should also note the amount of exercise the patient is doing. Exercise increases the vascular supply to the muscles, thereby improving muscle tone and helping to promote the early return to normal bowel functioning (see Chapter 16).

7. Decreased Mobility. During the Second World War, it was observed that patients who got up and walked around in the early postoperative period recovered sooner and had fewer complications than those who remained in bed for a week or so before being allowed to dangle their feet over the side of the bed and then progressed slowly to walking. Since then, early ambulation has become the general rule for surgical patients. However, the patient often needs a great deal of physical and psychological support from nursing staff in order to become mobile.

A careful assessment of the patient's motor functioning abilities is essential preoperatively, in order to identify existing and, wherever possible, potential problems the patient may have in regard to walking, sitting up in bed, or transferring from bed to a chair. Preparation for early ambulation begins with good preoperative teaching, which we will discuss later in this chapter. During surgery, the patient is often maintained in one position for a prolonged period of time. Anesthesia causes muscle paralysis. When the anesthetized patient is positioned, the muscles cannot contract against the stretching effects of certain positions. The patient may later complain of soreness in the muscles. He should be informed of the possible cause of it, and measures should be taken to relieve it. Often, movement is seriously curtailed in the postoperative patient, because of pain and his inability to move himself. The nurse must be alert to the patient's discomfort and assist him to move as much as possible, both for his comfort and to minimize the development of complications resulting from immobility (see Chapter 23). In most cases, the patient will receive physical therapy to assist in the maintenance of muscle tone and function. Often, it is a nursing responsibility to supervise and assist the patient with exercises suggested by the physical therapist.

The nurse should also be observant of the patient's difficulty, because of limited mobility or pain, in carrying out the necessary activities to maintain his bodily functions, such as problems with hygiene (e.g., because one arm has an intravenous infusion running into it), or problems in feeding himself, in using a bedpan, or in turning over in bed. It is a nursing responsibility to provide the help the patient needs.

8. Infection. Infection is an ever-present threat with any type of surgical procedure, and the most stringent precautions must be taken before, during, and after an operation to minimize this risk. Preoperatively, it is important to assess the patient's skin carefully. Is it in good general condition? Does it look well-nourished? Are there any breaks in the skin continuity that would give potential pathogens access to deeper tissues? Are there signs of infected areas on other parts of the body that could be potential sources for infection of the operative site? Does the patient have any predisposing conditions to infection, such as diabetes, obesity, or immunosuppression? Skin around the proposed operative area needs particular attention. Scratches, bruises, rashes, reddened areas, edema, or other abnormalities should be noted, the notations carefully documented, and a report made. In most cases, the skin is cleansed and shaved prior to surgery, with good clean, rather than sterile, technique. In orthopedic surgery, a sterile skin preparation is often done to minimize the possibility of pathogenic invasion of bone tissues that are being manipulated. Postoperatively, a strict watch must be kept on the incision site to detect signs of infection in or around the wound (see pages 596–597).

The nurse should also be alert to the possibility of generalized infection following surgery. Observations the nurse should make in regard to both generalized and localized infectious processes were discussed in Chapter 26. They include signs of redness, pain, swelling, unusual discharge, elevated temperature, and increased white blood cell count.

9. Pain. The nurse, in her initial assessment of the patient, assesses pain that he is currently having, or has had, prior to surgery. Preoperatively, the nurse should also ascertain the patient's expectations in regard to the pain he is likely to experience with his surgery.

Before coming in to a health agency, most patients have talked with someone who has had surgery—possibly even the type of operation they are scheduled to have. Usually, the pain element is discussed. The experience of other people will affect the person's expectations. Then, too, as we noted in Chapter 21, reactions to pain are highly individualized. It is helpful to find out just what the patient expects and, if possible, his previous experience and reactions to pain. The nurse should correct any misconceptions he has. She should also discuss with him his surgeon's usual postoperative orders for pain relief and reassure him that his needs for pain relief will be watched closely and responded to promptly.

Postoperatively, the patient's pain must be monitored closely. Strong analgesics are often needed in the first 48 hours (sometimes longer), with medications of a lesser intensity continued for a longer period. As we mentioned in Chapter 21, a number of factors may contribute to pain. With the postoperative patient, it may be that he is in an uncomfortable position—perhaps because of limitations on his mobility—and a position change may help. Too tight a dressing will also cause pain because of pressure, and the tight dressing may also be cutting off circulation. It is important, then, to observe the patient's position, to check the dressing for tightness, and to assess the condition of the skin in the surrounding area for warmth, color, and mobility to ensure that a dressing is not impairing circulation.

10. Disturbed Sensory Functioning. With any type of anesthesia, it is implicit that sensory functioning will be disturbed. Prior to surgery, it is imperative that the nurse have accurate baseline data on the efficiency of functioning of the individual's sensory abilities. This information should be part of the nurse's initial clinical appraisal and her history on the patient. Postoperatively, it is important to assess the functioning of sensory organs in the areas affected by the surgical procedure and those affected by the anesthesia. For example, in a patient who has had a spinal anesthetic, it is important to monitor the return of sensory functioning in the hips and legs (all areas below the site of insertion of the anesthetic agent). Similar monitoring is needed in an area that has been anesthetized by local anesthesia. Sensory functioning may also be disturbed as a result of a surgical procedure. If the procedure involved the nose or mouth, for example, vision, smell, or taste will be affected. The nurse should also be mindful of the possibility that neural pathways may have been disturbed, by accident or by design, during the course of surgery. She must, therefore, be observant of any deviations from the initial baseline data in regard to sensory functioning, so that these can be documented and reported as soon as noted, and adequate precautions can be taken to assure his safety.

11. Altered Mental Functioning. During the surgical process the individual's mental functioning is affected by a number of factors, including medications, anesthesia, and disturbances in his internal physiological processes. He will experience varying levels of consciousness as anesthesia is induced and as he recovers from it. We mentioned that some people have untoward reactions to sedation and to anesthetic agents. Older people are particularly sensitive to drug reactions, and there are now large numbers of older people undergoing surgery. There are also, of course, many other causes of disturbed mental functioning. (We mentioned that it may occur with excessive potassium depletion—a not uncommon happening in patients who have had major surgery.) The nurse should be watchful for signs of disorientation and confusion in all surgical patients. The confused and the disoriented patient and the patient with altered levels of consciousness have increased safety and protection needs, as we discussed in Chapter 24.

12. Anxiety or Depression. Anxiety is such a common accompaniment of surgery, that the nurse should always be alert to signs of it in her pre- and postoperative patients. One of the best ways to assess the patient's anxiety is to spend time with him, finding out what he knows about the pending (or performed) surgical procedure and how he feels about it. By maintaining a pleasant, relaxed atmosphere and spending enough time with the patient, the nurse can usually gain insight into the nature and extent of his anxieties. It is helpful to know what the surgeon has told the patient and to assess the patient's understanding of the surgeon's explanation. Often, the nurse can help to clear up misunderstandings by explaining in more detail or in simple terminology what others have told the patient.

The nurse should also be observant of the physical signs and symptoms, and the behavioral manifestations of anxiety. One can usually identify the person who is tense, but some people do not like to admit their fears and will cover them up with laughing and joking behavior. A discussion of the physiological and behavioral manifestations of anxiety as well as the individual's subjective perceptions of it, are included in Chapter 30, which the student may want to refer to at this point.

Some people react to stressful situations by becoming depressed rather than anxious. The nurse may see this in some preoperative patients, if they feel that their situation is hopeless and nothing can really be done about it. Following surgery, when the body's reserves are low, there is also a potential problem of depression. If the surgery has gone well, and the intervention has been successful, the person will usually experience a great feeling of relief when he is informed of the results. Sometimes, however, nurses assume that the physician has told the patient (he generally does), only to find that the patient has been experiencing considerable distress because everyone took it for granted that the patient knew the results, while in fact no one has told him. If the prognosis is poor, or if a malignancy has been discovered during the operation, the patient is likely to be very anxious and may well become quite depressed. It is mandatory for the nurse to know the surgical findings and to provide the emotional support the patient needs in his distress (see Chapters 30 and 31).

It is important for the nurse to remember, too, that the patient's family and the significant others in his life are also anxious and may become depressed. Keeping the family informed and providing them with thoughtful, caring attention to their needs is also a part of the nurse's role. It contributes significantly to the patient's emotional security if he knows that his loved ones are being looked after.

13. Lessened Capacity for Self-Protection. We have mentioned numerous times throughout this section that the nurse has a responsibility to protect the surgical patient because he is frequently not able to protect himself. The nurse should be alert to any or all of the problems we have discussed that decrease the person's ability to cope with his own safety needs. Particularly important to watch for are the signs of altered levels of consciousness, disturbed mental functioning, limited mobility, weakness on the part of the patient, and anxiety or depression. It is a fundamental responsibility of nurses to do all in their power to protect the patient from harm. Measures we discussed in Chapter 23 are particularly pertinent to the surgical patient and should be reviewed by all nurses caring for surgical patients.

PRIORITIES FOR NURSING ACTION

Situations that necessitate prompt action on the nurse's part are hemorrhage, shock, evisceration, and infection. *Hemorrhage* is always a medical emergency and the nurse should report her observations promptly if she encounters fresh bleeding or excessive oozing from a healing wound, so that action can be taken before the bleeding becomes excessive. If the nurse notes signs of gross bleeding, or signs that the patient is going into shock, immediate action is required. The beginning student should summon help at once. In this case, it is preferable, if possible, for the nurse to send someone else for aid and stay with the patient herself. He is usually apprehensive and needs support.

Shock may be caused by excessive bleeding, or by other factors disturbing the body's physiological balance before, during, or following surgery. It is always a medical emergency.

Evisceration is a visible separation of a wound that allows underlying viscera to protrude. Sometimes there is bleeding at the site of the

PRINCIPLES RELEVANT TO PRE- AND POSTOPERATIVE CARE

1. Surgery evokes a major stress reaction in the body.
2. A major assault on the body, such as surgery, lowers a person's ability to cope with other stressors.
3. Major surgery affects a person's ability to meet all of his basic needs.
4. The skin is the body's first line of defense against harmful agents.
5. Penetration of the skin by surgical incision provides a portal of entry for invading pathogens.
6. The very young and the very old are particularly vulnerable to the adverse effects of surgery, as are people with respiratory problems, cardiovascular disease, abnormal blood coagulation patterns, diabetes, or disorders causing vascular insufficiency.
7. The extremely fearful patient is a poor surgical risk.
8. Fear of the unknown is a potent factor in pre-surgical anxiety.
9. Information can often help to dispel fear.
10. Learning is most effective when a person needs and wants to learn.

protrusion. Usually there is localized pain. This situation is a medical emergency and requires prompt surgical intervention. The patient's physician should be notified at once. While awaiting his instructions, the nurse should cover the protruding viscera with sterile dressings soaked in normal saline. The area should never be probed, nor an attempt made to push the viscera back into the wound. The patient will need to be prepared for emergency surgery. If the beginning student observes evisceration, for example, while she is changing the dressing, she should summon help at once.

Signs of localized or generalized *infection* should also be drawn to the team leader's attention promptly, so that appropriate intervention can be initiated as early as possible to arrest the infection in the individual and to prevent its spread to other patients, visitors, and staff.

SPECIFIC NURSING MEASURES

Teaching

Good pre- and postoperative teaching helps to prepare the patient for surgery and makes the postoperative recovery period smoother and less hazardous for the patient. Numerous studies have documented the tangible benefits of preoperative teaching in making the patient less anxious both before and after surgery, in minimizing postoperative complications, and in hastening the individual's recovery. Many agencies have developed a structured format for teaching people who are having surgery, including the specific things they need to know, the skills that need to be developed, and the common fears

and anxieties that should be examined. Sometimes the teaching program is on a one-to-one basis. Sometimes it is done in groups, either before the person is admitted (when it may be done on an ambulatory basis) or after admission. Many good teaching aids have been developed, both within agencies and by health care supply houses and drug companies. Whatever type of program is used in the agency in which you are having clinical experience or, later, working, it is important that the content you use in your teaching be consistent with the policies of the agency and have the approval of the surgeon.

It cannot be overemphasized that a structured teaching program, whether carried out on an individual or group basis, is much more likely to be effective than one that is carried out on an impromptu basis as the need arises.

The process of developing and implementing a teaching program for surgical patients is the same as that for all other patients. Needed are:

1. *A good data base about the patient* (or patients, if a group is to be taught). Particularly pertinent to the process of teaching and learning are a knowledge of the patient as a person (such as his age, occupation, level of educational attainment, his family, his interests and hobbies), his health history, his previous experiences with surgery, and his understanding of and particular concerns about the surgical procedure he is to undergo.

It is helpful to involve the patient's family or significant others in the teaching program. They are the ones who are best able to provide the support and assistance the patient needs to supplement the nurse's teaching and to help him in utilizing it.

It is also important to assess the patient's

ability to learn, and to identify any problems that might interfere with his learning, such as poor eyesight, a hearing loss, extreme anxiety, or limited mobility.

2. *An assessment of his learning needs.* This process of assessment is similar to the pre-test many teachers give at the start of a course, or unit, to identify the extent of the student's previous knowledge or skill. It is important for the nurse to determine the patient's level of understanding of the surgical process and the type of surgery he is to have in order to determine what he needs to learn.

If there is not much time between the patient's admission and his departure for the operating room, the nurse will have to set priorities, that is, she will have to decide on the most important things that the patient needs to learn before surgery. She will also have to take into consideration the level of his anxiety. When the person's anxiety is high, and many things are happening to him all at once, he is not receptive to teaching, except that designed to meet his immediate needs.

3. *Identification of content.* On the basis of the assessment, specific topics that need to be included in the teaching program are identified. If some of the teaching is done prior to the patient's admission to a health agency, the agency's admission procedure should be explained. Other topics that usually need to be included are: (a) terminology the patient needs to know to converse intelligently with health personnel and to understand what they are talking about; (b) encounters the person is likely to have with other departments, e.g., the laboratory, x-ray, dietary, and physiotherapy departments; (c) preparation for surgery, e.g., skin preparation, enemas, medications, care of his valuables, and the consent form; (d) going to the operating room, e.g., sedation, the stretcher, safety precautions, and the anesthesia procedure; (e) usual experiences in the postanesthetic recovery room, e.g., waking up, the taking of vital signs, turning, deep breathing, coughing, intravenous infusions and blood transfusions, tubes and drains, and the checking of dressings; (f) returning to the nursing unit; (g) nature and extent of the pain he is likely to experience, measures taken to minimize the pain experience, and how to request pain relief; (h) specific exercises to be done pre- and postoperatively, e.g., turning, deep breathing, coughing, and exercises to maintain muscle tone or to strengthen specific muscles; (i) ambulation; (j) dressing changes; and (k) going home, e.g., expected length of stay; care of incision; dressings, medication, and exercises to be continued at home; activity level; home care services; and postoperative checkups.

In identifying specific content the student will find the questions, Who? What? When? Where? Why? and How? helpful to ask herself regarding the topics we have listed.[5]

4. *Development of specific behavioral objectives.* Identification of the content to be covered leads to the development of a list of expected patient behaviors, or outcomes. A set of specific behavioral objectives developed for one preoperative teaching program is shown below.

5. *Selection of teaching strategies and teaching aids.* The nature of the material to be taught and characteristics of the person or persons doing the learning help to determine the most

A PREOPERATIVE TEACHING PROGRAM

Specific Behavioral Objectives

At the end of the Pre-Operative Class, the patient and his family will be able to:

1. verbally define or describe, with at least 70 percent accuracy, the terms introduced at the beginning of the class.

2. verbally describe the usual expected encounters upon admission to the hospital to the time of surgery, with 70 percent accuracy.

3. verbally describe what usually takes place in the immediate postoperative period, with 70 percent accuracy.

4. correctly demonstrate the "stir-up" routine as shown by the nurse instructor, *i.e.*, cough, deep breathe and move legs.

5. ask questions comfortably.

6. use "Blow bottles" properly if that is to be a part of his post-operative course (could also be IPPB).

7. assist in teaching other patients in the class.

8. find the surgical waiting area.

9. state acceptance of patient participation in post-operative care and recovery.

10. state awareness of any special interest groups, agencies or rehabilitation centers that might be of assistance post-operatively.

11. state awareness of the hospital Social Services Department, its location, and the services that it offers.

Methods and Materials
Methods:
1. Lecture—short
2. Observation-tour
3. Discussion
4. Teacher-learner demonstration
Materials:
1. Blackboard
2. Sphygmomanometer, stethoscope
3. Blow bottles
4. Anti-embolism stockings
5. Special equipment ordered by physician
6. Posters, picture, graphs
7. Audio-visual equipment videotape films to be used with pt's television)

From Schrankel, D. P.: Preoperative Teaching. *Supervisor Nurse,* 9:82–90, May, 1978, p. 90.

appropriate methodology and assist in the selection of teaching aids. Suggested methods and material for preoperative teaching are listed below the specific behavioral objectives shown on page 588.

6. *Evaluation Techniques.* Ways of evaluating the extent to which learning has taken place are built into the behavioral objectives, if criteria have been carefully and realistically determined and included in the stated objectives. As with all types of teaching, the nurse must obtain feedback from the patient and must observe his utilization of the knowledge and skills he has gained in order to evaluate his progress.

Preparation of the Skin

In most agencies the area of the planned incision is shaved prior to surgery. The benefits of preoperative shaving versus the risks of increasing the potential for infection by shaving are currently being debated. Some agencies advocate other methods of removing hair, such as using depilatory creams.

Each agency usually has its own special procedures for preparation of the skin prior to surgery. We will, therefore, only offer general guidelines here on the area to be prepared, the equipment needed if shaving is to be done, and the methodology.

Area. Generally, the area that is prepared is larger than the area that is expected to be incised, in case the incision needs to be extended during the procedure. There is fairly general agreement on the extent of the skin preparation for commonly performed surgical procedures involving various parts of the body. Examples of areas that are usually prepared are shown on page 590.

Equipment. A dry or wet shave may be done. For a dry shave, the nurse will need a set of electric clippers, a pair of scissors (for cutting long hairs), tissues for wiping off excess hair, towels for draping the patient, and a good light to see by. If a wet shave is to be done, the nurse will need a good, sharp razor (a straight razor or a safety razor may be used). Disposable razors are in common use in many agencies. She will also need a liquid soap solution for cleansing the skin, cotton sponges and cotton-tipped applicators, a pair of forceps, a waterproof drape, and a covering towel. A basin is also needed for disposing of used sponges and applicators. Most agencies have prepackaged sets that contain all the equipment needed for a skin preparation.

Method. The nurse explains the procedure to the patient and the reasons for doing it. In most instances, it is easier to carry out the procedure when the person is lying flat in bed. An exception is made when the head or the neck is involved; then, it is usually easier to have the person sitting up. The area of the body to be prepared is exposed, and the patient is draped to protect modesty and to keep him warm. The waterproof drape and covering towel are placed under the patient to protect the bed clothing. The nurse then lathers the skin with the soap solution, using the forceps and sponges as needed. (This step is omitted in a dry shave.) A razor is then used to remove the hairs. The razor is best held at a 45-degree angle to the skin. A clean, close shave is desired, with no nicks or scratches that would allow infection to enter the operative area. Shaving is done against the grain of the hair shaft (in the direction in which the hair is growing). Following the shave, the area is rinsed and patted dry with cotton sponges. Cotton tipped applicators are used to clean out the umbilical cavity and other small areas such as the ear lobes. In some agencies, before putting away the equipment, the nurse has her team leader or the charge nurse check the preparation. Then the patient is made comfortable, the equipment is taken care of, and the procedure is documented in the patient's record.

Immediate Preoperative Care

The afternoon or evening prior to surgery (or, immediately prior, in the case of emergency surgery) the preoperative skin preparation is usually done, the patient is examined by the resident or intern, and is visited by the anesthesiologist, who may or may not carry out his own physical examination of the patient. It is now becoming more frequent for a member of the operating room nursing staff also to visit the patient the evening before surgery. The purposes of this visit are to assess the patient and plan his care, to get to know him, to explain the operative procedure, to tell him the expected time the surgery will take place, to answer his questions, and, it is hoped, to dispel some of his fears.

In many hospitals, the schedule of operations is prepared in the late afternoon for the next day's surgery and is sent around to the surgical nursing units.

If an enema has been ordered for the patient, it is usually given after the evening meal on the day prior to surgery. It is sometimes done in the morning for surgery scheduled in the afternoon, but this is not usually done because the slate

Examples of the Skin Areas to be Prepared for Surgery as Determined by the Type of Operation

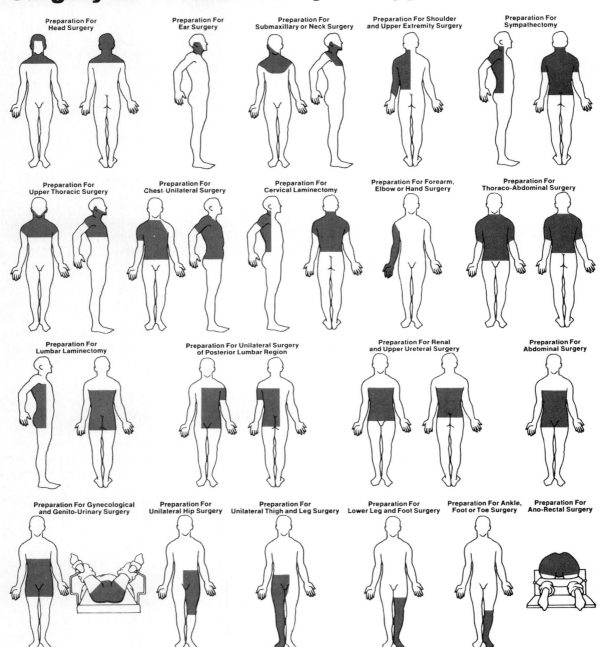

operative site prepping instructions with Betadine Surgical Scrub and Betadine Antiseptic Solution

After the skin area is shaved, wet it with water. Apply BETADINE Surgical Scrub and rub thoroughly for about five minutes. Then develop a lather and rinse off by aid of sterile gauze saturated with water. Pat dry with sterile towel. Paint area with BETADINE Solution (or spray area with BETADINE Aerosol Spray) and allow to dry. If self-adhering plastic drapes are to be used, you may apply these directly over the <u>dried</u> BETADINE Solution.

may be changed and the patient's surgery moved up on the schedule. A sedative is usually ordered for the patient at bedtime, to ensure a good night's rest prior to surgery. An order for nothing by mouth is usually enforced after midnight. A sign should be posted on the patient's bed (or some other place where all staff and visitors will see it) to ensure that the order is carried out.

The patient's skin, hair, fingernails, and toenails should be cleaned prior to surgery to decrease the amount of bacteria on the skin. If he has not had a bath the evening before, one is sometimes given the day of surgery. After the bath, or morning care, the patient puts on a freshly laundered hospital gown and, in some agencies, operating room stockings.

The patient's hair should be free of pins, barrettes, or other objects. Women patients are advised not to wear makeup or nail polish, to facilitate assessment of skin color. Jewelry and other valuables the patient may have at the bedside are removed for safekeeping, either in a locked cupboard on the nursing unit or in the hospital safe. The nurse sees that the patient voids and that the urinary bladder is empty before the preoperative medications are given. If the patient has dentures, these are removed and put in a container in the patient's bedside locker. The patient's vital signs are taken. The nurse checks to make sure the consent form has been signed and is on the chart before giving preoperative sedation.

The nurse who is looking after the patient preoperatively is usually responsible for giving the premedication ordered to induce drowsiness and to lessen secretions in the mouth and throat. Once the medication has been given, the patient should be kept in bed, with the side rails up as a safety precaution, and he should be left undisturbed until called for surgery.

The nurse, meanwhile, makes sure that everything that should have been done has, in fact, been done for the patient. She checks the medication orders to see if regular medications that have been ordered have been given (unless there were orders to withhold these) and charted. She makes sure that vital signs have been taken and recorded with a notation regarding any abnormalities. She notes whether an enema was ordered, or given, and the results noted, and that the time and amount of voiding have been recorded. If there were no results from the enema, the surgeon should be notified.

The nurse makes sure that the chart is complete, with all laboratory and other preoperative tests and investigations noted, and available results attached to the record.

Many agencies have developed a preoperative checklist to assist nursing staff in making sure that no detail has been omitted.

When the patient is called for surgery, the nurse assists the operating room escort to help the patient transfer to the stretcher unless the patient is going to the operating room in his own bed. The patient's chart, and x-rays if these are to accompany him, are collected from the nursing station. The nurse accompanies the patient to the operating room, where she reports to the nurse in the holding room or waiting room. On her return to the unit, she makes up the bed for his return (see Chapter 20).

Immediate Postoperative Care

Most patients are seen from the operating room directly to a postanesthetic recovery room for the special care and attention that is required in the immediate postoperative period. This care includes:

1. Assessing the patient's physiological status on arrival and at frequent intervals during his stay in the recovery area, including level of consciousness, vital signs, presence or absence of reflexes, and drainage from dressings, tubes, and collecting bags.
2. Carrying out immediate postoperative orders for infusions, medications, and treatments
3. Seeing that orders for x-rays or laboratory work are carried out promptly
4. Monitoring the administration of oxygen
5. Monitoring the administration of intravenous infusions and blood transfusions
6. Maintaining a safe physical environment for the patient's recovery
7. Providing emotional support and comfort for the patient[6]

The patient is transferred to the nursing unit when he is fully conscious, his vital signs are stabilized, and his physical condition is judged satisfactory. If his condition warrants more intensive nursing care than the nursing unit is able to provide, he may, instead, be sent to an intensive care unit. The nurse in charge of the unit to which he is being transferred is alerted to prepare for his arrival. A nurse and an escort accompany the patient to the unit, where they notify the charge nurse of his arrival. The operating room staff transfer the patient to his own bed, making sure that he is in a comfortable position and that all tubes, drains, suctioning equipment, and other equipment are in place and functioning. The operating room nurse shows the receiving nurse the position of the dressing and explains the placement of drains and their care. If the patient is still sleepy, he is usually best on his side, unless there are contraindications to this position. All safety precautions must be taken to ensure his safety. This includes putting the bed in the lowest position compatible with safe care and positioning the patient so that his airway is patent and secretions can drain easily from the mouth.[2] The recovery room nurse gives a verbal report on the patient's progress in the recovery room stay, reviewing the records kept and the patient's condition in the immediate postoperative period. She completes her notation on the patient's record, and the chart is then handed over to the nursing unit staff.

The nurse who receives the patient takes the patient's vital signs on arrival, assesses his level of consciousness, checks his dressing, and notes the position of drains.

She makes sure that the patient is warm, comfortable, and safe before she leaves his room. An emesis basin should be left at the bedside, within easy reach of the patient, and his call light attached to his gown. Constant vigilance is required to maintain his safety, and prompt attention must be paid to the patient's signal for help and to the earliest signs of discomfort or distress the nurse observes in the patient. We discussed points to watch for earlier in connection with assessment of the patient's ability to cope with basic needs pre- and postoperatively (pages 580–586). The nurse will want to review the operating room and recovery room records as soon as she is assured of the patient's immediate safety and comfort. There will be new, postoperative medication and treatment orders to be noted and implemented. Careful documen-

Postoperative exercises. (Adapted from Shaughnessy Hospital, Vancouver, Patient Information Pamphlet.)

1. Place one hand over stomach, take a deep breath in through nose, letting stomach rise. Blow out through pursed lips.

2. Place hand on ribs, breathe in, letting ribs push against your hands. Blow out through pursed lips.

Do each exercise 5 times per hour when awake, for the first few days, or until you are up and walking around.

Lying or sitting in bed: with knees bent, hold your hands or a pillow firmly over the incision for support. Take 5 deep breaths and then cough.

or

Sitting on side of bed: support incision, lean forward a little, keep feet on floor, take 5 deep breaths and then cough.

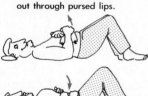
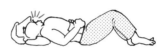
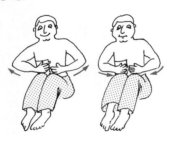

DEEP BREATHING

COUGHING

Bend and straighten one leg; then the other. Do 3 times a day, 5 times each.

Point your toes towards your head, then towards the foot of the bed. Make your feet go around in circles. Do 3 times a day, 5 times each.

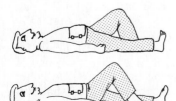
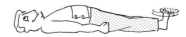

LEG EXERCISE

FOOT EXERCISES

MOVING IN BED

Change your position often, at least every 2 hours while awake. If you have difficulty moving because of your incision, here are some tips.

1. To move your body sideways: lie on your back, bend knees, lift your hips and shift them sideways; follow with shoulders.

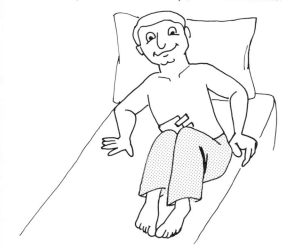

2. To roll onto your side: bend knees, support your incision with your hand and roll like a log.

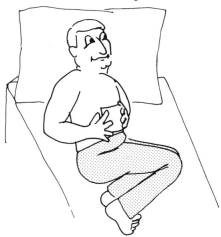

3. It is even easier if the bed rail is up. Reach across to hang on to the bed rail and pull yourself onto your side, rolling like a log.

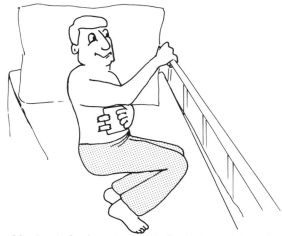

4. To sit up on the side of the bed: log roll onto your side, drop your legs over the edge of the bed and push up using your arms.

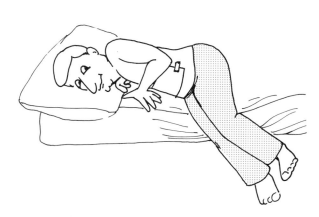

Moving in bed postoperatively. (Adapted from Shaughnessy Hospital, Vancouver, Patient Information Pamphlet.)

tation of the patient's time of arrival back in the nursing unit, and his condition on arrival, as well as all observations made subsequently and all nursing actions carried out, is essential.

In the early stages of his recovery, the patient will probably need reminding, and often assistance, to practice deep breathing and coughing and the other exercises taught preoperatively. Ambulation begins as soon as medically feasible, when the patient's vital signs are stable. Most surgical patients are up within the first 24 hours. Orders will be written by the physician regard-

ing ambulation—when it is to start, how long it is to be, and how often. It is a nursing responsibility to assist the patient to carry out these orders. Many patients are very apprehensive about getting out of bed so soon after surgery. They are afraid that their stitches will break open, that it will be too painful, or that they won't have the strength or will power. You can reassure them that there are several layers of stitching, that the incision site is well protected, and that a little tension on the suture line helps to promote healing. You can assure him that you will be there to support and assist him as need be. It is best to get the patient up while he is still comfortable and free of pain, but not under the effects of a recent medication that impairs his senses. One authority suggests that ambulation can often be tried an hour before the next pain medication is due.[7]

In preparing the patient for ambulation, the nurse gets his slippers or shoes, draws the curtains for privacy, and clears the pathway from bed to door of obstructions. Tubes are disconnected whenever possible. Some cannot be disconnected, and they must be secured by pins or tape.

Continuing Postoperative Care

The patient needs close monitoring during the first 48 hours following surgery. He is usually quite drowsy for the first day or so and requires special precautions to ensure that he is protected from all hazards, that his basic physiological needs are met, and that postoperative complications are prevented, insofar as this is possible, or picked up in an early stage so that prompt action can be initiated. The nurse should make sure that the patient is in a comfortable position and that he is free from pain. Pain tends to make the patient restless, and he could quite easily damage early tissue repair if he is not kept comfortable. The patient should not, however, be kept in the same position. His position must be changed frequently.

The nurse should assess the patient at frequent intervals to watch for signs or symptoms of the common problems that we discussed earlier in this chapter. In addition, the nurse must be constantly alert to see that intravenous infusions are kept running at the required rate and replenished as ordered before they run dry. She also needs to check the infusion site frequently to make sure that the infusion has not gone into the tissues. Equipment such as suctioning apparatus and drainage tubes must be checked to see that they are functioning well. The nurse also needs to keep a watchful eye on dressings for signs of leakage or oozing.

Intake and output must be monitored closely. If voiding has not occurred in the first 8 hours after surgery, this fact should be reported. A flowsheet for recording vital signs and other pertinent observations is helpful to ensure that the patient is checked at regular specified intervals and the nurse's observations noted and documented. The documentation is essential for legal reasons (see Chapter 7).

If the patient has a draining catheter in situ, he often carries the drainage bag with him as he walks. The IV infusion must be on a portable pole and may need to be transferred to one. All infusion fluids should be above the infusion site, and all drainage receptacles below the point where the tube exits from the body.

The bed should be low enough that the patient can easily reach the floor when he puts his legs over the side of the bed. It is often easier on the patient if the bed is in the high Fowler's position. Most patients like to wear their own bathrobe and slippers, and should be helped into these, or into hospital ones if they have not brought their own.

It is usually advisable for the patient to dangle his legs from the side of the bed for a few minutes before attempting to stand up. At this time, the nurse assesses the patient for dizziness. If he is able to proceed, he can use the nurse's shoulder or the side rail on the bed for support as he steps onto the floor. A chair should be conveniently placed by the bed so that he can sit down on it if he feels weak or dizzy. He should be well supported when walking, and may require the aid of two people if he is unsteady on his feet. Surgical patients usually have a tendency to bend over to protect their incision when they are walking. This, however, throws them off balance. It also hampers their breathing. They should be encouraged to stand up straight and look ahead at where they are going.

Ambulation is usually ordered for a given number of times per day, and it is important that these orders are scrupulously carried out. As the patient builds up strength, the length and time of his walks is gradually increased.

During the course of his convalescence, the patient may have stitches that need to be removed. This procedure is usually a medical one, although it is sometimes done by the nurse. Sometimes, the doctor wishes to do the first dressing change in order to observe healing of the wound. Often, however, changing dressings is a nursing responsibility.

Care of Wounds

1. *Skin and mucous membranes normally harbor microorganisms.* In order to decrease the transfer of organisms to a wound, handwashing is indicated before and after attending a patient. In addition, the use of an antiseptic upon and around a wound decreases the number of microorganisms and thus lessens the danger of infection.

2. *Microorganisms are present in the air.* Sometimes a wound is left exposed, particularly if it is a superficial one that has closed itself.

PRINCIPLES RELEVANT TO THE CARE OF WOUNDS

1. **Skin and mucous membranes normally harbor microorganisms.**
2. **Microorganisms are present in the air.**
3. **Moisture facilitates the growth of microorganisms.**
4. **Moisture facilitates the movement of microorganisms.**
5. **Fluids move through materials by capillary action.**
6. **Fluids flow downward as a result of gravitational pull.**
7. **The respiratory tract often harbors microorganisms, which can be spread to open wounds.**
8. **The blood transports the materials that nourish and repair body tissues.**
9. **Skin and mucous membranes can be injured by chemical, mechanical, thermal, and microbial agents.**

The majority of surgical incisions, however, and wounds involving deeper-lying tissues are protected by a sterile dressing. When the dressing is changed, precautions are taken to keep the time the wound is exposed as short as possible and the circulation of the air in the room at a minimum. These precautions have a twofold purpose: to protect the wound from possible contamination by air-borne bacteria in the atmosphere and to minimize the convection of microorganisms from the wound to the circulating air. When a wound is infected, or there is possibility that pathogenic bacteria (such as *Staphylococcus aureus*) are present in the atmosphere, these precautions are particularly important.

3. *Moisture facilitates the growth of microorganisms.* Dressings that are wet with drainage are more likely to foster the growth of organisms than are dry dressings. Often dressings are changed whenever they become soaked through to the top. If there is no order to change the dressing, it can be reinforced with additional dry sterile dressings to inhibit the transfer of organisms from the outside to the wound until the physician has been notified.

4. *Moisture facilitates the movement of microorganisms.* When a dressing becomes soaked through to the outside, the movement of microorganisms toward the wound is facilitated because the moisture provides a vehicle for their transport. Because the outside of a dressing is generally highly contaminated, the movement of organisms from the outside inward must be prevented. Maintaining dry dressings inhibits the multiplication and the transfer of organisms.

5. *Fluids move through materials by capillary action.* Loosely woven fabrics such as gauze provide a good surface for capillary action. The fluid is absorbed through the material as each thread in the material conducts the fluid away from the wound by the action of the surface

tension of the fluid and the forces of adhesion and cohesion. Adhesion and cohesion are forces that draw together.

6. *Fluids flow downward as a result of gravitational pull.* In a draining wound the area of greatest contamination is, in all probability, the lowest part, where the drainage collects. If it is desirable to promote drainage, a drain or packing is usually placed in the lowest part of the wound by the doctor.

7. *The respiratory tract often harbors microorganisms, which can be spread to open wounds.* When an open wound is exposed, measures are taken to prevent the spread of microorganisms from the respiratory tract. It is common practice in many agencies for nurses and physicians to wear masks while dressing wounds, and in some instances patients also wear masks. In any case, as a precautionary measure against contamination, it is advisable not to talk while a wound is exposed.

8. *The blood transports the materials that nourish and repair body tissues.* When dressing and bandaging a wound, care is exercised to ensure that circulation to the area is not restricted in any way. Bandages and dressings are never made restrictively tight, and they are applied starting at the distal portion of the body and proceeding to the proximal portion as a means of promoting venous flow.

9. *Skin and mucous membranes can be injured by chemical, mechanical, thermal, and microbial agents.* The disinfectants and medications used to cleanse and treat a wound and the surrounding tissue should be strong enough to be effective, but they should not irritate healthy tissue. Protective ointments such as sterile petrolatum can be used to protect the skin when it is necessary to use irritating disinfectants upon open wounds. Ointments such as zinc oxide are frequently used to protect the skin from irritating drainage.

To avoid mechanical injury at bony prominences that are to be bandaged, padding is provided to prevent irritation due to friction. Adhesive tape must be removed carefully; often, to avoid trauma, specially prepared solvents can be used to loosen the adhesive. Thermal injury can be avoided by the use of solutions at a temperature which is noninjurious to tissue. Room temperature is generally considered to be safe for most tissues.

Microbial injury can be largely avoided by practicing sterile technique in the care of wounds. All solutions, dressings, and equipment that come into contact with an open wound should be sterile.

Organisms Causing Wound Infection. There are several organisms that are commonly found in wound infections. Of the gram-positive group, *Staphylococcus aureus* and *S. albus* are found most commonly. These are spherical asymmetric bacteria that are normally found in the nose, skin, and feces. The alpha- and beta-hemolytic streptococci also cause many infectious processes. It has been estimated that 8 per cent of all people carry these bacteria in the nasopharynx.

The toxigenic clostridia are anaerobic spore-forming bacilli. They thrive in airless conditions, being found in the intestinal tracts of animals, in dust, and in soil. *Clostridium tetani*, the cause of tetanus, is a well known member of this family; many physicians automatically give prophylactic doses of tetanus toxoid to patients whose wounds have come in contact with soil.

Of the gram-negative bacteria, *Escherichia coli* and species of *Aerobacter* and *Alcaligenes* are frequently found in wounds. These, together with *Proteus* and *Pseudomonas,* are the principal inhabitants of the intestine. They can also often be isolated in the anogenital area, and are frequent causes of urinary tract infections.

General Considerations in Wound Care. The basic goals of nursing action in the care of patients with wounds are:

1. To promote tissue healing
2. To prevent the development of infection in the wound
3. To promote the comfort of the patient

Just as there is considerable variety in the kinds of wounds, so there is a variety in the care that they require. A wound may be closed by sutures, with no drainage resulting. This type of wound is often left with the original dressing in place until it is completely healed. Sometimes wounds are sprayed with a clear plastic material that seals the wound and eliminates the need for any dressings.

Observation of Wounds. The physician's instructions regarding wound care, and any specific precautions to be taken, will be written and included in the doctor's orders.

When a wound is examined, as, for example, while a dressing is changed, certain features of the wound itself and the discharge from it are carefully observed. The wound is observed for the approximation of its edges. Some wounds are closed by sutures or skin clips, others by the pressure of a bandage or butterfly tape. Steri-Strips are frequently used, or a butterfly tape can be made from a strip of adhesive tape narrowed in the middle and placed across the wound so that the adhesive part of the tape sticks to the patient's skin on both sides of the wound and draws the edges of the wound together. The adhesive side of the tape directly over the wound is usually covered so that it will not adhere to the wound itself. Gapping in a sutured or taped wound could delay healing and should be reported. Some wounds are not closed deliberately but are left to close naturally by second intention. A wound is also observed for signs of inflammation and infection, such as redness, swelling, pain, heat, and limitation of function of the afflicted part of the body.

The amount of discharge that is considered normal is dependent upon the site, size, and type of wound. Normally it is not unusual for a wound to exude some serous drainage postoperatively. (Serum is the clear portion of the blood.) A wound in the anogenital area can be expected to have more serous discharge than a wound of the face. Serous discharge is amber in color and contains water, blood cells, and some cellular debris.

Sanguineous drainage is red. ("Sanguineous" refers to blood.) Bright sanguineous drainage is composed of fresh blood; dark sanguineous drainage is composed of old blood.

Infected wounds often have a purulent discharge. "Purulent" is defined as containing pus. Pus can be white, yellow, pink, or green, often depending upon the infecting organism. It is usually thick and may have a distinctly unpleasant odor. In addition to the three basic kinds of wound discharge, there are combinations such as serosanguineous, seropurulent, and purosanguineous.

An accurate description of a wound's discharge must include the amount. Traditional descriptions, such as gross, moderate, and small are highly subject to individual interpretation and often relative to the site and type of wound. For example, the amount of drainage that would be considered moderate after perineal surgery would usually be considered abnormally large after an appendectomy. Because the use of these adjectives can be misleading, more exact measures are used. It is the policy in some agencies to describe the amount of drainage by the number of dressings that are soaked and drainage upon the dressing. An example of this kind of descriptive charting would be "serosanguineous drainage 7.5 cm. (3 inches) in diameter soaked through two gauze dressings."

In addition to a description of the wound and the drainage, other signs and symptoms are recorded—for example, stabbing pain near the wound, fever, headache, anorexia, hemorrhage, or other symptoms of generalized or localized infection.

Dressings. The frequency with which dressings are changed depends on the needs of the patient and the orders of the physician. An order might state that a wound is to be dressed at regular intervals (for example, twice a day), or it might leave the frequency with which a dressing is to be changed to the nurse's judgment. In the latter situation the dressing is changed when it is wet, but never more often than necessary, because each time a wound is exposed the chance of initiating an infection is increased.

Operative wounds may be sutured with a wide variety of nonabsorbable sutures, including those made of polyester, polypropylene, or silk, or with absorbable sutures made from surgical gut or a synthetic fiber. Wire sutures are occasionally used. Skin sutures are usually nonabsorbable. If a wound is expected to drain excessively, a drain or packing is inserted by the physician to facilitate this process. Soft and firm rubber drains as well as plastic drains are used for this purpose. Packing is usually made of a long strip of gauze, often impregnated with a disinfectant or antibiotic. Drains and packing are sometimes withdrawn a little each day to encourage healing from the depth of the wound toward the surface. Considerable drainage can be anticipated from wounds of this nature. Some drains are sutured in place, whereas others are freely movable. Soft rubber drains (Penrose drains) often have a sterile safety pin attached to the distal portion of the drain to prevent it from slipping completely inside the wound.

Wounds that are draining need to be changed whenever the dressings are wet. Not only is the drainage frequently irritating to the skin, but it also serves as a likely site for infection.

Preparation of the Environment. When a wound is to be exposed to the open air, every effort is made to decrease the number of micro-

organisms which could possibly come in contact with it. Consequently, windows and doors are closed to eliminate drafts, and curtains are drawn around the patient to provide privacy.

The bed unit is arranged for the convenience of the person changing the patient's dressings. Usually the bedside table or overbed table is cleared beforehand so that the nurse can put the dressing tray in a convenient place. Before wound care, the nurse washes her hands to reduce the number of microorganisms which are normally on her skin (see Chapter 26).

Preparation of the Equipment. The specific equipment required depends upon the kind of wound. The safest aseptic technique is carried out by using individual trays containing only the materials and equipment which can be discarded or sterilized after the wound is dressed. By not taking bottles and other articles from one patient to another the transfer of microorganisms by such vectors is eliminated.

For changing most wound dressings it is necessary to have a receptacle for the old dressings and gauze sponges (waxed paper bags permit such contaminated materials to be covered and disposed of easily, while the wax keeps the moisture inside the bag), a container of disinfectant, two or three forceps (tissue and artery forceps are often used), sterile dressings, and gauze sponges. For the care of some wounds it is also necessary to have sterile scissors either to shorten drains or to shape the dressings. The nurse will usually need adhesive tape as well.

After this equipment has been placed on a tray and protected from contamination (by covering it with a sterile towel, for example), it can be safely transported to the patient. Some agencies have standard sets ready for use; it is then necessary only to add the disinfectant and any additional equipment needed by a particular patient. If a mask is to be worn, it is usually put on before the equipment is arranged, and it is kept on until the wound care has been completed.

Preparation of the Patient. Prior to the dressing of a wound, the needs of the patient for information about the procedure are determined. If the patient will be seeing his wound for the first time, he may want some information about its appearance and what will happen during the dressing change. The details of the explanation depend upon the patient's needs. Often a wound has a meaning for the patient other than the obvious; for example, he might be worried about the appearance of a scar.

The patient can assist by lying still during the procedure in order that the wound and the equipment do not accidentally become contaminated. Some patients need to be advised not to talk and to keep their hands away from the wound area so that sterile technique is maintained. During the explanation, words such as "infection," "contaminated," and "dirty" are used with caution, since they may make the patient feel that something is wrong or may stimulate him to speculate about future complications.

Inexperienced people often ask whether changing a dressing or removing drains and sutures is painful. These people are frequently worried about their ability to cope with pain in a socially acceptable manner. Generally all of these measures are painless, with the exception of removing dressings that adhere to the skin surface. Dressings that do stick to the skin because of dried discharges can usually be removed with little discomfort by soaking them with sterile normal saline or sterile water.

Another possible source of discomfort is the use of a disinfectant with an alcohol base. Such applicants may feel cold to the patient and may possibly sting when they come in contact with an open wound. The use of a disinfectant without an alcoholic base is often advisable. Most agencies have a particular type of disinfectant that they recommend using in caring for wounds. If the procedure is going to be uncomfortable, patients are usually better able to cope with it if they have been given some warning so that their responses can be structured in advance.

Prior to the changing of a dressing, the patient assumes a position that is convenient and comfortable for him. It may be necessary to provide drapes for adequate warmth and privacy.

Procedure for Donning Sterile Gloves. Some agencies advocate the use of sterile gloves for changing a dressing and cleaning a wound; others prefer a "no touch" technique using sterile forceps. Whichever method is practiced, it is important that all equipment coming in contact with an open wound be sterile. If sterile gloves are to be worn during the dressing procedure, they are usually put on after the soiled dressings are removed. In preparing the dressing tray at the patient's bedside, then, the glove wrapper is laid on a clean, flat surface and unfolded. Many agencies now use disposable sterile gloves; most are now prepowdered. If they are not, the nurse will find a small packet of powder inside the glove wrapper (the powder makes it easier to slip on the gloves).

When the nurse is ready to don the gloves, she carefully lifts the powder packet from the wrapper, opens it, and carefully powders her hands. (If the gloves are prepowdered, this step is not necessary.)

The right-handed nurse usually puts on the left glove first. To do this, she grasps the *inside* of the folded cuff tip of the left glove with her right hand, lifts the glove from the wrapper, and slides her left hand into it. (It is easier if the fingers are kept straight.)

The nurse is then ready to don the second glove. Using the gloved left hand, she slips her fingers *under* the folded cuff edge of the right glove and lifts it from the wrapper. Then, being careful not to touch the skin of her hand or her uniform, she carefully slides her right hand into the glove, pulling the cuff up over the wrist with her left (gloved) hand, which is still under the cuff edge.

The cuff of the left glove may then be pulled up over the wrist (using the same technique of sterile surface to sterile surface), by slipping the fingers of the now gloved right hand under the folded cuff edge of the left glove and carefully pulling it up over the wrist.

When both gloves have been put on, the nurse can adjust the fingers in the same manner she would use in putting on a pair of gloves for street wear.

Procedures for Changing the Dressing. The equipment is arranged in a manner such that it is not necessary to pass soiled dressings and sponges over the sterile field. Generally the old dressing is removed with sterile forceps, the dressing is dropped into the wax paper bag, and the forceps are then placed in a discard container. The wound is then cleansed with a disinfectant. Five rules for cleansing a wound are:

1. Use a sponge only once, cleansing from the top of the wound to the bottom, and then discard the sponge. The cleanest part of the wound is at the top, where there is the least amount of drainage.

2. After cleansing the wound itself, work away from the wound to a distance of about 5 cm. (2 inches). The wound is the cleanest area; the surrounding skin contains more microorganisms.

3. When not wearing sterile gloves, keep the tips of the forceps lower than the handle. Ungloved hands contaminate the handle of the forceps and the solution on the tips will run down to the handle if the tips are held up; then upon lowering the tips the contaminated solution returns to the tips, contaminating the entire instrument.

4. Do not carry contaminated sponges over sterile areas. There is a danger that the contaminated solution will drop on sterile equipment.

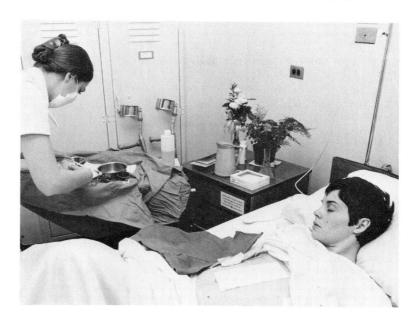

Strict aseptic technique must be maintained throughout the dressing procedure.

5. Do not reach over a sterile field. There is a danger that contaminants from the nurse's arms or uniform will drop onto the sterile field.

After a wound has been cleansed, it is irrigated if this has been ordered. Normally about 500 ml. of a sterile solution at room temperature is used for wound irrigation. If the irrigating solution is irritating to the skin, the surrounding areas should be protected beforehand by an ointment such as sterile petrolatum. During irrigation, the patient lies so that when the nurse administers the irrigating solution with a sterile syringe it flows freely over the wound and then into a receptacle. After an irrigation, the skin is patted dry with sterile sponges.

The new sterile dressing is placed over the wound with sterile forceps. It should be dropped in place rather than moved over the skin so as not to transfer microorganisms from the skin to the center of the wound and to avoid mechanical injury to the wound. When wet dressings are used, they are soaked in the prescribed solution, wrung out with artery forceps, and then placed on the wound. The outer dressing should extend at least 5 cm. (2 inches) beyond an open wound as a precaution against later contamination should the edges be accidentally turned back.

The dressings can be secured by adhesive tape, elasticized tape, waterproof tape, adhesive ties, binders, bandages, or plastic tape. The type of material and the method by which it is secured depend upon the site of the wound and the specific needs of the patient. For the patient who is allergic to adhesive tape, some other type of commercially prepared adhesive bandage can be used. Plastic tape is frequently used on the face because of its nonirritating quality. Waterproof tape keeps a wound dry; thus, it is especially useful next to a draining area. Adhesive ties are used when frequent dressing changes are necessary, since only the tie part needs to be undone when the dressing is changed; the adhesive portion does not have to be removed from the skin unless the tape becomes soiled.

When a dressing is to be secured by adhesive tape, painting the patient's skin with tincture of benzoin beforehand serves to protect the surface epithelium. It is also more comfortable for the patient when areas that have hair are shaved so that the tape does not stick to the hair on removal. Adhesive tape can be readily removed by using a solvent such as acetone to loosen the gum of the tape. Ether and benzene can also be used, but they are highly flammable and for this reason are not often kept near patients.

Binders. Binders can be used to retain dressings, to apply pressure, to support an area of the body, and to provide comfort. Binders are generally made of a heavy cotton material that is strong and durable. Scultetus binders are occasionally lined with flannel, which absorbs moisture and provides additional comfort. When the purpose of the binder is to provide support to abdominal muscles, a two-way stretch type of binder, similar to a girdle, is sometimes used.

Guides for the Application of Binders

1. Binders are applied in such a manner as to provide even pressure over an area of the body.

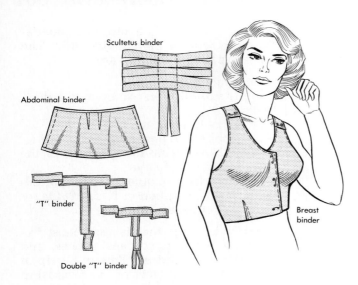

Types of binders.

2. Binders should support body parts in their normal anatomical position, with slight joint flexion.

3. Binders are secured firmly so that they do not cause friction and thereby irritate the skin or mucous membrane.

Types of Binders. There are five basic types of binders: T binder, straight abdominal binder, scultetus (many-tailed) binder, breast binder, and triangular binder.

The T binder is made of two strips of cotton attached in the shape of a T. The top of the T serves as a band which is then placed around the patient's waist. The stem of the T is passed between the patient's legs and is then attached to the waistband in front. In some T binders the cotton strip that goes between the patient's legs is split into two tails about 22.5 cm. (9 inches) from the end. These tails provide wider support to the perineal area and add to the comfort of the male patient particularly.

T binders are used chiefly to retain perineal dressings. Because of the profuse drainage that often occurs from this area, they are usually changed frequently.

The straight abdominal binder is a rectangular piece of cotton from 15 to 30 cm. (6 to 12 inches) wide, and long enough to encircle the patient's abdomen and overlap at least 5 cm. (2 inches) in front. This type of binder is used to retain abdominal dressings or to apply pressure and support to the abdomen.

The scultetus binder, which is also known as the many-tailed binder, is a rectangular piece of cotton, usually 22.5 to 30 cm. (9 to 12 inches) wide and 37.5 cm. (15 inches) long, with perhaps 6 to 12 tails attached to each side. It is usually used to provide support to the abdomen,

but it can also be used to retain dressings. It can be applied to the chest as well as the abdomen. The advantage of the scultetus binder is that it fits the contours of the body closely.

The breast binder is a rectangular piece of cotton shaped roughly to the contours of the female chest. It usually has straps that fit over the shoulders and pin to the binder in front.

Various forms of the triangular binder (sling) are used to support a limb, to secure a splint (as a first aid measure), and to secure dressings. The triangular binder is made of heavy cotton, is triangular in shape, and has two sides approximately 1 meter (40 inches) in length. It can be applied as a full triangle or, after it has been folded, in a variety of ways.

As a full triangle, the binder is used frequently to make a *large arm sling*. Folded into a broad bandage, it can be used as a *small sling* to support the patient's wrist and hand. A triangular binder can also support a person's arm in such a manner as to elevate the hand. This is called a *triangular sling*.

Triangular binders can also be used to retain

A large arm sling.

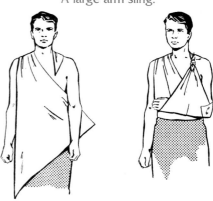

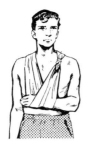

A small arm sling.

dressings on the elbow, hand, shoulder, hip, knee, and foot. For details on the application of binders the nurse should consult a bandaging or first aid book. There are also a number of multimedia aids now available to help students to develop skills in applying binders and bandages.

Problems Related to the Use of Binders. Binders are most often used for large areas of the body, and since they are not secured to skin surfaces, they have a tendency to slip out of position. A binder should be changed or reapplied as often as necessary to maintain its intended function of support, comfort, or the application of pressure. Soiling is also a problem with binders. Because a dirty binder can be a source of both irritation and infection, it is essential to see that soiled binders are changed promptly.

When a binder is applied it should be secured firmly, but the nurse should be careful that there is no interference with normal body functioning. An abdominal or breast binder that is too tight, for example, can restrict movements of the chest wall and interfere with respiration. In postoperative patients this could lead to serious complications. The nurse should be alert for signs of impaired respiration, such as shallow breathing, which could indicate that a binder is too tight and should be loosened.

A triangular sling.

Bandaging. A bandage is a piece of material that is used to wrap a part of the body. The purposes of applying a bandage are:

1. To limit movement
2. To apply warmth—for example, to a rheumatoid joint
3. To secure a dressing
4. To keep splints in position
5. To provide support—for example, to the legs to aid venous blood flow
6. To apply pressure in order to control bleeding, promote the absorption of tissue fluids, or prevent the loss of tissue fluids

The type of bandage that is used most frequently in hospitals, physicians' offices, and clinics is the roller bandage. This is a strip of material from 1.8 to 7.4 meters (2 to 8 yards) in length and varying in width from 1.25 to 15 cm. (½ to 6 inches). A roller bandage has three parts: the initial or free end, the body or drum, and the terminal or hidden end.

Materials Used in Bandaging. *Gauze* is one of the most frequently used materials for bandaging. It is a soft, woven cotton that is porous but not bulky, light in weight, and readily molded to any contour. Although gauze does not wash well and frays with repeated use, it is inexpensive and easily disposed of. The gauze is sometimes impregnated with various ointments such as petrolatum. Gauze is frequently used to bandage fingers and hands and to retain dressings on draining wounds.

Kling gauze and *Kerlix* gauze are woven so as to allow the gauze to stretch and thus mold to the body contours. The gauze has a crepe-like texture and tends to cling to itself, an attribute that helps keep it in place after it has been applied.

Flannel makes a soft and pliable bandage. It is heavy and keeps in the heat of the body; therefore it can be used to apply warmth to body joints.

Crinoline is a loosely woven gauze, coarse in texture and strong. Crinoline is impregnated with plaster of paris for use as a base for applying casts. It may also be impregnated with petrolatum for application to an open wound.

Muslin (factory cotton) is a strong heavy cotton that is not pliable. It is used to provide support, as for splints, or to limit movement.

Elasticized bandages made of cotton with an elastic webbing (Ace bandages) are often used as tensor bandages to apply pressure. They are expensive but can be washed and reused. Patients who require support for their legs immediately following surgery for varicose veins often use tensor bandages.

Elastic adhesive (Elastoplast) is a woven bandage with an adhesive side. It is applied to give support—for example, when dressings are being secured.

Plastic adhesive is a waterproof bandage with an adhesive side. It is somewhat elastic and can be used to apply pressure and at the same time keep an area dry.

Principles Relevant to Bandaging. *Microorganisms flourish in warm, damp and soiled areas.* A bandage is applied only over a clean area; if it is to be placed over an open wound, the wound is dressed aseptically beforehand. Skin surfaces are dry and clean and are not pressed together when bandaging. Adjacent skin surfaces may be kept separated by inserting a 5 cm. by 5 cm. (2 inch by 2 inch) piece of gauze between them. Bandages are removed at regular intervals and the skin surfaces are washed and dried. Soiled bandages are never reused.

Pressure exerted upon the body tissues can affect the circulation of blood. A bandage is applied from the distal to the proximal part of the body to aid the return of the venous blood to the heart. Bandages are always applied evenly so that they do not restrict circulation. They should be checked frequently to make certain that there is no interference with blood supply to the part.

Friction can cause mechanical trauma to the epithelium. A bony prominence of the body is padded before it is bandaged, so that the bandage does not rub the area and cause an abraded wound. Skin surfaces are separated to prevent friction and maceration.

The body is maintained in the natural anatomical position with slight flexion of the joints to avoid muscle strain. Bandages are applied with the body in good alignment to avoid muscle extension, which is fatiguing and produces strain. In particular, adduction of the shoulder and hip joint is avoided.

Excessive or uneven pressure upon body surfaces can interfere with blood circulation and therefore with the nourishment of the cells in the area. Bandage evenly and if possible leave the distal portion of the bandaged limb exposed so that any restriction in circulation can be detected. Signs and symptoms of restricted circulation are pallor, erythema, cyanosis, tingling sensations, numbness or pain, swelling, and cold.

When a bandage is applied over a wet dressing, allowances are made for shrinkage as the bandage becomes wet and subsequently dries.

Fundamental Turns in Bandaging. There are five fundamental turns in bandaging, and it is these turns that are used to make up the variety of bandages applied to the various parts of the body.

The *circular turn* is used to bandage a cylindrical part of the body or to secure a bandage at its initial and terminal ends. In a circular turn, the bandage is wrapped about the part in such a way that each turn exactly covers the previous

Spiral reverse bandage. (From Rambo, B. J., and Wood, L. A.: *Nursing Skills for Clinical Practice.* 3rd ed. Philadelphia, W. B. Saunders Company, 1982, p. 742.)

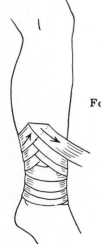

Folding bandage over to make spiral reverse turn.

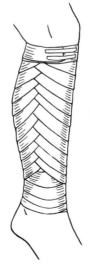

Spiral reverse bandage fits contours of extremity.

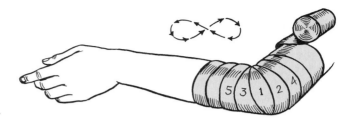

Figure-eight turn on the elbow.

one. Two circular turns are usually used to initiate and to terminate a bandage. For comfort the initial and terminal ends are not situated directly over the wound.

The *spiral turn* is used to bandage a part of the body that is of uniform circumference. The bandage is carried upward at a slight angle so that it spirals around the part. Each turn is parallel to the preceding one and overlaps it by two thirds of the width of the bandage. A spiral turn is used on parts of the body such as the fingers, arms, and legs.

The *spiral reverse turn* is used to bandage cylindrical parts of the body that are of varying circumference, such as the lower leg. To make a spiral reverse turn, the thumb of the free hand is placed on the upper edge of the initial turn, the bandage being held firmly. The roll is unwound about 15 cm. (6 inches) and then the hand is pronated so that the bandage is directed downward and parallel to the lower edge of the previous turn, overlapping it by two thirds of the width. The roll is then carried around the limb and another reverse is made at the same place so that the turns are in line and uniform.

The *figure-eight turn* is usually used on joints but may also be used for the entire length of an arm or leg bandage. It consists of repeated oblique turns that are made alternately above and below a joint in the form of a figure eight. After the initial circular turns are made over the center of the joint, the next turn is superior to the joint and the next is inferior to the joint. Thus the turns are worked upward and downward, with each turn overlapping the previous turn by two thirds of the width of the bandage.

The *recurrent turn* is used to cover distal portions of the body, such as the tip of a finger or the toes. After the bandage is anchored with a circular turn, the roll is turned and brought directly over the center of the tip to be covered. It is then anchored inferiorly, and alternate turns are made, first to the right and then to the left, over the original turn covering the tip so that each turn is held above and below. Each turn overlaps the preceding one by two thirds of its width. The bandage is secured by circular turns that gather in the ends.

Generally speaking, bandages for the hands, arms, and feet are made with circular, spiral, and spiral reverse turns. Bandages for the joints are made with figure eights, and bandages for the distal portions of the body are done with recurrent turns.

In addition, there are many special bandages, such as the thumb spica, ear and eye bandages, and skull bandages. It is suggested that the nurse consult a bandaging text for more detailed information.

A, Finger bandange with the tip covered; B, thumb spica.

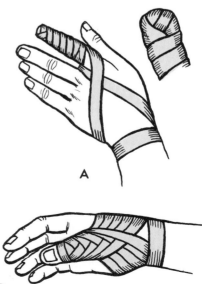

A

B

Recurrent turn on the hand.

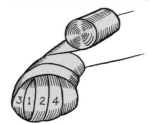

Guides to Bandaging

1. Face the person who is being bandaged.

2. Start a roller bandage by holding the roll of the bandage upward in one hand, the initial end in the other hand.

3. Bandage from the distal to the proximal and from the medial to the lateral.

4. Do not initiate or terminate a bandage directly over a wound or an area where the patient is likely to exert pressure, for example, the posterior side of the thigh.

5. Bandage evenly and firmly, overlapping the preceding turn by two thirds of the width of the bandage.

6. Use the bandage material that best serves the purpose of the bandage.

7. Cover a dressing with a bandage that extends past each side of the dressing.

8. Separate the skin surfaces and pad bony prominences and hollows to prevent friction and to apply even pressure.

9. Check the bandage and look for any signs of restricted circulation.

10. A bandage should be safe, durable, neat, therapeutically effective, and economical.

PLANNING AND EVALUATING NURSING INTERVENTIONS

The specific nursing interventions discussed in this chapter were concerned with changing dressings on a wound, applying binders, and the fundamental techniques of bandaging. The expected outcomes of these interventions are the comfort and safety of the patient. Questions the nurse might ask herself are:

1. Is the dressing, binder, or bandage accomplishing its purpose?

2. Is the patient concerned about his wound? Has his anxiety been allayed?

3. Has the dressing, binder, or bandage been applied so that there is no impairment to circulation?

4. Has the dressing, binder, or bandage been applied so that drainage, if desired, is unimpeded?

5. Has safe sterile technique been maintained?

6. Has each intervention been performed as comfortably as possible for the patient?

GUIDE TO ASSESSING THE SURGICAL PATIENT

1. What do you know about this patient as a person? about his family?

2. What is his basic health problem? his general health status? Why is he coming in for surgery? What operation is he to have? When? What type of anesthetic will be used? What laboratory tests and other investigations have been done preoperatively? What are the results?

3. What was done during surgery? Were tubes or drains inserted? What was the patient's immediate postoperative condition?

4. What is the status of his vital signs preoperatively? postoperatively?

5. What is his breathing like preoperatively? Does he have any chronic respiratory problems? Does he have a cold or other acute respiratory condition now? Postoperatively, is his airway clear? Are there signs of difficulties in breathing? respiratory distress? Is he positioned for optimum ease of breathing? drainage of fluids from the mouth? Can he cough? Can he breathe deeply?

6. What is the condition of the skin preoperatively? postoperatively? Are there signs of inflammation, local or general? Are there breaks in the open infected areas?

7. Does the patient report pain preoperatively? postoperatively? What is the nature, location, and intensity of his pain? Is his dressing too tight? Is he in a comfortable position? Can he move around by himself? Do the analgesics ordered relieve his pain?

8. What do the test results show regarding his fluid and electrolyte balance preoperatively? postoperatively? Is he on intravenous infusions? having blood transfusions? Are there signs of dehydration? Is there edema around the incision site, the infusion site, or other areas? Is he showing signs of muscle weakness? tremors?

disorientation? agitation? Are there indications of warm, reddened areas on the thighs? in other places?

9. What is the patient's nutritional status preoperatively? Is he on a special diet? Does he have particular food preferences? Is he permitted food and fluids postoperatively? If so, does he tolerate them well? Is he nauseated? vomiting?

10. What is the patient's normal voiding pattern? Does he have any long-standing, or acute, problems of urinary functioning? Does the preoperative urinalysis show any signs of abnormality, e.g., sugar in the urine? Has he voided before going to the operating room? Does he show any signs of bladder distention preoperatively? What was the intraoperative intake and output? Has he voided within 8 hours postoperatively? Is he voiding adequately? Does he have a catheter in situ?

11. What is his usual bowel pattern? Does he have any problems? Use any aids? Was an enema (or laxative) ordered preoperatively? If so, what were the results? Postoperatively, does he complain of gas pains? Does he show signs of abdominal distention? Can he pass flatus by rectum? Is he taking an adequate amount of fluids and, if tolerated, food to promote peristalsis? Is he getting sufficient exercise? Has he had a bowel movement? Are there orders for laxatives or an enema? Result?

12. What particular concerns does the patient have preoperatively? Does he seem tense, anxious, or depressed pre- or postoperatively? Have his fears been allayed? What were the results of his surgery? Is his prognosis good? Was there evidence of malignancy or irreparable condition during surgery? Are the family members upset?

13. What is the status of the patient's mental functioning preoperatively? Is he alert, well-oriented, capable of logical reasoning? extremely anxious? Postoperatively, what is his level of consciousness? Is he fully awake? Is he drowsy? disoriented? confused?

14. Are the sensory organs all intact and functioning normally prior to surgery? Does the patient have any chronic, or acute, problems with any of the senses? Postoperatively, has sensory functioning been regained in all areas affected by the surgery or anesthetic? Are there any deviations from his preoperative status in regard to any areas of sensory functioning?

15. Did the patient have complete range of movement in his limbs, trunk, and head and neck preoperatively? Can he move freely in bed? turn over? sit up? walk? Does he need any aids for or assistance with any of these activities? Postoperatively, are his movements restricted by any equipment, or by limitations placed on his activities? Does he need assistance to carry out the activities of daily living? When is he to start ambulating? How much support does he need? Is he carrying out exercises to improve muscle tone? to increase range of motion?

16. What are this patient's specific safety and protection needs?

17. What are his learning needs?

GUIDE TO ASSESSING WOUND HEALING

1. What type of wound does the patient have?

2. What phase of healing would you judge this wound to be in?

3. Is the wound healing normally?

4. Are there factors which might delay healing of the wound? For example, is the patient in poor nutritional status? Does he have an infection?

5. Does the patient show localized or generalized symptoms that would indicate the wound is infected? Are there signs of bleeding?

6. How would you describe the wound?

7. Does the wound require dressing? If so, how often? Are there special precautions to be taken or additional equipment required for doing the dressing?

8. Does the patient need a binder or bandage? If so, for what reason? What is the best type to use for this patient's needs?

STUDY SITUATION

Mr. John Smith is a 30-year-old law enforcement officer who is married, has four children, and is in excellent physical condition. He was admitted to hospital 3 days ago with a bullet wound to his right shoulder. The bullet has been removed, but since there may still be particles of foreign matter present, the physician has not sutured the wound. The physician's orders for Mr. Smith include:

1. Change dressing as necessary

2. Cleanse wound b.i.d. with preferred antiseptic

3. High protein diet

4. Force fluids

When you arrive to change his dressing, Mr. Smith complains of headache and a burning sensation in the region of his wound. You notice a yellow discharge seeping through the previous dressing. Mr. Smith also remarks that he feels hot, although there is a fresh breeze coming through the open window beside his bed.

Mr. Smith has been worried that he may not regain full use of his right arm, and since he is right-handed, he fears he may have to resign from active duty.

1. What would you do first when faced with this situation?

2. What might be causing the yellowish discharge from the wound?

3. What other observations might you expect to note in the area of Mr. Smith's wound?

4. What other observations might you note about his general condition?

5. How would you record your observations concerning Mr. Smith?

6. Are there any things you could do to assist in relieving his anxiety?

SUGGESTED READINGS

Aspinall, M. J.: Scoring against Nosocomial Infections. *American Journal of Nursing,* 78(10):1704–1707, October, 1978.

Boore, J. B.: Preoperative Care of Patients. *Nursing Times,* 73:409–411, March 24, 1977.

Croushore, T. M.: Postoperative Assessment: The key to Avoiding Common Nursing Mistakes. *Nursing'79,* 9(4):46–51, 1979.

Chalmers, H.: Return to Basics: 4. Pre-operative and Postoperative Care. *Nursing Mirror* Supplement, July 28, 1977, pp. i–iv.

Dziurbejko, M. M., and Larkin, J. C.: Including the Family in Preoperative Teaching. *American Journal of Nursing,* 78(11):1892–1894, November, 1978.

Finn, K. L.: Postoperative Ambulation. *Critical Care Update,* 7:22–26, December, 1980.

Hewitt, D.: Is the Pre-op Patient Terrified? *RN,* 42:44–47, September, 1979.

Lyons, M. L.: What Priority Do You Give Pre-op Teaching? *Nursing '77,* 7(1):11–12, January, 1977.

Mitchell, M.: Routine Postoperative Management and Immediate Recovery Room Care. *Nursing Care,* 9:30–31, June, 1976.

Postoperative Complications. *Nursing '81* 11(3):50–53, March, 1981.

Rayder, M.: A New Nurse Asks Why Preoperative Teaching Isn't Done. *American Journal of Nursing,* 79(11):1992–1995, November, 1979.

REFERENCES

1. Bennett, J. V., and Brockman, P. S. (ed.): *Hospital Infections.* Boston, Little, Brown and Company, 1979.
2. LeMaitre, G. D., and Finnegan, J. A.: *The Patient in Surgery: A Guide for Nurses.* 4th ed. Philadelphia, W. B. Saunders Company, 1980.
3. Lear, M. W.: *Heartsounds.* New York, Simon and Schuster, 1979.
4. MacBryde, C. M., and Blacklow, R. S. (eds.): *Signs and Symptoms: Applied Pathologic Physiology and Clinical Interpretation.* 5th ed. Philadelphia, J. B. Lippincott Company, 1970.
5. Schrankel, D. G.: Preoperative Teaching. *Supervisor Nursing,* 9:82–90, May, 1978.
6. Mitchell, M.: Routine Postoperative Management and Immediate Recovery Room Care. *Nursing Care,* 9:30–31, June 1976.
7. Finn, K. L.: Postoperative Ambulation. *Critical Care Update,* 7:22–26, December, 1980.

28

The Nurse Should Be Able to:

- Describe methods commonly used in health agencies for communicating medication orders
- Discuss the five "rights" in administering medications
- Discuss special problems and precautionary measures related to drugs pertaining to people in all age groups
- Compare the advantages and disadvantages of administering medications by the oral, subcutaneous, and intramuscular routes
- Prepare and administer medications, using adequate safety measures, by all of the following routes: orally, subcutaneously, intramuscularly, intradermally, topically, and by instillations into the ear, eye, nose, throat, vagina, and rectum.
- Record the administration of medications correctly, according to the policy of the agency in which she is working

MEDICATIONS

CHAPTER 28

INTRODUCTION

The use of medications to treat disease has been known throughout history. In recent years, however, the number of different medicines that are manufactured commercially for distribution has increased enormously. Hundreds of new drug products are introduced each year, yet relatively few of these are new chemical substances. Most new preparations that appear on the market are actually modified forms of drugs previously used, or new dosage forms of the same drug, or new combinations of drugs that have been used for some time. Pharmacists, as well as physicians and nurses, are continually challenged to keep up to date with these constantly changing products.

Sources of information available to nurses about new drugs include the agency pharmacy department, physicians, the professional nursing and medical journals, and information put out by the commercial drug firms. In many health agencies, the pharmacy department maintains an up-to-date *formulary* which lists and describes drugs currently used in the agency. Copies of the formulary are usually distributed to all nursing units, where they are readily available for reference. In addition, many head nurses like to keep a drug file on their nursing units with information about new drugs. The pharmacist is, of course, an excellent reference source, and the nurse should not hesitate to request information from him. Physicians too are usually very willing to explain the nature and purpose of new drugs they have prescribed for patients. With the multitude of new drug products constantly appearing on the market, it is difficult for anyone to keep informed about them all. The nurse should be aware of the sources of information available in her agency about new drugs and should make use of these.

Many drugs are marketed under their trade, or proprietary, names. Each drug usually has at least three names: its trade name, a chemical name, and an official or *generic* name. The trade *(proprietary)* name is the name given a drug by the manufacturer. Consequently, one drug may have several trade names, since the same drug may be manufactured by several drug companies, each one giving it a different trade name. The chemical name of the drug is a description of its chemical constituents. The official, or generic, name of a drug is the name under which it is listed in one of the official publications. A generic name is originally assigned by the individual or company that develops the drug. When the drug becomes official, it may be assigned a new generic name, in which case the original one is dropped. Official publications of drugs include the *United States Pharmacopoeia* and the *National Formulary* in the United States. In Canada, the equivalents are the *Vademecum International of Canada* and the *National Formulary* (Canadian); drugs are not termed "official" in Canada, but their generic names appear in these official publications. The World Health Organization publishes a guide, *Specifications for the Quality Control of Pharmacuetical Preparations*, which is an international pharmacopoeia listing important drugs used in many countries.

An increasing number of health agencies are adopting the practice of using the generic or official names of drugs for patient prescriptions. This practice not only eliminates much confusion about the nature of the drug prescribed, but means too that products of different drug companies can be used alternatively, unless the physician specifically requests that one company's product be used.

Drug standards provide for identification, purity, and uniformity of the strength of drugs. The *Pharmacopeia of the United States of America* (U.S.P.) lists drugs and defines the standards according to which a pharmacist in the United States must fill a prescription. The *Vademecum International of Canada* does the same for pharmacists in Canada. In this way the physician can always be assured of the uniform purity and potency of the medications that he or she orders. The World Health Organization publication has been a major step toward establishing international standards for drugs.

The administration of medications is a therapeutic nursing function that is chiefly dependent upon the orders of the physician. Some medication orders state the exact time for administration; others leave the time of administration to the nurse's judgment. For example, it is not unusual for ferrous sulfate to be prescribed three times a day after meals, whereas an order for 15 mg. (¼ gr.) of morphine subcutaneously is often written so that the nurse can give it when, in her judgment, the patient requires an analgesic.

ORDERING AND RECORDING MEDICATIONS

Medications are, in most instances, ordered or prescribed by a physician. In an ambulatory care setting, the physician usually writes the prescription on a form which the patient gives to the pharmacist. The prescription tells the pharmacist what medications the patient is to have, the dosage required, the amount to be supplied, how to prepare it, and the instructions the patient is to be given for taking them. In many places, the name of the drug and the unit dosage must be included on the label of the medication the patient receives.

In an inpatient facility, the prescription is usually in the form of a written order that is dated and signed by the physician, although some health agencies permit physicians to telephone orders to the nursing staff. In such cases, the physicians are usually required to countersign their orders within a definite number of hours. In an emergency situation medications are given on a verbal order that is later written and countersigned as needed. Generally speaking, written orders are considered to be the safest practice.

There are two types of written orders: the self-terminating order and the standing order. *Self-terminating orders* have a time limit on them. A stat. order is a self-terminating order that is to be carried out only once and immediately, for example, Demerol 100 mg. I.M. stat. (I.M. refers to intramuscularly). It is not repeated unless there are specific instructions to that effect. Another type of self-terminating order is an order in which the time limit is actually specified; for example, the physician writes, aspirin 0.65 g. (gr. $\bar{x}$) for six doses, or digitalis 0.1 g. (gr. $\bar{iss}$) June 12th and 14th. Sometimes a self-terminat-

ing order is dependent upon the condition of the patient, as when an order is written, aspirin 0.65 g. (gr. $\bar{x}$) q4h until temperature has remained below 100° F (37.8° C) for 24 hours. Some institutions have policies that place a time limit on orders regardless of how they are worded. For example, it is not unusual for a narcotic order to be effective for only 3 days, after which it is automatically discontinued unless the physician writes another order.

Standing orders are orders that are carried out indefinitely; for example, vitamin C 25 mg. b.i.d. (twice a day) oral. Some standing orders contain the direction "p.r.n.," which means "as necessary." The administration of a drug under a p.r.n. direction is left to the nurse's judgment.

An order should always include the name of the drug, the exact dosage, the route of administration, and the frequency of administration. If the physician wishes a medication to be given at a time other than the accustomed distribution time, this should also be specified. The nurse has an obligation to question any order that is ambiguous or that she feels is unsafe for a patient. In health agencies it is a customary practice for all of a patient's orders to be written on a doctor's order sheet, which may be kept in the patient's chart or in a central book. Hospitals employ different ways of flagging charts to indicate that a patient has new orders. The orders are then usually copied in the nursing unit Kardex system or nursing care plan and a medication card may be filled out. A medication card has the patient's full name, the name of the drug, the dosage, the route of administration (in some hospitals if the route is oral it is omitted), the frequency of the administration, and the times of administration. Frequently, the room number or location of the patient's bed is also written on the medication card. If the drug is ordered q.i.d. (four times a day), the exact times are added—for example, 0800 (8 A.M.), 1200 (12 noon), 1600 (4 P.M.), and 2000 (8 P.M.). Medication cards are kept in a central place in the nursing unit and are frequently grouped so that they are easily selected at the time of administration.

Although different methods of posting medication orders are used in various agencies, the nurse should remember that the original written order is the primary source of information. Whenever orders are copied, whether onto a Kardex file, a nursing care plan, or a medicine card, the possibility of error is present. The nurse who administers medications should always check the original orders to make certain that communication tools are accurate.

Agencies have different methods of indicating

that a medication has been discontinued. In hospitals it is common practice for "discontinued" to be imprinted across the physician's order once it is no longer in force and for the medication card to be discarded. In a public health agency the notation "discontinued" and the date are entered on the nursing care record. Communication tools such as medication cards and nursing care records should be regularly checked against the original orders in order to keep them up to date. In hospitals where orders change frequently this is generally done at least once a day.

Medications are recorded in the patient's chart immediately after they have been administered. They should be recorded by the nurse who administered them. The recording includes the name of the drug, the time it was administered, the exact dosage, the method of administration, and the signature of the nurse administering the drug. Some agencies also require that the status of the person administering the drug also be designated, as, for example, R.N. or S.N. (student nurse).

When a p.r.n. order has been administered a notation is also made as to why the patient took the medicine at that particular time. Recording should also include observations of the effect of the medication when these are, or should be, apparent. In some hospitals the nurse also indicates on the doctor's order sheet that stat. dosages have been administered.

The administration of narcotics and, in some places, barbiturates and other controlled drugs is recorded not only on the patient's chart but also on a special form which is kept separately. Narcotics and other controlled drugs are kept in locked containers in hospitals and their distribution is closely governed. The forms upon which narcotics are recorded vary from place to place, but usually the nurse records the name of the patient to whom the narcotic was administered, the drug and dosage, the date and time, the name of the physician ordering the drug, and the signature of the nurse administering the drug. Any narcotics that are wasted are also recorded with a notation that the drug was wasted. Narcotics, barbiturates, and other controlled drugs are counted at specific times—for example, at the end of each shift—and the number distributed plus the number remaining on hand must tally with the number assigned to the nursing unit or agency. This count is usually done by two nurses, the one coming on duty and the nurse who is "handing over" to her. This practice helps to protect both nurses. Narcotics, barbiturates, and other controlled drugs are under strict governmental control. Any

losses or inconsistencies in the count must be reported immediately.

SPECIAL PRECAUTIONS THROUGHOUT THE LIFE CYCLE

As a general rule, pregnant women are well advised not to take any medications, since most drugs will cross the placental barrier and affect the fetus. Recent studies have shown that many commonly used drugs can cause damage to the unborn child. Both a low birth weight in the infant and prematurity have been linked to smoking. Alcohol has definitely been linked with mental and physical abnormalities so characteristic they are termed *fetal alcohol syndrome*. There is also some evidence that the caffeine in ordinary tea and coffee, if consumed in large quantities, may cause abnormalities. It has also been suggested that acetylsalicylic acid, the principal ingredient of aspirin, can damage the fetus, even during the last trimester of pregnancy. The fetus is most susceptible to the effects of drugs, however, during early pregnancy when the brain and other organs are developing. Some drugs (such as alcohol, nicotine to a lesser degree, and heroin) may cause mental and growth deficiencies in the developing fetus. If the fetus has been affected by medications, there is usually no major "catch up" growth after birth. Narcotic addiction in a pregnant woman can cause an infant to be born addicted, with the newborn suffering withdrawal symptoms during its first few days of life. Drugs that are given to a woman during labor also cross the placenta and affect the newborn. Women who have been given general anesthetics during delivery usually find that their babies are drowsy for the first 2 to 3 days after birth (see Chapter 22).

Infants, because of their small size, require a smaller amount of medication than adults do. The dosage of medications for infants is usually ordered according to the infant's weight. Infants are often more sensitive to the pharmacologic effects of drugs—again because of their smaller size and more rapid absorption, metabolism, and excretion of ingested substances compared with adults. Most medications are given to infants orally, in liquid form. They may be administered by dropper, on a spoon, or with a medicine dispenser that is specially designed for children.

With older children, drug dosage is usually calculated in relation to height and weight, with weight being considered the more important factor. When a very exact correction of the dosage for size is necessary, surface area may be

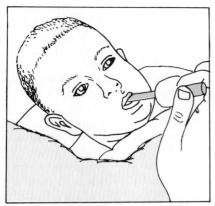

A dropper can be used to administer small doses of medicine to infants.

used, the area being estimated from both height and weight measurements.

Allergies to drugs often begin to develop in adolescents and young and middle-aged adults. The nurse should be particularly alert for allergic reactions in patients in these age groups. The problem of drug abuse, which is discussed at the end of this chapter, is also most prevalent among people of these ages.

With older persons, drug overdoses have become fairly common. They may result from a number of factors, such as:[1]

1. Too large a dosage being ordered for the person. There is a decline in kidney and liver functioning with aging, and often the body simply cannot process the drugs and excrete them as efficiently as it did before.

2. The prescription of a confusing drug program. Often, elderly people are taking a number of medications—a diuretic for hypertension, a drug for their heart condition, and perhaps one for the pain in their joints. Some of these may be taken once a day, or every other day, or two or three times a day. It all becomes very confusing for the older person, who may have difficulty reading the typing on the prescription bottle because of failing vision. He may not understand what he is supposed to take and exactly when he is to take it. The nurse often has to help the elderly patient to set up a simple orderly system for making sure that he gets the right drug at the right time and in the proper dosage. Dispensing a week's supply of pills into small envelopes for daily consumption and distributing them in egg cartons are methods of doing it.

3. Drug interactions in persons on multiple drug regimens. This not infrequently happens when an individual is being treated by more than one physician for different conditions. His general practitioner may have prescribed medications for his heart problem and other long-standing maladies, but the urologist who is treating him for a urinary tract obstruction may order other drugs and the two sets of drugs are not always compatible.

4. Idiosyncratic reactions to drugs because of the age factor. Older people often react poorly to certain drugs. The barbiturates and the tranquilizers are two groups of drugs that many older people do not tolerate well. The barbiturates often cause excitement in older patients instead of putting them to sleep, while the tranquilizers may cause mental disturbances such as delusions.

5. Intentional overdose, due to despondency. Suicide rates are highest among older people. Because the sedatives and tranquilizers are so commonly prescribed, they are readily available, and drug overdose is a common method of committing suicide among older people.

Nurses are often in the best position first of all, to identify problems the older person is having with his medications and, secondly, to do something about it. Her responsibilities include explaining the actions of various medications to the individual, reviewing with him the schedule for taking them, and helping him to set up a simple, straightforward medication regimen. She is also frequently the first person to observe untoward reactions to drugs in patients, and she should be alert to the side effects and possible reactions of drugs her patients are taking. Often the nurse is in the position of patient advocate, explaining to the physician the problems the patient is having and alerting him to drugs that have been ordered for the patient by other health professionals.

GUIDES FOR ADMINISTERING MEDICATIONS

The Type of Drug Preparation Often Governs the Method of Administration. Medications are distributed in a variety of preparations, and each type usually requires a specific method of administration. It may be that one preparation can be administered in several ways, and this is specified on the medication label. More often a preparation of a drug has only one method of administration, and if the drug must be administered by some other route, another preparation is required. Drugs are administered only by the route ordered by the doctor and specified on the medication label. For example, penicillin tablets are taken orally; a special solution of penicillin is given intramuscularly. It is a good practice to read the label carefully and also check the medication card for the route of administration.

The Route of Administration of the Drug Affects the Optimal Dosage of the Drug. The optimal dosage of a drug administered by mouth may not be the same as the optimal dosage when the drug is administered subcutaneously. Portions of drugs taken orally are excreted through the digestive tract instead of being absorbed into the cells; therefore, a larger dosage is generally required for oral administration than for administration by other routes.

The Safe Administration of Medications Requires a Knowledge of Anatomy and Physiology as Well as a Knowledge of the Drug and the Reason It Has Been Prescribed. A knowledge of anatomy and physiology is particularly important when medications are administered intramuscularly or subcutaneously. When drugs are administered intramuscularly, large blood vessels and nerves can be damaged if they are accidentally punctured.

A knowledge of the drug and its effects also helps safeguard against the administration of medication which could harm a patient. For example, if a patient has very slow respirations (e.g., 10 per minute), morphine can be contraindicated, because it can depress the respirations even more. This knowledge helps the nurse to make intelligent observations that assist in the assessment of the effectiveness of both the medication and the nursing care.

An understanding of the total plan of care for each patient and the desired therapeutic effect of the medications prescribed for him is essential. The nurse should know why the individual patient is receiving each medication so that she knows what effects to watch for in that patient.

The Method of Administration of a Drug Is Partially Determined by the Age of the Patient, His Orientation, His Degree of Consciousness, and His Health Problem. The disoriented patient may refuse to swallow his oral medication, or the nauseated patient may vomit his medicines after he has taken them. The unconscious patient is unable to take a medication orally, and a child may be too young to swallow a capsule. It is important for the nurse to report *any* difficulties that are encountered when administering a medication.

The Element of Error Is a Possibility in All Human Activity. Errors in the administration of medicines can be serious and, because the possibility of error is always present, special precautions are taken to avoid mistakes. If a nurse is ever in doubt about whether or not she should give a medication, she should consult a reliable source before going ahead. Most agencies have literature to which the nurse can refer, and physicians and pharmacists can also be consulted.

If an error is made, it is reported immediately either directly to the physician or to the nurse in charge, so that immediate steps can be taken to protect the patient from injury. The error is also analyzed to determine the exact cause in order to safeguard against another such error. Most hospitals also have unusual-occurrence forms which the nurse fills out to inform the agency administration of the details of the error (see Chapter 7).

Each Patient Has His Own Needs for Explanations and Support with Respect to the Administration of Medications. Medications are given to people, and the nurse will find, as in all of her nursing care, that each individual is different. Some people want to know about their medications; others prefer not to know about them. The amount of knowledge that a person requires is highly dependent upon individual circumstances. The seriously ill patient in a hospital may be too ill to care about any knowledge of the drug. The information that each person should have depends on his intelligence, age, education, illness, and emotional needs. The nurse is guided by both the patient and the physician as to the amount of information she provides.

GENERAL PRECAUTIONS

The administration of medications is a nursing function in most health agencies. In some hospitals the nurse administers all intravenous injections, but in others it is the physician's responsibility to administer specific medications, such as ergotamine, which is used to contract the uterus.

There is a wide variety in the medication policies that guide nursing action. But, regardless of policy, before the nurse administers any medication she must be sure that her action is safe for the patient. A sound basis for safe nursing practice is *knowledge.*

Traditionally, the "five rights" have served as guides to the administration of medications: the right *drug,* the right *dose,* the right *route,* the right *time,* and the right *patient.* These rights are no less true today than they were years ago; however, sound nursing practice involves more

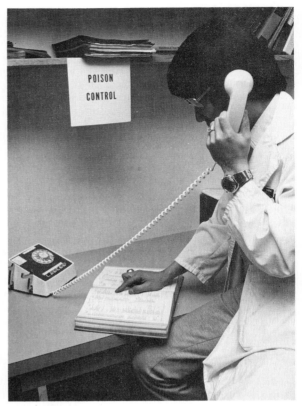

than just a knowledge of these. The nurse's information should extend to an identification of the individual problems of the patient and how she can help the patient resolve these problems. For example, will helping a patient to change his position and the provision of physical support facilitate the action of an analgesic?

Complementary to the administration of many medications is the provision of nursing care measures that serve to supplement the action of a drug. For example, giving the patient a back rub and straightening his bed might increase the effectiveness of a sedative, and drinking fluids can help prevent the crystallization of sulfonamides in the kidneys.

People vary in their reactions to specific drugs. The patient's reaction to any drug is important and should be recorded. Patients often require information about what reactions to report to the nurse or the physician. This is particularly true for the person who is taking medicine at home and does not have constant contact with health personnel.

A knowledge of the effects of a drug and its prescribed dosage is important for some patients. People often mistakenly believe, "If one tablet is good for me, two tablets are twice as good." Some people also need help to understand why they should take a prescribed dose and realistic explanation of the action and anticipated effects of the drug. Not only is this a need of hospitalized patients but also it is important for people who take medicines in their homes. All people taking medications at home should be aware of the nature of the drugs they are taking, why they are taking them, the dosage they are to take, and possible side effects of the drug. They should also be alerted to adverse signs and symptoms to watch for when they are taking these medications, and the dangers of altering the dosage or omitting to take medications.

Another area of nursing practice is concerned with idiosyncratic reactions to medications, overdoses of drugs, and the ingestion of poisonous materials. Many medical centers provide immediate information to laymen and physicians about the antidotes and emergency measures for the common poisons. Poison control centers are located in the emergency departments of many hospitals. An up-to-date list of the poison control centers can be obtained from the Superintendent of Documents, U.S. Government Printing Office, Washington, D.C. A list of poison control centers in Canada is contained in the *Vademecum International of Canada: Pharmaceutical Specialties and Biologicals* (up-

The poison control center is a source of information about the composition, action, and antidotes of poisonous materials. Its services are available to everyone in the community.

dated each year) and also in the *Compendium of Pharmaceuticals and Specialties of Canada*.

It is also a nursing responsibility to assist in evaluating the effectiveness of a medication and often in making judgments as to when a specific medication should be given. The need of a patient for some medications varies from time to time and, of course, needs vary from patient to patient. One patient may require frequent sedation, whereas another requires none.

Medications and the Patient

One of the most important factors in the administration of a medication is identification of the patient. Any method that accurately identifies a patient is satisfactory. Some hospitals provide each patient with an identification band. Many institutions suggest asking the patient his name before administering a medication. If this is the case, the nurse should not say, "Are you Mr. Smith?" nor should she rely on the patient answering to his name. In both situations, the

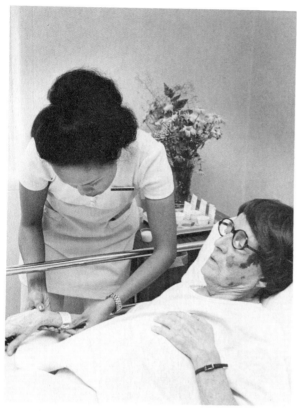

The identification band is one way the nurse can ensure that the right patient receives a medication.

patient may give an automatic affirmative answer. It is better to say, "What is your name?" The habit of relying upon bed numbers and even room numbers in order to identify people is also dangerous, for patients' rooms are changed and patients move to other units. In situations in which patients are continually reassigned to new rooms, identification is especially difficult.

After the nurse has accurately identified a patient, his need for explanation and support must be met. Often, simple explanations are reassuring to the patient; they can often help provide conditions of acceptance in the patient that can enhance the effectiveness of the drug. At this time the nurse can also provide him with information about the action of the medication in terms that he can understand. Patients usually like to feel they are participating in their therapy and have some control over situations. If the physician does not want the patient to receive information about a medicine from the nurse, it can be suggested that he confer with the physician about this subject.

If the administration of a drug is contingent upon some factor, such as the patient's pulse

rate, this is assessed first. With few exceptions the nurse stays with a patient until his medication has been completely administered. The exceptions are drugs that have been ordered to be left with a patient, for example, a drug that the patient has for immediate use as needed (such as nitroglycerin for cardiac pain), a cough medicine, or a drug that is contained in an intravenous infusion for gradual administration.

Refusal to Take Medications. Sometimes people refuse a medication, and often their reasons are valid. If a patient does decline to take a prescribed medication the nurse should find out why. Some of the possible reasons are:

1. The medicine is nauseating and makes him vomit.
2. He is allergic to the medicine. A record of the patient's allergies should be noted on admission. Sometimes this is not possible, however; for example, the patient may have been unconscious when he was brought in.
3. The medicine does not help him.
4. He thinks it is the wrong medicine.
5. He believes the physician has changed the order.
6. The needles with which the medicine is administered hurt him.
7. The medicine has an unpleasant taste.
8. He does not want it because of religious or cultural beliefs. A patient of the Hindu religion may refuse a hormonal preparation that contains extracts from cattle. A patient who belongs to the Jehovah's Witnesses sect may refuse a blood transfusion. Many people who believe in naturopathic remedies will refuse any medicine prepared from inorganic chemicals.
9. He does not understand the purpose of the medication and is afraid it will harm him.
10. The nurse wants to administer the medication at an inconvenient time, such as when his visitors are present.

The reason a patient refuses a medicine can often be satisfactorily dealt with by the nurse. For example, if it has an unpleasant taste it can usually be administered in a vehicle such as orange juice. The physician's order should be checked if the patient questions it. Perhaps there is a new order in the chart that has not been transcribed to his medication card. A patient's refusal to take a medication should always be reported to the physician or to the nurse in charge and recorded in the patient's chart. Under some circumstances it is best to notify the physician at once, particularly when a patient's condition is seriously affected by the omission of the medication, as when a patient with heart disease will not take digitalis.

Observing and Reporting

Immediately after a medication has been administered, the fact is recorded on the patient's chart. If the drug was administered at the nurse's discretion, the reason for the administration is also recorded.

After the administration of any therapeutic agent, the nurse observes the patient for his reaction. The criteria by which the nurse judges the effectiveness of a drug depend on the purpose for which it was administered. It can be the alleviation of pain, the reduction of fever, a decrease in swelling, or even the appearance of orange-colored urine. These are anticipated results and they reflect the effectiveness of the particular medication. The observations are recorded in detail on the patient's chart. Sometimes patients experience untoward reactions as a result of a medication—for example, nausea and vomiting, diarrhea or a skin rash. These observations are always reported promptly. If a reaction is severe, that is, if the patient is acutely uncomfortable or essential body functions are impaired, the physician is notified immediately so that measures to stop the reaction can begin.

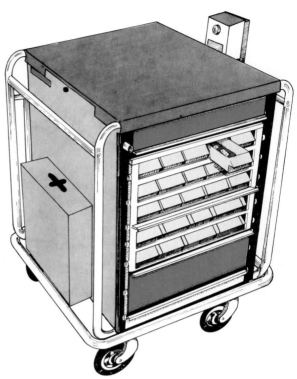

Medication carts provide separate drawers for each patient's medications. When giving a medication to one patient, the nurse can keep the drawers with medications for other patients closed to limit the spread of infection from one patient to another.

In a hospital, medications are usually prepared in a separate room adjoining the nursing station.

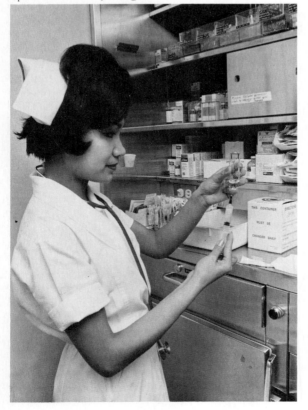

In severe allergic reactions the tissues of the throat may become so edematous that breathing is difficult. Prompt intervention at the earliest sign of an allergic reaction is required. These reactions are also recorded in detail on the patient's chart.

PREPARING MEDICATIONS

The first step in the preparation of any medication is to get the complete order and make sure it is understood. Sometimes agency policies or the orders themselves govern the administration of a specific drug or the special nursing measures that accompany its administration. For example, an order might read "withhold drug if pulse is below 60 beats per minute."

Before administering drugs, the nurse washes her hands to minimize the transfer of microorganisms and then she gathers the equipment she needs. In a hospital all the necessary equipment is usually kept in a medication room, near the nursing unit office yet separate from it so that medications can be prepared without disturbance. In the home, such equipment is generally

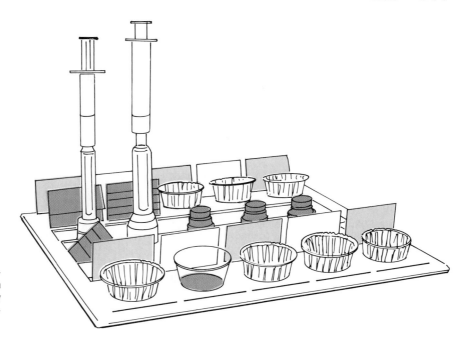

Trays are often used in hospitals instead of medication carts. Cards placed in the tray identify which patient is to receive each medication.

kept in one place, usually in a cupboard that is out of reach of children. Some hospitals use medication carts to deliver the medicines; others use trays, often with special slots so that the medicine card stands upright and can be read easily.

A hospital medication cupboard is usually locked, the key being kept by the head nurse, the nurse responsible for administering medications (if this system is used), or in a designated place in the nursing unit. Adjacent to the medication cupboard are usually a locked narcotic cupboard and a refrigerator. Drugs that lose their potency unless kept cold are kept in the refrigerator.

The nurse selects the medicine that was ordered by the physician. Drugs kept in a hospital are either stock or private (prescription). The former are the more commonly used medicines; the latter are especially prepared for a patient. Stock drugs are frequently grouped according to action; for example, all vitamin preparations are kept together. Another method of storing drugs is to arrange them alphabetically according to their generic or trade names. Either method facilitates finding a specific preparation quickly.

It has become an accepted safety practice in the preparation of medications to read the label three times on a bottle, tube, package, envelope, or the like. It is read (1) before the container is taken off the shelf, (2) before it is opened, and (3) just before it is placed back on the shelf. The nurse should read both the name of the drug and its strength, and pay particular attention to the route of administration by which the particular medicine is designed to be given.

Medications come in a variety of preparations; capsules, Spansules, lozenges, tablets, and liquids can all be given orally. A capsule contains a powder, oil, or liquid within a gelatinous covering; a tablet is a compressed powdered drug. Troches are oral preparations which are sucked. Vials and ampules contain either powdered or liquid medications for injection. A vial is a glass container with a rubber stopper, whereas an ampule is a sealed glass container. A suppository is a medication that is molded into a firm base in order that it can be inserted into a body orifice or cavity. An ointment is a semisolid mixture that is applied topically to mucous membranes or skin.

A medicine must be administered in the exact dose that is ordered by the physician. If small doses are required (for example, for children), the usual practice is to have these doses prepared accurately by a pharmacist. In situations in which the dose must be calculated, the safest practice is for a second nurse to check the calculations made by the first. The nurse should not estimate a dosage on her own initiative; it is not a safe practice to break an unscored tablet to get a dosage. The dose of a drug is ordered by the physician in consideration of the weight, age, sex, and physical condition of the patient. Thus, approximating dosages is a dangerous practice.

In order to avoid errors the nurse who prepares a medication should administer it herself immediately after she has prepared it. If prepared medicines are left unattended, the chances of the drug being misplaced or taken by another patient are increased. More to the point, the nurse is legally responsible for the medications she administers, and only if she has prepared a medication herself can she testify to the actual constituents of the medication and to its strength. The identification of a medication just by its appearance is a dangerous practice. If it happens that medications are distributed while a patient is in another department, his medication can be returned to the nursing unit and locked in the cupboard with the medication card which serves to identify it.

When a nurse is preparing a variety of medications for a group of patients, the medicines for one patient are separated from the medicines for another. Generally all medicines that are administered by the same route for one patient can be placed in the same container, except for specific drugs whose administration is dependent upon some specified criterion. For example, if digitalis 0.1 g. (gr. $\overline{iss}$) is to be withheld when the patient's pulse is below 60 beats per minute, this drug is put in a separate container from the other oral medications for that particular patient.

Only a pharmacist should label a container of drugs. Therefore when the nurse finds an unlabeled container or a label that has been partially obscured, the entire container is returned to the pharmacy for clarification. It is also considered a safety practice not to return medications to a container once they have been removed; they should be disposed of by flushing down a toilet or hopper. Some agencies require that a witness be present when narcotics (and sometimes other drugs as well) are disposed of. Drugs should not be transferred from one container to another.

METHODS OF ADMINISTERING MEDICATIONS

The most common method of administering medications is by mouth (orally). Not only is it simple but it is also the most economical way. Capsules, liquids, tablets, powders, and troches are all administered by mouth. Troches are usually sucked for their local effect. Sublingual administration involves placing the drug (for example, nitroglycerin) under the patient's tongue, where it is dissolved and absorbed.

Parenteral refers to the administration of drugs by a needle. Intramuscular, intradermal, subcutaneous, and intravenous injections are common means of parenteral therapy. Intracardiac, intrapericardial, intrathecal (intraspinal), and intraosseous (into bone) injections are less

common methods that may be used by physicians. All parenteral therapy involves the use of sterile equipment and sterile, readily soluble solutions. Generally those drugs that are administered parenterally are readily absorbed by the body. Intravenous therapy was discussed in Chapter 17.

Inhalation is the administration of a drug into the respiratory tract. Once the drug is inhaled it is almost immediately absorbed. Volatile and nonvolatile drugs can be inhaled, the latter by means of a vehicle such as oxygen. The administration of medications by inhalation was discussed in Chapter 18.

Instillation is a method of putting a drug in liquid form into a body cavity or orifice, for example the ears, the eyes, and the urinary bladder. Liquid medications can be instilled with a dropper (into the ear) or with a syringe (into the urinary bladder).

Medications are also applied to the skin and mucous membranes; this process is called topical application. Antiseptics, astringents, and emollients can be applied as liquids or ointments.

Drugs are generally administered for either their systemic or local effect. Systemic effect refers to the actions of the drug upon the entire body, whereas local effect is the effect upon one specific area, such as that of an ointment upon a particular area of the skin. Sometimes drugs that are administered for their local effect have systemic actions; for example, an untoward reaction such as a fever may result from the topical application of an ointment to an incision.

A suppository is used for insertion into a body cavity or orifice, such as the rectum or vagina. As the suppository gradually dissolves at body temperature, the drug is released and is absorbed through the mucous membrane. Although a suppository is sometimes used to administer drugs when a systemic action is desired, as, for example, a sedative, it is not considered as efficient as a medication administered by other routes. Suppositories are therefore used principally for their local action. They may be used, for instance, to administer an analgesic to the rectal area, or to stimulate peristalsis and bring about a bowel movement.

Oral Administration

Oral medications are absorbed chiefly in the small intestines, although they can also be absorbed in the mouth and the stomach. Medications administered sublingually are absorbed through the capillaries under the tongue. Drugs in liquid form, either upon administration or upon dissolution within the stomach, are absorbed through the gastric mucosa. Absorption of a drug is slowed by the presence of food in the stomach as well as by its administration in concentrated form. Dilution, an alcoholic base, and an empty stomach facilitate absorption.

Advantages and Disadvantages. The oral administration of medications has the advantages of convenience, economy, and safety. It is convenient in that it is a simple method of administration; it is economical in that oral preparations usually cost less to manufacture than many other preparations; it is safe in that its administration does not involve breaking through any of the body defenses—for example, the skin—as is necessary with injections.

The chief disadvantages of the oral administration of medications are their taste, gastric irritation, effect upon teeth, inaccurate measure of absorption, and limited use.

Drugs that are decidedly *unpleasant tasting* can stimulate nausea and vomiting. Drugs in liquid or partially dissolved form activate the taste buds more than drugs in tablet or capsule form; however, since cold is less stimulating than warmth, the taste buds can be partially desensitized by giving cold fluids or ice chips.

Some medications are particularly *irritating to the gastric mucosa*; others are destroyed by the gastric secretions. The latter are usually manufactured either with an enteric coating so that they do not dissolve in the stomach, or in a form to be given by parenteral administration. Irritation of the gastric mucosa can be minimized by administering a drug after a meal, while food is still in the stomach. Also, the more diluted the medicine is, the less irritating it will be to the mucosa. A medicine that is particularly irritating can sometimes be given with another drug or with food, such as bread, in order to modify its undesirable effect.

Some medications are *harmful to the teeth.* Drugs such as hydrochloric acid damage enamel, and liquid iron preparations often discolor the teeth. These undersirable effects can be avoided by giving highly diluted forms and by using a straw in order that the teeth do not come in contact with the liquid. It is also wise to have the patient rinse his mouth with water or a mouthwash after he takes these medicines.

Another disadvantage of the oral administration of medications is the relative inability to *measure their absorption accurately* in the gastrointestinal tract. Certain disorders affect absorption; for example, accelerated peristalsis will decrease absorption because of the drug's speedy propulsion through the gastrointestinal tract. Moreover, some medications are destroyed

to a variable extent by gastrointestinal secretions. In addition, the adequacy of the circulation of the blood to the tract affects the rate of absorption. If a person vomits after he has ingested a medicine, the amount of drug retained in his body is questionable. Generally the physician is consulted when this happens in order that he can assess the patient's need for a repeated dose of the medicine.

Oral medications are *limited in use* to patients who are able to swallow and retain them. The unconscious patient, the patient who is unable to swallow, and the vomiting patient are unable to take these medications. Patients who are restricted to taking nothing by mouth cannot be given oral medications. Some patients cannot take oral medications because of gastric suction and some find swallowing difficult because of surgery or paralysis. Frequently, it is the nurse who first becomes aware that a patient had difficulty in swallowing a medicine. She needs to communicate this fact to the physician so that a change in the order can be made to a more easily consumed drug. Tablets can be crushed and a scored tablet can be broken for easier administration, but the protective coverings of capsules or enteric-coated pills should not be removed to facilitate administration.

Preparation. In the preparation of oral medications for distribution, the nurse follows the general guides outlined earlier in this chapter. Oral drugs are generally distributed in disposable containers. Liquid medications are often given in plastic or waxed paper containers. The advantages of using disposable containers are obvious: their cleanliness is assured, and washing and sterilizing are eliminated. Medications should not be handled indiscriminately with the fingers. It is considered a cleaner practice to drop a tablet into the bottle cap or into an empty medicine container before transferring it to the container that the patient uses. If there is any doubt about administering a specific drug, the drug is kept separately from the other tablets for a specific patient.

When pouring liquids, the dose is measured from the bottom of the concave meniscus. Some liquids separate after standing in a bottle and need to be shaken before they are poured. Minims (0.06 ml.) and drops are not interchangeable measures. Special droppers or glasses, and, in some agencies, syringes, are used for measuring small amounts of liquid medications.

Administration. After the patient is appropriately identified, the nurse gives him his medications and stays with him until they have been taken. Sometimes the patient needs assistance to sit up or to turn on his side to swallow without choking. Usually people find it easier to take oral medicines with water or juice. If the consistency of a liquid is unpleasant, as, for example, mineral oil, patients often find it easier to take if the medicine has been chilled. With some exceptions, drugs are not left at a patient's bedside in hospitals. The exceptions are usually part of a planned program of teaching patients to self-administer drugs.

Subcutaneous Injection

Advantages and Disadvantages.   Some medications are best administered into the subcutaneous tissue by a needle. This route has the advantage of almost complete absorption, provided that the patient's circulation is good; therefore, an accurate measure of the amount of the drug absorbed is possible. Medicines administered in this manner are not affected by gastric disturbances (although it should be remembered that the medicines may themselves cause gastrointestinal disturbances), nor is their administration dependent upon the consciousness or rationality of the patient.

The chief disadvantage of this method is that by introducing a needle through the skin one of the body's barriers against infection is broken. It is therefore important that aseptic technique be used for all needle injections.

The Site of Injection.   The subcutaneous tissue is just below the cutaneous tissue or skin. It has fewer sensory receptors than the skin itself; therefore once a needle is through the skin an injection is relative painless. Some drugs sting upon injection, but an isotonic solution can usually be administered painlessly. The term isotonic refers to a concentration that is the same as a normal saline solution.

The exact site for a subcutaneous injection depends on the need of the specific patient and to some extent upon the policy of the institution. Since drugs administered subcutaneously (hypodermically) are usually given for their systemic effect, the site is irrelevant with respect to any local effect. Areas of the upper arms, anterior and lateral aspects of the thigh, and the lower ventral abdominal wall are suggested.[2] The skin and subcutaneous tissue should be in good condition, that is, free of irritation such as itching and free of any signs of inflammation, such as redness, heat, edema, tenderness, or pain. Areas where there is scar tissue should not be used. A common practice is to choose the outer aspect of the patient's upper arm, about one-third of the distance down between the

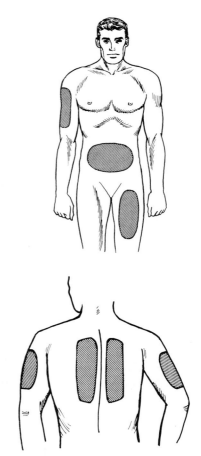

Sites that are commonly used for subcutaneous injections include the outer aspect of the upper arm, the loose abdominal tissue, the anterior aspect of the thigh, and the subscapular area of the back.

shoulder and the elbow. Other sites are the anterior aspect of the thigh, the loose tissue of the abdomen, and the subscapular region of the back. Actually the subcutaneous tissue in any area can be injected provided that is is not over bony prominences and is free of large blood vessels and nerves. If a patient is receiving a series of injections the sites are rotated and the

(From Wood, L. A., and Rambo, B. J.: *Nursing Skills for Allied Health Services.* 2nd ed. Vol. 3. Philadelphia. W. B. Saunders Company, 1980.)

Insulin Syringes

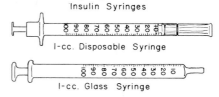

Insulin syringes (disposable or reusable) — U40, U80, U100 (Becton-Dickinson Co.)

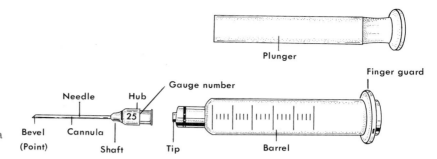

Diagram of needle and parts of a syringe.

site is charted each time so that two consecutive doses are not given in the same area. Sometimes a map is made of the skin areas to be used to indicate the sites for rotating injections, or a chart may be attached to the nursing care plan for the patient.

Equipment. Subcutaneous (hypodermic) injections involve the use of sterile equipment and supplies. These include a syringe, a needle, the medication, and a swab and disinfectant to cleanse the skin. Syringes vary in size from 1 to 50 ml. The 2-ml syringe, commonly used for subcutaneous injections, is calibrated in cubic centimeters. For the administration of insulin, special 1 ml. syringes are often used. Insulin syringes are usually calibrated in units to correspond to the strength of a particular insulin.

The 100-unit scale is most common, although some agencies still use a 40- or 80-unit scale.

A syringe has two parts, the barrel or outer part, and the plunger or inner part. Most syringes are manufactured so that their parts are interchangeable, but if they are not, the two pieces of a set bear corresponding numbers on the plunger and barrel.

Syringes are made of glass or plastic. The latter, which are usually disposable, are being used increasingly in hospitals, offices, and clinics. The maximum volume of solution that can be given comfortably by this route is thought to be 20 minims (less than 1.5 ml.). Certainly anything greater than 2 ml. will cause pressure on surrounding tissues and therefore be painful.

A needle has a hub and a shaft or cannula. The hub is the larger part that connects to the

For a subcutaneous injection the needle enters the skin at a 90-degree angle if a ½ inch needle is used, at a 45-degree angle if a ⅝ inch needle is used. The bevel of the needle is uppermost. The needle is inserted deeply into the subcutaneous tissue.

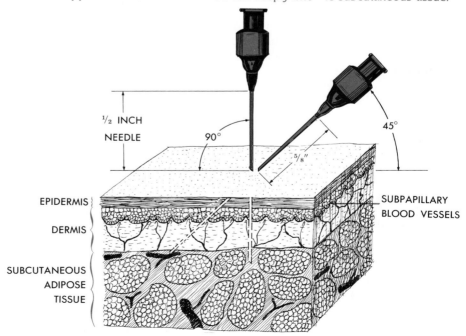

barrel of the syringe; the cannula is the long narrow part. At the end of the cannula is the bevel (point) or slanted portion where the fluid is ejected. A short or small bevel is used when there is a danger that a larger bevel would become occluded, as in intravenous injections in which the bevel could rest against the side of the vein. The longer bevel provides a sharper needle and is used for subcutaneous and intramuscular injections.

The needle used for a subcutaneous injection is usually 24, 25, or 26 gauge. The larger the number, the smaller the diameter of the needle. The length that is required varies from 1 cm. (3/8 inch) to 2.5 cm. (1 inch), depending upon the amount of subcutaneous fat and the degree of hydration of the patient. A longer needle is needed for the obese patient, a shorter needle for the dehydrated person. Generally a No. 24 needle 1.5 cm (5/8 inch) long is used for the average adult.

The needle used for any injection should be straight and sharp. As disposable needles are increasingly being used, the problem of the bent or dull needle is disappearing. If disposable needles are not used, the needles are checked for sharpness and the presence of barbs before they are sterilized. A needle may be checked for the presence of barbs by passing the tip lightly over a piece of absorbent cotton. If the needle does catch on the cotton, it may have a barb and will be uncomfortable for a patient. Needles that are bent should not be used, because of the possibility that they will break off in a patient. The weakest point in a needle is where the cannula joins the hub.

A word of caution on the use of disposable needles and syringes: After use they should be discarded in the designated containers, never where they can be obtained by addicts. Disposable needles and syringes should be bent after use so that they cannot be used again. These practices also help to protect the housekeeping staff from injury, since the bent needle point will not be as likely to penetrate garbage bags.

Two variations in the traditional means of administering injections subcutaneously are the injector syringe equipped with a spring which releases the needle for rapid insertion, and the jet injector by which the medication is introduced into the subcutaneous tissue by means of high pressure rather than through a needle. Although these methods are preferred in some instances, they have not replaced the usual subcutaneous injection by hypodermic syringe.

Preparation.   Medications for injection come in tablet, liquid, and powder forms. All these forms must be kept sterile during preparation and administration. If a drug in tablet form is to be administered subcutaneously, it is first dissolved in a sterile solution. The safest method is to carefully drop the tablet into a sterile container, draw up a measured amount of sterile solution into the syringe (sterile normal saline is less painful to the patient than sterile water), add the solution to the tablet to dissolve it and, finally, draw up the measured amount of medicated solution into the syringe ready for administration. Another method, which is being used increasingly, is to mix the tablet and the solution directly in the syringe.

Medications in a liquid form generally come in single dose ampules or multiple dose vials. To open an ampule, the nurse first taps it to shake all the medication to the bottom and then obtains a sterile cotton ball which she holds behind the neck of the ampule. Some ampules open directly upon pressure at the neck; others require filing. The cotton ball is used to protect the nurse's fingers when breaking the glass. After the ampule is opened, the needle is carefully inserted, the ampule is inverted, and the solution is drawn into the sterile syringe.

Multiple dose vials of medication have a sealed rubber cap at the top which makes them airtight. The cap is first wiped off with an antiseptic solution, the plunger of the syringe is drawn back to a point which indicates the volume of solution to be withdrawn, and then the needle is inserted through the rubber cap. Air is injected into the vial to equalize the pressure and thus facilitate removal of the solution. The vial is held upside down with the syringe at eye level in order to obtain an accurate measure of the drug. Incorrect holding of the vial may result in air being drawn into the syringe.

Injectable drugs that come as powders are dissolved in sterile solution before they are administered. Generally there are directions on the label as to the amount and kind of solution that is to be added to a vial. In order to maintain normal pressure inside the vial, air is removed in a volume that corresponds to the amount of solution that is inserted. If a large vial is used, it is often easier to insert a second sterile needle through the rubber cap to allow the free flow of air out of the vial as the fluid flows in.

Some drugs are prepared commercially in two-compartment vials. One compartment contains the powdered medication and the second contains the sterile liquid for dissolving the drug. The insertion of a sterile needle or pressure upon a rubber diaphragm releases the liquid to mix with the powder, which is then ready for injection. Some drugs are packaged this way because they are more stable in a dry state and thus can be kept for a longer period of time than the same drug in liquid form.

Whenever a powder or tablet is prepared for injection it should be completely dissolved before it is drawn into the syringe. Rotating a vial between one's hands is an effective way of mixing a powder and a liquid without creating bubbles on the top of the solution. Bubbles can make it difficult to ascertain an accurate measure of the drug.

Administration. When a subcutaneous injection is to be administered, a site is selected and cleansed with an antiseptic solution. The type of antiseptic used depends on the policy of the agency. Isopropanol in 70 per cent solution is used in many hospitals. The antiseptic solution is allowed to dry on the skin surface prior to insertion of the needle to prevent local irritation at the site of the injection.

When the skin is dry, air is expelled from the needle. The needle is then inserted through the skin. The angle of insertion depends on the size of the needle used. It is recommended that the injection be given deeply into the subcutaneous tissue. Therefore, if a 1.2 cm. (½ inch) needle is used, it is inserted at a 90-degree angle, that is, perpendicular to the skin surface. Injections with a 1.5 cm. (⅝ inch) needle are inserted at a 45-degree angle. Some authorities feel that the skin should not be drawn taut or pinched or pulled into a skin fold for the injection, but rather should be left in its natural state.[2] The nurse will find it easier to give the injection, however, if she lightly holds the area around the injection site.

After the needle is inserted, the plunger is drawn back in order to determine whether the needle is in a blood vessel. If no blood appears in the syringe, the solution is injected slowly, after which the needle is quickly withdrawn. If blood does appear in the syringe, the needle is immediately withdrawn and another medication prepared. After the needle is withdrawn the area is massaged gently with an antiseptic sponge to facilitate dispersion of the solution. If there is any sign of bleeding from the site of the injection, firm pressure over the area for a few minutes will usually stop the bleeding and thus prevent bruising.

Recording. A subcutaneous injection is recorded on the patient's record in the same way as any other medication but, in addition, the word "subcutaneous" or the abbreviation "H" follows the dosage of the drug to indicate the route. Sometimes the site of the injection is also recorded.

Intramuscular Injection

Advantages and Disadvantages. Intramuscular injection is the method of choice for the administration of some medications. Drugs which are irritating to subcutaneous tissue are often given by this route. In addition, a large amount of fluid can be injected into muscle tissue than into subcutaneous tissue. Absorption through a muscle is faster than through subcutaneous tissue because of the vascularity of the muscle area. The danger of damaging nerves and blood vessels, however, is greater.

The Site of Injection. Regardless of the site chosen, the area must be exposed adequately so that the nurse can see what she is doing. The selection of an area for an intramuscular injection depends on a number of factors: the size of the patient and the amount of muscle tissue

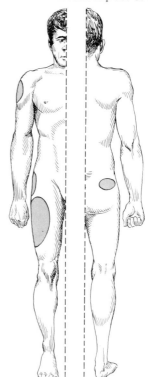

Four sites used for intramuscular injections are the deltoid muscle, the ventrogluteal site of the gluteus minimus and gluteus medius muscles, the dorsogluteal site of the gluteus maximus muscle, and the vastus lateralis muscle on the lateral aspect of the thigh.

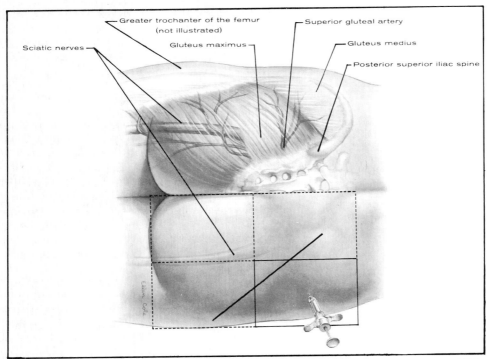

Greater trochanter of the femur
(not illustrated)

Superior gluteal artery

Sciatic nerves

Gluteus maximus

Gluteus medius

Posterior superior iliac spine

Intramuscular injection. With the patient lying in a prone position, the nurse can establish the dorsogluteal site as indicated. (Courtesy of Wyeth Laboratories, Philadelphia, Pa.)

available for injection, the proximity of nerves and blood vessels, the condition of the skin around the area, and the nature of the drug to be administered. The site should be anatomically safe; that is, an area should be chosen where the danger of hitting a nerve or large blood vessel is minimal. The tissues in the area should be free of bruising or soreness. There should be no abrasions on the skin, and areas with hardened tissue (such as scar tissue) should be avoided.

Various sites are suitable for intramuscular injections; areas in the buttocks, the thigh, and the upper arm are used most frequently. Generally it is best to rotate the areas when a series of injections is to be given. The gluteal muscles are thick and permit the injection of larger quantities of fluid. Also, the use of these muscles in many normal daily activities aids in the absorption of drugs administered by this route. Two sites in the gluteal muscles are commonly used: the dorsogluteal site and the ventrogluteal site.

The *dorsogluteal site* uses the gluteus maximus muscle. The site may be located by dividing the buttock into quadrants. The crest of the ilium and the inferior gluteal fold act as landmarks for describing the buttock. The injection is given in the upper outer quadrant of the buttock, 5 to 7.5 cm. (2 to 3 inches) below the crest of the ilium. By using this area, large blood vessels and the sciatic nerve are avoided. Another method for locating a safe gluteal site is to draw an imaginary line from the posterior superior iliac spine to the greater trochanter of the femur. This line runs lateral and parallel to the sciatic nerve, and consequently an injection lateral and superior to it is in a safe area.

When the *ventrogluteal site* is used the injection is made into the gluteus minimus and the gluteus medius muscles. To locate the ventrogluteal area, the nurse has the patient lie on his back or his side. She then places her hand on the patient's hip with her index finger on the anterior superior iliac supine, and stretching her middle finger dorsally, palpates the crest of the ilium and presses below the iliac crest. The injection site is the triangle that is formed by her index finger, her middle finger, and the crest of the ilium. The ventrogluteal site is being used increasingly because there are no large nerves or blood vessels in the area; also there is usually less fatty tissue than in the buttocks. If the patient's gluteal muscles are tense, he can flex his knees to relax them for the injection.

The *vastus lateralis* muscle on the lateral aspect of the thigh is also being used more

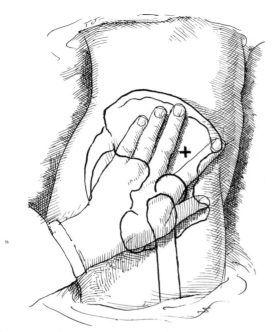

Locate the triangle for injection by placing the left index finger on the anterior iliac spine and the middle finger just below the iliac crest. (From *What's New*. Abbott Laboratories, No. 211, Spring, 1959.)

frequently for intramuscular injections. The area is free of major blood vessels and nerve trunks, and the vastus lateralis muscle provides a good long area when numerous injections have to be given. The muscle extends the full length of the thigh from mid-anterior to mid-lateral and is approximately 7.5 cm. (3 inches) wide. The injection may be given anywhere from approximately 10 cm. (4 inches) above the knee to approximately 10 cm. below the hip joint.

The *deltoid muscle* of the arm is also used for intramuscular injections. This site is two to three fingerbreadths down from the acromion process on the outer aspect of the arm. In most people this is a smaller muscle than the gluteal muscle and therefore is not capable of absorbing as large a volume of medicine comfortably. The essential danger in this area is that of harming the radial nerve.

Equipment. The equipment required for an intramuscular injection is similar to that used for a subcutaneous injection. The quantity of solution to be administered varies from 2 to 10 ml. In many agencies, however, nurses are permitted to inject no more than 5 ml. in any one injection; therefore, if more than 5 ml. is ordered, the amount is given in two injections. A 2-, 5-, or 10-ml. syringe is used with a No. 19 to 22 gauge needle 2.5 to 5 cm. (1 to 2 inches) long. The

gauge of the needle to be used depends on the viscosity of the drug and the sensitivity of the patient. The length of the needle depends on the size of the patient's muscle and the amount of adipose tissue that is present. It is desirable to inject the drug into the center of the muscle. A No. 22 needle 3.75 cm. (1½ inches) long is commonly used for an adult.

Preparation. The drug is prepared for administration in the same way as for a subcutaneous injection. Some authorities recommend that a small air bubble be left in the syringe to force the last of the drug out of the needle into the muscle and thus prevent any solution from being left in the subcutaneous tissue when the needle is removed. There is probably considerable merit to this practice, particularly with drugs that are known to be irritating to subcutaneous tissue.

Administration. For an intramuscular injection to the gluteal muscle, the patient lies in a prone position with his toes internally rotated in plantar flexion. In this position the gluteal muscles are relaxed and there is good visualization of the injection site.

The selection of the area for an injection is determined by four factors: Is it anatomically safe? free of bruises or sore areas? free of hardened areas? free of abrasions on the skin?

The muscle is palpated and the skin is wiped as for a subcutaneous injection. The skin is held taut and the needle is inserted at a 90-degree angle to the distance required to reach the center of the muscle. When the needle is inserted smoothly and firmly, this is a relatively painless procedure. The skin is then released and the plunger is withdrawn in order to make sure the needle has not entered a blood vessel. Keeping the needle in place, the solution is injected slowly into the muscle tissue. The needle is then removed quickly, and the area is massaged gently with the disinfectant sponge to aid in dispersion of the solution.

In the air bubble method mentioned, it is common practice to draw a small bubble of air into the syringe before the solution is injected. The bubble rises to the top of the solution when the syringe is inverted for the injection. The air then helps to clear the needle of fluid before the needle is withdrawn. This prevents dripping of the fluid as the needle is being withdrawn through the subcutaneous tissue.

When administering particularly irritating drugs into muscle tissue, the Z-track method is used. In this method the site is selected and then the skin is pulled firmly toward the lateral

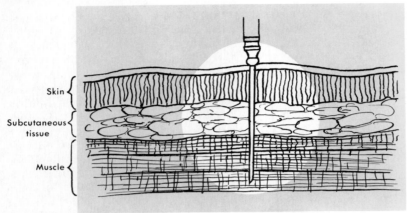

Skin

Subcutaneous tissue

Muscle

For an intramuscular injection the needle is inserted at a 90-degree angle into the center of the muscle.

aspect of the buttock. The injection site is reassessed and cleansed with disinfectant solution, and then the needle is inserted at a 90-degree angle to the desired depth. The plunger is then pulled back slightly to determine whether the needle has entered a blood vessel. If blood appears, the needle is withdrawn and another site is selected. If no blood appears, the solution is injected slowly. After injecting the solution, the nurse waits for 10 seconds to allow the medication to disperse. She then withdraws the needle and allows the stretched skin to return to its normal position. Then the area is massaged with a cotton ball. This method helps keep the drug in the muscle and away from the subcutaneous tissue.

With careful technique, complications from intramuscular injections can be avoided. Abscesses, nerve injuries, cysts and necrosis of tissue do occur as a result of intramuscular injections; however, the use of aseptic tech-

nique, individual establishment of landmarks for injection sites, and the alternating of sites help to avoid these unpleasant results.

As more research is done in the field of intramuscular injections, the nurse may well find traditional techniques being modified in many agencies in the light of new research findings.

Recording. After the administration of an intramuscular injection, the drug, dosage, and method of administration are recorded. The abbreviation "I.M." is frequently used to indicate the route. The site of administration is often recorded also.

Intradermal Injection

An intradermal injection is the injection of a small amount of fluid into the dermal layer of the skin. It is frequently done as a diagnostic

Diagram of Z-track method of intramuscular injection. The correct technique converts the needle track into a zig-zag, which prevents leakage into tissues.

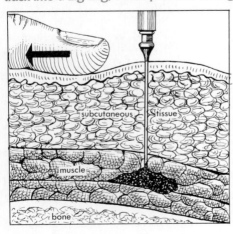

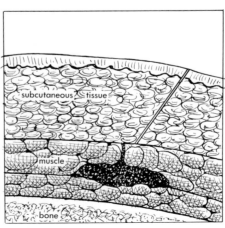

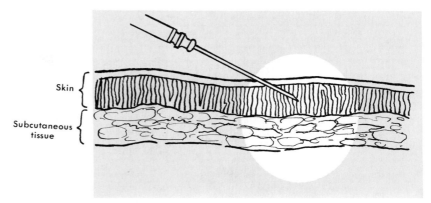

For an intradermal injection the needle is held at a 15-degree angle, bevel upward, and inserted into the dermal layer of the skin.

measure, as in tuberculin testing and allergy testing. The areas of the body commonly used are the medial aspect of the forearm and the subscapular region of the back.

A 1-ml. syringe (or a tuberculin syringe) and a 26 gauge needle 1 cm. (⅜ inch) in length are commonly used. A tuberculin syringe is calibrated in tenths and hundredths of a cubic centimeter in order that minute doses can be measured. The needle is inserted at a 15-degree angle with the bevel up, and the fluid is injected to produce a small bleb just under the skin.

Topical Application

Medications may be applied to the skin or mucous membranes in the form of lotions, ointments, or liniments. Lotions are liquid preparations that are usually applied to protect, soothe, or soften surface areas, to relieve itching, or to check the growth of microorganisms. Ointments are preparations with a fatty base, such as lard, petroleum jelly, or oils. They may be applied to the skin or mucous membranes where they are melted by the heat of the body and absorbed. Ointments are frequently used for antiseptic or antimicrobial purposes. Liniments are liquids that are applied to the skin by rubbing. They are frequently used to warm an affected area; this dilates the superficial blood vessels and also helps to relax tight muscles.

Lotions or Liniments

Equipment. The application of lotions or liniments is often a clean, rather than a sterile, procedure in a home situation. In a hospital or other inpatient facility, however, it is advisable to use sterile cotton balls or gauze to apply the liquid and to use a sterile glove on the hand being used for the application. The nurse will then need a medicine tray, the bottle of lotion or liniment, packages of sterile 5 × 5 cm. (2 × 2 inch) gauze, or sterile cotton balls, and a sterile glove for this procedure.

Administration. The area where the lotion or liniment is to be applied is exposed, making sure that the patient is kept warm and not unduly exposed. The bottle is opened and the cap is placed upside down on the tray. The package of gauze or container of cotton balls is opened and the nurse then puts on the sterile glove. Using the gloved hand, she picks up the gauze or cotton ball. Then, holding the bottle of lotion in her ungloved hand, she pours the required amount onto the gauze, being careful not to spill the liquid over the label. (It is wise to hold the label facing outward to avoid this.) The lotion or liniment is then applied to the affected area. Lotions are not rubbed in; liniments are. The procedure is repeated until all of the affected area is covered. The nurse observes the area carefully for changes in color, swelling, the appearance of a rash, or other observable signs.

Ointments

Equipment. As with lotions and liniments, it is advisable in an institutional setting to use sterile equipment for the application of an ointment. A sterile glove is not needed since the ointment is applied with a sterile tongue depressor. The equipment required is a medicine tray, the jar or tube of ointment, sterile tongue depressor(s), sterile gauze, and tape, if the area is to be covered after application of the ointment.

Administration. The area is exposed; the jar or tube is opened and the cap placed upside down on the tray. The nurse then removes the tongue depressor from its wrapper, being careful to keep the distal end sterile. The ointment is then squeezed or scooped onto the tongue depressor and applied to the area with gentle but firm strokes. The tongue depressor is never returned to the jar for additional ointment. A new one is used instead. The nurse again observes the skin for changes such as color, rash, or swelling. A sterile dressing is applied as indicated to keep the ointment from soiling the bed or patient's linen.

Recording. After the administration of a lotion, a liniment, or an ointment, the drug and the method of administration are recorded. The nurse also records her observations of the condition of the area to which the medication was applied and any changes she noted (as described above.

Instillations

Instillation means to introduce small amounts (drops) of a medication into a body opening. Common sites for instillations are the ear, eye, nose, throat, vagina, and rectum.

Instillations into the Ear. Liquid medications are instilled into the ear cavity usually for one of two purposes: to insert a softening agent so that earwax can be removed easily or to introduce an antibiotic suspension in cases in which the ear canal or the eardrum is infected.

Equipment. The medication to be inserted should always be warmed before being inserted into the ear. A temperature of 105°F (40.6°C) is recommended. Cool solutions are uncomfortable and may cause dizziness or nausea because the equilibrium sense receptors in the semicircular canals are stimulated. The bottle of ear drops may be placed in a small open container of warm water for a few minutes before it is to be used. The temperature of the solution may be tested by dropping a small amount on the inner aspect of the wrist. If it feels comfortable (that is, neither hot nor cool), the solution should be comfortable for the patient.

The nurse will need a medicine tray, a sterile medicine dropper, the bottle of medication, and some sterile cotton balls. Many preparations for individual use come with an attached dropper.

Administration. This procedure is best done with the patient in a sitting position with the ear into which the drops are to be instilled nearer the nurse. The medication is drawn up into the medicine dropper. The nurse then straightens the auditory canal. One method of doing this is as follows: With her left hand on the lobe of the ear, the nurse grasps the upper portion of the auricle between her middle and index fingers and pulls gently with an upward and backward motion to straighten the auditory canal of an adult. For a child, the lobe is pulled downward and backward. The tip of the dropper is inserted into the external ear canal, with care being taken not to injure the delicate ear tissue. The medicine is injected by compressing the bulb on the dropper. The external meatus is plugged with a sterile cotton ball to keep the medicine from escaping, unless drainage from the ear is being promoted, in which case the meatus is not plugged.

Recording. After the administration of the medication, the time, the medication, the amount instilled, and the affected ear are recorded, with a notation also made if a cotton ball was inserted.

Instillations into the Eye. Liquid medications in the form of eye drops, or eye ointments, are instilled into the eye for any one of several reasons: to soothe the eye if it is irritated, to dilate the pupil for any eye examination, to apply an anesthetic, or to combat infection.

Equipment. The administration of eye drops or an eye ointment requires a medicine tray, the bottle of medication with an eye dropper (most eye medications come in bottles with their own dropper) or the tube of ointment, and cotton balls or tissues. Medications for the eye are ordered individually for each patient; they should never be used for another patient.

Administration. The patient may be in a sitting position or supine position for this procedure. If the patient is sitting up, the nurse will find it easier to stand behind the patient to instill eye drops. The nurse asks the patient to look upward; this helps to keep the dropper from touching the cornea if the patient blinks and also helps him to keep his eye from moving while the drops are being instilled. The nurse pulls the lower eyelid down toward the cheek, using her left index finger and thumb (if she is right-handed), to expose the lower fornix (spot indicated on the diagram above). The medication is dropped onto the lower fornix. Excess drops may be wiped off the cheek with a cotton ball or tissues. In removing the eye dropper from and returning it to the bottle, the nurse takes care not to touch the outside of the bottle with the dropper, to avoid contaminating it.

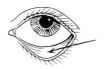

The desired site for instillations of a medication into the eye is the midpoint of the lower fornix. (From Wood, L. A., and Rambo, B. J.: *Nursing Skills for Allied Health Services.* 2nd ed. Vol. 3. Philadelphia, W. B. Saunders Company, 1980.)

If an ointment is to be applied, a thin ribbon of the ointment is laid along the entire length of the fornix. Ointment that is at room temperature is easier to apply. To end the ribbon cleanly, the tube is twisted with a lateral movement of the wrist. The patient's eyelids should be closed gently after the application. Having the patient roll the eyeball around with the lid closed helps to ensure that the medication covers the entire exterior eyeball. The eyelid is gently dried with a cotton ball or tissue to remove excess medication.

In the case of some medications, such as atropine, care must be taken that it does not get into the lacrimal (tear) duct. To avoid this possibility, the nurse can place her thumb over the inner canthus.

Recording. When the eyedrops or ointment has been instilled, the nurse records this on the patient's record, noting the time, the amount, and strength of the medication, and which eye (right, left, or both) received the medication.

Instillations into the Nose. The usual purpose of instilling medication into the nose is either to heal infections or to shrink swollen membranes.

Equipment. For this procedure, the nurse needs a medicine tray; the medication; a dropper (most nose drops come in a bottle with attached dropper), an inhaler, or an atomizer; and disposable tissues or a towel.

Administration. The dorsal recumbent position is considered the best position for the instillation of nose drops. A pillow under the shoulders permits the head to drop back, allowing the medication to flow deep into the nasal cavity. The patient may also be positioned with his head over the edge of the bed; if this position is used, the nurse supports the patient's head with one hand to avoid undue strain on his neck muscles. The patient's head may be positioned either in a straight line from the neck (Proetz position), or with the head deflected to one side (Parkinson position). The former is usually advised if the medication is being used to treat the ethmoid and sphenoid sinuses; the latter is used in treating for the frontal and maxillary sinuses.

To avoid touching the outer or inner surfaces of the nose, the nurse holds the dropper slightly above the nostril to inject the drops, directing

Positions for the instillation of nose drops. (From Wood, L. A., and Rambo, B. J.: *Nursing Skills for Allied Health Services.* 2nd ed. Vol. 3. Philadelphia, W. B. Saunders Company, 1980.)

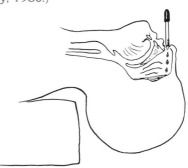

Proetz position

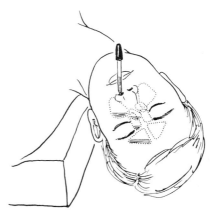

Parkinson position

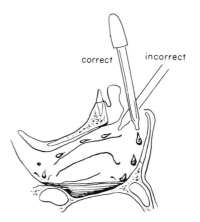

correct   incorrect

the tip toward the midline of the superior concha of the ethmoid. This deflects the medication toward the back of the nasal cavity. The patient is instructed to lie in a recumbent position for 5 to 10 minutes to allow the medication to be absorbed.

When an inhaler or an atomizer is used instead of a dropper, the same procedure is used. The patient is instructed to breathe through his nose while keeping his mouth open during the treatment.

Instillations into the Throat. The throat may be either sprayed or painted in applying an antiseptic or an anesthetic.

Equipment. For spraying or painting a throat, the nurse will need a medicine tray, a tongue depressor, the bottle of medication and, if the medication is to be painted on the tissues, cotton-tipped applicators.

Administration. The best position for this procedure is for the patient to be sitting up and the nurse standing directly in front of the patient, so that she can look down into the throat. A good light is essential for this procedure.

The nurse asks the patient to tilt his head backward (or she helps him to do this) and to open his mouth. She uses her left hand to hold down the tongue with a tongue depressor, and applies the spray or medication, using either an atomizer for spraying or cotton-tipped applicators for painting the tissues.

Recording. After the throat has been sprayed or painted, the nurse records the time, the name and strength of the medication used, and the method of administration.

Instillations into the Vagina. Medications are usually instilled into the vagina to combat infection. They may be applied in the form of a suppository or an ointment. Ointments for use in the vagina usually come in a narrow tube with an attached plunger.

Equipment. The nurse needs sterile or one-use gloves and the medication. A perineal pad may be used to absorb any leakage.

Administration. The patient is positioned in the dorsal recumbent or side-lying position with the legs spread far enough apart to enable the nurse to see the vaginal opening. The patient is draped so that only the perineal area is exposed. Using her left hand to hold open the vagina, the nurse inserts the suppository or tip of the tube applicator into the vagina. If a tube applicator is

used, the plunger is pressed down to expel the ointment. A perineal pad is applied to keep the medication from soiling the patient's clothes.

Instillations into the Rectum. A rectal suppository is inserted with the patient in a side-lying position with the upper leg flexed. With a gloved hand, the nurse inserts the suppository just past the internal anal sphincter, to prevent expulsion.

TOLERANCE AND ADDICTION

When some medications are taken over a long period of time, the effect of the drug diminishes and the patient requires continually larger doses. This reaction to a medicine is called *tolerance*. Narcotics are among the drugs for which patients frequently develop such a tolerance.

Addiction refers to the habitual use of a drug. Usually the person is physically and psychologically dependent upon the drug.

Addiction may become a problem when people receive narcotics for pain or barbiturates or other transquilizers to treat psychological problems over a prolonged period of time. Surveys show that the most widely used drug (other than alcohol) is the tranquilizer diazepam (Valium).

An awareness of which drugs are most likely to result in tolerance and addiction is important. At the first indication that a drug is not acting as it did previously, or at the first indication of dependency upon a particular medication, the physician should be notified. Often alternative medicines can be administered as a preventive measure.

Illegally Used Drugs

While drug abuse can result from the use of drugs for therapeutic purposes, it is a more widespread problem among those who use drug illegally. Experimentation with drugs such as marijuana, hashish, psilocybin ("magic mushrooms"), and alcohol is often done by young people under the influence of a peer group. It may constitute both a new experience and an "escape from reality" for the user.

There is a considerable lack of public understanding about the effects of drug abuse. Professional controversy exists regarding the consequences of the use of "soft" drugs such as marijuana, both in regard to the direct effects of these drugs and in regard to the question of whether use of "soft" drugs leads to use of "hard" drugs. Attempts are under way by several groups to decriminalize the possession and use of marijuana. However, it is clear that marijuana, like alcohol, can severely impair the user's ability to drive and can lead to automobile accidents.

Health professionals may come into contact with drug users in an "overdose unit" in the emergency unit of a hospital. The effects of "hard" drugs such as cocaine, heroin, and LSD (lysergic acid diethylamide) are dealt with there. These drugs are mind-altering and mood-changing. The sense of being "high" on these drugs is usually followed by a "low" or hangover of some type, which may be difficult for the individual to cope with himself. Someone may be needed to "guide" or "talk down" the individual on an LSD "trip" who is hallucinating badly and experiencing a distorted sense of reality.

As we mentioned in Chapter 4, drug overdose has become a leading cause of death among teen-agers. Drug overdoses often seen in emergency units include both accidental overdoses of illegal drugs and deliberate attempts at suicide, which may involve the use of either illegal drugs or sedatives prescribed for other family members. The combination of sedatives with alcohol is particularly dangerous.

Several of the drugs that are widely used illegally may also have uses in medical therapy. Cocaine and morphine are used as anesthetics, and it has been proposed by some people that heroin, which like morphine is derived from opium, should be used to alleviate pain in terminally ill patients. Marijuana is currently being administered to some cancer patients to lessen the nausea and vomiting that often accompany radiation therapy and chemical therapy. Marijuana has also been proposed as a treatment for the eye disease glaucoma.

It is interesting to note the difference between some Eastern cultures and our Western one in regard to drug and alcohol use. In Western cultures, we tend to look upon the drunk lying in the gutter with ridicule but tolerance, and we put the person who uses drugs in jail. In most states in India, the use of alcohol is severely restricted by law, and one may have to sign a form saying that he is an alcoholic in order to purchase a drink in a bar. On the other hand, pleasure boats ply some Indian rivers offering weekend excursions where people can experience the joys of smoking hashish.

GUIDE TO SAFE MEDICATION ADMINISTRATION

1. Does the patient have any allergies?
2. How old is the patient?
3. What medications have been prescribed for the patient?
4. Why is the patient receiving these medications?
5. What observations should the nurse make relative to the effect of these medications on the patient?
6. Are specific nursing measures indicated because of the action of drugs contained in these medications?
7. How are the patient's medications to be administered?
8. What precautions should be taken in administering these medications? Are there special precautions that should be taken because of the patient's age, physical condition, or mental state?
9. Do any of the medications require special precautionary measures in their administration?
10. Does the patient have learning needs relative to his medicinal therapy?
11. Does the patient or his family require specific skills or knowledge in order to continue medicinal therapy at home?

GUIDE TO EVALUATING THE EFFECTIVENESS OF MEDICATIONS

1. Is the patient taking the medicines that have been prescribed?
2. Have the medications been administered safely?

3. Does the patient show signs or symptoms which indicate that the medications are effective (or ineffective)?

4. Has the administration of the medications been accurately reported on the patient's record? Have pertinent observations been recorded and reported to appropriate personnel?

STUDY SITUATION

In the health agency in which you are having clinical experience, find out the following information:

1. The method by which medications are ordered for patients.

2. Communication tools used to facilitate the execution of these orders by nurses, e.g., Kardex file, medication cards, etc.

3. The location of medications on a nursing unit, storage facilities, and system for arranging medications.

4. The equipment used for preparing and administering medications.

5. Safety precautions taken in the preparation and administration of medications.

6. The approved method of recording medications by various administration routes, including narcotic and controlled drugs.

7. Reference material on drugs.

8. Pertinent agency policies regarding the administration of medications.

SUGGESTED READINGS

Allen, M. D.: Drug Therapy in the Elderly. *American Journal of Nursing,* 80(8):1474–1475, August, 1980.

Amdur, M. A., and Cohen, M.: Medication Groups for Psychiatric Patients. *American Journal of Nursing,* 81(2):343–345, February, 1981.

Anders, J., and Moeller, P.: Topicals: What to Use, How to Apply. *RN,* 44:32 September, 1982.

Asperheim, M. K., and Eisenhauer, L. A.: *The Pharmacological Basis of Patient Care.* 4th ed. Philadelphia, W. B. Saunders Company, 1981.

Cardoni, A. A.: Drug Information Sources. *Nursing '78,* 8(5):56–64, May, 1978.

Coyle, N.: Analgesics at the Bedside. *American Journal of Nursing,* 79(9):1554–1557, September, 1979.

Drugs and Alcohol. American Journal of Nursing, 76:65, January, 1976.

Evans, M. L., and Hansen, B. D.: Administering Injections to Different-aged Children. *American Journal of Maternal-Child Nursing,* 6:194–199, May-June, 1981.

Falconer, M. W., et al.: *The Drug, the Nurse, the Patient.* 6th ed. Philadelphia, W. B. Saunders Company, 1978.

Foerst, H.: Drug-prescribing Patterns in Skilled Nursing Facilities. *American Journal of Nursing,* 79(11):2000–2004, November, 1979.

Giving Medications. Nursing '80 Photobook. Horsham, Pa., Intermed Communications, Inc., 1980.

Gotz, B. E., and Gotz, V. P.: Drugs and the Elderly. *American Journal of Nursing,* 78(8):1347–1351, August, 1978.

Hayter, J.: Why Response to Medication Changes with Age. *Geriatric Nursing,* 2:411, November-December, 1981.

Lenhart, D. G.: The Use of Medications in the Elderly Population. *Nursing Clinics of North America,* 11:135–144, March, 1976.

McCaffery, M.: Patients Shouldn't Have to Suffer—Relieve Their Pain with Injectable Narcotics. *Nursing '80,* 10(10):34–39, October, 1980.

McCaffery, M.: Relieve Your Patients' Pain Fast and Effectively with Oral Analgesics. *Nursing '80,* 10(11):58–64, November, 1980.

Newton, D. W., and Newton, M.: Route, Site, and Technique: Three Key Decisions in Giving Parenteral Medication. *Nursing '79,* 9(7):18–25, July, 1979.

Youngren, D. E.: Improve Patient Compliance with a Self-medication Teaching Program. *Nursing '81,* 11(3):22–23, March, 1981.

REFERENCES

1. Gotz, B. E., and Gotz, V. P.: Drugs and the Elderly. *American Journal of Nursing*, 78(8):1347–1351, August, 1978.

2. Pitel, M.: The Subcutaneous Injection. *American Journal of Nursing*, 71:79, January, 1971.

29

The Nurse Should Be Able to:

- Explain the role of sexuality in human life
- Describe the structure and functioning of the male and the female reproductive systems and male and female sexual response
- Discuss major factors affecting sexual needs
- Discuss changes in sexual needs throughout the life span
- Outline pertinent points to cover in the nursing history regarding an individual's sexuality
- Describe observations to be made in the physical appraisal
- List common problems interfering with sexual functioning
- Identify situations requiring immediate intervention and take appropriate action
- Apply relevant principles in planning and implementing nursing interventions
    a. to meet patients' learning needs in regard to sexual functioning
    b. to cope with male-female problems in the nurse-patient relationship
- Evaluate the effectiveness of specific nursing interventions

Section Four   PSYCHOSOCIAL NEEDS

SEXUAL NEEDS

CHAPTER **29**

INTRODUCTION

"So God created man in his own image . . . male and female created he them. And God blessed them, and said unto them, Be fruitful, and multiply, and replenish the earth. . . ."[1] Thus does the King James version of the Bible describe the beginnings of the human race.

According to Navaho Indian legend, Changing Woman (the Navaho chief deity) was the Creator who gave life to First Man and First Woman. They, in turn, created the universe and mankind.

Darwin's theory of the gradual evolution of man from more primitive forms of life offers a more scientific, although less colorful, explanation of the origin of the human species. Still, religion, legend, and science all appear to be in agreement on the fundamental nature of human sexuality. That is to say, in man, as in other higher animals, there are both a male and a female form to the species, with sexual reproduction being necessary for procreation.

With very few exceptions, each of us is born into this world as either a distinctly male or a distinctly female being. Our sex is determined at the time of conception, through union, in the fertilized ovum, of a pair of sex chromosomes derived one from each parent.

Once the sex of an embryonic human being is established, the die is cast for subsequent development of all those characteristics, both genetic and socially acquired, that differentiate the male from the female in human society. These include not only the more obvious physical differences in structure and functioning of the male and the female bodies but, also, differences in growth and development patterns between boys and girls, as well as differences in the social roles of men and women.

Even at birth, the physical differences are readily apparent. The externally located penis and testes make it easy to identify the newborn boy, while the presence of a recessed vagina clearly marks the infant girl. Except for the primary sex characteristics, however, there is little difference in appearance between boys and girls in early childhood. Indeed, with today's hairstyles and common modes of dress, it is sometimes difficult to tell which is which.

It is not until adolescence that the differences in body structure become accentuated. Then—suddenly, it seems—the budding papillae on the chest of a little girl begin to develop into mature breasts; the hips begin to broaden; hair begins to appear in the pubic and axillary regions; and the girl's menstrual cycle commences.

With the adolescent boy, the shoulders start to broaden and the genital organs enlarge. In addition to the pubic and axillary hair that begins to sprout on the bodies of both sexes, the teen-age boy watches anxiously for hair to appear on his upper lip, and a beard to develop. About this time, too, his voice starts to change, fluctuating from tenor to bass, and finally settling about an octave below the pitch of the average female voice.

In adulthood, men generally have a larger body frame than women, and they are usually taller, heavier, and stronger, although this is not always the case. The average man is approximately 10 per cent bigger than the average woman. He has longer bones, which provide better leverage, and wider shoulders, which give greater strength in the upper body. His lungs and his heart are bigger than those of his female counterpart, and he has a slower, more powerful heartbeat. The average male has more muscle than the average female, and the male hormone, testosterone, adds bulk to the muscle fibers. Women, on the other hand, have more body fat than men, and they seem to have greater ability to call on their extra reserves of energy, which gives them greater endurance in sports such as swimming.

The male embryo is slower to develop in utero than the female, and this lag generally persists through childhood. Girls usually experience their prepubertal growth spurt earlier than boys, with the result that girls in the pre-teen years are often taller than boys of the same age. Girls also mature earlier than boys as a general rule, and they usually enter adolescence approximately 2 years younger. The male's maturation is inclined to be less predictable than the female's, and there is a wider variation among boys than among girls in this regard.

Psychologists tell us that traditional distinctions between masculine and feminine personality traits are rapidly blurring in Western society. More women, it seems, are showing traits such as assertiveness, venturesomeness, competitiveness, and self-assurance today than there were a generation ago, when these were considered highly masculine characteristics. At the same time, more men are openly· revealing that they have feelings of nurturing, artistic creativity, and intuitiveness—traits that were formerly considered feminine.

Yet, there is still a marked difference in almost all organized societies between male and female social roles. More women than ever before are in the labor force, and the number of single-parent families has increased phenomenally in the past 20 years. The sex stereotyping of a good many occupations has been broken down by human rights legislation, and the women's liberation movement has done a great deal to eliminate many of the more blatant forms of sex discrimination. Still, in most parts of the world men are looked upon as the protectors and providers in the family, with women having the major responsibility for looking after the home and raising the children.

A girl's perception of her sex-typed role is usually more advanced than a boy's and, with the earlier maturation of girls, they are often ready earlier than boys to become sexually active. With adolescence, there is an awakening of interest in members of the opposite sex, for both boys and girls, as the sexual organs mature and the hormonal secretions begin to flow.

The sex drive, or *libido*, is a very powerful motivating force in human beings, since it is necessary for survival of the species. Maslow, in his hierarchy of human needs, ranked it among the basic physiological needs. Kalish, in his adaptation of Maslow's hierarchy, put it in the second level of priority, subservient only to the needs for individual survival, that is, the needs

for food, air, water, temperature maintenance, elimination, rest, and pain avoidance.

Despite the basic nature of sexual needs, the topic of human sexuality has, until fairly recently in North America, been a taboo subject—not to be discussed in mixed groups—and it has been all but ignored in nursing and medical education programs. The Kinsey reports on sexual behavior in the human male (1948)[2] and the human female (1953),[3] followed by the research of Masters and Johnson into human sexual response (in the 1960's), did much to encourage open discussion of human sexuality. Another forward step was establishment of the Sex Information and Education Council of the United States. In May 1964 SIECUS was chartered as a nonprofit educational organization. Among its goals are those of establishing human sexuality as a health entity and dignifying it by openness of approach.[4]

In the years since SIECUS was established, some people feel that perhaps the pendulum has swung too far in the other direction, as we are confronted on all sides by blatant advertising about sex. Sexual activities the very mention of which would have shocked our grandparents and perhaps even our parents are being shown on stage and movie screen, and feminine hygiene practices once never mentioned in public are matter-of-factly discussed in radio and television commercials.

Whether there is now too much or still too little openness about sex is a moot point. What is important for nurses is the acceptance of sexuality as a health entity, and the need to consider an individual's sexual needs as an integral part of a holistic approach to health care. Nurses today need to be well-informed about the changing sexual needs of individuals throughout the life cycle, and knowledgeable about health problems related to sexual functioning, in order to incorporate consideration of the patient's sexual needs into their practice. A good place to start is to briefly review the anatomy and physiology of sexual functioning.

ANATOMY AND PHYSIOLOGY OF SEXUAL FUNCTIONING

Sex Differentiation

Human body cells, with the exception of the sex cells, contain 23 pairs of *chromosomes*. Twenty-two of these are homologous pairs; that is, they are alike and they bear *genes* for the same traits. The twenty-third pair are the sex chromosomes. Females have two similar sex chromosomes, which are called X *chromosomes*. Males, on the other hand, have 2 dissimilar sex chromosomes. One is an X; the other has been designated a Y chromosome.

During the process of maturation, the gametes, or sex cells (the male sperm and the female ovum) divide and the number of chromosomes each carries is reduced by half (to 23). The mature ovum always contains one X chromosome, but the mature sperm may contain either an X or a Y. If an ovum is fertilized by a sperm carrying an X chromosome, the resultant embryo will be female and ovaries will develop. If it is fertilized by a sperm carrying a Y chromosome, a male embryo results and the gonads (sex organs) develop as testes.

A major function of the Y chromosome is to ensure that male testes develop in the embryo. The hormone *testosterone* is secreted in the embryonic testes and stimulates formation of the male external genitalia, duct system, and accessory sex organs. Testosterone is also responsible for sexual differentiation of the brain. In the absence of testosterone, the female reproductive organs develop.

Hormonal Control of the Reproductive System

The master gland controlling the sex hormones of both men and women is the hypothalamus. This gland secretes gonadotropin-releasing factor, which stimulates the anterior pituitary to secrete gonadotropic hormones. The follicle-stimulating hormones (FSH) are responsible for stimulating production of the ova and the sperm. The luteinizing hormone (LH) stimulates production of the male and the female hormones. The hypothalamus is sensitive to external stimuli, such as physical stress, emotion, and marked changes in time zone. In turn, these can affect the functioning of pituitary and the testes and ovaries. In women athletes, for example, menstruation may temporarily cease under the considerable stress of competitive sports.

The male hormones are collectively known as androgens. The principal male hormone is testosterone, the functions of which are to:

1. Induce sexual differentiation during embryonic development
2. Stimulate growth of the genitalia and secondary sex characteristics
3. Maintain the process of spermatogenesis
4. Promote growth through protein anabolism
5. Increase the sex drive

The principal female hormones are the estrogens and progesterone. The estrogens are secreted by the ovarian follicle, by the corpus luteum, and, during pregnancy, by the placenta. Their functions are to:

1. Stimulate growth of the uterus and vagina and development of secondary sex characteristics at puberty
2. Induce repair of the endometrium following menstruation
3. Promote growth of the duct system of the mammary glands
4. Increase motility of the uterus and its sensitivity to oxytocin
5. Accelerate matrix formation in bone

The functions of progesterone, which is secreted by the corpus luteum and, during pregnancy, by the placenta, are to:

1. Convert the partially thickened endometrium during the postovulatory period to a secretory structure suitable for implantation of the fertilized ovum
2. Promote growth of the mammary gland alveoli
3. Decrease motility of the uterus

Hormone production in the male is not cyclic, as it is in women. Nor does the production of the male sex hormones decrease dramatically at a male climacteric, although it may decrease gradually in later years. Women have high levels of sex hormones during the reproductive period of life and low levels during childhood and after menopause.

The Male Reproductive System

The function of the male reproductive system is to produce mature spermatozoa and deposit these in the body of the female for the purpose of fertilization of the ovum. Components of the system include the organs that produce the germ cells and the various hormones, a duct system to transport the cells to the exterior, and the various accessory structures that facilitate the process. The male organ of copulation, the penis, is used to inject sperm into the body of the female.

Testes. The male organs which produce the germ cells are a pair of oval organs called the *testes*. As is the case with many mammals, human male germ cells cannot survive in temperatures that are either too hot or too cold. The internal body temperature is too high for the process of spermatogenesis and, shortly before birth, the testes descend from the abdominal cavity into the *scrotum*, a pouch that hangs behind the penis and is suspended from the pubis. Normally the muscles are relaxed and the scrotum is pendulous but, in cold temperatures, they contract to bring the testes up to the peri-

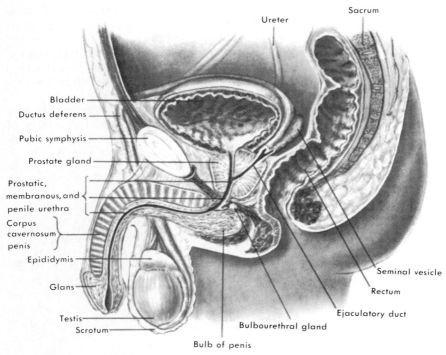

Ureter

Sacrum

Bladder

Ductus deferens

Pubic symphysis

Prostate gland

Prostatic, membranous, and penile urethra

Corpus cavernosum penis

Epididymis

Glans

Testis

Scrotum

Bulb of penis

Bulbourethral gland

Ejaculatory duct

Rectum

Seminal vesicle

The male pelvis (sagittal section). (From Dienhart, C. M.: *Basic Human Anatomy and Physiology*. Philadelphia, W. B. Saunders Company, 1979.)

neum between the thighs in order to keep them warm.

Each testis consists of about 250 wedge-shaped lobes, each of which contains one to four narrow, coiled tubes, known as the *seminiferous tubules*, which produce the spermatozoa. Also located in the testes are *Sertoli's cells*, which supply nutrients to the sperm, and the *interstitial cells of Leydig*, which produce the male hormones.

Duct System. The process of spermatogenesis takes about 60 days in the seminiferous tubules. After that, the sperm require another 2 weeks in the epididymis to become motile and capable of fertilizing an ovum.

As the sperm cells travel from the testes to the urethra, several glands contribute secretions that help to nourish and maintain the viability of the sperm. First along the route are the *seminal vesicles*. These membranous pouches lie behind the bladder and secrete a thick, nutrient-containing fluid that mixes with the germ cells. The *prostate gland*, which lies below the bladder and surrounds the first part of the urethra, secretes a thin, milky, alkaline fluid that aids in maintaining the viability of the sperm cells. Finally, the *bulbourethral (Cowper's) glands*, a pair of pea-shaped structures that lie alongside the lower portion of the urethra, secrete a mu-

cous lubricating substance that is slightly alkaline during sexual stimulation. This is thought to help neutralize the acid in any urine remaining in the urethra.

Semen. During the process of ejaculation, approximately 2 to 6 ml. of *semen,* or *seminal fluid,* are secreted, the amount depending on the length of time between ejaculations. Each discharge of semen contains several hundred million sperm, plus the secretions from the accessory glands and mucus, picked up from glands along the urethra. The average normal sperm count is about 120 million per ml. Semen is thick and milky when first secreted but rapidly becomes watery on standing because of the action of hydrolytic enzymes from the prostate.

Penis. The male organ of copulation is the *penis*. It varies in size in different individuals, but is usually about 15 cm. by 2.5 cm. (6 inches by 1 inch) when in a state of erection. It is attached to the anterior and lateral walls of the pubic arch in front of the scrotum. The penis consists of three longitudinal columns (cavernous bodies) of erectile tissue bound together by fibrous bands and covered by skin. Normally, the penis is a flaccid structure. During sexual arousal, the cavernous bodies become filled with blood and the penis becomes *turgid* (stiff) and erect. The flow of blood into the cavernous sinuses is under the control of the autonomic nervous system. The enlarged conical structure at the end of the penis is called the *glans penis*. The glans contains the external orifice of the urethra. The glans is covered by a fold of retractable skin, the *foreskin* or *prepuce*, which is often removed by circumcision shortly after birth.

The Female Reproductive Tract

The function of the female reproductive system is to produce mature ova, to receive the male sperm, and to furnish a suitable environment for nurturing the fetus until it is ready to be born. Components of the system include the organs that produce the germ cells, a transport system that carries them to a suitable location for fertilization by the sperm and, thence, to a suitable place for implantation, and a storage area where the developing embryo can be nourished and protected. The system also includes a birth canal for the mature embryo and a mechanism for suckling the infant after it is born.

Ovaries. The organs producing the female germ cells are the *ovaries*. These are a pair of small, oval organs located in the pelvic region of the abdominal cavity. They are suspended from the lateral pelvic wall by a portion of the broad ligament. The ovaries produce both eggs and hormones. At birth, the ovaries contain a woman's full, lifetime complement of approximately 400,000 *primordial follicles* (primitive ova), of which probably 350 to 500 will develop into graafian follicles during the woman's reproductive years.

A few years before puberty starts, the ovaries begin to secrete greatly increased amounts of hormones. These include the estrogens, progesterone, and some androgens (male hormones).

The process of oogenesis takes place in the ovaries. Approximately once every 28 days, a mature ovum is produced.

Fallopian Tubes (Oviducts). The *fallopian tubes*, or *oviducts*, are two small intraperitoneal structures that are approximately 10 cm. (4 inches) long and extend from the uterus to the ovaries. They open into the uterus, approximately two thirds of the way down on either side, but have no attachment to the ovaries. Instead, the distal end (closest to the ovaries) has a long fringe consisting of finger-like projections that curve in a bell shape around the ovaries. The tubes are attached to the broad ligaments. Their purpose is to transport mature ova to the middle third of the tube, where fertilization takes place, and to carry the fertilized ovum to the uterus for implantation, or the unfertilized ovum for discharge in the menstrual

Median section of the female pelvis. (From Dienhart, C. M.: *Basic Human Anatomy and Physiology*. Philadelphia, W. B. Saunders Company, 1979.)

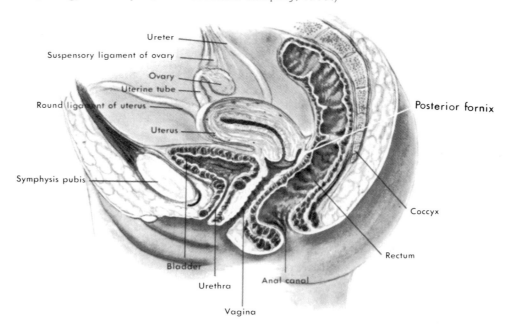

flow. The ovum is transported through the tubes by a series of peristaltic waves and ciliary action. Transport takes about 3 to 4 days.

Uterus. The *uterus* is a thick-walled, hollow, muscular organ located in the pelvic portion of the abdominal cavity, between the rectum and the bladder. The lining of the uterus consists of a specialized mucous surface, the *endometrium,* which is the primary site for implantation of the fertilized ovum.

Cervix. The *cervix* is the neck of the uterus, and it protrudes into the vault of the vagina. It is a rounded, rather firm, conical body, roughly 2 to 2.5 cm. in diameter. It has a narrow canal in the center, the cervical canal, which joins the vagina with the uterine cavity.

Vagina. The *vagina* is a muscular tube lying between the bladder and the rectum. It is approximately 10 cm. in length and 4 cm. wide. It functions as a passageway for sperm to enter the uterus and for menstrual flow to be discharged and it forms part of the birth canal. During coitus, the erect penis is inserted into the vagina where ejaculation normally occurs. Sperm are deposited at the external opening of the cervix and swim through into the uterus.

Vulva. The external female genital organs are collectively known as the vulva. The *mons pubis* is a rounded soft cushion of adipose tissue, which is located over the symphysis pubis. It is covered with hair. The *labia majora,* which are like the male scrotum, consist of longitudinal folds of skin. They cover and protect the opening to the vagina, the urinary meatus and the labia minora. The *labia minora* are narrow folds of skin and fibroareolar tissue which extend from the clitoris to the fourchette. Their purpose is to protect the vaginal opening.

The *clitoris* is the female organ corresponding to the male penis. It is a short, erectile organ just below the arch of the pubis and above the urinary meatus. It is highly sensitive to tactile stimuli.

The *vestibule* is an ovoid area between the labia that contains the vaginal opening, the urethral orifice, the hymen, and the openings of several ducts. The *hymen* is a tough, elastic mucosa-covered septum across the vagina in virgins. It may be partial, or completely absent. Occasionally it completely covers the vaginal opening, a condition called *imperforate vagina,* or *imperforate hymen.*

Mammary Glands (Breasts). The mammary glands are accessory sexual structures in the female. Their purpose is to secrete milk to nourish the newborn infant. Each breast contains compartments, or lobes, that are separated by adipose tissue. Each lobe is made up of lobules which contain milk-secreting cells called alveoli, which appear in grapelike clusters in the lobules. The milk is conveyed to storage areas (ampullae), and thence to the lactiferous ducts which terminate in the nipple.

Menstrual Cycle. Menstruation is the periodic uterine bleeding which is the shedding of the secretory endometrium of the uterus when fertilization of the mature ovum does not take place. The first menstrual period, which occurs at puberty, is called the *menarche.* Menstruation continues until the *menopause,* approximately 40 years.

Menstruation takes place approximately 14 days after ovulation. The first day of bleeding is considered the first day of the menstrual cycle. The average cycle lasts for 28 days, although the normal range is from 24 to 32 days. Average duration of the menstrual period is 5 days, and the average blood loss is 70 ml. The cycle consists of three phases:

1. Menstrual—shedding of the superficial two thirds of the endometrium.
2. Proliferative—from the fifth day to the time of ovulation—the endometrium is regenerated with an eight- to tenfold thickening while the follicles begin to grow.
3. Secretory—from the day of ovulation to 3 days before the next menstrual period—the endometrium develops into a secretory type of tissue for reception of the fertilized ovum

Menopause. Menopause occurs usually between the ages of 45 and 55. It is most often gradual, with menstrual periods becoming irregular and with differences in amount of flow over a few years. Two major symptoms that women find distressing during the menopause are: (1) Flushes—a reddening of the skin involving the head, neck, and upper part of the thorax which may last for minutes or for hours; and (2) Flashes—brief intense periods of heat over the entire body. These are both circulatory disturbances that are related to the decreasing production of estrogen by the ovaries.

Sexual Response

Physiologists divide the human sexual response into four phases: excitement, plateau, orgasm, and resolution. Essentially, there are two principal physiological changes that take place in both male and female during the sexual response:

1. Vasocongestion. The primary response, in sexual stimulation, is the engorgement of blood vessels (chiefly the venous vessels) in the sexual organs.

2. Myotonia. The vasocongestion is accompanied by increased muscular tension in the organs necessary to carry out the sexual act.

Excitement Phase. Sexual arousal is brought about in women primarily by the touching and caressing of various body parts. Some areas of the body are more sensitive to sexual stimulation than others. These are called the "erogenous zones" (after Eros, the Greek god of love). The breasts and external organs, especially the clitoris, are most responsive. In the sexually aroused woman, the glans of the clitoris becomes bigger, the shaft enlarging in length and diameter. The vaginal barrel also expands, becoming wider and longer. The wall of the vagina becomes purplish, due to vasocongestion, which also causes the appearance of a fluid that traverses the vagina, lubricating it to make penetration easier. (The process has been likened to that of sweating.) In multiparous women there is a flattening and separating of the labia majora and extension of the labia minora.

Meanwhile, the extragenital organs are also aroused. The nipples become erect, breast size increases, the areolae become engorged, and venous patterns on the breast are obvious. Sometimes there is a "sex flush" in the form of a maculopapular rash that appears in the epigastric region and the breasts. The heart begins to beat faster and blood pressure increases as sexual tension mounts. There may also be an involuntary tensing of the intercostal and the abdominal muscles. A man may be sexually aroused as a result of mental or visual images, as well as by direct stimulation of the penis. The penis rapidly increases in size as blood vessels within the erectile tissue become engorged. The normally flaccid organ becomes erect and stiff. Valves in blood vessels located at the base of the penis close, thus preventing blood from leaving the vessels and keeping the penis erect. The scrotal sac becomes elevated and there is a tensing and thickening of the scrotal skin. Involuntary muscle tension occurs and the heart rate and blood pressure levels increase as sexual excitement mounts.

Plateau Phase. During the plateau phase, a woman's uterus becomes fully elevated and the barrel of the vagina becomes larger. Increased vasocongestion causes the labia minora and the outer third of the vagina to increase in size. The labia minora show a vivid color change from bright red to wine colored. The Bartholin glands secrete a small amount of mucoid material and the clitoris retracts against the symphysis pubis. The muscles of the pelvic floor retract, producing a tentlike effect to accommodate insertion of the penis.

In a man, the penis increases in circumference and the testes become bigger and move closer to the perineum. Muscle tension is increased; the man experiences hyperventilation; his heart beat is greatly accelerated and his blood pressure becomes markedly elevated. These vascular changes are much more marked in a man than in a woman. At the height of his sexual excitement, and just prior to ejaculation, the urethra closes at the neck of the bladder, thus preventing urine from being discharged, and two or three drops of mucoid material are secreted from Cowper's glands to lubricate the passage of semen.

Orgasm. In both men and women, orgasm is characterized by a series of strong muscular contractions. In the female, there are usually five to 12 contractions occurring at 0.8 second intervals. They occur in the uterus, beginning at the fundus and proceeding to the lower segments, and in the muscles of the pelvic floor where the muscles surround the lower third of the vagina. Contractions of the anal sphincter also occur.

In a man, there are clonic contractions along the length of the urethra to expel the semen and force it beyond the glans penis. The epididymis, the vas deferens, the seminal vesicles, and the prostate gland also contract. The contractions usually begin at 0.8 second intervals, becoming less frequent as most of the semen is expelled. The ejaculatory process usually takes only a matter of seconds.

Resolution. The resolution phase involves both a relaxation of the muscles and a loss of vasocongestion. The latter is called *detumescence.* In the man the loss of vasocongestion is rapid at first. In the woman, the clitoris returns to a normal position within 5 to 10 seconds after orgasm.

While the woman can be sexually aroused again almost immediately after orgasm, the man has a period of from 10 to 45 minutes during which he cannot be restimulated. This *refractory period* is usually shorter in younger men and increases with age, although not as much as was once suspected.

FACTORS AFFECTING SEXUAL FUNCTIONING

Probably there is no other area of human functioning that is affected by so many factors

S.F. maybe decreased b/c of medications, depression, disorders, diease, + surgical procedures.

as sexual functioning. Of primary importance are the changing sexual needs of the individual throughout his life span. These are affected by an individual's age and his stage of physical and psychosocial development. In addition to age, other biological influences, such as genetic factors, injury, and disease, affect the development and functioning of the reproductive organs. Then, too, there are social, moral, and psychological factors that must be taken into account in any discussion of sexual needs.

ctors:
= elopment

Biological Factors

Age and stage of physical development are very important considerations in sexual functioning. Although the primary sex characteristics, that is, the physical structures necessary for reproduction, are present at birth, it is not until adolescence that these organs mature and become capable of functioning. Normally, the reproductive period for women lasts about 30 to 40 years and, with onset of the menopause, the female ovaries cease to function and the reproductive organs begin to atrophy. In men, the testes continue to produce spermatozoa until old age, but there is a slowing down of all aspects of sexual functioning and a gradual atrophy of the organs of reproduction with the aging process.

The primary biological agents controlling sexual functioning are the genes and the hormones. Initial differentiation of the sexual organs is determined in utero by the XX or XY chromosome combination of the newly formed embryo. Subsequent development of these organs is controlled by hormonal secretions. Defects in the sex chromosomes or disturbances in balance of the hormones regulating sexual development and functioning, then, may give rise to problems in the growth and development of the sexual organs, or in their functioning.

The human reproductive system, like other systems in the body, is also susceptible to both injury and disease. The breasts and the uterus in women and the prostate gland and testes in men are particularly prone to the development of tumors. The reproductive organs are also very vulnerable to infection. The intimacy of sexual contact between partners facilitates the transfer of infection from one partner to another, and the reproductive tract, in both men and women, provides an open passage for the conduct of infectious agents from the outside of the body to the internal organs of reproduction. Then, too, a person's general state of health will affect his sexual functioning. Under conditions of good

health, a woman's sexual functioning is affected by the cyclic changes in hormone production that were discussed earlier in the chapter. Generalized infections may affect the sexual organs. Mumps and liver disease, for example, are known to cause atrophy of the sex organs in males. In adult males, mumps may involve inflammation of the testes (orchitis), which causes the damage.

Sexual functioning may be disrupted because of pharmacologic agents, severe depression, medical disorders such as systemic, endocrine, and local genital and vascular diseases, and certain surgical procedures.

Social, Moral, and Psychological Factors

Every organized society from the beginning of time has exerted controls on sexual behaviors. Although the sexual drive is considered basic and instinctual for survival of the species, sexual behavior is primarily learned. Ethical norms regarding what is right and what is wrong in the way of sexual activity in a given society are taught early in childhood, and these exert a powerful controlling influence on behavior.

Although the standards, or norms vary considerably from one culture to another, every society has certain sexual taboos. One of the most powerful of these, which anthropologists tell us is found in all cultures, is the prohibition of incest, that is, sexual intercourse between members of the same family—between father and daughter, between mother and son, or between siblings. Sexual taboos are frequently enforced by legal controls. Marriage is a legal institution established for protection of the family, and in most countries a legal age has been set below which an individual cannot enter into marriage without his or her parents' consent. Certain sexual acts are considered criminal. These include rape, which is the violent sexual attack of one person by another; child molesting, which involves sexual activity by an adult with a child; and indecent exposure, which is exposure of the genitalia in public or without the consent of those to whom the display is made. In many parts of the world, including some states in the United States, homosexual activity is still considered a crime.

Religion has traditionally exerted an important influence on what is considered right and wrong in the way of sexual activity. The Judeo-Christian religions have traditionally sanctioned sexual intercourse only in monogamous marriages and taught that the principal objective of marriage is the production of children.

Psychological factors also have a tremendous bearing on sexual functioning. Ignorance about sexual matters, social attitudes toward sexual activity outside marriage, fear of unwanted pregnancy, and numerous other factors have all contributed to shrouding this normal biologic function with feelings of guilt, repression, and inadequacy. But social attitudes towards sexual functioning have undergone considerable change in Western cultures in the past two decades. There is increasing acceptance of homosexuality and, in many states, the laws prohibiting it have been repealed. There is much openness about people engaging in sexual relationships outside marriage, with people living together and being accepted by family and friends as a social unit in the absence of a marriage certificate. There has been much talk about the "new morality," and certainly many of the traditional social controls have been lifted. The right of women to sexual satisfaction in their relationships with men is recognized, as opposed to the woman's being regarded as the submissive partner, participating in sexual activity only to fulfill the man's sexual needs. The widespread use of effective birth control agents has freed women from the fear of unwanted pregnancy. This development, increased knowledge about her own body's functioning, and the conciousness-raising about their rights by the women's liberation movement have all contributed to a sexual revolution for women.

SEXUAL NEEDS THROUGHOUT THE LIFE CYCLE

The biological purpose of the sex drive is reproduction of the species, but human sexual needs include much more than just the physical need to propagate the race. Involved is a very complex set of interrelationships between people. These include the need to develop and live out one's life as a male or a female being in the society of which one is a part, the need to establish and maintain close, reciprocal relationships with other persons, and the need to mate and produce children.

Sex differentiation begins in utero, as we have already mentioned, with the sex organs beginning to appear in the second month of gestation. They are all intact, albeit immature, by the time the infant is ready to be delivered. Just before birth the testes of the male infant descend from the abdomen into the scrotal sac. At birth, the genitals of both sexes are usually red, swollen, and painful, with girl babies sometimes having a small amount of bloody discharge as the hor-

mone levels adjust. Sometimes, problems occur at the time of conception, or later in utero, that affect the sex organs. These include:

(1) abnormalities in the sex chromosomes, such as an extra X or Y chromosome

(2) *cryptorchidism*, or undescended testicles, which may require surgery or treatment by hormones if they do not descend spontaneously during the first year of life

(3) ambiguous genitalia, or *hermaphroditism*, when the external genitalia are not clearly of one sex or the other

Freud postulated that an infant derives his first sexual pleasure from enjoying his own body and that of his mother. He likes to explore his mother's body, and enjoys the warmth, taste, touch, and rhythm of it. If the relationship that develops between mother and infant is positive, as it is in most instances, the baby's feelings of love, trust, and self as a sexual being are nurtured. These are the feelings that furnish the basis for risk-taking and extending oneself to others in future relationships.

One of the most important of the developmental tasks of childhood is *gender identification*. *Gender identity* refers to the self-concept of maleness and femaleness. Not only must the child learn his or her appropriate gender—that he is a "boy" or she is a "girl"—but he or she must learn the appropriate sex role. The term *gender role* includes all those things that a person does that indicate that he or she is a boy or man, or a girl or woman. It is indicated by a person's mannerisms, deportment and demeanor, and preferences in regard to play activities and recreational interests, and it will be evident in daydreams and fantasies, performance on projective tests, and responses to indirect questioning. It is said that gender role is imprinted during the first 3 years of life. By the time a child is 3 years old, the male child labels himself as a boy, and prefers associating with his father, while a female child labels herself a girl and associates herself with her mother. Close identification with the parent of the same sex (or a parent substitute) is important in early childhood. Children, however, need the role models of both mother and father (or substitutes) in order to develop their own sexual identity and later relationships with members of the opposite sex.

Sex roles are well internalized during the early years of school. By the age of 9 to 10 years, segregation of the sexes is almost complete. Boys play mainly with other boys, and girls with other girls. Their play activities differ, with boys going in for more sports—soccer, baseball, football,

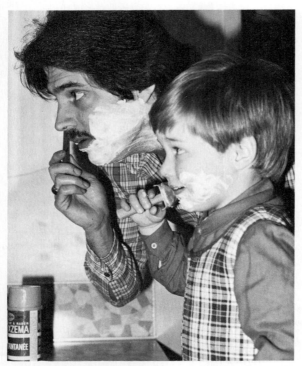

In developing gender identity, a boy often imitates his father.

and the like—whereas girls tend to participate in activities like skipping rope, dancing, and skating. There are, of course, exceptions to prove the rule, and it is becoming more common to see boys and girls on the same baseball team.

Children explore and derive pleasure from their own bodies, including the genital area. *Masturbation* (stroking and stimulating one's own genital area) is quite common throughout childhood. Children are also usually very curious about sexual matters. There is a need for them to learn facts and gain an understanding of the cooperative nature of sexuality. Sexual molestation within the family is a problem that can be difficult to deal with; school health nurses may come across victims of this among their students.

The levels of sexual hormones in boys (androgens) are low until about the age of 8 years, and in girls estrogen begins to appear about the age of 9 years. Changes in sexual anatomy and physiology are more profound during adolescence than at any other time in the life cycle. The reproductive organs develop rapidly and the secondary sexual characteristics begin to appear. In boys the changes include: axillary sweating; increased testicular sensitivity to pressure; enlargement of the testes; reddening and stippling of the scrotum; increase in penis length; appearance of axillary, pubic, and facial hair; voice change; nocturnal emissions ("wet dreams"); increase in height; and broadening of the shoulders. In girls the changes include: appearance of the breast bud, menarche, the appearance of pubic and axillary hair, broadening of the hips, and axillary sweating.

The early ovarian cycles are usually anovulatory; that is, the ovaries do not produce an ovum. During the early years of menstruation, some girls have problems, such as *dysmenorrhea*, which is difficult or painful menstruation, and

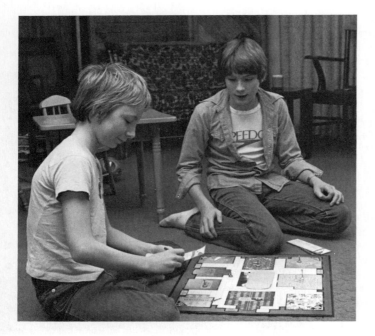

In later childhood, play is often segregated by sexes.

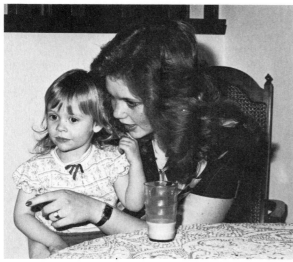

Many teen-age girls enjoy baby-sitting, which provides an opportunity to prepare for the adult role of motherhood.

menstrual irregularity. *Amenorrhea* is the absence of menstruation. Often, girls have difficulty coping with the mood changes as their bodies adjust to the rhythm of the menstrual cycle; for example, premenstrual tension often gives rise to tears at the slightest provocation.

Adolescents have to come to terms with the new physical appearance they acquire with development of the secondary sex characteristics— developments that are occurring at a younger age these days. The average age of physical maturation has decreased from 16 to 13 years over the past century. Adolescents must also cope with the sexual stirrings they feel in their bodies. By this age, sexual identity is usually firmly established, but the adolescent also has to achieve a satisfactory social role based on sex. This means essentially learning to be comfortable in heterosexual relationships as the individual prepares for marriage and family life.

Most adolescents have strong feelings about what activities are appropriate for each sex. Even today, with the changing adult male and female roles, teen-age girls and boys tend to be traditional about sex roles. Baby-sitting is still considered girls' work, whereas boys work at gas stations or other "male-image" work.

In many primitive societies, the transition from childhood to adulthood is marked by formal rites of passage. Pubescent boys may be removed from the parental home and instructed in the manly arts of hunting, fishing, and self-defense, with bravery, endurance, and skill with weapons being encouraged. Return to the community is marked by an elaborate ceremony. Ceremonies also are often held for girls at the

onset of the menarche. Sometimes, slash marks are made on the face to signify physical maturation, or with girls, markings may be made on the skin between the breasts. With the encroachment of Western civilization into virtually every part of the world, many of these traditional ceremonies are disappearing.

Many religious denominations, too, have ceremonies that mark the passage into adulthood, as for example, the Jewish bar mitzvah and the Roman Catholic and Episcopalian confirmation ceremonies.

Adolescents tend to be sexually active, a development that appears to be taking place at an earlier age these days in all segments of society. Usually, the sexual drives can be channeled into sports, studies, or hobbies. However, teenagers today are exposed to a considerable amount of sexual information through television, movies, magazines, and other media. There has also been much more permissiveness about sexual activities, so that many more teen-agers are experimenting with sex at an earlier age. These trends have led to a marked increase in the incidence of venereal disease, with over half of the cases in the United States and Europe involving people in the 15- to 24-year-old group. There have also been alarming increases in pregnancies among teen-agers and in abortions performed on adolescent girls. These pregnancies are related in many cases to ineffective contraceptive methods. Surveys show that most teenage girls want more detailed and explicit information about sex. Although there seems to be an abundance of literature about sex available, the vital details are often missing.

Marriage and starting a family are important goals for most young adults.

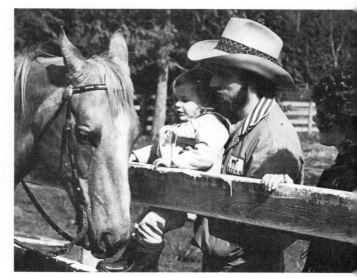

Early adulthood is the time when the biological urge for sexual satisfaction reaches its peak, with men usually having the stronger sex drive. For both men and women, there is a need to achieve a sense of intimacy in sexual relationships, and mating and beginning a family are major goals for most young adults. Living together has gained increasing acceptance as a prelude to marriage, although the basic pattern is still marriage-oriented. The desire to have children prompts many couples to marry legally, even after living together. Indeed, there now seems to be a swing back to regarding marriage—and even virginity—as a desirable state of affairs.

People who do not achieve sexual intimacy with others report a need for close relationships with others. Often, close reciprocal relationships with family, friends, or co-workers are developed.

Among the common problems in this age group are the sexually transmitted diseases and unwanted pregnancy. Also, with the increased permissiveness and open discussion about sexuality, young adults are often concerned about their sexual performance, and more are seeking professional advice about their sexual functioning.

A woman's reproductive life usually lasts less than half her life span. Although there is decrease in fertility and a gradual decrease in sexual function in the middle years, this is often the time of greatest sexual drive and satisfaction for women. Menopause brings its attendant problems of "hot flashes" and "flushes" and, sometimes, mood swings due to decreased hormonal levels. There is atrophy of the vagina, also due to decreases in hormones, that can cause irritability and increased susceptibility to infections. Women are also prone to tumors of the breast and the uterus. Many have problems with a prolapse of the uterus, especially if the muscles of the pelvic floor have been weakened by childbirth. Fibroid growths are also common in the uterus, especially in unmarried women of middle age.

Men are often very concerned about sexual adequacy at this stage of life. As we mentioned in Chapter 13, they will often seek reassurance in extramarital sex with younger partners. Benign or cancerous tumors in the prostate gland are common among men in the late middle years. Older men and women must adjust to the physiological changes that have taken place in their bodies. Older men often worry about sexual potency, which is to many a symbol of masculinity and personal worth. Women worry about the loss of attractiveness, which may threaten

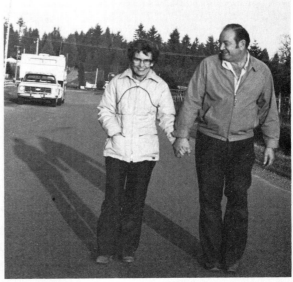

Middle age can be an enjoyable time, when children have left home and individuals reach career peaks.

their marriage and their self-esteem. However, many couples who overcome their worries about these problems find middle age to be a most rewarding time of life, as they complete the task of raising their children to adulthood and as they reach career peaks. There is still a need for sexual satisfaction through physical sexual relationships, and a need for touching and caressing.

PATTERNS OF SEXUAL ACTIVITY

It has been suggested that "Any sex behavior that is mutually enjoyable, expresses affection, hurts no one and is not offensive to an unwilling observer could be considered normal."[5] Patterns include:

1. Heterosexual activity, which may involve genital coitus, extragenital coitus, and noncoital contacts. Noncoital contacts include such physical activities between a man and a woman as hand holding, kissing, petting, "heavy petting," and mutual masturbation.

2. Homosexual activity, which involves sexual contact between two persons of the same sex. Sexual gratification comes, in this case, from body contact, embraces, manual stimulation of genital areas by the partner, and orogenital or anogenital intercourse. It should be noted that homosexuality was quite widely practiced in ancient Greece. Although there are still laws against homosexuality in some states, repressive enforcement of these has been relaxed.

3. Autosexual activity, which involves sexual activity with oneself. *Masturbation* is one form of autosexual activity. In men, it is usually accomplished by stroking the shaft of the penis. Masturbation in women may take the form of stimulation of the clitoris with the hand or fingers, rhythmic motion of the thighs, or insertion of a finger or a foreign body into the vagina with rhythmic motion. At one time, people thought that masturbation was wicked and would lead to mental illness. Now, however, it is widely considered a normal prelude to other forms of sexual activity.

4. Nocturnal orgasm. Sexual dreams are experienced by many people, particularly if other forms of sexual activity are not permitted, or if the need for sexual expression is great. Sometimes, these dreams end with orgasm being experienced. There may be an ejaculation of semen, as in the "wet dreams" that are common with adolescent youths.

ASSESSMENT ✓ *1) history 2) physical appraisal 3) test + exams*

Assessment of the patient's sexual status forms a part of the general assessment of an individual's health. In the adult, there are usually three parts to sexual assessment. They include: (1) history of sexual functioning, (2) physical appraisal of the genital organs, and (3) laboratory tests and examinations. Because these are different for men and women, they will be discussed separately.

Assessment of the Female Patient

History. The female sexual history includes observations about the person's general body stature. While taking the history one can note whether the person has a feminine body build, that is, smaller, lighter, more curvaceous, and with less muscle mass than a man's. Information should be gathered about the occurrence of female reproductive disorders, such as cancer of the breast or uterus, in the family, particularly in the individual's mother. The patient's obstetric history and record of surgical operations should also be noted. Does she have children? Are they all living? What are their ages? How many pregnancies, and how many live births has she had? Has she had any abortions? Were they spontaneous or induced? Has she had any surgery involving the reproductive tract, as, for example, a hysterectomy (removal of the uterus)? Questions should be asked about the woman's menstrual pattern. What was the age of menarche? Did she experience any problems at menarche? How long does the menstrual period last? What is the interval between menses? Does the woman have pain during her menses? If the woman is in the appropriate age group (over 40), information should be gathered about the menopause—whether it has taken place yet, the age at which it took place, and whether it was natural or brought about by surgery or radiation. Then, too, information should be obtained about the presence of abnormal vaginal discharges.

The nurse should also be aware of the individual's marital status and sexual relationships with others. This is often a highly sensitive area, and the nurse should not probe if the patient does not want to give information about her sexual relationships.

As part of the sexual assessment, the nurse should also gather information about the patient's knowledge of her own health care. Has she had a pelvic examination and a Papanicolaou test (Pap smear) done recently? Does she do a monthly breast self-examination? Is she using contraceptives? If so, what is she using? She should also, of course, ask the woman if she is having any problems now.

Physical Appraisal. The female physical appraisal involves examination of the external genitalia and an internal (pelvic) examination. To assure proper evaluation of vaginal discharges, the woman should be instructed not to have a douche in the 24-hour period prior to the examination. It is wise to have the woman void immediately prior to the examination, since a full bladder distorts the position of the pelvic organs. This also makes palpation easier and eliminates the danger of incontinence. Several positions are suitable for the examination. These include the lithotomy position, the left lateral prone position (Sims's position), and the knee-chest position (see illustration on page 163). A standing position may also be used to evaluate hernias, uterine prolapse, relaxation of vaginal walls or pelvic supports, and stress incontinence. This is followed by inspection and palpation of the external genitalia—the pubic area, vulva, labia, clitoris, urinary meatus, and perineum. Normally, the vulva is darker in color than other skin areas, and the mucous membranes are dark, pink, and moist. Abnormalities that should be noted include tenderness, irritations, or lesions of the skin, discoloration, lumps or swelling in any area, abnormal size or adhesions of the clitoris, and unusual discharges from the vagina. A small amount of clear or whitish discharge is normal.

A speculum is inserted into the vagina to enable the examiner to see the cervix and vaginal walls. If the speculum is metal it should be warmed prior to use. The speculum should be lubricated prior to insertion. The examiner is looking for lesions, discoloration, or unusual discharges from either the vaginal walls or the cervix, abnormalities in size or position of the cervix, and signs of infection, damage, or growths in either area.

While the speculum is in place, the cervix may be scraped to obtain a sample of tissue for a Pap smear. At this time, too, a smear of vaginal discharge may be taken for microscopic examination and for a culture to test for gonorrhea. If this procedure is to be undertaken, the speculum should be moistened only by water.

Frequently, a bimanual vaginal examination is done to palpate the organs in the lower abdomen. The examiner inserts the index and middle fingers of one hand into the vagina and uses the thumb on the lower abdominal wall. In this way, the uterus, fallopian tubes, and ovaries can be felt. They are checked for size, shape, consistency, mobility, and tenderness. Abnormalities include unusual growths, pelvic pain, evidence of inflammation (pain or swelling), or abnormal placement.

Sometimes a rectovaginal examination is done to get more information about the tone and alignment of the various pelvic organs. In this case, the examiner inserts one gloved finger into the vagina and one into the rectum.

Women can do a self-examination of the cervix and vagina, using a speculum, a long-handled mirror, and a strong flashlight or other directional light.

Laboratory Tests and Examinations. The most common laboratory tests performed in connection with sexual functioning are the pregnancy tests, the cytology tests for cancer, the smears and cultures taken to identify infectious agents, and the blood tests for syphilis. X-ray procedures, body scans, and thermography are used to detect tumors.

Pregnancy Tests. The two most commonly used tests for pregnancy today are the urine tests and the B scan. X-rays may be taken in certain cases, as when a multiple pregnancy is suspected, for example. A sensitive infrared thermometer may also be used to detect increases in the skin temperature over the breast, which becomes elevated very early in pregnancy, usually by 4 weeks. A fetal electrocardiogram is also sometimes done. It can detect fetal heart tones by approximately 10 weeks gestation, but is not 100 per cent reliable until about 20 to 22

weeks.[6] The most commonly used urine tests for pregnancy are the agglutination (or immunological) tests. These test for the presence of the gonadotrophic hormone, HCG, which is produced from the trophoblast (embryonic cells) in the uterus. HCG is significantly raised by about 4 weeks after conception (or 6 weeks after the last normal period). These tests are considered to be 98 per cent accurate, although a false positive or false negative result may occur if the reagents have deteriorated, the glassware is not clean, there are errors in technique, or the test is done too early. Menopause or drugs, such as chlorpromazine, may also affect the accuracy of the test, giving a false positive. An early morning urine specimen is collected for the test because the urine is more concentrated then. The specimen should be free from blood and other debris.

Fetal heart tones can be detected by ultrasound machines such as the Doptone and Sonicaid from about the sixth week onward, but they are not completely reliable until about 10 weeks. Their use has largely been replaced by the B scan. With a compound B scanner, the outline of the fetal sac can be determined as early as the sixth week of pregnancy, and the embryo shortly afterwards.

Papanicolaou Test. This test is used to detect changes in the cervix that indicate the presence of cancer or a condition that may lead to cancer. It is usually done routinely for women over the age of 18 years during a periodic physical examination. Having the test done once a year is recommended for women after the age of 40 years. A small amount of tissue is scraped from the cervix during the pelvic examination. The sample is placed on a sterile glass slide, covered with another slide, and sent to the laboratory.

Serological Tests for Syphilis. Routine screening of people for syphilis is done by means of a blood test, for which 5 ml. of venous blood are withdrawn from a vein in the antecubital space. A number of serological tests are now being used in place of the Wassermann test, which was used for so many years that people still call the test a "Wassermann." The most commonly used test today is the Venereal Disease Research Laboratories (VDRL) Test, which is easily quantitated.

Assessment of the Male Patient

History. The male sexual history is usually combined with the history and examination of the urinary system. As the history is being taken, the examiner notes the general body stature. Is it that of a male, with broad shoulders and more muscle mass than a woman? He also notes the secondary sex characteristics, such as the distribution of facial and axillary hair, pitch of the voice, and development of the genitals. The family history of male genitourinary disorders is noted, as is the person's marital history or history of sexual relationships, as well as current relationships. Questions are asked about any discharges, or sores, the patient has noticed and any pain he has experienced in the genital area. The male physical appraisal includes an examination of the penis and the scrotum, the inguinal region (for hernias), and the rectum and the prostate gland. The penis and the scrotum are examined by inspection and palpation. To examine the penis, the prepuce of the uncircumcised male is retracted around the head of the penis. The prepuce should retract easily; difficulties in retraction should be noted. A small amount of thick white secretion is normal from the urethral opening, which should be located at the tip of the penis.

Abnormalities that may be noted include: *Phimosis*; in which the prepuce adheres to the penis; *paraphimosis*, which is inflammation of the prepuce; edema, which may indicate fluid retention; healed scars or active lesions on the penis—for example, an indurated painless ulcer may be indicative of syphilis; and excessive discharge—a thick, purulent discharge is often seen in gonorrhea, whereas a thin, mucoid one may indicate inflammation of the urethra.

The scrotum is usually held in the palm of the hand for examination. Normally, the testes are asymmetrical, the left usually being slightly lower than the right. Their size varies; approximately 2 cm. in diameter at the larger end is average. Normally the testes feel firm on palpation. Abnormalities the examiner is looking for include: atrophy, which may be indicative of mumps orchitis or liver disease; scrotal cysts; and varicoceles, which are localized cystic enlargements of the spermatic cord or epididymis.

An examination of the inguinal canal region is usually done with the patient standing. The examiner inserts a gloved finger into the rectum. An inguinal hernia may protrude into the anal canal. For an examination of the prostate and the rectum, several positions may be used. The patient may lie on his left side with the knees drawn up to the abdomen, or in a supine position with his legs spread apart. He may be in a standing position, bending forward so that his elbows rest on the bed or table. A knee-chest position may also be used, with the patient's head turned to one side.

Inspection of the external area is done and the internal organs are palpated through the rectum.

The examiner is looking for obstructions of the prostate gland, which may be caused by benign hypertrophy, or other masses, or he may be able to note atrophy of the gland. If infection is suspected, smears and cultures may be done. A smear may be taken from the urinary meatus, or a culture from an open lesion.

COMMON PROBLEMS

Now that there is more openness about all aspects of sexuality, including sexual problems, postgraduate courses in sex education and counseling are being offered for health professionals who wish to incorporate this aspect of health care into their practice. People are also being trained in sex therapy, which has rapidly become a specialized area of practice for professional nurses, physicians, psychologists, and social workers. The first level professional nurse, without the benefit of such additional training, has a responsibility in her general assessment of the patient to screen for sexual problems and dysfunctions. She may also be involved in limited sex education. Indeed, the student nurse will probably find that she is looked upon as a source of information about sexual matters by her peers who are not nurses.

Common problems in sexual functioning that a nurse is likely to encounter in practice and that she should be alert to in her general assessment of the patient include those affecting the structure or physiological functioning of the sexual organs, those involving sexual performance, and those involving deviant sexual behavior. We have mentioned a number of these problems in the section on sexual needs throughout the life cycle. Most will be covered in greater detail in more senior courses such as pediatric nursing, obstetric and gynecologic nursing, and urologic nursing. We will, therefore, concentrate here on two of the more common problems that first year nursing students may be expected to identify and do something about. These include: (1) a lack of basic information about sexual functioning and the maturational and disease processes affecting it, and (2) sexual problems in the nurse-patient relationship, which include embarrassment in discussing sexual matters, and potentially embarrassing nursing procedures involving the urogenital tract.[7]

PRIORITIES FOR NURSING ACTION

An acute vaginal infection that requires emergency treatment is the toxic shock syndrome, which has been traced to the use of superabsorbent tampons by women during the menstrual cycle. The causative agent of the infection has been identified as *Staphylococcus aureus,* which is the organism that has been responsible for many types of hospital infections (see Chapter 26). This particular vaginal infection appears to be very virulent, with affected women often showing a high fever, vomiting, and diarrhea. This may progress, with a rapid drop in blood pressure, to a loss of consciousness and clinical shock (see Chapter 17). The particular brand of tampons implicated in a number of cases of toxic shock has been removed from the market. Women are, however, urged to use all tampons with care and to change them frequently to minimize the possibility of infection. The vagina, with its dark, warm, and moist interior, provides an excellent breeding ground for the growth of bacteria and, during menstruation, organisms are provided with a highly nutritive medium.

Then too, if the nurse notes evidence suggestive of any of the venereal diseases in her clinical assessment of the patient, this observation should be reported without delay to the patient's physician so that further investigation can be done and treatment can be instituted as soon as possible if it is needed. Particular signs to be watchful for are a purulent discharge from the urethra in men or the vagina in women and open sores (lesions) on the genitals.

Other priority situations that a nurse may encounter when working in the emergency department of a hospital, or in the community, are rape and the sexual abuse of children. In both cases, the police will need to be notified (if the victim was not brought in by them), since both are criminal acts. The individuals will probably need treatment for shock and should be seen by a social worker or some other person qualified in doing a psychiatric assessment.

Hemorrhaging from the vagina is always a priority matter, and women can die from a vaginal hemorrhage if treatment is not instituted promptly. Prompt medical intervention, often of a surgical nature, is imperative.

Post-abortion infection has become a less widespread problem since the legalization of abortion in the United States, but it is still an emergency when it occurs. In illegal abortions, it is often caused by the use of unsterile equipment or poor technique by the person performing the operation. Women with post-abortion infection usually show all the signs of an acute infection, with a high temperature, severe pain in the pelvic region, and a copious discharge of purulent material. People with post-abortion infections require prompt medical intervention. Again, surgery is frequently indicated, often in addition to drug therapy.

GOALS FOR NURSING ACTION

The principal goals of nursing action in regard to the sexuality of a patient are:

1. To help the individual to gain the knowledge and skills needed to safeguard his own sexual health
2. To assist in the detection of illness, abnormality, or other disorder causing sexual dysfunctioning in the individual
3. To carry out therapeutic measures related to the restoration of normal sexual functioning in the individual

PRINCIPLES RELEVANT TO SEXUALITY

1. **Human sexuality provides for reproduction of the human species.**
2. **Sexual fulfillment is a very basic human need.**
3. **Sexuality pervades virtually every aspect of life from birth to death.**
4. **All human cultures have sanctions, often legal as well as moral, controlling expression of the sexual drive.**
5. **Individuals have strong cultural, religious, and esthetic convictions regarding the expression of human sexuality.**
6. **Moral values concerning appropriate sexual behavior have undergone considerable liberalization in most Western cultures in recent years.**
7. **Successful gender identification in early childhood is important for an individual's health and well-being throughout life.**
8. **Actual or potential damage to the integrity of an individual's sex organs poses a considerable threat to his self-esteem.**

SPECIFIC NURSING INTERVENTIONS

Teaching

Nurses, as knowledgeable and trusted health professionals, are often approached by friends and relatives, as well as patients, to explain sexual matters. Despite the blatant advertising about sex these days, there is still a considerable amount of ignorance on the part of the public in general regarding the basic anatomy and physiology of the reproductive tract, the sexually transmitted diseases, and effective contraceptive methods. We are not suggesting that the student nurse set herself up as a sex counselor for her friends, nor as a teacher to all on sexual matters. However, she should be able to give accurate information to people on the three topics mentioned above.

The specific learning needs of the patient, and the level at which information should be presented, are highly dependent on the person's age, his developmental stage, and his social activity. Is the person dating, about to be married, or about to become a parent? Children usually want to know where they came from, and they are very curious about their own bodies and the differences between themselves and members of the opposite sex. Their questions should be dealt with truthfully, matter-of-factly, and at their level of understanding. Most young children are satisfied, for example, with an answer such as "You grew inside Mommy in a special place for babies" to their question of "Where did I come from?" Adolescents usually want to learn about the menstrual cycle and the changes that are taking place within their bodies, including the emergence of the secondary sex characteristics. They also usually want information about dating, petting, sexual intercourse, and contraception. Those who have become sexually active should also be aware of the common venereal diseases, how these are spread, the signs and symptoms of them, and how to protect themselves from these diseases.

Some of this information is being taught in school classes in many parts of the country. The topic is still a highly controversial one, however, and the nurse should be aware of public opinion in the community and school policy before explaining aspects of human sexuality, such as contraceptive methods, to high school students.

Young adults who are about to marry or commence living together may also be in need of information about contraceptive methods. If they decide to have a family, they will need counseling in regard to parenthood—from pregnancy through the infant's first year of life.

Young adults should be aware of the need for tests and examinations for disease processes involving the urogenital tract, such as a regular Pap test for women, and regular checkups for men.

Women should be taught how to do their own breast examinations to discover nodules or tumors in the early stages, when they are still most amenable to treatment. The technique is illustrated on page 652.

Men should learn to examine their testes. The technique is ideally performed after a warm bath or shower, when the skin of the scrotum is most relaxed and the contents of the scrotal sac can be felt most easily. Each testicle should be examined with the fingers of both hands gently probing the soft flesh. If any hard lumps are found, they should be brought to a physician's attention promptly. It should be noted, however, that not all such lumps are cancerous.

Women in their middle years often need counseling and reassurance during the menopause, as do men during their climacteric, so that they understand what is happening in their bodies. People in this age bracket should also be aware of the early warning signs of common health problems related to sexual functioning that affect people in the middle years, and what to do about these problems. Middle-aged and older people may need sexual counseling in regard to their specific health problems, for example, sexual activity following a heart attack or following removal of a breast. Although it is not likely that first year students using this book will become involved in teaching situations such as these, we have included some articles in the Suggested Readings at the end of this chapter for those who want to pursue these topics further.

Birth Control Methods

Oral Contraceptives. The widespread use of oral contraceptives, more commonly known as "the pill," has revolutionized birth control methods and, by and large, freed women from the fear of unwanted pregnancy. Two types of oral contraceptives are commonly used, a *combination pill*, which contains both estrogen and progestogen, and a tablet containing a progestogen only. The combination pills are taken on a cyclic basis; that is, the person takes the same dosage every day for 20 or 21 days, skips 7 days, then repeats the cycle. Basically, these pills suppress the hypothalamic–anterior pituitary–ovarian system. Thus, they prevent the normal cyclic ovarian production of hormones and suppress ovulation. The pills also produce a thick cervical mucus that is hostile to sperm. They

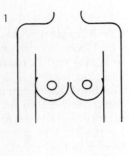

1. Sit or stand in front of your mirror, with your arms relaxed at your sides, and examine your breasts carefully for any changes in size and shape. Look for any puckering or dimpling of the skin, and for any discharge or change in the nipples.

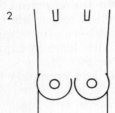

2. Raise both your arms over your head, and look for exactly the same things. See if there's been any change since you last examined your breasts.

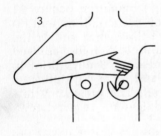

3. Lie on your bed, put a pillow or a bath towel under your left shoulder and your left hand under your head. (From this Step through Step 8, you should feel for a lump or thickening.) With the fingers of your right hand held together flat, press gently but firmly with small circular motions to feel the inner, upper quarter of your left breast, starting at your breast-bone and going outward toward the nipple line. Also feel the area around the nipple.

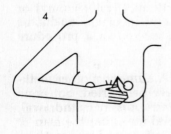

4. With the same gentle pressure, feel the lower inner part of your breast. Incidentally, in this area you will feel a ridge of firm tissue or flesh. Don't be alarmed. This is perfectly normal.

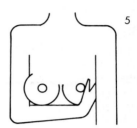

5. Now bring your left arm down to your side, and still using the flat part of your fingers, feel under your armpit.

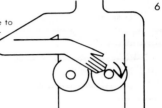

6. Use the same gentle pressure to feel the upper, outer quarter of your breast from the nipple line to where your arm is resting.

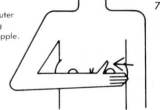

7. And finally, feel the lower outer section of your breast, going from the outer part to the nipple.

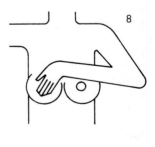

8. Repeat the entire procedure on the right breast.

Your own doctor may want you to use a slightly different method of examination. Ask him to teach you that method. Examine your breasts every month, just after your period. Be sure to continue these checkups after your change of life. If you find a lump or thickening *leave it alone* until you see your doctor. Don't be frightened. Most breast lumps or changes are not cancer, but only your doctor can tell.

Method for self-examination of the breasts. (Redrawn from Canadian Cancer Society pamphlet, "Breast Self-Examination," 1974.)

are considered 100 per cent effective if taken regularly. The progestogen-only tablets contain a low dosage of progestogen, and hence are often called the "mini-pill." Taken continuously, they do not suppress ovulation but produce changes in the cervical mucus and endometrium that inhibit implantation of the ovum. The pills do have some side effects. They may give rise to a pseudopregnancy, sometimes with nausea and vomiting. Fluid retention and headaches may also occur. Sometimes there are changes in the menstrual cycle, the usual change being that the duration is shortened. Dysmenorrhea is usually reduced. Women on the pill sometimes experience breakthrough bleeding, or "spotting." With the mini-pills there is often unpredictable bleeding. High oral doses or injections of estrogens may be used as postcoital contraceptives, often called the "morning after" pill. To be effective, they must be given within 72 hours of unprotected intercourse, and they can only be given once in a single menstrual cycle.

Contraceptive Injections.
Injectable progestogen products are available on the market and some are in fairly common use. They are very effective contraceptives, and only need to be administered two to four times a year. Unfortunately, they cause serious disruption in the menstrual cycle and, for this reason, have not achieved widespread use as yet.

Mechanical Barriers and Spermicides.
The condom (sheath, skin, safe, rubber, or prophylactic) is considered to be 80 per cent effective. It is applied to the erect penis before it is inserted into the vagina. In addition to its birth control function, the condom provides some prophylaxis against venereal disease.

A diaphragm must be fitted by an experienced person, and the woman taught to insert and remove it herself. In order to be effective the diaphragm must cover the cervix and it has to fit snugly. A woman needs to be refitted for a diaphragm after a pregnancy or if her weight changes drastically. A diaphragm may be inserted up to 2 hours before intercourse. It is used with contraceptive jelly or creams spread liberally on both sides of the barrier. Foams are not considered to be effective when used in conjunction with a diaphragm. The diaphragm should be left in place for 6 hours after intercourse. It can be cleaned with a mild soap and water after use, dusted with plain talcum powder, and kept in a container.

Spermicides come in the form of creams, foams, or jellies. They may be used with the condom or diaphragm for up to 90 per cent effectiveness. They are inserted into the vagina shortly before intercourse. The woman is advised not to douche for 4 to 6 hours after intercourse, because douching removes the spermicide.

Intrauterine Devices.
The intrauterine device, or IUD, is also known as the loop. It consists of a small piece of plastic or metal and is inserted into the uterus by a trained professional. Most types have a tail, called "strings," that protrudes out of the cervix. IUDs have been 95 to 98 per cent effective in all women who have used them. No one is quite sure why the IUD is effective. The currently accepted theory is that it initiates a foreign body reaction in the endometrium that renders it hostile to sperm and makes implantation impossible. Some types have a tiny copper coil, and it is known that low doses of copper are spermicidal. In most women, there is increased menstrual bleeding and cramping following insertion of the loop. Some women using the IUD have had intermenstrual spotting.

Rhythm Method.
The rhythm method requires no mechanical or chemical aids. It is based on two well-known facts: (1) ovulation occurs 14 days prior to the onset of menstruation; and (2) the length of viability of the sperm and of the ovum is 48 hours. A couple is therefore advised to abstain from intercourse for 3 days prior to the expected ovulation and for 3 days after—a total of 7 or 8 days in all. The pregnancy rate with the rhythm method is about 14 per cent.

Sterilization.
Sterilization may be accomplished in the woman by tubal ligation or by the removal of either the uterus (hysterectomy) or the ovaries (oophorectomy). In a man, the ductus (vas) deferens may be severed in a procedure known as a vasectomy.

Unreliable Methods.
A number of other methods of birth control have been tried, but none are effective. Coitus interruptus, or withdrawal, is not a satisfying method for either the man or the woman and is not effective because there are sperm in the pre-ejaculate of the man. Douching immediately after intercourse is considered to be a losing battle, because fertilization is likely to have already taken place. The insertion of tampons, sponges, deodorant suppositories, and lubricating jellies into the vagina is also ineffective.

Breast feeding sometimes inhibits the ovulatory cycle, but this does not provide a reliable method of contraception. Menstruation often resumes during lactation. In addition, women may conceive during the first cycle after ovulation resumes, before the bleeding that would occur at the end of the cycle. Thus, the woman who is breast feeding may become pregnant before she realizes that the temporary period of infertility has ended.

Venereal Diseases. Diseases that are transmitted by sexual contact are called venereal diseases, after Venus, the goddess of love in Roman mythology. In recent years, there has been an alarming increase in the incidence of venereal diseases, which has been blamed on such factors as increased permissiveness in regard to extra-marital sex and the rise in homosexuality. The most prevalent of the venereal diseases are syphilis and gonorrhea, with gonorrhea now ranked as the most common communicable disease in North America.

Syphilis is caused by the spirochete *Treponema pallidum*, a corkscrew-shaped microorganism. It is passed from one person to another by intimate bodily contact, usually sexual. The incubation period is 10 days to 3 months, with an average of 3 weeks. Syphilis is an insidious disease which progresses through a number of stages. It may be so mild that it is overlooked until it reaches vital body tissues, such as the blood vessels, heart, brain, and nerves. The disease begins with a sore, or *chancre*, which is most commonly seen in the genital area, although it may appear in any body orifice, for example, in the mouth or on the lips. A diagnosis of syphilis is made on the basis of two laboratory tests. One is direct observation of the spirochetes on a slide made with a drop of fluid taken from the chancre. The other is the blood test. One of the unfortunate aspects of the disease is that it may be passed from an infected mother to an infant in utero. However, this is preventable if the disease is diagnosed and treated early in pregnancy. In its early stages syphilis responds well to penicillin. Persons who have had sexual contact with the infected individual (contacts) are also treated with penicillin as a preventive measure.

Gonorrhea is caused by the bacterium *Neisseria gonorrhoeae*, a bean-shaped organism that is transmitted by direct mucous membrane contact, which is usually sexual. It can, however, be picked up from contaminated objects within 24 hours after the object is infected. The organism grows rapidly. It has an incubation period of 2 to 14 days, with an average of 3 to 5 days. In 90 per cent of women and 10 per cent of men, the disease is without symptoms in the early stages. An acute infection may, however, cause a thick, purulent, heavy discharge from the va-

gina in women, from the urethra in men, or from the pharynx if the infection was transferred by oral sex.

Gonorrhea can often be diagnosed by microscopic visualization of the organisms in a drop of the purulent discharge. A culture may also be taken from the discharge and sent to the laboratory for growth of the gonococcal organism. In addition to the discharge, there may also be a burning pain on urination and frequency of urination.

If the infection progresses, other genital organs may be affected and, if left untreated, systemic disease such as arthritis and endocarditis, as well as sterility in men, may result. During its passage through the birth canal, an infant may pick up organisms from an infected mother. The eyes are most commonly affected; therefore, silver nitrate drops are instilled into the newborn's eyes as a preventive measure. Gonorrhea responds well to treatment by penicillin. Both the infected person and all known contacts should be treated at the same time to prevent reinfections occurring. Research is currently in progress to develop a gonorrheal vaccine but, so far, none has emerged.

Another disease that is passed from person to person by sexual contact and can cause sores on the genital organs is *genital herpes simplex*. The virus causing this disease is related to the herpes virus that causes cold sores and fever blisters on the lips and the nostrils. Genital herpes gives rise to a similar type of blister, which erodes and leaves a small, shallow ulcer. In 90 per cent of the people who are infected, the disease does not give rise to symptoms; the remaining 10 per cent may have a mild to a severe attack. In vulnerable persons, the blisters usually appear within 3 to 7 days after exposure, with itching and an extensive genital rash often being the first indication. The sores are itchy and painful. This discomfort may be accompanied by pain on urination and by generalized symptoms in some cases. Usually the ulcers will heal themselves and the symptoms will disappear within 2 to 6 weeks. There is no known cure for the herpes; treatment is directed at relief of the itching and pain, and keeping the sores dry and clean to prevent secondary infections from developing. A person never gets completely rid of the organism from his system, and the blisters may reappear if the person is under physical or emotional stress. Antiviral agents are being developed to combat the disease, which has reached epidemic proportions in North America.

Other infectious agents may cause an inflammation of the urethra in men and of the vagina in women. In men, a causative agent is identified in only about 10 per cent of the cases, and the disease is usually classified as a non-gonococcal urethritis (NGU). In women, the most common cause of vaginitis is *Trichomonas vaginalis,* which is transferred through sexual contact from the man, who is usually asymptomatic. The resultant vaginal discharge has an offensive odor. In severe cases there may be a large amount of frothy, yellowish-green discharge. In pregnant women, women with diabetes, and those who have been taking some types of contraceptive pill, the fungus *Candida albicans* which is a normal inhabitant of the large intestine, may cause an infection in the vagina. The condition is called *vaginal thrush.* The discharge is usually watery and may have flecks of a white, curdlike material. Both *Trichomonas* infections and vaginal thrush respond well to treatment with drugs, metronidazole and nystatin, respectively, which are available on prescription.

Three other conditions that may affect the genital organs should also be mentioned, because the nurse, in her clinical appraisal, may note them. One is *genital warts,* which are caused by a virus and may be transmitted by sexual contact from one person to another. The wart begins as a tiny swelling anywhere from 1 to 6 months after contact, and develops into a cauliflower-like growth. The warts are usually treated with chemicals or with cautery (the use of a caustic substance or a hot instrument to destroy tissue). *Crab (pubic) lice* are small insects that resemble crabs and are found most profusely in the pubic hairs around the genitals. They may spread to other hairy areas of the body, but do not normally invade the hair on the head. Lice can be picked up from a toilet seat where one or more may have dropped from the pubic hair of an infested person. *Scabies* is caused by the female itch mite, a tiny insect that passes rapidly from one individual to another when people are in crowded unsanitary conditions without facilities for washing themselves or their clothes adequately. The female itch mite burrows a tunnel under the skin in order to lay her eggs. It is this burrowing that causes the individual to itch and scratch. The burrows may be found in the skin between the fingers, the wrist area, the armpits, and the genital areas. The condition is usually treated with benzyl benzoate or another organic sulfur compound.

Reporting. The venereal diseases, like other communicable diseases, are reportable. A physician in private practice or in a public clinic who diagnoses a person as having a venereal disease is required by law to report the case to the local Department of Health. Treatment may be given by a private physician or by public clinic. Treatment is given free of charge in public clinics. The local health department has a responsibility to follow up persons named as sexual contacts by the person with a diagnosed infection, in order to control spread of the disease.

Dealing with Male-Female Problems in the Nurse-Patient Relationship

The open knowledge and acceptance of sexual needs as an integral part of a person's health needs is still fairly recent in North American society. It is no wonder, then, that the topic is still fraught with much embarrassment. When it comes to asking questions about sexual matters during the nursing history, it may be the student, the patient, or sometimes both who are uncomfortable. Sexual needs are now being discussed openly in nursing school classes (they were not only a decade ago) and this helps to put students more at ease with the topic. Students who still have difficulty should discuss the matter with their teacher.

Older people who were brought up in an era when the discussion of sexual matters was taboo, except as a confidential matter between husband and wife or between themselves and their physician, are often acutely uncomfortable if a nurse attempts any discussion about sexual relationships. People of cultures that differ from that of North America are also often affronted by it, for example, those from Oriental cultures, especially if they have been brought up in traditional families. In India, a great many women will still not go to a male doctor, nor will the husbands permit their wives to be examined by a male physician. It is important, often, that patient and nurse (or doctor) be of the same sex in order to promote an open climate for the discussion of sexual problems. A guiding rule for the nurse is that if the patient does not want to discuss the subject, he should not be pressed. The nurse should recognize the patient's right to privacy and leave the topic. The person may feel more comfortable about discussing it later, or he may not.

Nursing procedures involving the male or female urogenital tract, or causing exposure of the genital organs (even the bed bath), are potential sources of embarrassment for both nurse and patient. It is important to acknowledge the patient's feelings and respect his dignity in order to maintain his feelings of self-esteem. Unnecessary exposure shoud be avoided in all instances. A good idea is to try to think of yourself in the patient's place. What would you want done by the nurse to protect your own privacy, or that of your father or mother?

Another problem female nurses often encounter is the male patient who makes sexual advances towards them. A male patient may expose himself unnecessarily or he may not try to conceal an erection, or try to pinch the nurse's bottom as she goes by. The problem arises particularly with patients who are in hospital for a long period of time. Older patients who are resident in long-term care facilities may have no other opportunity for sexual contacts and may make advances to a nurse. Young men who are hospitalized for a lengthy period are likely to feel sexually aroused at times by nurses of the opposite sex. It is important for nurses to accept the need for sexuality in their patients, and to try to channel it into socially acceptable forms of behavior. A calm, professional manner and matter-of-fact dealing with situations will help to restore a balance between overfriendliness on the one hand and cold impersonality on the other in the nurse-patient relationship.

Irrigation

Irrigation is the washing out of a body opening by letting liquid flow in and out of the opening. The *douche,* or *vaginal irrigation,* is a washing out of the vagina. Douches for general cleansing purposes may be purchased on the consumer market, or they may be made up in the home by combining a tablespoon or two of vinegar in a quart of warm water. Some women prefer to douche routinely after intercourse, although postcoital douching is not a method of birth control. Douches cleanse the vaginal area of normal bacterial flora, removing any offensive or irritating discharge. Douching may be done to apply heat or cold, as in the treatment of inflammation or hemorrhage, to treat vaginal infections, or to cleanse preoperatively.

Douching is not advised more often than twice a week unless ordered by a physician. because

the vagina is normally self-cleansing and self-lubricating. It should not be done during menstruation, the late stage of pregnancy, or the postpartum period. There is a danger in using a solution that is too hot, because delicate mucous membrane tissue can be easily burned. For purposes of cleanliness, other deodorants or suppositories may be used. Most authorities recommend not douching for 24 to 48 hours before a vaginal examination, because it will remove secretions and specimens of discharges that may be necessary for diagnostic procedure.

The preferred method for douching at home is to use a bag with tubing and douche tip or catheter. While lying in the bathtub, the woman gently inserts the catheter or tip, the bag being held 2 or 3 feet above the level of the hips. The fluid enters, distending the vaginal area and cleansing it, and escapes. The woman continues filling and emptying the vagina until all the solution is used. Using force during douching with an appliance such as a bulb syringe is contraindicated because of the danger of introducing microorganisms into the cervix.

Administering a Douche to a Patient. The patient should be asked to void before the douche is begun, to reduce pressure of the bladder on the vagina. The patient lies on her back in bed, on a bedpan, or in a bathtub using a waterproof support. The irrigating container is placed at a level just above the patient's hips so that the solution flows easily, assisted by gravity. It should be noted that increasing the distance from the level of the fluid to the outlet in the tubing increases the force of the irrigating fluid; undue pressure may drive the solution, and any contaminants that are present, into the cervical opening. The vulva is cleansed, with the labia being separated to allow the solution to wash the area. The nozzle is inserted gently into the vagina and directed down and back. The nozzle is rotated in the vagina, cleansing all surfaces. The tube is then removed, and the perineal area is washed and dried, with care being taken to remove any debris displaced by the douche, which may cause odor and irritation.

GUIDE TO ASSESSING THE STATUS OF SEXUAL FUNCTIONING

1. Is the individual male or female? How old is he or she?

2. If the patient is a child, are all of the primary sexual characteristics, i.e., recessed vagina in the case of a girl, penis and testes in a boy, intact? Are there any abnormalities that you can see, or that have been noted? Does the child show

characteristic feminine traits or masculine traits? Which parent does the child associate with or prefer? Does the child identify himself or herself as a "girl" or "boy"?

3. If the person is an adolescent, what changes of sexual maturation have occurred? If the patient is a girl, consider budding breasts, pubic and axillary hair, and onset of the menstrual cycle. In a boy, consider facial, pubic, and axillary hair; voice change; broad shoulders; developed genitals (penis and scrotum); and nocturnal emissions (wet dreams).

4. If the person is an adult, what is the body build like—masculine or feminine?

5. If the person is a woman, what was the age of menarche? Were there any problems? What is the interval between periods? Is the period painful? If applicable, what was the age of menopause? Was it natural or induced? Does she have children? How many? What are their ages? Were there problems with any deliveries? How many pregnancies has she had? Were there any miscarriages or abortions? Has she had surgery on the reproductive tract? Is there a family history of disorders of the reproductive tract? What is her marital status and the current status of her sexual relationships?

6. If the person is a man, is there a family history of genitourinary disorders? What is his marital status and the current status of his sexual relationships?

7. Has the individual noticed, or can the nurse observe, discharges or sores in the genital area? tenderness? redness? pain? swelling? abnormal lumps or masses?

8. Have laboratory tests or examinations been done for this patient, such as serological tests for syphilis, smear or culture for gonorrhea, or pregnancy tests? If so, are the reports back yet? What do they indicate?

9. What problems does the person have now in regard to sexual functioning?

10. How much knowledge does the patient have now in regard to such matters as anatomy and physiological functioning of the reproductive system? venereal diseases? contraceptive methods?

11. Does the individual undertake a regular breast self-examination or examination of the testes?

GUIDE TO EVALUATING THE EFFECTIVENESS OF NURSING INTERVENTION

1. Has the patient gained the knowledge and skills necessary to promote healthy sexual functioning? to prevent unwanted pregnancy? to protect against venereal diseases? to identify the early signs and symptoms of commonly occurring disorders of the reproductive tract and take appropriate steps to obtain treatment?

2. Are you comfortable in asking patients questions pertaining to their sexual functioning? in teaching matters related to sexual functioning? Does the patient show embarrassment or distress at the questions? If so, what action did you take to put him or her at ease? Did you feel that it was appropriate?

3. If the patient is a woman, has she learned how to carry out a breast self-examination? administer a douche? insert a vaginal suppository? If the patient is a man, has he learned how to examine his testes for abnormal lumps or masses?

STUDY SITUATION (1)

Mr. Ivanovitch, a 70-year-old patient in extended care with a leg injury, complains to you constantly that he is lonely, demanding your attention. He is a divorced alcoholic who likes to play cribbage. He starts to make overtures, then makes direct passes at you, saying "I just want a woman." Apparently, it is fairly typical of his cultural background to be direct.

1. How do you deal with his behavior?

2. What are some of the ways to redirect his attention?

3. Are there community resource groups you can call on?

STUDY SITUATION (2)

Miss Lyons, 18, is a very unkempt girl who shows up repeatedly in the outpatient department for treatment of venereal disease. Her records indicate she is slightly retarded and has a fifth-grade education. She lives with her family. Her seven brothers and sisters have various learning disabilities. Her father is an occasional laborer; her mother stays at home. Both parents are alcoholics. Apparently she is engaged in prostitution.

1. What can be done to assist her in improving her situation and breaking out of the rut she is apparently in?

2. Who are some of the resource people who could be contacted?

3. What are some of the factors affecting her case?

4. Do you think she should be sterilized?

5. Do you think prostitution should be legalized? Why?

SUGGESTED READINGS

Boston Women's Health Book Collective: Our Bodies, Our Selves. New York, Simon and Schuster, 1971.

Burger, D.: Breast Examination. American Journal of Nursing, 79(6):1088–1089, June, 1979.

Cohen, S.: Programmed Instruction. Patient Assessment: Examination of the Male Genitalia. American Journal of Nursing, 79(4):689–712, April, 1979.

Falk, G., and Falk, U. A.: Sexuality and the Aged. Nursing Outlook, 28(1):51–55, January, 1980.

Frank, D. I.: Sexual Counselling to a Mastectomy Patient. Nursing '81, 11(1):64–67, January, 1981.

Griggs, W.: Sex and the Elderly. American Journal of Nursing, 78(8):1352–1354, August, 1978.

Henshaw, B.: Providing Holistic Patient Care as a Sex Educator. Nursing '79, 9(6):10–11, June, 1979.

Hickman, B. W.: All about Sex . . . despite Dialysis. American Journal of Nursing, 77(4):606–607, April, 1977.

Kandell, N.: The Unwed Adolescent Pregnancy: An Accident? American Journal of Nursing, 79(12):2112–2114, December, 1979.

Krozy, R.: Becoming Comfortable with Sexual Assessment. American Journal of Nursing, 78(6):1036–1038, June, 1978.

McCarthy, P.: Geriatric Sexuality. Journal of Gerontological Nursing, 5(1):20–24, January-February, 1979.

Murray, B. L. S., and Wilson, L. J.: Testicular Self-Examination. American Journal of Nursing, 78(12):2074–2079, December, 1978.

Nelson, S. E.: All about Sex Education for Students. American Journal of Nursing, 77(4):611–612, April, 1977.

Puksta, N. S.: All about Sex . . . after a Coronary. American Journal of Nursing, 77(4):602–605, April, 1977.

Roznoy, M. S.: The Young Adult. Taking a Sexual History. American Journal of Nursing, 76(8):1279–1282, August, 1976.

Stanford, D.: All about Sex . . . after Middle Age. American Journal of Nursing, 77(4):608–610, April, 1977.

Stockard, S.: Caring for the Sexually Aggressive Patient: You Don't Have to Blush and Bear It. Nursing '81, 11(11):114, November, 1981.

Yoselle, N.: Sexuality in the Later Years. Topics in Clinical Nursing, 3:59–70, April, 1981.

REFERENCES

1. Genesis 1:27–28.
2. Kinsey, A. C., et al.: *Sexual Behavior in the Human Male.* Philadelphia, W. B. Saunders Company, 1948.
3. Masters, W. H., and Johnson, V.: *Human Sexual Response.* Boston, Little, Brown & Company, 1966.
4. Barnard, M. U., et al.: *Human Sexuality for Health Professionals.* Philadelphia, W. B. Saunders Company, 1978.
5. McCary, J. L.: *Human Sexuality.* 3rd ed. New York, D. Van Nostrand, 1978.
6. Beischer, N. A., and Mackay, E. V.: *Obstetrics and the Newborn.* Sydney, Australia, W. B. Saunders Company, 1976.
7. Watts, R. J.: Dimensions of Sexual Health. *American Journal of Nursing*, 79:1568–1572, September, 1979.

30

The Nurse Should Be Able to:

- Discuss the importance of security and self-esteem to the well-being of an individual during his lifetime
- Describe the main tasks in maintaining security and self-esteem at different stages of the life cycle
- Identify factors contributing to security and self-esteem
- Assess the patient's status in regard to security and self-esteem
- Identify actual or potential problems of anxiety and depression in patients
- Identify situations requiring immediate nursing and/or medical intervention and take appropriate action
- Apply relevant principles in planning and implementing
    a. to promote the patient's security and self-esteem
    b. to prevent potential problems of anxiety or depression
    c. to assist patients in coping with anxiety and depression
    d. to assist patients to meet their spiritual needs
- Evaluate the effectiveness of nursing interventions

SECURITY AND SELF-ESTEEM NEEDS

CHAPTER
30

INTRODUCTION

Maslow believed that many problems people have today in our impersonal society are the result of failure to fulfill their very basic needs for security and self-esteem.[1] Man is a social being who needs the company of other people to feel at home in this world. His security is very much a cultural need, then, being dependent on his feeling safe and comfortable in his relationships with other people as well as physically safe from harmful factors in the environment.

A person's sense of security is derived from a number of different elements. An individual has to have his physiological needs met, first of all. A person does not feel very secure if his stomach is empty and he does not know where his next meal is coming from or if he is constantly in pain. In addition to having his physiological needs met, a person also has to feel that he can go about his daily activities without fear, that he is safe in his home at night, and that his children can play safely in the neighborhood in which he lives. These are very basic components of a safe physical environment that are essential for a person's security.

But physical safety is not enough. A person also needs a sense of belonging to the human race and a feeling that he is part of a particular segment of it. He also needs the love and companship of other people, although sometimes a pet will provide his owner with the love and affection he needs. An individual also needs attention and recognition from others—an acknowledgement that he is an accepted member of society. Communication is, therefore, an essential element of security, whether expressed in words or nonverbally, for without communication a person is not aware of his status in relation to others. One last essential element in a person's security is a realistic concept of himself. In the final analysis, an individual's security—or lack of it—stems primarily from how he sees himself in relation to others as being superior, inferior, or equal to them, liked or not

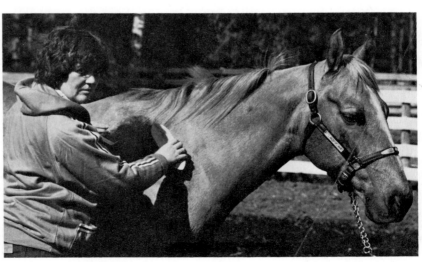

Pets provide their owners with love and companionship.

Security:
physiological needs met
— fear
Sense of belonging
attention
perception of self
communication

661

liked, respected or not respected, wanted or unwanted, and accepted or rejected. Self-esteem, the feeling one has about oneself, involves a critical evaluation of oneself. How do I measure up physically, socially, psychologically, and in my behavior to the standards and values I have chosen for myself? A person is constantly judging himself in relation to the standards he himself has established. Although he may not be aware of his self-evaluation on a conscious, verbalized level, he experiences it as a feeling about himself. He feels "good" about himself if, in his opinion, he has done something well, or he may feel small and miserable because he never seems to be able to do things right.

It has been said that a person's self-esteem is the key to his behavior. It influences his thinking processes, his emotions, his desires, his values, and his goals. Self-esteem has two interrelated aspects. One is self-confidence, that is, the feeling that he is a competent person and has the ability to do things. The other is self-respect, the feeling that what he is doing, or has done, is "right" according to his values. Cheating on an examination, for example, is not acceptable behavior in most people's value system; therefore, even if you manage to obtain a high grade on a paper by cheating, you will probably never feel good about it because you will have lost some of your self-respect.[2]

Part of a person's self-esteem is derived from how he perceives his physical being. This is called his "body image" and reflects both the mental picture a person has of himself, and his attitudes towards his body and its various parts and functions. A person develops a conception of his physical appearance from sensory input over the years. As an infant, he begins to notice his hands and his feet and other parts of his body that he can see, and he explores his own body and that of his mother, using touch, smell, taste, sight, and hearing. As he gets a little older, he begins to associate the reflection he sees in the mirror with himself, and then he hears other people telling him that he is a "good looking boy" or perhaps "the spitting image of his grandfather." He also looks at other people and he thinks, "Perhaps I look a bit like that," and he gradually builds up a mental image of himself. Because the bony prominences of his body, such as the elbows and the knees, and the body openings are most in contact with other objects, they serve as the most immediate points of reference in orienting a person to his environment and are particularly important in body image. A person's attitudes toward his body and its parts and functions are largely a product of his socialization. A child absorbs without question the attitudes of his parents regarding

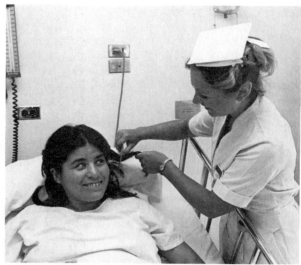

By looking after a patient's grooming needs, the nurse shows that she recognizes the patient as a person.

"clean" and "unclean" parts of the body, the appropriate state of cleanliness of his body generally, and whether it is good to be fat or lean.

People who are ill or, for one reason or another, have sought the help of health professionals, are always at least a little insecure and sometimes very much so, particularly if their world has been turned upside down by a sudden illness or accident that requires hospitalization. In health agencies, personnel sometimes are so busy taking care of the technical aspects when the patient is seriously ill that they tend to forget that there is a person attached to all the tubes and wires. A primary responsibility of the nurse is to look after the person—to help him to feel secure, and to support both his confidence in himself and his respect for himself as a person. These are part of the *caring* aspects of the nurse's role and, many would say, the most important part of all. "It may well be that nursing, in particular, holds the key to maintenance of humane, individualistic care for people and their health problems. And this capacity must be zealously enlarged."[3]

DEVELOPMENT OF SECURITY AND SELF-ESTEEM THROUGHOUT THE LIFE CYCLE

During pregancy many women say that they have never looked or felt better, and they feel a sense of satisfaction and completion that they have not known before—a new appreciation of being a woman. They feel a responsibility to care for the child within. This experience usually unifies a man and a woman. She is carrying his child—together they have created this new life.

The woman's needs now may become secondary to those of her unborn child. She is planning more and more for the coming birth. During this period some men feel excluded from the attention they are used to receiving. Both men and women need reassurance at this time. Women have to deal with clumsiness and ungainly proportions and a sense that their earlier self-image has been distorted and their equilibrium disturbed. They need to know that they are still attractive and that the changes in appearance are normal. They should be encouraged to see the beauty of the body during pregnancy, as exemplified by the many paintings and sculptures focusing on the subject of motherhood. A woman can invest her emotions in the care of the fetus better when she feels secure and protected by her husband. There is a desire for deeper intimacy during this period of life, and a new sense of family develops.

Some single women have children on their own, because of a desire to be close to someone and to have someone with whom they can share love. Single pregnant women need a supportive environment such as a nuclear family, a cooperative housing arrangement, or an extended family environment.

Prenatal classes are invaluable for both the mother and her partner; the latter also needs the reassurance and support of his peers. The birth of a child causes a major change in the lives of a man and woman. Some couples are deciding to have home births these days, with a midwife* present to deliver, because they feel it is important to be surrounded by their natural environment at the time of birth. Complications in the process of childbirth may, however, require medical intervention or an emergency trip to the hospital ward for surgical intervention or other specialized services. Home birth is a rather controversial matter at present. Many hospitals, however, now have a "birthing room" that is furnished like a home bedroom rather than the former delivery room. The atmosphere is more informal and fathers are welcome to attend the birth. After birth, the family must be reorganized to accommodate the new member; the roles of husband and wife alter in respect to each other. There are new responsibilities, additional financial considerations, and the well-being of the helpless infant to take into account. The first few weeks are usually anxious ones, often frustrating for both mother and father as they adopt new roles and adjust to the new arrival. One

*The practice of midwifery is not legal in Canada.

danger for a couple is that they will direct all their attention to the newborn, and none to each other.

The individual's feelings of security and sense of self-esteem develop from the moment of birth. Considerable emphasis is now put on the importance of parental bonding during the first few hours after birth, and throughout the first week, to give the infant a sense of security. No longer is the father barred from the delivery room in most North American hospitals. If there is no "birthing room," a separate room is usually set aside where the mother, father, and baby can get to know each other immediately after birth. The quality of the contact—with an emphasis on touching and caressing—is considered more important than the quantity of interaction. The voice of the mother is very important, giving positive reassurance to the infant of her presence.

Erikson felt that one of the major developmental tasks of infancy is the development of trust—in oneself, the environment, and the people in it. At first, the infant does not distinguish between himself and his environment. He can, however, sense and respond to feelings of approval or disapproval on the part of his mother or nurse. Approval leads to a sense of well-being, and disapproval causes discomfort; psychologists feel that these experiences are implanted forever in the human personality. At 3 months, the child begins to explore his sense of self. He watches his hands and his feet with great interest and he examines other areas of his body. At 4 months, he is aware of himself as distinct from the rest of the world and also begins to explore this world, using mother as a security base. Infants who have developed security in their attachment to mother are more likely to actively explore the world around them, although they will cry and fuss if she leaves them and show happiness when she returns.

Anxious infants may be more passive, showing less curiosity and less interest in exploring their environment than secure ones. "Stranger anxiety" is a common trait at 6 to 10 months, the time when infants distinguish between mother and others.

An infant's emotional security rests to a considerable extent on the relationship that develops between mother and baby. If it is a positive relationship, a rapport is established that permits interaction on a nonverbal basis, with the mother responding empathetically to her infant's needs. If the mother-infant relationship is cold, inconsistent, or rejecting, mistrust and insecurity are built into the personality of the infant. Parents who respond promptly to their infant's cries have happier, calmer, and more outgoing children as a general rule. Inconsistency or lack of response to the infant's needs leads to infant anxiety, which is manifested by crying and clinging behavior.

During the toddler stage, a child gains new motor skills, learns to walk, and extends his range of activities to investigate different aspects of his surroundings. His verbal and intellectual abilities develop at a rapid rate. He begins to comprehend and test out the meaning of the word "no." For the first time he learns that there are restrictions and limitations on his behavior. This is a time when the house needs to be childproofed, so that the restrictions and limitations can be kept to the minimum needed for his safety. Some mothers tend to overprotect their children and want to control their behavior too much. During the toddler stage and until about age 4, the principal developmental task is to gain a sense of autonomy without developing doubt or a sense of shame. Thus, the child needs to learn to negotiate the stairs (under Mother or Father's watchful eye) when he is ready to do so, without too many admonishments about being careful. A sense of the positive will greatly enhance the situation. The toddler's burgeoning communication skills enhance the development of self. His first and most deeply learned perception of himself is a composite reflection of how significant persons around him—his parents (or others taking a parental role), siblings, and grandparents—perceive him.

The preschooler needs to learn initiative and to develop skills that build self-confidence. It is important for him to be given the opportunity to try new things and to receive the support of his parents while doing so. The self-confidence that is gained is reflected in the child's sense of eagerness, his spontaneity, and the "bounce" in his step. The development of routine times for meals, bedtime, and outings helps to provide security for the child because it develops a sense of expectation with reinforcement. During the preschool stage the child is beginning to develop a conscience. Until approximately age 7, however, children are still very egocentric in thought. As they mature, they begin to think more about other people's needs and wishes.

When the child enters school, he is suddenly confronted with an expanding circle of people and new activities. He must learn how to interact and cooperate with others. He also has a wider range of roles to emulate as teachers and older students provide models to choose from. He learns how others, i.e., teachers, students, and principal, evaluate his strengths and how they care for him as a person. He learns the difference between work and play and to enjoy work for the rewards it brings. If he feels a sense of

inferiority or mediocrity, he may tend to withdraw and be discouraged. The school may provide reinforcement for his self-esteem through recognition of his achievements, which can often offset an adverse atmosphere at home. On the other hand, problems at school may counteract the benefits of a supportive home environment. The chief task of this age group is to develop a sense of industry rather than inferiority to others.

The adolescent stage begins at approximately 12 years and lasts until about 18. During the rather self-conscious time of puberty, the individual gradually achieves a sense of identity and belonging, usually through the stabilizing influence of his peer group. Adolescence is a period of great ambivalence in Western society, with both the desire to be free of authority forms, most importantly parents and school, and the need to be dependent upon them for emotional and financial support. The adolescent is dealing with who he is and what he wants to work at and do with his life. His major task is to gain a sense of identity. Failure to resolve this may lead to confusion, depression, or an identification with a group or cult that supplies an identity. It may also lead the individual to seize the first job or mate that offers him a sense of identity, or else to opt out through the use of alcohol and drugs to ease the difficult transition from adolescence to adulthood.

Positive reinforcement is vital during this period. One goal of education is to reinforce the adolescent's identity through teamwork and the development of skills that can support him through his life. In order to achieve a secure identity, young people need a sense of community in which they can exchange learning skills and support each other, especially since a vast number are now being raised in single-parent homes. Parents today are tending not to put high expectations on young people to achieve material success (as defined by the last generation), recognizing that life is much more complicated than it used to be and that other values are important, such as a sense of purpose in life.

The young adult is mainly concerned with developing more intimate relationships with others. Without these he experiences a feeling of isolation. Intimacy has usually centered on marriage, although many now accept extramarital relationships or a career and close friends as alternatives. It is necessary for the individual to have a firm sense of identity at this point, although in this rapidly changing world, people often have a strong sense of isolation and feel insecure. Rapid changes in our institutions and in our economic situation have an effect on human roles and greatly affect a person's sense

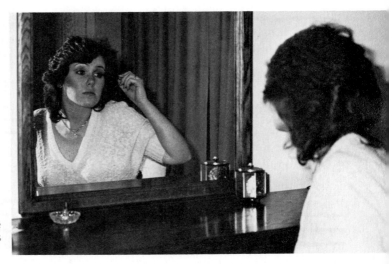

How well a person looks after her appearance is often a good indication of how she feels about herself.

of security. "The feeling that our lives 'count' comes from healthy relationships with the surrounding society—family, corporation, church, or political movement. It also depends on being able to see ourselves as part of a larger, even cosmic, scheme of things."[4]

There is a tendency to view oneself during young adulthood as being "indestructible" and able to burn the candle at both ends. This attitude often leads to accidents and to the physical and mental state colorfully called "burn out." These in turn may alter the self-image and adversely affect self-esteem. Damaged self-esteem and feelings of helplessness contribute to many of the suicides and homicides committed by people in this age group. The more stabilized young adult, however, who is married or in an intimate relationship with another and has a career under way tends to see his life as more secure, productive, and self-actualized.

Erikson felt that during middle age, there is a need to focus on a sense of generativity as opposed to stagnation in one's life, socially, at work, and in the community. He felt emphasis should be placed on a person's ability to pass on wisdom to the young and on innovation, rather than simply going through life in a mechanical routine. Men often tend to become more concerned with feelings and less aggressive in their middle years; women feel more free as their children become less dependent. A person's sense of security comes from the "home" one has created and the abilities one has developed. Men may be concerned with loss of physical prowess, and some may engage in extramarital affairs to try to dispel this concern. Women may experience doubt about their appearance and continued attractiveness, particularly if their husbands stray. Somatic disorders frequently develop in response to psychic stress and anxiety. Gastric ulcers, diarrhea, colitis, bronchial asthma, hyperventilation, and diabetes insipidus are among the health problems that are thought to have a strong psychosomatic component.

The middle years focus on a new type of freedom: freedom from the obligations of childraising, one of the most difficult jobs in the world. As someone was overheard saying: "When my youngest child finally gets married and leaves home, I'm going to be standing in the last row of the church, celebrating!" Essentially, middle age is a time for stock-taking and reevaluation. One has developed a sense of order in this world and a sense of how one's life is an aspect of history.

During the older years, there is increased attention to the maintenance of dignity to preserve the sense of self-esteem. Emphasis is being put on people's need to remain in their homes surrounded by their friends, relatives, and belongings until they reach a point where this is no longer possible. Homemakers, home care nurses, and other community services are beginning to make this easier.

During old age, security is ensured partially through financial means such as pensions, savings, and retirement plans and partially through the ability to adapt, often to the situation of being dependent upon others. Many older people retain an ability to enjoy things without much money, a skill they developed from earlier experiences during the depression years of the 1930's or the war years of the 1940's when people had to entertain themselves.

The main task during this period, according to Erikson, is the maintenance of integrity as opposed to despair: accepting what has been, feeling useful, and receiving respect. Old age is a period for looking back; the self-concept is related to past experience. When the future has little to offer, the mind tends to focus on earlier years.

The problem of dependency upon others for support and assistance may weigh heavily upon a person's sense of integrity. Depression may follow the loss of spouse, friends, home, and income coupled with a feeling of rejection of society. Help in dealing with daily situations is usually welcome, along with visits from friends and relatives. The problem of decreased mobility may create more of a sense of isolation, although many communities have transportation systems geared to the elderly. Our society has been chiefly concerned with cultivation of the sense of independence rather than group effort, with a resultant selfishness as opposed to selflessness. This has contributed to the alienation of the elderly and is reflected in the high percentage of suicides among the older population. In many cultures, older people are regarded as the venerable generation; to live longer is to be respected and to share your wisdom with others. Many recommendations on improving the lot of the elderly in North America are made in the book *Toward Healthy Aging*; the book recommends reemploying the elderly in service areas such as "recreational counselling, paraprofessional legal advice, health and social service, cottage industry and handicraft production."[5]

According to Fromm: "The development of the self is never completed; even under best conditions only part of man's potentialities is realized."[6]

According to one Texan, there are basically three things everyone needs during growth and development: "Everyone needs someone to love, something to do, and something to look forward to."

FACTORS AFFECTING SECURITY AND SELF-ESTEEM

Of primary importance in both the development and the maintenance of a person's security and self-esteem are the significant people who inhabit his social world. You will have noticed in the previous section the importance of the family in helping an individual to grow up comfortable and secure with his environment and with himself. One of the roles of the family is to provide help and support to its members in times of trouble. The strong shoulder of a grown-up son is very comforting for the grieving widow, and many a young mother has been relieved to see grandmother, with her years of experience in child-raising, arrive to assist when the new baby is brought home from the hospital.

It is a nice, secure feeling to know that there is a brother, sister, cousin, or close friend who will answer a call for help. It is the family, or significant others, who provide an individual with the support he needs to make his way in the outside world.

In the early, formative years, it is usually mother or father who bolsters the child's confidence in himself with words of encouragement like "You can do it" or "We know you can" and who pick up the shattered ego when the child's team does not win by saying, "Never mind—you played well anyway." Later, it is the girl friend or boy friend or the wife or husband who provides the support that encourages a person to reach his maximum potential. Everyone needs someone to praise and admire the thing he does, to believe in him, and to minimize his faults. An understanding friend often provides this type of support, sometimes more than the family. A close network of friends who provide support and companionship for each other often develops among older women in a community who have been widowed or who, for one reason or another, are living out their life alone. In our highly mobile North American society today, the predominant family pattern is the nuclear family of mother, father, and children. Grandparents, uncles, and aunts are often far away, and hence the friendship network becomes more important.

In many parts of India, and in some other Eastern countries, the extended family still prevails, with young couples usually returning to the parental home of the groom after marriage to start their new life. Their children, then, are brought up among cousins, uncles, and aunts as well as parents and grandparents. This arrangement provides a built-in system for the security of all family members and works well as long as relationships are good. One's place in the family is well understood in the hierarchical scheme of the extended family. The father is supreme, and he expects and receives symbolic deference from his wife and children. He is served first at mealtime, and often the wife will eat her meal afterwards. The young son's wife is expected to assist her mother-in-law in household chores. For young women who want to work outside the home, child care is provided by grandmother or by aunts and cousins who share the household. Children are loved and petted by all. The traditional extended family provides the older woman with protection from loneliness, and gives her a sense of purpose and a respected position within the family. She also may wield a considerable amount of power in the household, since she is often the one who carries the keys to the larder and other supplies, frequently on a ring at her waist. Increasingly, however, young couples are wanting their autonomy, as well as privacy and freedom from the control of parents—even in traditional cultures such as the Indian one. There is also an economic necessity to keep the family small these days, and this fact, combined with the increasing migration of young people to the cities, is contributing to the demise of the extended family in most parts of the world.

Fortunately, many traditional customs and mores are surviving, and these help an individual to maintain a sense of the continuity of life. There is an order that is reassuring, for example, in the fact that Thanksgiving comes at the same time every year, a few weeks before Christmas, and that Easter is celebrated in the spring at a time that was decreed centuries ago. The ceremonies that mark life events, starting, for example, with the circumcision of the male Jewish child a few days after birth and the baptism of the Roman Catholic infant, and continuing through the marriage ceremony and the death service, are all important in that they help family members to develop a sense of continuity. The ceremonies also contribute to meeting self-esteem needs for the participants and their families, since the event is being marked in the approved manner, according to one's cultural group. We are indeed fortunate in Canada and in the United States to have a mosaic in which ethnic groups have maintained their own cultural identity, with many of their traditional customs being passed down from generation to generation. We celebrate the Chinese New Year and Ukrainian Christmas and enjoy the German Oktoberfest in different parts of the country. These events all help people whose roots are elsewhere to feel more at home in a land that is far from their native land.

Many of the ceremonies and traditional events are religious in nature, as you may have noted. Religion has always provided man with a refuge from the uncertainties and vicissitudes of life. It is reassuring to feel that there is an order to the universe and that a Supreme Being is in charge to whom an individual can go for comfort, support, and guidance. The stress of living in today's fast-paced world, with all of the uncertainties brought about by rapid change, has no doubt contributed to the remarkable return of people to the churches that we have been witnessing in recent years. People seem to be looking for a semblance of order and a meaning to life to renew their faith and sense of safety and security in the world. Many people say they want something to "hang onto"; many find it in their religion.

Other factors in a person's lifestyle besides religion also contribute to his security. These include his educational attainment, his employment, and his socioeconomic status. Today, a person usually has to have a minimum of a high school education to even begin to compete in the job market. To enter most professions and occupations requires post–secondary school training (as with nursing, for which a 2-year community college course is a minimum requirement). A high school diploma, then, provides a certain amount of security for a person in regard to obtaining a job; a certificate or diploma from a college program or a university degree provides more. The attainment of a certificate, diploma, or degree also adds immeasurable to a person's self-esteem. It is a significant achievement and rightly deserves recognition.

A person's job, how he feels about it, the pleasure he receives from it, and the companionship and respect he obtains from his coworkers make a difference in whether an individual feels comfortable and secure in his daily living. A warm, supportive atmosphere at home can often nullify the damaging effects of a work environment that is filled with stress. More and more, however, employers are finding it advantageous to make the workplace more conducive to developing their employees' self-esteem. They are fostering a cooperative team spirit that gives people the feeling that they are an important part of the organization, and not just a cog in the machinery. It has been demonstrated in numerous studies that these factors are often more important than money in attracting and retaining good workers and in increasing productivity.

Money, or the lack of it, is important, however, to a person's security. Hence, pension funds and retirement savings plans have been developed so that a person can put away a certain amount of income for the time when he can no longer work. An economic recession puts untold stresses and strains on family life, especially if there is not enough money to pay the mortgage and all the other bills and buy shoes for the children for school. The uncertainty of not knowing whether there will be a job tomorrow can be very devastating to an individual's security.

Changes of any sort in a person's life will upset his equilibrium, and some may produce stress that can lead to illness. (see Chapter 2). Situations may arise, too, that cause a person to experience doubt and uncertainty. These include both the maturational crises (or passages, to use Sheehy's term) that we talked about in Chapter 13, and the hazardous events that happen in the course of a lifetime, such as accidents and illness. Accidents are a likely occurrence at least once in a person's life. A person may fall and break an arm, for example, or he may be involved in a motor vehicle accident. We have mentioned that being hospitalized is an event that makes almost everyone fearful and insecure.

Often, these hazardous events will cause changes in a person's appearance. A scar on the face may result from an accident, or a woman may have a breast removed in an operation to remove a cancerous growth. An illness may also result in alterations of body functioning. A person who has had a myocardial infarction may not be able to carry on with his favorite recreational activities for a while, especially if these are active sports. He will be disturbed by the changes in his body. Alterations in body image can seriously upset a person's equilibrium.

COMMON PROBLEMS

Human beings have a variety of adaptation mechanisms that help them to maintain equilibrium in all areas of functioning. In the case of emotional functioning, specifically for fear and insecurity, there are mechanisms both within the body and in a person's mental processes that help him to cope with threats of real or imagined danger. In Chapter 2 we discussed the flight-fight reaction; this is the body's physiological response that prepares a person to contend with fear by either removing himself from the cause (flight), or by overcoming it by standing his ground and fighting it. The defense mechanisms we discussed in Chapter 2 also help an individual to deal with real or imagined threats to his self-concept by adjusting his thinking to cope with these dangers.

When the fear extends over a long period of time, or is sufficiently intense, the normal mechanisms are unable to restore a balance, and problems arise in the individual's physical, mental, or social functioning.

The two most common problems that arise are anxiety and depression. Anxiety is considered to be a modified form of fear. Almost everyone has experienced it. Nurses, as well as patients, have anxieties. Depression is a morbid sadness or melancholy. A person whose security is threatened and who feels helpless in the situation may react with depression rather than anxiety. Thus, often the same stressors that cause anxiety in some people may give rise to sadness and melancholy in others. When the depression is caused by a situation or event that would normally cause a person to be sad, for example, the death of a spouse or a good friend, it is called a "reactive depression." Sometimes the term "situational depression" is used instead of "reactive depression."

Sources of Stress for the Sick

Many insecurities that patients experience could be prevented if potential sources of fear were eliminated. Others, if not preventable, can often be minimized by nursing intervention. Some of the most common sources of stress are: interference with the fulfillment of basic needs, developmental crises, and other life changes.

Interference with the Fulfillment of Basic Needs. A basic source of stress is actual, potential, or imagined interference with a person's ability to satisfy his basic needs. Physiological needs, as we have mentioned several times, take precedence over all other needs because they are essential for survival. Hence, people who are physically ill are usually frightened; something is wrong with their physiological functioning. Among the most frequently cited causes of anxiety in this regard are fear of pain, death, or disfigurement; loss of an organ or of strength; and inability to return to a normal life. Another source of anxiety that has been found among many hospitalized patients is fear of a bad reaction to medications.[7]

When people are ill, their basic body processes become a source of major worry. A healthy person takes for granted his breathing, the functioning of his heart and circulatory system, his intake of food and fluids, his elimination of wastes, and his ability to perform a multitude of activities using his motor abilities. When he is ill, the fact that something is interfering with these vital processes causes them to assume major importance. The sick person becomes very anxious and wants to know what his temperature, pulse rate, and blood pressure are, the results of his physical examination, laboratory, x-ray and other tests, what they found when he was operated on and so forth. His meals, his urinary output, and his bowel movements cause him daily concern.

Fear of the unknown is one of the principal sources of stress for people who come to a health agency. This would seem to bear out Kalish's suggestion that the need for knowledge, as exemplified by man's curiosity, is the second most important of the basic needs. Health practitioners have not always been fully aware of the patient's need for information, but it has come through in a loud, clear voice in the Patients' Bills of Rights (see Chapter 7). The incorporation of teaching plans in the POMR initial and sub-

basic needs upset,
STRESS: crises, (developmental)
life changes.

SECURITY AND SELF-ESTEEM NEEDS 669

sequent care plans for patients acknowledges the importance of giving the patient adequate information, and helps to ensure that he receives it.

Boredom and inactivity, or a lack of sufficient sensory stimulation in the environment, will also cause a person to be anxious. Kalish included the need for stimulation as one of the items in his discussion of basic human needs (see Chapter 13). The bored individual becomes restless; he wonders what to do, feels he should be doing something, and becomes anxious that he is not. If boredom or inactivity persists too long, the individual will become apathetic. This aspect of boredom was discussed more fully in Chapter 22.

Safety and security are next on the hierachy of human needs, and threats to these constitute a very real source of stress for sick people. They worry about their physical safety. Will they fall from the high bed? roll off the stretcher? receive the wrong medication? experience more pain than they can tolerate? They also worry about how hospital staff are going to react to them. For example will the nurse be angry at them? They may also worry that they won't be able to control their emotions.

Threats may also exist with respect to a person's financial security. People worry about having sufficient money to cover health expenses. A person may fear that a health problem will interfere with his ability to earn a living. The possibility of altered family structures, or changes in social relationships caused by illness, also threaten the security a person has in knowing who he is and his place in the scheme of things.

If the individual is hospitalized, he usually experiences stress because of the change in his environment. When people are in unfamiliar surroundings, they become anxious. The patient will worry until he knows where to find things, how to operate the various mechanical devices attached to his bed, and why the other things in his immediate environment are there. The patient is accustomed to routines, which provide him with security in his normal existence. These are disrupted, and he must adjust to changes in his sleeping habits, meal and bath times, and other aspects of daily living. The presence of strangers and the lack of familiar faces will also contribute to his anxiety until he knows that he can safely trust the people who are giving him care.

A lack of fulfillment of the basic need for love and belonging was discussed in Chapter 2 as a factor contributing to illness. Among hospitalized patients, the need to feel part of a group, to feel that people like them and accept them and their illness, has been cited as one of their most common concerns.[8] People often find companionship and acceptance in a group with other people with the same health problem. Common fears and anxieties can be shared and somehow do not seem as bad. New knowledge and skills can also be shared, and the group members can support each other.

Nor should we forget that threats to a person's self-esteem interfere with another of man's basic human needs. The loss, or potential loss, of independence, for example, poses a very real threat to a person with a health problem. It can cause him to lose his self-esteem and to think that other people will not respect him. It is important therefore to make sure that nothing the nurse does or says causes the patient to think that he is any less a person because of his health problem.

Potential or actual interference with achievement of self-actualization is another frequent cause of worry among people who are ill or think they have a health problem. Illness can interfere with a person's career, or with fulfillment of his need to make the best of his potentialities in any sphere. The loss or threatened loss of the ability to use one's hands, for instance, would be a major blow to a pianist or the person who uses his hand(s) in pursuing one of his principal interests in life. Similarly, the person whose hobbies are mainly outdoor ones that require motor skills, such as skiing or riding, would be very anxious about being able to continue with these activities if his health problem, actual, potential, or imagined, threatens the loss of his motor functioning abilities.

Developmental Crises. At certain times in a person's lifespan, major changes take place as he makes a transition from one developmental stage to another. We discussed these extensively in Chapter 13. Often referred to as "developmental crises," they cause the person to experience a considerable degree of insecurity as he wonders if he can cope with the demands that will be made upon him in the next stage of his development.

Other Life Changes. In addition to those linked to particular stages in a person's development, other changes in a person's life also cause stress. In one study assessing patients' perceptions of stressful life events, the most common situations causing stress were grouped as follows:

Changes at work
Changes in the health of self or family

Moving
Financial changes
Births (in addition to birth of the first child)
Arguments
Death (of a family member or close friend)
Involvement with law authorities
Marital situations
Changes regarding children
Changes at school
Other[9]

The results of this study indicated that the patients, all of whom were receiving care in an emergency unit, had had a greater number of life changes in the 6 months prior to their admission to the unit than are usually found in normally, "healthy" individuals. This finding would tend to lend support to the theory that change, and the anxieties associated with it, can be a major factor contributing to illness.

ASSESSMENT

In order to identify actual or potential problems of anxiety or depression, the nurse needs information about the individual's health status, information about him as a person, his stage of physical and psychosocial development, and about his lifestyle. In regard to his health status, she considers such questions as: Does this person have a recognized health problem, or does he think that he has a health problem? If so, is it one in which pain is a factor? Is death a possible consequence of the problem? Is disfigurement or loss of an organ a possibility? Is there a possibility that the person thinks these may occur? Does he perhaps perceive his health problem (actual or imagined) as leading to a loss of strength, or interfering with his ability to pursue his normal lifestyle? Is there a possibility of surgery or might he think there is? (Surgery, even the most minor, usually brings on anxiety.)

The nurse also needs to know something about the person as an individual. What are his personality characteristics? How has he coped with stress in the past? Where does he stand in relation to fulfillment of his basic needs? Is he concerned with self-actualization at this point in his life, or is he struggling to make enough money to provide himself (and, if he is married, his family) with the basic essentials of food, shelter, and security? Is his career the most important thing in his life? his home? his wife? his children? his outside interests?

The nurse considers also his age and his stage of physical and psychosocial development. Is there a possibility that he is going through a crisis time in his life? The nurse should also be aware of the individual's marital and family status. Who are the members of the family constellation? Where does this person fit into the family structure? Is he the head or a dominant member of the household? Is he in a dependent role in the family? Who are the other members of the family? If the patient does not live with his family, does he live with someone else? Who are the significant others in his life? What is this individual's occupation? What is his socioeconomic status? What are his hobbies and his interests? What are his immediate concerns? Another matter to consider is whether there have been any major changes in the person's life recently. If so, how many changes has he undergone? What sort of changes were they? Did they necessitate major readjustments in his life?

Some of this information will be available to the nurse from data she or other persons have gathered about the patient in the initial assessment interview and observations. Some she may learn from the physician's notations on the patient's records and his plans for diagnostic and therapeutic care, as well as other information that is on the patient's progress record. The social worker, if he or she has been called in, usually writes a lengthy social history on the patient, which is often helpful to the nurse in identifying actual or potential sources of anxiety or depression. The nurse supplements the information she has gathered from other sources by talking with the patient. As we noted in Chapter 10, most people will talk quite freely about things that are concerning them if the nurse has established a climate in which the patient feels free to communicate, and if she takes the time to be an attentive listener. In trying to identify sources of anxiety or depression, it is sometimes helpful to ask direct questions, such as about changes that have occurred in a patient's life, or other matters she feels are significant in relation to this particular individual.

Identifying the Problem of Anxiety

The threat of danger causes certain physiological reactions to take place within the body. These vary to a certain extent in different individuals according to their physical makeup, although many are commonly seen in the majority of anxious people. Anxiety also brings about changes in a person's behavior. The nature of these behavioral changes depends on a number of factors, such as the severity of the anxiety, the individual's basic personality structure, and the ways in which he has learned to cope with anxiety in the past. The physical condition of the patient affects his ability to tolerate anxiety.

Something that may constitute only a minor worry when one is well may create an overwhelming anxiety when the body's defenses are lowered.

● Through her observations of an individual, the nurse can often tell if he is anxious. The individual's verbalizations of his feelings, and statements he makes in regard to physical or mental symptoms he is having, also help the nurse to identify anxiety as a problem this person is having.

Physiological Manifestations. The principal physiological mechanism operating in anxiety is the fundamental "alarm reaction" as the body attempts to protect itself from harm (see Chapter 2). It was originally believed that the reaction was due to the outpouring of epinephrine into the blood stream in response to strong emotion. However, this theory does not account for all the physical signs and symptoms that occur in people with anxiety. It is believed that these are the result of stimulation of the autonomic nervous system. The sympathetic portion of the system is most usually affected, although, if the stimulus is sufficiently intense, the parasympathetic portion will be affected as well. Thus, the anxious individual may show evidence of muscular tension, which is a result of sympathetic nervous system stimulation, and, at the same time, have diarrhea due to increased gastric motility resulting from overactivity of the parasympathetic system.[10]

Almost everyone has had experience with some of the physical signs and symptoms of anxiety. There are varying degrees of anxiety, ranging from a mild apprehension to overwhelming panic. In its mild form, anxiety may be beneficial in that it has the effect of putting the body into an alert state and motivating the individual to take some action to alleviate it. Few people would study or get assignments completed on time if there were not a certain amount of anxiety involved. Unresolved anxiety, however, or anxiety in more than mild degree can be harmful.

Among the most easily observable physical signs of anxiety in an individual are the circulatory changes that take place. The action of the heart is strengthened and accelerated. The person's blood pressure may be elevated by 10 mm. of mercury or more above normal. The nurse may find that his pulse rate may be as much as 30 per cent above normal. A person's respiratory pattern is often disturbed as well. It may be increased in rate and depth, or may become irregular. There may be a marked pallor of the skin or sometimes a flushing of the face. Often the skin surfaces are cold.

Muscular tension is almost invariably present. In some people this may be observed in a taut expression of the face or in a clenching of the fists. Some people assume a very rigid posture. At times muscular tension is revealed by a tremor of the hands; in a facial, arm, or shoulder tic; or in a generalized shivering or trembling of the body. The tightening of the abdominal muscles and the "butterflies" in the stomach that one commonly experiences with anxiety are the result of muscular tension. The tension headache is another common symptom of anxiety.

People seek relief from muscular tension in a number of ways: by biting their nails, drumming their fingers on the table, or pacing up and down, for example. Restlessness and overactivity are usually fairly reliable indications that the individual is anxious.

Many people perspire excessively when they are in anxiety-provoking situations. It may be the palms of the hands or the soles of the feet that are most affected. This increased perspiration combined with a coldness and pallor of the skin (due to lessened peripheral circulation) results in the typical cold and damp hand of the very anxious individual.

Changes in the patient's voice and speech patterns should be noted as possible indications of anxiety. Some people talk very rapidly or constantly when they are anxious and sometimes the voice becomes very loud or high-pitched. The voice may quaver. In other persons there may be a hesitancy of speech; they may appear to be having difficulty finding the words they want to use. Stammering and stuttering are not uncommon in people with anxiety.

In anxiety, *mental activity is usually increased*. When the anxiety is mild, this may mean that the individual is simply more alert and better able to think clearly. As anxiety mounts, however, a person's perceptual awareness decreases. He becomes unaware of things in his immediate surroundings, except possibly a single thing on which his attention focuses. The anxious person often has difficulty concentrating on anything outside that one thing. His attention span is usually short and he may be unable to answer even simple questions. The very worried parents who bring a sick child into the emergency unit are sometimes so distraught that they cannot remember their own address.

With increasing anxiety, the heightened mental activity may hinder a person from getting rest, and insomnia (inability to get to sleep) frequently results. If the anxious person does manage to get to sleep, he is often troubled by nightmares.

Gastrointestinal symptoms often accompany anxiety also. The "knot" or "butterflies" in the

Anxiety: deny, talk too much, anger, hostility, crying, joke-laugh

stomach may progress to nausea and vomiting. Often people say they cannot face the thought of food when they are going to take an exam or have an important interview. Some people vomit before every exam they take. Diarrhea, as we mentioned above, is also a common symptom in anxiety. Often people have urinary frequency as well, as many a nervous traveler waiting for his plane to depart has found.

Behavioral Manifestations of Anxiety. People react to threatening situations in a variety of ways. The behavioral manifestations of anxiety in people who are sick usually reflect the ways in which they have learned to cope with life's dangers in the past. While some people can talk easily about their fears, and openly express these to the nurse, others may be saying, "I am frightened" in less easily recognizable forms. Some people attempt to *deny* the existence of anxiety. They ask no questions and frequently make a point of keeping conversation off the subject of their illness. In our culture, many men feel that it is unmanly to say that one is afraid, particularly to a woman. Men not infrequently (and sometimes women too) cover up their feelings of anxiety with *loud assurances* that they are not frightened, and they may *joke and laugh* in their attempts to minimize the seriousness of their condition.

Some people react to the threat of danger with *anger and hostility*. They may criticize the care they are receiving and be loud and insistent in their demands for special treatment. People who react in this way often engender hostility on the part of the staff, who label them consciously or unconsciously as "difficult" patients. There is an old saying that goes, "When in danger, when in doubt, run in circles, scream and shout." It is perhaps well for the nurse to remember this when she encounters a patient who is being very "difficult." If she can accept this type of behavior as being indicative of the patient's anxiety and not take it as a personal attack on herself, she will be in a better position to take positive measures to help the patient.

Crying is another way in which some people react to anxiety. Many nurses are embarrassed to find a patient in tears and find it difficult to know what they should say or do. Attempts to reassure the patient that everything is going to be all right are not usually effective in helping the patient to cope with his feelings. Crying often denotes a feeling of helplessness and inability to handle one's problems. The tears serve to relieve tension, and the nurse can perhaps be most helpful by staying with the patient and being ready to listen when the crying episode is over.

The Patient's Subjective Perceptions. As already mentioned, some people can verbalize their anxieties, others cannot. The nurse may find, however, that the patient may tell her about some symptoms he is having which, put together with her own observations, may confirm her suspicions that the individual is anxious. Pertinent observations which the patient may make relate to the physiological manifestations of anxiety described above. He may say, for example, that he has a headache that starts at the base of his neck (frequently caused by tension in the shoulder and neck muscles). He may complain that he just can't sit still, or that he can't concentrate on anything. He may describe a knot or butterflies in his stomach, or complain that he has a cramping pain, accompanied by frequent loose stools. He may tell her that he has to urinate frequently. The nurse must be careful not to jump to conclusions about these symptoms. Of course, they could very well be caused by something other than anxiety. They should, however, be reported in her observations about the patient in conjunction with her objective findings.

Identifying the Problem of Depression

Depression and anxiety both cause certain physiological reactions to occur within the body. They also both give rise to specific behavioral manifestations. The two sets of responses are quite different, however. The observant nurse should be able to distinguish between these problems in her patients in most cases. Sometimes, however, a person will show manifestations of both anxiety and depression, in what is called an "agitated depression." It is as if everything were in slow motion. The person is less active, his movements are slow, and his reaction time is longer. He is less responsive to any form of stimulation and he talks less; his speech is slower than normal. The severely depressed person may be totally unresponsive.

Gastrointestinal functioning also slows down, and he tends to become constipated. The individual loses interest in food. He usually has no appetite and will tell you that he just does not enjoy food any more. As a result, he will probably lose weight. A loss of anywhere from 5 to 20 pounds is not unusual. Men tend to lose their sex drive when they are depressed, and women may have a cessation of menses.

Behavioral Manifestations of Depression. There are three basic feelings that depressed persons experience as part of their depression. They do not want to socialize, and in fact do not really

[handwritten note at top:] no socialization ↓ self esteem + worthlessness Depression: hurt themselves or destroy

want to do anything. They have feelings of worthlessness and loss of self-esteem. They also want to hurt themselves and even destroy themselves because they feel they are not worthy to live.

Depression is so prevalent among the population that it is said to be the "common cold" of mental illness. It is often hidden by the individual who may wear a mask of joviality to cover his sadness, or it may masquerade as physical illness. Negative emotions have a deleterious effect on body functioning, and anger, hostility, and depression can all cause physical changes that give rise to disease processes. Nurses will encounter people who are depressed on all units of an inpatient facility, and among the people who are living in the community. She should be particularly watchful for it in young people who are having difficulty finding themselves during the teen years and early adulthood, in people who are going through the middle-age turmoil, and in old people.

Even if he has accomplished a great deal in his lifetime, the depressed individual often speaks of his achievements as meaningless. He never did anything that really amounted to much, he is likely to say. The depressed individual usually finds it difficult to concentrate and hard to remember things. He may forget his appointment at the clinic, or he may feel that it is too much effort to go. Often, activities are begun but not completed. The person either loses interest or just does not have the energy to finish.

The depressed individual usually walks with a stooped, slouching gait, his head down near his chest, often shuffling along. He usually wants to make himself as small as possible because he feels miserable within himself. He is also not much concerned about what he wears. It is such an effort just to get out of bed in the morning. He may begin to neglect his appearance, and not bother to take a bath or shave. A depressed woman may not bother with makeup. Most depressed people find that the worst time of the day is when they are waking up from sleep. They may describe their feelings in terms such as "blue," "down," "low," "sad," or even "depressed." Others may complain of being irritable. Often, people say they feel "hopeless," "worthless," or "no good." Or, they may say, "I can never do anything right!"

The table below lists several comparative observations that are helpful in distinguishing between anxiety and depression.

ESTABLISHING PRIORITIES FOR NURSING ACTION

Dealing with the Anxious Patient

Anxiety may be mild, moderate, or severe, or it may turn into panic. In establishing priorities, the nurse assesses the level of the patient's anxiety by observing the degree of severity of the physiological and behavioral manifestations he is showing. It has been suggested that nurses sometimes project their own anxieties onto the patient, and thus may assess that the patient is experiencing more severe anxiety than he actually is. It is wise, therefore, to use objective criteria in assessment. Particular observations to note are: evidences of greatly increased muscular tension, as seen in trembling hands and frequent position changes; increased perspiration, and a cold, clammy feeling of the hands; markedly decreased perceptual awareness and

✔DISTINGUISHING BETWEEN ANXIETY AND DEPRESSION

Anxious Patient	Depressed Patient
1. Talk and movements at normal speed or faster than normal	1. Talk and movements slower than normal
2. Readily discusses his symptoms or other topics; animated in discussion; discussing his problems frequently leads to improvement or change in behavior	2. Reluctant to discuss his emotional, social, or physical problems; talks in monotone and repetitively; discussion does not lead to changes in behavior
3. Retains interest in some things	3. Marked decrease or loss of interests
4. Able to enjoy some things, such as watching television or talking with others	4. Difficulty in enjoying things
5. Likely to feel worse in the evening, and better after sleep or rest	5. Usually feels worse in the morning, or after any sleep
6. No weight loss (except in patients with anorexia nervosa); eats constantly or intermittently; usually enjoys at least some food	6. Decreased appetite for and enjoyment of food, often with loss of weight
7. Diarrhea or loosening of bowel movements is common	7. Usually constipated

Adapted from Crary, W. G., and Crary, G. C.: Depression. *American Journal of Nursing*, 73(3):472–475, March, 1973.

PRINCIPLES RELEVANT TO ANXIETY

✓

1. It is easier to allay a known fear than anxiety from an unknown source.
2. People generally feel less anxious when they know what is going to happen to them.
3. Anxiety is lessened when people feel they have some control over their situation.
4. Loneliness aggravates anxiety.
5. A feeling of depersonalization contributes to anxiety.
6. Physical activity helps to relieve muscular tension.
7. Anxiety can often be relieved by diversional activity.

inability to concentrate; marked increases in pulse rate and disturbances in breathing; and disturbances in sleep patterns.[11]

Severe anxiety may become *panic,* in which the person is unable to say or do anything that is meaningful. His behavior may be completely out of context—he may laugh when he should be crying—and his thoughts and speech become incoherent. The person who has "panicked" needs someone who is calm to stay with him, to take charge of the situation, and to tell him what do do. He cannot think for himself at this point.

The nurse often encounters people in a state of panic in the emergency room unit. A calm, reassuring manner, simple directions on what to do, and, often, the familiar routine of offering a cup of tea or coffee will help to calm the person. Calming a person who is in a panic is always a matter of immediate priority. Severe anxiety is something that needs to be dealt with on a priority basis also.

In determining measures that will allay anxiety, the nurse must take into account the fact that her plan of care has to be individualized to suit each patient. No two people are alike in regard to the nature of their anxieties, their reactions to these, or the type of help they need in overcoming them. There is therefore no easy set of rules for the nurse to follow. The guiding principles given below, may, however, be helpful.

Dealing with the Depressed Patient

● The subject of depression will be treated in more detail in psychiatric nursing courses. The beginning student, however, should be alert to the possibility that a depressed patient may try to injure himself, or to commit suicide. Sometimes, a person will actually signal his intention. He may say, "I wish I could do away with myself" or "I'd like to kill myself," and may even discuss ways of doing so. The nurse should always be watchful of any patient who seems to be getting more depressed. She may notice that the physiological and behavioral manifestations are becoming more pronounced. It is important to remember that the depressed patient is not always on a psychiatric unit—he may be on a surgical or a medical ward. The patient's physician should be alerted if the nurse suspects that the patient is becoming more depressed, so that psychiatric counseling and appropriate therapy can be instituted promptly. Often, mood-elevating drugs are given. Meanwhile, the nurse should make sure that the environment is safe from objects that the patient might use to injure himself or take his own life. Sharp instru-

✓PRINCIPLES RELEVANT TO DEPRESSION[12]

1. A person who is depressed will show changes in his physiological functioning, in his feeling state, and in his behavior.
2. Depression alters a person's cognitive functioning.
3. Prolonged or deep depression may cause general metabolic retardation, mental confusion and/or dullness.
4. Emotions tend to be contagious.
5. Emotions are influenced by a person's physiological state.
6. A depressed person usually has very low self-esteem.
7. A depressed person may not want to live because he feels unworthy.

Anxiety: minimize it   cope w/it   depression: prevent for injury
alleviate it   support pt. physiologica
                depression: help overcome depression

SECURITY AND SELF-ESTEEM NEEDS 675

ments and drugs, for example, should not be left out. It is also a good idea to check frequently to make sure the patient is all right.

GOALS FOR NURSING ACTION

Dealing with the Anxious Patient

Nursing action for the individual who may develop anxiety is directed toward preventing it. For the person who is already anxious, nursing action may aim at one of three things: (1) alleviating his anxiety, (2) minimizing it, or (3) helping him cope with it.

Dealing with the Depressed Patient

Nursing interventions for the depressed patient are directed toward three principal goals: (1) preventing the patient from injuring himself or taking his own life, (2) supporting and maintaining the patient's basic physiological processes, such as nutrition and elimination, and (3) helping the person to overcome his depression.

SPECIFIC NURSING INTERVENTIONS

Dealing with the Anxious Patient

In deciding on specific nursing interventions to prevent anxiety, to minimize or alleviate it,

Often the comforting presence of someone who is sympathetic can help to allay some of the anxiety a patient feels in a stressful situation.

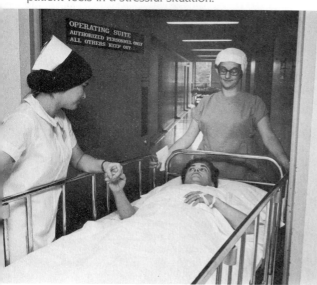

or to help the person to cope with anxieties that cannot be eliminated, the nurse is guided by her assessment of the individual patient, his particular problems, and her understanding of potential or actual sources of anxiety he may have. She also considers whether she can do something to help this person herself, or whether he needs the help of another member of the health team. If we review some of the interventions the nurse may undertake in applying the principles noted above, we will find some that she might consider in the care of specific patients:

1. *It is easier to allay a known fear than anxiety from an unknown source.* We have already discussed some of the ways the nurse can gather information to help her to identify the sources of a patient's potential or actual problem of anxiety. The nurse always verifies with the patient that her interpretation of the source of his anxieties is consistent with his perceptions in this regard. The nurse may think that the patient is very worried about the treatment he is going to have tomorrow, for example, when in actual fact he is not worried about that at all; he may instead be anxious about his daughter, who has not come in to see him as she had promised.

It is important to remember, too, that talking with the patient can also be therapeutic. It gives the patient an opportunity to explore the causes of his anxieties, to discuss them with someone and perhaps to work out his own solutions to some of the things that are worrying him.

The beginning nurse, however, should not feel that she can be a skilled counselor at this stage in her career. If the nurse does not feel comfortable in dealing with a patient's anxieties, or feels he needs more highly skilled counseling than she is able to provide, she should not hesitate to call in someone else. Nor should she feel guilty in doing so. Her instructor, or the head nurse on the ward, may be able to help the patient. If a psychiatric nursing specialist is available, this person is often able to help people with their anxieties more effectively than someone without that orientation. She may also be able to provide that nurse with help in her approach to the patient. Some patients need the counseling services of a psychologist or psychiatrist, and the patient should be referred for these services.

2. *People generally feel less anxious when they know what is going to happen to them.* Providing information is important both in preventing and in allaying anxiety. If a patient knows what is going to be done during a laboratory test, he usually is less apprehensive about

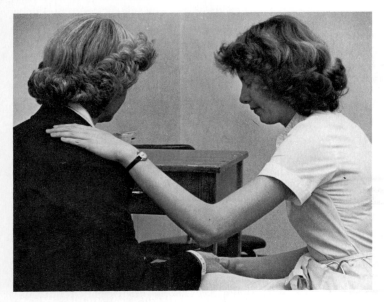

Anxiety is a common problem for both patients and their families. Here, a nurse comforts a woman being admitted to the hospital for diagnostic tests.

it. Similarly, the patient who has been told that a certain procedure may hurt a little is better able to face the pain. Teaching plans that identify information the patient needs should form a part of every nursing care plan.

3. *Anxiety is lessened when people feel they have some control over their situation.* Enlisting the patient's cooperation and having him participate in his care whenever possible help to give him this feeling. Giving the patient a voice in the scheduling of his activities, or the way some procedure should be done, is one way of helping him to feel he still has some control over events. The nurse might confer with him about the time for his bath, for example, or the time he prefers to have treatments done. When would be the best time to change his dressing, for example?

4. *Loneliness aggravates anxiety.* People need someone to whom they can talk and with whom they can share their feelings. A large part of the nurse's role is providing this kind of emotional support for patients. Talking with the patient is important, but feelings can also be shared without words, and sometimes words are not necessary. It is helpful to the patient simply to have someone who is sympathetic present. Some people feel more comfortable in talking over their anxieties with non-medically oriented personnel. The nurse should not overlook the contributions that such members as the chaplain and the social worker can make in helping patients with their anxieties.

5. *A feeling of depersonalization contributes to anxiety.* When the person feels that he has lost his identity, that he is just a health agency number or an interesting "case," his confidence in the care he is receiving is diminished. It is important to help the patient to retain the feeling

that he is a respected person in his own right. Referring to the patient by name, not by bed number, and taking an interest in him as an individual are among the many things a nurse can do to reassure him that he is in good hands.

6. *Physical activity helps to relieve muscular tension.* Exercise within the patient's limits of tolerance is a good way of relieving the muscular tension accompanying anxiety. Relaxation exercises also help. The assistance of the physical therapist is often helpful in teaching patients relaxing exercises or suggesting other measures to reduce muscular tension.

Two simple exercises from Yoga, which the nurse may find useful herself, are the sponge and eye exercises.

SPONGE*

I. *Benefits:*

The Sponge—
- promotes deep *muscular relaxation.*
- deeply *relaxes the nervous system.*
- restores *peace of mind.*
- results in a reduction of *anxiety* of "nerves" through the release of tension.
- is a marvellous *energy-recharger.*

II. *Technique:*
1. Lie on the floor, legs slightly apart, arms limply by your side. (A)
2. Point your toes away from you and hold for 5 seconds. Relax.
3. Pull the toes up towards the body, bending at the ankle. Hold. Relax
4. Pull your heels up two inches on the floor

---

*Reprinted from Kareen Zebroff: *The ABC of Yoga.* Vancouver, B.C., Fforbez Enterprises, Ltd., 1971.

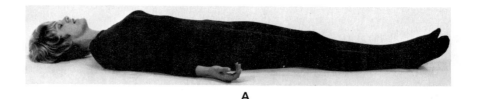

A

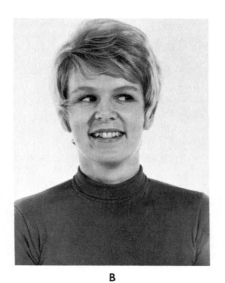

B

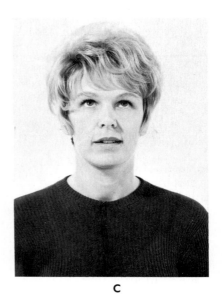

C

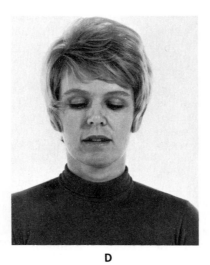

D

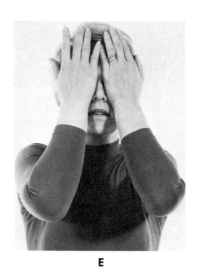

E

A, Sponge. *B–E,* Eye exercises. (From Zebroff, K.: *The ABC of Yoga.* Vancouver, B. C., Fforbez Enterprises, Ltd., 1971.)

and then straighten the legs, pushing the back of the knees firmly against the floor. Hold. Relax.

5. Point the toes toward each other and pull the heels under and up, keeping the legs straight. Hold. Relax.

6. Pinch your buttocks together. Hold. Relax.

7. Pull your abdomen in and up as far as possible. Hold. Relax.

8. Arch the spine back, pushing the chest out. Hold. Relax.

9. With arms straight by your side, palms down, bend the fingers up and back toward the arm, bending at the wrist. Hold. Relax.

10. Bend the elbows and repeat step 9, bending the hands back toward the shoulders. Hold. Relax.
11. Make a tight fist of your hands, bring the arms out to the sides and move the arms up perpendicular to the floor. Move very slowly, resisting the movement all the while to make the pectoral muscles of the bust stand out.
12. Pull the shoulderblades of the back together. Hold. Relax.
13. Pull the shoulders up beside the ears. Hold. Relax.
15. Bring the tongue to the back of the roof of the mouth. Hold. Relax.
16. Purse your lips, wrinkle the nose and squeeze the eyes tightly shut. Hold. Relax.
17. Smile with the lips closed and stretch the face. Hold. Relax.
18. Yawn very slowly, resisting the movement.
19. Press the back of the head against the floor. Hold. Relax.
20. Frown, moving the scalp forward. Hold. Relax.
21. Go through the eye exercises.
22. Pull your head under and against the shoulders without moving anything else.
23. Relax, melting into the floor, for up to 10 minutes. (A.)

III. *Dos and Don'ts:*

DO hold each holding position for at least 5 seconds.

DO relax after each holding position, by flopping back into place after each flexing position.

DO NOT worry or think of unpleasant things as you relax at the end of the Sponge. Rather, keep your thoughts to a minimum, on pleasant things, and dispassionately watch them wander past without trying to become involved.

The Sponge is called the Dead Man's Pose or Corpse in the Sanskrit language. Really, it is a deep relaxation pose where your body has a chance to assimilate what it has learned, at its leisure. Seldom do we take the time simply to relax. We may read, watch TV or sleep. Just because we lie down does not at all mean we are relaxing our deep-seated neuromuscular tensions. The body has to relearn how to do that. After some weeks of the deliberate Sponge technique you will find that you can relax without going through all the steps.

EYE EXERCISES*

I. *Benefits:*

The Eye Exercises—
• relieve *tension, fatigue,* and *strain* of the eyes.
• strengthen the *eye* muscles.
• relieve *headaches.*

---

*Reprinted from Zebroff, K.: *The ABC of Yoga.* Vancouver, B.C., Fforbez Enterprises, Ltd., 1971.

• give eyes a clear, *shiny* look.
• give a general feeling of *relaxation.*

II. *Technique:*

1. Sit in a comfortably cross-legged position; look straight ahead.
2. Look as far to the right as is possible without moving the head. Hold 5 seconds.
3. Look to the left. Hold. (*B.*)
4. Look up under the eyebrows. Hold. (*C.*)
5. Look down past nose. Hold. (*D.*)
6. Now imagine a giant clock with the 12 just under the eyebrows and the 6 on the floor immediately in front of you.
7. Look at each digit of this clock for one second, so that your eyes are moving jerkily.
8. Repeat, moving counterclockwise.
9. Cover your eyes with the palms of both hands for 30 seconds, to rest them. (*E.*)

Variations:

1. a. Look far away out the windows. Try to look miles toward the horizon. Hold.
   b. Slowly bring your gaze back and look cross-eyed at your nose. Hold.
2. Use your imagination: e.g., describe semi-circles or diagonals with your eyes.

III. *Dos and Don'ts:*

DO these exercises any time you are very tired or feel that your eyes have been strained, instead of just squeezing the eyes up in the customary fashion.

DO rest the eyes by closing them between each set of exercises.

The eyes are our most important sense and yet people neglect them greatly by taking them for granted. Eye strain and resulting headaches can be greatly reduced through exercising the eye muscles.

If exercise is not feasible or permissible, nursing interventions, such as a soothing backrub or massage, can frequently help to relieve tense muscles.

7. *Anxiety can often be relieved by diversional activity.* If a person has nothing to occupy his time or attention, he tends to become introspective and to brood on his troubles. Reading, watching television, and playing cards are activities that are usually available in hospitals to divert patients from a constant preoccupation with their illnesses. Women often like to knit, crochet, or do embroidery, and people of both sexes seem to like macramé; these activities should be encouraged. Frequently, the occupational therapist can make suggestions and help

to interest patients in activities that divert their attention from themselves.

Tranquilizers. Drugs of the tranquilizer group frequently are ordered to help to reduce anxiety. Among those most commonly used are Valium, Stelazine, Librium, and Mellaril. These are given as directed. The nurse should be alert to the possible side effects of tranquilizers in her patients. The most common side effect is drowsiness, but patients may show other reactions as well, such as headache, dizziness, nausea and vomiting, constipation, or mental disturbance. Because the side effects are usually specific for each drug, the nurse should acquaint herself with those associated with the drug ordered for her patient.

Particularly vulnerable are elderly patients, who sometimes experience a marked decrease in blood pressure after the administration of these drugs. It is not uncommon for elderly patients to develop symptoms of excitement or mental confusion when they are receiving tranquilizers.

Dealing with the Depressed Patient

Protecting the Patient from Self-injury. Constant vigilance is needed to protect the severely depressed patient from injuring himself or committing suicide. Patients who are seriously depressed are usually placed on a psychiatric nursing unit so that the specialized care they require is available. If they are on a general ward, often a private duty nurse or one staff nurse may be assigned to care for the patient. The nurse who has a depressed patient among her regular caseload should be particularly careful to make sure that the patient takes all of his medications under her watchful eye. There should be no opportunity for him to collect a large number of sleeping pills or other drugs. In tidying up the drawer of the bedside table each day, it is important to make sure that medications are not collecting there. Sharp instruments, and glass articles that could be broken to provide the person with an instrument with which to hurt himself, should not be left where the depressed patient can get them. The medication cupboard on the ward should be kept locked at all times, unless a nurse is actually in the process of dispensing medicines. This is a good general rule, in any case. One should not go off to answer a patient's signal light and leave the medication cupboard keys dangling from the door or leave the door open. If the person is known to be suicidal, all potential sources of self-injury, such as belts and shoe laces with which a person could strangle himself, are removed. There should also be a check on the patient at irregular but frequent intervals. Depressed patients who wake up in the early morning hours (when a person's body processes are at their lowest ebb) often need someone to talk to, and the nurse should take time to stop and chat for a few minutes with them. Occasionally, an individual will need to be physically restrained to keep him from injuring himself. This is most likely to be seen in the Emergency Unit, where a person may be coming out of the effects of a drug; LSD, for example, is noted for causing suicidal tendencies in people as they are recovering from its effects.

Maintenance of Physiological Processes. Because of his inactivity, the depressed person's nutritional status may suffer. He often has no appetite and must be tempted to eat. It is amazing how appetite will perk up in mildly depressed people if they have company to share their meals. The nurse should be alert to the problem of constipation in depressed people because of the slowing down of gastrointestinal functioning and the inactivity (see Chapter 16). These people need to be encouraged to take a sufficient amount of fluids. The slowing down of physiological functioning also causes a tendency for urine to be retained in the bladder overly long, and bladder infections could result from a combination of inadequate intake of fluids and stasis of urine. Because the person tends to sit a lot, he may develop edema in the dependent limbs, or in the sacral area (see Chapter 17).

A depressed person often needs help with hygiene and grooming, since it is too much effort for him alone. Often, assisting a person in improving his personal appearance will help to lift a mild depression. A new article of clothing may also stimulate an individual, helping with mild depression.

Helping the Patient to Overcome Depression. People who are lonely often get depressed. Everyone needs the stimulation of other people (or a pet) to keep him alert and responsive. One of the things the nurse can do for a lonely person is to encourage him to participate in group activities. Loneliness is a common accompaniment of old age, particularly if a person outlives his contemporaries. Community centers have a wide variety of activities for seniors, as do the Young Men's and Young Women's Christian or Hebrew Associations in most communities. Indeed, these places have become the "drop-in centers" for older people in many places. Many long-term care facilities now employ activity aides who help to get residents interested in doing things with other people. Often, there are also transportation aides, so that patients who are not mobile on their own can be taken by wheelchair to activities or special programs. We discussed types of interventions to counteract loneliness earlier in this chapter.

Unlike the anxious patient, the person who is depressed may not like to talk over his problems with the nurse—or with anyone—because talking really does not help him. Still, the presence of the nurse, with her touch on his arm or her arm around his shoulder, often goes a long way towards making a person feel that someone still cares for him. Many times depression will lift, however, when a companion who shares his interests can be found for him. It pays to discover your patient's interests, and to try to match him with someone else who is interested in the same things, such as finding a cribbage partner for an old gentleman. Music therapy is being used quite extensively now to assist in overcoming depression. Happy lively music will, as you are aware yourself, lift your spirits. Many people come out of depressed moods when they start to pick out a tune on a musical instrument. Activity is one of the best antidotes for depression, if you can get the person to take part in things again.

However, one should not try to force the severely depressed patient into activities to "cheer him up." Sitting beside the person and giving him quiet companionship is often helpful in gradually drawing the individual into responding. Very often the person needs to work through a problem, as in the case of a woman who has had a mastectomy and must adjust to her altered figure. Many patients need the help of a psychiatric nursing specialist or a psychiatrist to help them to overcome their depression. One should not forget the vital role of good nutrition and regular exercise both in helping to prevent depression and in helping people overcome it. Some of the most enthusiastic marathon runners took up the sport to overcome the effects of depression. All report that a person feels a real "high" when he is reaching his maximum potential in running. You very seldom see depressed athletes. Vigorous exercise also helps to promote sleep, so that a person rests better. It encourages good nutrition and promotes a more regular daily schedule. There is something to be said for the old adage of a "healthy mind in a healthy body."

Some persons who are depressed may need stronger therapy to lift their moods, however. Electroconvulsive therapy (electric shock) is sometimes used as a treatment for depressed patients. This therapy produces a grand mal seizure in the patient such as a person with epilepsy might have. Often a sedative is given about a half hour before the treatment, and usually an intravenous injection of a muscular relaxant, such as suxamethonium chloride, is given just a little while before the treatment. The muscular relaxant lessens the severity of the contractions the person has during the convulsion. The sudden jolt of electricity passing through a person's brain has the effect of lifting a depression. This is believed to result because the treatment increases the level of norépinephrine in the brain; a deficiency of this substance has been correlated with the symptoms of depression. Electroconvulsive therapy has proved to be an effective therapy in combination with psychotherapy for many depressed patients. The person usually sleeps immediately after the treatment, and he may be confused for a few hours afterward. The therapy is given up to three times a week for a period of a few weeks.[13]

Also, some drugs are used as antidepressants. The rationale for their use, as with electric shock treatment, is an increase in the level of norepinephrine in the brain. Drugs such as Marplan (isocarboxazid), Nardil (phenelzine sulfate), and Tofranil (imipramine hydrochloride) are among the commonly used antidepressants. Some of these drugs may cause untoward symptoms, such as restlessness, insomnia, headache, jaundice, and postural hypotension. The nurse should be aware of the possible side effects of the particular drug that is being used.

PROVIDING SPIRITUAL COUNSEL

Most people have some type of religious philosophy. In spite of the highly publicized trend toward secularism in the twentieth century, various studies show that from two thirds to nine tenths of the population of the United States profess a belief in a Supreme Being. Moreover, at a time of illness many nonprofessing persons look for spiritual guidance and consolation.

The spiritual needs of patients involve answers to such questions as: Who am I? What am I like? What kind of world is this? These highly personal questions often become urgent at a time of illness, when the patient finds himself with time to think about himself and the world about him. Shut off from everday concerns, some patients tend to question their entire system of values.

Some people look for an answer to why they are ill. They may look for moral significance to their illness and hope that religious doctrine will provide the solution. Other patients look for spiritual guidance to assist them in accepting their new role in the family. For example, the husband who normally supports his family but has become dependent upon his wife's earnings while he is ill may face a severe test. The acceptance of such changes in established roles and life patterns can be one of the most difficult adjustments a person must make.

Sometimes a person's values in life change with illness; often his horizons grow smaller, and his bed becomes his domain. Spiritual beliefs can help such a patient to accept his illness and plan for the future. They can help him maintain a realistic perspective of himself and his relationship to the world about him. They can give him that inner strength which is closely interwoven with emotional health and physical well-being.

Religion is a social as well as a spiritual institution within society. Most societies have developed some form of religion, which then serves as an integrative force within the society. Traditionally, the established religions have been concerned with ethics and moral behavior. Many established religions, however, have broadened their activities to include other areas, such as recreation centers for all age groups. Such centers offer the people of the community opportunities to find new interests and to join groups with which they can identify and in which they feel accepted.

Most churches have special programs for youth groups designed to help adolescents and young people with their particular problems as well as programs for older people to help them with their special problems. "Drop-in centers" and other variously named gathering places are operated by a number of denominations. Some of these are intended to cater to the needs of young people, and others are designed to serve people of all ages.

Spiritual Beliefs and Illness

Spiritual beliefs, then, often help a patient at a time of stress. Some patients look to religious philosophy to explain illness; others look upon illness as a test of faith. Viewed in this light, illness and injury are usually accepted with forbearance and pose little threat to religious belief.

Still others interpret disease as God's punishment. "What have I done to deserve this?" they may ask. People who believe this interpretation attach a moral significance to disease, and they reason that because they have sinned they are being punished. They often believe that through prayers, promises, and penance the cause of the disease will be treated. To them the physician

treats only the symptoms. When a patient who believes this gets well, therefore, it is an indication that as a sinner he has been forgiven. On the other hand, should he die, his family either accepts his death as God's punishment or finds it to be unacceptable and unjust.

There are situations in which religious beliefs can be a hindrance to therapy and to helath. Some religious groups tend to exalt faith and to disregard science. For example, many practicing Jehovah's Witnesses are by doctirne not permitted to have blood transfusions. The Church of Christ, Scientist, teaches spiritual healing; thus, when a practicing Christian Scientist seeks a physician's help, he may feel guilty because the prayers to relieve his symptoms were inadequate. He rarely blames his beliefs for the lack of cure, even when these beliefs may have caused him to delay his visit to a physician and his condition has worsened considerably during this time.

Generally speaking, religion helps people to accept illness and plan for the future. It can help a person to prepare for death, and it can also strengthen him during life. For example, the Christian belief of eternal life can help a patient face death more serenely. On the other hand, the Christian religion offers an interpretation of life that is based upon love and thus can also strengthen a person in his daily life.

A discussion of illness and religious philosophy would not be complete without mentioning faith healing. This is an area that has received considerable publicity and research. There are religious organizations that are active in faith healing, for example, some evangelical groups. Although claims that support divine healing as the sole factor in any reported cure are difficult to prove, one cannot rule out religion as an integral part of patient therapy.

Generally nurses and physicians recognize the importance of spiritual counsel as a part of a patient's therapy, and pastors recognize the close relationship between spiritual, emotional, and physical needs.

Identifying the Spiritual Needs of the Patient

Spiritual needs, as we have noted, often become particularly apparent during a time of illness. In the hospital, it is usually the nurse who recognizes patients who would like spiritual guidance, and it is also the nurse's responsibility to make available to the patient the sources of spiritual help.

Some patients bring articles with them that have a religious significance, and from these a nurse often can gain some idea of the importance that religious belief holds for a particular patient. For example, a Roman Catholic patient might have a rosary or a medal; an Episcopalian might have a prayer book.

Nurses should remember that there are patients who are not associated with any particular religious group. To them, spiritual need and spiritual belief are highly personal matters. Others are frankly agnostic, and for them any religious appeal would probably have a negative effect. Still others find the visits of a religious representative to be a source of discomfort rather than comfort; for example, a person might not like the particular hospital chaplain or the religious denomination that he (or she) represents. A nurse should cautiously assess the patient's attitude toward religion and his spiritual needs before she proffers suggestions or help.

Some patients who may want spiritual counseling include:

1. *Those who are lonely and have few visitors.* The perceptive nurse will hear a patient express loneliness in obscure ways as well as in obvious terms. The patient who continually has his signal light on to call the nurse may really be saying "I am lonely. Please stay with me." The nurse can also identify the lonely patient by making her rounds of the nursing unit during visiting hours. At this time she has an opportunity to meet patients' families and she can note those who do not have visitors. Patients whose homes are in distant communities may be lonely because their families and friends are far away.

2. *Those who express fear and anxiety.* Some people will state frankly that they are afraid. Others express their fears by their questions, silence, body tension, or facial expression. The taut, pale face and the anxious eyes often express fear as emphatically as words.

3. *Those whose illnesses are directly related to emotions or to religious attitudes.* Because of guilt feelings, occasionally related directly or indirectly to religious doctrine, some people might develop physical symptoms of illness. An example is the single woman who becomes pregnant and, as a result, feels that she faces religious and social condemnation.

4. *Those who are undergoing surgery.* People who face operations are often afraid, and their fear is not necessarily related to the seriousness of the operation. Many people fear anesthesia, body disfigurement, pain, or even body exposure, but above all they fear death during surgery.

5. *Those who may have to change their pattern of life as a result of illness or injury.* Some people take great pride in their independence, and the prospect of any degree of dependence upon others is frightening. Some people worry about their changing roles within their families or their ability to earn a living. Illness and injury often necessitate abrupt changes in established living patterns that must be met by both the patient and his family.

6. *Those who seem to be preoccupied with the relationship of religion and their health.* Such patients may be seeking the reason for their illness in religious doctrine or may be trying to explain their illness in terms of religious philosophy.

7. *Those who are unable to have a clergyman visit or who would not normally receive pastoral care.* People who come from distant communities may not know a pastor in the immediate area. Other patients may not belong to religious groups in the community, but at a time of illness they may want spiritual counsel.

8. *Those whose illnesses have social implications.* For example, the person who has had disfiguring surgery may feel that the hospital chaplain represents social acceptance or social rejection, and acceptance by the community may be important to his future plans.

9. *Those who are dying.* Facing death, the patient may be filled with uncertainty and worry about his family. Spiritual guidance can often help him to meet death, and it can help his family accept his death and plan for the future.

The Nurse and Spiritual Guidance in the Hospital

The nurse can play an important role in providing the patient with spiritual support. One of her most important activities is identifying people's spiritual needs. To do this effectively the nurse must take time to listen to the patient and to ascertain his emotional status. Usually a patient is not looking for answers from the nurse; he is looking for acceptance and help while he thinks out answers for himself.

Pastors appreciate referrals from nursing personnel and usually welcome the nurse's observations regarding the patient's spiritual needs. Most members of clergy prefer to look after these needs themselves, however, and nursing responsibilities are usually limited in this regard.

If the nurse feels competent and comfortable in helping to meet the patient's spiritual needs, she can assist him by helping him to read from the Bible, if he so desires. For example, if the patient is unable to read himself, the nurse can read to him. If the patient can do his own reading, the nurse can arrange privacy for him. Most hospitals provide Bibles, either at each bedside or at the nursing station or hospital library.

In addition to the Bible and prayer books, a

great deal of religious literature is available. Religious tracts, for instance, are published by many groups. Since tracts are often designed to meet specific needs, particular tracts can be selected to meet particular circumstances.

Prayers are the fourth area in which the nurse can help patients. Prayer takes many forms; to many it is a means of reaching God. However, prayer does not always involve a sense of mutuality; for example, in Buddhism, Gautama is regarded as unconscious and inaccessible.

One patient may prefer to pray silently, and to him prayer is a highly personal activity. Another may like the nurse to say a prayer for him, and this becomes a source of considerable comfort. Prayers need not be long; a simple, sincerely stated prayer can be as comforting as a lengthy one.[14] A simple evening prayer that can be readily learned by the nurse is:

O Lord, support us every hour of our lives until the evening comes and our work is done. Then grant us your mercy, holy rest, and peace at last, through Jesus Christ our Lord. Amen.

If the nurse does not feel comfortable praying with the patient or reading to him from the Bible, it is quite acceptable for her to suggest that someone else do this. Most clergymen are happy to assist the patient in these matters, and the nurse may refer the patient to the pastor of his faith.

There are many people in the United States and Canada who subscribe to faiths other than the ones we have mentioned, for example, persons from Viet Nam or the Middle Eastern countries. It is helpful to have on file the name of someone who is familiar with the individual's religion, e.g., a social worker or a resident in the community from the same country or region who is willing to make hospital visits to provide spiritual comfort.

The Hospital Chaplain

The hospital chaplain may be a minister, priest, rabbi, or other member whose chief charges are the patients in a hospital. Large hospitals frequently have full-time chaplains representing several faiths. The Protestant faith is usually represented by ministers of various denominations, for example, Episcopalian, Methodist, Baptist, and Congregationalist. The Roman Catholic faith is represented by the priest, the Jewish faith by the rabbi. Small hospitals may not have chaplains but, like their larger counterparts, they extend liberal visiting privileges to the representatives of the established religions in the community.

When the hospital chaplain or pastor comes to see a patient, he or she usually checks with

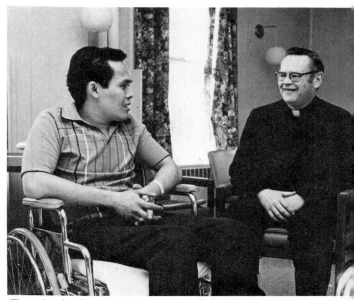

The chaplain's visit is a source of comfort to many patients.

the nurse to make sure the visit is convenient for the patient. At this time the nurse is afforded an opportunity to give him information that may help him in counseling the patient. She can also tell him the names of other patients who want him to visit. Hospital chaplains and community pastors are generally available day or night, and they often leave their telephone numbers with the nurse so that they can be called at any time. It could be imperative, for example, to call a priest quickly for a dying Roman Catholic patient.

Some hospitals have chapels in which religious services are held regularly for the patients and their families. The services are usually conducted by the hospital chaplain or by the pastors from the community. Patients who would like to attend these services should be helped to do so if it is possible. They may involve rearranging nursing care activities.

The hospital chaplain is an important member of the health team. He is often described as a physician of the soul. His knowledge and his spiritual guidance are important adjuncts to medical care. The hospital chaplain can help people clarify their anxieties and accept illness. The community pastor often maintains liaison between the hospital patient and his family and can lend his support when the patient returns home. He can also assist sometimes by interpreting medical instructions for the patient.

Many hospital chaplains attend health team conferences and contribute to the plans for the patient's therapy and his discharge.

Another service provided by the chaplain is as a source of information for other members of the health team. For example, his knowledge of religious dietary preferences can be helpful to the dietitian when she plans a patient's menu. The importance of baptism in Roman Catholic doctrine is particularly relevant for nurses in the delivery room. The hospital chaplain can also provide spiritual advice to members of the hospital staff. Counsel at a time of stress can often help a nurse to be more effective in helping patients and their families.

The hospital chaplain also administers the sacraments to patients in the hospital. Through the sacraments, both the patient and his family receive spiritual strength and solace. The specific sacraments of the Roman Catholic, Hebrew, and Protestant faiths are discussed in the following section.

Specific Religious Customs

The Jewish Faith. Most patients who belong to the Jewish faith belong to the reform, conservative, or orthodox groups. Not all Jewish people follow the same practices, so the nurse will need to be sensitive to the patient's individual wishes. Generally the Jewish patient who follows orthodox doctrine will adhere most closely to certain dietary and religious customs. The patient himself, his family, or the rabbi will assist the nurse regarding doctrinal customs.

The rabbi is the pastor of the Jewish congregation. Many Jewish patients like to have their own rabbi visit them when they are ill. He provides spiritual counsel to the patient and his family.

To the Hebrew people the act of *circumcision* is a religious rite. It marks the entrance of the male child as a potential citizen to the community. It should take place on the eighth day after birth of a male child; at the conclusion of the ceremony the child is named. Circumcision is called Brith Milah in Hebrew. The elaborateness of the ceremony depends on the preferences of the family. Ten Jewish men must always be present, including all the male members of the infant's family. Following the circumcision there may be a reception for the members of the family and their friends. The nurse will be instructed in advance by the rabbi or the mohel (one who performs the circumcision) as to what equipment will be required for the ceremony.

Upon the death of a Jewish patient, the rabbi should be notified if the family is not present. He will arrange for the patient's burial. There is no need to be concerned about baptism, since the Jewish faith does not practice this rite.

The orthodox Hebrew patient may follow certain dietary regulations. Jewish doctrine forbids the eating of certain foods, including any part of the pig. In addition, certain other foods may be eaten only when they are specially prepared. The permitted foods are called kosher. They include the meat of animals that are ruminants and have divided hoofs, such as cows and sheep. Kosher fowl are fowl that are not birds of prey, and kosher fish are fish with scales. Example of kosher fowl are chicken and duck; salmon and sardines can be classed as kosher fish. All shellfish, such as clams, oysters, and lobster, are prohibited. Meat dishes may not be eaten at the same meal with dishes containing milk, cream, or butter.

In order for meat to be considered kosher the animals must be slaughtered and the meat prepared in a special manner. No special precautions are required for vegetables. If a hospital is not prepared to provide kosher meat, other protein foods such as vegetable protein products can be substituted. Often a patient's family will arrange to provide kosher food if the patient is anxious about this. The nurse will need to instruct the family regarding any special dietary requirements for the patient.

There are other dietary regulations that apply at the time of the Passover. At this time a Jewish patient may refrain from eating leavened food, for example, bread. The rabbi can arrange to have special Passover matzo (unleavened bread) brought to the patient. Any Hebrew patient can be excused from strict dietary customs when he is ill. If the patient is concerned about this, the nurse can notify the rabbi and he will explain this to the patient.

The Roman Catholic Faith. The Roman Catholic faith recognizes several sacraments that have particular importance for nurses. In the Roman Catholic Church, God is conceived to be a God of mercy and grace, which are mediated through the church. The sacraments are signs and seals of God's expression to His people, and through them a person attains a state of grace, which is necessary for salvation. *Baptism* is the first of the sacraments to be administered to an individual. Because it is necessary for an infant to be baptized in order to receive salvation, it is very important to see to it that an infant in danger of death is baptized. According to Roman Catholic doctrine, an infant has a soul from the minute of conception; therefore a fetus at any stage of development must be baptized if it is born.

A nurse can perform a baptism by pouring water on the head of the child and at the same time saying, "I baptize thee in the name of the Father and of the Son and of the Holy Spirit." There are forms used in hospitals to record baptism of an infant, one of which is integrated into or attached to the patient's record; the duplicate is sent to the pastor of the family.

Holy Communion is another sacrament of the Roman Catholic Church. Patients are allowed water and medications prior to communion, as well as essential medical procedures up to the time of receiving communion. The patient should not take solid food or liquids other than water for an hour before receiving communion.

When Holy Communion is requested by the patient, the Catholic chaplain of the hospital is called, or a priest from the church which serves the hospital. In either instance, a clean towel is used as a cover on top of the bedside table, on which the nurse places a glass of water and a spoon. Hospitals usually have a communion set on each floor which is taken into the patient's room and left for the use of the chaplain or visiting priest. Privacy is to be observed for the patient and the priest during the communion service.

The *Anointing of the Sick* is a sacrament that is performed for many patients. Formerly known as Extreme Unction or last rites, it used to be given only to the person who was in danger of dying. Now, however, it is interpreted as an aid to healing and a source of strength. It may therefore be received by a patient one or more times for each illness, and may be received several times in a lifetime.

It is felt that this sacrament should be administered when the patient is conscious, although it can be administered to the unconscious patient. It can be performed any time of the day or night. The priest anoints the eyes, ears, nostrils, lips, hands, and feet with oil, for which cotton balls should be provided. Hospitals have a form for the priest to sign after he has administered this sacrament; the form is then attached to or integrated into the patient's record.

Even if a patient of the Roman Catholic faith dies without receiving the Anointing of the Sick, a priest should be called. He can administer the sacrament immediately following death, thus providing a source of comfort to the patient's family.

With the revisions in dietary practices for Roman Catholics, meat may be eaten on Friday, except during the season of Lent. Hospitals usually have a choice of meat or fish on the Friday menu and, during Lent, on the Wednesday menu also. The patient is free to select·whichever he or she wishes, unless there is a special diet prescription.

The Protestant Faith. The Protestant faith includes many denominations; Methodists, Baptists, Presbyterians, Episcopalians (Anglicans), and Congregationalists are but a few of the larger groups. Most Protestant patients prefer the chaplain of their own church, but in an emergency the chaplain of another denomination can often help.

The sacrament of *baptism* is performed in most Protestant denominations. Some denominations practice baptism in infancy; others baptize at the age of understanding, often when a child is 12 years old. For a few Protestants, baptism is a necessity before death.

Some Protestant denominations hold *Holy Communion*, and for many patients this can be a strengthening spiritual food. For this sacrament the clergyman requires a table in the patient's room to be cleared and furnished with a clean white cloth. It is preferable if the patient can assume a sitting position and, of course, privacy should be provided during the service. In communion the patient partakes of wine and bread; the wine represents the blood of Christ and the bread represents the body of Christ. Some Protestants consider this rite to be a cleansing of the soul from sin.

A few Protestant churches, the Episcopal Church for example, are placing increasing emphasis upon anointing, and for this rite privacy is important.

Some Protestants have dietary customs. Some are vegetarians and some do not drink tea or coffee—for example, members of the Mormon Church. Other people do not smoke or drink alcoholic beverages because of religious doctrine. During Lent, some Protestants practice a variety of dietary restrictions. Generally speaking, however, most Protestant's eating habits are not restricted by religious doctrine.

GUIDE TO ASSESSING ANXIETY AND DEPRESSION

1. What do you know about this patient as an individual? How old is he? What does he do for a living? What family does he have?

2. What is the patient's health problem?

3. What are some of the possible sources of stress this patient may have?

4. Does the patient express any fears or worries verbally?

5. Does the patient appear to treat his illness very lightly? That is, does he laugh and joke a lot about his condition?

6. Is there evidence that the patient has been crying?

7. Is the patient demanding, complaining, or hostile toward the staff?

8. Does the patient show physical signs or symptoms of anxiety or depression? For example, is his pulse rate above normal in the absence of a known physical cause for it? Is there evidence of muscular tension? What is the patient's appetite like? Is he constipated? Does he have diarrhea? What is his appearance like? his gait? his posture?

9. Are his talk and movements slowed down? speeded up?

10. Does he talk easily about his social or emotional problems and physical symptoms, or is he reluctant to talk? Does he talk in a monotone?

11. Does talking seem to help him?

12. Is he interested in a variety of topics?

13. Can he enjoy reading a book or watching television?

14. Is his mood better in the morning? in the evening?

15. Is the patient lonely?

16. Does the patient have activities to occupy his time?

17. What resource people might be able to help this patient?

18. Is religion important in the patient's system of values?

19. Does the patient feel spiritual counsel would help his health and well-being? Or does the patient indicate that he does not want assistance with spiritual needs?

20. Does the patient have specific spiritual needs with which members of the health team can be of assistance?

GUIDE TO EVALUATING THE EFFECTIVENESS OF NURSING INTERVENTIONS

1. Have the physical and behavioral manifestations of anxiety or depression lessened, or disappeared? For example, is the anxious patient's facial expression more calm and relaxed? Is his muscular tension reduced? Is his agitation less? Is the depressed patient more animated? Does he take more interest in his appearance? Does he socialize more with others?

2. Are the person's speech and voice patterns more normal?

3. Does he sleep well at night?

4. Does he say that he is feeling better?

5. Is he eating well? Has he gained weight?

6. Have distressing symptoms that he has had, such as diarrhea, constipation, urinary frequency, urinary retention, or headache, disappeared?

7. Has the chaplain, rabbi, or priest been notified if he is needed?

8. Does the patient have access to the Bible or other religious literature in accordance with his wishes?

9. Is the patient accorded the privacy and facilities required to fulfill his religious needs?

STUDY SITUATION

Julie Allen is an attractive, 22-year-old airline stewardess. She thoroughly enjoys her job and the benefits she receives through working for an airline. Although planning to be married next month, Julie intends to continue working for another few years before raising a family. In a routine physical examination, Julie's physician detected some evidence of tissue changes which could be indicative of early cervical cancer. He has suggested that she be admitted to hospital for further diagnostic tests. Julie is very upset.

1. For what reasons would Julie be upset? *young, not married, no children, enjoys life, has goals*

2. What physical manifestations of anxiety might the nurse observe in Julie? *denial, crying laughing*

3. When Julie is admitted to the nursing unit in the afternoon before surgery, she is very restless and talks constantly. She follows the nurse around and laughs and jokes about her work as an airline stewardess. She tells the nurse she just cannot sit in her room and it is too early to go to bed. What can the nurse do to help Julie? *Provide an activity, tell pt. of test + procedures, explain r+r, listen,*

SUGGESTED READINGS

Chestnutt, J.: He's 34, a Quadriplegic and Gets Along Just Fine. *American Journal of Nursing*, 76(8):1278, August, 1976.

Esberger, K.: Body Image. *Journal of Gerontological Nursing*, 4:35–38, July-August, 1978.

Hein, E., et al.: Providing Emotional Support to Patients. *Nursing '77*, 7(5):39–41, May, 1977.

Hudson, M.: She's 22 and Dealing with a Catastrophic Illness. *American Journal of Nursing*, 76(8):1273, August, 1976.

Kowalsky, E. L.: Encounters with Grief. A Lost Lifestyle. *American Journal of Nursing*, 78:418–420, March, 1978.

Pollitt, J.: Symptoms of Stress. Part 1. Types of Stress and Types of People. *Nursing Mirror*, June, 1977.

Pollitt, J.: Symptoms of Stress. Part 2. The Effects of Stress. *Nursing Mirror*, June, 1977.

Pumphrey, J. B. (consultant): Recognizing Your Patients' Spiritual Needs. *Nursing '77*, 7(12):64–68, December, 1977.

Rouhani, G.: Understanding Anxiety. *Nursing Mirror*, March, 1978.

Slobada, S.: Understanding Patient Behaviours. *Nursing '77*, 7(9):74–77, September, 1977.

Smith, E. C., et al.: Reestablishing a Child's Body Image. *American Journal of Nursing*, 77(3):445–447, March, 1977.

Stoll, R. I.: Guidelines for Spiritual Assessment. *American Journal of Nursing*, 79(9):1574–1577, September, 1979.

REFERENCES

1. Maslow, A. H.: *Motivation and Personality*. 2nd ed. New York, Harper and Row, 1970.
2. Branden, N.: *The Psychology of Self-esteem*. Los Angeles, Nash Publishing Corporation, 1969.
3. National Commission for the Study of Nursing and Nursing Education: Summary Report and Recommendations. *American Journal of Nursing*, 70:279–294, February, 1970.
4. Toffler, A.: *The Third Wave*. New York, Bantam Books, 1981.
5. Ebersole, P., and Hess, P.: *Toward Healthy Aging*. St. Louis, C. V. Mosby Company, 1981.
6. Fromm, E.: *Man for Himself*. New York, Holt, Rinehart and Winston, 1947.
7. Volicer, B. J.: Patients' Perceptions of Stressful Events Associated with Hospitalization. *Nursing Research*, 23:235–238, May-June, 1974.
8. Berni, R., and Readey, H.: *Problem-Oriented Medical Record Implementation*. St. Louis, C. V. Mosby Company, 1974.
9. Andersen, M. D., and Pleticha, J. M.: Emergency Unit Patients' Perceptions of Stressful Life Events. *Nursing Research*, 23:378–382, September-October, 1974.
10. Guyton, A. C.: *Human Physiology and Mechanisms of Disease*. 3rd ed. Philadelphia, W. B. Saunders Company, 1982.
11. Lagina, S. M.: A Computer Program to Diagnose Anxiety Levels. *Nursing Research*, 20:484–492, November-December, 1971.
12. Nordmark, M. T., and Rohweder, A. W.: *Scientific Foundations of Nursing*. 3rd ed. Philadelphia, J. B. Lippincott Company, 1975.
13. Falconer, M. W., et al.: *The Drug, the Nurse, the Patient*. 6th ed. Philadelphia, W. B. Saunders Company, 1978.
14. Westberg, G.: *Nurse, Pastor and Patient*. Philadelphia, Fortress Press, 1955.

31

The Nurse Should Be Able to:

- Discuss the five stages of dying
- Discuss her own reactions to death and dying
- Assess the needs of the dying patient and his family
- Plan and implement appropriate nursing interventions to assist the patient and his family to meet their needs
- Evaluate the effectiveness of nursing interventions

TERMINAL ILLNESS

CHAPTER

31

INTRODUCTION

Inextricably involved in nursing is the preservation of life, the alleviation of suffering, and the restoration of health. Our society exalts health, life, and youth. Death is a subject that generally is avoided; even when it is imminent, it is frequently denied. Yet death is a not infrequent occurrence on hospital wards or among the sick in the community. Nurses and physicians, by the very nature of their work, encounter the presence of death more often than most people do in the normal course of their lives.

The frequency of the encounter does not, however, make it easy to deal with. The care of the terminally ill patient and the comforting and consoling of the patient's family, whether death is sudden or follows a lengthy illness, presents one of the most difficult situations in nursing practice. It is particularly distressing for the young student who has possibly never been face to face with the realities of death before in her life. However, the five stages of dying (described below) are typical stages of individual or group adjustment to any calamity. Flunking a test, auto accidents, divorce, breaking up with a loved one, environmental disasters, and loss of a limb or a vital body part are a few examples of common occurrences "handled" in the same way as physical death. Thus, the student's own natural feelings of grief over the loss of the patient are something she has to work through in much the same way as the patient and his family do. It is helpful, then, if she understands the nature of the process of grieving so that she is better able to handle her own reactions and to help the patient and his family to meet their needs.

THE STAGES OF DYING

In her book, *On Death and Dying*, Elisabeth Kübler-Ross suggests that there are five stages that most people go through when they learn that they are going to die. These are: denial, anger, bargaining, depression. and acceptance.[1]

The first stage is one of nonacceptance. This is not happening to them! Surely, there must be some mistake. Often the patient seeks reassurance from the nurse and questions her regarding what the doctor has said. While the decision of what to tell the patient belongs to the physician, and the nurse accepts his guidance in this area, she should know what the patient and his family have been told so that she can provide support. Throughout the denial state, the nurse must accept the fact that the patient is not yet ready to acknowledge the seriousness of his illness. Some patients maintain this denial up to the point of impending death, and continue to talk optimistically of future plans and of what they are going to do when they get better. Nursing personnel often mistakenly admire this type of behavior, considering that the patient is being "very brave," although in fact, it is usually more difficult for this patient when the time comes when he can no longer deny that death is near. Many patients, however, are aware of their prognosis, even though they have never been told in words, and yet they may pretend not to know. Often, they maintain a façade of cheerfulness for the benefit of their families, whom they sense are uncomfortable talking about death, or because they feel that they are expected to behave in this manner by the hospital staff. For these patients, it is frequently a relief to drop the façade in the presence of someone who understands what they are going through. It should be pointed out, however, that most patients appear to prefer to hold onto some hope—that a new cure may be found or a miracle happen, even though they do not rationally expect one.

Once the person has passed the stage of denial, he usually goes through an understandable period of anger and hostility. Why should this be happening to him? What did he do to deserve this punishment? At this point, the patient often lashes out at those nearest to him—the physicians, the nurses, the hospital, his family. He may be highly critical of the care he is receiving. If the nurse is aware that there is nothing personal in his attack, that he is in reality angry at God and whatever fates there be rather than at those who are caring for him, it is easier for her to have patience and tolerate his behavior. The patient's family will usually go through this stage of anger and hostility also, and may take out their feelings on the staff. It is helpful to remember that this too is a normal reaction and one that the nurse should not counter with defensiveness or hostility.

The third stage of dying is often one of bargaining. From early childhood, one is taught that good behavior is rewarded and bad actions are punished. Therefore, promising to be very good may bring about a reversal of the decision that death is due. The nurse may hear the patient say that he would do anything—repent his sins, make up for previous errors — if he can just live a little longer or, perhaps, have a day free of pain. The nurse is probably personally familiar with the bargaining process; she has perhaps stated to herself or prayed that if she could just pass this exam she would faithfully study every night in the future.

When the patient realizes that his bargaining efforts are of no avail, he usually enters into a depressed phase. This again is a normal reaction, as the individual contemplates all that he has held dear in life and mourns its loss. During this stage the patient may be very concerned about how his family is going to manage when he is gone, and he may be anxious to "put his affairs in order." Sometimes it is difficult for him to discuss these matters with members of his family, who frequently react very emotionally to any talk of death. In this case, a third party such as the chaplain, a social worker, or a close friend of the patient may be the best person to deal with these practical concerns. During this stage of depression, the patient may not want to talk a great deal. He may wish to see only those nearest and dearest to him. Because of his withdrawal, however, the nurse should not take it for granted that he wishes to be left entirely alone. The presence of someone who sympathetically cares for him is reassuring. Many hospitals permit a member of the family to stay with a patient who is seriously ill, or family members to visit as often as they wish. A terminally ill patient is often placed in a single room so that the patient and his family may have privacy. Yet often this contributes to the patient's sense of isolation. By stopping in to see the patient at frequent intervals, if he has no family members with him, or spending time with him as her schedule permits, the nurse can help to overcome the patient's feelings of isolation.

The final stage of the dying process comes when the patient has accepted that he is going to die soon and he is prepared for it. By this time, the patient is usually tired but at peace. At this stage, it is the patient's family who usually require the most support. Patients' families react to death and dying in a variety of ways. They too go through the same stages as the patient does, but not always at the same time. When relatives are with a terminally ill person, they are often at a loss as to what to say and how to act. It is not uncommon to see even imminent death denied by a family. The nurse can often help the family by such actions as ensuring them privacy, permitting them access to the patient, and showing them small kindnesses in ministering to their comfort as well as to the patient's.

It is important to the family that they feel the patient is receiving the best care possible. Helping the patient to die in a dignified and peaceful manner is perhaps one of the most valuable contributions the nurse can make to the comfort of both the patient and the members of his family.

At times, it is up to the nurse to tell the family that a patient has died. It is best told to the family group in privacy. The nurse should anticipate that they will be upset and will look to her for supportive understanding. Many agencies have a small prayer room or a chapel where the nurse may take grieving families so that they can be alone for a while. With all cultural groups, there are certain rituals that are performed at the time of death, and these help the family to work through their grief. The nurse should be aware of these rituals and make provisions to ensure that they can be carried out. Often, family members will want to go in and pay their last respects to the dead person, and this should be permitted. Some ethnic groups expect that members of the immediate family will be very vocal in their outpouring of grief. With others, a more stoical behavior is expected. Regardless of the cultural background, however, the death of an immediate family member is one situation in which crying is considered not only permissible but helpful in the grieving process.

The Dying Person's Bill of Rights, shown on page 691, summarizes the needs of the terminally ill patient.

THE EXPERIENCE OF DEATH AND DYING

Kübler-Ross, after considerable experience in counseling patients on death and dying, decided

THE DYING PERSON'S BILL OF RIGHTS*

I have the right to be treated as a living human being until I die.

I have the right to maintain a sense of hopefulness, however changing its focus may be.

I have the right to be cared for by those who can maintain a sense of hopefulness, however changing this might be.

I have the right to express my feelings and emotions about my approaching death in my own way.

I have the right not be deceived.

I have the right to have help from and for my family in accepting my death.

I have the right to die in peace and dignity.

I have the right to retain my individuality and not be judged for my decisions which may be contrary to beliefs of others.

I have the right to participate in decisions concerning my care.

I have the right to expect continuing medical and nursing attention even though "cure" goals must be changed to "comfort" goals.

I have the right not to die alone.

I have the right to be free from pain.

I have the right to have my questions answered honestly.

I have the right to discuss and enlarge my religious and/or spiritual experiences, whatever these may mean to others.

I have the right to expect that the sanctity of the human body will be respected after death.

I have the right to be cared for by caring, sensitive, knowledgeable people who will attempt to understand my needs and will be able to gain some satisfaction in helping me face my death.

*This Bill of Rights was created at a workshop on "The Terminally Ill Patient and the Helping Person," in Lansing, Mich., sponsored by the Southwestern Michigan Inservice Education Council and conducted by Amelia J. Barbus, associate professor of nursing, Wayne State University, Detroit.

to record her patients' experiences in a book she called On Death and Dying. Another author, Raymond Moody, also organized the testimony of many people who had technically died and come back to life. The title of his book is Life after Life.[2]

Testimony regarding the death experience follows a similar pattern. The person describes the accident or hospital scene: he has had the heart attack or other injury, leaves his body, and can see himself below (as if he were floating on an astral plane). He can see people working trying to revive him, and he experiences their concern. Often at this point he returns to his body and comes to consciousness. He may have already been pronounced dead. Many report that while they were unconscious they were moving through a tunnel toward a light; there were figures around them that they could recognize and even communicate with. Sometimes they were told that it was not time for them to die, and they returned to life. This type of experience seems to have an effect on the type of life the individual leads afterward. He appears to have a renewed vitality and a sense of purposefulness in living. One man reported that during a heart attack, when he was under surveillance in an intensive care unit, he died and returned to his body 16 times.

There may be an accompanying feeling of regret on waking up in this life. One person reports of her experience: "I only recall that I moved through a space which was all light and love, toward the source of it. I received the message 'There's something you have to finish; you're going back.' I really didn't want to go back—but I felt myself coming down to my body again."* Records of this type of experience are not new. There is a book called The Tibetan Book of the Dead that was written to guide the dying through the passage of death hundreds of years ago.

Some Western critics attribute the experience of floating above the body while unconscious to the effects of anesthetic drugs. However, there is no adequate physiological explanation of why each person experiences the same effects or pattern of events. There seems to be a direct continuity between what a person experiences during lifetime and experiences in the next dimension (upon death).

COUNSELING CHILDREN AND RELATIVES

Dr. Ross's first experiences with death came from her early visits to the Nazi concentration camps. As a young woman traveling in Europe after the war, she saw the inscriptions made by children on the walls of the buildings where they were imprisoned. They drew butterflies. . . . It was their simple statement about death and the freedom of the spirit. Ross resolved to become a doctor. Many years later, while working

*Recounted personally to the author.

in the United States, she received calls asking her to counsel dying children and their relatives. She became a specialist in this area, setting up an office in her kitchen, where children would feel most at ease. During appointments, she talked with the children over a cup of hot chocolate, with a fire going in the background. They talked about death, and the children drew pictures of the form they felt they were going to take. She used the analogy of the children from the camps, the butterfly leaving its cocoon, to explain the process of dying. The children seemed to accept the concept of dying easily; their main concern was for the relatives they were going to leave—how would they cope without them? In such a manner, Dr. Ross was able to facilitate greater understanding on the subject of death for both patients and professionals. Many have gone on to work in the same area of counseling.

THE SPIRITUAL NEEDS OF THE TERMINALLY ILL PATIENT

Terminally ill patients have many needs: emotional, spiritual, and physical. Perhaps the need that can best guide the nurse is the need of a patient to die gracefully. In describing a way to acquire a positive approach to death, Cicely Saunders advises us "to look continually at the patients, not at their need but at their courage, not at their dependence but at their dignity."

In gaining the strength and courage to face death with dignity many people find their religious beliefs of inestimable assistance. Often patients and their families seek support from representatives of their religious faith. Even patients who profess not to believe in a Superior Being may find the visits of a chaplain comforting. The nurse is frequently the person who first identifies the spiritual needs of the patient, and she may be called upon to act as a liaison between the patient and the chaplain. Many hospitals maintain a list of clergyman of the different faiths who may be called if the patient does not have his own spiritual counselor, or the hospital may have its own chaplain. Nurses too may feel the need to talk over their feelings about death and the dying patient with someone and often find the chaplain a helpful person in this regard.

THE PHYSICAL NEEDS OF THE TERMINALLY ILL PATIENT

The physical needs of the dying person are similar to the needs of any seriously ill patient.

Unless death occurs suddenly, there is usually a progressive failure of the body's homeostatic mechanisms as the individual becomes weaker. The following changes take place:

1. Loss of muscle tone
2. Progressive cessation of peristalsis
3. Slowing of blood circulation
4. Labored respirations
5. Loss of the senses

Loss of muscle tone is usually manifested in the patient's inability to control defecation and urination. The sphincter muscles of the rectum and bladder relax, and as a result there is involuntary micturition and defecation. A retention catheter may be required, and absorbent pads can be used to help the patient keep dry and comfortable. Since patients are often embarrassed about their inability to control these functions, it is important that the nurse be discreet and understanding in her care. Deodorants are frequently used to keep the air in the patient's room fresh and free from unpleasant odors.

Involuntary micturition and defecation predispose the patient to decubitus ulcers. By helping the patient to keep dry and clean and to change his position regularly, the nurse can usually prevent these complications.

Because of the progressive loss of muscle tone the dying patient finds it increasingly difficult to maintain his position in bed without support. If the patient is conscious, Fowler's position is usually indicated in order to increase the depth of ventilation of the lungs. If he is unconscious, a semiprone position promotes the drainage of mucus from his mouth. Family members may become anxious when they see the patient positioned in this manner, and it is wise to explain to them the reasons for it. Regardless of the position that the nurse judges to be most beneficial, the patient will need supportive measures, such as pillows, to maintain it (see Chapter 20). If possible, the various parts of the body should be kept out of dependent positions to prevent the pooling of blood.

The inability to swallow (dysphagia) is also characteristic of the loss of muscle tone in the dying patient. Mucus tends to accumulate in the patient's throat, and as a result the air passing through it causes a typical gurgling sound, "the death rattle." Throat suctioning usually helps to keep his airway patent.

There is a *progressive diminution in peristalsis* of the gastrointestinal tract of the dying patient. His desire for food is usually minimal, but he may want frequent sips of water. His mouth may be dry, owing to dehydration and perhaps to a slight fever, which sometimes precedes death. Good oral hygiene is essential.

Because of the reduced peristalsis, flatus accumulates in the stomach and intestines, often distending the patient's abdomen and causing nausea. More than a few sips of water at a time can, as a consequence, cause vomiting. Dying patients are often given nourishment and fluids parenterally, but rarely are sips of fluid contraindicated.

As *blood circulation slows,* the patient's extremities appear cyanosed or mottled and feel cold and clammy to the touch, although he probably perceives warmth and his temperature is above normal. When circulation is considerably decreased, the effectiveness of the administration of analgesics, intramuscularly or hypodermically, is decreased. As a consequence, the patient may require analgesics in an intravenous solution.

Respiratory embarrassment is alleviated by throat suctioning, by positioning (such as Fowler's position), and by the administration of oxygen. Aside from its effect on the patient, respiratory difficulty is one of the most distressing signs that his family has to witness.

There are also *alterations in the senses* of the dying patient. His vision frequently becomes blurred, and as a result the patient prefers a lighted room, rather than the darkened room that so often comes to mind. His eyes may need special attention also. Frequently secretions tend to gather, and these should be removed with absorbent cotton dipped in normal saline to prevent crusting. Sometimes, however, the eyes become dry and it may be necessary to instill some sterile ophthalmic ointment onto the lower conjunctivae to keep them lubricated.

Hearing is considered to be the last sense to leave the body; hence the patient who cannot respond verbally often understands what people are saying. When people talk to a dying person, they should take care to speak distinctly in a normal voice. Whispering is to be avoided, because it may disturb the patient to realize that people are talking and yet he is unable to understand what they are saying.

Varying degrees of consciousness precede death: *Drowsiness* is a state of sleepiness, *stupor* is a state of unconsciousness from which one can be aroused, and *coma* is an unconscious state from which one cannot be aroused. The patient may remain conscious and rational until the moment of death, or he may become unconscious or confused several days or even weeks prior to death.

For the comfort of the dying patient and his family, the patient's room is kept clear and tidy. As mentioned, frequently the dying patient is given a private room on the nursing unit of the hospital so that he and his family may have privacy.

Some patients experience pain while they are critically ill. Generally in such cases the physician orders an analgesic to prevent discomfort. Analgesic drugs are generally considered to be more effective if they are given regularly every 3 to 4 hours rather than only when pain becomes unbearable and the patient requests them. Some analgesics have the unfortunate side effect of clouding the consciousness. Consequently the patient may ask that they be withheld near the time of death so that he can think and talk clearly. The nurse is guided by the physician's orders, but in most instances, the physician and the nurse follow the patient's wishes in this respect.

HOSPICES AND HOME CARE FOR THE DYING

In Chapter 5, we talked a little about the *hospice* as a new type of health agency that has been rapidly developing in recent years. The hospice provides palliative care for people who are dying. It includes the provision of both physical care and emotional support for patients and their families, including both inpatient care and home care services. The hospice has developed in response to a need on the part of patients and their families for an alternative to the hospital, to help people to die with dignity. More and more people are deciding that they want to stay at home during their last illness; many want to die at home. The hospice provides the services needed to help people to stay in their own homes as long as possible. These services include nursing care in the home and counseling for the individual and his family as well as the opportunity to move into the hospice facility if necessary to control symptoms or to wait for death.

The general goals of hospice care include:
1. Control of physical symptoms, primarily the control of pain
2. Reduction of the sense of isolation
3. Maintenance and control of decisions that influence treatments, care provided and lifestyle preferences
4. Contined contact with the family through the bereavement period[4]

Primary nursing care is usually practiced in a hospice (see Chapter 6), and patients are encouraged to participate as much as possible in their own care. The hospice movement's goals are to promote peacefulness and serenity in dying. Although it is a fairly recent development

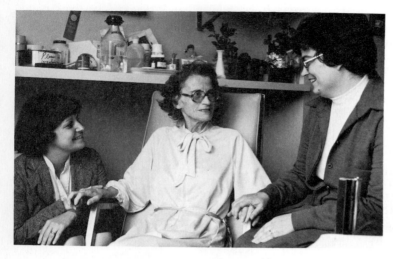

Listening to patients warmly and affectionately is important for palliative care team members Sister Judith Soulière, left, and Sister Linda Lazarus, right. (Photo by M. L. van Schaik. Reprinted from *RNAO News, 37*(1):9, March-April, 1981.)

in health care, it has already contributed a great deal toward helping people to die with dignity and grace.

EUTHANASIA AND "LIVING WILLS"

Euthanasia means an easy or painless death, the word being derived from the Greek words meaning "good death." The term is often used synonymously with "mercy killing," a concept that has caused a considerable amount of controversy over the years. There are, basically, two forms of euthanasia. *Passive*, or *negative*, *euthanasia* means the withholding of life-preserving techniques. It involves an omission (or failure to do something). *Active*, or *positive*, *euthanasia* is the initiation of life-shortening measures and involves taking deliberate action to end the person's life, or a commission (in the words of the Anglican church).

The issue is an ethical one which has not been fully resolved as yet. It revolves around two fundamental beliefs, the right of an individual to decide his own time and means of dying and the equally strongly argued premise that all measures must be tried before death is accepted as inevitable. Often, it becomes a matter of "to treat or not to treat." Passive euthanasia is much more widely accepted than active life-shortening measures and, often, in hospitals and long-term facilities, directions will be left for care that prolongs life, particularly of an older person, only if the individual and/or his family wish it.

In the past 10 years or so, there has been a strong "grass roots" movement to guarantee the right of an individual to determine the nature of his own death, insofar as this is possible. The movement has been successful to the extent that,

beginning in January 1977 with California, several states have passed legislation that enables people to express in writing their wishes regarding care during terminal illness. These laws are variously known as "Living Will," "Natural Death," or "Right-to-Die" legislation. Basically, they protect the right of the individual to die and not be kept alive by medications, artificial means, or "heroic measures." The person must make his wishes known while he is still in full command of his senses ("of sound mind," in legal terminology). In the case of a person who is incompetent—for example, because he is in a coma or in a vegetative state—a "decision-maker" may try to determine what the individual would have wanted, and act for him. The traditional decision-makers in cases such as these are the family and the patient's physician.

Some of the laws incorporate the format for a document that must be used by persons wishing to express their directives regarding care during terminal illness; some "suggest" a form, while others leave that matter up to the health agency or the individual. The organization Concern for Dying has prepared a "Living Will" that can be used for this purpose. A copy of their form is shown on page 696.

SIGNS OF IMMINENT DEATH

Certain signs are indicative of the imminence of death. The patient's reflexes gradually disappear and he is unable to move. His respirations become increasingly difficult; Cheyne-Stokes respirations may occur. Typically his face assumes a pinched expression, and often a faint cyanotic pattern becomes discernible in the skin of his face. The patient's skin feels cold and clammy and his pulse accelerates and becomes weaker. With increasing anoxia, the pupils become dilated and fixed. Low blood pressure, an elevated temperature, and a rapid respiration rate are often seen.

SIGNS OF DEATH

Death is considered to have occurred when the patient's respirations and heart have ceased to function for several minutes. Usually breathing stops first; the heart stops beating a few minutes later.

In this day of cardiac massage and mouth-to-mouth resuscitation, it is not unusual for a patient to "die" only to revive and walk out of the hospital.

Nursing personnel should note for the medical record the exact time that respirations cease and the heart stops beating. A physician pronounces the patient dead.

For the purpose of human transplants, it has become necessary to have a more precise definition than the cessation of respiration and heart beat as the absolute signs of death. The absence of brain wave activity as measured by the electroencephalogram is usually used to confirm that death has occurred.

CARE AFTER DEATH

In caring for the body of the patient after death, whatever procedures are carried out are performed with dignity and respect. In some religious faiths, only family members are permitted to care for the body of the deceased. Generally, however, this is a nursing responsibility. Although each agency usually has its own specific procedures, there are some general guidelines for the care of the body after death which are fairly universal.

The body is generally placed in a supine position in bed with one pillow under the head. The head is slightly elevated to prevent postmortem hypostasis of blood, which could discolor the face. The body is positioned immediately after death and before rigor mortis sets in.

Rigor mortis, a stiffening of the body after death, is a result of a chemical action within the muscles in which glycogen is coagulated and lactic acid is produced. It generally occurs shortly after death, progressing from the jaw down the trunk to the extremities. Once rigor mortis has set in, the body remains rigid for 1 to 6 days.

When relatives wish to see the body, the nurse first tidies the room and removes extraneous equipment. The body should appear clean, comfortable, and peaceful. A slightly shaded room affords a comforting effect.

In some hospitals it is the policy to insert dentures immediately after death; other institutions send the dentures with the body to the morgue, where they are inserted later by the mortician. In most institutions, rings are removed; if a ring cannot be removed it is taped in place and a notation is made on the patient's chart and on the form that goes with the body to the morgue.

The preparation of the body by the nurse involves the application of pads to the perineal area or the insertion of packing into the rectum and vagina. Rarely is it necessary to bathe the body; this procedure is carried out by the mortician. It is, however, necessary to cleanse the body of any blood or drainage that may have accumulated after death.

At most hospitals bodies are labeled twice: one label is attached to the ankles, the other to the shroud in which the body is wrapped. If the ankles and wrists are to be tied together, they should be well padded in order to prevent bruising. In some areas it is the practice to treat the body as if the patient were still living, and no shroud is used. When the preparation of the body is complete, the body is taken to the hospital morgue. If the hospital does not have a morgue, the mortician should be notified to come for the body.

The patient's valuables and clothes should, whenever possible, be sent home with the relatives. If there is no one present who can assume responsibility for these, valuables should be placed in the hospital safe and the clothes labeled and stored until such time as the family collects them.

The family of the deceased may be asked by the physician to sign a permission for an autopsy (postmortem examination). Under some circumstances an autopsy is required by law. For example, when a patient dies within 24 hours of admission to a hospital or when he dies as a result of injury or accident, some states require an autopsy. It is usually not the nurse's responsibility to secure permission for an autopsy. She may, however, be called upon to explain to the family the reasons for the autopsy.

The death certificate is signed by the physician and then sent to the local health department. If the deceased has a communicable disease, special regulations are observed regarding the care and disposition of the body.

To My Family, My Physician, My Lawyer and All Others Whom It May Concern

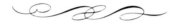

Death is as much a reality as birth, growth, maturity and old age—it is the one certainty of life. If the time comes when I can no longer take part in decisions for my own future, let this statement stand as an expression of my wishes and directions, while I am still of sound mind.

If at such a time the situation should arise in which there is no reasonable expectation of my recovery from extreme physical or mental disability, I direct that I be allowed to die and not be kept alive by medications, artificial means or "heroic measures". I do, however, ask that medication be mercifully administered to me to alleviate suffering even though this may shorten my remaining life.

This statement is made after careful consideration and is in accordance with my strong convictions and beliefs. I want the wishes and directions here expressed carried out to the extent permitted by law. Insofar as they are not legally enforceable, I hope that those to whom this Will is addressed will regard themselves as morally bound by these provisions.

Signed _____

Date _____

Witness _____

Witness _____

Copies of this request have been given to _____

_____

_____

_____

The Living Will prepared by the organization Concern for Dying. In addition to the basic form of the will, the organization notes the following:

"Declarants may wish to add specific statements to the Living Will to be inserted in the space provided for that purpose above the signature. Possible additional provisions are suggested below:

1. a) I appoint _____
      to make binding decisions concerning my medical treatment.

                                        OR

   b) I have discussed my views as to life sustaining measures with the following who understand my wishes

      _____

      _____

      _____

2. Measures of artificial life support in the face of impending death that are especially abhorrent to me are:
   a) Electrical or mechanical resuscitation of my heart when it has stopped beating.
   b) Nasogastric tube feedings when I am paralyzed and no longer able to swallow.
   c) Mechanical respiration by machine when my brain can no longer sustain my own breathing.
   d) _____

3. If it does not jeopardize the chance of my recovery to a meaningful and sentient life or impose an undue burden on my family, I would like to live out my last days at home rather than in a hospital.

4. If any of my tissues are sound and would be of value as transplants to help other people, I freely give my permission for such donation."

(Reprinted with the permission of Concern for Dying, 250 West 57th Street, New York, New York, 10107.)

GUIDE TO ASSESSING NURSING PROBLEMS OF THE TERMINALLY ILL

1. Is the patient aware of his prognosis?

2. What have the patient and his family been told about his prognosis?

3. Does the patient have any special requests?

4. Does the patient wish to have a chaplain visit him?

5. Is the patient in pain?

6. Is he lonely?

7. What problems do the family have which the nurse can help to resolve?

STUDY SITUATION

Mr. John Edwards is in a hospital with a malignancy that the doctors consider terminal. He is 93 years old and has three sons and seven grandchildren. Mr. Edwards has been in a stuporous state and upon waking he complains of pain.

1. What are some of the nursing needs of this patient?

2. What is stupor?

3. What needs of the family could be met by the nurse?

4. Which other members of the health team might be able to assist Mr. Edwards and his family?

5. How can you evaluate Mr. Edwards' nursing care?

SUGGESTED READINGS

Ames, B.: Art and a Dying Patient. *American Journal of Nursing,* 80(6):1094–1097, June, 1980.

Dobihal, S. V.: Hospice: Enabling a Patient to Die at Home. *American Journal of Nursing,* 80(8):1448–1450, August, 1980.

Freeze, B. M.: Brief Life. *Nursing '79,* 9(4):88, April, 1979.

Goffnett, C.: Your Patient's Dying—Now What? *Nursing '79,* 9(11):26–33, November, 1979.

Greishaw, S.: My, These Are Beautiful Flowers. *American Journal of Nursing,* 80(10):1782–1783, October, 1980.

Keeling, B.: Giving and Getting the Courage to Face Death. *Nursing '78,* 8(11):38–41, November, 1978.

Kelleher, K. L.: Go Gentle. *Nursing '79,* 9(7):16–17, July, 1979.

Kochmar, T.: Caring for the Mother of a Stillborn Baby. *Nursing '80,* 10(4):70–73, April, 1980.

Martin, A.: Hospice Nursing: Walking a Fine Line. *Nursing '81,* 11(2):29–30, February, 1981.

McNairn, N.: Helping the Patient Who Wants to Die at Home. *Nursing '81,* 11(2):66–69, February, 1981.

O'Connell, A. L.: Death Sentence: An Invitation to Life. *American Journal of Nursing,* 80(9):1646–1649, September, 1980.

Olson, J.: To Treat or to Allow to Die. *Journal of Gerontological Nursing,* 7(3):141–147, March, 1981.

Paige, R. L.: Living and Dying. *American Journal of Nursing,* 79(12):2171–2172, December, 1979.

Putnam, S. T., et al.: Home as a Place to Die. *American Journal of Nursing,* 80(8):1451–1453, August, 1980.

Rebele, M. E.: When We Tried to Get Close to Carrie, She Pushed Us Away. *Nursing '79,* 9(8):52–55, August, 1979.

Sharer, P. S.: Helping Survivors Cope with the Shock of Sudden Death. *Nursing '79,* 9(1):20–23, January, 1979.

Sherry, D.: The Bond. *Nursing '79,* 9(9):5–14, September, 1979.

Toth, S. B., and Toth, A.: Empathetic Intervention with the Widow. *American Journal of Nursing,* 80(9):1652–1654, September, 1980.

Wald, F. S.: Terminal Care and Nursing Education. *American Journal of Nursing,* 79(10):1762–1765, October, 1979.

REFERENCES

1. Kübler-Ross, E.: *On Death and Dying*. New York, Macmillan Company, 1969.
2. Moody, R.: *Life after Life*. Harrisburg, Pa., Stackpole Books, 1976.
3. Saunders, C.: The Last Stages of Life. *American Journal of Nursing*, 65:70, March, 1965.
4. Walborn, K. A.: A Nursing Model for the Hospice: Primary and Self-Care Nursing. *Nursing Clinics of North America*, 15(1):205–217, March, 1980.

GLOSSARY

abduction. movement away from the central axis of the body.

ablative surgery. the removal of a diseased or damaged organ.

abortion. the spontaneous or artificially induced expulsion of an embryo or fetus before it is viable.

abrasion. an area of the body rubbed bare of skin or mucous membrane.

abscess. a localized collection of pus in a cavity formed by the disintegration of tissue.

acapnia. a condition of decreased carbon dioxide in the blood.

acceptance. the ability to be nonjudgmental, understanding, and respectful of another's point of view.

accountability. the status in which one accepts responsibility and can be expected to answer for and explain one's professional actions.

acetone. a colorless liquid with a pleasant ethereal odor. It is found in small quantities in normal urine and is used as a solvent for fats, resins, rubber, and plastics.

acidosis. a condition in which there is an excessive proportion of acid in the blood and a reduced reserve of alkali (bicarbonate).

acne. an inflammatory disease of the sebaceous glands.

acromion process. the outward extension of the spine of the scapula, forming the point of the shoulder.

active exercise. exercise in which the muscles actively contract.

active transport. mechanism that transfers electrolytes from the cells to the extracellular fluid and vice versa to achieve balance.

actual problem. a problem that is causing the patient to have difficulty at the present time.

acupuncture. the practice of inserting long, fine needles into particular sites of the skin in order to cure disorders, relieve pain, or anesthetize an area of the body for surgery.

acute. having a short and relatively severe course.

adaptation. condition in which the brain no longer perceives the available stimuli because the receptors are not picking up enough stimuli or are picking up too much of the same stimulus.

addiction. the state of being given to some habit, as a drug habit.

adduction. movement toward the central axis of the body.

adhesion. a fibrous band or structure by which parts may abnormally adhere.

adipose. of a fatty nature.

adrenal gland. endocrine gland located atop the kidney.

adrenocortical hormone. a hormone secreted by the cortex of the adrenal gland.

adynamic ileus. paralytic ileus.

affective learning. the development and acquisition of attitudes and opinions.

agitate. to excite the mind or feelings; to move with irregular, rapid, or violent action.

air-fluidized bed. a bed which uses the flotation principle to provide uniform support to all parts of the body.

air hunger. respirations that are abnormally deep and accompanied by an increased respiratory rate.

alarm reaction. mobilization of the body's defense forces in response to physiological or psychological stress.

albuminuria. the presence of protein in the urine, in the form of white blood cells.

aldosterone. a hormone secreted by the cortex of the adrenal glands; a mineralocorticoid.

alkalosis. a condition in which there is an excess of alkali, such as bicarbonate, in the blood.

alternating pressure mattress. an air- or water-filled mattress, areas of which are alternately deflated and inflated with a resultant continual change of pressure upon the various parts of the body.

alveolus(i). an air sac of the lungs formed by the terminal dilatations of a bronchiole.

ambient oxygen. the oxygen that is available from the atmosphere.

ambulate. to move about; to walk from place to place.

ameba. a minute one-celled animal organism of the phylum Protozoa.

amenorrhea. absence of menstruation.

amino acid. the structural unit of protein.

amniotic sac. a protective membrane filled with fluid that surrounds the developing embryo in the uterus, providing warmth, moisture, and relative freedom of movement.

ampule. a sealed glass container.

anabolism. the synthesis of compounds by the cells.

anaerobe. a microorganism that grows in the absence or near absence of oxygen.

analgesic. relieving pain; a pain-relieving agent.

anatomical position. the position of the human body standing erect, with all body parts in good alignment.

anemia. a condition in which the blood is deficient in hemoglobin or red blood cells.

aneroid. containing no liquid.

anesthesia. loss of feeling or sensation.

anesthetic bed. a bed prepared to receive a patient immediately after surgery.

anion. a negatively charged ion.

anogenital. pertaining to the area around the anus and genitalia.

anorexia. loss of appetite.

anoxemia. a decrease in the amount of oxygen in the blood below normal physiological levels.

anoxia. a decrease in the amount of oxygen in the tissues below normal physiological levels.

antecubital. situated in front of the cubitus or forearm.

antibiotic. a chemical substance produced by microorganisms that has the capacity to destroy or inhibit the growth of other microorganisms.

antibody. a substance formed in the body in response to an antigen.

antidiuretic hormone. a hormone produced by the hypothalamus gland that inhibits the secretion of urine.

antigen. a substance that stimulates the production of antibodies within the body.

antihelminthic. destructive to worms.

antipyretic. an agent that reduces fever.

antisepsis. the prevention of sepsis by inhibiting the growth of microorganisms.

anuria. the absence of urinary excretion from the body.

anus. the distal orifice of the alimentary canal.

anxiety. an emotional response to danger of unknown origin.

aortic receptor. a nerve ending in the aortic arch which is sensitive to changes in blood pressure.

apathy. lack of feeling or emotion.

aphasia. the state of being unable to speak at all.

apical beat. the beat of the heart as it is felt over the apex.

apical-radial pulse. the results of taking the apical and the radial pulses at the same time on the same watch.

apnea. a period of cessation of breathing.

apomorphine. an alkaloid that is a powerful emetic and relaxant.

appendicitis. inflammation of the vermiform appendix.

appetite. desire for food.

arachnoid membrane. a membrane between the pia mater and dura mater surrounding the brain and spinal cord.

arachnoidal granulations. the capillary-like projections of the arachnoid membrane.

areolar connective tissue. loose connective tissue widely distributed in the body.

Aschheim-Zondek test. a pregnancy test in which urine from a female is injected into mice.

ascites. abnormal accumulation of fluid in the peritoneal cavity.

asepsis. freedom from infection—that is, from pathogenic organisms.

asphyxia. suffocation; a condition in which there are anoxia and an increase in carbon dioxide tension in the blood and tissues.

aspiration. the act of breathing or drawing in; the removal of fluids or gases from a cavity by suction.

assault. a threat to do bodily harm to another.

assessment. the collection and analysis of information leading to the identification of problems.

asthma. a condition marked by periodic attacks of dyspnea, with wheezing and a sense of constriction.

astringent. an agent that causes contraction and arrests discharges.

asymmetrical. not symmetrical; lack of correspondence in paired organs.

atelectasis. incomplete expansion of the lungs at birth or collapse of the adult lung.

atherosclerosis. a condition in which there is an accumulation of fatty deposits on the walls of medium-sized and large arteries.

atrioventricular valve. the valve between the atrium and the ventricle of the heart.

atrophy. a wasting away or diminution in the size of a cell, tissue, organ, or other part.

attendant. a person who assists with care, such as dressing and feeding patients and looking after their personal hygiene.

auditory. pertaining to the sense of hearing.

auscultation. observation by listening for body sounds.

autocratic teaching style. teacher-dominated method of conducting classes in which all decisions are made by the person conducting the class.

autonomic. self-functioning; independent.

autonomy. the condition of being functionally independent.

autopsy. a postmortem examination.

bactericidal. capable of destroying bacteria.

bacteriostatic. capable of inhibiting the growth or multiplication of bacteria.

bacterium(a). any microorganism of the order Eubacteriales.

Balkan frame. a frame made of wood or metal that extends lengthwise over the bed and is supported at either end by a pole.

barbiturate. a salt or derivative of barbituric acid used as a sedative.

barrier technique. medical aseptic practices to control the spread of pathogenic bacteria and contribute to their destruction.

basal metabolism. the rate of energy expenditure of the body at rest.

basic need. a need that is necessary for the individual's health and well-being.

basilic vein. superficial vein of the arm.

battery. the unlawful beating of another or the carrying out of threatened physical harm.

behavior. deportment or conduct.

Bence-Jones protein test. examination of urine to detect bone tumors.

binder. a type of bandage.

biological clock. the physiological mechanism that governs the rhythmic occurrence of certain biochemical, physiological, and behavioral phenomena in plants and animals.

biopsy. the removal and examination of tissue or other material from the living body.

Biot's respirations. irregular respirations as to speed and depth; pauses may be associated with a sigh.

bleb. a skin vesicle filled with fluid.

blister.   a collection of fluid in the epidermis causing an elevation of the outer layer (stratum corneum).

body temperature.   the internal temperature of the human body.

boil.   furuncle; a painful nodule in the skin caused by bacteria and often having a central core.

bolus.   a mass of food ready to be swallowed or a mass passing along the intestines.

bonding.   the attachment that occurs between parent and newborn.

botulism.   food poisoning caused by the organism *Clostridium botulinum.*

brachial pulse.   the pulse located on the anterior surface of the arm, just below the elbow, where the brachial artery passes over the ulna.

Bradford frame.   a canvas, stretcher-like device supported by blocks on the foundation of the bed. It is used to immobilize patients who have injured spines.

bradycardia.   a very slow heart beat, reflected in a pulse of under 60 beats per minute.

bradykinin.   chemical substance released by damaged cells which excites pain receptors.

bradypnea.   an abnormal decrease in the respiratory rate.

bronchoscopy.   inspection of the bronchi with a lighted instrument (bronchoscope).

bronchus(i).   one of the two main branches of the trachea; also the divisions of the main bronchi within the lungs.

burette.   a graduated glass tube.

cachexia.   a general physical wasting, often associated with chronic disease.

calculus(i).   a stone formed in various parts of the body, such as the gallbladder or kidney.

calorie.   a unit of heat. One small calorie is the amount of heat required to raise the temperature of 1 gm. of water $1°$ C. A large calorie is the amount of heat required to raise the temperature of 1 kg. of water $1°$ C.

calyx (calyxes or calices).   a cup-shaped organ or cavity; in the kidney, one of the recesses in the pelvis.

cannula.   a tube for insertion into the body, often made of a hard substance, and the lumen of which contains a trochar during the insertion.

canthus.   the angle formed at either end of the eye by the upper and lower eyelids.

carbohydrate.   an organic chemical compound composed of carbon, hydrogen, and oxygen, found in most plants, fruit sugars, and natural starches.

carbuncle.   a boil.

cardiac sphincter.   the band of circular fibers situated at the opening of the esophagus into the stomach.

carminative.   a medicine that relieves flatulence.

carotid receptors.   nerve endings located in the carotid sinuses and carotid bodies that are sensitive to changes in blood pressure, excess blood CO_2, and blood pH.

carrier.   an individual who harbors disease organisms in his body and yet does not manifest symptoms but who can pass on the infection.

cast.   coagulated protein in the urine, passed from the lumen of the kidney tubules.

CAT scan.   computed *axial tomography*; a sophisticated form of radiography in which a series of cross-sectional images are combined by computer to present a three-dimensional image.

catabolism.   a destructive process within the cells in which complex substances are converted into simpler substances.

cathartic.   a medicine that hastens bowel evacuation.

catheter.   a tube used to withdraw fluid from body cavities (such as urine from the bladder or blood samples from major vessels or heart chambers) or to introduce fluids (as in intravenous feedings or in injecting radiopaque material for angiocardiography).

cation.   a positively charged ion.

cementum.   true bone that protects root of a tooth.

central pain.   pain arising from injury to sensory nerves, neural pathways, or areas in the brain concerned with pain perception.

cephalic vein. a superficial vein on the thumb side of the arm.

cerebral cortex. the outer layer (gray matter) of the largest part of the brain (cerebrum).

cerebrospinal fluid. the fluid that surrounds the brain and spinal cord.

certification. a mechanism for ensuring the quality of a practitioner's competence in a specialized area at a level higher than licensure.

ceruminous. secreting wax.

cervix. a necklike structure; the lower narrow portion of the uterus.

Cheyne-Stokes respirations. respirations with rhythmical variations in intensity occurring in cycles, often with periods of apnea.

child molesting. sexual activity or contact forced upon a child by an adult.

chill. involuntary contractions of the voluntary muscles, with shivering and shaking.

cholangiography. radiography of the bile ducts.

cholecystography. radiography of the gallbladder.

chordotomy. surgical division of the anterolateral tracts of the spinal cord.

choroid plexus. a network of capillaries found in the ventricles of the brain which produce the cerebrospinal fluid.

chronic. persisting over a long period of time.

cicatrization. a healing process that leaves a scar.

cilium(a). a minute hairlike process attached to the free surface of a cell, as in the nose.

cinefluorography. the production of a motion picture record of a sequence of fluoroscopic images.

circadian rhythm. a rhythmic repetition of certain things in living organisms at approximately the same time each 24 hours.

circumcision. removal of all or part of the foreskin of the penis.

circumduction. circular movement, as of a limb or an eye.

cisterna. a closed space serving as a reservoir.

cisterna magna. an extension of the subarachnoid space below and behind the corpus callosum.

cisternal puncture. the insertion of a needle into the cisterna magna.

clarification. the act of making clear one's impressions on a particular point.

clavicle. the collar bone. It articulates with the sternum and the scapula.

clinic. a community or hospital agency providing services for promotion of health, prevention of illness, and care and treatment of the sick on an ambulatory basis.

clinical nursing specialist. A nurse who has expanded her nursing knowledge and skills in one particular branch of nursing.

clean. denoting the absence of disease-producing microorganisms.

closed bed. an empty bed, to which no patient has been assigned.

cognition. the process by which we become aware through thought or perception, including reasoning and understanding.

cognitive learning. acquisition of knowledge.

cohesion. a force that unites particles.

COLD. chronic obstructive lung disease.

collagen. an albuminoid supportive protein found in connective tissue.

colostomy. the surgical creation of an opening between the colon and the surface of the body.

colostrum. thin, yellow, milky fluid secreted by the mammary gland a few days before or after parturition.

coma. a state of unconsciousness from which an individual cannot be aroused.

combustible. inflammable; liable to take fire.

comfort. ease of body or mind.

commode. a portable toilet-like structure.

communicable disease. a disease capable of being transmitted from one person to another.

compensation. attempting to make up for real or imagined inferiorities by becoming highly competent in a sphere of endeavor.

compress. a pad or cloth that is folded and applied to press upon a body part.

concave. rounded inward or hollowed.

concurrent disinfection. ongoing measures to control the spread of infection during the time the patient is considered infectious.

conditioned. learned through repetition of a stimulus, as in Pavlov's experiment.

condom. a sheath used to cover the penis for birth control.

conductive heat. heat transmitted to the body by contact with a heated object, such as a hot water bottle.

confusion. mental state of appearing bewildered and perplexed, and/or making inappropriate answers to questions.

congenital. present at birth.

congestion. an abnormal accumulation of blood in a part.

consciousness. the normal state of awareness.

constant data. information that is not expected to change during the period of care.

constipation. abnormal delay in the passage of feces.

constructive surgery. the building or correction of a body part by surgical means to improve function or appearance.

contact. a person who is known to have been sufficiently near an infected person to be exposed to the transfer of infectious organisms.

contaminate. to soil or make unclean.

context. the environment; the portions of a discourse that precede or follow a word or words.

contracture. a shortening or distortion of muscle tissue.

contrast medium. a substance deliberately introduced into a person's body to provide greater visualization of body parts or organs on x-rays.

convalescence. the stage of transition from illness to health.

convection. transmission of heat in liquids or gases.

conversion reaction. a condition in which emotional disorders are experienced as physical symptoms.

conversive. pertaining to a change in the state of energy, as from electricity to heat.

conversive heat. heat developed in the tissues by a current of electricity or by some form of radiant energy.

COPD. chronic obstructive pulmonary disease (also same as COLD).

corneal reflex. closing of the eyelids as a result of irritation of the cornea.

counterirritant. an agent applied to the skin to produce a reaction that relieves irritation.

covert. hidden; covered.

cradle. a frame placed over the body of a bed patient for protecting the injured parts from contact with the bedclothes.

creatinine. nitrogenous waste excreted in the urine.

crime. a legal wrong, generally committed against the public.

cultural shock. stress caused by exposure to customs and social values at variance with one's own.

culture. those aspects of society which include knowledge, beliefs, art, morals, laws, and customs.

curative aspects. pertaining to diagnostic, therapeutic, and rehabilitative measures in health care.

curative surgery. surgery performed to arrest a pathological process by removing its cause.

custom. a practice that is common to many or to a place or class or that is habitual to an individual.

cyanosis. bluish tinge in the skin and mucous membranes frequently associated with respiratory distress.

cyst. a sac, usually containing a liquid or semisolid material.

cystitis. inflammation of the urinary bladder.

cystoscopy. examination of the urinary bladder with a lighted instrument.

dandruff. dry, scaly material shed from skin of the scalp.

data base. the sum total of information gathered in the admission work-up of a patient.

debilitated. enfeebled; lacking strength.

deceleration. the state of moving at decreasing speed.

decubitus ulcer. a bedsore.

deep pain. pain arising from deeper structures of the body, such as muscles, tendons, and joints.

defamation of character. the damaging of an individual's reputation by written or spoken statements.

defecation. the evacuation of feces.

defense mechanism. an individual's reaction to disturbances in psychosocial equilibrium, manifested by changes in intellectual behavior.

dehiscence. the breaking open of a wound.

dehydration. removal of water from the body or tissues.

delirious. suffering from mental confusion, incoherence, and physical restlessness.

democratic teaching style. method of teaching in which learners participate in decisions regarding goals and nature of learning experiences, and accept some responsibility for direction of teaching and learning activities.

denial. refusing to acknowledge a problem or forbidden motive.

dependency. having to rely on others for the satisfaction of basic needs.

dependent nursing function. the carrying out by the nurse of a decision made by another health professional.

depression. a feeling of sadness or melancholy.

deprivational stress. stress produced by a lack of some factor essential for the well-being of an organism.

dermis. the inner, thicker layer of the skin.

detergent. an agent that purifies or cleanses.

detrusor muscle. the three layers of smooth muscle of the urinary bladder.

developmental crises. major changes in an individual's life as he reaches certain stages in his physical and/or psychosocial development.

diabetes. a hereditary disease in which the body is unable to burn up its intake of sugars, starches, and other carbohydrates because of the deficiency of insulin.

diacetic acid. acetoacetic acid; an acid excreted in the urine.

diagnosis. the determination of the nature of a disease.

diagonal toe bed. a bed made up to expose the leg or foot of the patient, at the same time providing warmth and adequate covering for the rest of the body.

diaphoresis. profuse perspiration.

diarrhea. undue frequency of the passage of feces, with the discharge of loose stools.

diastolic blood pressure. the pressure in the arteries when the ventricles of the heart are relaxed.

diathermy. the generation of heat in the tissues by the application of high frequency electric currents.

dietitian. a person educated in the use of diet in health and disease.

differentiation. distinguishing of one thing or disease from another on the basis of differences.

diffusion. process whereby molecules and ions distribute themselves equally within a given space.

digital. pertaining to the fingers.

diplopia. double vision; seeing two objects when there is only one.

disassociate. to separate; to detach from association.

discipline. a field of study.

disease. a cluster of abnormalities in functioning, producing recognizable signs and symptoms.

disinfection. the destruction of disease-producing microorganisms.

disorientation. a state of mental confusion; a lack of awareness of time, place, or person.

displacement. redirecting aggressive feelings and actions toward a substitute.

distal. farther from a point of reference or point of attachment.

distention. the enlargement of the abdomen due to the internal pressure of gas or liquid or other causes.

diuresis. the abnormal secretion of urine.

diuretic. a substance that increases the secretion of urine in the kidneys.

doctor's order sheet. a written record of the orders given by the physician for the patient's treatment.

dorsal. pertaining to the back; posterior.

dorsal recumbent. supine; lying on one's back.

dorsalis pedis pulse. the pulse felt on the dorsum of the foot in a line between the first and second toes, just above the longitudinal arch.

douche. a washing out of the vagina.

drowsiness. readiness to fall asleep.

drug. a chemical compound used for diagnosis or therapy or as a preventive measure.

duodenum. the first part of the small intestine.

dysphagia. difficulty in swallowing.

dysphasia. difficulty in speaking.

dyspnea. difficult breathing.

dysmenorrhea. painful or irregular menstruation.

dysuria. difficulty in voiding or pain on voiding.

ecchymosis. extravasation of blood into the tissues.

ecology. the study of the relationship between living organisms and their environment.

ectoderm. the outermost of the three primary germ layers of the embryo.

edema. the presence of excessive amounts of fluid in the extracellular spaces.

edentulous. without teeth.

effacement. shortening and thinning of the cervix during first stage labor.

efferent. carrying outward from the center.

egocentric. centering all one's ideas on oneself.

electrocardiogram. a graphic tracing of the electrical current produced by the contraction of the heart muscle.

electroencephalogram. a record of the electrical impulses produced by the brain.

electrolyte. a compound which in an aqueous solution is able to conduct an electrical current.

elopement. the act of running away clandestinely.

emaciated. excessively lean.

embolus. a clot in a blood vessel which has been transported from another vessel.

embryonic stage. the period after the zygote has attached itself to the uterine wall, during which the cells multiply, forming three layers.

emergency surgery. surgery performed on an urgent basis in response to an immmediate threat to a person's life or well-being.

emesis. vomiting.

emollient. softening or soothing.

emphysema. a condition in which the pulmonary alveoli are distended or rupture as a result of air pressure.

EMT. Abbreviation for Emergency Medical Technician, a person with formal preparation in resuscitation and basic life support skills.

emulsion. a liquid which is distributed throughout another liquid in small globules.

enamel. the hard, inorganic substance covering the crown of a tooth.

endemic. present at all times among a particular people or within a particular country.

endoderm. the inner layer of the embryo in the uterus, which becomes the digestive system.

endogenous. developing from within.

endogenous spread. the transfer of microorganisms from one area of a person's body to another.

endoscopy. the visual examination of the interior of a body cavity by means of a scope.

endothelium. the layer of squamous cells which lines the blood vessels.

enema. a liquid to be injected into the rectum.

enteric coated. coated with a substance that prevents medications from dissolving until reaching the intestines.

enteroclysis. the injection of a nutrient or medicine into the bowel.

enuresis. incontinence of urine during sleep.

environment. the sum total of the external surroundings and influences.

environmental equilibrium. the balance achieved by an organism in its interactions with the surrounding environment.

environmental technologist. a worker primarily concerned with the improvement, control, and management of man's environment.

epidemic. attaching many people in a region at the same time; widely diffused and rapidly spreading.

epidermis. the outer, thinner layer of the skin.

epididymitis. inflammation of the epididymis, the oblong body containing a duct, attached to the testicle.

epinephrine. a hormone produced by the medulla of the adrenal gland or prepared synthetically; a vasopressor.

epistaxis. nosebleed.

equilibrium. a static or dynamic state of balance between opposing forces or actions.

erythema. redness of the skin due to congestion of the capillaries.

esophagus. the canal extending from the pharynx to the stomach.

estrogen. the principal female sex hormone, produced in the ovary.

etiology. the study of the causes of disease.

eupnea. normal, regular, or effortless breathing.

evaluation. determining whether the expected outcomes have been attained or not.

evaluative response. reacting to statements by imposing one's own values on another individual.

eversion. a turning outward.

excoriation. the loss of superficial layers of skin.

excreta. waste materials excreted by the body.

exhibitionism. impulsive, compulsive exposure of the genitalia to achieve sexual satisfaction; may be accompanied by masturbation to orgasm.

exogenous. developing from outside.

expectorate. to bring mucus up from the lungs or trachea.

expiration. the act of expelling air from the lungs (breathing out).

explicit policy. a written governmental plan of action on which health programs are based.

extended care facility. an agency whose primary purpose is the care of people with long-term illnesses.

extension. the act of straightening a limb.

extracellular. situated outside the cells.

extravasation. the escape of blood from a vessel into the tissues.

extrinsic rewards. those that come from an outside source, e.g., praise, encouragement, or small tokens such as stars or candy.

exudate. a substance produced and deposited on or in a tissue by disease or a vital process.

false imprisonment. the unjustifiable detention of an individual without a legal warrant.

family nutritionist. a member of a community health agency who is primarily concerned with matters of food and its relationship to health.

fantasy. the use of daydreaming to temporarily escape from reality.

fastigium. the high point of a fever.

fats. organic compounds composed of carbon, hydrogen, and oxygen, found in nature in animals and in plant seeds.

fear. an emotional response to a known and identifiable danger.

feces. excreta discharged from the intestines.

femoral pulse. pulse which may be taken at the point in the middle of the groin, where the temporal artery passes over the pelvic bone.

femur. the leg bone extending from the pelvis to the knee.

fetal stage. the period of gestation from 8 weeks to birth, during which systems formed in the embryonic stage increase in complexity and maturity.

fever. an elevated temperature.

fibrin. a protein substance that forms an essential part of a blood clot.

fibroplasia. the formation of fibrous tissue.

Fishberg concentration test. a special urine test to determine specific gravity.

fissure. a deep cleft or groove.

fistula. an abnormal passage leading from an abscess or hollow organ to the body surface or from one hollow organ to another.

flatulence. distention of the stomach or the intestines with air or gases.

flatus. gas in the intestines or stomach.

flexion. the act of bending.

flight-fight reaction. the body's response to immediate (real or imagined) danger.

flowsheet. a special form that details a specific intervention or group of related interventions to be done on a regular basis and documents the results thereof.

fluoroscopy. examination of structures of the body such as the stomach by means of roentgen rays and a fluorescent screen.

flushing. a redness of the skin, particularly noticeable in the face and neck.

fomite. a substance other than food that can harbor microorganisms.

footboard. a device placed toward the foot of the patient's bed as a support for his feet.

forgetful. suffering from a temporary loss of memory.

fossa navicularis. a widened area of the lumen of the male urethra just superior to the meatus; a depression on the internal pterygoid process of the sphenoid bone.

Fowler's position. the sitting position in which the head gatch of the patient's bed is raised to at least a 45-degree angle.

fracture board. a support placed under the patient's mattress to give it added rigidity.

free clinic. a clinic providing readily accessible health services on a free or nominal charge basis for people living in poor neighborhoods.

fremitus. vibration of the chest.

frequency. in reference to voiding, abnormally short intervals between times of voiding.

friable tissues. tissues that are more easily pulverized or crumbled than normal healthy tissues.

friction. the force which opposes motion.

Friedman test. a test for pregnancy which involves the injection of urine into rabbits.

frontal plane. the plane that divides the body into dorsal and ventral sections.

fulcrum. the fixed point of a lever.

functional pathology. referring to diseases which have no apparent physical basis.

gastrocolic reflex. mass peristalsis of the colon stimulated be the entrance of food into the stomach.

gastroenteritis. inflammation of the stomach and intestines.

gastroscopy. the examination of the stomach with a lighted instrument.

gavage. feeding through a stomach tube.

gender role. all those things that a person does that indicate that he or she is a male or female.

general adaptation syndrome. the generalized response of the body to any agent that causes physiological stress.

genitalia. the reproductive organs; generally, the external reproductive organs.

geriatric nursing. the nursing care of older people.

germinal stage. the period from fertilization to 2 weeks, during which the zygote develops

gingivae. the gums in the mouth.

glaucoma. a condition in which there is increased tension within the eyeball.

gliding. movement in one plane, as in sliding.

glomerulus. a tuft of capillaries such as that of the nephron of the kidney.

glossopharyngeal nerve. the ninth cranial nerve; the nerve serving the tongue and pharynx.

glottis. the vocal apparatus of the larynx.

glycerol. glycerin; a byproduct of the breakdown of fats.

glycogen. a polysaccharide stored in cells after the breakdown of carbohydrate.

glycosuria. the presence of glucose in the urine.

Good Samaritan law. a law designed to protect a person from malpractice suits arising from care given at the scene of an emergency.

granulation. fleshy projections formed on the surface of a wound that is not healing by first intention.

gravity. the force that pulls objects toward each other; on earth, the dominant gravitional pull is toward the center of the earth.

Guérin's fold. a fold of mucous membrane occasionally seen in the fossa navicularis of the urethra.

gustatory. pertaining to the sense of taste.

gynecology. the branch of medicine that deals with diseases of the female reproductive tract.

halitosis. foul odor of the breath.

hallucination. distortion in sensory perception.

hallucinogens. drugs that produce sensory experiences not existing in the external world.

health. a positive state of being which includes physical fitness, mental (or emotional) stability, and social ease.

health educator. person primarily responsible for the development of health education programs in the community.

Health Maintenance Organization. organization of private physicians providing a comprehensive range of health services on a fixed contract basis.

health status indicators. statistical information about illness and death, usually compiled on an annual basis by national governments.

health team. all those who participate in providing health care services.

hectic (septic) fever. an intermittent fever with wide variations in temperature elevation but in which the temperature falls to normal during each 24 hour period.

hematemesis. the vomiting of blood.

hematuria. the discharge of blood in the urine.

hemiplegia. the loss of motor functions on one side of the body.

hemoglobin. the red pigment of the red blood cell which carries oxygen.

hemoglobinuria. hemoglobin in the urine.

hemophilia. a hereditary blood disease in which the blood lacks elements necessary for normal clotting.

hemoptysis. the spitting up of blood or of blood-tinged sputum.

hemorrhage. bleeding; the escape of a large amount of blood from the blood vessels.

hemorrhoid. enlarged, often infected veins and sinuses at or near the anus.

hemothorax. a collection of blood in the thoracic cavity.

herbalist. a nonmedical practitioner of the healing arts who makes use of herbs (plants) to treat disease.

Hering-Breuer reflex. the reflex that limits respiratory inspirations and expirations.

hermaphrodite. a person with ambiguous genitalia; that is, one whose external organs are not clearly of one sex or the other.

heterosexuality. sexual attraction or activity between male and female.

hierarchy. an arrangement in a graded series.

histamine. a chemical substance found in all animal and vegetable tissues, liberated when cells are injured.

holism. the concept of the individual as a whole, including physical, social, and emotional components.

homeostasis. tendency to uniformity or stability in body states; dynamic equilibrium.

homosexuality. sexual attraction or activity between persons of the same sex.

hospice. an institution for care of the terminally ill.

hospital. an institution whose chief purpose is to provide inpatient services for the care of people with health problems.

host. an animal or plant that harbors or nourishes another organism.
human biology. the science of human life.
humidity. the degree of moisture in the air.
hunger. an uncomfortable feeling that indicates a need for nourishment.
Huntington's chorea. a hereditary disease characterized by progressive degeneration of the nervous system.
hyaluronidase. an enzyme that initiates the hydrolysis of the cement material (hyaluronic acid) of the tissues.
hydration. the act of combining with water; the state of having adequate body fluids.
hydraulic. pertaining to the action of liquids.
hydrostatic. pertaining to fluids in a state of equilibrium.
hydrostatic pressure. the pressure of liquids.
hygiene. the science of health and its preservation; practices conducive to good health.
hyperalgesia. excessive sensitivity to pain.
hypercalcemia. an excessive amount of calcium in the blood.
hyperemia. excessive blood in any part of the body.
hyperextension. extension beyond the normal range of motion.
hyperglycemia. an increased concentration of glucose in the blood.
hyperkalemia. an excessive amount of potassium in the blood.
hypernatremia. an excessive amount of sodium in the blood.
hyperplasia. an abnormal increase in the number of cells in a tissue or organ.
hyperpnea. an abnormal increase in the rate and depth of respirations.
hypersomnia. uncontrollable drowsiness.
hypertension. persistently high arterial blood pressure.
hyperthermia. an abnormally high body temperature; fever.
hypertonicity. a state characterized by excessive tone or activity.
hypertrophy. an abnormal increase in the size of an organ or tissue as a result of an increase in the size of the cells.
hypervolemia. an abnormal increase in blood volume.
hypnotic. a drug that acts to induce sleep.
hypocalcemia. a decrease in the amount of serum calcium.
hypochloremia. a reduced concentration of chlorides in the blood.
hypodermoclysis. the introduction of fluids into the subcutaneous tissues.
hypogastric nerve. the nerve trunk of the autonomic nervous system that serves the abdominal viscera.
hypoglycemia. a reduction in the amount of glucose in the blood.
hypokalemia. a reduction in the amount of potassium in the blood.
hyponatremia. a decrease in the amount of sodium in the blood.
hypotension. abnormally low arterial blood pressure.
hypothalamus. part of the diencephalon of the brain, from which fibers of the autonomic nervous system extend to the thalamus, neurohypophysis, and so forth.
hypothermia. an abnormally low body temperature.
hypoxemia. a reduction in the oxygen content of the blood.
hypoxia. a reduction in the oxygen content of the tissues.
hysterectomy. surgical removal of the uterus.

identification. modeling oneself upon the image of another person.
ileostomy. the surgical creation of an opening between the distal portion of the small intestine and the surface of the body.
immunity. the condition of being protected against a particular disease.
impacted bowel. the condition in which there is an accumulation of feces in the rectum, pressed firmly together so as to be immovable.
impaction. the condition of being firmly lodged or wedged.
implementation. the carrying out of the specified measures outlined in a plan.
implicit policy. a health plan demonstrated by the actions of a health department, though not formally expressed.
inattentive. unable to focus the mind on an idea or some aspect of the surroundings.

incoherent speech.   speaking in such a way that one's meaning is not clear (to people speaking the same language).

incontinent.   unable to control urination and/or defecation.

independent nursing function.   the carrying out, or delegation by the nurse, of a decision made by herself in respect of the care of a patient.

industrial hygienist.   a person whose main concern is the detection and control of environmental hazards in the work situation.

infant mortality.   the death of infants under one year of age.

infection.   the invasion of the body by disease-producing microorganisms and the body's reaction to their presence.

infestation.   invasion of the body by arthropods, including insects, mites, and ticks.

inflammation.   a condition of the tissues in reaction to injury.

informed consent.   consent, preferably in writing, obtained from a person to whom the risks, alternatives, and benefits of a proposed therapy or procedure have been explained in terms the person can understand.

infusion.   the therapeutic introduction of a fluid into a vein or part of the body.

inguinal hernia.   the protrusion of an organ or tissue through an abnormal opening into the inguinal canal.

inhalation.   the drawing of air or other substances into the lungs.

inhalation therapist.   a technician who is skilled in the performance of diagnostic procedures and therapeutic measures dealing with the respiratory tract.

inpatient.   a patient who is confined to a hospital; pertaining to health services rendered to such a patient.

insertion (of a muscle).   the place of attachment of a muscle to the bone that it moves.

insomnia.   the inability to sleep.

inspection.   observation by use of the sense of sight.

inspiration.   the act of taking air into the lungs.

instillation.   the dropping of liquid into a cavity such as the ear.

insulator.   a material or substance that prevents or inhibits conduction, as of heat.

intercostal.   located between the ribs.

interdependent nursing function.   the carrying out by the nurse of a decision made by herself in consultation with other health professionals.

intermittent (quotidian) fever.   fever that falls to normal at some time during a 24-hour period.

intern.   a graduate of a basic professional program (medicine, nursing, and so forth) who is receiving a planned program of clinical experience, usually in order to complete requirements for licensure.

interstitial.   located between the cells of tissue.

interview.   a talk with a purpose.

intracellular.   located within the cells.

intradermal.   located within the dermis.

intramuscular.   located within the muscle tissue.

intraosseous.   located within the bone.

intrathecal.   located within the spinal canal.

intravascular.   located within a vessel.

intravenous.   located within a vein.

intravertebral.   intraspinal.

intrinsic rewards.   rewards that are internal, e.g., feelings of satisfaction.

intubation.   the insertion of a tube.

invasion of privacy.   the exposing of an individual or his property to public scrutiny without his consent.

inversion.   a turning inward.

inward rotation.   a turning of a bone upon its axis toward the midline.

irradiation.   exposure to x-rays, radioactive matter such as radium, or ultraviolet rays.

irrational.   confused as to time, place, or person; not possessing normal judgment.

irritant.   an agent applied to the skin to produce a reaction.

ischemia.   localized anemia due to an obstruction to the inflow of blood.

isolation.   the separation of one person, material, or object from others.

isometric exercise. exercise in which muscle tension is increased but the muscles are not shortened and the body parts are not moved.
isotonic. pertaining to equal tone or pressure; pertaining to solutions having equal osmotic pressure.
isotonic exercise. exercise in which muscles are shortened and body parts are moved.

jargon. technical terms used in a particular line of work that are not in common use outside the field.
jaundice. a condition in which yellowish pigment is deposited in the skin, tissues, and body fluid.

keratin. a scleroprotein substance in hair, nails, and horny tissue.
ketone. a compound containing the carbonyl group.
17-ketosteroid. a type of hormone classed as an androgen and excreted in the urine. It is partially produced in the adrenal cortex and partially derived from testosterone.
kilogram. a unit of weight equal to 1000 grams or approximately 2.2 pounds.
kinesiology. the science of motion.
Kussmaul's breathing. air hunger; dyspnea occurring periodically without cyanosis.

labor. the sequence of events through which the baby is expelled from the uterus.
labored breathing. breathing that involves the active participation of accessory inspiratory and expiratory muscles.
laissez faire teaching style. teaching in which the learners control and direct their own learning experience.
languor. listlessness; lassitude.
lanugo. a thick, downy hair on newborn infants.
laryngeal stridor. a coarse, high-pitched sound which accompanies inspiration.
lassitude. weariness; fatigue; languor.
lateral. relating to the side; situated away from the midline.
lavage. therapeutic washing out of an organ such as the stomach.
lesion. an open area or break in the skin surface.
lethargy. abnormal drowsiness; state of being lazy or indifferent.
leukocyte. white blood cell.
lever. a rigid bar that revolves around a fixed point.
liability. responsibility.
libel. the damaging of an individual's reputation by a written statement.
licensed practical nurse. one who is licensed to perform standardized nursing procedures and treatments, working under the direction of a registered nurse or physician.
licensed vocational nurse. the designation given to licensed practical nurses in some states of the United States.
licensure. approval by an appropriate authority that permits a person to offer to the public his skills and knowledge in a particular jurisdiction.
life expectancy. the average number of years that a person of a given age may be expected to live.
lifestyle. the way of life of an individual, dictated in part by circumstances and in part by active decision.
ligament. a band of connective tissue that connects bones or supports organs.
linea nigra. a vertical line of dark pigment appearing between the navel and pubic area during pregnancy.
local. restricted to one spot or part.
local adaptation syndrome. the body's localized reaction to stress affecting a specific part or organ.

lumbar puncture. the introduction of a needle into the subarachnoid space in the lumbar section of the spinal cord for diagnostic or therapeutic purposes.

lumen. the cavity of a tubular organ.

lymph nodes. an accumulation of densely packed lymphatic tissue.

lymphatic. pertaining to or containing lymph.

lysis. the gradual fall of an elevated temperature.

major surgery. surgery involving considerable hazards to the patient because of widespread physiological effects.

malaise. a vague sense of debility or lack of health.

malignancy. a tendency to progress in virulence.

malnutrition. a disorder of nutrition.

malpractice. improper or injurious action on the part of a professional practitioner.

mandatory licensure. legislation requiring a professional nurse to hold a valid, current license in the state (province) in which she is employed in order to be able to practice.

manometer. an instrument for measuring the pressure of liquids or gases.

massage. systematic stroking and kneading of the tissues.

mastication. the process of chewing food in preparation for swallowing and digestion.

masturbation. autosexual activity; for example, stimulation of the penis or clitoris by stroking.

meatus. an opening.

medial. pertaining to the middle; situated toward the midline.

medical asepsis. practices which are carried out in order to keep microorganisms within a given area.

medical diagnosis. a physician's opinion as to the nature of a patient's illness.

medical laboratory technologist. a person responsible for collecting, treating, and analyzing many of the specimens needed for laboratory tests used in the detection and treatment of illness.

medicament. an agent used in therapy; medicine; drug.

medicine. any drug or remedy.

medulla oblongata. the part of the rhombencephalon which attaches to the spinal cord and contains a number of the vital centers.

menarche. the beginning of the menstrual function.

meniscus. a crescent-shaped structure; the surface of a liquid column.

menopause. the ending of the menstrual function, also called "change of life."

menstruation. the monthly flow of blood from the female genital tract.

mesoderm. the middle layer of the fertilized ovum (zygote), which forms the skeletal, muscular, and circulatory system during the embryonic stage of pregnancy.

metabolism. the sum of all physical and chemical processes by which living substance is produced and maintained.

microorganism. an organism that can be seen only by means of a microscope.

microwave. an electromagnetic wave of high frequency and short wavelength.

micturition. voiding.

minerals. inorganic elements or compounds occurring in nature.

minim. a unit of volume equal to 1/60 part of a fluid dram.

minor surgery. surgery involving less hazard and fewer generalized physiological effects than major surgery.

miter. to square a sheet at a corner when making a bed.

mold. a type of fungus.

morbid. pertaining to disease.

morbidity data. information relating to the frequency of illness within a specific population.

morning sickness. the experience of nausea and vomiting during pregnancy, commonly first thing in the morning.

mortality. the quality of being subject to death.

mortality rate. the death rate.

Mosaic Law. writings attributed to Moses.

mucoid. a moist, viscid protein substance.

mucous membrane. the membrane that lines passages and cavities of the body which communicate with the air.

myelography. the x-ray examination of the spinal cord by using a contrast medium.

myocardium. heart muscle.

narcolepsy. a condition marked by an uncontrollable desire for sleep or by sudden episodes of sleep occurring at intervals.

narcotic. a drug that relieves pain or induces sleep or stupor.

nasopharynx. the upper part of the pharynx continuous with the nasal passage.

naturopath. a nonmedical practitioner of the healing arts who makes use of physical forces such as heat and massage to cure disease.

nausea. stomach distress accompanied by an urge to vomit.

necrosis. localized death of tissue.

need. something an individual perceives as being useful or necessary.

negligence. failure to take appropriate action to protect the safety of the patient.

neighborhood health center. a center providing comprehensive health services for the residents of a given community in their own neighborhood.

neonatal mortality. the death of infants within 28 days of birth.

neoplasm. any new and abnormal growth.

Neo-Synephrine. phenylephrine hydrochloride, an adrenergic drug which produces vasoconstriction.

nephron. functional unit of the kidney.

nervousness. state of being easily excited, irritated, jumpy, uneasy, or disturbed.

neurogenous. arising in the nervous system.

neuron. functional unit of the nervous system.

nitrogen mustard. an agent used therapeutically to inhibit the growth of abnormal new cells, such as white blood cells in leukemia. It is very irritating to tissues.

nocturia. excessive urination at night.

nonverbal communication. the conveying of feelings or attitudes by such behavior as facial expressions, gestures, and so forth, rather than with words.

norepinephrine. a hormone produced by the adrenal medulla.

norm. a fixed or ideal standard.

nuclear medicine. the branch of medicine that deals with the use of radioisotopes in diagnosis and treatment.

nurse practitioner. a nurse functioning in an expanded role by providing primary health care in the community.

nurse's aide. person who is usually trained on the job to perform tasks ranging from those principally of a housekeeping nature to assisting in the care of patients.

nursing action. those measures that nurses carry out to help patients in the achievement of health goals.

nursing assistant. the designation given to practical nurses in some provinces in Canada.

nursing audit. the examination of a nurse's charts for redundancy, evidence of poor judgment, and lack of explicitness in the definition of problems, and/or the failure to carry out appropriate nursing interventions.

nursing care plan. a plan of care for a patient.

nursing diagnosis. an assessment of those needs of patients that a nurse can help to meet through nursing action.

nursing history. a written record of information about a patient obtained by the nurse through interview and observation.

nursing intervention. action taken by the nurse as a result of the identification of specific problems.

nursing orderly. a male member of the nursing team who assists in the personal care of male patients and who may perform simple nursing tasks.

nursing process. the series of steps the nurse takes in planning and giving nursing care.

nutrient. nourishing; a substance affording nourishment.

obese. corpulent; excessively fat.

object permanence. the understanding, usually developed during the second year of life, that objects continue to exist even when they are not directly perceived.

objective symptom. evidence of a disease process or dysfunction of the body that can be observed and described by other people.

obstetrics. that branch of medical science which deals with birth and its antecedents and sequelae.

occult. hidden.

occupational health nursing. the employment of nurses in various work settings to provide care, health counseling, maintenance, and protection services for employees.

occupational therapist. a member of the health team who assists patients to develop new skills or to regain skills lessened or lost through illness.

official health agency. a government agency concerned with the prevention of disease, the promotion of health, and the detection and treatment of illness.

olfactory. pertaining to the sense of smell.

oliguria. secretion of a diminished amount of urine.

open bed. a bed that has been prepared for an incoming patient.

ophthalmoscope. an instrument used to examine the interior of the eye.

optimal health. the highest level of functioning attainable by an individual.

optional surgery. surgery that is not essential to preserve a person's physical well-being, but that may be important to his self-esteem.

oral. concerning the mouth.

organic. of, relating to, or containing living organisms.

organic pathology. pertaining to disease processes which can be identified physically, as, for example, tumors or communicable diseases.

oriented. aware of time, place, and person.

orifice. entrance or outlet of any body cavity.

origin (of muscle). the fixed end or attachment of a muscle.

oropharynx. that division of the pharynx between the soft palate and the epiglottis.

orthopnea. the inability to breathe except when in a sitting position.

osmosis. passage of a solvent through a membrane from a lesser to a greater concentration of two solutions.

osmotic pressure. the minimum amount of pressure that will prevent osmosis between two solutions separated by a semipermeable membrane.

osteoporosis. abnormal rarefaction of bones, seen most commonly in the elderly.

otoscope. an instrument used to inspect the ear.

outpatient. a patient who comes to a hospital only for the time necessary for treatment, rather than being confined to the hospital; pertaining to health services rendered to such a patient.

outward rotation. a circular motion directed away from the midline.

overbed cradle. see cradle.

ovulation. the discharge of an ovum from the ovary.

pain. unpleasant sensation resulting from the stimulation of specialized nerve endings.

pain perception. the ability to perceive pain.

pain reaction. the behavioral response to pain.

palliative. affording relief but not cure.

palliative surgery. surgery performed to lessen distressing symptoms without removing the cause of a pathological process.

pallor. a lack of color.

palpation. examination by using one's fingers (sense of touch).

pandemic. widespread epidemic disease.

panic. a severe state of anxiety in which the individual is unable to say or do anything meaningful.

Papanicolaou smear. a cytologic test in which cells are taken from the cervix for examination, chiefly to detect malignancy.

papillary reflex. tactile response of the skin.

paracentesis. the removal of fluid from the peritoneal cavity.

parallel play. the period (about age three) during which children play side by side but take little notice of each other.

paralysis. loss or impairment of motor or sensory function due to neural or muscular disease.

paralytic ileus. (adynamic ileus). obstruction of the intestines resulting from an inhibition of motility of the gastrointestinal tract.

paramedic. emergency personnel with formal training in advanced emergency care and life support skills.

paraplegic. paralyzed from the waist down.

parasite. a plant or animal that lives upon or within another living organism.

parasympathetic nervous system. the craniosacral part of the autonomic nervous system.

parenteral. by injection, rather than through the alimentary tract.

paresthesia. an abnormal sensation without objective cause; for example, numbness or tingling in any or all parts of the limb or other body parts.

Parkinson's disease. a chronic condition marked by muscular rigidity and tremor.

parotid glands. salivary glands situated near the ear.

parotitis. inflammation of the parotid glands; mumps.

passive exercise. exercise in which the muscles do not actively contract.

patent. open; unobstructed.

pathogen. a disease-producing microorganism or material.

pathogenic. capable of producing disease.

pathology. the branch of medicine that deals with the nature of disease.

patient. a person who seeks professional help or advice concerning his health.

patient advocate. someone who speaks on the patient's behalf and who can intercede in his interest.

patient profile. a brief account of the patient's assets and liabilities in relation to health.

patient's record. a written record of a person's medical history, examinations, tests, diagnosis, prognosis, therapy, and response to therapy while he is a patient.

pediculosis. infestation with lice.

pedophilia erotica. child molesting.

peer. one of equal standing.

peer review. a formal process of evaluating medical care or practice by a committee of knowledgeable medical professionals.

pelvis (of kidney). funnel-shaped cavity of the kidney.

perception. the conscious, mental registration of a sensory stimulus.

percussion. eliciting sounds or vibrations by tapping or striking the body to aid in diagnosis.

perineum. the area between the anus and the posterior part of the genitalia; entire anogenital area.

periosteum. fibrous membrane surrounding bone.

peripheral. outward or toward the surface.

peristalsis. wormlike movement by which the alimentary tract propels its contents along.

peritoneal cavity. the potential space between the layers of the peritoneum.

peritoneum. the serous membrane lining the abdominal cavity.

peritonitis. inflammation of the peritoneum.

permissive licensure. the situation in which a professional nurse is free to choose whether or not to register for a license.

personal information. information of a specific nature about a person's feelings, attitudes, behaviors, or details of his personal life.

perspiration. the secretion of fluid by sweat glands of the skin.

petechia. a pinpoint spot of blood in the skin or mucous membrane.

Petri dish. a shallow glass receptacle for growing bacterial cultures.

phantom pain. pain believed to be caused by a pain "memory," after the cause of the pain has been removed, as pain in amputated limbs.

pharmacist. a person responsible for the preparation and dispensing of drugs and other substances used in the detection, prevention, and treatment of illness.

phenolsulfonphthalein. a chemical used to test the function of the kidneys.

phlebitis. inflammation of the veins.

phlebotomy. an opening into a vein made in order to remove blood.

photophobia. an extreme sensitivity to light.

physical therapist. a member of the health team who assists in assessment of patients' functional ability and carries out therapeutic and rehabilitative measures dealing particularly with the musculoskeletal system.

physician. a person who has successfully completed a basic course of medical studies, concerned with preventing, diagnosing, and treating human illnesses, and is authorized to practice medicine in a given jurisdiction (state, province, or country).

physician's assistant. a trained person, usually employed by a physician, who performs, under the physician's supervision, many tasks considered a part of medical practice.

physiological. concerning body function.

physiology. the science that deals with the function of living organisms and their parts.

piggy-back set. intravenous equipment used for the intermittent administration of a drug into an intravenous infusion.

placenta. the "afterbirth"; the tissue attached to the uterine wall by which the fetus is nourished by its mother's blood.

planning. developing a course of action to help the patient.

plantar flexion. a reflex in which an irritation of the sole of the foot contracts the toes; extension of the foot away from the body.

plaque. film of mucus and bacteria that forms on the teeth.

plasma. the fluid portion of blood.

pleura. the serous membrane lining the thoracic cavity.

pleural cavity. the potential space between the plurae.

pneumothorax. the accumulation of gas or air in the pleural cavity.

poliomyelitis. a virus disease which when serious can involve the central nervous system, with resultant paralysis.

polydipsia. excessive thirst.

polyethylene. a lightweight plastic resistant to chemicals and moisture and having insulating properties.

polypnea. an abnormal increase in the respiratory rate.

polyuria. excretion of an increased amount of urine.

POMR. problem-oriented medical records; a method of recording information about patients that is based on the scientific problem-solving process.

popliteal. concerning the posterior surface of the knee.

population density. the number of persons per square mile of a given area.

posterior fornix (of the vagina). a vaultlike space at the back of the vagina.

post-neonatal mortality. the death of infants from 28 days of age up to, but not including, one year of age.

posture. the relationship of the various parts of the body at rest or in any phase of motion.

potential problem. a problem that may arise because of the nature of the patient's health problem, or because of the nature of the diagnostic or therapeutic plan of care.

precordium. the region over the heart or stomach.

preoptic center. the nerve center anterior to the optic center.

prepubic urethra. the part of the male urethra inferior to the pubis.

preventive. directed at averting the occurrence of something.

primary care. the initial health care given to an individual.

primary nursing. the method of allocating nursing responsibility whereby each patient is assigned on admission to a specific nurse, in whose care he remains for the duration of his hospital stay.

principle. a concept, scientific fact, law of science, or generally accepted theory.

private duty nursing. the employment of nurses on a one nurse–one patient basis in cases of acute illness.

problem.   anything with which the patient needs help.

problem list.   a summary of all the known health problems of the patient.

proctoclysis.   Murphy drip; the slow injection of a large amount of liquid into the rectum.

proctoscopy.   examination of the rectum and the anus by means of a lighted instrument.

progesterone.   a hormone produced by the corpus luteum of the ovary.

prognosis.   medical opinion as to the outcome of a disease process.

progress notes.   information concerning the monitoring, plan modification, and follow-up phases of the problem-oriented process.

projection.   ascribing one's own unacceptable feelings or attitudes to other people.

proliferation.   growth by rapid reproduction.

pronation.   turning down towards the ground.

prone.   lying on the stomach (face down).

prophylactic.   preventive.

prostate.   a gland that surrounds the male urethra just below the bladder.

prostration.   extreme exhaustion.

protein.   a complex organic compound containing carbon, hydrogen, oxygen, and nitrogen found in nature in animals and plants.

proteinuria.   the presence of protein in the urine.

protoplasm.   the living substance of cells.

proximal.   closer to the point of reference or to the point of attachment.

prudence.   the habit of acting after careful deliberation.

pruritus.   intense itching.

psychiatry.   the branch of medicine that deals with disorders that are mental, emotional, or behavioral.

psychology.   the science of mind and mental processes.

psychomotor learning.   the development of motor skills.

psychosomatic.   concerning the mind and the body.

puberty.   the period of sexual maturation in humans, marked by menarche in females and the production of sperm in males.

public health inspector.   a worker concerned with the elimination or control of factors in the environment that may endanger health.

pulse.   the throbbing of an artery as it is felt over a bony prominence.

pulse deficit.   the difference between the apical rate and the pulse rate.

pulse pressure.   the difference between the systolic and diastolic blood pressures.

pulse rate.   the number of pulse beats per minute.

pupil.   the opening in the center of the iris of the eye.

purulent.   containing pus.

pus.   the thick liquid product of inflammation, composed of leukocytes, liquid, tissue debris, and microorganisms.

pyemia.   a general septicemia in which there is pus in the blood.

pyloric sphincter.   the thickened layer of circular fibers that surround the opening between the stomach and the duodenum.

pyrexia.   fever.

pyrogen.   a fever-producing substance.

pyuria.   pus in the urine.

quadriplegic.   paralyzed from the neck down.

Queckenstedt's sign.   in a normal person, when the veins on either side of the neck are compressed, the pressure of the cerebrospinal fluid rises.

quotidian fever.   intermittent fever.

radial pulse.   the pulse located on the inner aspect of the wrist on the thumb side, where the radial artery passes over the radius.

radiation.   treatment with x-rays, radium, or other radioactive matter.

radiologic technologist.   a person who performs diagnostic or therapeutic measures involving the use of radiant energy.

radiopaque. not permitting the passage of roentgen rays.

rales. the term used when bubbling sounds can be heard in the air cells or bronchial tubes during breathing.

rapport. a relationship marked by accord or affinity.

rationalization. giving socially acceptable reasons for one's behavior.

reaction formation. attempting to remove a subconscious and forbidden motive or desire by vigorously attacking it.

reciprocal. given in return; mutual.

reconstructive surgery. the repair of damage to appearance or function caused by disease or trauma in a previously intact anatomical structure.

recording. the communication in writing of essential facts in order to maintain a continuous history of events over a period of time.

recreation specialist. a person responsible for developing recreation, sports, or physical fitness programs in the community.

rectum. the distal portion of the large intestine.

referred pain. pain perceived in one area of the body when the stimulus for its origin is in another area.

reflex. an involuntary movement or action; an automatic response to stimuli.

regimen. a regulated pattern of activity.

registered nurse. a person who has successfully completed a program of nursing studies and is authorized to practice in a specific jurisdiction (state, province, or country).

regression. reverting to a previously acceptable, but no longer appropriate, form of behavior.

rehabilitation. the restoration of function of ill or injured at their full capacity.

relapsing fever. a fever in which there is one or more days of normalcy between febrile periods.

REM sleep. the stage of sleep in which dreaming is associated with mild, involuntary muscle jerks and rapid eye movements.

remittent fever. a fever with marked variations but in which the temperature does not reach normal.

renal. relating to the kidney.

renal dialysis. the process whereby blood is continually removed from an artery and allowed to circulate through a channel with a thin membrane, which removes the impurities from the blood before it is returned to the patient through a vein.

repression. unconsciously forgetting problems or experiences.

resident. a qualified medical practitioner who is in residency in a hospital, usually while preparing for practice in a medical specialty.

residual volume. the amount of air remaining in the lungs after a forceful expiration.

respiration. the means by which the individual's lungs exchange gases with the atmosphere.

respiratory technologist. a person who performs diagnostic procedures and therapeutic measures in the care of patients with respiratory problems.

resuscitation. restoration to life or consciousness.

retching. an unproductive attempt at vomiting.

retention (of urine). a condition in which urine is accumulated in the bladder and not excreted.

rickettsiae. minute rod-shaped microorganisms of the family Rickettsiaceae.

rigor mortis. the stiffening of a dead body.

roentgen. the unit of measurement of x-radiation.

role. the pattern of behavior that is expected of an individual in a particular group or situation.

rotation. turning in a circular motion around a fixed axis.

rubefacient. reddening of the skin; an agent that reddens the skin.

ruga(e). a ridge, wrinkle, or fold.

sacrament. a formal religious act.

sadomasochism. obtaining sexual gratification from acts of cruelty, or from being hurt or degraded.

sagittal plane.   the plane that divides the body into right and left sections.

sanguineous.   pertaining to blood.

saphenous veins.   superficial veins of the legs.

scab.   the crust of a sore, wound, ulcer, or pustule.

scapegoating.   directing feelings or actions of hostility towards one particular person or group of persons.

sclerosis.   an induration or hardening.

scored.   marked with significant notches, lines, or grooves.

sebaceous.   secreting oil.

sebum.   the secretion of the sebaceous glands.

secretion.   a product of a gland.

secularism.   indifference to religion.

sedative.   tending to calm or tranquilize; a sedative agent.

self-esteem.   an individual's feeling that he is a worthwhile human being.

semantics.   the study of meaning in language.

semicircular canal.   an organ within the temporal bone which functions to give the sense of equilibrium.

semilunar valves.   pulmonary and aortic valves of the heart.

senility.   the feebleness of body and mind incident to old age.

sensitivity.   responsiveness to various stimuli; frequently used to refer to the responsiveness of bacteria to specific antibiotic agents.

sensory deficit.   a partial or total impairment of any of the sensory organs.

sensory deprivation.   a lack of alteration of impulses conveyed from the sense organs to the reflex or higher centers of the brain.

sensory overload.   an overabundance of sensory stimulation.

septic.   due to or produced by putrefaction.

septic fever.   hectic fever.

serum.   the clear portion of an animal liquid; the liquid part of blood as distinct from the solid particles.

sex role inversion.   total identification with, and preference for adopting, the role of the opposite sex.

shock.   a condition of acute peripheral circulatory failure.

sigmoidoscopy.   examination of the sigmoid colon with a lighted instrument.

sign.   an objective symptom that can be detected through special examination.

significant others.   a term used to encompass family and friends—all those persons who are important to a patient.

Sims's position.   a lateral position in which the patient is placed in a semiprone (sometimes called 3/4 prone) position.

slander.   the damaging of an individual's reputation by a spoken statement.

sleep.   a period for the body and mind during which volition and consciousness are in partial or complete cessation, and the bodily functions are partially suspended.

sleep deprivation.   loss of sleep.

slipper pan.   a bedpan with one end flattened for ease of slipping under the patient.

slurring.   sliding or slipping over utterances that would normally be heard and understood.

smear.   a specimen for microscopic study prepared by spreading the specimen across a glass slide.

SOAP format.   the method of writing the narrative aspect of the patient's progress notes. S stands for subjective (the patient's expression of the problem); O, objective (clinical findings); A, assessment; P, proposed plan of action.

social worker.   a member of the health team who assists in evaluating the psychosocial situation of patients and helps them with their social problems.

sociology.   the science of social institutions and relationships.

somnambulism.   habitual walking in one's sleep.

sordes.   a collection of bacteria, food particles, and epithelial tissue in the mouth.

spasm.   involuntary contraction of a muscle or a group of muscles.

speculum.   an instrument for opening to view a cavity or canal.

sphincter.   a ringlike muscle that closes a natural orifice.

sphygmomanometer.   an instrument used to measure blood pressure in the arteries.

spinothalamic tract.   the neural pathway along the spinal cord to the thalamus.

split foam rubber mattress. a mattress divided horizontally into three sections, which is generally used for debilitated patients and those unable to move.

spore. the reproductive element of a microorganism.

sprain. the wrenching of a joint, resulting in injury to its attachments.

sputum. matter ejected from the respiratory tract, often from the lungs.

stadium acmes. the high point of a disease.

stammering. hesitant speech.

stasis. stagnation of fluid such as blood.

stenosis. a narrowing or constriction.

sterile. free from microorganisms.

sterilization. the destruction by heat or chemicals of all forms of bacteria, spores, fungi, and viruses.

sternum. the breastbone.

stertorous. characterized by noisy breathing.

stethoscope. an instrument used to transmit sounds, as the heart beat.

stomatitis. inflammation of the oral mucosa.

stool. the fecal discharge from the bowels.

stopcock. a valve for stopping or regulating the flow of fluids or gases.

strain. the overstretching or overexertion of muscles; a group of organisms within a species or variety.

stressor. any factor that disturbs the body's equilibrium.

stretch marks. streaks appearing on the breast and abdomen during pregnancy.

stricture. an abnormal narrowing of a passage or canal.

stroke volume output. the amount of blood ejected by the heart with each beat.

structured interview. a conversation controlled and directed by the interviewer.

stupor. partial or nearly complete unconsciousness.

stuttering. spasmodic repetition of the same syllable when speaking.

subarachnoid space. the space beneath the arachnoid tissue.

subcutaneous. beneath the skin.

subjective symptom. evidence of disease or bodily dysfunction that can be perceived only by the patient.

sublimation. channeling unacceptable motives into acceptable forms of behavior.

sublingual. situated under the tongue.

subscapular. situated below the scapula.

sulfanilamide. a drug used in infections.

superficial pain. pain arising from stimulation of receptors in the skin or mucous membranes.

supination. turning upwards.

supine. lying on the back.

suppository. a medication that is molded into a firm base so that it can be inserted into a bodily orifice or cavity.

suppression. the sudden stoppage of a secretion, excretion, or normal discharge; consciously putting out of one's mind problems or unpleasant experiences.

suppuration. the formation of pus.

supraoptic. pertaining to the area above the eye.

supraorbital. situated above the orbit of the eye.

surgery. the deliberate and planned alteration of anatomical structures to arrest a pathological process, alleviate it, or eradicate it.

surgical asepsis. practices carried out to keep an area free of microorganisms.

suture. a surgical stitch.

sympathetic nervous system. the thoracolumbar branch of the autonomic nervous system.

symptom. evidence of a disease process or a disturbed body function

synapse. juncture of nerve cells; to form such a juncture.

syncope. a faint.

syndrome. a group of symptoms that commonly occur together.

synthesis. the process of putting together parts of a whole.

systemic. pertaining to or affecting the body as a whole.

systolic blood pressure. the pressure of the blood in the arteries at the time of ventricular contraction.

tachycardia. an accelerated heart beat, with a pulse rate of over 100 per minute.

tachypnea. abnormal increase in the respiratory rate.

tactile. pertaining to the sense of touch.

tartar. film formation on the teeth.

temporal pulse. the pulse felt anterior to the ear at the mandibular joint, where the temporal artery passes over the temporal bone.

tenacious. adhesive.

tenesmus. ineffectual and painful straining at stool or urination.

teratogenic. pertaining to influences during pregnancy that result in damage to the fetus.

terminal disinfection. measures taken to destroy pathogenic bacteria in an area that has been vacated by a patient with an infection.

testator. a person who makes a will.

testosterone. the principal male hormone, which is responsible for the appearance of secondary sex characteristics.

tetany. tonic spasm of the muscles.

thalamus. part of the diencephalon of the brain; one of its functions is the relay of sensory impulses.

therapeutic environment. an environment which helps a patient grow, learn, and return to health.

therapy. treatment that is remedial.

thermal trauma. injury involving the presence of harmful levels of heat or cold.

thermography. a diagnostic technique that senses and records temperatures emanating from the surface of the body.

thoracentesis. the insertion of a cannula into the pleural cavity

thrombosis. the formation or development of a blood clot.

thyroxine. a hormone produced by the thyroid gland.

tidal volume. the amount of air normally inhaled and exhaled.

tinnitus. buzzing or ringing in the ears.

tissue turgor. the condition of normal tissue fullness and resilience.

tolerance. the ability to endure without ill effect.

tonsillectomy. surgical removal of the palatine tonsils.

tonus. the slight continuous contraction of muscle.

topical. pertaining to local external application.

tort. a legal wrong committed by one person against the person or property of another.

tourniquet. an instrument to compress blood vessels in order to control circulation.

toxemia of pregnancy. a disease occurring in late pregnancy and characterized by hypertension, edema, and proteinuria.

toxin. any poisonous substance of microbic, vegetable, or animal origin.

trachea. the windpipe; the tube extending from the larynx to the bronchi.

tracheotomy. a surgical incision into the trachea.

traction. the act of drawing, as in applying a force along the axis of a bone.

transition. a period of change.

transsexual. a person who undergoes surgery and hormone treatment to physically change to the opposite sex.

transudation. the passage of serum or other fluid through a membrane.

transverse plane. the plane that divides the body into superior and inferior sections.

transvestism. a desire to wear the clothing of the opposite sex.

trauma. injury.

tremors. quivering or involuntary, convulsive muscular contractions.

Trendelenburg's position. the position in which the patient is lying on his back with the foot of the bed elevated.

trocar. a sharp-pointed instrument often used with a cannula.

troche. lozenge.

tumor. an abnormal mass of tissue that arises from cells of preexistent tissue and possesses no physiologic function.

ulcer. a break in the skin or mucous membrane with loss of surface tissue.

ultrasound. sound waves that have a frequency above the range that can be heard by the human ear; diagnostic procedures using such sound waves.

ultraviolet. pertaining to rays whose wavelengths lie between those of the violet rays and the roentgen rays.

umbilicus. the site of attachment of the umbilical cord in the fetus.

unresponsive. making no response to sensory stimulation.

urban. relating to or characteristic of a city.

urea. the final nitrogenous product of the decomposition of protein. It is formed in the liver and carried by the blood to the kidneys, where it is excreted.

urea frost. the appearance on the skin of salt crystals left by evaporation of the sweat in cases of acute renal failure.

uremia. a condition in which the urinary constituents are found in the blood.

ureter. the tube that carries the urine from the kidney to the bladder.

urethra. the canal that conveys the urine from the bladder to the body's surface.

urgency. a compelling desire to void.

urinalysis. examination of the urine.

urobilin. a brownish pigment normally found in feces.

urticaria. a temporary condition of raised edematous patches of skin or mucous membrane that are itchy.

uterus. the muscular organ of the female reproductive tract in which the fetus grows and is nourished.

vagina. the canal in the female reproductive system extending from the cervix to the vulva.

variable data. information concerned with the current status of the patient, such as temperature, which is liable to vary with changes in the patient's health status.

vasoconstriction. a narrowing of the lumen of the blood vessels, particularly the arterioles.

vasodilation. an increase in the size of the lumen of the blood vessels, particularly the arterioles.

vector. an organism that transmits a pathogen.

ventral. anterior; situated toward the front when in anatomical position.

ventricle. a cavity, such as those of the brain or heart.

ventriculography. x-ray examination of the ventricles of the brain after the insertion of a radiolucent medium.

vermin. external animal parasites, such as lice.

vernix. thick, cheesy substance composed of sebum and desquamated epithelial cells, which covers the skin of the fetus.

vertigo. dizziness.

vesicant. an irritant that is used to produce a blister upon the skin.

vestibule. a space or cavity at the entrance to a canal.

vial. a glass container with a rubber stopper.

virulence. the degree of pathogenicity of a microorganism.

virus. a submicroscopic pathogen.

viscera. plural of viscus.

visceral pain. pain arising from the viscera.

viscosity. the quality of being sticky.

viscus (viscera). any large interior organ such as the stomach.

vital capacity. the amount of air that can be expired after an inspiration.

vital signs. indications of basic physiological functioning as evidenced by an individual's temperature, pulse, and respirations.

vitamins. organic chemical substances, widely distributed in natural foodstuffs, that are essential to normal metabolic functioning.

voiding. evacuation of the bladder.

volatile. tending to evaporate rapidly.

voluntary health agency. a private, nonprofit health agency that is established and supported by people in a community.

vomitus. emesis; matter ejected from the stomach via the mouth.

voyeurism. watching others' sexual activities in order to achieve sexual gratification.

warmth. a genuine liking for people.

wheezing. difficult breathing accompanied by whistling sounds.

xiphoid process. the inferior part of the sternum.

x-rays. the visualization of parts of the body by roentgen rays.

x-ray technologist. See radiologic technologist.

yeast. a minute fungus, particularly *Saccharomyces cerevisiae*.

zygote. the cells of the fertilized ovum.

APPENDIX 1

PREFIXES AND SUFFIXES IN MEDICAL TERMINOLOGY

Prefix	Meaning
adeno-	gland
arthro-	joint
chole-	bile
chondro-	cartilage
colpo-	vagina
cranio-	skull
entero-	intestine
gastro-	stomach
hystero-	uterus
laparo-	loin, flank
litho-	stone
masto-	breast
myo-	muscle
nephro-	kidney
neuro-	nerve
osteo-	bone
phleb-	vein
pneumo-	air
pyelo-	pelvis of kidney
salpingo-	tube
teno-	tendon
thoraco-	chest
trachel-	neck

Suffix	Meaning
-ectomy	a cutting out or excision
-oscopy	examination by means of a lighted instrument
-ostomy	formation of a fistula or opening
-otomy	a cutting or an incision
-pexy	fixation
-plasty	molding
-rhaphy	a suturing of

APPENDIX 2

Procedures for Testing for Sugar in Urine

Several different methods may be used to test for excess sugar in the urine. In the Clinitest* method, 5 drops of urine are mixed with 10 drops of water and a Clinitest tablet is added. The color of the solution after 15 seconds is compared to a color chart provided by the manufacturer. Six different shades ranging from dark blue to orange are shown on the chart. The instructions must be followed exactly and only the proper color chart used for comparison. The color chart reports percentages of sugar in the urine according to the following scale:

Negative
Trace   ¼%
+   ½%
+ +   ¾%
+ + +   1%
+ + + +   2%

CLINITEST* TABLET PROCEDURE

1. ● Use a clean receptacle
   ● Hold Clinitest dropper in upright position
   ● Place 5 drops urine in Clinitest test tube
   ● Rinse dropper
   ● Add 10 drops water

2. ● Add one Clinitest tablet
   ● Do not shake test tube
   ● Wait 15 seconds after boiling stops

3. ● Shake test tube gently
   ● Compare solution color with color chart
   ● Record results

IMPORTANT: You must carefully observe the solution in the test tube while reaction takes place and during the 15-second waiting period. Rapid "pass-through" color changes may occur, caused by amounts of sugar over 2%. Should the color rapidly "pass through" green, tan and orange to a dark greenish-brown, record as over 2% sugar without comparing final color development with the color chart.

---

*Clinitest is a Trademark of Ames Division, Miles Laboratories, Incorporated, Elkhart Indiana.

Reagent Strip Tests for Glucose and Ketone (Acetoacetic Acid)

Commercial reagent strips can be used to test for glucose and ketone in urine. Reagent strips are chemically treated strips or tapes that react when exposed to a specific substance, such as urine. Strips from different manufacturers react differently and instructions must be followed carefully for the specific test you are doing. The following instructions are for Keto-Diastix.* The color chart shown here is only a sample. The manufacturer's color chart for glucose is light green to brown and for ketone is light pink to maroon.

DIP-AND-READ TEST FOR GLUCOSE AND KETONE (ACETOACETIC ACID)

IMPORTANT: DO not touch test areas of strip. Store at temperatures under 30°C (86°F). Do not store in refrigerator. Do not remove dessiccant. Remove only enough strips for immediate use. Replace cap promptly and tightly.

DIRECTIONS: **MUST BE FOLLOWED EXACTLY.**
1. Dip a reagent end of strip in FRESH urine and remove immediately. (Alternatively, wet reagent areas of strip by passing through urine stream.)
2. While removing, draw the edge of the strip against the rim of the urine container to remove excess urine.
3. Compare reagent side of test areas with corresponding color charts at the times specified.

CAUTION: Ketone levels reading "Moderate" or greater may depress the color development of glucose test area.

Glucose—*read at exactly 30 seconds.*

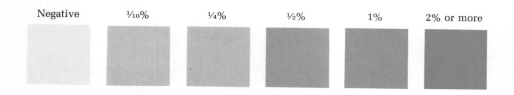

| Negative | 1/10% | 1/4% | 1/2% | 1% | 2% or more |

Ketone—*read at exactly 15 seconds.*

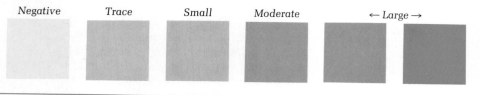

| Negative | Trace | Small | Moderate | ← Large → |

---

*A Registered Trademark of Ames Division, Miles Laboratories, Inc., Elkhart Indiana.

INDEX

Note: Page numbers for illustrations are in *italic* type. Tables are indicated by (t).

Illness *(Continued)*
  impact on family, 29
  maintenance of health after, 29
  nourishment in, 286
  reactions to, 27, 122
  safety needs and, 511
  sleep problems in, 426
  spiritual beliefs and, 681
  state of, 27–29
  stress of, sources of, 668–670
  terminal, 689–699
    health care in, 29
Immunity, 712
  acquired, 553
  active, 553
  in childhood, 245
  innate, 553
  passive, 554
Immunization, 245
  programs for, 54
  schedule for, 557
Immunosuppression, wound healing and, 579
Impaction, fecal, 331, 712
Imperforate hymen, 640
Implementation, 712
Implicit policy, 712
Imprisonment, false, 104
Incoherent speech, 160, 713
Incontinence, fecal, 332, 713
  urinary, 309
Indigestion, 18, 276
  diagnosis of, 282
  psychosocial stressors and, 278
Industrial First Aid, 77
Industrial hygienist, 76, 713
Industrialization, impact on health problems, 33
Indwelling catheter, 320
Infant(s), accident prevention for, 512–513, 513(t)
  administering medication to, 610
  anxiety in, 663
  fluid and electrolyte balance in, 355
  major health problems of, 41
  medication dosages for, 611
  medication for, administration of, 612
  metabolic rate of, 355
  mortality of, 38, 39(t), 713
  motor development of, 242, 488, 488
  newborn, 241–243
    body temperature of, 401
    bowel function of, 328–329
    infections in, 556
    nutritional needs of, 267
    respiratory function of, 375
    skin care for, 534
    sleep needs of, 427
  psychosocial development of, 235
  reactions to pain, 453
  reflexes of, 243
  restraints for, 521
  security needs of, 663
  sensory perception of, 469
  urinary function in, 305
Infection, 552, 713. See also *Infectious disease(s)*.
  body's reaction to, 554
  control of, isolation procedures in, 568–569(t)
    nursing interventions for, 559–571
    through life cycle, 556–558
  cycle of, 552, 552
  early signs of, 558
  endogenous spread of, 556
  fungal, 552
  nosocomial, 551, 554–556

Infection *(Continued)*
  portals of entry of, 553
  potential for, assessment of, 570(t)
  prevention of, 550–571
    principles of, 559(t)
    teaching patients about, 566
    techniques for, 564
  respiratory, in infants and children, 375
  risk of, in surgical patient, 584–585
  susceptibility to, factors affecting, 554
  urinary function and, 308
  viral, 552
Infectious agents, body's reaction to, 553–554
  reservoirs for, 552
  vehicles for transmission of, 552, 555–556
Infectious disease(s), changing patterns of, 5, 33, 551. See also *Infection*.
  environment and, 35
Infectious process, 552–554
Infestation, 713
  parasitic, 333, 333(t)
Inflammation, 17, 554, 713
Influenza, 39, 40
Information, analysis of, in nursing assessment, 123. See also *Data; Data base*.
  collection of, 114–123
    interview in, 185–187
    forms for, 115, 117–119
    methods of, 115
    physiological data in, 120
    purpose of, 114
    sources of, 114
  giving of, to patient, 180
  reporting of, to health care team, 187
Informed consent, 102, 104, 105, 713
Infrared lamps, use of, 414
Infusion, 713
  interstitital, 367
  intravenous. See *Intravenous infusion*.
Inguinal hernia, 713
Inhalation, 713
  steam, 415, 415
Inhalation therapist, 713
Inhalation therapy, 385–390
  aerosol, 390
  carbon dioxide in, 389
  oxygen, 386–389
  principles of, 387
Injection, dorsogluteal, 624, 624
  intradermal, 626, 627
  intramuscular, 625–626. See also *Intramuscular injection*.
  intravenous. See *Intravenous infusion*.
  subcutaneous, 620–623
    equipment for, 620–621, 621
    preparation of medication for, 622–623
    sites of, 620
  ventrogluteal, 624
Injector syringe, 622
Injury, effects on motor function, 489. See also *Trauma*.
Innate immunity, 553
Inpatient, 713
Insertion, of muscle, 483, 713
Insomnia, 18, 428, 713
Inspection, 140, 713
Inspiration, 147, 713
Instillation, 713
Insulator, 713
Insurance, 50
Intellectual development, Piaget's theory of, 234–235